NURSING THE PHYSICALLY ILL ADULT

East Roding School of Nursing,
Barking Hospital,
Upney Lane,
Barking,
Essex.

Editors

JENNIFER R.P. BOORE
BSc (Hons) PhD SRN SCM RNT
Professor of Nursing and Head of Department of Nursing and Health Visiting, University of Ulster, Coleraine, UK

RUTH CHAMPION
BA (Hons) MSc SRN SCM DipN RNT
Designate Director of Nursing Studies, Oxfordshire Health Authority; former Principal Lecturer, Department of Health Studies, Sheffield City Polytechnic, Sheffield, UK

MARION C. FERGUSON
MA SRN SCM HV TutCert CertFEd
Former Director of Nursing Studies and Honorary Research Associate, Department of Social Policy, Royal Holloway and Bedford New College, London, UK

NURSING THE PHYSICALLY ILL ADULT

A TEXTBOOK OF MEDICAL-SURGICAL NURSING

Edited by

JENNIFER R.P. BOORE

RUTH CHAMPION

MARION C. FERGUSON

Churchill Livingstone

EDINBURGH LONDON MELBOURNE AND NEW YORK 1987

CHURCHILL LIVINGSTONE
Medical Division of Longman Group UK Limited

Distributed in the United States of America by Churchill Livingstone Inc., 1560 Broadway, New York, N.Y. 10036, and by associated companies, branches and representatives throughout the world.

First published 1987

ISBN 0-443-02148-1

British Library Cataloguing in Publication Data
Nursing the physically ill adult : a textbook of medical surgical nursing.
1. Nursing.
I. Boore, Jennifer R.P. II. Champion, Ruth III. Ferguson, Marion C. 610.73 RT41

Library of Congress Cataloging in Publication Data
Nursing the physically ill adult.
Includes index.
1. Nursing. 2. Surgical nursing. I. Boore, Jennifer R.P. II. Champion, Ruth III. Ferguson, Marion C. [DNLM: 1. Nursing Care. 2. Surgical Nursing. WY 100 N9795]
RT41.N892 1987 610.73 87-11602

Produced by Longman Singapore Publishers (Pte) Ltd.
Printed in Singapore

Preface

This book is addressed to students of nursing who already possess some understanding of its practice and who have some knowledge of biomedical and social psychological processes. It is not intended primarily for beginning students but rather for those in the second and subsequent years of undergraduate courses and for those undertaking post-experience studies.

There are a number of features of the book that are fundamental to its approach and focus.

Firstly, we feel strongly that there is a need in the UK for a book with a new approach — an advanced, research-based text which prompts as many questions as it attempts to answer. Such an approach is, we feel, essential to the development of effective nursing practice. It draws on literature from the fields of nursing and medicine, the paramedical disciplines and the biological and psychosocial sciences. Currently such literature, while available, is dispersed amongst the many books, journals and reports linked with these disciplines. This book attempts to bring some of this together. It also recognises that much nursing knowledge is not yet systematically validated or developed and that there is an urgent and continuing need to explore, practise and document nursing in such a way as to increase understanding of its nature and effectiveness.

Secondly, in developing the nursing framework upon which the book should be based, we considered that a functional approach, based on the work of Henderson (1966), which is also the basis of the model developed by Roper, Logan and Tierney (1980 and 1985), would be the most useful and realistic. The framework focuses on normal activities of living which, while universal in their application, are modified in their expression by a wide range of physical, psychological and cultural factors. During episodes of illness these activities are further modified by physiological disturbances, treatment regimes and generally speaking the 'care' environment. Thus this framework, while it recognises fundamental physiological needs, places the individual within his or her cultural context.

It was our intention that this framework be utilised by contributors in their consideration of the effects of disordered body systems on individuals and as a guide to their exploration of nursing approaches. However, it soon became apparent to us that it was not possible to impose such a framework on contributors drawn both from the UK and Australia given the different backgrounds and experiences, and subsequent understanding of nursing models. Therefore the chapters vary considerably in their use of an identified nursing framework as a basis for their consideration of nursing practice.

Thirdly, we have focused on the physically ill adult in the knowledge that a considerable amount of nursing practice concentrates on those patients who present with some physical and physiological disturbances. In so doing we have moved away from a strict 'medical' model (a traditional disease orientation) by taking on board issues related to the prevention of those disturbances, and exploring what is required for effective care during episodes of disturbance including maximising the chances of recovery and rehabilitation. Other aspects of nursing, for example health promotion in general, care of other groups such as children or those suffering from disturbed patterns of relationship, belief or thought, are the focus of other books. In addition, this book is one for 'generalists' rather than specialists. The amount of detail on any one topic is limited to that which will provide the basis for understanding general care issues. Nurses who wish to develop their knowledge and expertise in specific fields will want to consult more specialized works.

Fourthly, the book is intended as a stimulus to the enquiring student of nursing to challenge ideas presented, as well as current nursing practice. We hope that readers will add to their knowledge by further exploration of relevant and wide-ranging literature and dialogue with other nurse practitioners and those involved in all aspects of health care. Systematic enquiry into nursing practice will help to put nursing knowledge on a sound footing when focusing on the health care needs and experiences of individuals.

After an initial introductory chapter the book is divided into three unequal sections. The introduction develops some of the themes of this preface. Section One focuses on causation and manifestation of disease, both challenging the concept of causation and including traditional pathologies. This section concludes with an exploration of three concepts which are fundamental to the understanding of any physiologically disturbed person — stress, pain and shock. Section Two details the principal modes of therapy utilised in the treatment of physically ill adults. Section Three, the most substantial section, examines the nature and implications of disturbances of physiological function. The organisation of these chapters originates from an examination of features affecting cellular and total body function, rather than that of body systems per se. For example, there are chapters which explore disturbances of control mechanisms, protective mechanisms and the maintenance of the internal environment. Thus while most chapters relate closely to specific body systems, others cross system boundaries. In all the chapters there has been an attempt to explore issues of nursing concern and to draw out the implications for nursing practice.

1987 J.R.P.B. R.C. M.C.F.

REFERENCES

Henderson V 1966 The nature of nursing. Macmillan, New York

Roger N, Logan W, Tierney A 1980, 1985 The elements of nursing. Churchill Livingstone, Edinburgh

Contributors

Jennifer R. P. Boore

BSc (Hons) PhD SRN SCM RNT

Professor of Nursing and Head of Department of Nursing and Health Visiting, University of Ulster, Coleraine, UK

Surgery and the implications for nursing
Disturbances of nutrient supply (other disorders of the gastrointestinal tract)

Ruth Champion

BA(Hons) MSc SRN SCM DipN RNT

Designate Director of Nursing Studies, Oxfordshire Health Authority; former Principal Lecturer, Department of Health Studies, Sheffield City Polytechnic, Sheffield, UK

Disturbances of physical and chemical transport mechanisms

Marion C. Ferguson

MA SRN SCM HV TutCert CertFEd

Former Director of Nursing Studies and Honorary Research Associate, Department of Social Policy, Royal Holloway and Bedford New College, London, UK

Aetiology of disease and disorder

Frances E. Abramowich

RN BScN MSc MACE FCNA

Head of Nursing, Gippsland Institute of Advanced Education, Churchill, Victoria, Australia

Disturbances of protective mechanisms — the skin (skin disease)

Sarah Denison Andrews

SRN NDN PNT DNCert DNT PGCEA

Lecturer in District Nursing, South Bank Polytechnic, London, UK

Disturbances of protective mechanisms — the skin (leg ulcers)

Pat Ashworth

MSc SRN SCM Oph&ENT NDip FRCN

Senior Lecturer in Nursing, Department of Nursing and Health Visiting, University of Ulster, Coleraine, UK

Shock
Disturbances of maintenance of the internal environment — oxygenation and carbon dioxide excretion

Virginia L. Bonawit

RN PhD

Senior Lecturer, School of Nursing, Lincoln Institute of Health Sciences, Melbourne, Victoria, Australia

Aetiology of disease and disorder

Margaret Clarke

BSc(Hons) MPhil SRN RNT

Director, Institute of Nursing Studies, University of Hull, Hull, UK

Psychological therapies and the alleviation of stress
Disturbances of neurological control mechanisms

Jill A. David

RGN HV BSc(Hons) MSc(Pharm)

Director of Nursing Research, The Royal Marsden Hospital, London, UK

Drug therapy
Disturbances of protective mechanisms — the skin (pressure sores)

Cecilia Edward

BSc DipN(Lond) RGN SCM RNT

Clinical Supervisor, Department of Molecular and Life Sciences, College of Technology, Dundee, UK

Disturbances of temperature control

Gail Ewing
BSc PhD RGN SCM
Research Nurse, Medical Research Council, Dunn Nutrition Unit, Cambridge, UK

Disturbances of maintenance of the internal environment — excretion of unwanted substances (stoma care)

Ian W. Francis
BPharm MPS
Principal Lecturer, Human Physiology and Pharmacology, Department of Biological Sciences, Sheffield City Polytechnic, Sheffield, UK

Appendix — the physiology of pain

Bernadette M. Hannigan
BA PhD AIMLS
Lecturer in Biology, University of Ulster, Coleraine, UK

Degenerative and neoplastic processes

Chris Henry
SRN HV BEd MEd PhD
Senior Lecturer in Physiology/Health, Department of Health Studies, Sheffield City Polytechnic, Sheffield, UK

The nature and meaning of signs and symptoms (a psychological perspective)
Psychological therapies and the alleviation of stress

Rosamund A. Herbert
MSc BSc SRN
Lecturer in Nursing Studies, Department of Nursing Studies, King's College London, London, UK

The nature and meaning of signs and symptoms (a physiological perspective)

David A. Hill
BSc MCSP DipTP
Head of Department of Occupational Therapy, University of Ulster, Coleraine, UK

Physical methods of therapy (specialist physical therapy)

David J. Holme
MPhil MIBiol FIMLS
Principal Lecturer, Department of Biological Sciences, Sheffield City Polytechnic, Sheffield, UK

Infection and immunity

Susan M. Holmes
BSc SRN MRSH
Research Officer, Division of Nursing Studies, Department of Biochemistry, University of Surrey, Guildford, UK

Dietary therapy and nutritional care
Disturbances of nutrient supply (nutritional disorders)

Michael G. Irving
BSc PhD
Senior Lecturer, School of Science, Griffith University, Brisbane, Australia

Disturbances of hormonal control mechanisms

Gary S.A. James
BSc(Hons) RGN RNMH
Senior Nurse (Research), Hull Health Authority, Hull, UK

Disturbances of maintenance of the internal environment — excretion of unwanted substances

Simon Kay
BA FRCS
Senior Registrar, Plastic Surgery, University Hospital of South Manchester and Booth Hall Children's Hospital, Manchester, UK

Disturbances of protective mechanisms — the skin (burns)

Alison L. Kitson
BSc(Hons) DPhil RGN
Project Co-ordinator, Standards of Care, Royal College of Nursing, London, UK

Physical methods of therapy (routine therapies)

Julie K. Laverick
BSc(Hons) SRN HVCert
Health Visitor, Hull Health Authority, Hull, UK

Radiotherapy

Janet M. Marks
BSc SRN
Currently training as Student Health Visitor

Trauma and repair

Susan Mason
B Nurs SRN HVCert NDNCert
Senior Sister, Burns Unit, Booth Hall Children's Hospital, Manchester and doctoral research student, University of Manchester.

Disturbances of protective mechanisms — the skin (burns)

Patrick Gerald McKenna
BSc PhD MIBiol FIMLS
Senior Lecturer in Biology and Director of Biomedical Sciences Research Centre, University of Ulster, Coleraine, UK

Degenerative and neoplastic processes

Susan E. Montague

BSc(Hons) SRN HVDip RNT

Visiting Lecturer, South Bank Polytechnic, London

The nature of stress and its relationship with physical illness

Alan Pearson

PhD MSc RGN ONC RNT DipNEd DANS FRCN

Professor of Nursing and Dean of the School of Nursing, Deakin University, Geelong, Victoria, Australia

Disturbances of protective mechanisms — the musculoskeletal system

Jenny M. Piercy

BA(Hons) RGN SCM DipN CEd RNT

Senior Lecturer in Nursing Studies, School of Health and Applied Sciences, Leeds Polytechnic, Leeds, UK

Disturbances of fluid and electrolyte balance

Bernard Rhodes

BA(Hons) PhD SRN RNT

Principal Lecturer, Department of Health and Community Studies, Leeds Polytechnic, Leeds, UK

Trauma and repair

Pam Smith

MSc BNurs

Senior Nurse (Research), The Middlesex Hospital, London, UK

The nature and meaning of signs and symptoms (a sociological perspective)

Beatrice Sofaer

PhD BA SRN SCM RCT

Lady Davis Postdoctoral Fellow, Henrietta Szold Hadassah Hebrew University School of Nursing, Jerusalem, Israel

Pain: helping to meet the challenge from a nursing point of view

Patricia Wilkie

MA RGN

Research Fellow, Department of Psychology, University of Stirling and Department of Medicine, University of Glasgow, UK

Genetic factors in disease

Jenifer Wilson-Barnett

PhD SRN FRCN

Professor of Nursing Studies and Head of Department of Nursing Studies, King's College London, London, UK

Medical diagnosis and the implications for nursing

Note

Our knowledge in clinical nursing practice and related biological sciences is constantly changing. As new information obtained from clinical experience and research becomes available, changes in treatment and in the use of drugs become necessary. The editors, the contributors and the publishers of this volume have, as far as it is possible to do so, taken care to make certain that the doses of drugs and schedules of treatment are accurate and compatible with the standards generally accepted at the time of publication. Readers are advised, however, to consult carefully the instruction and information material included in the package insert of each drug or therapeutic agent that they plan to administer in order to make certain that there have been no changes in the recommended dose of the drug or the indications or contraindications for its administration. This precaution is especially important when using new or infrequently used drugs.

Contents

1 Introduction

REFLECTIONS ON NURSING

This introduction sets out to explore the nature of nursing and nursing knowledge in the context of sociological and political perspectives. Thus, it is more by way of a reflective essay on nursing than a definitive statement, and is intended as a backcloth against which the more specific and prescriptive material contained within subsequent chapters can be viewed.

The major theme of this book is the care of adults with disturbances of physiological functioning. In considering how such a state might manifest itself and may be repaired and/or eased, Henderson's model of daily living activities, discussed in her book *The Nature of Nursing* (Henderson, 1966), provides the initial framework. Interest in using this model lies in its irresistible attraction as a guiding principle which focuses directly on individuals' physiological and behavioural reponses to their respective illnesses.

ACTIVITIES OF LIVING

In Britain, Roper, Logan & Tierney (1980 and 1985), developing their ideas from the Henderson model, demonstrate how activities of living as interpreted by nurses can provide a basis for a tighter conceptualization of nursing care. They examine a selection of such activities and suggest how, in each case, a person's functional ability can be aided towards optimal performance. The activities with which they are concerned are those thought essential for human living and are modified by physical and psychological factors, and by a vast range of social variables which interlink with one another to produce specific population patterns of existence. In the context of illness other factors impinge, such as the nature of the illness itself, the treatment regime instituted and the environment within which the health care is mediated. The importance of interrelating sociological and illness factors is amply demonstrated by documentary evidence such as the Black Report (Townsend & Davidson, 1982). This not only demonstrates that social patterns of illness exist but also highlights illness' double nature, rooted as it is within the social fabric of any society and invariably displaying specific and highly individualistic physiological signs and symptoms.

RETHINKING NURSING AND THE PROBLEM OF NEEDS

The conceptualization of nursing as being concerned with such things as 'activities of living' is a fundamental breakthrough in nurse thinking since the Nightingale era. This elucidation clarifies where, in the twilight between illness, disease, disease and health, nurses have a function which is less to do with assisting doctors, much more to do with contributing to health care, and ultimately very much to do with assisting patients to improve their state of health. The premise that there is little agreement on what constitutes a state of health is acknowledged, and nurses will be guided by their respective understanding of the term from within the society in which they work.

In re-thinking nurses' contribution to illness-care, Henderson's approach to nursing was influenced by the work carried out at the Institute for the Crippled and Disabled in New York. In this context, rehabilitative efforts concentrated on the development of patients' ability ultimately to lead independent lives, an important consideration which Henderson found lacking in traditional hospital programmes. In hospitals she observed that patients' passivity was both engendered and nurtured. On the basis of the work of the Institute, Henderson developed a list, primarily physiologically-based, of activities of daily living concerned, for example, with eating, drinking, eliminating and sleeping. Thus, by focusing on functional behaviour with disease as an influencing factor rather than as the centre of attention, Henderson was responsible for shifting the whole emphasis of thinking about nursing care. This optimal functional approach also has the potential to initiate health promotion programmes and, therefore, redirects nursing attention away from its traditional concern with ill health.

Recently nursing has been much concerned with 'basic human needs', utilising Maslow's hierarchic model of need and motivation (Maslow, 1970). While Maslow's assumption about relevant, though not fixed, hierarchical positions still awaits scientific confirmation, and while consensus about the nature of needs is likewise still in a state of jeopardy and equivocation, a general concept of need must remain central to any welfare policy. For the moment, however, for nursing, as Roper, Logan & Tierney (1985) point out, activities of living have an edge over needs in that they are observable and lend themselves to objective measurements. Though the debate about identifying basic needs is thereby in no way obsolete it can only be refined and further developed in collaboration with others, health professionals and the lay public (Doyle & Gouch, 1984).

THE NURSING ENVIRONMENT — AN IMPRECISE CATEGORY

While nurses will nurse to the best of their abilities given their own understanding of themselves and their patients, and given access to nursing knowledge to apply to their practice, often the best of their intentions will defy execution. It seems that, in spite of often excellent nurse teaching and the provision of educational facilities, well worked-out plans do not come to fruition. What is it that interrupts those plans? The 'cri de coeur' is about an apparent gap between theory and practice. Many studies strongly underpin the 'gap theory', for example, Bendall (1975), Birch (1975) and Melia (1983 a & b). Martin (1984) and Folta & Deck (1966), however, attempt to develop an explanatory model elucidating some of the forces responsible for the divergence between what 'is' and what 'ought to be'. Martin addresses his study to managers in hospitals, be they nursing, medical, paramedical or institutional administrators. He introduces his book with the cardinal concern:

> This is a book about failures of caring in hospitals. It seeks to illuminate the problem posed by the question, "How is it that institutions established to care for the sick and helpless can have allowed them to be neglected, treated with callousness and even deliberate cruelty?".

The fact that this study deals specifically with mental health care institutions is not saying that institutions caring for the physically ill are exempt. The studies by Stockwell (1972), Evers (1980) and Webb & Wilson-Barnett (1983) indicate that institutional care for the physically ill is also deficient. Patients are neglected. Standards of care leave much to be desired. In particular Evers and Webb & Wilson-Barnett highlight how the health care system both overlooks and denies distinctive gender-related needs, observations supported by the studies of Oakley (1981) and Barrett & Roberts (1978), who investigated how women fare when entering the health care system in Britain.

Martin's (1984) uncomfortable and thought-provoking study directs the readers' attention to organizational conflicts and diverse sub-groups' interests. These organizational and subgroup conflicts are also clearly outlined by Tuckett (1976) in his chapter on hospitals, an excellent introduction to the complex triangular interrelationship between organization's formal structure, the people who work within it and who, apart from being members of the organization, are also members of their wider society and are implicated in its values. Adequate funding is clearly an important issue when considering hospitals in trouble. However, a major component of the problem is that associated with the way in which resources are obtained and distributed.

In turn, resource allocation arises from deeply entrenched notions of power and privilege, supported by an accompanying system of patronage and reward.

Nursing is part of this system, and as such requires a close and constant analysis for change if it is to have the substantive effect which might enhance nursing policy and practice. Folta & Deck (1966), both nurses, in developing their sociological framework for patient care (which although first published in 1966, has not been superseded) provide a sound theoretical model for potential conflict resolution within hospitals and other health care institutions. The model is a guide towards the identification, not only of where individuals under stress might exhibit levels of psychopathology, but where an organization under stress can also show signs of perversion.

Lack of fit between theory and practice, the 'gap theory', is not necessarily unique to nursing. It may also stem in part, as Clinton (1981) argues, from the values of the wider society which apportions priority resources in line with an ideology of a market economy which marginalizes those in need of care and protection. The Clinton study would support the adaptation of Folta & Deck's framework as a source of analysis of much of nursing practice. In the context of a critical review of the literature on 'good' and 'bad' patients, Kelly & May (1982) conclude that an interactionist conception of the nurses' role, rather than an identification of features specific to such patients, may be a more appropriate way to analyze such situations. This interactionist interpretation conceives the patient as active in legitimizing the nurse's role. Thus, patients who confirm the nurse's role are 'good' patients whereas those who deny such legitimation are 'bad' patients.

Such a conceptualization of the nurse's role might contribute to understanding the nature of nurses' anxiety which Menzies (1970), in her by now classical study, recognized as being responsible for much of nursing's own organizational pattern. In her study of first year student nurses, Parkes (1985) found that they reported considerable stress. This stress related to interpersonal conflicts with other nurses, to insecurities about their practical competence and to lack of adequate support from and guidance by senior nurses. It is all too easy to blame the victim, whether it is the patient who does not comply, the nurse who is unwilling and incompetent, or the doctor who is both insensitive and imposes style and order. Even if the apparently offending person is removed, situations do not change substantially, even if they change pro forma for a period. What these studies indicate is that before raising a trigger mechanism of re-direction, actual organizational patterns and situations require an in-depth analysis with the legitimate participation of all concerned.

Uncritical acceptance of an interactionist model points to the power of the individual patient in influencing the way in which nurses can express their role and undertake nursing care. The application of the nursing process and a deliberate consideration of the individual's activities of living focus on the individuality or uniqueness of the person who is a patient, as it should, given a nurse's professional commitment. Yet, embedded in executing this commitment is the need to address issues of a collective nature. For example, those of class, gender and race divisiveness, of the organization of work procedures and of the demands and consideration of priorities within health care. Because these are expressed collectively they demand collective action. Mauksch & Miller (1981), in discussing nursing, see that much of its professional expertise lies in risk-taking. This they identify as involving a calculation of the worth of taking risks. Professional commitment combining a consideration of a patient's individuality with the recognition of the need to pursue collective solutions, is an exercise in professional risk taking.

ABOUT THE INTERRELATIONSHIP OF THE SOCIAL AND THE PHYSIOLOGICAL

A knowledge about body systems is deeply implanted in much of traditional nursing practice. However, for nursing, the basis for such knowledge was never explored nor its methodology examined. In part, this was because the basis for this knowledge was not made available to nurses and in part because it was not considered important. Nurses were content to live by experience, handed on from one generation to the next. Indeed, they were proud to be building nursing knowledge on yesterday's experiences without requiring scientific legitimation because of their strongly held belief that experience was fundamental. Nursing has moved on and, as indicated earlier, there now exists a considerable body of knowledge of and about many aspects of nursing care. But because nursing research is still seen as a somewhat esoteric exercise, and research in other related areas is often not recognized as significant for the nursing problem in hand, such research is left on the bookshelves and disintegrates to dust in archives rather than being properly integrated into the nursing knowledge accepted, utilised and seen as essential for the provision of care.

A sound knowledge of the body's disease and symbiotic physiological functioning in its cellular detail provides overall understanding of how, physiologically, the body acts as a unity. By breaking this knowledge up into its component parts, without losing sight of the whole, the practitioner will encompass the functioning of the complete physiological entity.

To discuss illness, however, only in terms of physiological norms and deviations is taking a very limited, though useful, view. By this means illness can be classified, categorized and recognized in other countries and on other continents. But illness and health have another reality, and these broader dimensions and concepts are relative and do not lend themselves to simple definitions. Engel (1962), in his discussion on health and disease, points to the reductionist nature of conceptualization when discussion is focused primarily on changes within the cells as a basic component of disease. He argues for a much broader formulation, disregarding the substantive assumption that disease is a thing in itself, unrelated to the patient. By applying a multifunctional concept, disturbances or failures can be seen at all levels of organization and their relationship considered. This enables cellular, biochemical, organic, psychological and social dimensions to be linked and interrelated with one another. In recognizing a patient's and nurse's individuality in the clinical encounter, the implications of the existence of cultural variables require notice and need to be acted upon. This includes aspects of what is considered 'ill' in each culture or society, when cultural interpretation of symptoms follows normative roles.

Studies by Berkanovie (1972), Pill & Stott (1982), Baumann (1961), Apple (1960) and many others indicate that a lack of congruence between patients' perception of illness and doctors' diagnosis of disease is common. The now classical study by Koos (1954) about the health of people in Regionville demonstrates how processes of recognizing states of ill health are determined from within specific cultural milieu, and differ according to class, age, religious affiliation, educational standard and other factors. What finally happens at the doctor's surgery is no more than a bureaucratic exercise (Strong, 1977) and partially, as Stimmson & Webb (1975) and Oakley (1981) argue, a battle of wits between doctor and patient. While the doctor likes to impose diagnostic categories, the would-be patient angles for a patient-centred diagnosis. The vulnerability of an individual in an illness situation is clearly illustrated by consideration of the nature of the cultural variables which are operating. Bury's (1982) sensitive essay on chronic illness as a biographical disruption spells out how patients suffering from rheumatoid arthritis learn to negotiate their handicap in order to save face in their daily encounters. Charmaz's (1983) study of chronically ill persons with varied diagnoses demonstrates how patients' former self-images disintegrate when new equally-valued ones are not developed concurrently. In her sample, people discuss how their disease has led to being a burden on others, to leading restrictive lives, to being discredited and experiencing social isolation. The citing of such studies related to chronic illnesses is not to argue that those experiencing more acute disruptions as a result of illness do not suffer similar injustices. Though medically there may be a clear cut division between what constitutes chronic as opposed to acute illness, in real-life this division has little meaning.

The fundamental ethos of nursing is a process that takes account of the totality of the human being. This presupposes that whilst the physical conditions are of importance to the nurse, so is the nature of the social-psychological environment in which individuals are deeply rooted and from which, if they are torn away, disruptive elements subsequently result. If, through disability of one sort or another, such separation should occur, the implications for patients are considerable and must of necessity become the object of concern. The biomedical model which has been challenged underpins a much taken-for-granted approach to illness and disease in society. This assumes that disease can be freely accounted for by deviation from the norm of measurable (somatic) variables and that it can be dealt with as an entity independent of social behaviour.

Whilst nurses have no problem in recognizing the limitations of this model, the consideration of an individual's daily living activities when nursing a patient will be only the first step in transcending the biomedical model. Nurses' physical and constant closeness to their patients demands that aspects of patient behaviour are not seen as mere behavioural aberrations but rather as important and significant indicators of being sick, being under stress, and feeling none too well.

To comprehend fully a patient's despair and discomfort, nurses need to develop additional concepts, frames of reference and skills. These are needed in order to provide insights to link the world of the biomedical perspective with those of patients' experiences when they report on their own understanding of their illnesses. Kestenbaum (1982), by outlining a phenomenological approach, directs much of future nursing orientation towards a recognition and acceptance of the patient's experiences as a valid input into his/her own biography. High level interviewing and observational skills are required, coupled with an understanding of physiological, psychological, social and cultural determinants of health and illness behaviour, if nurses are to begin to appreciate the experience of patients or to understand the effect that illness has on their activities of living. Often, nurses' insistence on relying primarily on technical information and procedure overlooks and misses important cues which are essential to this understanding of patients. The way and manner in which a patient will talk about his or her illness, under what conditions such discussion occurs, how the illness affects him or her and close friends and relatives — all this and more constitutes the clinical data of illness without which even the best of high technology medicine cannot expect to work. The specific knowledge thus acquired does not only relate to a mere accumulation of data from separate areas of concern. It relates to the juxtaposing of this data, linking and recognizing its connections. In this way observed behaviour can be matched to laboratory documentation and a patient's verbal account of his or her perspective need no longer be disregarded as irrelevant to care.

The inclusion of a patient's perspective into consideration of nursing and medical care constitutes the adoption of a biopsychosocial approach in preference to a biomedical model. This has implications for nurse teaching and research, and brings with it its own additional stress.

The complexity of a biopsychosocial model makes it difficult to determine specifically which part of nursing, which part of biomedicine and which part of the social, cultural environment was indeed the causative agent responsible for the easing of the patient's concern. Thus the nurse may feel robbed of determining which of her or his individual contributions led to a patient's recovery. If the recovery is successful, the process of dying eased, the living with chronic illness helped to become a possibility by adopting a biopsychosocial approach, no single health professional will ever be sure which, if any, of their methods enhanced a solution. Does it matter?

Resource issues force the question to be addressed. What becomes important is that approaches are adopted that do promote health, that do facilitate recovery and resumption of self care, that do prevent further deterioration or limitation of functional restoration, and that do promote comfort and dignity in disability, illness or dying. Whether these approaches are unique to nursing or develop into more professionally interchangeable modes of operation remains to be seen. What is certain is that the search for effective health care practice cannot ignore the contribution of all those involved in its provision. It cannot ignore the psychological, social and cultural factors which inevitably involve the practitioner in constant enquiry into the nature of his or her practice. This includes the systematic documentation of the structures, processes and outcomes of health care episodes. Thus knowledge and understanding will develop with practice and the effective nurse will be the nurse who espouses this philosophy.

REFERENCES

Apple D 1960 How laymen define illnesses. Journal of Health and Human Behaviour 1:219–225

Barrett M, Roberts H 1978 Doctors and their patients. Social control of women in general practice. In: Smart C, Smart B (eds) Women, sexuality and social control. Routledge and Kegan Paul, London

Baumann B 1961 Diversities in conception of health and physical fitness. Journal of Health and Human Behaviour 2:39–46

Bendall E 1975 So you passed nurse. Royal College of Nursing, London

Berkanovie E 1972 Lay conception of the sick role. Social Forces, 51(1):53–64

Birch J 1975 To nurse or not to nurse. Royal College of Nursing, London

Bury M 1982 Chronic illness as a biographical disruption. Society of Health and Illness 4(2):167–182

Charmaz K 1983 Loss of self. A fundamental form of suffering in the chronically ill. Sociology of Health and Illness 5(2):168–195

Clinton M E 1981 Unpublished PhD Thesis, University of East Anglia

Doyle L, Gouch J 1984 A theory of human needs. Critical Social Policy, Summer, 6–38

Engel G 1962 Psychological developments in health and disease. Saunders, Philadelphia

Evers H 1980 Care or custody? The experiences of women patients in long-stay geriatric wards. In: Hutter B, Williams G (eds) Controlling women: the normal and the deviant. Croom Helm, London
Folta R, Deck E S 1966 A sociological framework for patient care. Wiley, New York
Henderson V 1966 The nature of nursing. Macmillan, New York
Kelly M, May D 1982 Good and bad patients. A review of the literature and a theoretical critique. Journal of Advanced Nursing 7:147–156
Kestenbaum V 1982 The humanity of the ill. University of Tennessee Press, Knoxville
Koos E L 1954 The health of Regionville. Columbia University Press, New York
Martin J P 1984 Hospitals in trouble. Blackwell, Oxford
Maslow A 1970 Motivation and personality. Harper and Row, New York
Mauksch J G, Miller M H 1981 Implementing changes in nursing. Mosby, St Louis
Melia K 1983a Students' view of nursing. Nursing in the dark. Nursing Times 79(21):62–63
Melia K 1983b Students' view of nursing. Doing nursing and being professional. Nursing Times 79(22):28–30
Menzies J 1970 The functioning of a social system of defence system of defence against anxiety. Tavistock, London
Oakley A 1981 Becoming a mother. Penguin, Harmondsworth
Parkes K 1985 Stressful episodes reported by first-year student nurses. Social Science and Medicine 20(9):945–953
Pill R, Stott N 1982 Concepts of illness causation and responsibility. Social Science and Medicine 16:43–52
Roper N, Logan W, Tierney A 1980 & 1985 The elements of nursing, 2nd edn. Churchill Livingstone, Edinburgh
Stimmson J, Webb C 1975 Going to the doctor. Routledge and Kegan Paul, London
Stockwell F 1972 The unpopular patient. Royal College of Nursing, London
Strong P 1977 Medical errands. In: Davis A, Horobin G (eds) Medical encounters. Croom Helm, London, 38–54
Townsend P, Davidson N 1982 Inequalities in health. Penguin, Harmondsworth
Tuckett D 1976 The organisation of hospitals. In: Tuckett D (ed) An introduction to medical sociology. Tavistock, London
Webb C H, Wilson-Barnett J 1983 Hysterectomy. A study in coping with recovery. Journal of Advanced Nursing 8:311–319

SECTION ONE

Disease causation and effect

This section examines the causation and manifestation of physiological disease. While the first chapter challenges the assumption that underlies the 'medical model' approach to disease — that there is always a clear and exclusive relationship between physiological disturbances and identifiable pathological processes — it takes into consideration that disease itself takes place within a social context which has implications for the patient as well as for the nature of the disease.

The next four chapters examine the pathological processes which underlie much disease and some of these chapters also discuss the nursing implications of that pathology. Whereas some physiological disturbances result in the person exhibiting and experiencing 'signs and symptoms', the presentation and experience of these are not standard. While there may well be some commonality related to physiological disturbances, social and psychological factors impinge in such a way that each person will experience illness differently, and thus express illness in terms of 'signs and symptoms' in a different manner. Chapter 7 on 'signs and symptoms' is divided only for analytical purposes into three sections (biological, psychological and sociological) and pinpoints a way of seeing, in that 'signs and symptoms' may be differently interpreted by people of different professional/occupational, psychological and social orientations. This chapter needs to be considered as a whole to obtain a broad understanding of the meaning of 'signs and symptoms' for the individuals concerned.

The remaining three chapters in this section on stress, pain and shock are included here as they can be both causes of physiological disturbance and results of disease. In these chapters the nursing management is discussed in some detail in addition to the underlying theoretical considerations.

2

Aetiology of disease and disorder

THE PROBLEM — WHY EXAMINE IT?

The cause-effect relationship in illness and disease is complex in the sense that it concerns a 'chicken and egg' situation. Whereas at one level the pathophysiological process can be recognized as the 'cause' and the resulting disease as the 'effect', at another level the pathophysiological process itself can be seen as an effect of other causations. For example, atheroma can be seen as the 'cause' of ischaemic heart disease but itself is in part caused by factors associated with life style.

Disease causation, however, is a cornerstone of medical studies. Of what interest is it to nurses? Nursing practice may be said to focus on the behaviour of patients as it relates to their illness. Another focus of nursing practice is the health seeking behaviour of people. An examination of the World Health Organization's (1947) definition of health as 'a state of complete physical, mental and social well-being' implies that not only does the range of disorders demanding medical and nursing intervention include physical problems, it has broadened to include behavioural and social problems.

Goldstein (1983) discusses the problems inherent in this definition for health planning, especially the lack of criteria enabling the observer to determine if health is improving or deteriorating. Current interpretations of positive health such as physical fitness, personal growth and social development are difficult to measure.

He suggests that the need for health planners to set goals in operational terms leads more naturally to a definition of health as '... a state associated with absence of disease, of symptoms associated with mental illness and of social dysfunctions such as social alienation, drug abuse and antisocial behaviour.' This allows the standard of health of the community to be expressed in terms of incidence and prevalence of various diseases and conditions. Once this is done, one of two approaches can be used, setting health goals in terms of per cent reduction in deaths or days of illness to be achieved, or ranking diseases or conditions in terms of their contribution to loss of life, loss of function or capacity to work and using economic cost as a guide to priority setting of preventive measures. He also notes that the contribution of disease to suffering is an aspect which needs to be considered but there is no satisfactory way of measuring this.

The maintenance of health is now a commitment of the medical and nursing professions. Effective practice therefore demands that the environmental effects on health are explored to discover causative agents. There may be difficulties associated with the degree to which a positive definition of health can be dealt with practically, but it cannot be denied that the promotion and maintenance of health and a healthy environment is an ever increasing component of medical and nursing practice.

Social concern with health can be considered under the following four headings:

- mortality, morbidity and health indices
- ethical issues
- environmental aspects
- structural/political aspects.

Mortality, morbidity and health indices

These refer to research into the incidence of ill health:the number of deaths and their attributed causes; the number of people treated in the health care system; those who, although ill, are not treated, either because they do not enter the health care system or because they suffer from disorders with which the present system is unable to cope. Among other things, this body of research addresses itself to establishing criteria for 'health' and health behaviour. The present criteria largely comprise mortality and morbidity statistics which, while valuable, do not measure aspects of positive health nor the process of becoming ill.

In a study to assess prevalence of various symptoms in a health centre population (Hannay, 1979) 23% of all the subjects interviewed had medical symptoms which would be considered serious but which were not referred for professional help.

What motivates people to seek medical care has been the subject of much study and thought. Attempts have been made to discover:

1. Personal characteristics or belief systems of people who delay or do not seek help
2. Trigger mechanisms, societal and other pressures which bring people into the health care system
3. The kinds of decisions required, including how people try to explain their symptoms, e.g. the cause and likely outcome, which leads to the decision to seek help or not (Mechanic, 1976).

Ethical issues

These question the nature of quality of life and distribution of health care, for example, costly high technology for the few as opposed to cheaper health measures for the many, which ultimately may be more effective.

Environmental aspects

These address the identification of attributes in the environment (pollutants, stress and fatigue) contributing to less than optimal well being or to eventual illness.

Structural/political aspects

These examine the organization of society, which includes the economic structure, to determine the barriers to attainment and maintenance of health.

CAUSE: THE CONCEPT

'A cause is an act, event or state of nature, which initiates or permits, alone or in conjunction with other causes, a sequence of events resulting in an effect' (Rothman, 1976). That events have a cause we take as given. One can speculate on whether it is possible to prove a cause-effect relationship, but not upon the existence of the law of causality. It is a norm of our reasoning (Dilman, 1973).

In a formal sense the conditions for cause are:

- The cause must be a necessary element in bringing about the effect such that if the cause is absent, the effect will be absent. This is called necessary cause.
- The cause must be sufficient to bring about the effect such that if it is present, the effect will be present. This is called sufficient cause (Riegelman, 1979).

Koch's postulates exemplify a simple linear cause-effect relationship. Briefly summarized, they state: in all cases of a given disease the same microorganism must be recovered and must be able to be grown in pure culture; the micro-organisms from this pure culture, when innoculated into a susceptible animal, must be able to reproduce the disease; in addition it must be able to be recovered from the experimentally infected animal and grown again in pure culture.

These postulates established the criteria for the rigorous cause-effect relationship between agent and disease. However, Koch himself recognized causative agents of some diseases, e.g. typhoid and leprosy, to which his criteria could not be applied. Since his time, the existence of a healthy carrier state has been recognized. In addition, viral diseases and disorders involving the immunological mechanisms do not fit these criteria (Evans, 1977).

Valuable ways of looking at the cause-effect relationship come from epidemiology. Riegelman (1979) discusses the clinical concept of contributory cause which is based on the following criteria:

- the cause precedes the effect
- altering only the cause, alters the effect.

He points out that retrospective and prospective studies are ways of trying to establish a cause-effect relationship. However this, in practice, is extremely difficult to do.

Riegelman suggests that if, in clinical practice, the requirements for necessary and sufficient cause had been adhered to very few causes of disease already identified could, in fact, have been identified. Rothman (1976) deals with the concept of sufficient cause in terms of a constellation of phenomena which, acting together, make up a sufficient cause. He points out that the constellation of causes making up the sufficient cause may vary but, if there is one unvarying member of every constellation of sufficient causes for a given disease, then that one member constitutes a necessary cause. For example, in tuberculosis, the mycobacterium tuberculosis is always present and is the necessary cause, but the disease may not manifest itself unless other members of the constellation, e.g. undernutrition and overcrowding, occur with it. Further, the constellation of other causes may vary with individual circumstances, e.g. in some cases stress, advanced age or alcoholism may make up the complete constellation.

René Descartes proposed that man consists of a material body,open to scrutiny, and a non-material soul, which is not open to study. This mind-body dichotomy became a very powerful tool in the reductionist approach to the study of the human body. This has proved very fruitful for medicine, but has also resulted in psychiatry and psychology growing separately from the mainstream of medicine. There are now attempts to reconcile this dichotomy to fit our modern concept of health (Shontz, 1975). The concept of psychosomatic illness and the development of psychosomatic medicine date from the late 1920s. Psychosomatic disease is organic pathology brought on at least in part by psychological forces. Traditionally conditions such as asthma, high blood pressure and ulcers were regarded as diseases of psychosomatic origin.

One of the most significant contributions to a unifying concept of illness causation was the development of the concept of stress by Selye (1956). This is discussed in detail in Chapter 8. It is clear that the brain can be viewed as an endocrine organ that can alter our ability to deal with a variety of illnesses (Rosch, 1979). The hypothalamus of the brain plays a major role in the regulation of body metabolism through control of most endocrine activity. The limbic system,i.e. those areas of the brain involved in the experience of emotion, has many links with the hypothalamus and through these influences body function. The resulting changes in metabolism, including depression of the immune system, as a result of the individual's response to a stressful situation can play a part in the development of illness. Lazarus (1976) wrote about the individual's perception of the situation as critical in determining whether or not stress would result.

Totman (1979), dealing with the idea that social factors or events can cause illness, also discusses individual perception of events or impinging stimuli. He emphasizes the importance of ascertaining the significance of the event or stimulus to the individual — what is significant to one person may not be to another. If an event is to provoke a reaction it must be significant to the individual experiencing it. He proposes a model of events leading to the onset of symptoms; his thesis is that the social world is subject to constructive interpretation in the same way as the physical world, and this interpretation involves a comparison of what is with what ought to be. Within a given culture, there are social norms. Actions are interpreted in the light of their relationship to these norms.

The structure on which the interpretation of the social world rests is a system of information about goals and objectives which society recognizes. This structure is hierarchical. It proceeds from general or universal categories to categories specific to an individual's group with which he identifies, and finally to the individual. In addition to understanding actions in terms of the information about what ought to be, the individual also approves or disapproves. Values, beliefs and preferences form prescriptive rules. A given action is compared with these rules until consistency is achieved. As there is a strong need to register consistency, rules need to be consolidated. This can be done by engaging in goal-directed activity, involving at least some effort, or by conversation in which a verbal commitment particular to our beliefs is made. The likelihood of abnormal sensations, (symptoms), appearing is increased in the absence of frequent registration of consistency. Resistance to disease remains high if a person's values and beliefs are consistent with his group and he has sufficient opportunities to become involved in socially approved activities. The concept of life events as causal agents of illness is a current well debated topic. In this context, Totman's model is a useful one.

Totman also attempts to explain another phenomenon which is relevant to current ideas about illness. This refers to the apparent effectiveness of some treatments in some individuals when the treatment itself can be shown to be neither physically nor chemically effective against a given illness. He explains this phenomenon on the basis of the cognitive dissonance theory. This states that after a person makes a decision, he will work on justifying that decision and will be in a state of tension called 'cognitive dissonance' until the justification is internalized. This suggests that when a person commits himself to a course of treatment, often involving effort or unpleasantness, he justifies his commitment by becoming better.

The foregoing discussion on the cause-effect relationship in illness has made it clear that causation must be seen as multifaceted. It is therefore clearly inappropriate to approach illness management on the basis of there being a simple linear relationship between cause and effect. Weiner (1978) points out some generalizations which must be encompassed by a newer more complex model of disease or illness. They are:

- predisposing factors to disease or illness are not necessarily the same ones which initiate or sustain it
- genetic polymorphism plays a role in disease
- age and sex of the individual determine the response to the disease

- phenotypic expression of a disease is a product of the interaction of the host's adaptive-defence response and the disease agent.

These generalizations come from observations on the nature of slow virus disease. If individual variations in factors such as level of intelligence, conditioning, social and psychological milieu are considered in the light of these generalizations, this model of illness is useful.

CAUSE/EFFECT? ILLUSTRATIVE EXAMPLES

It has been noted that the focus of nursing intervention is largely on the behaviour of patients as it relates to their illness, and people in relation to the maintenance of their health. Environmental factors both internal, e.g. biorhythms, and external, e.g. physical, social and economic, have been the subject of research in relation to their causative role in illness, injury and inability to maintain a state of well being. Awareness of the research findings is important for nurses in developing an understanding of their role.

INTERNAL ENVIRONMENT — BIORHYTHMS

Biorhythms can be studied in terms of the effect of disruption of normal circadian rhythms on the maintenance of health or propensity to illness. They can also be viewed from the standpoint of the influence that circadian and other biological rhythms have on behaviour, mood, efficiency and the effectiveness of treatment regimens.

General aspects

Most organisms exhibit rhythmical variations in behaviour and metabolic functions influenced by geomagnetic forces, rotation of the earth around the sun (seasonal), lunar cycles, and rotation of the earth on its axis (daily). The best understood are those rhythms with an approximate 24 hour period, called circadian, from the Latin, *circa* (around) *dies* (day). Cycles shorter than this are referred to as ultradian and longer cycles as infradian. Examples are shown in Table 2.1. The period is the length of time the entire cycle occupies. The frequency is the reciprocal of the period, e.g. for circadian rhythms, once in 24 hours. The phase is a specific point on a cycle, often used to compare one cycle with another.

When isolated from external cues, most people will demonstrate circadian rhythms rather longer than 24 hours and different rhythms may show different periodicities. For example, after about 15 days in an isolation unit designed to ensure that no external cues are available, body temperature showed a rhythm of 25.1 hours and sleep/wakefulness a rhythm of 33.4 hours (Wever, 1975). Most circadian rhythms have both endogenous and exogenous components. There appear to be two internal regulators (or oscillators), but rhythms of many other factors are subservient to these two. Under normal circumstances these endogenous rhythms are entrained, or adjusted, to a 24-hour rhythm, by external cues or zeitgebers (Minors & Waterhouse, 1981).

Table 2.1 Examples of bodily rhythms in humans

Ultradian (less than 20 hours)	Circadian (20–28 hours)	Infradian (more than 28 hours)
Alternating periods of REM/non-REM sleep Cardiac cycles Growth hormone secretion during sleep	Cyclic fluctuations in: body temperature heart rate blood pressure urine secretion serum corticosteroid levels eosinophil values sleep and wakefulness	Menstrual cycle

Comfort (1978) discusses the possibility of a biological clock concerned with ageing and suggests the hypothalamus as a site and the rate of tryptophan (a precursor of neuroamines) synthesis as a possible mechanism. He also discusses the evidence from experiments on rats and mice in which the caloric intake of the animals was reduced by feeding them only two days out of three, resulting in a doubling of the life span.

In addition to the above, there is some statistical evidence which suggests that there may be seasonal variations in peak periods of births, suicides and accidental deaths and puerperal depression (Natalini, 1977) although it is difficult to ascertain if these peaks are expressions of geophysical, microbiological or sociocultural influences, or a combination of these.

Biorhythm effects on performance and mood — effects of disruption of biorhythms

Lanuza (1976) discusses the relationship between circadian rhythms of body temperature and mental efficiency and performance (measured by sorting tasks, mathematical calculations and measures of alertness). In people who are active during the day and sleep at night, the body temperature begins to increase just before or just after waking and reaches a peak in the late afternoon. Mental efficiency and physical performance peaks coincide with that of the body temperature. Studies on periodicity of mood and affect reported by Stephens (1976) on a group of male tertiary students showed, in general, an increase in positive moods and a decrease in negative moods from midday to late afternoon. A group of younger (secondary) students found that anxiety, stress and inability to cope were more pronounced in late afternoon. Studies on 'larks', people who feel better earlier in the day, and 'owls', people who feel better later in the day, correlating body temperature and feelings of introversion and extroversion indicated that the more introverted group of subjects was characterized by a rise in body temperature earlier in the day.

Menstrual cycle

Stephens (1976) also notes that some studies done on the menstrual cycle correlate plasma levels of monoamine oxidase (inactivators of adrenergic and serotoninergic neurotransmitters), ovarian hormones and mood during the menstrual cycle in normal and depressed women. The findings indicate that oestrogens appear to suppress monoamine oxidase levels and it is postulated that the high premenstrual accident and suicide rates may be a consequence of low plasma oestrogen levels at this time, leading to high monoamine oxidase activity and subsequent effect on the noradrenaline and serotonin (neurotransmitters which affect mood) levels.

Taylor & Watson (1977) discuss the results of an investigation undertaken to determine if women who report especially severe symptoms of premenstrual tension have objectively worse symptoms than other women or exhibit a lower tolerance to them. In their study, 90% of the women reported depression, irritability and tension as the commonest psychological symptoms. The commonest physical symptoms were headache, breast discomfort, abdominal distension and weight gain. Among the possible causes identified was poor progesterone output from the corpus luteum. Low levels of progesterone were found in 40% of the subjects and administration of progesterone brought relief from the mental disturbances, oedema and weight gain, but not from breast discomfort.

Disturbances of sleep-activity pattern

A number of studies have been undertaken on the effect that shifting the normal sleep-activity pattern has on normal circadian rhythms, mood and performance. The evidence from these studies shows that, in general, when a reversal of the normal sleep-activity cycle persists, the body's circadian rhythms eventually reverse. Some rhythms adjust in about 5 to 7 days, others take up to about 14 days. Some individuals never completely adjust (Hawkins & Armstrong-Esther, 1978). Studies by Folkard & Haines (1977) and Lobban & Nessling (1977) on full time and part time night nurses measuring body temperature, renal excretion patterns and performance indicate that, among nurses who normally work nights, long term adjustment takes place in the full time, but not in the part time, nurses.

The effect of rotation of the shifts worked has also been studied. Slow rotation allows some degree of circadian rhythm adaptation to occur while with rapid rotation (2 mornings, 2 afternoons, 2 nights followed by days off) no adaptation of body temperature rhythm was seen (Knauth & Rutenfranz, 1976). The circadian rhythm remained entrained to the 'usual' day hours of living. Of particular interest is the fact that those who were more tolerant of rapid shift rotation had more stable circadian rhythms than those who were less tolerant. The more tolerant workers, who had less digestive troubles, less fatigue and fewer sleep disturbances, were found to have circadian rhythms of large amplitude. These adjust more slowly than low amplitude rhythms and appear to increase tolerance to shift work (Andlauer & Reinberg, 1979).

The usefulness of the kinds of studies cited above in determining policies of shift rotation is obvious. Eaves (1980) for example, suggests that quickly changing rotas might ameliorate some of the circadian rhythm disturbances experienced by nurses on night duty because very rapid changes in rotas would prevent a shift or partial shift in circadian rhythms with the constant need to readjust.

While sleep loss and extra sleep can affect behaviour, in general it appears that normal waking efficiency depends more on maintaining regular sleep-activity cycles than on the absolute amount of sleep. An attempt has been made (Leddy, 1977) to separate the influence of sleep time per se and social routine, to determine which is the dominant factor; the results of this study were not conclusive but it is an area worth pursuing.

Circadian rhythms in daily life

Another area of research on the effects of biorhythms on daily life is suggested by a study (Hoskins, 1979) which examined body temperature, level of activation and interpersonal conflict in married couples. It was hypothesized that desynchrony in circadian rhythms of body temperature and activity levels between partners resulted in a higher level of interpersonal conflict. The results were not conclusive, perhaps because of compensatory and complementary behaviour exhibited by the couples. However, ordinary observation suggests that widely divergent sleep-activity cycles are a potential source of interpersonal strife among individuals living in close proximity.

Disturbances in rhythms due to rapidly changing time-zones results in jet-lag with feelings of fatigue and general discomfort. While motivation can overcome the fatigue, undesirable effects soon after travel can be minimized by planning meetings etc. at a time which fits into both the old and the new time-zone. Adaptation to the new time-zone is more rapid when moving west than when travelling eastwards as it is easier to adapt to a delay in time than to an advance (Minors & Waterhouse, 1981).

Biorhythms in giving care

As biorhythms affect so much of human functioning, they need to be taken into account when planning and executing therapeutic regimes (Yura & Walsh, 1978). Tom (1976) discusses in some detail the assessment of biorhythms, and Table 2.2 shows the objective and subjective data that she suggests can be obtained from the patient. This information can then be used to plan the patient's care to conform to his/her own circadian rhythm. The stress involved in adaptation can thus be minimized.

In the elderly the amplitude and level of many rhythms are reduced and there is an increase in the variability of the timing (Minors & Waterhouse, 1981). Disturbed sleep can result from changes in the sleep-wakefulness cycle and from the need to micturate because of the increased volume of urine produced at night. These changes in rhythm need to be taken into

Table 2.2 Tool for assessing circadian rhythms (Tom, 1976)

Objective data	Subjective data
1. Daily peaks and troughs on TPR and BP graphic records. 2. Urinary excretory patterns (quantity and frequency in relation to time of day) 3. Consistent behaviour patterns (cheerful, alert, energetic, verbose or irritable, quiet, less alert, and lethargic) in relation to time of day. 4. Environment, e.g. lighting schedule, activity-rest schedule, meal times, presence of clocks or other time cues.	1. Would you consider yourself a 'day' person or a 'night' person? 2. If you had your choice, would you go to bed after midnight or much earlier? 3. What time do you usually go to bed? Get up in the morning? 4. How does it make you feel when you are forced to change these habits, e.g. by your job, by long-distance travel or hospitalization? 5. Do you feel sociable and cheerful or antisocial and grumpy when you first get up? If you are grumpy and irritable, how long does this last? 6. Do you have a 'best' or 'worst' time of day? What makes you classify it as 'best' or 'worst'? 7. Do you have any physical complaints that you notice? Do these correlate with when you feel 'best' or 'worst'? 8. How many meals do you eat per day? What times do you usually eat them? When do you eat your largest meal? 9. How often do you usually urinate during a day? Do you get up at night to void?

account when planning care. Hall (1976), in her work with elderly, chronically ill patients, found that the five patients she studied had two peaks in body temperature during the day. The troughs corresponded to periods of sleep, at night and during the afternoon. When the rehabilitation programme was planned so that spells of activity corresponded to periods of increased alertness near peak temperature times more satisfactory progress in achieving goals was achieved.

Chronopharmacology is a developing field that addresses itself to the determination of the effect of drugs in relation to the times when they are administered. Studies on both animals and humans indicate that circadian rhythms affect the susceptibility to a wide variety of drugs such as antibiotics, antihistamines, corticosteroids and antihypertensives. The pituitary adrenal axis, for instance, is more susceptible to suppression from exogenous corticosteroids during the phase of reduced adrenocortical function. The adjustment of the timing of the dosage of these drugs, especially in chronic corticosteroid therapy, is important (Smolensky & Reinberg, 1976). If adrenal suppression is desired (as in adrenal hyperplasia) then these drugs should be given in divided doses throughout the day. Otherwise, morning administration is preferable.

THE WORKPLACE

Interest in industrial health and safety has risen sharply in the past few years. This is due to the increasing public awareness of health hazards within the workplace and to the incidence of injuries, disabilities, deaths and occupational disease. Ashford (1976) cites the following estimates of the National Safety Council for the USA—14 000 deaths and 2.2 million disabling injuries annually — and the Department of

Health, Education and Welfare estimate of 390 000 new cases of occupational disease and as many as 100 000 injuries each year, as an example.

Iveson-Iveson (1979) brings out the importance of community knowledge, awareness and co-operation in regard to the Safety and Health at Work Act if it is to be successfully implemented. Ashford (1976) makes the observation that the focus in the past has been on industrial safety and not on health. He suggests that both are important and further, that industrial health care not only includes disease prevention but likewise the promotion of health in the work environment. Western Europe leads other developed nations in research and effective approaches to occupational health. In these countries physicians and occupational health nurses play an important part, together with the health inspectors, in the team approach to setting and maintaining standards. Sweden led in research into stress related aspects of the work environment (Ashford, 1976). The study of ergonomics is also contributing to knowledge about health in relation to the adaptation of the machine and its working environment both to the individual and to groups of workers.

Environmental hazards

Examples of environmental hazards of the workplace are numerous. They include the familiar chemical and particulate pollutants causing diseases like pneumoconiosis, asbestosis, liver damage from chemicals like PVC, and various cancers. The category also includes the less publicized hazards like noise, vibration and ultraviolet and ionizing radiation. Vibration, for example, can cause microvascular changes leading to increased sensitivity to spasm in the hands of persons operating pneumatic drills and similar tools (WHO, 1972). Noise is a major health hazard not only in the workplace but in the home and leisure environments. Progressive, irreversible neurosensory deafness occurs when one is exposed to sustained relatively high noise levels. The response to noise varies with individuals, with age, and with the pitch and length of time of exposure and therefore standards are difficult to set. The range of loudness of noise in the human environment is variable. Safe limits, where they are set, are usually around 80 to 90 decibels for a continuing level of noise. It is noteworthy that not only is the noise of much industrial machinery above this level but a kitchen in which several appliances are running simultaneously also exceeds this level, traffic noise and a noisy office can approach it and discotheque music is about 120 db.

Work related accidents

Work related injuries and accidents are responsible for great personal and economic loss. Some conditions such as low back pain are very common, result in much misery and work time lost, and yet are not taken very seriously (Timbs, 1978). The causes of accidents have been the subject of much research.

Accident proneness. A number of hypotheses have been developed, some involving personality characteristics, of which an example is the concept of accident proneness. Ashford (1976) reviews some research findings on industrial accidents and points out that the relationship between personal factors and accidents is relatively weak, whereas age and inexperience are significant contributing factors. Smith (1977) notes that, in the absence of anxiety, attitude and group pressure are important determinants of safety awareness. Some studies on accident causation have been carried out in a specific context and the findings may be important for that context, but not necessarily generally applicable. Banta & Kosnosky (1978) for example, present a case study of a trainee pilot which illustrates the possible connection between a 'perfectionist' personality and channelization of attention. Over-correction and denial of error result in judgemental errors because the individual lacks an overview of the situation.

Fatigue. Cameron (1974) discusses the concept of fatigue, a subject often studied in terms of its impact on industrial productivity and safety. He suggests that the feelings of discomfort, irritability and restlessness and the deterioration of performance described as 'fatigue' can be accounted for by a 'reactive inhibition' effect. This reactive inhibition effect can occur with extended activity, but also with prolonged periods of anxiety and fear, and with sleep deficit. The conclusion that may be drawn is that fatigue is not a unique phenomenon but can be defined as a 'generalized response to stress over a period of time', the time dimension being the unique feature. This time dimension is useful in that it allows researchers to abandon the practice of quantifying fatigue in performance terms and to measure its severity in terms of the time required for recovery.

Health and safety

It is hoped that research on accident causation will place increasing emphasis on environmental factors causing stress and accidents. The contribution of ergonomics may shift the blame for accidents away from the worker and focus attention on the ways in which management should provide a safe and healthy work environment.

Ashford (1976) discusses four essential conflicts which impede progress toward better health and safety in the workplace:

- the clash of self interest between management and workers
- the lack of data on the health hazards in the workplace
- the problem of who should pay for improving health and safety aspects in the workplace
- the lack of interaction between industries and public bodies about industrial health related issues.

The Health and Safety at Work Act of 1974 in Britain promoted the concept of shared responsibility for health and safety between management and worker. While this concept appears attractive, the reality may work to the disadvantage of the worker; the nebulous gain of 'health' being bartered for the loss of autonomous work practices and the potential loss of productivity and financial bonuses. Loss of productivity is also clearly of major concern to management. Thus the shared nature of the responsibility might result in abrogation of this responsibility and the ignoring of agreed rules about safety in the interests of productivity.

Though there exists a fair amount of data relating to health and work and to safety and working conditions (Doyle, 1981; Kinnersly, 1980), it remains necessarily incomplete and in no way considers potential hazards of the newer and newest industrial processes or work situations. Debate on 'standards' in relation to 'safety and health' is often acrimonious and invariably the burden of proof remains with the victim. 'Cause' is more difficult to prove, particularly when considering the unequal relationship between that of management versus that of an individual worker.

Who should pay for improving health and safety aspects in the workplace?

Work not only involves hazards to the worker (Doyle, 1981; Kinnersly, 1980) — a vast number of work processes likewise also involve potential hazards to the public, as is exemplified in current public debate on the dispersion of radioactive material or the removal of lead from petrol. Reducing such hazards involves the whole society which includes those who own or manage the means of production. Who, for example, should pay for the removal of sulphur dioxide from industrial waste gases? Responsibility for the production of a cleaner environment is pushed hither and thither between those representing government and those who own or direct industrial development. Equally, the argument over energy production is complex. Though the dangers associated with coal production, in terms of health and safety of the individual miners, are considerable, yet its continuous production is mandatory both as a form of energy and as an insurance of sustained employment. The nuclear fuel debate runs along similar lines. While its production offers a potential risk to the health of a large section of the population, it has an important potential contribution to economic development in developing countries.

The lack of interaction between industries and public bodies about industrial health related issues

There is clearly inadequate interaction between institutions concerned with the general environment and those concerned with the industrial environment. As an example, DDT is an ecological danger. Its replacement with parathion reduces the danger to animals and the public at large, but creates a high risk for those who handle it.

Mathews (1983) discusses the current procedures for collection of data relating to occupational health in Australia. Some of the sources are national and some are from individual states and represent a variety of data bases, only a few of which refer directly to occupation (e.g. statistics on industrial accidents and diseases from insurance companies who deal in workers' compensation insurance). Mathews' proposals for change include: a national cancer register including occupational histories; inclusion of the occupational histories of both parents on birth registrations as a way of providing information on occupation-related fertility; routine post-mortem examination and recording of occupational history on death certificates; a regular public health survey; and the institution of national bodies responsible for collecting, linking and analysing data, conducting investigations, and promulgating standards for the recording and notifying of injury and disease in the workplace.

THE HOME AND COMMUNITY ENVIRONMENT

The home

Housing standards are an important influence on health. A very large proportion of the world's population live in substandard housing where filth and disease vectors abound, and the physical conditions contribute not only to discomfort, such as inadequate warmth, but also to stress due to overcrowding. Gray (1978) points out the problem of drawing a direct connection between poor housing and physical illness but suggests that when poor housing is seen in the light of its effect on existing illness or on well-being a clearer connection can be seen (Townsend & Davidson, 1982). The home is potentially hazardous under the best conditions of housing with the introduction of new potent cleaning compounds, more personal grooming aids, as well as paints, pesticides and the like. Not only are many of these compounds toxic if ingested, but the long term effects of low level exposure are largely unknown. However, there are indications that there may be serious effects on health (WHO, 1972).

Home accidents are a major problem. An international study initiated by the World Health Organization in 1964 in Europe showed that accidents in the home accounted for 1–2% of all deaths, 20% of all accidental deaths among men and 50% among women. The groups most at risk were children, the aged and the physically and socially handicapped. The largest proportion of accidents were falls, followed by fires (WHO, 1972). Wynn-Davies (1977) points to the increase in accidents as new and unfamiliar leisure time activities are introduced.

The community

Road accidents are also a major cause of concern and give rise to a number of studies seeking to identify causes. Some of these have concentrated on the personality characteristics of drivers (Jamieson et al, 1971), while others have examined factors such as fatigue and the driver's ability to cope under conditions of illness or even minor discomfort (Hopkins, 1978). Studies have shown a strong association between blood alcohol concentration and road accidents to pedestrians (Irwin et al, 1983). McDermott & Hughes (1983) point out the disproportionately high representation of probationary drivers among road casualties and the higher proportion of inexperienced to experienced drivers found driving with blood alcohol concentrations over the legal limit. McLean (1983) suggests that given the combination of driver inexperience and alcohol consumption as a major contributing factor in motor vehicle accidents, specific countermeasures such as prohibition of motor vehicle operation by probationary drivers after ingestion of even a small amount of alcohol may be useful. The complexity of the driving task has been stressed and there is a need to take an ergonomic approach to the problem. Achieving a better fit of the vehicle to road conditions and a better fit of the vehicle to passenger will decrease the vulnerability of both passengers and pedestrians (Jamieson et al, 1971).

Socio-demographic factors in relation to accidental death and injury have been studied as have the characteristics of the individuals at risk. Brown & Davidson (1978) looked at the accident risk to children of a random sample of women living in a former inner London borough in association with social class and psychiatric history of the mother. They found that a highly increased accident risk to children was associated with working class status and a history of psychiatric disorder (usually depression) in the mother. The increased accident risk to the children was not explained on the basis of poor supervision but was perceived by these authors to be more likely to stem from increased anxiety and insecurity in the children resulting in a behaviour which led to more accidents. Nixon & Pearn (1978), in an Australian study, showed a relationship between migrant status, large families, late birth order and a high risk of childhood drowning accidents.

ECONOMIC ENVIRONMENT

Poverty

The health of disadvantaged groups, whose health behaviour contributes through succeeding generations to the perpetuation of a poor health status and seems refractory to public education and health measures, is a source of ongoing and growing concern. In order to examine the effects of poverty on health it is important to have some understanding of the phenomenon of poverty. This includes the attitudes towards it, attempts to explain its existence, a working definition and an idea of the magnitude of the problem of poverty. The dominant ideology which is fundamental to the ordering of priorities will affect attitudes to poverty. These attitudes will determine not only the amount and distribution of the money spent but also the access to health care facilities. In addition, they also influence health care delivery, even on an individual level, because of the often judgemental attitudes of health professionals.

Kosa et al (1969) outline four possible attitudes to poverty:

- a fatalistic acceptance of poverty within an immutable social order — poverty is then not perceived as a problem.
- poverty is recognized but not considered amenable to change — and therefore charity is offered as a token solution.
- poverty is a result of mismanagement of one's affairs and is thus blameworthy.
- poverty is a problem which can be and is solved by social legislation. Thus poverty should not exist in developed nations.

Peter Townsend (1979) in his comprehensive work *Poverty in the United Kingdom* develops the concept of poverty. He discusses theories of poverty which essentially deal with either characteristics of the poor themselves or social/economic explanations. The former refers to that concept commonly known as 'the cycle of deprivation' which accepts that values peculiar to the poor ensure a continuation of the state of poverty. The economic or social structure theories attempt to explain poverty on the basis of the distribution of income. Townsend points out that historically, poverty has been expressed as an absolute minimum level of needs below which people are 'poor', leading to the promulgation of fixed 'poverty level' income. He suggests that in order to arrive at a more meaningful definition of poverty we need to measure all types of resources, public and private, that are unequally distributed and contribute to an individual's standard of living. In addition it is necessary to define the style of living shared and approved by a given community, at a given time, and find the income point at which families do not significantly share in this style of living, e.g. the customs, activities and diet. He introduces the concept of a threshold level of income below which deprivation increases disproportionately to the decrease in income level.

Poverty and health

The effect of poverty on health is often looked at from the standpoint of standard epidemiological indicators of health status, e.g. mortality rates, morbidity rates, incidence and prevalence of diseases and infant mortality. Townsend notes that in the UK there is little indication of narrowing of the gap between social class I and social class V in indicators such as infant mortality. Some statistics gathered from various national health surveys in the US reveal that 60% of the children of the poor have never seen a dentist, 30% of their parents have one or more chronic diseases, the incidence of all forms of cancer is inversely related to income, the poor have four times as many heart problems, six times as many cases of hypertension, arthritis and rheumatism, eight times as many visual impairments and more psychiatric illnesses than the more affluent (Kane et al 1976). Similar statistics exist in the UK (Townsend & Davidson, 1982).

Illness can lead to poverty because of the cost of care (particularly in the USA) the loss of income from work and loss of potential to work. Conditions of poverty do not allow good recovery from illness or the freedom from more pressing concerns of survival to pursue preventive medicine and health maintenance care. Whether poverty directly causes illness is contentious, but there is good evidence that the poor utilize the health care system less and less efficiently than the more affluent. There have been many suggestions why this may be so. These include differences in the perception of illness, lack of confidence in the health care system, poor communication between health professionals and the poor, impersonal attitudes, problems with transport, being away from work, child minding and the like (Bergner & Yerby, 1976).

Suggestions concerning health care delivery and the approach of health professionals to the poor made by people involved with disadvantaged communities are valuable. Hughes (1976) discusses the efficacy of direct personal intervention with mothers in a poor city environment characterized by bleak physical surroundings, depression and apathy. At a 'low key' level of persuasion, the mothers were shown how to relate better to their children through the introduction of limited joint outings. The mothers were able to share experiences with each other and the children explored new play environments. She suggests that this is the type of activity in which a health visitor can engage. Such involvement, however, is problematic, because while it might promote temporary diversion from everyday pressures, it may also serve to deflect attention from the root problem.

Studies on Australian aboriginal communities (Samisoni & Samisoni, 1978; Dinnell, 1976) identify not only the problem of poverty and poor housing, but the additional burden of the imposition of European values, with the resultant breakdown of traditional societal values and viable social networks. Improvement does not seem to come about by formal education programmes or by making the health care system more available. What is suggested is an improvement of the living conditions and more involvement of the aboriginal community in their own health care. The problem of how much involvement or control the community should have, especially as it relates to programmes for the poor, is a much debated issue in the US. Hochbaum (1976) suggests that more research is needed to determine the effects of community control and consumer participation in health planning.

THE SOCIAL ENVIRONMENT

Roles

A conference on women's health held in Queensland, Australia in 1975 to celebrate International Women's Year (Commonwealth Department of Health, 1978) demonstrated how stereotyping of male and female roles can influence the health status and health behaviour of women. The following issues were highlighted:

- The need for women to form self-help groups to share information about disorders such as premenstrual tension (PMT). This relates especially to the less than sympathetic response of physicians and the tendency to minimize the problems associated with PMT or to label it as 'psychosomatic'.
- The problems associated with establishing and maintaining physical exercise and sporting programmes for women in an atmosphere which casts women in a passive 'feminine' role.
- Women (in their role as carrying responsibility for family nutrition) are the target of guilt-provoking advertising in relation to foods, food supplements and vitamin products, when the nutritional value of the products advertised is not known.
- Problems women encounter in the workplace, where equipment and facilities are not geared to their size or strength.
- The 'fashion plate' image women are expected to maintain which prevents them from adopting sensible footwear.

An interesting counterpart to literature on women and health is the effect that the sterotyped male role has in precipitating the increased anxiety, depression and symptoms of physical illnesses many men experience between the ages of 40–50.

Hauser (1980) suggests that there is little evidence for a biological basis for this so called male middlescence, but men are required to maintain totally inappropriate behaviour in terms of aggressiveness in business, upward mobility and sexual performance which do not correlate with reality. Middle age is often a time of re-ordering of priorities, changes in family circumstances, making way for younger people in the workforce, and ageing and death of friends. Hauser feels that the conflict between role expectations and reality is worth examining further as a source of this anxiety and depression.

Life change

There has been recent interest in determining whether any direct effects on health can be shown to be due to major life changes. The several studies cited below relate to this question and indicate some approaches to it. A US study (Pesznecker & McNeil, 1975) attempted to discover the relationship between the variables of health habits, social assets and psychological well-being, and life changes and alterations in health status. A life change refers to an event which changes one's life in a significant way, e.g. change in job status, marriage, divorce. The study revealed that the magnitude of life change was the best predictor of health status and that the other variables were weakly correlated with the maintenance of health. Andrews et al (1978) conducted a study among adults (mean age 42) in typical families in a residential suburb of Sydney, Australia to determine the relationship between various social factors and physical and psychiatric illness. The variables studied included stressful life events, occupational rank, migrant status, availability of a social support system, maturity of coping mechanisms and adverse childhood experiences. The results showed that 46% of adults reported a chronic physical condition and 24% psychiatric impairment. Life events, stress, adverse childhood experiences and poor social support were related to both physical and psychiatric illness. Low occupational status was associated with poor physical health and poor coping style with psychiatric illness. However, age was the best predictor of adult physical illness. In summary, 20% of physical and 37% of psychiatric impairment was associated with social factors. These authors point out that there is a difficulty in separating social factors from factors of poor health behaviour, e.g. smoking and excess drinking, so the interpretation of these data is not simple. In addition, they suggest that the mere demonstration of association between social factors and illness is of little value for public health, and research ought to be directed toward identifying factors which enable people to cope with social stresses.

Similarly, a study by Andrews & Tennant

(1978) demonstrates the difficulty in drawing direct causal links between social factors and illness. The authors report that a review of the literature on the relationship of episodic psychological stress to the onset of physical illness, in which the effect of major disasters, the impact of cumulative life event stresses and the consequence of conjugal bereavement were examined, revealed that there was no weight of evidence to show that psychological stress leads directly to physical illness. However they did report that it may lead to life style changes which increase the risk of poor health, complicate existing illnesses or lead to illness behaviour.

A number of studies cited by Hinton (1967) indicate an increase in mortality rate for widows and widowers. He notes that the death rate in this group is greater than in the general population, even after one excludes death by suicide or conditions attributable to self neglect. For example, there seems to be a tendency for a higher mortality from physical conditions such as cardiac disorders.

Herbert (1978) looked at the relationship between life change and the seriousness of illness in female university students and found a significant relationship between the number of life changes and the seriousness of the illness. It is noteworthy that this finding occurs in a young relatively healthy population. Piper et al (1978) examined the relationship of life events which caused change and distress to a specific physical illness, gastric ulcers, and found no difference in the life change and distress scores between controls and gastric ulcer patients, although the amount of change and distress was increased with increased age, when there was no increase in the number of events.

Occupational stressors in relation to the risk of illness are discussed by Adams (1976) and several stressors are identified such as role ambiguity and conflict, too much or too little work, too little meaningful participation, too little or too much responsibility for others and poor support system in work relationships. Kobasa (1979) conducted an interesting study relating certain personality traits to the illness-provoking effect of stressful life events. Two groups of executives were identified, one with a high stress/high illness score, the other with a high stress/low illness score. The personality characteristics markedly present in the latter group were more control, more commitment and an interest in change as a challenge. This brings to light the generally recognized observations that there are some individuals who survive extremely stressful circumstances and remain in good physical and mental health. It also seems to open another avenue of investigation, namely the mitigating effects of personality on the relationship between stress and illness.

CONCLUSION

The evidence presented relating various forms of stress, social structure, economics or personality structure to illness or accidental injury rests upon demonstrating a positive correlation between these variables and the incidence or onset of illness. Positive correlation between variables, however strong, can never be construed as establishing a cause-effect relationship. However, if one waited until a direct cause-effect relationship was established to intervene, many illnesses would not be treated.

NURSES' RESPONSIBILITY

In the developed countries, nurses make up a large part, if not the majority, of workers in the health care system. Mackenzie (1979) cites the following figures for the UK from the DHSS annual report for 1976: in England alone there was a total of 338 997 staff in nursing and midwifery (including part time equivalents) compared to 54 679 doctors. The voice of the nursing profession has traditionally not been well heard in matters of social and health care legislation. This must be remedied. In order for the views of nurses to be taken seriously they must be well informed and gain an overview of the living environment including economic and societal structure. In addition, it is necessary that relationships with individual patients be free of uninformed, biased judgements which hamper one's effectiveness. This can only be achieved if nurses know something about their patients in terms of the context in which they live, work and seek help from the health care system. Nurses cannot be effective members of the health care system if they are not conversant with contemporary political, social and ethical issues. If nurses cannot be seen to be effective and influential members of the health care system the nursing profession will continue to have a low profile and a weak power base. Thus, needed reforms may be a longer time than is proper in coming to fruition.

REFERENCES

Adams J 1976 Stress and the risk of illness. In: Transition: understanding and managing personal change. Martin Robertson, London

Andlauer P, Reinberg A 1979 Amplitude of the oral temperature circadian rhythm and tolerance to shift work. Chronobiologia Supplement 1 : 67–73

Andrews G, Tennant C 1978 Being upset and becoming ill: an appraisal of the relation between life events and physical illness. Medical Journal of Australia 1:324–327

Andrews G, Tennant C, Hewson D, Schonell M 1978 Relation of social factors to physical and psychiatric illness. American Journal of Epidemiology 1081 (1): 27–35

Ashford N A 1976 Crisis in the workplace: occupational disease and injury. MIT Press, Cambridge, Mass.

Banta G, Kosnosky D 1978 Case report of an obsessive-compulsive personality: a precursor to accident proneness. Aviation Space and Environmental Medicine 49 (6):827–828

Bergner L, Yerby A 1976 Low income and barriers to the use of health services. In: Kane L, Kastler J, Gray R (eds) The health gap. Springer, New York

Brown G, Davidson S 1978 Social class, psychiatric disorder of mother, and accidents to children. Lancet 1 (8060):378–381

Cameron C 1974 A theory of fatigue. In: Welford A (ed) Man under stress. Taylor & Francis, London

Comfort A 1978 Comfort for the aging. Australian Nurses Journal 7(9):32–36

Commonwealth Department of Health 1978 Women's health in a changing society. Australian Government Publishing Service, Canberra

Dilman I 1973 Induction and deduction. Basil Blackwell, London

Dinnell G P 1976 Aboriginal health. Australian Nurses Journal 5:29–32

Doyle L 1981 The political economy of health. Pluto Press, London

Eaves D 1980 Time for a Change. Nursing Mirror 150(6): 22–24

Evans A J 1977 Limitation of Koch's postulates. Lancet 2: 1277–1278

Folkard S, Haines S M 1977 Adjustment to night work in full and part time night nurses. Journal of Physiology 267:23–24

Goldstein G 1983 Goals and priorities in prevention: the challenge of chronic disease and disability. Community Health Studies VII (I): 54–59

Gray J A M 1978 Housing, health and illness. British Medical Journal 2:100–101

Hall L 1976 Circadian rhythms, implications for geriatric rehabilitation. Nursing Clinics of North America 11(4):631–638

Hannay D R 1979 The symptom iceberg. Routledge & Kegan Paul, London

Hauser M J 1980 Male middlescence. Occupational Health Nursing 2:18–24

Hawkins L H, Armstrong-Esther C A 1978 Circadian rhythms and night shift working in nurses. Nursing Times Supplement 74: 49–52

Herbert D 1978 Life changes and seriousness of illness in female college students. Psychological Reports 43:1297–1298

Hinton J 1967 Dying. Penguin, Harmondsworth

Hochbaum G M 1976 Consumer participation in health planning. In: Kane R, Kastler J, Gray R (eds) The health gap. Springer, New York

Hopkins P 1978 Causes and prevention of road accidents. Nursing Times 74:1594–1596

Hoskins CN 1979 Level of activation, body temperature and interpersonal conflict. Nursing Research 28(3):154–160

Hughes J 1976 The cycle of deprivation. Health Visitor 49: 266–267

Irwin S T, Patterson C C, Rutherford W H 1983 Association between alcohol consumption and adult pedestrians who sustain injuries in road traffic accidents. British Medical Journal 286:522

Iveson-Iveson J 1979 How to stay healthy: environmental hazards. Nursing Mirror 149 (21) : 22

Jamieson K G, Duggen A W, Twedell J, Pope L I, Zvirbulis V E 1971 Traffic crashes in Brisbane. Australian Road Research Board Special Report 2:255–277

Kane R, Kastler J, Gray R (eds) 1976 The health gap. Springer, New York

Kinnersly P 1980 The hazards of work, 7th edn. Pluto Press, London

Knauth P, Rutenfranz J 1976 Experimental shift work studies of permanent night and rapidly rotating shift systems, Vol I. Circadian rhythm of body temperature and re-entrainment at shift change. International Archives of Occupational and Environmental Health 37:125–137. Cited in Minors D S, Waterhouse J M (eds) Circadian rhythms and the human. Wright, Bristol

Kobasa S 1979 Personality and resistance to illness. American Journal of Community Psychology 7 (4):413–423

Kosa J, Antonousky A, Zola I (eds) 1969 Poverty and health. Harvard University Press, Cambridge

Lanuza D 1976 Circadian rhythms of mental efficiency and performance. Nursing Clinics of North America 11 (4): 583–594

Lazarus RS (1976) Patterns of adjustment. McGraw Hill, New York

Leddy S 1977 Sleep and phase shifting of biological rhythms. International Journal of Nursing Studies 14 (3):137–150

Lobban M, Nessling R 1977 Twenty–four hour pattern of renal excretion in full and part time night nurses. Journal of Physiology 267:24–25

Mackenzie W J M 1979 Power and responsibility in health

care. Oxford University Press, Oxford
McDermott F T, Hughes E S R 1983 Driver casualties in Victoria 1978–80: predominant influence of driver inexperience and alcohol. Medical Journal of Australia 1:609–611
McLean A J 1983 Alcohol drugs and road accidents. Medical Journal of Australia 1:596–597
Mechanic D 1976 The growth of bureaucratic medicine. Wiley, New York
Minors P S, Waterhouse J M 1981 Circadian rhythms and the human. Wright, Bristol.
Natalini J 1977 The human body as a biological clock. American Journal of Nursing 77 : 1130–1132
Nixon J, Pearn J 1978 An investigation of socio-demographic factors surrounding childhood drowning accidents. Social Science Medicine 12 (5A) : 387–390
Pesznecker B L, McNeil J 1975 Relationship among health habits, social assets, psychologic well-being, life change and alterations in health status. Nursing Research 24:442–447
Piper D, Greig M, Shinners J, Thomas J, Crawford J 1978 Chronic gastric ulcer and stress. Digestion 18:303–309
Riegelman R 1979 Contributory cause: unnecessary and insufficient. Postgraduate Medicine 66 (2):177–179
Rosch P J 1979 Stress and illness. Journal of the American Medical Association 242:427–428
Rothman K 1976 Causes. American Journal of Epidemiology 104(6) :587–592
Samisoni M T, Samisoni J I 1978 The health of aboriginal and islander children of urbanized communities. Australian Nurses Journal 7 (11):44–47
Selye H 1956 The stress of life (revised 1976). McGraw-Hill, New York
Shontz F C 1975 The psychological aspects of physical illness and disability. Macmillan, New York
Smith J M 1977 The occupational psychologist and health and safety. Occupational Health 29 : 150
Smolensky M H, Reinberg A 1976 The chronotherapy of corticosteroids: practical application of chronobiologic findings to nursing. Nursing Clinics of North America 11(4):609–614
Stephens G 1976 Periodicity in mood, affect and instinctual behaviour. Nursing Clinics of North America 11 (4):595–607
Taylor R W, Watson J M 1977 Premenstrual tension. Nursing Mirror 145 (7) : 39–40
Timbs O 1978 Attack on back pain. Occupational Health (London) 30:119–122
Tom C K 1976 Nursing assessment of biological rhythms. Nursing Clinics of North America 11 (4):621–630
Totman R 1979 Social causes of illness. Souvenir Press, London
Townsend P 1979 Poverty in the United Kingdom. Penguin, Harmondsworth
Townsend P, Davidson N 1982 Inequalities in health. Penguin, Harmondsworth
Weiner H 1978 The illusion of simplicity. American Journal of Psychiatry 135 supplement: 27–33
Wever R 1975 The circadian multi-oscillator system of man. International Journal of Chronobiology 3 : 19–55. Cited in Minors D S, Waterhouse J M 1981 Circadian rhythms and the human. Wright, Bristol
World Health Organization 1947 The constitution of the World Health Organization. WHO Chronicle 1:29–43
World Health Organization 1972 Health hazards of the human environment. WHO, Geneva
Wynn-Davies B 1977 Lethal leisure. Nursing Mirror 145(7):13–14
Yura H, Walsh M B 1978 Human needs and the nursing process. Appleton-Century Crofts, Connecticut

3

Genetic factors in disease

INTRODUCTION

The study of genetics is of increasing importance not only to the nursing and medical professions but to all members of our society. More is now known about the basic facts of inheritance since Gregor Mendel's work with garden peas and the rediscovery of his work simultaneously in Holland, Austria and Germany at the beginning of the 20th century. A growing understanding of the universal nature of the biochemical structure and functioning of living organisms has brought about an awareness of the crucial role of genes in living organisms. With the control of many infectious disorders being achieved by improvements in standards of living, public health measures and the use of antibiotics, genetic disorders have increased in relative importance in infant mortality statistics and in both infant and adult morbidity.

Genetic disorders affect all systems of the body and vary enormously in their severity and in their risk of occurrence or recurrence. Some, such as Duchenne muscular dystrophy, are very disabling and lethal, those boys affected seldom surviving beyond their teens; some are lethal at birth, for example anencephaly; while others, such as polydactyly, are unlikely to affect expectation of life and may only create minor inconvenience to an affected person. Some genetic disorders are easily diagnosable at birth, e.g. the skeletal abnormalities, achondroplasia and cleft palate, while other disorders, of variable age of onset, e.g. myotonic dystrophy and Huntington's chorea, are unlikely to be diagnosed until middle years. Some genetic disorders due to mutant genes of large effect are inherited and transmitted in different but relatively straightforward patterns according to Mendelian principles of probability. And others, as Clarke (1970) indicates, are often caused by a subtle interaction between genetic and environmental factors so that it is essential also to understand something of polygenic inheritance.

Patients suffering from or associated with genetic disease are to be found in most hospital wards and also in the community. They are not, however, segregated into a specific ward or unit. Frequently the emphasis is on the medical or surgical management of the condition, e.g. in haemophilia and polycystic kidney disease, and the genetic nature of the condition and the implications that this creates are ignored or left in the background. With knowledge of genetic disease and the implications of the disease, nurses are in a position to identify patients who may be in need of information and to offer appropriate counselling both to patients and to their families.

Genetic disease is frequently associated with inaccurate, distorted information, myth and old wives' tales. Sadly, this is sometimes true of nurses and doctors as well as the lay public. With more knowledge and better understanding, nurses will be able to clarify misunderstanding, dispel myths and therefore help minimize fear and anxiety.

This chapter begins with sections on the genetic structure, the different forms of transmission and the variety of genetic disease and continues with sections on treatments available, prenatal diagnosis and genetic counselling.

SCOPE OF THE SUBJECT

Human genetics is a relatively new and expanding subject of study. General and easily read introductions to the subject are Milunsky (1980), Harper (1981) and Weatherall (1982) who discuss the medical aspects of human genetics, while the different approaches to genetic counselling are well covered by Kessler (1979), Sorenson et al (1981) and Lubs & de la Cruz (1977). Some of the advances in genetics and ethical issues are discussed in a well-written popular paperback by Harsanyi & Hutton, (1983).

Genetic engineering involves the process of changing the genetic material of a cell, through numerous complex manipulations. It is hoped that this will lead to practical applications in the diagnosis and treatment of inherited disease. Advances in this field are discussed by Williamson (1981). This subject raises ethical issues and moral dilemmas, some of which are considered in Birch & Abrecht (1975), in 'Life and Death before Birth' (Council for Science and Society, 1978) and in Thomas (1986). Articles on these subjects appear in numerous medical and other journals and newspapers, particularly the American Journal of Human Genetics and the Journal of Medical Genetics.

GENETIC STRUCTURE

A human being originates in the union of two gametes, the ovum and the spermatozoon, each containing 23 single chromosomes. These cells contain all that the new individual inherits organically from his or her parents. The hereditary elements are the genes which are discrete regions arranged linearly on the chromosomes present in the nucleus of each cell. Genes contain the vital hereditary material DNA — deoxyribonucleic acid. Chromosomes are basically long strands of DNA composed of a succession of many thousands of genes arranged in linear order.

The nucleus of the human cell contains 23 pairs of chromosomes, one of each pair being derived originally from each parent: 22 of the 23 pairs are the same in both males and females and are called the autosomes. One pair, the sex chromosomes, is different. The female has two X chromosomes usually depicted XX, while the male has one X chromosome which is the same as the two in the female but its partner is the much smaller Y chromosome, described XY.

GROWTH AND DEVELOPMENT

Reproduction and growth involve the multiplication of cells. In order to multiply, cells undergo cell division. One divides into two, two into four, four into eight and so on. The word 'division' is possibly misleading as it implies halving. It is known that cell division is accompanied or preceded by the formation of new cell components so that the products of cell division, the daughter cells, are identical to the parent cell. The process of cell division is complex (see Roberts, 1977 for a detailed explanation). But put simply, as the cells divide and the new individual grows and develops, the full number of 46 chromosomes, 23 pairs, in the nucleus of each cell is maintained with the exception of the gametes which contain 23 single chromosomes.

As growth and development is brought about by cell division, assimilation of material leading to expansion, and cell differentiation, any factor that affects these processes will influence growth. These factors could be either internal or external. Internal factors affecting growth include the actions of the genes and the relative quantities of different hormones present in the fetus. These two are connected in that the genes influence growth through the intermediary of the hormones. But hormones are also influenced by environmental factors, e.g. lack of iodine in the diet can result in cretinism. Iodine deficiency has this effect because it is needed for the synthesis of thyroxine, the hormone that regulates the metabolic rate.

External factors include many environmental influences such as temperature, light, atmospheric pollution and diet. Normal growth and development depend on an extremely complex and fine interaction between internal and external influences (Kalter & Warkany, 1983).

Genes are of particular importance in the early period of growth as it is during this period that the detailed characteristics of shape and function of every kind come to maturity and result in a unique new person. Every one of the thousands of genes is the initiating point of one of the many thousands of biochemical activities which, when they occur at the right time and place, result in the creation of a healthy individual, or which in other cases result in genetic abnormality.

GENETIC DISORDERS

Genetic or inherited diseases are frequently categorized as:

- those due to single genes of large effect
- those due to chromosomal aberrations
- those with multifactorial causation.

DISORDERS DUE TO ABNORMALITIES OF SINGLE GENES

Single genes may give rise to highly distinguishing differences in an individual. A classical example of a constitutional change due to a single genetic abnormality is albinism. Similarly, such metabolic disorders due to single gene defects as phenylketonuria and galactosaemia, produce chemical aberrations discernible at the laboratory level as well as constitutional findings seen by inspection and physical examination. On the other hand traits or constitutional factors such as height, intelligence and blood pressure are believed to be due to the action of many genes. The inheritance of these traits is said to be 'polygenic' or 'multigenic' in origin.

Genetic disorders due to single genes can be inherited in one of the following four ways:

- autosomal dominant
- autosomal recessive
- X-linked
- Y-linked.

It is important to understand these modes of inheritance, as it is this information which indicates the likelihood of an individual being affected or having an affected child. The study of family trees or pedigree charts will help in this understanding (see Figs. 3.1–3.5). Family pedigrees are constructed to help in the making of a genetic diagnosis because they show the pattern of the disorder through and down the

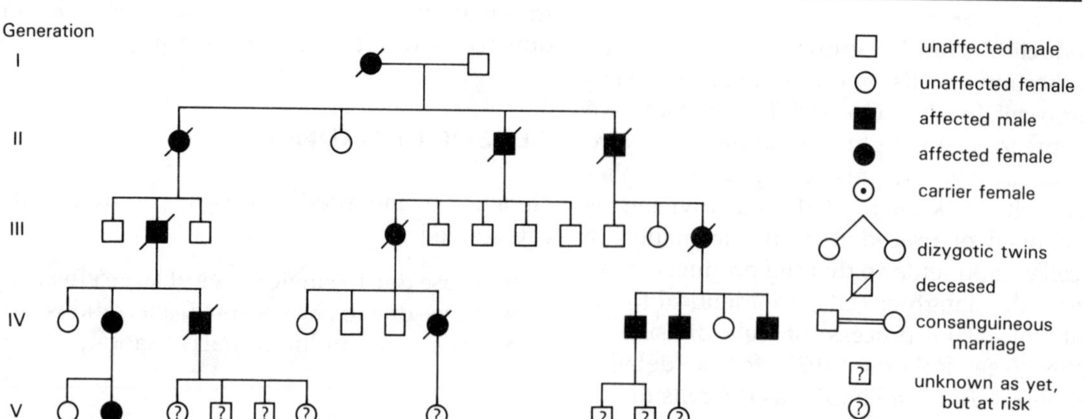

Fig. 3.1 Pedigree pattern of autosomal dominant inheritance — a family with Huntington's chorea.

generations. They are also useful as a means of highlighting the impact of disease in particular families.

Autosomal dominant inheritance (AD)

Inheritance pattern

Figure 3.1 shows the pedigree of a family affected by a condition inherited in an autosomal dominant way. This mode of inheritance is characterized by the presence of a single gene on one of a pair of matched autosomal chromosomes. Therefore, a person with an autosomal dominant trait possesses one abnormal (mutant) gene which causes the disorder or trait as well as one normal gene. Such a person is described as being heterozygous for the gene. In disorders transmitted in an autosomal dominant fashion, the following pattern usually occurs:

- males and females are equally affected
- each affected person has an affected parent
- every child of an affected person has a 50–50 chance of being affected by the disorder (assuming that only one parent is affected).

This is the most usual pattern, but there are exceptions or situations where this does not appear to occur. For example, an affected person may not always have an affected parent, as sometimes a disorder seems to appear suddenly in one generation when no one else in previous generations has apparently been affected. There are several possible explanations for this:

- The disorder could have arisen as a result of a new mutation — a spontaneous change in which the abnormal gene is not inherited but created afresh on the chromosome. New mutations are, however,relatively rare (Roberts, 1977).
- It could also be that a parent did have the disorder but was so mildly affected that it was not detected and diagnosed. Some genetic disorders present problems for diagnosis, and whether the disorder was diagnosed or not could depend on where the person lived, the availability of resources and the person's age. Further, although the accurate recording of information on death certificates has greatly improved in recent years, the cause of death may not be the inherited disease, and the fact that the deceased was affected by a particular genetic disorder may not have been recorded.
- Finally, an affected person may not know about his or her parents because he or she was adopted or had lost contact with them.

It is important to remember that in genetics it

is a question of chance or probability at each conception whether or not the new conceptus receives the deleterious gene. In the case of autosomal dominant inheritance the probability is 50–50 or one in two. An affected person may be lucky enough to have a family with no affected children. The larger the family, the more opportunities there are for the transmission of the deleterious gene. On the other hand, in some families all the children may be affected, and in others none.

Age of onset

Some disorders transmitted in an autosomal dominant fashion are diagnosable at birth, e.g. those involving skeletal malformations, achondroplasia and cleft palate and the eye disorder, retinoblastoma. Others have what is known as a variable age of onset. This means that the disorder does not normally appear until adulthood and cannot be diagnosed until a series of symptoms is present. Depending upon the condition this may be at any time in adulthood. In these disorders, of which Huntington's chorea is perhaps the best known, there is no definitive predictive test for those 'at risk' (Hayden, 1981; Thomas, 1982). Such autosomal dominant disorders of variable age of onset present many very difficult and delicate problems for those offering genetic counselling and these will be discussed later.

Variable severity

Autosomal dominant inherited disorders, besides showing variability in age of onset, may also demonstrate variability in their severity. For example, Harper (1979) describes a family with myotonic dystrophy AD where an infant child presented with a severe neuromuscular problem. The parents were stated to be healthy but further inquiry showed the maternal grandfather to have been affected by myotonic dystrophy since middle life. To 'miss a generation' is not compatible with autosomal dominant transmission. On further investigation it was discovered that the mother was indeed affected, but virtually asymptomatic.

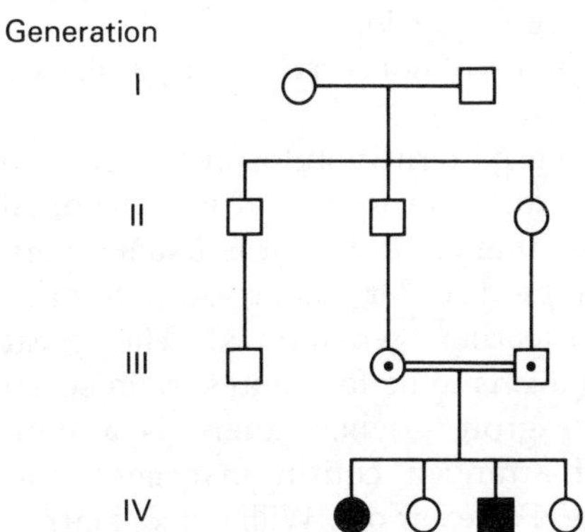

Fig. 3.2 Pedigree pattern of autosomal recessive inheritance — consanguinous marriage.

Autosomal recessive inheritance (AR)

Figure 3.2 shows the pedigree of a family with an autosomal recessive disorder. As in the case of autosomal dominant inheritance, disorders transmitted in an autosomal recessive fashion affect both males and females. In autosomal recessive inheritance both parents of an affected individual are normally* asymptomatic, heterozygous carriers of the disorder in that they both have one abnormal gene and one normal gene and do not present symptoms. It should be noted, however, that the asymptomatic carrier of some conditions can be identified by biochemical testing. An affected symptomatic individual is homozygous for the disorder — that is, the disorder only appears when the gene is present in a double dose. All children of such a person must receive the abnormal gene and will therefore be heterozygous carriers. If they mate with another heterozygous carrier for the same disorder then they have a chance of having an affected child. The risk to the conceptus at each conception when both parents are heterozygous carriers of a particular disorder is as follows:

- 1 in 4 chance of being affected

* In discussing forms of inheritance and transmission, examples given are for the more common situations. On the rare occasions when two persons affected by the same disorder and attributed to the same gene, or an affected person and a carrier, mate, the outcomes are not discussed. See Roberts & Pembrey (1978).

- 1 in 2 or 50–50 chance of being a heterozygous carrier
- 1 in 4 chance of not carrying the gene.

The pedigree pattern in autosomal recessive inheritance is different from that in autosomal dominant inheritance, in that it is usually very unlikely that the disorder will be found to have appeared in earlier generations. The great exception to this is to be found in certain social and religious groups where there is a high incidence of arranged cousin marriages and intermarriage. For example, Williams & Harper (1976) have described in a genetic study of Welsh gypsies the presence of many members of a large family with phenylketonuria. There was extensive consanguinity and all the cases were derived from a single carrier common ancestor.

Consanguinity

With rare recessive disorders, the parents of affected individuals are often related, the reason being that cousins are more likely to carry the same genes because they received them from a common ancestor. The chance that first cousins will carry the same genes because they receive them from a common ancestor is 1 in 8. The chance that two unrelated persons carry the same gene is usually much less than 1 in 8 but the exact figure will depend on the frequency of that gene in the general population and the ethnic origin of the individuals. For example, there is a high frequency of Tay-Sachs disease amongst Ashkenazi Jews amongst whom it is estimated that 9 in 30 carry the gene (Kaback & O'Brien, 1973). Members of such groups are highly likely to have had a common ancestry and therefore share the same genes. It is suggested that Ashkenazi Jews are descended from those who fled to northeast Europe after the sacking of Jerusalem in AD 70 (Milunsky, 1980). Similarly, in the USA, it is estimated that 1 in 10 of the black population carry the gene for sickle cell anaemia (Weatherall & Clegg, 1981).

Cystic fibrosis is the most common autosomal recessive disorder known in Caucasian populations, affecting approximately 1 in 2000 births. It is very rare amongst Negroes and Orientals and is most common in Northern Europeans (Bergsma, 1973). In the United Kingdom approximately 1 in every 22 persons carries the gene. The chance of two persons, both heterozygous carriers for this disorder, mating is much greater than for rarer conditions with lower gene frequency such as alkaptonuria, the gene for which is carried by only 1 person in every 500 in the general population (Committee on Mutagenicity of Chemicals in Food, 1981).

The rarer the recessive disorder, the greater is found to be the frequency of consanguinity among the parents of affected persons. It is estimated that the frequency of first cousin marriages in the general population in the UK is about 0.5%: that is, about 1 in every 200 marriages is between first cousins. In cystic fibrosis, the frequency of consanguinity is a little greater than in the general population. In the very rare disorder alkaptonuria more than one quarter of parents are first cousins, and in albinism it is estimated that approximately 1 in 20 are first cousins. As mentioned above, the chance of first cousins carrying the same gene is 1 in 8, having received the gene from one or other of their common grandparents. Therefore, if there is a family history of a recessive disorder such as cystic fibrosis or phenylketonuria, the chance of two cousins having affected offspring is considerably greater than in the case of unrelated parents (Emery, 1983).

Because of the nature of the problems, the profoundly deaf and those with severe impairment of sight are often educated together and it is, therefore, not surprising that similarly affected persons should marry. If two persons homozygous for the same recessive disorder were to have children, all their children would be affected. However, cases are known where all the children born to deaf-mute parents have normal hearing. The explanation must be that the parents were not homozygous for the same gene and that different genes may cause very similar disorders.

Sex-linked inheritance

Sex-linked inheritance refers to the pedigree pattern of genes carried on either of the sex

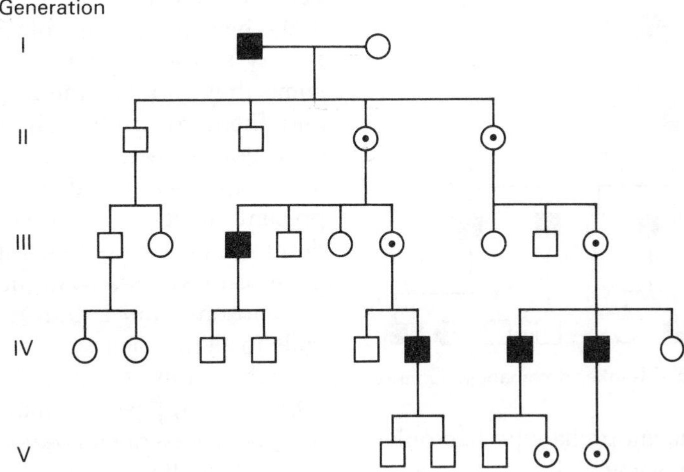

Fig. 3.3 Pedigree pattern of X-linked recessive inheritance — a family with haemophilia.

chromosomes. Both males and females have two sex chromosomes. In the female they are the same, represented as XX. In the male one is the same as in the female, X, while the other is smaller, not found in the female, and is referred to as the Y chromosome. Thus males have an XY sex chromosome constitution.

In the female each ovum carries one or other of the X chromosomes but in the male each sperm carries either an X or a Y chromosome, so there is an almost equal chance or probability of either an X-bearing sperm or a Y-bearing sperm fertilizing the egg, with the result that the number of male and female births is almost equal.

Some genetic disorders are associated with these X and Y sex chromosomes. Y-linked inheritance refers to the pedigree pattern of genes carried on the Y chromosome and X-linked inheritance refers to the pedigree pattern of genes carried on the X chromosome.

X-linked inheritance — X-recessive (XR) and X-dominant (XD)

As with autosomal disorders, there are both dominant and recessive X-linked traits and disorders. An X-linked recessive trait (see Fig. 3.3) is determined by a gene carried on the X chromosome. A disorder inherited in this way normally only affects males, whose sex chromosome constitution is XY. It follows, therefore, that all sons of an affected male will be unaffected (as they cannot receive the deleterious gene in the X chromosome from their father) but all daughters will be carriers (receiving one X chromosome from their mother and the other, with the deleterious gene, from their father). The risk at each conception for a woman who is a carrier of an X-linked recessive disorder is as follows:

- 1 in 4 chance of having an affected son
- 1 in 4 chance of having a carrier daughter
- 1 in 4 chance of having a non-carrier daughter
- 1 in 4 chance of having a son unaffected by this condition.

Sex-linked recessive disorders, therefore, normally only affect males. Very occasionally a woman may be affected by an X-linked recessive disorder. There are several explanations for this:

- She may be homozygous for the gene because her mother was a carrier and her father was affected.
- She may have an abnormal sex chromosome constitution. There have been, for example, cases described of

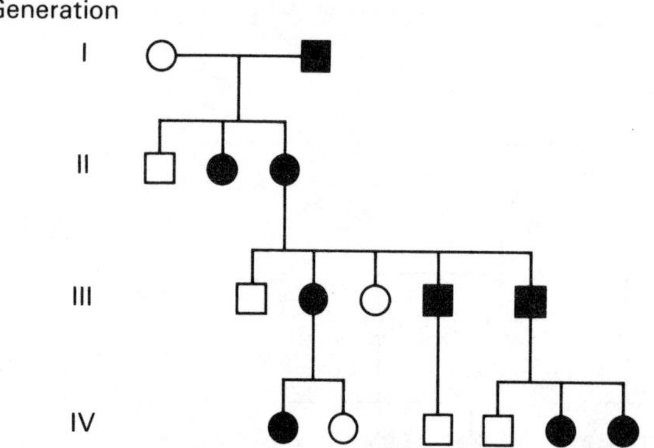

Fig. 3.4 Pedigree pattern of X-linked dominant inheritance.

women with haemophilia who had only a single X chromosome.

- Another possibility is that she may be a manifesting carrier, i.e. a manifesting heterozygote. In this situation the condition is not as severe as in an affected male or a homozygous female (Emery, 1983; Roberts & Pembrey, 1978).

X-linked dominant disorders (see Fig. 3.4) are very rare and require little discussion. In X-linked dominant inheritance, the pattern of transmission is that an affected male transmits the disorder to all his daughters while his sons are unaffected. And each female and each male child of an affected woman has a 50–50 chance of being affected.

Y-linked or holandric inheritance

Another form of sex-linked inheritance is that of genes exclusive to the Y chromosome (see Fig. 3.5). The mode of transmission of a Y borne gene is very simple. As women have no Y chromosome they cannot inherit or transmit the gene and therefore cannot show symptoms of the condition. The male has only one Y chromosome; the gene is therefore impaired and if present must be expressed. The question of dominance or recessiveness cannot arise. The gene simply follows the path of the Y chromosome and is transmitted by an affected male to all his sons who, in turn, will transmit it to all their sons.

Several supposed instances of Y borne genes have been described but invariably they depend on single pedigrees and, therefore, considerable doubt must remain. McKusick (1975) and Stern (1973) describe one condition, hairy ear rims, which has been demonstrated with reasonable probability to be transmitted on the Y chromosome. This is a physically harmless condition characterized by a growth of hair on the outer rim of the ear and is common in certain parts of India.

CHROMOSOMAL ABERRATIONS

Chromosomal disorders are due to the lack, excess or abnormal arrangement of chromosomes. There are two types of chromosomes: those concerned with sex determination, known as the sex chromosomes, and the remainder, which are referred to as the autosomes. Normal

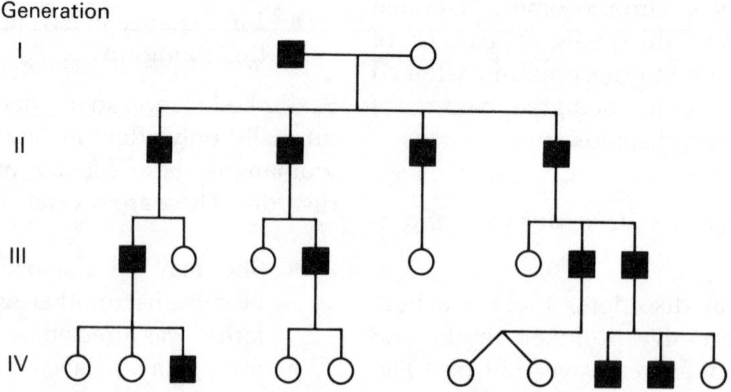

Fig. 3.5 Pedigree pattern of Y-linked or holandric inheritance.

human cells have 23 chromosome pairs, that is 46 chromosomes in all. A sex cell, however, whether sperm or ovum, contains only 23 chromosomes, one half of the full set. A cell formed by the union of a sperm and an ovum will then normally contain a full complement of 46 chromosomes. But if, for example, two sperms, instead of one, fuse with an ovum, then the fertilized ovum will contain 69 chromosomes instead of the normal 46.

De Grouchy (1976) calculated that chromosomal disorders are a possible cause of fetal wastage in up to 50% of pregnancies in the immediate post conceptual period. After formation of the placenta a further 10–15% of pregnancies may be lost and 60% of those are found to have chromosomal abnormalities.

Chromosomal abnormalities can be divided into those involving the autosomes and those involving the sex chromosomes. They can be further subdivided into numerical and structural abnormality. Structural abnormalities are extremely complex and very varied in their effects. Numerical abnormalities involve the loss or gain of one or two chromosomes (aneuploidy) or even sometimes the gain of a whole chromosome set. The latter condition is referred to as polyploidy and appears to be lethal in man, as does the loss of an autosome (monosomy) (Emery, 1983). It appears that even the very small autosomes carry so many important genes that the loss of such a chromosome is fatal.

Autosomal disorders

The addition of an extra autosome, trisomy, has been described in several disorders in man. One of the best known of these is Down's syndrome, popularly known as mongolism. Individuals with Down's syndrome have a very characteristic appearance with a roundish head and almond-shaped eyes. They frequently have an increased susceptibility to infection and often congenital heart disease. They suffer from varying degrees of mental retardation and have a low expectation of life (see Smith & Wilson (1973) for a very useful discussion on the child with Down's syndrome). This condition is most frequently caused by the presence of an extra chromosome in the G(21–22) group.*

When Down's syndrome was first shown to be due to an extra G group chromosome it was not possible to distinguish these two chromosomes, and by convention it was assumed that the chromosome pair relevant to Down's syndrome was No. 21. Some 95% of those with Down's syndrome have 47 chromosomes, being trisomic for chromosome No. 21. In these cases the extra chromosome is discrete and unattached. In a small percentage of children with Down's syndrome the extra No. 21 chromosome is attached (translocated) to a chromosome from group D or G so that the child has 46 chromosomes, one of which contains genetic material from 2 chromosomes.

The importance of these differences in the cause of mongolism is that it may affect the information given to parents regarding their risk of having another similarly affected child. It is essential that knowledge of the chromosomal situation and, wherever possible, the karyotype, of the affected child and both parents is established before information about risk to subsequent children is given. The calculation of these risks is extremely complex and is well described in Chapter 8 of Stevenson & Davison (1976).

There is a marked increase in the incidence of Down's syndrome with maternal age. From ages 20–30, the risk increases from 1 in 2000 live births to 1 in 900. By age 35 the incidence has risen to 1 in 350, and by 40 it is 1 in 110. At age 46 the risk is 1 in 25. However, it is estimated that the cause of at least one-fifth of all Down's syndrome births is for reasons other than maternal age (Roberts & Pembrey, 1978). It is, therefore, recommended that, regardless of the chromosome situation, all women who have had a child with Down's

---

* The chromosome pattern is called a karyotype. This term is applied to a systematic array of the chromosomes of a single cell prepared by very detailed drawing or photography. As it is not always possible to distinguish between individual chromosomes, they are often divided into groups A–G depending on their size. Cytological techniques continue to improve and it is hoped that it will eventually be possible to identify chromosomes more precisely.

syndrome should be offered prenatal diagnosis (see p. 47).

Abnormalities of the sex chromosomes

While many chromosomal abnormalities cause death of the early embryo or fetus and some cause death of the newborn child, e.g. Patau's and Edward's syndrome, abnormalities in the number of sex chromosomes appear to have less lethal effects than abnormalities in the autosomes. In the late 1950s investigations found that not all males have an XY sex chromosome constitution, nor all females an XX sex chromosome constitution. In Klinefelter's syndrome it was found that these males had an extra X chromosome, and cases have been described with an XXXY constitution. In Klinefelter's syndrome pubertal hypogonadism frequently leads to tall stature, deficient maturation of male secondary sexual characteristics with disturbance of sexual function, osteoporosis and frequently truncal obesity. There is also some evidence of emotional disturbances and certain behavioural problems, but whether this is due directly to the genetic abnormality is unclear as patients with these abnormalities are investigated more frequently than those without (Opitz, 1973).

Recently, there has been considerable discussion about men with an XYY sex chromosome constitution (Jacobs, 1969). Some studies of the male residents in institutions for the mentally subnormal and male prisoners have demonstrated that about 3% have an XYY constitution compared with approximately 1 in 1000 or 1 in 2000 in the general population, depending upon the method of calculation (Bergsma, 1973). These men seem to have a tendency to demonstrate aggressive and antisocial behaviour. On the other hand, it is estimated that many men with this constitution do not present such behaviour so caution must be exercised. Prospective studies on male XYY subjects are being carried out in Edinburgh.

However, the presence of an extra Y chromosome and the type of publicity surrounding the studies raise, as Heller (1973) suggests, many basic social, legal and ethical questions for which there is no easy answer. For more detailed information about the XYY chromosome see Strong et al (1966),Welch et al (1967), Price & Whatmore (1967) and Witkin (1976).

Females with three or even four X chromosomes, instead of the normal XX constitution, have been described. They may sometimes be mentally retarded, but frequently they appear to be normal females. A sex chromosome constitution of XO instead of XX is found in Turner's syndrome in which the affected female has primary amenorrhoea and a lack of pubertal sexual development. There are often many other abnormalities including congenital heart disease, usually coarctation of the aorta, small stature and transverse folding of the skin at the back of the neck at birth (Roberts & Pembrey, 1978).

MULTIFACTORIAL CAUSATION

This type of inheritance is, as the name implies, dependent not on a single gene for which the individual is homozygous but on many other factors, such as the environment and/or a number of genes. The genes responsible are usually all genes of varying but small effect and with varying dominance. It is not always possible to distinguish which are the inherited components responsible for the condition and which are the environmental ones. The term polygenic has a meaning similar to 'multifactorial', but differs in that it only refers to the genetic component of a character controlled by many genes.

Pattern of inheritance

Clarke (1970) points out that it is easy to understand that traits which are controlled by many genes show continuous variation, whereas those which are controlled by single genes show clear cut 'either/or' differences. It is simple to visualize the fact that many genes control human stature — most people are not 'tall' or 'short' but are placed on a continuum with few at either of the extremes. A graph of heights shows a normal curve. There are, of course, racial and sex differences and differences based on nutrition. And it must be remembered that any attempt to assess the relative contribution of heredity and environment refers to one time and one place. In another geographical area, where conditions are different, the balance may be greatly altered. Similarly, when environmental conditions change, the relative importance of heredity usually changes as well.

The calculation of the part played by genes in multifactorial inheritance is complex and based on statistical mathematics. Roberts & Pembrey (1978) give a very clear and relatively simple introduction to the principles which are based on the resemblance between relatives. A parent passes on to a child half of his or her chromosomes, and so half of his or her genes. Parent and child always have exactly half their genes in common. When the child has a child of his own, he transmits on average one-half of the genes derived from that particular parent, so grandparent and grandchild have on average one quarter of their genes in common. This is halved again in the next generation so that great grandparent and great grandchild have on average one-eighth of their genes in common. Put another way, each person has two parents, four grandparents and eight great grandparents, and these are the proportion of genes handed on to him, on average, by each. With siblings the proportion of genes in common is on average one half.

Beyond this the matter is complicated and there are a variety of approaches used in attempting to understand the genetics of a condition in multifactorial inheritance. These may include studies comparing the incidence in different racial groups, studying the incidence of the disorder amongst relatives, studying the association of the disease with other characteristics such as blood group, studying certain pathological components of the disorder in relatives and comparing the incidence in identical and non-identical twins.

Twin studies

Twin studies are sometimes used in an attempt to isolate the genetic factor in certain conditions. The assumption is that most twins, particularly identical twins, share the same environment. Similarities between identical twins may thus reflect their sharing the environment as much as their identical genetic structure. If it were possible to study identical twins reared apart, then genetically determined traits present in one twin should also be present in the other, regardless of environment. As one can imagine, it is relatively unusual for identical twins to be reared separately, although some work is discussed by Chen (1979) and Holden (1980). In one study reported in Emery (1983) in which 19 pairs of identical twins were reared separately, the data showed clearly that each pair of twins differed little in height but there was considerable difference in weight. This suggests that heredity plays a bigger part in determining stature than it does in determining weight.

Another approach to twin studies is that of Wilson & Harpring (1972) who have been studying the effects of genes on early development in children by comparing fraternal and identical twins.* They examined the children at 6-week intervals during the first two years of life for the development of mental and motor skills. Wilson & Harpring showed that these areas of development in very young children are unpredictable, and that these skills increase in no discernible order. The rates of change were also not uniform. A child's progress could differ significantly from one age to another. However, what is interesting from Wilson & Harpring's findings is that identical twins progressed at almost the same rate while no such correlation existed among fraternal twins. The trend was so pronounced that Wilson & Harpring could predict the state of development of one identical twin simply by examining the other. They could not, however, predict future development for either twin alone.

Incidence within families

In disorders caused by a single gene there is, as

---

* Human twins are of two kinds, fraternal or dizygotic and identical or monozygotic. Dizygotic twins arise from two separate fertilized ova. In monozygotic twins a single fertilized ovum splits into two very early in development and two separate embryos are thus produced. Identical twins are always of the same sex.

has been already shown, a clear pattern of inheritance. However, there are many common congenital abnormalities which appear to be 'familial' but where the pattern of inheritance is not consistent with that for a single gene. In these circumstances, among the relatives of an affected person the incidence of the disorder is much higher than the general population, but lower than it would be in single gene causation. Further, the incidence falls off quickly when one moves from first degree relatives — parents, siblings and children — to uncles, aunts and cousins, and more quickly than would happen with disorders due to a single gene. For example with hare lip, first degree relatives show approximately 30 times the frequency in the general population. If this followed the pattern for single gene inheritance, the corresponding incidence in second and third degree relatives would be 16 times and 8 times respectively. They actually turn out to be only 6 times and 2 times the incidence in the population at large (Roberts & Pembrey, 1978).

The pattern for the common disorder of infants, pyloric stenosis, is even more complex. In the first place, 5 times as many boys are affected as girls. Brothers and sons of affected men show a frequency of 10 times the population average; sisters and daughters of affected men 25 times; and sisters and daughters of affected women 100 times (Carter, 1969). Pyloric stenosis is characterized by persistent vomiting after feeds. Mortality used to be very high until the introduction of the successful Ramstedt operation.

Disorders showing multifactorial causation

Other common congenital malformations believed to be multifactorial in causation and following a similar pattern include spina bifida and anencephaly, hare lip, cleft palate, and congenital dislocation of the hip and the commoner forms of congenital heart disease.

Cardiovascular disorders

The most common cause of death in the majority of Western industrialized societies is disease of the heart and blood vessels, and there has recently been a considerable increase in the incidence of such disease. Both genetic and environmental factors play a part and it is suggested that a possible explanation for the recent increase in incidence could be due to environmental changes which have come too quickly to be countered by genetic changes. Some of the environmental factors reflect life style and include cigarette smoking, lack of exercise, obesity from extra calorie intake and possibly also an excessive intake of saturated fats and refined carbohydrates.

Steptoe (1981) suggests that individuals are more likely to suffer from atherosclerotic disease when they are at risk for more than one of the factors described in the Pooling Project. This project combined results from five longitudinal studies of middle-aged white males. Some 8300 subjects were incorporated into the project and followed up for an average of 8.6 years. Over this period 650 originally disease-free men suffered either a fatal or non-fatal myocardial infarction or sudden cardiac death. The study showed that vulnerability increased progressively with a rise in systolic blood pressure, an increase in lipid concentration in the blood and with heavy smoking. It divided the population into quintiles (20%s) of combined risk on diastolic pressure, cholesterol count and smoking. People in the highest 20% were nearly six times more vulnerable than those in the lowest. In this project the 20% in the highest multiple risk quintile sustained 40% of major first coronary events. However, there are clearly other factors at work.

The Doll & Hill (1964) pioneering study of smoking habits in British physicians revealed a 30% higher cardiac mortality amongst self-reported cigarette smokers. This association has been subsequently confirmed by other studies. Oliver (1976), using a different data base, calculated that although people at risk on the three major factors sustain eight times more cardiac disease over a decade than those not displaying these characteristics, the incidence is still only 17%. Thus, 83% of the 'high-risk' subjects survive throughout that time. However, the incidence of coronary atherosclerosis is rare in the Third World countries. As Carter (1969) points out, this is not due to genetic racial difference, since atherosclerosis and deaths from ischaemic heart disease rapidly appear when such people adopt Western European habits as, for example, Bantus in Johannesburg or people of African descent in the cities of the United States. It may be possible in the future to identify those who are genetically at special risk and help them to be protected.

Mental disorders

While several single gene and chromosomal abnormalities are associated with mental retardation, conditions resulting in mental retardation have more frequently both an environmental and a genetic factor. It is estimated that 0.3–0.4% of the childhood population of the UK are mentally retarded (Weatherall, 1982). Brown (1979) suggests that there is a strong social class difference between the mildly retarded child, with a high incidence of these in 'social classes' 4 and 5, and the profoundly mentally retarded (those with an IQ of less than 50), in whom no social class difference is found. Carter (1981) who analyzed three large surveys to assess the different causes of mental retardation in children and teenagers, found that Down's syndrome was the commonest single cause.

Schizophrenia is the diagnostic label currently given to a condition expressing itself as a disorder of feeling through inappropriate behaviour and an increasing withdrawal from interpersonal contacts. It is the principal diagnosis in chronic mental illness and affects 1% of the population (Lancet, 1970). In the UK there are approximately 80 000 patients diagnosed as schizophrenic in mental hospitals. Most studies suggest that while environmental factors play a part, there is also a genetic contribution to the aetiology of schizophrenia (Heston, 1970; Kety & Wender, 1980; Kidd & Cavalli-Sforza, 1973). However, the nature and extent of this contribution is unclear. It is possible that schizophrenia represents a variety of different disorders and causes and consequently different patterns of inheritance can be expected.

This section on multifactorial inheritance can be concluded by noting that polygenic determination is more likely if the condition is relatively common, the incidence in relatives is low, the incidence falls off rapidly as one passes to more distant relatives, the incidence in relatives rises as the manifestations become more severe and the risk rises following the birth of two affected children.

RANGE OF DISORDERS

There are many genetic disorders affecting all systems of the body. Both McKusick (1975) and Bergsma (1973) provide a full catalogue with descriptions, references, calculations of risks for siblings and children, and incidence and prevalence rates of some 2000 disorders which are genetically transmitted. Carter (1977) lists the more common single gene determined conditions of childhood. These catalogues illustrate the enormous variety of conditions due to mutant genes. These range from such conditions of the urological system as polycystic kidneys to the enzyme deficiencies, such as phenylketonuria, the degenerative disorders of the central nervous system such as Huntington's chorea and disorders affecting the senses. Table 3.1 lists a few of the more common genetic disorders, giving their mode of transmission and the incidence (number of cases among a group of births) or prevalence (number of cases in the total population) where available. Major systems of the body which are affected are also described.

The diversity, seriousness and extent of genetically transmitted disorders may seem overwhelming to those commencing a study of the subject. Wilkie & Sinclair (1977), between January 1974 and June 1976, interviewed 104 patients with high risk (greater than 1 in 10) conditions who had attended a genetic clinic in the area. They were all from the southeast of Scotland. More than 30 different disorders were represented, but for half the disorders there was only one individual involved. Table 3.2 shows the range of these disorders, the mode of transmission and the numbers in each group. These figures only include the more serious genetic disorders. The total number of different

Table 3.1 Common genetic disorders

Name of disorder	Mode of trans-mission	Occurrence or prevalence	Major clinical features
Achondroplasia (classical)	AD	Unknown	Dwarfism
Albinism (several types)	AR	1 in 39 000 (Caucasian)	Decreased pigment in skin, hair and eyes. Nystagmus and photophobia.
Alport's syndrome (with sex limitation to males)	AD	Unknown	Haematuria, proteinuria and sometimes pyuria. Decreased renal function with renal failure in males 20-30.
Aniridia	AD	1 in 100 000 – 1 in 200 000 population	Absence of all or part of iris.
Becker muscular dystrophy	XR	Unknown	Progressive weakness and wasting of pelvic and pectoral muscles.
Brachydactyly	AD (if genetic)	Rare	Shortening of fingers.
Colour blindness (total)	AR	Rare	No colour vision
Congenital deafness	AR but also XR & AD	Unknown but 10% unilateral deafness related to hereditary factor	Deafness
Cystic fibrosis	AR	1 in 2000 live births	Affects exocrine glands. Production abnormal secretions resulting in pancreatic insufficiency, chronic pulmonary disease, cirrhosis of liver.
Cystinosis	AR	Unknown	Defect in water reabsorption resulting in polyuria and polydipsia. Affected children show severe growth retardation.
Duchenne muscular dystrophy	XR	1 in 100 000 live births	Progressive weakness of vital musculature. Enlargement of calf muscles. Death in teens usually from pulmonary infection.
Ehlers-Danlos syndrome	AD	Unknown	Abnormality of collagen causing tissue frailty.
Factor VIII deficiency—haemophilia A	XR	1 in 2500 live births	Reduction of clotting factor. Bleeding in and around joints leads to permanent damage and restriction of movement.
Factor XIX deficiency—haemophilia B	XR	1 in 2500 live births	
Galactosaemia	AR	Unknown	Digestive difficulties. Retarded physical and mental development, liver enlargement and infection.
Goitrous cretinism	AR	Unknown	Early signs include lethargy and feeding difficulties, leading to growth retardation in untreated cretin.
Homocystinuria	AR	Unknown	Skeletal abnormalities including genu valgum, pes cavus. Osteoporosis, ectopia lentis and frequently some mental retardation
Huntington's chorea	AD	1 in 18 000 population	Chorea and dementia. Choreiform movements of limbs, trunk and face, gait clumsy, speech indistinct.
Leber congenital amaurosis	AR	1 in 33 000 live births	Severe sight defect.

Table 3.1 (continued)

Name of disorder	Mode of trans-mission	Occurrence or prevalence	Major clinical features
Maple syrup urine disease	AR	Unknown but rare	In first week of life feeding difficulties, vomiting and shrill cry. Followed by convulsions, coma, respiratory difficulties and death.
Marfan's syndrome	AD	1 in 60 000 in most populations	Skeletal abnormalities, ectopic lentis, and abnormality of aorta.
Myotonic dystrophy	AD	Unknown	Wasting and weakness of facial and neck muscles and distal limbs.
Neurofibromatosis	AD	1 in 3300 live births	Cutaneous tumours which may be widespread. Severity depends on site of tumours. Cafe au lait spots.
Osteogenesis imperfecta congenita	AD	Unknown	Infant born dead or survives only a short time. Multiple fractures and skeletal deformities.
Phenylketonuria	AR	1 in 14 300 live births in USA	Irritability, epileptic seizures and vomiting during first weeks of life. Mental retardation if untreated.
Polycystic kidney disease (adult)	AD	Unknown	Progressive renal insufficiency.
Polyposis coli	AD	Unknown	Multiple polyposis of large bowel. Frequently undergo malignant changes. Intestinal obstruction.
Retinitis pigmentosa	XR, AD & AR	1 in 200 of world population	Initially night blindness followed by deterioration in sight.
Retinoblastoma	AD	1 in 20 000 live births	Tumour in retina of one or both eyes.
Spherocystosis	AD	Some estimate 1 in 4500 population	Haemolytic anaemia ameliorated by splenectomy.
Von Willebrand's disease	AD	Unknown	Prolonged bleeding time. Epistaxis and excessive bleeding after dental extraction and minor traumas.
Waardenburg's syndrome	AD	1 in 4000 live births	Deafness and infection of tear ducts.
Xeroderma pigmentosum	AR	Unknown but high in racial groups with high consanguinity	Photosensitivity and photobia to ultraviolet light. Development of premalignant and malignant skin lesions.

Table 3.2 Range of disorders seen at a genetic clinic over a 2-year period

Name of disorder		Mode of transmission	Number
Christmas disease	bleeding disorders	XR	4
Haemophilia		XR	36
Von Willebrand's		AD	2
Albinism		AR	1
Blindness (unspecified)	disorders of sight	AD, XR & AR	9
Buphthalmos		not known	1
Congenital cataract		AD & AR	2
Congenital nystagmus		not known	1
Macular degeneration		XR & AR	3
Retinitis pigmentosa		XR, AR & AD	8
Retinoblastoma		AD	1
Becker muscular dystrophy		XR	1
Duchenne muscular dystrophy		XR	5
Myotonic dystrophy		AD	8
Peroneal muscular atrophy		AD	1
Brachydactyly		AD	1
Cerebellar ataxia		AD	1
Cleft lip & palate		AD	2
Deafness (unspecified)		AR	2
Down's syndrome		XR & unknown	2
Huntington's chorea		AD	5
Hydrocephalus		Unknown	2
Lobster claw deformity		XR	1
Marfan's syndrome		AD	4
Moebius' syndrome		AR	1
Nephrogenic diabetes insipidus		XR	1
Neurofibromatosis		AD	4
Oculopharyngeal muscular dystrophy		AD	1
Polycystic kidney (adult)		AD	4
Polyposis coli		AD	2
Spherocytosis		AD	1
Waardenburg's syndrome		AD	1

genetic disorders represented among the people attending such a specialist clinic at any one time would be greater.

The fact that so many different disorders are featured raises problems of diagnosis for general practitioners and those not working in specialist units. Medical genetics has never featured largely in the medical curriculum, and because of the distribution of the disorders most general practitioners are unlikely to have patients with even the more common genetic disorders. Nursing staff will care for those patients in the specialist units, e.g. obstetrics and paediatric units, renal units and departments specializing in disorders of the blood. Frequently patients, such as those suffering from cystic fibrosis and haemophilia, continue to be followed up from a specialist unit so that general practitioners may not be directly involved in their care.

GENETICS AND CANCER

A malignant tumour consists of an abnormal proliferation of cells. Such tumours invade the surrounding tissues and often, in the later stages of the disease, metastasize. A major factor in malignancy is increased and uncontrolled growth of cells. As growth is under gene control, it implies that genes are involved in all cancers (Emery, 1983). It is still unknown how a cell or group of cells starts to change. For cancerous changes to begin a cell must be ready for change (the genetic factor) and an external factor, a triggering agent or carcinogen, sets it off. A carcinogen can be a chemical or a virus or radiation. In some cancers it appears that the primary cause is environmental, e.g. cancer of the bladder amongst aniline dye workers, cancer of the skin amongst dye workers and lung cancer due to cigarette smoking (Doll, 1971; Doll & Peto, 1976).

In the majority of cancers there is no clearly defined environmental cause, nor is there any clear-cut mode of inheritance. In certain cancers, in particular cancer of the stomach and the breast, genetic factors seem to play an important part (Lynch, 1969). Studies involving calculations of the frequency of the disease in near relatives of affected persons, blood group studies and the use of animal analyses are still not conclusive. In 1959 Macklin, comparing families of breast cancer patients with controls, found the incidence of breast cancer in first degree relatives of the patients to be approximately three times that of the control population, and this finding has been confirmed by other investigators (Lynch, 1969). However, Mendelian inheritance patterns have not yet been identified.

Some cancers are more common in certain national groups, but the reason is not necessarily genetic. For example, breast cancer is six times more common in Europeans than in Japanese (Petrakis, 1977). This may be a true racial difference and therefore a genetic difference in cancer proneness: but it may also be that it is only a reflection of differences in fertility and infant feeding habits. Skin cancer is more common in Australian whites than in the native Aboriginal population, presumably because the melanin in the skin of the Aborigines prevents the penetration of ultraviolet radiation (Petrakis, 1977).

In some cancers it seems that the primary cause is an abnormal gene (Harnden, 1979). In the condition polyposis coli, which is transmitted in an autosomal dominant fashion, the entire large bowel is lined with numerous polyps. There is a very high risk of carcinomatous changes taking place in these polyps and, if untreated, approximately 90% of affected persons die from cancer of the bowel. In the condition neurofibromatosis, which is transmitted in an autosomal dominant fashion, tumours appear in the peripheral and central nervous system. Almost every part of the central nervous system has been affected by this disease process. An early diagnostic feature is the presence of cafe-au-lait spots which may be present at birth. They may increase in size and number with age and tend to occur on the unexposed areas of the body. This disorder is well illuminated in Howell & Ford's (1980) *The True History of the Elephant Man,* which describes the cruelty of the condition and 19th century society's equally cruel response to it.

In retinoblastoma, an autosomal dominant condition, malignant tumours of the retina occur. The most common presenting sign is a white 'cat's eye reflex' in the pupil and the next is strabismus. The average age in the USA at the time of tumour diagnosis is 17 months. The tumour is highly sensitive to radiation and other chemotherapeutic agents, but early diagnosis is vital as once the tumour has extended outside the eye into the orbit, the chances of cure are slim and no patients who are known to have metastatic retinoblastoma have survived. In the skin condition xeroderma pigmentosum, transmitted in an autosomal recessive fashion, there is early photosensitivity and photophobia to the ultraviolet range of light and the development of premalignant and malignant skin lesions in light-damaged areas. A useful review of the genetic aspects of cancer is Bodmer (1982).

MANAGEMENT OF GENETICALLY INHERITED DISORDERS

Some of the major forms of transmission and inheritance of genetic disorders, as well as the relationship between genes and the environment as factors in the cause of disease, have been examined. Clearly there are implications of genetic disease for a number of groups of people. These include the affected individual, parents of an affected child, those at risk of having an affected child and those at risk of developing the disorder themselves, as in autosomal dominantly transmitted disorders of variable age of onset.

TREATMENT OF THE AFFECTED PERSON

Some genetic disorders may be successfully and effectively treated by surgery. For example, for children with cleft palate and hare lip, surgery can repair the lip and palate and plastic surgery reduce scarring. Affected children may require prosthetic replacement of teeth and orthodontic treatment and in some cases speech therapy. For the majority, treatment should be finished by mid-teens (Ross & Johnston, 1972). In hereditary spherocytosis, characterized by chronic haemolytic anaemia, splenectomy is invariably effective allowing the affected person to reach a normal expectation of life (Jandl & Cooper, 1972).

Other disorders may be treated by drug therapy or a combination of drugs and dietary control.

Haemophilia is a disorder of the blood due to a deficiency of one of the clotting factors, Factor VIII or Factor IX. Those who have between 5% and 50% of the factor are affected mildly. They may bleed after major physical trauma and dental extraction. Indeed in some cases, with the most mildly affected, it is not until difficulties occur in stemming post-extraction haemorrhage that the diagnosis is made. Those who have 1% to 5% of the factor are affected moderately and may bleed excessively after minor physical trauma. But for those who have less than 1% of the normal levels of the factor, the situation is more problematic. They are severely affected and bleed spontaneously into various sites of their bodies including muscles and, in particular, the joints – knees, elbows and ankles. It is important to remember that the main physical problems of moderately and severely affected patients are not the stemming of bleeding from external cuts and wounds but the regular, spontaneous bleeding into the joints, leading to very painful crippling of such joints. Haemorrhagic episodes are treated with concentrates of the appropriate factor obtained from human plasma. Fresh frozen plasma may be used when no concentrates are available. The duration of treatment, interval between treatments and dosage depend on the location and extent of the bleeding (Forbes & Lowe, 1982).

The autosomal recessively transmitted disorder, cystic fibrosis, is a generalized disorder affecting the exocrine glands of the body, with production of abnormal secretions resulting in pancreatic insufficiency, chronic pulmonary disease and cirrhosis of the liver. Affected children are treated with pancreatin as well as control of salt ingestion, pulmonary therapy and antibiotic therapy; their life expectancy remains low, although some now attain maturity.

In the autosomal recessive condition, phenylketonuria, there is a deficiency of the enzyme phenylalanine hydroxylase without which phenylalanine cannot be converted into tyrosine. Instead it accumulates in the blood and is converted into phenylpyruvic acid and this, in turn, into phenyllactic acid and phenylacetic acid. One or more of these substances has toxic effects and produces phenylketonuria, a condition in which there is usually severe mental deficiency and sometimes epilepsy. Much of the cerebral damage may be prevented if the condition is diagnosed and, from an early age, the child is given a diet very low in phenylalanine.

These are only a few examples of genetic disorders that can be treated with considerable effectiveness, and steady advances are being made in this area.

Palliative management

However, in other genetic disorders there is no satisfactory treatment although some help can be given for the symptoms as they appear. An example is Huntington's chorea, a disorder characterized by chorea and, frequently, eventually dementia, lasting 10–20 years from the variable age of onset. At first the chorea may be minimal but, as the condition progresses, it becomes more pronounced and many patients present with ceaseless writhing, jerking and twisting of different parts of the body. Disturbance of gait is very common, and affected persons are often thought to be drunk. These patients have some difficulty in articulation (dysarthria) and dysphagia is common. Personality changes are very common (Hayden, 1981). Drugs can be used to give some control of the chorea but there is, as yet, nothing that can stop the progression of the disorder.

Similarly, in the autosomal dominant disorder myotonic dystrophy, treatment is palliative. In myotonic dystrophy there is progressive deterioration of muscle fibres due to an unknown defect or defects in them. There is wasting and weakness of facial and neck muscles and of distal limbs. It is unusual for those affected to reach normal expectation of life, and death usually occurs prematurely from pulmonary infection or cardiac failure.

Nevertheless, regardless of the effectiveness and success of the treatment, at the moment an affected individual cannot be 'cured', as they retain the deleterious gene for the rest of their life and therefore the ability to pass it on to the next generation.

DETECTION OF HETEROZYGOTES

It is now possible in several conditions to establish whether a woman is a carrier for a particular condition. In the eye disorder retinitis pigmentosa, there is a gradual degeneration of the retina which may result in severe loss of vision. The disorder may be transmitted in XR, AR and AD forms. In the X-linked form the condition in males is indistinguishable from other forms. However, in heterozygous women there are minor manifestations demonstrating their carrier status. Nephrogenic diabetes insipidus is an X-linked recessive disorder characterized by failure to thrive and attacks of hyperpyrexia, and mental deficiency is common. The condition can be controlled, if diagnosed at an early age, by the maintenance of fluid and electrolyte balance. The heterozygous female can be easily detected by her inability to produce a normally concentrated urine. In Duchenne muscular dystrophy two-thirds of heterozygous women have an elevated serum creatine kinase and, thus, a significantly raised level is the most reliable single test for carrier status. Also, in haemophilia a proportion of heterozygotes can be detected, with varying certainty, depending on the level of Factor VIII activity (Forbes & Lowe, 1982). However, there is considerable overlap in the quantities of these substances in the blood of heterozygotes with the levels found in the normal population. At the moment, screening for heterozygous carrier status is likely to be reserved for those suspected of being at risk because they have a relative affected by a particular disorder, or because they belong to an 'at risk' racial or social group.

PRENATAL DIAGNOSIS

All expectant parents wish for a healthy baby. Until recently it has been impossible to detect abnormality early in pregnancy. Now, as a result of advances in prenatal diagnosis, it is possible to diagnose certain abnormalities before the birth of the child. For prospective parents, such investigations can demonstrate that their baby does not have certain abnormalities and they can therefore be reassured. If the results of the tests are positive, and the fetus is affected by a specific disorder, then the parents can have the choice of terminating that pregnancy if they wish.

In recent years advances in prenatal diagnosis in the form of amniocentesis, ultrasound and radiographic examinations have made it possible to detect antenatally certain of the chromosomal disorders and inborn errors of metabolism, as well as the multifactorial defects of spina bifida and anencephaly. Amnioscopy has provided a means of obtaining fetal blood for the diagnosis of many of the hereditary anaemias.

Prenatal diagnosis can be either late or early. Late prenatal diagnosis usually involves X-ray diagnosis in the last trimester, and the concern is then usually with the obstetric management of the patient. However, the following discussion focuses on the early detection of fetal abnormality, ie before 20 weeks gestation.

Various techniques are used in diagnosing abnormality early in pregnancy. Clinical examination is, of course, used but it is virtually impossible for the obstetrician to diagnose any fetal abnormality before the 20th week. Ultrasound is now a normal part of the management of every pregnancy and is used to confirm that the patient is pregnant, to test for multiple births and to discover the position of the fetus. Early in pregnancy ultrasound can only pick up gross fetal abnormality, e.g. anencephaly. The position of the placenta within the uterus is relatively easily identified by ultrasound and this is helpful in locating the optimal site for amniocentesis.

Amniocentesis

Amniocentesis involves obtaining fluid and cells from the amniotic sac. Under local anaesthesia, a fine needle is inserted aseptically into the amniotic cavity to a depth and angle determined by the ultrasound examination. Usually 20 ml of fluid is removed. If the specimen is bloodstained, or difficult to obtain, a further attempt is made in a week's time. Amniocentesis is preferably carried out between the 16th and 18th weeks of pregnancy and, depending on the nature of the tests being carried out, the results can take up to 28 days to return from the laboratory.

Fetoscopy and fetal blood sampling

Some genetic conditions cannot be diagnosed from the amniotic fluid alone. Attempts are now being made to find reliable and safe techniques for obtaining samples of blood from the fetus or its placental circulation. When the placenta lies on the anterior wall of the uterus a needle can be inserted, under ultrasound guide, and a specimen of blood obtained. This technique is usually referred to as transabdominal intraplacental aspiration. Fetal and maternal cells must then be separated and the appropriate laboratory tests carried out.

When the placenta lies on the posterior wall it is more difficult to obtain fetal blood as the fetus is inevitably, to a greater or lesser extent, in the way. In these circumstances fetoscopy enables the obstetrician to obtain a direct view of the placenta using a fibreoptic telescope, thus making it easier to obtain a specimen of fetal blood. Fetal blood samples are already being used in the prenatal diagnosis of alpha and beta thalassaemia and sickle cell disease, and research is advancing in the diagnosis of haemophilia and Duchenne muscular dystrophy (Valenti, 1978).

Indications for prenatal diagnostic testing

There are four main areas in which prenatal diagnosis may be considered:

- when a mother is at risk of having a child with a chromosomal abnormality
- when there is a risk of a child with a neural tube defect
- when there is a risk of a child with one of the biochemical disorders
- where fetal sexing may be beneficial, as when the mother is a carrier of one of the more serious XR disorders.

More specifically, the Clinical Genetics Society (1978) Working Party on Prenatal Diagnosis in Relation to Genetic Counselling suggests that the following are at present the main indications for prenatal diagnosis:

- risk of recurrence of open neural tube defects
- risk of chromosome aberration at maternal age 35–39 and 40 years and over
- risk of chromosome abnormality in pregnancies in which the patient has had a previous child with trisomic Down's syndrome
- risk of open neural tube defect associated with raised alphafetoprotein in maternal serum (see below for an explanation of this)
- risk of recurrence of a detectable metabolic disease.
- risk of chromosome aberration resulting from parental translocation.
- risk of a male fetus with 50% chance of being affected with a severe X-linked recessive disease where the mother is a carrier.

Prenatal diagnosis of neural tube defects

Brock & Sutcliffe (1972) in Edinburgh demonstrated that the normal fetal blood constituent, alphafetoprotein, was present in greatly increased amounts in the amniotic fluid when the fetus had anencephaly. Since then it has been established that a raised level of alphafetoprotein in amniotic fluid at about 17 weeks' gestation, in the absence of fetal death or marked fetal blood contamination, is usually diagnostic of such lesions as anencephaly and open spina bifida. In the United Kingdom, however, over 90% of children with neural tube defects are the first affected child in the family. Offering amniocentesis to such parents may prevent the birth of a subsequent affected child, but it would be quite impracticable to screen by amniocentesis the entire antenatal population.

Brock and his colleagues demonstrated that a raised maternal serum alphafetoprotein at 15 to 18 weeks' gestation may be a useful screening test for open neural tube defects. Closed neural tube defects cannot be detected by this method.

There is, however, some overlap in the maternal serum levels between those carrying affected and unaffected fetuses. The majority of cases (4 out of 5) where there is elevated serum alphafetoprotein are not due to a neural tube defect, but to some other condition or a technical artifact. Nevertheless, the test of serum does provide a measure which indicates whether further investigations should be carried out. In the Edinburgh study reported by Brock, before considering amniocentesis for patients with raised maternal serum levels, clinical and ultrasound examination excluded some women whose gestational dates had been under-estimated, and whose serum alphafetoprotein became normal with a raised dating. Amnio-centesis was not performed on any patient who showed clinical signs of threatened abortion at the time of alphafetoprotein determination, as it has been shown that this may elevate the value. The Working Group on Screening for Neural Tube Defects (1979) reported that, in favourable circumstances, it has been possible to screen about 90% of the 'at risk' pregnant population at the correct time (16 to 20 weeks' gestational age) and 80% of the cases of open neural tube defects have been successfully detected. The Working Party suggests that it is very probable that the number of severely disabled children would be reduced by a nationwide screening programme.

There have been strong recommendations, the most recent being the DHSS Report *Inequalities in Health Care* (Townsend & Davidson, 1982), for a national programme for the detection of open neural tube defects by maternal serum alphafetoprotein screening. Part of the success of such a service to prevent the births of children with open neural tube defects will depend on women being persuaded to book in early for antenatal care, and on their willingness to undergo termination of the pregnancy.

Prenatal diagnosis and chromosomal abnormalities

All the numerical and many of the structural chromosomal anomalies can be detected by culture of cells obtained by amniocentesis. The most common indication for such an analysis is the risk of trisomic Down's syndrome which is caused by an additional chromosome 21. The incidence of Down's syndrome is increased with maternal age and also varies from area to area. Hagard & Carter (1976) quote an overall incidence of Down's syndrome of 1.67 per thousand births. Expectation of life of those with Down's syndrome is reduced, although there is now evidence of increasing life expectancy. Many of those affected by Down's syndrome require long-term care. Brotherston (1978) estimates that 12% of the 7000 patients in hospitals for the mentally handicapped in Scotland have this disorder and that possibly rather more are cared for in the community, so that there are likely to be more than 2000 affected individuals in Scotland.

There has been considerable discussion about the age at which routine antenatal screening for Down's syndrome should be offered to women who are not known to be 'at risk' of having such a child. Many studies, including those of Polani (1978) and Mikkelsen & Nielsen (1976), show an increase in risk beyond a maternal age of 35 and in particular beyond the age of 38. In Passarge's (1978) study based on data from the Federal Republic of Germany it was estimated that if antenatal screening for trisomy 21 were carried out on all mothers aged 40 and over, some 23% of fetuses with trisomy 21 would be detected in utero. If mothers aged 39 to 35 are successively included the percentage increase in detection of trisomy 21 in utero decreases with each descending year of maternal age. It is generally accepted that antenatal screening for Down's syndrome should be offered routinely to women of 40 or over. If the age is reduced to 35 the benefit over cost ratio is reduced, but still may be economically justified.

Prenatal diagnosis for biochemical disorders

It is now possible to detect antenatally certain genetic metabolic diseases which result in severe handicap, and for which there may be no satisfactory treatment. At present the exact nature of the primary biochemical abnormality, including in most cases the specific enzyme deficiency, is known for approximately 130 genetic disorders. For about 60 of these the abnormality has been demonstrated in cultured skin fibroblasts from patients. Similar diagnostic tests can also be applied to culture of amniotic fluid cells, since their basic complement of enzymes is, for the most part, qualitatively similar to that of skin fibroblasts. Patrick (1978) reports that these tests have been successfully used for the prenatal diagnosis of 30 metabolic genetic disorders including galactosaemia, homocystinuria, maple-syrup urine, Lesch-Nyhan and Tay-Sachs diseases. All these conditions are rare and not all laboratories can carry out a comprehensive diagnostic service. The identification of an 'at risk' individual is problematic. However, where groups as opposed to individuals are known to be 'at risk', for example the Ashkenazi Jews of Eastern European origin in relation to Tay- Sachs disease, prenatal screening can be undertaken routinely.

Amniocentesis and fetal sexing

Sex can be determined by the presence of the Barr body* on the amniotic cells, though usually nuclear sexing results are checked by direct chromosome studies. Prenatal sexing is usually limited to situations where the mother is known to be a carrier, or suspected of being a carrier, of one of the more serious X-linked recessive disorders, e.g. Duchenne muscular dystrophy and perhaps haemophilia. Establishment of the sex of the fetus does not establish the diagnosis of the disease since, with heterozygous carriers, both affected and non-affected male fetuses may be conceived. In some disorders, e.g. Lesch-Nyhan disease and recently haemophilia, it is possible by an examination of the cells obtained in the amniotic fluid to identify an affected fetus. With many other X-linked recessive conditions it is, as yet, only possible to tell the parents whether the fetus is male or female. In some cases, therefore, a non-affected male fetus will be aborted. Although in the more serious disorders the parents may wish to prevent the birth of an affected child, to take such a decision is likely to cause considerable anxiety and distress to the parents.

In a similar way, the wife of a man affected by an X-linked recessive disorder could seek antenatal sexing of the fetus so that female fetuses who will be carriers can be aborted, thus stopping the transmission of the gene in that family. This is a much less likely situation, as males suffering from lethal or the more life-threatening conditions are unlikely to become sexually active. On the other hand, some families may feel very strongly that it is not right to pass on the disorder to the next generation. The ability to choose exists.

Parental anxiety

In the previous sections the main indications for prenatal diagnosis have been discussed. Another indication for prenatal screening which should be included is that of parental anxiety. It may be that the parents have already had a child with a handicap of unknown origin or they have a relative with congenital malformation. Bartsch (1978) found that many of the parents presenting with high anxiety and requesting amniocentesis had very close contact with handicapped children, often because they worked with them.

Termination of pregnancy

As a result of the prenatal investigations described in the preceding paragraphs, prospective parents can be told whether or not there is fetal abnormality. When the results are negative, the parents can be reassured that a number of conditions are not present. When the results are positive, prospective parents have the choice of terminating the pregnancy and, thus, preventing the birth of a handicapped child. While undoubtedly everyone wishes a 'normal', 'perfect' baby, it is unwise to assume that all parents would wish termination of an abnormal fetus. Forbes & Markova (1979) report a worldwide resistance on the part of female carriers of haemophilia to fetal sexing and

* It has been found that a high proportion of female nuclei contain a sex chromatin body applied to the inner surface of the nuclear membrane. Recently, to distinguish this sex marker from the fluorescent marker for the Y chromosome, it has been customary to refer to the sex chromatin body as an X-chromatin or Barr body after its co-discoverer (Roberts & Pembrey, 1978).

termination of pregnancy when it is offered. It is possible that attitudes may be different when serious abnormalities can be detected in the first trimester of pregnancy.

It is therefore extremely important that before amniocentesis is offered there should be a discussion about the procedure, its benefits and limitations and the possible outcomes. The discussion might include the following points:

- the reason for carrying out the procedure, emphasizing that there is little point in having amniocentesis unless termination of the pregnancy in the presence of an abnormal fetus is being considered
- the risk that a normal pregnancy will miscarry as a result of the amniocentesis, albeit this risk is small
- explanation of the procedure, emphasizing the sensations involved
- the length of time to wait for the results
- the limitations of amniocentesis; tests can only be carried out for a limited number of abnormalities and the procedure does not guarantee a normal baby
- parents can, if they wish, know the sex of the fetus.

Siggers (1978) recommends that these points should preferably be discussed with parents before conception because:

- couples may not have thought through the possible consequences of having amniocentesis and the various courses of action they need to consider in the light of particular amniocentesis results
- they may have misunderstood the limitations of prenatal diagnosis
- insufficient time may remain to carry out particular diagnostic tests.

Many might regard Siggers' suggestion as idealistic, but there are sound practical grounds for giving it careful consideration, and there is evidence of increasing interest in the idea of preconception clinics (BMJ Editorial, 1981). However, at the moment the reality of the situation is that amniocentesis is likely to be offered to women who are already pregnant.

Nursing staff have an important part to play in helping expectant parents to understand what is happening during the period when prenatal investigations are being carried out. They are in a unique position to listen to and to allay fear and anxiety. Prospective parents may be concerned about amniocentesis, its possible outcome and about termination. It is easy to explain the procedure of amniocentesis, but it may be more difficult to allay fear about the possible damage to the fetus should the amniocentesis results be negative and the pregnancy be allowed to continue. Anxiety is likely to be reduced if there is an opportunity for both the father and the mother to discuss these issues and time should be set aside for this.

All parents want a healthy baby and many are likely to be relieved that the birth of an abnormal child can be prevented by prenatal diagnosis and selective abortion. But the realization that the fetus is abnormal makes termination of the pregnancy an immediate and real issue for the parents involved. Most couples facing a pregnancy termination will do so with mixed emotions. These emotions will vary in their range and intensity and may depend on circumstances, such as marital status, religion and the degree of support received from family, friends and the caring professions. The parents' assessment of the situation is likely to vary according to whether they already have healthy children or whether this is their first child, and especially if the mother is older with fewer opportunities to have further children. Their approach to the problem may also be modified if they already have a handicapped child, or have had a previous pregnancy terminated because of an impaired fetus. Any of these factors may influence their attitude, not only to termination of pregnancy, but also to prenatal diagnosis, and may require discussion with the medical and nursing staff.

In this area of care there is a natural tendency to focus on the mother. She is the 'patient' when investigations are carried out. However, it is important to include the father of the child in discussions about what is happening. He is likely to be concerned and should be involved in all discussions and decisions to be taken as a result of prenatal investigations.

THE 'NEW GENETICS' AND GENE MARKERS

The techniques of prenatal diagnosis that have been described have relied on either the analysis of amniotic fluid cells or on fetal blood sampling. From the recent development of techniques for isolating and analyzing DNA has arisen the new genetics with a change in emphasis from the analysis of human genetic disease at the clinical, cellular and biochemical levels, to the molecular level (Weatherall, 1982).

Gene mapping or restriction endonuclease mapping has become a major tool in analyzing human genetic disease. DNA is obtained from available tissue, often peripheral white blood cells, is purified and is treated with a particular restriction enzyme. By using a series of different enzymes which cleave the DNA, it is possible to build up what are called restriction enzyme maps of the area of the gene.

The advent of this restriction enzyme technology has suggested a completely new approach to defining potentially large numbers of polymorphic marker loci. Polymorphism is defined as the existence in the same habitat at the same time of two or more distinct forms of the species. What can now be done is to define a series of restriction fragment length polymorphisms scattered throughout the genome and then attempt to determine linkages with specific genetic disorders. Several approaches to defining restriction fragment length polymorphisms are described by Gusella et al (1979 & 1983). Using one of these approaches and once specific probes have been obtained, it is then necessary to carry out detailed family studies. This involves developing a pedigree and then taking blood samples from affected, unaffected and at risk members of a family affected by the disorder being studied. By studying affected and unaffected family members, it is then possible to see whether one form of the marker is transmitted with the abnormal gene.

Gusella et al (1983) found one of a series of DNA sequence polymorphisms, which was used as a genetic marker in family studies, to be linked to the Huntington's chorea gene on chromosome 4. It has been suggested that this discovery is the most important application of molecular genetics to medicine as yet (Harper, 1983). It means that the marker discovered by Gusella could possibly be used as a predictive test for those families shown to be heterozygous for the marker. However there are problems. This is not the gene itself that has been identified but a marker or indicator of where the gene may be located. Therefore, information from this is an estimate of prediction.

The precise distance between the marker and the gene needs to be established so that the error rate of prediction can be calculated. When this problem is overcome, it should be possible to offer a prediction for those family members who are at 50% risk of having inherited the gene as well as to carry out prenatal diagnosis since the polymorphism should be detectable in fetal DNA samples taken from chorion biopsy specimens or amniotic cells. The result of this work is that for those who are at high risk of inheriting Huntington's chorea, for which there is neither cure nor simple diagnostic test, the possibility of diagnosis of the asymptomatic individual and of the fetus is becoming a reality.

Such scientific advances often create their own particular problems. Will individuals wish to be tested when there is still neither cure nor effective treatment? Should such a test be offered at all? If such a test is to be offered, how are people to be prepared for it and who will do this work? Will those at risk individuals wish to know a positive result? Previous studies have shown that between 10–40% of family members may choose not to be tested (Barrette & Marsden, 1979; Tyler & Harper, 1983). It is extremely difficult to live with the risk of developing Huntington's chorea. But in the uncertainty of not knowing, there is always room for optimism. The person does have a 50–50 chance that he will not develop the disease. A predictive test moves that uncertainty and leaves no room for 'it may never happen'. For those who have a negative result, it is marvellous news. But will those found to be positive be able to cope with the burden of the information?

It is clear that a major implication of predictive testing for a disorder for which there is as yet no cure is the need for highly skilled counselling prior to the taking of the test (Merz, 1985). It is necessary to ask whether the test should be available to all or whether some people may be considered unable to deal with the information and therefore unsuitable for testing. Wexler (Merz, 1985) believes that all those at risk over the age of 18 who wish the test should be allowed to have it and this view is shared by Thomas (1982) who believes that early certainty about the gene would be easier to bear than the present protracted uncertainty. It is necessary to develop training programmes for staff so that pre-test counselling and the giving of test results can be carried out in a sensitive manner appropriate to each individual.

Recombinant DNA technology also offers a new approach to the pathogenesis of adult polycystic kidney disease (APKD) in which the underlying biochemical defect is still unknown. Reeders et al (1985) have isolated a gene marker for APKD and assigned it to the short arm of chromosome 16. 183 members of nine families from northern Europe were investigated. The reliability of the marker used by Reeders et al was calculated at approximately 95%. The authors estimated that diagnosis of asymptomatic at risk family members will be possible in about 93% of cases. Adult polycystic kidney disease can be diagnosed in the adult by ultrasound but has the disadvantage that sensitivity depends on age (Sahney et al, 1983). An accurate marker test would enable at risk family members to be offered earlier diagnosis and prenatal diagnosis. We do not know whether individuals would make use of such a test. This apect should be the subject of further investigation.

The application of gene markers to clinical medicine does create very searching questions that must be faced. However, in the long run, these advances give the very real possibility of identifying and analyzing the deleterious genes themselves and of subsequently isolating their gene products. It is hoped that in the future a more radical approach to treatment would follow.

GENETIC COUNSELLING

DEFINITIONS

In the previous sections the possibilities for treatment of, and prenatal diagnosis for, genetic disease have been examined. This information is the essential background to genetic counselling. There have been many definitions of this term and in recent years there has been a change of emphasis in its practice. Epstein (1979) states that 'the principal purpose of genetic counselling is the prevention of genetically determined disorders. This is usually accomplished by the provision of information concerning risks of occurrence or recurrence'. Authors such as Davis (1979) and Murray (1976) endeavour to present accurate medical, genetic and social facts related to the conditions under consideration, as well as a full discussion of all the options available to the individual and their likely consequences. The WHO Scientific Group (1972) suggested that 'the role of the genetic counsellor should be to assist the physician with diagnosis, to estimate the recurrence risk, to interpret this information to the patient in meaningful terms to help the patient reach and act upon an appropriate decision'. Here a new element is introduced, that of helping the patient decide what to do with the information that is provided.

Perhaps one of the clearest definitions is that of the Ad Hoc Committee on Genetic Counselling (1975). This committee of American and Canadian physicians and scientists describe genetic counselling as 'a communication process which deals with the human problems associated with the occurrence, or the risk of occurrence, of a genetic disorder in a family. This process involves an attempt by one or more appropriately trained persons to help the individual or family:

- comprehend the medical facts, including the diagnosis, the probable course of the disorder and the available management
- appreciate the way heredity contributes to the disorder and the risk of recurrence in specified relatives
- understand the options for dealing with the risk of recurrence
- choose the course of action which seems appropriate to them in view of their risk and the family goals and act in accordance with that decision

- make the best possible adjustment to the disorder in an affected family member and/ or to the risk of recurrence of that disorder.'

In this definition the emphasis is now on counselling — 'communication process ... to help the individual or family comprehend ... appreciate ... understand ... choose ... act ... make the best possible adjustment'. It could be argued that there has been a shift in emphasis from prevention as the main objective of genetic counselling to counselling and education. There is also an increasing awareness of the complexity of the problems.

In the past children have been born, not without concern as to how normal they might be, but without the ability to make reproductive decisions on the basis of probability statements of how normal a child might be.

Sorenson et al (1981) remind us that those receiving genetic counselling are experiencing a series of life events of major importance:

- some may be considering their desire to be parents for the first time, or again
- some may be considering their willingness to live with a child with a congenital defect or disorder
- some may be having to consider the fact that their relative — child, spouse, or other close relative — has a progressive illness for which there is no cure
- some may be having to consider that they themselves are suffering from a progressive illness
- some may have come to realize that they have already passed on an inherited defect
- some may be considering for the first time that they themselves may or may not develop, some time in the future, a serious progressive disorder.

The majority will have to examine their own ability to restructure their lives in terms of events and compromises that most have never previously had to consider. The ways in which people make decisions in such circumstances, and live with their decisions, are central to genetic counselling.

The outcome of genetic counselling may have considerable implications for the society of the future, in addition to the as yet unborn child. In the current genetic counselling situation, the concern is with an individual or family who have presented with a problem. This individual may be an affected person, the parent of an affected child, a heterozygous carrier, or an individual 'at risk' of developing an autosomal dominant disorder of variable age of onset. For all these people the implications of information given in genetic counselling may be very different.

'CONTENT' OF GENETIC COUNSELLING

Information

It is not sufficient merely to give the patient the name of the disorder. There is considerable evidence (Sorenson et al, 1981) that there is a variety of information that patients wish from genetic counselling and this can be loosely divided into medical and socio-medical. Individuals concerned wish to know the cause of the disorder, why it happened, the course of the illness and its prognosis. Both the type and availability of treatment should be discussed as this could influence where people live, e.g. centres for the treatment of such conditions as haemophilia and polycystic kidney disease are likely to be situated in major teaching hospitals only. The risk of occurrence or recurrence of having an affected child is important information. In addition to discussion it is particularly helpful if the information about the nature of the disorder, risk of recurrence or occurrence and treatment can be given to the individuals concerned in written form, as retention of information under stress is poor (Ley & Spelman, 1967). The individual can be given a letter, perhaps similar to that sent to the general practitioner, describing the factual information, but this may not be appropriate to their needs. Some departments produce their own leaflets indicated in Miller & Lubs' (1980) *The Inheritance of Haemophilia.* Some self-help groups such as the Muscular Dystrophy Group, the Haemophilia Society and the Huntington's Chorea Association produce informative and useful booklets. Nurses working in this area have an important role in giving information, facilitating understanding and in subsequent support.

Explanation of risk

Until recently, the majority of studies of genetic counselling emphasized the importance of explaining the transmission of the disorder and the risk to patients and their children. Indeed the 'success' of the counselling was measured in terms of how correctly the individual retained the information about risk and probability when asked at a later date. However, to understand the concept and language of risk and probability theory when applied to oneself is difficult (Pearn, 1973). A 50–50 chance interpreted as 'it may not happen' or 'it may happen' is relatively simple, although the way the information is phrased and whether the emphasis is put on the 'may not' or on the 'may' could well affect the person's perception of the risk.

A similar problem arises with a probability of a 1 in 4 chance at each conception of having an affected child. The statement of risk is usually phrased in that way, but it can equally well be turned round and phrased as a 3 in 4 chance at each conception of having an unaffected child. Once more the emphasis is important. There is also a tendency to abbreviate this information to 'a 1 in 4 chance of having an affected child'. Perhaps because the phrase 'at each conception' is so often omitted, some misunderstandings have arisen. It is not uncommon to hear parents state that, if the first child is affected the next three will be all right. It is important to remember that the risk is the risk at each conception.

The work of both Pearn (1973) and Sorenson et al (1981) demonstrate how difficult it is to know how risk is interpreted. What is a high risk to one person may be a medium or low risk to another. Because of this difficulty Sorenson et al suggest that it may be better to explain risk to patients in numeric terms, rather than using the more subjective non-numeric terms.

Information about risk and probability is clearly an important part of the information given in genetic counselling. It should, however, be kept in perspective as it is only part of the information given to individuals to enable them to reach decisions about their future.

The 'at risk' individual

It has already been seen that the implications of genetic disease will vary according to the relationship of the individual to the disorder. The situation of an individual at risk of developing an autosomal dominant disorder of variable age of onset for which there is no satisfactory treatment, e.g. Huntington's chorea, highlights the skills required of the counsellor, as well as the conflict of aims in genetic counselling. Unlike the debate about whether the cancer patient should or should not be told of their diagnosis, in this situation it is not known whether or not an individual will develop the disorder. There is no certainty of diagnosis. The advantage of informing an individual of their risk is that it may help them to make plans for the future, and possibly reduce suffering. The disadvantage of telling such individuals of their risk is that, on average, half of this group will never develop the disorder.

Nevertheless, they are all being asked to live with the knowledge that they *may* develop the disorder, and with the discomfort and uncertainty that this knowledge inevitably brings to their lives. As a result of this knowledge, 'at risk' individuals may find it more difficult to make relationships with the opposite sex, to be accepted for training schemes or jobs (particularly in times of relative job shortage and high unemployment) and to be accepted for life insurance at reasonable rates.

It is often helpful to see the 'at risk' individual together with other members of the family to discuss the different problems facing each individual, as the uncertainty under which the 'at risk' individual lives creates pressure for himself and his family (Wexler, 1979). It is also important to realize that 'at risk' persons may be patients for conditions unrelated to the inherited disorder or they may be visitors to an affected family member. In these situations nurses have an excellent opportunity to show tact and understanding and offer an opportunity for discussion. The counselling of 'at risk' individuals requires very skilled handling and it raises problems for which there are no easy solutions.

COMMUNICATION PROBLEMS IN GENETIC COUNSELLING

For many people the situation surrounding the need for genetic counselling creates anxiety. It is, therefore, all the more important that the information given to these individuals is clear. Several studies of doctor-patient communication suggest that considerable shortcomings exist in the communication process between patient and doctor (Korsch & Negrete, 1972). This can lead to a feeling of mutual dissatisfaction and often the effectiveness of the health care provided is diminished. As yet, there has been no published work of a detailed study of the communication process in genetic counselling.

Leonard et al (1972) interviewed parents of children with genetic disorders to assess their knowledge of the disease and the genetic risks involved, as well as other biological and genetic information. The authors concluded that about half of the parents 'had any kind of comprehension that could make the information helpful to them' and that 'some parents who did give correct answers denied their validity or said that they did not apply to themselves. Others confessed to a lack of comprehension of the correct answers that they had given and some exhibited a lack of perception of the meaning of the risk'.

Sibinga & Friedman (1971) investigated parental understanding of phenylketonuria by questionnaires, and found that only 15 out of 79 parents gave correct answers. Half of the parents displayed a considerable tendency to distort their answers. In this study the education of the parents was not related to their understanding. Sorenson (1974) calculated that between 21% and 75% of couples failed to remember or acquire the genetic information provided. This would suggest that there is a gap between the goals genetic counsellors intend to reach and the goals being accomplished with respect to communication of factual information.

There are several possible explanations for this. The information itself may be unclear: the subject is complex and considerable care is needed to isolate the relevant points and to put them over in a straightforward manner. The process of giving the information may not be such that the individual can make the best use of it; the interview may be too short; the patient may have had to wait too long; the counsellor may have been rushed; the patient may have been distracted by noise or interruptions. These are some of the more practical considerations. There are also psychological factors that must be considered if genetic counselling is to be effective.

Stress in genetic counselling

It has already been suggested that the circumstances surrounding the need for genetic counselling may be very stressful. Studies of individuals facing important life stresses indicate that, in general, there are recognizable stages of coping (Horowitz, 1976; Nelson-Jones, 1982). At first there is a response of protest or resistance that one's world has changed. The individual may attempt to deny and block out reality. The individual is likely to cry a lot. As the impact of the stress sinks in, a period of disorganization occurs in which the person's inner sense of the world begins to alter. Lastly, a period of reorganization ensues, in which a new way of looking at and coping with the world is developed, and this often requires a change of behaviour (Horowitz, 1976).

In genetic counselling, e.g. following the birth of an abnormal child or after the confirmation of a serious diagnosis, the individual's thoughts tend to dwell on certain themes:

- The fear of repetition. If it happened once, it could happen again. In many genetic diseases, this fear may have a realistic basis. The thought of repetition may be feared as much as the event itself.
- Anger and faultfinding. Frequently individuals will say 'why has this happened to me?', and assign blame to anyone who might be at fault. This could include a parent, an affected child, the doctor or a spouse (especially in X-linked disorders). However, the defective gene, the cause of the problem, may be carried by the person concerned. The individual can only 'blame' himself or herself.

- Shame and helplessness: stressful situations such as the diagnosis of a genetic disorder engender a feeling of helplessness arising from the realization of the lack of control over one's own life. This realization is often experienced as shame.

THE NURSES' ROLE

Following the diagnosis of a genetic disorder, nurses can play an important role in helping the individual to cope with the diagnosis. They can be an important source of information regarding the disorder, the course, possible problems, burden and management. They can also provide information about relevant community agencies and support groups. The person needs this information in order to make relevant decisions. By imparting information empathetically, being aware of the individual's needs and providing the most relevant information, nurses as counsellors show that they understand and care.

Nurses can also help the person involved to deal with some of the feelings discussed previously by spending time listening, being positively supportive at times when the individual needs to express his or her anger, frustration or guilt, and reiterating forgotten information. It is also important for the nurse to recognize that the feelings that the person is experiencing may disorganize their ability to make decisions.

Nurses can also help to prepare the individual for future possible problems. There is considerable evidence to suggest that when an individual is made aware of, or anticipates, an impending crisis or stress, the coping process is easier (Janis & Mann, 1976). Thus the couple may be helped if they can begin to consider, for example, the possibility of abortion when being offered an amniocentesis.

Individuals may need to change their behaviour or way of life as a result of the information given in genetic counselling. For some, the diagnosis may mean a much shorter life for themselves, as in disorders such as Marfan's syndrome, Huntington's chorea and neurofibromatosis. For parents where the diagnosis is Duchenne muscular dystrophy or cystic fibrosis it may mean a life with much pain or disability, or lack of hearing or sight for their child. Plans for children or more children may have to be changed and another way of life, involving voluntary childlessness, be found.

Nurses can help by conveying to patients that it is normal to feel emotions such as sadness, anger or guilt. By doing so they go a long way to easing the pain and restoring the patient's self-esteem.

THE TEAM APPROACH

The application of knowledge about genetic disease now requires a multidisciplinary team approach with laboratory resources, diagnostic facilities and the skills of different disciplines, both medical and non-medical. Such facilities are found in genetic advisory centres of which there are several in the United Kingdom, mostly associated with university teaching departments, but some associated with departments of obstetrics and paediatrics. Patients with genetically transmitted diseases will not be concentrated in any one hospital department. Genetic counselling offers to those who receive it an opportunity to choose different courses of action. Sometimes it will be very easy to make a decision, but in other situations decisions cannot be reached quickly. This has implications for genetic counselling in that it can be a long-term process involving many counselling sessions at home, in hospital clinics or in a general practitioner's surgery. In these situations it is important that individuals have continuity of contact. Wilkie & Sinclair (1977) found that general practitioners felt that they, along with health visitors and perhaps social workers, were the appropriate people to offer such long-term support and counselling, but this may depend on the nature of the disorder, the available resources and the geographical area. General health care practitioners involved in genetic counselling also require further education and training.

In the United Kingdom, genetic counselling

has traditionally been offered by doctors. There is now increasing support and scope for non-medically-qualified counsellors particularly skilled in counselling techniques (Powledge, 1979; Black, 1980; Sorenson et al, 1981) who can provide what Fraser (1976) describes as 'supportive' counselling so essential in genetic health care. Nurses clearly have a role here both in hospital and community services.

Finally, nurses have an important part to play in general health education about genetic disease. Considerable ignorance, fear and stigma exist about handicaps and diseases which are genetically inherited. More education and discussion, not only with the general public but in schools of nursing, is essential in order to help the ever-increasing number of people discovered to be involved with genetically transmitted diseases.

REFERENCES

Ad Hoc Committee on Genetic Counselling 1975 Report of the American Society of Human Genetics. American Journal of Human Genetics 27:240–242

Barrette J, Marsden CD 1979 Attitudes of families to some aspects of Huntington's chorea. Psychological Medicine 9:327– 336

Bartsch F K 1978 Indications, technique and limitations of amniocentesis. In: Scrimgeour J B (ed) Toward the prevention of fetal malformation. Edinburgh University Press, Edinburgh

Bergsma D 1973 Birth defects atlas and compendium. The National Foundation March of Dimes Williams & Wilkins, Baltimore

Birch C, Abrecht P 1975 Genetics and the quality of life. Pergamon Press, Oxford

Black R B 1980 Support for genetic services: a survey. Health and Social Work, 5 (1):27–34

Bodmer W F 1982 Cancer genetics. Cancer Surveys 1:1–15

British Medical Journal 1981 Editorial. British Medical Journal 283:685

Brock D J H, Sutcliffe R G 1972 Alphafetoprotein in the antenatal diagnosis of anencephaly and spina bifida. Lancet 2:197–199

Brotherston Sir J 1978 Implications of antenatal screening for the health service. In: Scrimgeour J B (ed) Toward the prevention of fetal malformation. Edinburgh University Press, Edinburgh

Brown J 1979 Inherited causes of mental retardation. In: Proudfoot A T (ed) Heritable factors in disease. Royal College of Physicians, Edinburgh

Carter C O 1969 Genetics of common disorders. British Medical Bulletin 25(1):52–57

Carter C O 1977 The relative contribution of mutant genes and chromosome abnormalities to genetic ill health in man. In: Scott D, Bridges B A, Sobels F W (eds) Progress in genetic toxicity. Biomedica Press, Amsterdam

Carter C O 1981 Genetics of mental handicap. International Colloquium on Childhood Mental Deficiency. Paris, France, 21–23, October Colloques Inserm vol 105

Chen E 1979 Twins reared apart: A living lab. New York Times Magazine, 9 December

Clarke C A 1970 Human genetics and medicine. Institute of Biology, Studies in Biology 20

Clinical Genetics Society 1978 The provision of services for the prenatal diagnosis of fetal abnormality in the United Kingdom. Eugenics Society Supplement No. 3

Committee on Mutagenicity of Chemicals in Food, Consumer Products and the Environment 1981 Guidelines for the testing of chemicals for mutagenicity. HMSO, London

Council for Science and Society 1978 Life and death before birth CSS London

Davis J G 1979 A counsellor's viewpoint. In: Capron A M (ed). Genetic counselling. Facts, values and norms. Birth defects. Original article Series XV(2). The National Foundation March of Dimes. Alan R. Liss, New York

De Grouchy J 1976 Human chromosomes and their anomalies. In: Baltrop D (ed) Aspects of genetics in paediatrics. Fellowship of Post Graduate Medicine, London

Doll R 1971 The age distribution of cancer implications for models of carcinogenesis (with discussion). Journal of Royal Statistical Society series A 134:133–166

Doll R, Hill A B 1964 Mortality in relation to smoking: 10 years observation of British doctors. British Medical Journal 1:1399–1410, 1460–1467

Doll R, Peto R 1976 Mortality in relation to smoking: 20 years observations of British male doctors. British Medical Journal 2:1525–1536

Emery A E H 1983 Elements of medical genetics, 6th edn. Churchill Livingstone, Edinburgh

Epstein, C J 1979 Foreword. In: Kessler S (ed) Genetic counselling. Psychological dimensions. Academic Press, New York

Forbes C D, Lowe G D 1982 Unresolved problems in haemophilia. MTP Press, Lancaster

Forbes C, Markova I 1979 An international survey of genetic counselling in haemophilia. Ethics in Science & Medicine 6:123–126

Fraser F C 1976 Genetics as a health–care service. New England Journal of Medicine 295:486–488

Gusella J, Varsanyi-Brelner A, Kao F T, Jones C, Puck T T, Keep C, Orkin S, Housman D 1979 Precise localisation of human beta-globin gene complex on chrosome II. Proceedings of the National Academy of Sciences, USA 76 10:5239–5242

Gusella JF, Wexler NS, Connelly PM et al 1983 A polymorphic DNA marker genetically linked to Huntington's disease. Nature 306:234–238

Hagard S, Carter F A 1976 Preventing the birth of infants with Down's syndrome: a cost benefit analysis. British Journal of Preventive Social Medicine, 30(1):40–53

Harnden D G 1979 Genetics and cancer. In: Proudfoot A T (ed) Heritable factors in disease. Royal College of Physicians, Edinburgh

Harper P 1979 Patterns of Mendelian inheritance. A clinician's guide. In: Proudfoot A T (ed) Heritable factors in disease. Royal College of Physicians, Edinburgh

Harper P S 1984 Practical genetic counselling 2nd edn. Wright, Bristol

Harper P 1983 A genetic marker for Huntington's chorea. British Medical Journal 287:1567–1568
Harsanyi Z, Hutton R 1983 Genetic prophecy. Beyond the double helix. Granada, London
Hayden M H 1981 Huntington's chorea. Springer, New York
Heller J H 1973 Human chromosome abnormalities as related to physical and mental dysfunction. In: Bresler J B (ed) Genetics and society. Addison–Wesley, London
Heston L L 1970 The genetics of schizophrenia and schizoid disease. Science 167:249–256
Holden C 1980 Identical twins reared apart. Science 207:1323 –1327
Horowitz M J 1976 Stress response syndromes. Jason Aronson, New York
Howell M, Ford P 1980 The true history of the elephant man. Penguin, Harmondsworth
Jacobs P A 1969 Structural abnormalities of the sex chromosomes. British Medical Bulletin 25(1):94–98
Jandl J N, Cooper R A 1972 Hereditary spherocytosis. In: Stanbury J B, Wyngaarden J B, Frederickson D S (eds) The metabolic basis of inherited disease, 3rd edn. McGraw Hill, New York
Janis I L, Mann L 1976 Coping with decisional conflict. American Scientist 64:657–667
Kaback M M, O'Brien J S 1973 Tay–Sachs' prototype for prevention of genetic disease. Hospital Practice 8:107–116
Kalter H, Warkany J 1983 Congenital malformations (2 parts). New England Journal of Medicine 308(8):424–431, 308(9):491–497
Kessler S 1979 Genetic counselling. Psychological dimensions. Academic Press, New York
Kety I S, Wender P H 198O Psychiatric genetics. Studies of adoptees and their families. Annual Meeting of the Association of Research in Nervous and Mental Disease, New York
Kidd K K, Cavalli–Sforza L L 1973 An analysis of the genetics of schizophrenia. Social Biology 20:254–265
Korsch B M, NegreteV P 1972 Doctor–patient communication. Scientific American 227:66–74
Lancet 1970 Genetics of schizophrenia (Editorial) Lancet 1 :26
Leonard C O, Chase G, Childs B 1972 Genetic counselling. A consumer's view. New England Journal of Medicine 287:433–439
Ley P, Spelman M S 1967 Communicating with the patient. Staples Press, London
Lubs H A, de la Cruz F (eds) 1977 Genetic counselling. Raven Press, New York
Lynch H T 1969 Genetic factors in carcinoma. Medical Clinics of North America 53(4):923–939
Macklin M T 1959 Comparison of the number of breast cancer deaths observed in relatives of breast cancer patients and the number expected on the basis of mortality rates. Journal of the National Cancer Institute 23:1179–1189
McKusick V 1975 Mendelian inheritance in men. Catalogs of autosomal dominant, autosomal recessive and X–linked phenotypes, 4th edn. Johns Hopkins University Press, Baltimore
Merz B 1985 Markers for disease genes open new era in diagnostic screening. Journal of the American Medical Association 254:3153–3159
Mikkelsen M, Nielsen 1976 Cost benefit analysis of prevention of Down's syndrome. In: Boué A (ed) Prenatal diagnosis. INSERM, Paris
Miller C H, Lubs M L 1980 The inheritance of haemophilia. Medical and Scientific Advisory Council
Milunsky A 1980 Know your genes. Penguin, Harmondsworth
Murray R F 1976 Psychosocial aspects of genetic counselling. Social Work in Health Care 2(1):13–23
Nelson-Jones R 1982 The theory and practice of counselling. Psychology. Holt, Rinehart and Winston, New York
Oliver M 1976 Dietary cholesterol, plasma cholesterol and coronary heart disease. British Heart Journal 38:214–218
Opitz J M 1973 Klinefelter syndrome. In: Bergsma D (ed) Birth defects atlas and compendium. The National Foundation March of Dimes. Williams & Wilkins, Baltimore
Patrick A D 1978 Biochemical studies on amniotic fluid and its cells. In: Scrimgeour J B (ed) Toward the prevention of fetal malformation. Edinburgh University Press, Edinburgh
Passarge E 1978 Screening populations for genetic disease. In: Scrimgeour J B (ed) Toward the prevention of fetal malformation. Edinburgh University Press, Edinburgh
Pearn J N 1973 Patients' subjective interpretation of risks offered in genetic counselling. Journal of Medical Genetics 10:129–134
Petrakis N L 1977 Breast secretory activity and breast cancer epidemiology. In: Mulvihill J J, Miller R W, Fraumeni J F (eds) Genetics of human cancer. (Progress in cancer research and therapy vol 3). Raven Press, New York
Polani P E 1978 Future developments in antenatal screening and diagnosis. In: Scrimgeour J B (ed) Toward the prevention of fetal malformation. Edinburgh University Press, Edinburgh
Powledge M 1979 Genetic counsellors without doctorates. In: Capron A M (ed) Genetic counselling. Facts, values and norms. Birth defects. Original Article Series XV(2). The National Foundation March of Dimes. Alan R Liss, New York
Price W H, Whatmore P B 1967 Behaviour disorders and the pattern of crime among XYY males identified at a maximum security hospital. British Medical Journal 1:533–536
Reeders S T, Breuning M H, Davies K E, Nicholls R D, Jarman A P, Higgs, D R, Pearson P L, Weatherall D J 1985 A highly polymorphic DNA marker linked to adult polycystic kidney disease on chromosome 16. Nature 317: 542–545
Roberts J A, Pembrey M E 1978 An introduction to medical genetics, 7th edn. Oxford University Press, Oxford
Roberts M B V 1977 Biology: a functional approach. Wilson, London
Ross R B, Johnston M C 1972 Cleft lip and palate. Williams & Wilkins, Baltimore
Sahney S, Sandler M A, Weiss L, Levin N W, Hricak H, Madrazo B L 1983 Adult polycystic kidney disease: presymptomatic diagnosis for genetic counselling. Clinical Nephrology 20:89–93
Sibinga M S, Friedman J 1971 Complexities of parental understanding of phenylketonuria. Paediatrics 48(2):216–224
Siggers D C 1978 Prenatal diagnosis of genetic disease. Blackwell Scientific, Oxford
Smith D W, Wilson A A 1973 The child with Down's syndrome: Causes, characteristics and acceptance. Saunders, Philadelphia
Sorenson J R 1974 Genetic counselling. Some psychological considerations. In: Lipkin M, Rowley P T (eds) Genetic responsibility. Plenum Press, New York
Sorenson J R, Swazey J P, Scotch N A 1981 Reproductive pasts, reproductive futures. Genetic counselling and its effectiveness. Alan R Liss, New York

Steptoe A 1981 Psychological factors in cardiovascular disorders. Academic Press, London
Stern C 1973 Principles of human genetics, 3rd edn. Freeman, Oxford
Stevenson A, Davison B C 1976 Genetic counselling. Heinemann, London
Strong J A, Whatmore P B, McClement W F 1966 Criminal patients with XYY sex chromosome complement. Lancet 1:565–560
Thomas S 1982 Ethics of a predictive test for Huntington's chorea. British Medical Journal 284:1383–1385
Thomas S 1986 Genetic risk. Penguin, Harmondsworth
Townsend P, Davidson N 1982 Inequalities in health. Penguin, Harmondsworth
Tyler A, Harper P S 1983 Attitudes of subjects at risk and their relatives towards genetic counselling in Huntington's chorea. Journal of Medical Genetics 20:179–188
Valenti C 1978 Fetal blood sampling in early pregnancy. In: Scrimgeour J B (ed) Toward the prevention of fetal malformation. Edinburgh University Press, Edinburgh
Weatherall D J 1982 The new genetics and clinical practice. Nuffield Provincial Hospital Trust, London
Weatherall D J, Clegg J B 1981 The thalassaemia syndrome, 3rd edn. Blackwell Scientific, Oxford
Welch J P, Borgaonkar D S, Herr H M 1967 Psychopathy, mental deficiency, aggressiveness and the XYY chromosomes. Nature 214:500–501
Wexler N S 1979 Genetic Russian roulette. The experience of being at risk for Huntington's chorea. In: Kessler S (ed) Genetic counselling, psychological dimensions. Academic Press, New York
WHO 1972 Genetic disorders: prevention, treatment and rehabilitation. Report of a WHO Scientific Group. WHO Technical Report Series No. 497:1–46
Wilkie P, Sinclair S 1977 Report of the genetic register system acceptability study. Department of Social Administration, University of Edinburgh
Williams E M, Harper P S 1976 Genetic study of Welsh gypsies. Journal of Medical Genetics 14(3):172–176
Williamson R (ed) 1981 Genetic engineering, Academic Press, New York
Wilson R, Harpring E 1972 Mental and motor development in infant twins. Development Psychology 7(3):277–287
Witkin H A 1976 Criminality in XYY and XXY men. Science 193:547–555
Working Group on Screening for Neural Tube Defects 1979 Report to the Standing Medical Advisory Committee. HMSO, London

4

Trauma and repair

INTRODUCTION

In order to survive, the human species has to contend with many environmental forces capable of damaging tissues, destroying structural integrity and disrupting organic processes. Despite attempts to minimize hazards in occupational, domestic and social spheres of life the incidence of trauma in the modern world has reached epidemic proportions. In Britain 4 million people attend Accident Departments each year and trauma is the major cause of death in people under the age of 40 years (Crockard, 1981a).

It is apparent that many of the injured would not survive without protective, biological mechanisms capable of reacting immediately to noxious stimuli, limiting the effects of injury and subsequently restoring damaged areas.

As trauma is such a global concept, embracing any type of injury to any part of the body, it is neither possible nor desirable to attempt to deal in detail with a large number of specific injuries in this chapter. A broad overview of some common problems will be presented and general principles will be discussed but the main emphasis will be on those mechanisms common to all forms of injury.

TYPES OF TRAUMA

AETIOLOGICAL FACTORS

Biological injuries may be caused by the

application of physical force. This may be in the form of penetrating or non-penetrating force, internal torsion or shearing of structures, barotrauma due to sudden pressure changes, and acceleration-deceleration forces. All of these are common in road accidents, industrial accidents and modern warfare. Tissues may also be damaged or destroyed by a range of chemicals, particularly acids and alkalis, by ionizing radiations and by extremes of heat or cold — burns, scalds, electrical currents or frostbite. Table 4.1 indicates the range of causes and effects of tissue damage.

COMMON INJURIES

Skeletal

Fractures of bone are common in all age groups, although the elderly are more susceptible due to the metabolic changes which occur with ageing. Adolescents, however, are more likely to engage in activities which expose them to risk, e.g. playing rugby or motor cycling.

A break in the continuity of bone is a wound in a dynamic, living tissue and will evoke responses analogous to those seen in soft tissue injury, with the addition of the laying down of calcium hydroxyapatite during the re-ossification process. Loss of structural support and function are immediately evident in limb fractures, and early immobilization and fixation are necessary to provide support, prevent further damage, relieve the pain of muscle spasms and enhance healing. Fractures may be complicated by nerve or blood vessel involvement and compounded by the presence of an open wound. Some fractures may be stable but the movement of unstable fractures may produce further complications. Serious neurological impairment may be caused by unstable vertebral fractures and suspected cases should be moved very carefully with head, shoulders and pelvis moving together (Evans, 1984).

Head injury

Some degree of brain damage should be anticipated whenever there has been a blow to the skull. A fracture may or may not be present, but if present it may be depressed onto the underlying brain. Control of superficial bleeding by direct pressure may exacerbate brain damage.

Bleeding within the cranial cavity may be extradural, subdural, subarachnoid or intracerebral and will be accompanied by some degree of vasogenic and cytotoxic oedema (Sharr, 1984). Even if the bleeding is self-limiting, a haematoma may continue to act as a slowly expanding space-occupying lesion by osmosis. Raised intracranial pressure will impede cerebral perfusion and may cause herniation of the brain — particularly midbrain herniation through the tentorium with compression of the oculomotor nerve (Ch. 18).

In such cases intravenous mannitol may be prescribed to reduce the pressure. Steroids (dexamethasone) may be given, although Sharr is of the opinion that they are of little use in traumatic oedema. Positive pressure ventilation is recommended by many to ensure adequate gas exchange at the cerebral level, even when there is no indication of respiratory impairment. This practice is not considered justified by Crockard (1981b). It seems advisable not to place the patient in a head dependent position for any reason,and to avoid overhydration.

Loss of consciousness renders the patient totally dependent on carers for life support, protection from further injury and maintenance of functional potential. Assessment of the level of consciousness using the Glasgow Coma Scale (Teasdale et al, 1975) is probably the best guide to the patient's condition, despite the availability of direct intracranial pressure measuring devices (Lindsay, 1984).

Computerized tomography has vastly improved the medical management of those with a head injury and localized blood or blood clots may be quickly evacuated via a burr hole.

Chest injury

Injury to the chest cavity, whether penetrating or not, often involves collapse of a lung due to the entrance of fluid, gas or blood into the normally sub-atmospheric pleural space

Table 4.1 Tissue damage — causes and effects

Cause		Effect
Infection	Localized General	See Chapter 5.
Agents which burn	Direct heat	External burns affect skin. Severe burns may also affect deeper tissues
	Radiation	
	Electrical current	Burn may be deeper than appears.
	Sun	May burn skin and also cause heat exhaustion and sunstroke.
	Chemicals	May cause severe skin burns. Present a particular hazard to eye if splashed onto conjunctiva.
Cold		May cause frostbite on body extremities. Elderly and young infants are particularly at risk of hypothermia (lowering of body temperature).
Poisons	Contact	Some substances irritate the skin, causing rashes and dermatitis.
	Bites and stings	Some insects and snakes inject poisons. These may cause a severe local reaction and occasionally a general body reaction.
	Inhaled	Some gases irritate the lining of the respiratory passages. Others interfere with oxygen intake by the body.
	Swallowed	Some chemicals corrode or irritate the lining of the upper digestive tract.
	Drugs and alcohol	Overdoses affect nervous system in a variety of ways, including blocking neural pathways and inducing sleep and respiratory depression. Some cause overexcitability, others interfere with cell metabolism.
Tissue anoxia	Generalized	Occurs when the body is unable to obtain sufficient oxygen via the respiratory system, e.g. drowning, gassing, suffocation, blockage of respiratory passages.
	Local	Specific tissues may be deprived of oxygen when blood supply is interrupted or decreased, e.g. thrombus, embolus, atherosclerosis, physical pressure. Gross haemorhhage may deprive tissues of oxygen by lowering the number of circulating erythrocytes.
Violence	Crush injury	Crushing by a heavy weight may injure large areas of muscle, internal organs and bone.
	Fractured bones	May be caused by direct or indirect force. See Chapter 21.
	Joint injuries	Caused when joints forced into abnormal positions. *Strain:* no soft tissue damage. *Sprain:* muscle, ligament or tendon is torn. *Dislocation:* bones of joint move out of position. *Subluxation:* partial movement only.
	Head injuries	If the head is hit by an object or moves rapidly and is brought to a sudden stop, injuries may include: *Fracture* of the skull; *Bleeding* from a blood vessel in the brain, on the brain surface, or under the skull; *Contusion:* bruising and swelling of the brain; *Concussion:* loss of consciousness brought about by movement of the brain stem.
	Skin wounds	are described as: *Incised:* a clean cut by a sharp instrument. *Lacerated:* a jagged cut. *Punctured:* caused by a sharp, pointed instrument. *Stab:* deep wound caused by knife–like object. *Abrasion:* the skin is scraped or excoriated. *Avulsion:* a flap of skin and tissue is lifted. *Contusion:* bruising of tissue. The skin may or may not be broken. *Amputation:* part of a limb is removed.

resulting in some degree of respiratory impairment. This will become progressively worse with mediastinal shift if there is a tension pneumothorax with a 'sucking wound' of the thorax acting as a one-way valve. Such wounds should be sealed immediately — Vaseline gauze and pressure pad are quite effective. Fluid removal to permit lung expansion requires an underwater seal drain (Hurt, 1985). In some cases the patient may be disturbed by the presence of surgical emphysema — the presence of air in the subcutaneous tissues which, though harmless, can grossly distort the body image.

Laceration of heart or lung may be caused by rib fracture, and cardiac function may be impeded by cardiac tamponade — the pressure exerted by a collection of blood in the pericardial sac. This may be detected by a raised jugular venous pressure, hypotension and possible arrhythmia. Pericardial aspiration is necessary and a sealed drain may have to be employed.

Multiple rib fractures may produce a free segment which moves paradoxically with the respiratory cycle. This may be sufficient to negate the inspiratory tidal volume and is, therefore, a serious situation. Positive pressure ventilation by mouth-to-mouth or Ambu bag will be necessary in severe cases until ventilation facilities are to hand. Ventilation provides internal splinting for the floating segment and is the treatment favoured in most cases. Some recommend surgical fixation in order to limit the need for ventilatory support (Davidson & Caves, 1981).

Abdominal injury

The organs of the abdominal cavity have little skeletal protection but the mobility of some of them decreases their vulnerability to some extent. Fixed organs are highly susceptible to penetrating objects. The assessment considerations include ascertaining:

- if the wound is penetrating or not
- if foreign bodies are likely to be in the cavity
- if they are signs of hypovolaemic shock
- if there are indications of the rupture of a hollow organ.

The latter may evoke abdominal rigidity and peritoneal inflammation, and peristalsis may cease. In kidney trauma there will be some impairment of renal function and there may be the added problem of clot retention. Conservative treatment may be advocated and clot retention may be avoided by 3-way bladder irrigation.

Cardiovascular support is the main priority in all cases and circulatory function should be assessed regularly by estimation of blood pressure, pulse, central venous pressure, renal output and clinical appearance. Peritoneal lavage may be undertaken to determine abdominal contents and abdominal girth should be noted.

In most cases an exploratory laparotomy will be done and surgical repair attempted. Repair of the spleen is rarely done, splenectomy being considered safer. Colonic injuries may require a temporary colostomy. Drainage tubes will be used in excision and repair beds and a T tube used following hepatic-biliary damage (McPherson, 1985).

Pelvic injury

The organs of the pelvic cavity may be pierced by a missile with a downward trajectory, involved in pelvic fractures or perineal trauma. Muscular organs tend to react with strong spasm which may help to decrease blood loss and spillage. In bladder injury, nevertheless, urine may be discharged intraperitoneally or subperitoneally. If there is suspicion that the urethra is damaged or severed, i.e. because of the site of bruising or wound, urethral pain, meatal blood and the inability to pass urine, urethral catheterization should not be attempted. A suprapubic catheter will be a temporary necessity until urethral repair can be carried out. Long term problems of prostomembranous urethral injury are impotence and stricture (Mundy, 1983).

Soft tissue injury

The soft tissues of the body may be injured by

any of the factors discussed. Of particular relevance in nursing is ischaemic tissue destruction caused by prolonged pressure e.g. decubitus ulcers, and the fact that most wounds encountered in nursing practice are iatrogenic.

THE RESPONSE TO TRAUMA

THE SPECIFIC RESPONSE TO TRAUMA

Inflammation

Inflammation is the local response to any form of injury although it is associated with many general, systemic features.This response is something of a 'two edged sword' in that it is central to protective and reparative processes yet it causes pain and loss of function, and is the mechanism underlying the adverse effects of many diseases, e.g. arthritis, nephritis, vasculitis. The general features of redness, pain, swelling and heat have been known for nearly two millenia, loss of function being added to the list by Hunter in the 18th century. It would appear that until this century the phenomenon was mainly seen as pathological, although Hunter makes mention of 'salutory effects'.

The observed and experienced features of inflammation are due to the vascular, fluid and cellular changes which occur mediated by an array of chemical substances. When foreign, antigenic materials, mainly microorganisms, are introduced by breakdown of the skin barrier the immunological system augments many facets of the inflammatory process in addition to producing antibodies.

In brief, the swelling observed in inflammation is due to the collection of fluid in the tissues. The heat is due to the increased blood flow through the area and can only reach that of the body's core temperature. This hyperaemia also accounts for the red appearance. Pain is produced by the increase in tissue tension and also by the direct action of some of the chemical mediators of the inflammatory response, e.g. bradykinin.

The events in inflammation

Although the inflammatory-reparative process is essentially a single phenomenon it has many components and it is customary to divide it into different stages for descriptive purposes. Bruno (1979) divides it into three phases — the defensive, the reconstructive and the maturative. Johnson (1984) describes the three stages as — the inflammatory, the proliferative and the remodelling. Others describe four phases — traumatic inflammation, destruction, proliferation and maturation (see Schumann (1982) for other descriptive terms). All, however, impose somewhat arbitrary divisions and here we shall attempt to follow a sequence of events with acknowledgement of considerable overlap between them.

Initially, blood will be lost from damaged vessels; in severe haemorrhage, hypovolaemic shock is inevitable and is of prime concern in all cases, once it has been established that respiration and cardiac function are maintained (see Ch. 10). With less severe bleeding and where first aid measures are applied, platelet adhesion to damaged vasculature and vessel retraction will be followed by activation of the coagulation cascade culminating in the production of fibrin. Within the vessel this constitutes a thrombus, preventing further bleeding, while in the damaged tissue space the fibrin forms a network within the haematoma. In wounds with little tissue loss, and where cut edges can be brought into apposition without undue tension, this fibrin clot will bridge the defect. In other cases it will accumulate on the floor and edges of the denuded area.

Vascular and fluid changes. The inflammatory response begins immediately with vasoconstriction, which may be neurogenic or effected by thromboxane, but which is quickly followed by vasodilatation and slowing of the blood flow. This is effected by histamine, 5-hydroxytryptamine and prostaglandins produced by platelets and mast cells. Other substances such as bradykinin are involved (Williams, 1984) and along with histamine and 5-hydroxytryptamine increase vascular permeability which permits fluid to move more easily into the tissues.

Increased blood flow to the damaged area and increased vascular permeability cause an increase in local extracellular fluid, which is most rapid during the first twenty-four hours. At first the fluid exudate is serous in nature, but later proteins also leak into the tissues, increasing the osmotic pressure in the tissues and encouraging further exudation from the blood vessels. The resulting local oedema is responsible for the swelling at the site of the injury, and also gives rise to pain.

Cellular response. Within the blood flow the polymorphonuclear leucocytes leave the axial (central) stream to occupy the plasmatic zone adjacent to the vascular endothelium (pavementing) and then actively migrate through the intercellular junctions of the wall into the tissue spaces. How they cross the basement membrane is not known (Robbins & Cottran, 1979).

Polymorphonuclear leucocytes predominate in the early stages of acute inflammation, being attracted by a number of substances (termed chemotaxins) produced by organisms, cells and the complement system. These polymorphs are actively phagocytic and in the process may destroy viable host cells as they attempt to deal with attached antigens. These cells are capable of extracellular killing, they activate complement and produce a chemotaxin.

The complement system is composed of 9 major plasma proteins but there are possibly 24 distinct fragments when the whole system is activated (Barrett, 1983). Traditionally two pathways have been described; the classical, activated by antigen-antibody reactions, and the alternative, activated by several substances including plasmin (Pesce & Dosekun, 1982). The latter may be viewed as a non-immunological pathway for the opsonization and lysis of bacteria in the early stages of injury before antibody production is underway. Activation of complement C3–5, 6, 7, 8 and 9 causes lesions in cell membranes and destabilization of the cells. C5a is a powerful chemotaxin.

The next leucocyte to appear in the inflamed region is the monocyte. Earlier looked upon as merely a larger scavenger cell, particularly useful in chronic inflammation, its role is now known to be essential to the affector and effector arms of the immune system, as well as for macrophage activity necessary for the subsequent repair of tissues (Pesce & Dosekun, 1982; Davies, 1984). The blood monocyte belongs to the macrophage system along with the tissue histiocyte, the liver Kupffer cell and the alveolar macrophage. This system was previously referred to as the reticuloendothelial system.

The immunological system may be active from the beginning of injury if the patient already possesses some immunity against the specific invading organism. If immunity does not already exist the system must initially identify the specific antigen. The macrophage has the cardinal role of processing and presenting antigen determinants to the cells of the immune system, the lymphocytes (Ch. 5).

In the damaged tissues the macrophages engulf foreign material and cell debris, both important for subsequent repair. A number of monokines are produced to assist, e.g. complement proteins, lysozyme, elastase, collagenase, neural proteases, as well as others, one of which stimulates lymphocyte activity, another which is a procoagulant and another which is an endogenous pyrogen.

Pyrexia. As the name indicates it is the endogenous pyrogen which is thought to be the main factor in causing pyrexia by affecting hypothalamic heat regulating centres via prostaglandins (Foreman, 1984). It has long been considered that this thermogenesis is either a toxic side effect of trauma and sepsis or a defence mechanism against organisms whose metabolism may be disturbed at the higher temperature. Recent work suggests that it may also be significant in the post-traumatic metabolic state (Beisel, 1983).

It is, however, often associated with general malaise, with raised energy expenditure and potential fluid and electrolyte disturbance. Very high temperatures are also considered dangerous to human cells and it may be valid to attempt to decrease it if it rises more than 2° Celsius (Ch. 27).

Erythrocyte sedimentation rate (ESR). The ESR is significantly raised when there is inflammation or tissue destruction, due to the increased level of fibrinogen in the blood. It is therefore used as a valuable aid in assessing the progress of inflammatory conditions.

Management of inflammation

Any tissue injury, however caused, will invoke inflammation and the symptoms of inflammation will therefore be present in many differing conditions. Two of the effects of inflammation will be of most concern to the patient, pain and swelling. These two together may also cause loss of function.

Pain is caused by irritation of nerve endings due to increased local pressure from the oedema present, and also to the presence of pain producing chemicals. In lower concentrations these chemicals may produce increased sensitivity or itching; the damaged area will be tender to touch. This increased nerve excitability is antagonized by aspirin. Occasionally the nerve endings may be irritated to such an extent that muscle spasm results, and the pain arising from this may be eased by the application of local heat.

Aspirin and several newer compounds including indomethacin are effective inhibitors of inflammatory oedema.Their action depends upon the suppression of production of prostaglandins, compounds which sensitize blood vessels to the action of chemicals which increase vasodilatation and permeability. These anti-inflammatory drugs are widely used in the long term treatment of such conditions as rheumatoid arthritis, when they may give rise to toxic reactions including gastric irritation. For a full discussion of the actions of these drugs see Simon & Mills (1980).

The choice of treatment for local inflammation must depend upon whether a continued or heightened response is desirable, as for example when infection is present, or whether the response could reasonably be reduced to decrease pain or prevent further damage resulting from oedema, for example in a joint sprain. Gentle warmth increases vasodilatation and enhances the inflammatory response while cold increases vasoconstriction and dampens down the response. Care must be taken in the application of heat as there is danger not only of burns but of reflex vasoconstriction.

Corticosteroid therapy. Cortisone, hydrocortisone and many related derivatives are commonly used to suppress the inflammatory response at many differing sites in the body. This they do when present at concentrations above the normal physiological level, inhibiting the intracellular synthesis of histamine, and therefore reducing both the vascular and cellular inflammatory responses. Oedema and pain are both lessened and further damage to surrounding tissue is reduced. Resistance to infection is also decreased, however, and this may necessitate special precautions in the nursing management of the patient receiving corticosteroid therapy. The nursing implications of corticosteroid administration are discussed more fully in Chapter 19.

METABOLIC RESPONSE TO TRAUMA

The body's response to severe trauma, including surgery, is dependent upon the secretion of adrenal hormones, especially adrenaline and glucocorticoids, the magnitude of the response depending upon the severity of the injury. This general stress response is elicited under any stress situation, including emotional stress, and is discussed in detail in Chapter 8.

The result of the hormonal response to trauma is a rise in oxygen consumption in the body and an increased blood circulation making energy producing substances more readily available to body tissue. It follows that patients whose hormonal response is inhibited, for example, by corticosteroid therapy, morphine or hypothermia, will have a reduced ability to respond to severe stress (Taylor, 1978).

Phases in the response

The ebb phase

In the immediate post-traumatic phase the body's resources are mobilized and conserved to maintain plasma volume to ensure adequate perfusion of vital organs. Short-term glucose stores and fatty acids are used as substrate for energy as protein breakdown occurs at the site of injury and begins on a more general scale. Incomplete oxidation of glucose within the tissue leads to a rise in lactic acid and acidosis may result. In this period, metabolism is decreased, and it has been termed the ebb phase

(Cuthbertson, 1979). This phase is usually short lived — about 24 hours maximum — and is succeeded by the flow phase.

The flow phase

In this period the resting metabolic expenditure increases and a catabolic state is present, with an inhibition of the peripheral anabolic effects of insulin and a high rate of gluconeogenesis stimulated by stress hormones such as the catecholamines, glucagon and cortisol (Cahill, 1984). In this phase the patient will exhibit negative nitrogen balance as tissue breakdown exceeds synthesis. It has been postulated that this proteolysis is governed by prostaglandins and monokines; being proportional to the degree of trauma, sepsis and inflammation (Reeds & James, 1983). Essentially the picture is that of fuelling reparative processes at the expense of body tissues elsewhere — primarily from peripheral and visceral proteins. How long this can continue depends upon the pre-traumatic nutritional state and the demand.

House (1978) reports a study of 32 elderly patients following surgery. She states that catabolism may continue for 5–6 days following trauma in the elderly and that nitrogen lost may total 10–20 gram per day. Each gram lost is the equivalent of 6.25g of edible protein. Attempts were made to reduce the severity of the negative nitrogen balance by feeding protein supplements, and this was to some extent successful, but even so only two patients achieved a positive balance by the end of 7 days.

In some patients (especially those burned), catabolism may be reduced by increasing the environmental temperature and thus reducing heat loss from the body. The necessity for increased body heat production is therefore decreased (Hanson, 1978).

Secretion of ADH and aldosterone result in water and sodium retention; the urine volume falls and the body may become overloaded. Gain in weight from fluid retention may mask weight loss through catabolism. Potassium is released when tissues are injured, and urinary potassium may rise. There may be a brief period of negative potassium balance.

Management

The severely injured patient will usually need fluid replacement and an intravenous infusion is set up routinely. As catabolism is under hormonal control, and anabolism of tissues is also reduced in the first few days, weight loss will occur but can be minimized by adequate nutrient intake via the most appropriate route (Ch. 14).

If parenteral feeding is required, all necessary nutrients must be included in the regime, but the emphasis must be on a high nitrogen intake and sufficient calories to meet the demands of the increased metabolic rate.

The more severe the trauma or infection the greater the energy and protein required. Hanson (1978) states that the patient's energy expenditure may be raised to 25% above normal in cases of multiple fractures, or up to 50% in major infections, while in major burns the metabolic rate may be doubled (Elwyn, 1980).

TISSUE REPAIR

WOUND HEALING

Following injury, the body tissues differ in the extent to which they are capable of regenerating parenchymal cells and restoring their normal structure and function. Three types have been described (Bruno, 1979; Robbins & Cottran, 1979); labile cells which retain the power of division and complete regeneration, e.g. epithelium and bone; permanent cells which cannot regenerate, e.g. neurones and cardiac cells; and stable cells which have the capacity to regenerate providing the structural framework of the tissue or organ is intact, e.g. liver and kidney cells. If regeneration is not possible or is incomplete, scar formation ensues.

Healing involves the migration of epithelial cells and fibroblasts into the wound area. Initiation of epithelial proliferation and migration may be due to loss of contact inhibition or some as yet unknown substance. A monokine has been identified which stimulates fibroplasia and another has been shown to promote angiogenesis — the growth of capillary buds and the formation of new blood vessels (Pesce & Dosekun, 1982). A wound may reduce in size in the early stages but the mechanism of this contraction is not yet understood. Some favour the theory of collagen maturation and contraction, others maintain that collagen is not a contractile protein and that wound contraction is brought about by special myofibroblasts.

Fibroblasts produce new ground substance — mainly mucopolysaccharides, and collagen fibres. The precursor tropocollagen is synthesized on the ribosomes of the rough endoplasmic reticulum with hydroxylation of lysine and proline. Without vitamin C these hydroxylations cannot occur (Berlinger, 1982). The insoluble collagen is secreted from the cell following peptide cleavage by procollagen peptidase. Wounds heal by proliferation of these cells and their products,regeneration, and revascularization. Epithelium eventually covers the surface, tensile strength is regained over the next few months, vascularity decreases and collagen fibres align and mature. In sutured wounds only 3–5% of the original tensile skin strength is attained within two weeks, 20% is achieved in three weeks and about 35–50% in a month. They never regain more than 80% of intact skin strength (Schumann, 1982).

Incised wounds

If the wound involves little loss of tissue, is not infected, and the severed tissues lie close to each other, the wound will heal by first intention or primary union. Immediately following the injury, plasma and some blood cells exude from the edges of the damaged area and a fibrin clot is formed which binds the edges together.

Epidermal cells at the periphery of the wound respond by undergoing rapid mitosis, and the new cells so formed migrate across the surface of the wound, this movement being made possible by the presence in the cells of contractile fibres. The visible gap in the skin is quickly closed.

Under the regenerating epidermis, polymorphonuclear lymphocytes and then macrophages enter the area and remove bacteria and debris, while the fibroblasts invade and begin to form collagen, one of the main constituents of connective tissue. Capillary blood vessels and lymphatic vessels proliferate by means of buds growing from their endothelial lining which eventually meet, join and establish new vessels. All these processes are well under way within three days.

The rapidly forming new tissue, composed mainly of fibroblasts, collagen fibres and vascular tissue is called granulation tissue, and it is this which forms the scar left after a wound. When healing is complete the fibres in the tissue contract, and the scar shrinks. In clean incised wounds which heal rapidly there is little granulation tissue formed and therefore only a small scar is left.

Wounds with tissue loss

Where there is loss of tissue at the site of the wound, caused either by the injury itself or by subsequent infection,the edges of the wound cannot be quickly bound together and a scab forms. There is growth of granulation tissue from the base of the wound, which is later covered by epidermal tissue from the periphery. The wound is said to be healing by second intention or granulation. As this type of wound usually contains necrotic tissue, phagocytic cells are present in large numbers and are usually effective in preventing infection. If, however, infection does occur or there are foreign bodies present, healing may be delayed.

Wounds healing by second intention contain much more granulation tissue than those healing by first intention, and therefore more collagen. As this scar tissue shrinks it may pull on surrounding tissue and cause deformity and malfunction.These wounds also contain less vascular tissue than those healing by first intention, and this may contribute to delayed healing and ulcer formation.

In large shallow wounds there is mitosis not only of epidermal cells around the periphery of the wound, but also of cells surrounding remaining hair follicles and sebaceous glands. The migration of cells is vitally important if such wounds are to heal quickly. With very superficial skin lesions (e.g. blisters) the epidermis would normally reform in 5–7 days, and it has been shown (Winter, 1978) that in shallow wounds over 90% of new epidermis originates from hair follicles. Areas of the body having a thick covering of hair are known to heal more rapidly than other areas.

If hair follicles have been destroyed during the injury the area will require a skin graft as, at a rate of movement of 1 mm in 4 days, epidermal cells moving only from the periphery of the wound would take weeks or months to cover a large wound.

Healing of specific tissues

Bone

Bone is a highly plastic material; its structure is constantly changing in response to mechanical stimuli and it therefore heals well, new patterns of tissue linking and remoulding the site of injury. Hyaline cartilage also regenerates easily.

At the site of a broken bone there is bleeding from damaged local blood vessels and a haematoma forms. Granulation tissue grows into the haematoma and fibroblasts produce collagen which binds the broken ends together. Osteoblasts proliferate and osteoid tissue is laid down. The new tissue so formed can be clearly seen on X-ray, and is called callus. It unites the broken bone but lacks the strength of true bone, which is not gained until the ossification process (laying down of calcium and phosphate salts) is complete. As ossification proceeds, the trabecular pattern is laid down according to compression and tensile forces operating on the bone.

If a fracture is allowed to set out of alignment, the trabecular pattern of the bone will alter according to the new stresses imposed upon it and the new bone will be misshapen. Careful and correct alignment of a fracture must therefore be carried out before the ends of broken bone are united.

Vitamins A, D and C are thought to be necessary for the efficient healing of bone. Vitamin A is required for the organisation of rebuilding activity, vitamin D for deposition of calcium and phosphate salts, and vitamin C for collagen production.

Delayed union of bone may occur because:

- the space between the broken ends of bone is too great for the callus to unite them
- the callus is damaged by movement or weight bearing
- foreign tissue such as muscle is caught between the broken bone ends
- there is infection present
- the blood supply is inadequate
- there are important deficiencies in diet.

In the case of some delayed unions no obvious cause presents itself.

Muscle

Muscle cannot proliferate by cell division, but individual muscle fibres may regenerate if only partially destroyed. Regeneration involves outgrowth of new tissue from the living stumps of damaged fibres, but is dependent upon the retention of the original sheaths of connective tissue which guide the growth of the new fibres. Muscle extensively damaged in such a way as to retain these sheaths, by, for example, toxic conditions or local bruising, may fully recover. If the area of damage is too large, however, fibrosis may impede the growing stumps by obliterating the framework of sheaths, and full functional recovery is unlikely.

Tendons

Tendons consist of bundles of connective tissue and are therefore readily healed by the collagen laid down by fibroblasts. Severed tendons require suturing to hold the two parts together until the repair process is complete.

Articular cartilage

This heals slowly and damaged areas are replaced by fibrous tissue.

Serous membranes

The cells surrounding the damaged area multiply rapidly and may succeed in restoring the area to a healthy state. If the injury is too large fibrous tissue forms and this may cause adhesions, which frequently follow inflammation.

Mucous membranes and glands

These are easily repaired and the loss of function of gland tissue is also compensated for by hypertrophy of remaining healthy tissue. The extent of regeneration or hypertrophy is related to the body's requirement, and large areas of damaged tissue can be replaced.

Liver

Up to two-thirds of the liver may regenerate if necessary. Remaining cells proliferate and the regenerated tissue is structurally and functionally normal. Growth hormone is necessary for liver regeneration and thyroxine and cortisone facilitate healing.

Blood vessels

New capillaries are constantly being formed by outgrowths from existing capillaries to replace older ones which are reabsorbed. Larger blood vessels appear to have little or no capacity for regeneration.

Lymphatic system

In damaged tissue, lymphatic capillary vessels regenerate by growth from existing healthy vessels. They tend to grow more slowly than blood capillaries and their growth may be delayed by dense scar tissue. The extent to which larger vessels may regenerate is still unknown.

Partially removed lymph nodes may regenerate from remaining healthy tissue, but if the node is completely removed it will not reform.

Central nervous system

It is thought that the brain and spinal cord have no regenerative capacity, but experimental work continues.

Peripheral nervous tissue

When a peripheral nerve is cut, those parts of the nerve axons nearest the cell bodies have the power of regeneration.

The axon and its sheath distal to the cell body degenerate and Schwann cells multiply and fill the endoneural tubes. The proximal stump of the axon sends out buds of new nervous tissue, some of which reach the old endoneural tubes and grow down them. If conditions are favourable, new growth may appear after a week and continue at a rate of 3–4 millimetres per day, eventually forming motor and sensory endings and restoring function (Le Gros Clark, 1975).

Regeneration may be delayed by dense scar tissue or if a large portion of the nerve is lost. Also, fibrous tissue may be laid down in the denervated muscles and prevent the new nerve from establishing functional endings.

Painful swellings or scars may result when regenerating nerves attempt to grow through dense scar tissue. Such swellings are called neuromata.

Abnormal healing

Keloid scarring

In some people the fibroblasts so important in the normal healing process may produce an excess amount of fibrous tissue. This gives rise to an enlarged scar or occasionally to a large tumour-like growth of tissue known as a keloid, which occurs mainly in the dark-skinned races and occasionally becomes malignant (Westaby, 1985).

Delayed healing

The common causes of non-healing of a wound are infection and poor circulation. The body's own defences are well equipped to deal with invading bacteria, but may on occasion be insufficient to repel the attack, especially if the infection is deep in a wound which has a poor blood supply. Necrotic tissue forms an ideal medium for bacteria to thrive in, and the lack of oxygen prevents the body's white blood cells from functioning efficiently. As long as there is infection, pus, or dead tissue in a wound, healing will not be complete, and hence the necessity to ensure that all wounds are kept clear of these during the healing process.

Poor circulation is responsible for two other examples of wounds which commonly present problems of delayed healing; varicose ulcers and pressure sores. These are discussed in detail in Chapter 20.

Healing may be delayed in the elderly person because:

- their nutritional state before injury may be poor, and following injury it may be difficult to encourage them to take an adequate and balanced diet
- vascular changes may reduce the supply of oxygen and nutrients at the site of the injury.

It is when treating a wound which refuses to heal normally that the nurse's flexibility of approach is most important. The cause of non-healing must if at all possible be identified, and the method of treatment chosen accordingly. The newest products to come onto the market claim some success with problem wounds, their development having been aimed at producing an optimum microenvironment for the operation of the body's own defence and healing mechanisms.

As the temperature of the skin varies according to the vascularity of the underlying tissue, thermographs may be used as an aid to diagnosing and prescribing treatment for sores, and detecting pre-gangrenous conditions.

NURSING THE INJURED PATIENT

IMMEDIATE CARE

In the immediate post-traumatic phase, the following require attention:

- decreased tissue perfusion and oxygenation
- structural defect
- potential infection
- pain
- anxiety.

Tissue perfusion and oxygenation

Tissue perfusion depends upon maintenance of the blood pressure and is dealt with in the chapter on shock (Ch. 10). In essence, blood losses must be made good or plasma expanders and electrolyte solutions given. Large volumes of crystalline or colloid solutions will be necessary in the burnt patient in a relatively short time. Renal function should be carefully monitored.

Indications of respiratory impairment and therefore of impaired gas exchange must be dealt with and positive pressure ventilation will be necessary if blood gas levels are unsatisfactory.

Wound management

Surgical exploration will be necessary for deep-lying injuries and surgical repair of surface wounds may be carried out. Wounds more than six hours old should be considered infected and it is inadvisable to deal with them by primary closure. Wound toilet and debridement should be done, the wound loosely packed and left for several days during which the wound develops resistance to infection (Westaby, 1985). Examination of the wound will be done later to see if there is any sign of infection and non-viable tissue. After freshening of the wound edges it may be closed if all is clear.

In open wounds the bleeding should be controlled by pressure, cautery or ligation. Foreign materials and dead tissue should be removed and the wound closed if possible. This may not be possible in areas of extensive tissue loss or infection. Patients should be protected against tetanus with a booster dose of toxoid or, in rare instances, human antitoxin. A depot penicillin may be given.

Fractures may require closed or open reduction and usually some form of immobilization. If traction is employed the resultant vector of the system and its counter-traction must be maintained to give the essential degree of stability to the fracture site. Figure 4.1 shows the vectors of one such system (Draper, 1984).

Relief of pain and anxiety

Initially, and if not contra-indicated, pain may be

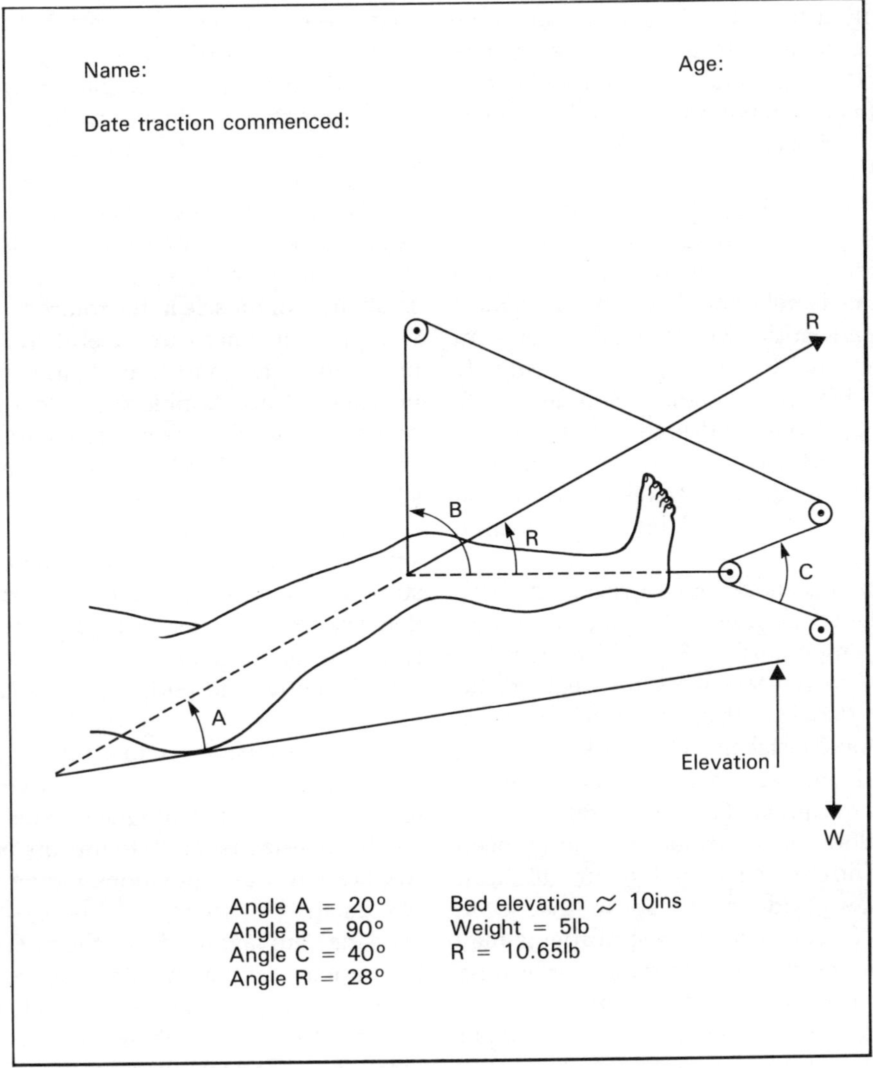

Fig. 4.1 A diagram for use in the maintenance of Hamilton-Russell traction.

relieved with inhalations of Entonox or opiates may be prescribed. Thermal comfort and stability will lessen the pain of the injury site, and careful, considerate handling will prevent unnecessary pain. Relief of pain, explanation of management and treatment and good emotional support will help to ease anxiety.

LONGER-TERM CARE

After the initial phase, the major aim of care is to promote healing and this involves all aspects of care. Maintenance of an adequate nutritional status is essential, but relief of anxiety and measures to relieve emotional stress are also important as are other general measures to enhance healing. The specific management of the wound may either enhance or hinder healing.

Nutritional care

As discussed earlier the catabolic phase is an effort to provide energy and materials for repair. The resultant hyperglycaemia and ureagenesis may cause fluid loss initially, along with some loss of potassium (Drugs and Therapeutic Bulletin, 1980) compounded by fever and excess sweating. Insulin rebound, stress hormones, ADH and aldosterone may produce fluid retention. This reliance on body tissues will be detrimental to healing if it continues, and exogenous supplies of energy and protein ought to be provided to attempt to restore nitrogen balance. If this is not done, after about 3–5 days nutritional deficiencies will occur which prevent healing and render the patient relatively immunodeficient (Cunningham-Rundles, 1982; Keusch, 1982). Continued high levels of stress hormones, particularly cortisol, suppress aspects of the inflammatory response, inhibit macrophage activity and inhibit the production of collagen.

As part of the endeavour to regain positive nitrogen balance the patient should be nursed in an ambient temperature of 30° Celsius. This has been shown to have benefits for healing and metabolism (James, 1980). Despite fever no measures should be taken which evoke shivering and create increased energy expenditure, or which lower the ambient temperature.

Protein-calorie malnutrition has long been associated with infection and failure to heal. There is now evidence to show that even moderate deficiencies of specific nutrients may have adverse effects. Of importance for healing are zinc, iron, vitamin C and vitamin A, along with a number of trace elements such as copper and selenium (Chandra, 1981; Beisel, 1982; Chandra & Dayton, 1982). Return to a good intake of nutrients as soon as possible seems desirable. Chandra et al (1982) report how immuno-deficiency in elderly patients was corrected by dietary supplementation.

Artificial feeding

Initially the oral route should be used, but anorexia and poor absorption may prevent this. There is evidence that, even in the traumatised patient, nitrogen balance can be achieved by enteral feeding using fine-bore tubes and feeding systems with non-expensive preparations such as Caloreen and Complan with additives. Diarrhoea may be a problem if hyperosmolar feeds are given or if feeds are given in bulk. A slow drip system is preferable. However, it may not be possible to achieve an intake of 3600 kcal, 120 g of protein and 4 litres of fluid by enteral feeding, and peripheral or central intravenous feeding may be prescribed (Karran & Foster 1980). Leverue et al (1984) have demonstrated that total parenteral nutrition reduces the catabolism of muscle in the injured

Peripheral lines are useful for parenteral nutrition in the short term. Unfortunately, they provoke thrombophlebitis, particularly if hyperosmolar glucose solutions are given. The incidence of this has been reduced by the use of silver cannulae rather than catheters and by short-term use (Johnston, 1980). Catheters advanced along the subclavian vein into the superior vena cava have the advantage of delivery into a faster flow, and hyperosmolar solutions can be given.

Both central and peripheral lines run the risk of introducing infection via the skin puncture site and it is customary to send catheter tips for microscopy, culture and sensitivity tests on removal. The best technique for site care has not yet been established (Thompson et al, 1983). Application of povidone-iodine daily is advocated by some, occlusive, transparent dressings are favoured by others. Some redress the puncture site daily, others leave well alone. A recent study on the use of OpSite on wounds suggests that it may enhance some aspects of the protective inflammatory response (Holland et al, 1984). It may, therefore, be useful for covering such sites. Feeding lines should be changed every 48 hours and blood or plasma should not be given through them. When using a dual delivery system, care should be taken not to allow solutions and emulsions to backflow and air should not be allowed to be drawn into the system.

The debate continues about the best form of parenteral nutrition in the catabolic patient. It is agreed that a supply of amino acids is essential to achieve nitrogen balance, but the amino acid profile and the source of non-protein calories has not yet been agreed. It has been proposed that infusion of the branched chain amino acids —

leucine, isoleucine and valine — is just as useful as giving a wide range (Clark, 1981) but this does not seem to be generally accepted.

Glucose is necessary for the utilization of infused amino acids but there is some evidence that it is inefficiently used once an obligatory level has been exceeded (Rogaly et al, 1982). Better results may be obtained by using fat infusions to make up the required energy. Fats produce more energy per gram than glucose and do not provoke thrombophlebitis.

On the available evidence it seems justifiable to supply the nitrogen by a wide spectrum of amino acids and to give the non- protein calories in a dual system of glucose and fat emulsions to which water soluble and fat soluble vitamin preparations may be added, e.g. Multibionta, Solivito, Vitlipid. Trace elements may be supplied by addition of Addamel. Insulin is usually necessary. In fact Munro (1979) has claimed that the beneficial effects on protein balance are attributable to the anabolic effects of the insulin and not to the glucose per se. Continued assessment of the patient receiving enteral or parenteral nutrition should include 24 hour urinary urea, daily body weight (if bed scales are available), fluid balance record, temperature record and blood glucose estimations.

Psychological aspects of care

It has been noted that every effort should be made to reduce anxiety and minimize stress. These concepts are dealt with in detail elsewhere (Chs 8 & 12) but full and open communication, whenever feasible, is recommended to establish rapport and trust, to allay anxiety. The injured patient has been suddenly and dramatically ensconced in a new and strange environment, outside of his/her control and often his/her understanding. Environmental stressors such as lights, noise and disturbances should be identified and dealt with. Pain and discomfort should be promptly relieved — better still, anticipated and prevented. These efforts are aimed at reducing psychological distress and inhibiting levels of the circulating stress hormones and impairment of the immune response, thus reducing the risk of development of overt infection (Boore, 1978).

General measures

A number of general measures which may enhance healing can be used with the patient. The need for nutritional factors has been discussed, but adequate oxygenation and transport of required materials to the healing tissue is necessary and mobility is important also.

Oxygenation of tissues

The patient in bed recovering from injury may not be breathing as deeply as normal and the supply of oxygen to the tissues may be reduced. This is unlikely to be markedly lower in a patient who was relatively fit before the trauma, but in a patient with a chronic chest condition this could reduce healing. Deep breathing and coughing exercises will enhance lung expansion and oxygenation of the blood, with the added benefit of reducing the risk of chest infection

Transport

The circulation transports all the required materials for healing and dealing with infection. Tissues with a good blood supply, e.g. face and scalp, heal well, while those with a poor supply heal slowly. In the dermis new tissue originates from connective tissue associated with vascular tissue and in deep wounds where vascular tissue, is destroyed healing may be impaired. The nurse must take steps, therefore, to maintain as good a blood supply as possible to the injured area.

A good blood volume can be maintained by ensuring an adequate fluid intake and the circulation can be stimulated by exercises. Excessively oedematous limbs may be elevated to decrease some of the tension and improve blood flow, and tight restrictive bandages should be avoided. If perfusion of an injured limb is impaired or suspect it should be monitored by palpation of pulses and/or the use of a Doppler Ultrasound flowmeter.

Movement

The strength of a wound in the early stages of healing is much lower than the strength of surrounding tissues, and if strain is put on the wound by excessive movement the newly formed granulation tissue may tear. By the fourteenth day following a clean surgical incision, the wound should have a strength of about one quarter that of the surrounding tissue. Remodelling (that is selective laying down and removal) of collagen at the wound site continues for some months, during which time the new tissue gains in strength. As remodelling is influenced by the forces acting on the wound, after a two week period of immobility a gradual increase in activity of the injured part should be encouraged.

Although injured tissues require stability, rest and support, general immobilization is conducive to calcium and phosphorus loss from the skeleton and nitrogen loss from muscle. It seems advisable to recommend passive (Cuthbertson, 1979) and active exercises as soon as possible.

Wound management

The broad aim of wound management is to provide conditions which will promote wound healing. Several aspects must be considered:

- the wound must be free of dead and infected tissue before healing can begin
- protection against external agents which may retard healing, e.g. microorganisms or clothing rubbing, is necessary
- provision of an environment conducive to wound healing is required.

Part of the protection of the wound from microorganisms is achieved through general management of the environment and procedures. A high standard of cleanliness of the ward and of the patient's immediate environment, i.e. bed linen and clothing, is important. This is particularly so when a wound dressing is not applied. Careful handwashing between patients and the use of aseptic technique when performing dressings helps to prevent pathogenic bacteria coming in contact with the wound.

Debridement and selection of appropriate dressings are the other major aspects of management to be considered.

Debridement

Necrotic tissue must be removed in order to allow healing to occur and three approaches to this can be used — surgical, chemical or enzymatic debridement (Torrance, 1983).

Some necrotic tissue can often be cut away fairly easily so that chemical or enzymatic methods can function more effectively. Large areas of necrotic tissue may be excised in theatre in preparation for grafting, but bacteraemia has been reported following surgical debridement of pressure sores (Glenchur et al, 1981).

Chemical debriding agents such as hypochlorite solutions (e.g. eusol), hydrogen peroxide, Aserbine or Malatex are often used. However, many of these can impede growth of new tissue while desloughing another area. Barton & Barton (1981) also suggest that some of these substances (and they mention hypochlorite solutions) may cause release of endotoxins from Gram negative bacteria in the wound and lead to renal failure.

Proteolytic enzyme preparations can be used to break down the necrotic tissue. Varidase Topical contains the enzymes streptokinase and streptodornase which cause fibrinolysis and breakdown of cell nuclei of dead tissue. The necrotic area is liquefied without damage to healthy tissue. The use of this preparation in the treatment of necrotic pressure sores is discussed by Torrance (1983). It can be prepared as a gel and applied directly to the wound or gauze soaked in the liquid preparation can be applied. A non-porous dressing such as Opsite applied over this will keep the dressing moist. Normal saline is used to clean the wound when the dressing is changed once or twice a day.

Properties of dressings

There are many types of dressing available and the selection of an appropriate dressing for the particular wound is an essential part of wound management. The dressing chosen can enhance or retard healing.

Lawrence (1983) has described a number of properties that a wound dressing should possess. The dressing should be:

- simple to apply and conformable to body contours
- able to absorb wound exudate adequately
- strong enough to provide mechanical protection but not rigid such that movement is impaired or abrasive such that movement irritates the wound
- non-toxic
- free of material that might be shed into the wound
- non-adherent to the wound surface
- bacteria-proof
- compatible with topical therapeutic agents
- able to produce a wound environment that permits healing to occur as rapidly as possible.

Most of these characteristics require little discussion but some need further consideration.

Absorbency. Some wounds produce considerable amounts of exudate and absorbent dressings have been in use for a considerable time. 'Strike-through', when the absorbed moisture reaches the outside of the wound dressing, allows bacteria ready access to the wound and must not be allowed to persist. Replacement of the outer layers of the dressing prior to strike-through will provide protection against bacterial access. Sometimes, when large amounts of exudate are produced, the application of a drainage bag can simplify wound management and allow measurement of the drainage.

Non-adherence. Dressings can adhere to wounds through exudate entering the dressing and drying and by epidermal growth into the mesh of the dressing material. In either case removal of the dressing will detach the regenerating epithelium or granulation tissue and delay healing.

Environment for wound healing. Turner (1979) suggests that, in addition to the characteristics identified above, a wound dressing should:

- maintain high humidity at wound/dressing interface
- allow gaseous exchange and thus maintain oxygen levels and hydrogen ion concentration
- provide thermal insulation to wound surface.

The identification of these characteristics as important factors in wound dressings is a result of the work carried out on wound healing. Winter (1972) has shown that prevention of drying of a wound reduces the loss of dermis through dehydration. This is illustrated in Figure 4.2 showing the enhanced healing of burns dressed with vapour-permeable occlusive dressings. In addition, migrating epithelial cells can move about three times more rapidly through the exudate between the dressing and the wound than they move through tissue underlying a scab (Fig. 4.3).

Types of dressings

Wound dressings can be examined in three main groups:

- absorbent dressings
- materials which attempt to emulate the properties of skin
- special materials for difficult wounds.

Absorbent dressings. These are designed to remove exudate and the results of infection, but they often adhere to the wound and can result in pain and tissue damage as they are removed. They have to be changed frequently. The use of a non-adherent material between the wound and the absorbent dressing helps to reduce tissue damage, but few of these materials are totally non-adherent.

Although the value of a moist environment in promoting wound healing is becoming recognized, absorbent dressings are still used, with or without a non-adherent surface. Prepacked airstrip dressings used for first-aid, but also for dressing some surgical wounds, is one example of an absorbent dressing.

Tulle gras, with absorbent dressing on top, is a non-adherent type of dressing and Melolin is another example. Melolin consists of a thin sheet

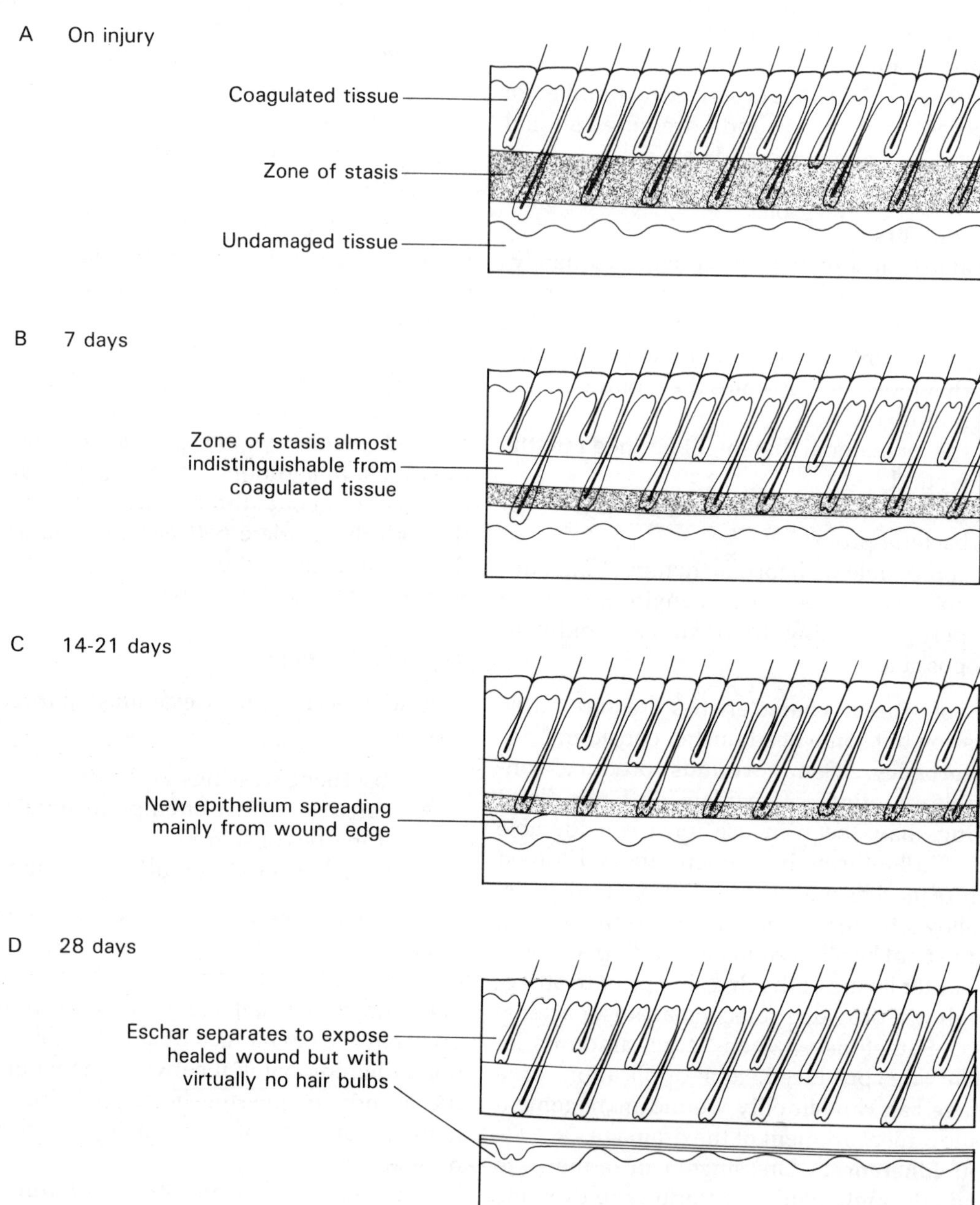

Fig. 4.2 Diagram illustrating the healing of experimental burns in guinea-pigs covered either with freely permeable dressings (A to D) or vapour-permeable occlusive material (E to H).

Under non-occlusive cover the zone of stasis gradually becomes indistinguishable from coagulated tissue. Both layers comprise the eschar which eventually separates.

Occlusive cover can reverse stasis such that the tissue recovers. Any hair bulbs in this layer subsequently recover (Lawrence, 1983).

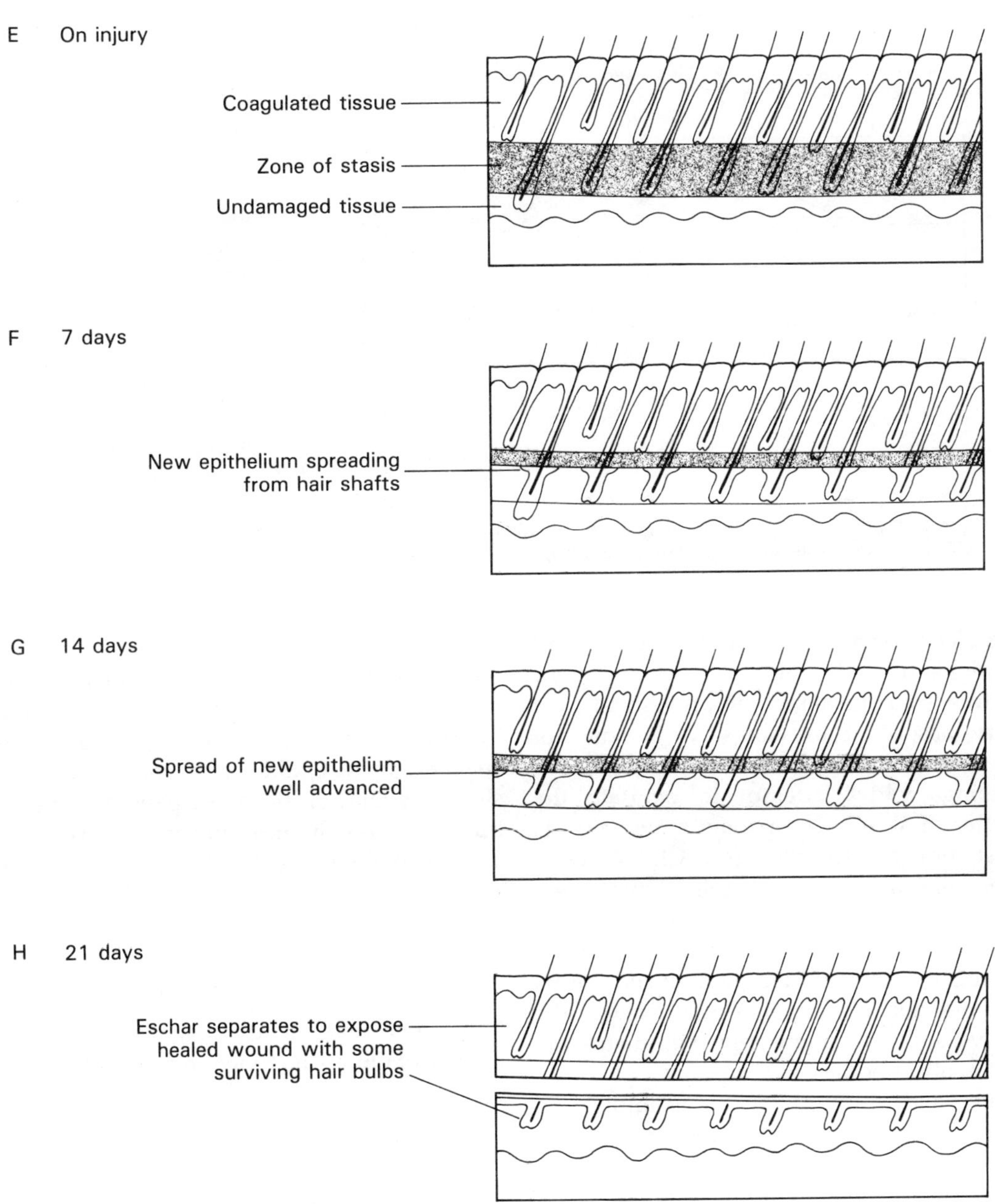
E On injury
Coagulated tissue
Zone of stasis
Undamaged tissue
F 7 days
New epithelium spreading from hair shafts
G 14 days
Spread of new epithelium well advanced
H 21 days
Eschar separates to expose healed wound with some surviving hair bulbs

Fig. 4.2 continued

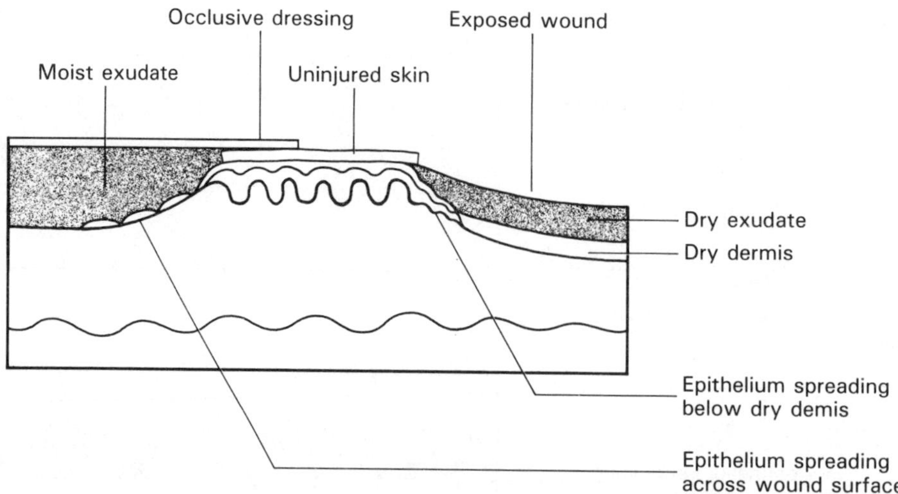

Fig. 4.3 Diagram illustrating the migration of epithelium in wounds of skin covered with either occlusive or permeable dressings (Lawrence, 1983)

of Terylene film with numerous small perforations backed with an absorbent pad. While this is a considerable improvement over ordinary absorbent dressings, it is still not completely non-adherent

Dressings which attempt to emulate the properties of skin. The patient's own skin is the best form of protection (see Ch.20) and a number of dressing materials have been developed in an attempt to emulate the properties of skin. Porcine skin is available in fresh, frozen or freeze-dried (lyophilized) forms and as epidermal or dermal skin. However, it is expensive and, to some extent, stimulates the formation of antibodies.

OpSite and Granuflex are examples of synthetic materials which have been developed. These are both occlusive materials. OpSite is a very thin transparent polyurethane sheet backed with adhesive and is permeable to gases and water vapour. Granuflex is described as a polymeric hydrocolloid. It is a foam 2–3 mm thick with adhesive on one side and a very thin plastic sheet on the other. This absorbs some exudate and the foam dissolves around the wound. Both these materials retain the exudate and thus keep the wound moist and the patient is able to bathe without disturbing the wound.

May (1983) has compared the use of OpSite with Scarlet Red impregnated gauze and with porcine skin in the treatment of skin donor sites in patients with burns. In each case a wound covered with OpSite was compared with a similar wound on the same patient at the same time treated with one of the other two materials. The mean wound healing time was as follows:

OpSite	6.8±0.8 days (sample size 78)
Scarlet Red impregnated gauze	9.6±2.2 days (sample size 48)
Porcine skin	12.0±1.0 days (sample size 30)

May stated that the advantages associated with the use of OpSite include the fact that:

- there is bacterial and fungal exclusion by mechanical protection
- there is a promotion of rapid re-epithelialization due to retention of moisture, electrolytes and metabolites, and to the fact that epithelial cells traverse the exudate more rapidly than through an eschar or fibrin clot
- protection of the wound is promoted by white cell action and the viability of the white blood cells is maintained by the significant levels of oxygen transmitted through the dressing

- protection of the wound is also obtained from increased levels of immunoglobulins — specifically IgM
- these dressings have low cost
- the dressings have high mobility for physical and occupational therapy
- there is an improved cosmetic result from the use of these dressings, particularly with regard to the flatness of the epidermal surface that results
- the dressings allow visual inspection of wound healing.

However, he also identified some limitations of OpSite:

- it requires a perimeter of intact, dry skin
- the location and area of dressings are restricted
- there is often a haematoma or seroma of significant volume
- many times there is fluid leakage under the dressing
- the dressing only protects wounds of patients with adequate immunological responses.

It is possible to drain excess fluid with a syringe and needle, preparing the site with alcohol and covering the hole made with a small patch of OpSite.

Although the assessment of pain is not easy May also found that significantly less pain was associated with the use of OpSite.

Barton & Barton (1981) recommend the use of occlusive dressings in the treatment of pressure sores, provided that infection can be controlled.

Special materials for difficult wounds. Infected wounds and cavities or ulcers where granulation tissue is developing are often difficult to deal with, and new materials offer some advantage over the old absorbent dressings.

Two very similar dressing materials, dextranomer (Debrisan) and cadexomer iodine (Iodosorb), are available which can be used in the management of infected wounds. These are composed of small, spherical, polysaccharide beads which absorb water and small molecules while large molecules and particles pass between the beads. In an infected wound, bacteria are removed from the wound surface. Dextranomer has been shown to be effective in the treatment of infected wounds (Soul, 1978) but in a moist wound it becomes saturated within a few hours and bacterial growth occurs. Cadexomer iodine is very similar to dextranomer but slowly releases iodine which kills the bacteria as they are removed from the wound. It appears to have considerable advantages over dextranomer (Lawrence, 1983). Both these materials are washed out of the wound and fresh material applied as necessary. A yellow brown colour indicates that active iodine is still present in cadexomer iodine.

Silastic foam dressings have been found to be particularly useful in the management of open granulating wounds (Wood et al, 1977; Harding & Richardson, 1979). In the past, wounds such as that left after excision of a pilonidal sinus have been packed with ribbon gauze, often soaked in eusol (a hypochlorite solution) and paraffin. The removal of such dressings is painful and often damages the regenerating tissue. Other disadvantages related to the use of eusol have been discussed above. The foam dressing is formed by mixing a resin and the catalyst and pouring it into the cavity to be dressed where it solidifies within two minutes. It enables any drainage to escape, is easily removed, washed in antiseptic solution, rinsed and replaced after the wound has been cleaned. Patients can care for their own wounds and pain is minimised. Granulation is not inhibited in any way as the pressure exerted by this dressing material is not great. As the wound heals, new dressings need to be formed every one or two weeks. Obviously this material cannot be used where the wound opens into another organ or cavity.

Selection of dressing

A number of factors have to be considered in the selection of dressings. The type of wound and factors which will enhance healing are of major importance and have been discussed when considering types of dressing available. The implications of the dressing for the patient and his or her life style is also important. If it is a dressing that can be readily changed by the patient then earlier discharge from hospital may be possible than with another type. The acceptability of a dressing may also influence the choice. While it is useful for the medical and nursing staff to be able to observe the wound through the dressing, the patient may be less happy and, in some circumstances, may not come to terms with it.

CONCLUSION

Nursing of the injured patient requires circulatory support in the first instance, control of bleeding, protection from further injury and infection, and relief of pain and stress. Subsequent interventions are aimed at maximizing the beneficial effects of the inflammatory-reparative response and preventing nutritional imbalance and functional complications. Wound management is an essential part of this. As soon as possible, exercises are undertaken to restore the function of injured parts and physiotherapy and occupational therapy referrals should be made as appropriate.

Acknowledgement

We are grateful to Dr J.C. Lawrence, MRC Burns Research Group, Birmingham Accident Hospital and The Medicine Group (UK) Ltd for permission to include Figures 4.2 and 4.3 in this chapter.

REFERENCES

Barrett J T 1983 Textbook of immunology, 4th edn. C V Mosby, St Louis
Barton A, Barton M 1981 The management and prevention of pressure sores. Faber, London
Beisel W R 1982 Single nutrients and immunity. American Journal of Clinical Nutrition 35:417–468
Beisel W R 1983 Mediators of fever and muscle proteolysis. New England Journal of Medicine 308:586–588
Berlinger N T 1982 Wound healing. Otolaryngologic Clinics of North America 15(1):29–34
Boore J 1978 Prescription for recovery. RCN, London
Bruno P 1979 The nature of wound healing. Nursing Clinics of North America 14 (4):667–682
Cahill G F 1984 Insulin and trauma: some thoughts. Clinical Nutrition 2:169–172
Chandra R K 1981 Immunodeficiency in undernutrition and overnutrition. Nutritional Reviews 39(6):225–231
Chandra R K, Dayton D H 1982 Trace element regulation of immunity and infection. Nutritional Research 2:721–733
Chandra R K, Joshi B, All B, Woodford G, Chandra S 1982 Nutrition and immunocompetence of the elderly: effect of short term supplementation on C.M.I. and lymphocyte subsets. Nutrition Research 2:223–232
Clark R G 1981 Parenteral nutrition. In: Howard A, McLean Baird I (eds) Recent advances in clinical nutrition 1. Libbey, London
Crockard H A 1981a The trauma problem. In: Odling-Smee W, Crockard A (eds) Trauma care. Academic Press, London
Crockard H A 1981b Head injury. In: Odling-Smee W, Crockard A (eds) Trauma care. Academic Press, London
Cunningham-Rundles S 1982 Effects of nutritional status on immunological function. The American Journal of Clinical Nutrition 3:1202–1210
Cuthbertson D P 1979 The metabolic response to injury and its nutritional implications: retrospect and prospect. Journal of Parenteral and Enteral Nutrition 3(2):108–129
Davidson K G, Caves P 1981 Injuries to the thorax. In: Odling-Smee W, Crockard A (eds) Trauma care. Academic Press, London
Davies P 1984 The mononuclear phagocyte. In: Dale M M, Foreman J C (eds) Textebook of immunopharmacology. Blackwell Scientific, Oxford
Draper J 1984 An investigation into the application and maintenance of Hamilton-Russell traction on three orthopaedic wards. Unpublished BSc thesis, Leeds Polytechnic
Drugs and Therapeutic Bulletin 1980 Drug and Therapeutic Bulletin 18(22):85–88
Elwyn D H 1980 Nutritional requirements of adult surgical patients. Critical Care Medicine 8:9–20
Evans D K 1984 Injuries of the cervical spine. Surgery 1(4):76–79
Foreman J C 1984 Pyrogenesis In: Dale M M, Foreman J C (eds) Textbook of immunopharmacology. Blackwell Scientific, Oxford
Glenchur H et al 1981 Transient bacteraemia associated with debridement of decubitus ulcers. Military Medicine 146(6):432– 433. Cited by Torrance C 1983 Pressure sores: aetiology, treatment and prevention. Croom Helm, London
Hanson G C 1978 The acute metabolic management of the critically ill patient. In: Hanson G C, Wright P L (eds) The medical management of the critically ill. Academic Press, London
Harding K, Richardson G 1979 Silastic foam elastomer for treating open granulating wounds. Nursing Times 75(39):1679– 1682
Holland K T, Davis W, Ingham E 1984 A comparison of the in–vitro antibacterial and complement activating effect of 'OpSite' and 'Tegaderm' dressings. Journal of Hospital Infection 5:323–325
House S M 1978 Post traumatic nitrogen metabolism in the elderly. Nursing Times 74:1457–1459
Hurt R L 1985 Thoracic trauma. Surgery 1(16):381–387
James W P T 1980 Protein turnover in injury. In: Karran S J, Alberti K G M (eds) Practical nutritional support. Pitman Medical, London
Johnson A 1984 Towards rapid tissue healing. Nursing Times 80(48):39–43
Johnston I D 1980 The complications of access to the

circulation. In: Karran S J, Alberti K G M (eds) Practical nutritional support. Pitman Medical, London

Karran S J, Foster K J 1980 Choosing the method of nutritional support. In: Karran S J, Alberti K G M (eds) Practical nutritional support. Pitman Medical, London

Keusch C T 1982 Immune function in the malnourished host. Paediatric Annals 11(12):1004–1014

Lawrence J C 1983 Laboratory studies of dressings. In: Lawrence J C (ed) Wound Healing Symposium held at the Queen Elizabeth Postgraduate Centre, Birmingham, October 1982. Medicine Publishing Foundation, Oxford

Le Gros Clark W E 1975 The tissues of the body, 6th edn. Clarendon Press, Oxford

Leverue X, Guignier M, Carpentier F, Serre J C, Caravel J P 1984 Effect of parenteral nutrition on muscle amino acid output and 3-methylhistidine excretion in septic patients. Metabolism 33(5):471–477

Lindsay K W 1984 Clinical assessment after brain damage. Surgery 1(4):80–84

McPherson S 1985 Liver trauma. Surgery 1(16):369–373

May S R 1983 Physiological activity from an occlusive wound dressing. In: Lawrence J C (ed) Wound Healing Symposium held at the Queen Elizabeth Postgraduate Centre, Birmingham, October 1982. Medicine Publishing Foundation, Oxford

Mundy A R 1983 Injuries of the lower urinary tract. Surgery 1(3):67–70

Munro H N 1979 Hormones and the metabolic response to injury. New England Journal of Medicine 300:41–42

Pesce A J, Dosekun A K 1982 Interrelationships between the immune systems, complement, coagulation and inflammation. Clinic Physiologic Biochemistry 1:92–116

Reeds P J, James W P T 1983 Protein turnover. Lancet 1(8324):571–574

Robbins S L, Cottran R S 1979 Pathologic basis of disease, 2nd edn. Saunders, Philadelphia

Rogaly E, Clague M B, Carmichael M J, Wright P D, Johnston I D A 1982 Comparison of body protein metabolism during TPN using glucose or glucose and fat as the energy source. Clinical Nutrition 1:81–90

Schumann D 1982 The nature of wound healing. AORN Journal 35(6):1068–1077

Sharr M M 1984 Mechanics of raised intracranial pressure. Surgery 1(8):187–190

Simon I E, Mills J A 1980 Nonsteroidal anti-inflammatory drugs (Parts 1 and 2). New England Journal of Medicine 302:1179–1185, 1237–1243

Soul J 1978 A trial of Debrisan in the cleansing of infected surgical wounds. British Journal of Clinical Practice 32:172–173

Taylor K M 1978 Injury and wound sepsis — hypothalamic and pituitary changes in relation to injury. Annals of the Royal College of Surgeons of England 60(3):229–233

Teasdale G, Galbraith S, Clarke K 1975 Acute impairment of brain function 2. Observation record chart. Nursing Times 71:972–973

Thompson D R, Jones G R, Sutton T W 1983 A trial of povidone-iodine for the prevention of cannula thrombophlebitis. Journal of Hospital Infection 4:285–289

Torrance C 1983 Pressure sores: aetiology, treatment and prevention. Croom Helm, London

Turner T 1979 Today's products and wound management. Nursing Mirror 149(25):suppl.

Westaby S (ed) 1985 Wound care. Heinemann, London

Williams T J 1984 Mechanisms of inflammatory oedema formation. In: Dale M M, Foreman J C (eds) Textbook of immunopharmacology. Blackwell Scientific, Oxford

Winter G D 1972 Epidermal regeneration studied in the domestic pig. In: Maibach H I, Rovee D T (eds) Epidermal wound healing. Year Book Medical Publishers, Chicago

Winter G D 1978 Wound healing. Principles and management. Nursing Mirror 146 (10): special supplement

Wood R A B, Williams R H P, Hughes L E 1977 Foam elastomer dressing in the management of open granulating wounds: experience with 250 patients. British Journal of Surgery 64:554–557

5

Infection and immunity

INFECTION (Mims, 1980)

Infection is the invasion of the host by microorganisms which subsequently multiply in the host's tissues, but the ability of a microorganism to cause disease depends upon its pathogenicity. Some microorganisms are said to be frank pathogens because they are the causative agents of particular diseases; *Clostridium tetani,* for instance, is the cause of tetanus. Patients whose defence mechanisms have been depleted for one reason or another may develop infections by opportunistic pathogens, for example *Escherichia coli.*The symptoms of an infection by an opportunistic pathogen vary depending upon the nature and site of the infection. *E. coli,* for instance, may be the cause of infections in sites which vary from urinary tract to gastrointestinal tract.

Some microorganisms are known as non-pathogens since they rarely or never cause human disease. However, microorganisms in this category must be treated cautiously because bacteria are adaptable and it is possible for many non-pathogens to become opportunistic pathogens, if the conditions are appropriate.

Normally the external surfaces of the body are very resistant to the entry of microorganisms. The skin is a dry, impermeable horny layer, often with very acid secretions, while most of the internal surfaces have a continuous layer of living cells bathed in fluids containing a range of protective agents which include antibodies

Table 5.1 Sites of infection

Microorganism	Disease	Attachment site
Influenza virus	Influenza	Respiratory epithelial cells
Vibrio cholerae	Cholera	Intestinal epithelium
Salmonella typhi	Enteric fever	Intestinal epithelium
Corynebacterium diphtheriae	Diphtheria	Mucosal epithelium
Bordetella pertussis	Whooping cough	Respiratory epithelium
Plasmodium vivax	Malaria	Human red blood cells

and cytolytic enzymes such as lysozyme. Mucin is also secreted — this is a gel which acts as a waterproofing agent as well as aiding lubrication. In many situations it will mechanically trap foreign particles and bacteria which are then washed away in the secretion.

SPREAD OF MICROORGANISMS

Microorganisms can gain entry to the body in several ways. Some have specific mechanisms for attaching to cells and sometimes are able to penetrate the layer of cells (Table 5.1).Bites of infected insects provide a very easy access to the tissues and many diseases such as malaria, plague and typhus are initiated in this way. Many infections commence as a result of preliminary damage to the external or internal surface of the body. However, some microorganisms can cause disease without penetrating the body tissues by producing soluble, toxic substances which are absorbed. *Vibrio cholerae,* for instance, secretes a toxin which is absorbed from the intestinal tract.

Once microorganisms have penetrated to the tissues it is most likely that they will enter the local lymphatic system and drain via the lymph nodes and the thoracic duct to the blood. Although this is the stage at which they will encounter immune system cells and possibly be eliminated, it may also result in the dissemination of the infective organism. This spread of pathogenic microorganisms throughout the body can be very rapid (Table 5.2).

Some microorganisms, particularly the viruses, grow within cells (intracellular); if these are mobile cells, e.g. blood cells, the infection will be carried to other parts of the body. These microorganisms cannot replicate until they have entered a susceptible cell and as a result the route of infection is of major significance. Influenza virus replicates at epithelial surfaces but cannot infect blood cells and as a result is unlikely to cause an infection by entry to the body via the blood or the lymphatics. Other viruses need to reach the susceptible target tissues rapidly (the central nervous system in the case of polio virus) and hence spread via the blood and lymphatics.

Table 5.2 Transport of microorganisms in blood

Transport mode	Viruses	Bacteria	Protozoa
Free in plasma	Polio Yellow fever	*Pneumococcus* *Anthrax*	Trypanosomes
In leucocytes	Measles Smallpox	*Mycobacteria* *Brucella*	Leishmania
In red blood cells	Colorado tick fever	*Bartonella*	Malaria

Table 5.3 Exotoxins

Microorganisms	Disease	Type of toxin	Action	Effect
Clostridium tetani	Tetanus	Neurotoxin	Blocks action of inhibitory neurones	Muscle spasm
Corynebacterium diphtheriae	Diphtheria	Cytotoxin	Inhibits cell protein synthesis	Nerve paralysis Heart damage
Shigella dysenteriae	Dysentery	Enterotoxin	Induces fluid loss from vascular and intestinal vessels	Diarrhoea Neurological disturbances
Vibrio cholerae	Cholera	Enterotoxin	Activation of adenyl cyclase	Water loss Diarrhoea
Bacillus anthracis	Anthrax	Cytotoxin	Increases vascular permeability	Oedema Haemorrhage
Straphylococcus aureus	Pyogenic infections	Cytotoxin	Lysis of blood neutrophils	Necrosis at site of infection

Those microorganisms that replicate outside cells (extracellular) tend to multiply local to the initial site of infection or, as a result of drainage, in the body fluids. However, such organisms are particularly vulnerable to the antimicrobial mechanisms of the body e.g. phagocytosis, complement and antibodies.

MECHANISMS OF TISSUE DAMAGE

One of the first symptoms of an infection is a general feeling of malaise and this is often felt before any characteristic symptoms of the disease are seen. Toxins of one form or another have generally been implicated as the cause but it is possible that it is one of the side-effects of the production of interferon by the body.

Most viruses directly damage the cells in which they replicate, the effects generally being confined to the infected cells, and toxic microbial products are not usually liberated to damage other cells. The effect is caused primarily by the diversion of the cellular DNA and RNA to viral use and may result in damage to membrane functions, lack of products which are essential for other cells or tissues, or the direct death of the cell. Intracellular bacteria also cause direct damage to cells, these usually being the phagocytic cells.

The major effects of infections are caused by microbial toxins, which can be either exotoxins or endotoxins. Exotoxins are proteins produced and secreted by the living microorganism and they cause damage to local cells and hence to the tissues (Table 5.3). Most can be destroyed by heat (heat labile) and are among the most potent toxic substances known. Cytotoxins constitute a wide range of proteins acting against a variety of cellular functions. The enterotoxins stimulate the hypersecretion of fluid and electrolytes from the intestinal epithelial surfaces and some can also cause smooth muscle contraction resulting in abdominal cramp. The neurotoxins act on the nervous system, often preventing impulse transmission.

Endotoxins are derived from the outer layer of a bacterial cell wall and, although small amounts may be released from the living microbe, in general they are only liberated on the death of the cell. They are usually lipopolysaccharide in nature and cannot be degraded by heating. Although they are less toxic than exotoxins, they are significant in the development of toxic effects of an infection. Endotoxins act as potent pyrogens, causing the general symptoms of fever. Many are also capable of provoking major changes in the vascular system varying from hypo- to hypertension. They are very potent activators of the complement pathway, resulting in the consumption of large amounts of complement proteins with a resulting impairment to the effect of antibody action against cells.

In addition to these direct effects of microbial

growth on the host cells, material released from dead microorganisms acts as a potent stimulator of the inflammatory processes. Excessive inflammation also causes damage to adjacent cells and often produces the characteristic symptoms of the disease. Also, the process may result in excessive stimulation (hypersensitivity diseases) or positive suppression (immunodeficiency diseases) of the immune processes of the host.

MICROBIAL STRATEGY FOR AVOIDING IMMUNE MECHANISMS

Once microorganisms have gained access to the tissues, the main defence mechanisms of the body involve phagocytic cells, complement, antibodies, cell-mediated immunity and interferon. While these are extremely powerful defensive agents, nevertheless many microorganisms are capable of defeating or avoiding them, at least for a time. It is estimated that there are over 400 different microorganisms that are capable of infecting man.

The presence and effectiveness of phagocytic cells is an extremely important aspect of the immune state, and congenital abnormalities of the phagocytic processes lead to a significant increase in microbial infections. The most invasive microorganisms are able to minimize the effectiveness of the phagocytic cells to a greater or lesser degree in a variety of ways. Some microorganisms can inhibit the migration of the motile phagocytic cells by an antichemotactic factor, so reducing the ability of the host to concentrate blood neutrophils and monocytes at the sites of infection. Some organisms release soluble products which are capable of killing phagocytic cells: the staphylococci and streptococci are particularly effective in this way, and wholesale destruction of blood neutrophils results in the formation of large amounts of pus, giving the name pyogenic to this type of infection.

The external structure of some microorganisms inhibits phagocytosis, the presence of a capsule around a microorganism being particularly significant. Many strains of bacteria lose their virulence when, often as a result of being grown under artificial conditions, they lose the ability to form a capsule. The pneumococcal and anthrax bacteria are specific examples. Most microorganisms, including those with capsules, are far more easily ingested by phagocytic cells when they have been coated with antibodies or complement proteins, a process known as opsonization.

A variety of microorganisms can cause immunosuppression in the host, particularly those microbes which multiply in macrophages and lymphoid tissues. In some instances the immunosuppression is general in nature, but some viruses are capable of depressing the immune responsiveness specifically with regard to their own antigens.

Microorganisms can avoid the effects of antibodies in various ways. Some viruses and many parasites change their antigenic nature either over repeated replications, as in the case of some viruses, or over the various stages of their replicative cycle, as with the parasites. In such situations, by the time enough specific antibody has been formed the antigenic makeup of the microbe has changed. Alternatively many parasites shed large amounts of surface antigen which effectively neutralizes circulating antibody before it reaches the microbe.

Microorganisms infecting cells which then do not exhibit much membrane-bound foreign antigen tend to avoid stimulating the immune response. Others are capable of hiding or capping membrane antigens with antibodies and the resulting complexes are shed from the cell, so diverting the action of the non-specific features of immunity. Some microbes persist in cells which face external surfaces and their products are secreted into spaces external to the tissues, e.g. into saliva, gastric juice, etc. As a result the virus cannot easily be reached by either antibody or cytotoxic cells.

IMMUNITY

LEVELS OF PROTECTION (Richards, 1976)

The production of antibodies is only one way in which an animal can protect itself from

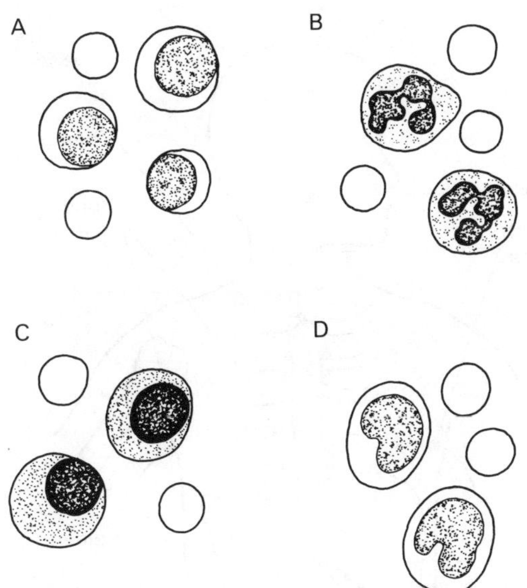

Fig. 5.1 White blood cells. The cells are represented, together with red blood cells, as they are often seen in blood smears after having been stained with a Romanovski stain such as Leishman. (A) Lymphocytes are small cells with spherical, deeply-staining nuclei and a limited amount of clear blue cytoplasm. (B) Polymorphonuclear leucocytes are phagocytic cells with highly segmented nuclei and an abundant cytoplasm containing many lysosomal bodies. (C) Plasma cells are the antibody-producing cells and are rarely seen in peripheral blood smears, being found mainly in the lymphoid tissues. The cytoplasm of a plasma cell is deeply-staining due to the presence of large amounts of RNA necessary for the synthesis of protein. (D) Monocytes in the blood are the circulating and often juvenile forms of the tissue macrophages. They are motile, phagocytic cells and often show a 'ground glass' cytoplasm containing variable numbers of lysosomes.

substances or microorganisms which are potentially harmful, and in the overall protective process there are three different levels of organization.

Mechanical protection

The first barrier is provided by the mechanical protection of intact skin and membranes, together with the secretion of mucus from many internal membrane surfaces. Foreign particles or cells are trapped in secretions and by the action of ciliated cells can be removed from the potentially vulnerable area and be either destroyed, as in gastric juice, or discharged from the body, as in nasal secretions. Many of the secretions of the body are either bactericidal or bacteriostatic. The acidity of the skin and gastric secretions, due to the presence of various acids, can often either inhibit or kill microorganisms. For instance, the susceptibility of the soles of the feet to fungal infection is due to the lack of sebaceous glands and their acid secretion, and the initial access of the microorganism is made easier when the skin is waterlogged, hence the incidence of verruca infections at swimming pools. Many secretions contain the enzyme lysozyme which is a mucolytic enzyme capable of degrading the glycoproteins of some bacterial cell walls, causing the destruction of the microorganism. This enzyme is synthesized by many cells and is present in most tissue fluids, cerebrospinal fluid being a major exception.

Inflammatory response

If the mechanical protections of the body are breached, the inflammatory response provides a second line of defence. This also is non-specific in nature and is mediated initially by substances released from the tissues or cells damaged as a result of either trauma or the toxic effects of the infective agent. A group of substances known generally as vasoactive amines, of which histamine is an example, are released primarily from the tissue mast cells and cause an increased blood flow through the tissue by inducing dilatation of the blood vessels. This is the cause of the increase in redness and temperature seen in inflamed tissues. These substances also increase the permeability of the blood vessels, resulting in fluid seeping from the blood into the tissues (oedema).

These symptoms are known as 'humoral effects' because they are caused by substances in the body fluids (humours). In addition to these humoral effects, a major aspect of inflammation is the involvement of large numbers of phagocytic cells, particularly the polymorphonuclear leucocytes (Fig. 5.1). These are motile blood cells formed in the bone marrow and drawn to the site of inflammation by the action and effects of substances released by damaged cells in the early stages of the inflammatory response. The

Table 5.4 Blood leucocyte count

	Normal adult	Acute infection
Total count: (x 10^{12} per litre)	3.5–7.5	15.0
Differential count:		
Neutrophils	40–75%	79–90%
Lymphocytes	20–45%	10–20%
Monocytes	2–10%	5%
Eosinophils	1– 6%	2%
Basophils	1%	1%

process of attracting motile cells is known as chemotaxis. The phagocytosis of micro-organisms by these cells usually results in the death of the microorganisms by the action of the hydrolytic enzymes produced by the cells and stored in the lysosomes of the cytoplasm. However, the process also eventually results in the death of the cell, due probably to the leakage of the hydrolytic enzymes into the cell cytoplasm during the phagocytic process. The large number of these cells which die results in the formation of pus.

This process of active phagocytosis involving many cells is known as acute inflammation. During this process the bone marrow is stimulated to produce more blood cells and the number of circulating white blood cells increases significantly (Table 5.4). If the infection is not eliminated quickly, the reserves of the bone marrow become depleted, the number of circulating phagocytic blood cells begins to decline, and the process moves into a stage known as chronic inflammation.

The immune response

The third major line of defence, the immune response, is initiated during the inflammatory response and involves another group of cells known as lymphocytes (Fig. 5.1). These are also found in the blood, usually in lower numbers than the polymorphonuclear leuco-cytes, but are particularly abundant in those tissues known as lymphoid tissues (Fig. 5.2). These include the lymph nodes, spleen, tonsils, thymus and the bone marrow, as well as areas of tissue in the digestive and bronchial tracts. Although lymphocytes are morphologically very similar to each other, they include cells with many varied functions all of which are involved in some aspect of the immune response.

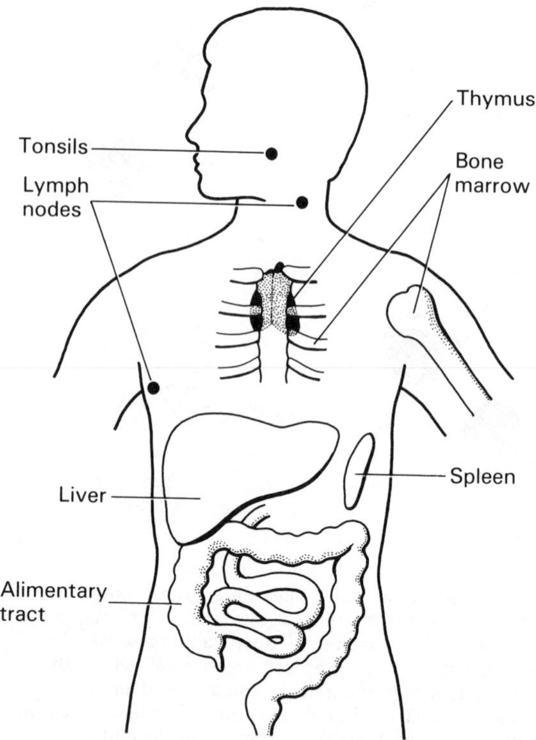

Fig.5.2 Sites of lymphoid tissues.

The immune response can be broadly divided into two main aspects. Humoral immunity is involved with the production of antibodies which are carried throughout the body in the body fluids. Cell-mediated immunity involves the production of cells (one variety of lymphocyte) which are capable of destroying the invading or foreign cell by direct action rather than through the action of antibodies. In order to illustrate the differences between the two aspects of immunity, it can be said that the rejection of tissue transplants is due primarily to the effects of cell-mediated immunity, while the protection against smaller agents such as toxins produced by bacteria is afforded mainly by antibody production. There is, however, considerable overlap and interaction between the two mechanisms of the immune response.

The ability to resist infection varies considerably from one species to another and from one individual to another. Man is not usually susceptible to the disease known as distemper to which dogs are prone, however the reverse is true of diphtheria. Within species there are often marked differences, for instance North American Indians are more susceptible to tuberculosis than Caucasians, and people with a genetic condition known as sickle cell trait (which results in the production of some abnormal haemoglobin) show an increased resistance to some forms of malaria. In most instances the reasons for such variations are unknown, but seem to lie in major genetic differences.

In man, differences in the ability to resist infection are often associated with age, the young and the old being the most susceptible. Variations in nutritional and hormonal states can also significantly influence all aspects of the resistance mechanisms, particularly the immune response.

ACQUIRED IMMUNITY (Drutz & Mills, 1984)

Enhancement of the immune response resulting in both humoral immunity (production of specific antibodies) and cell-mediated immunity (production of sensitized lymphocytes) results in acquired immunity, as distinct from naturally occurring or innate immunity. The process may be *active* as a result of the stimulation of the immune system of the individual in a normal manner, or it may be *passive* which implies the transfer of the products of an immune response in one individual to the recipient. This occurs naturally in the transfer of antibodies across the placental membrane from the maternal blood to the fetus, or artifically by the injection of an 'antiserum'. A third method of inducing an immune state is by an *adoptive* process, in which lymphocytes capable of responding to an antigen are introduced into an individual and repopulate

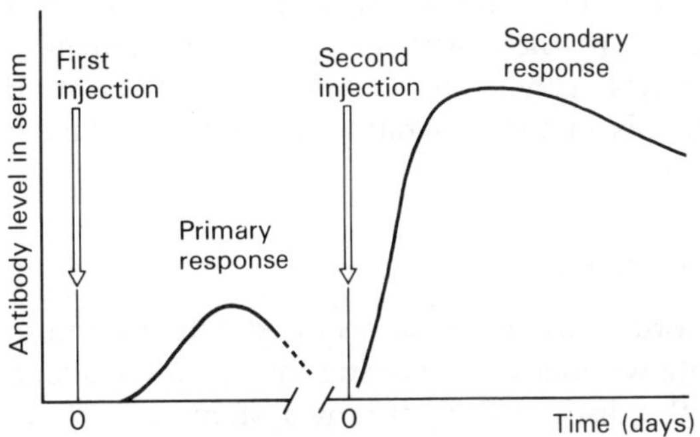

Fig.5.3 Kinetics of the immune response. The injection into an animal of a second dose of an immunogen several weeks after a first injection will result in a response which is more rapid and more intense than the first.

the lymphatic tissues, as in bone marrow transplants.

The immune system of an individual is stimulated when a substance or cell known as an *immunogen* gains access to the tissues, and to the lymphoid tissues in particular. The word 'antigen' is often used synonymously with 'immunogen', although strictly speaking some antigens can only react with an antibody but do not themselves stimulate the immune system to produce that antibody. One fundamental requirement of an immunogen is that it must be 'foreign' or 'non-self' as far as that individual is involved. The precise way in which the immune system can recognize 'self' and 'non-self' is one of the major questions in immunology.

The process of stimulating the immune system to produce either antibodies or sensitized lymphocytes is known as 'immunization' and, regardless of the precise nature of the immunogen, the process consistently shows certain features. The introduction of an immunogen not previously encountered initiates a 'primary response' in the person. Subsequent exposure to the same immunogen stimulates a 'secondary response'. Figure 5.3 illustrates the major differences between the two forms of response. One feature which explains some of the differences between these two responses is the development of a 'memory' after the first encounter with an immunogen which not only significantly reduces the time needed to respond to that immunogen but also increases the rate of response. It is this understanding which is the basis of many immunization regimes either for antibody production in animals or for generating an immune state in man.

Vaccination

In order to induce an acquired active immune state without encountering the causative agents of the disease, the immune system needs to be stimulated to produce a memory bank which will react against the causative agent with the kinetics of a secondary response whenever it is encountered. It is for this purpose that the concept of vaccines was developed. The immunogen must be as similar to the causative agent as possible without having its disease-causing property. Various types of preparations may be used, depending upon the nature of the causative organism. *Vaccines* are cultures of the microorganism which have been killed by either heat, radiation or chemicals. These are used in a series of immunization procedures designed to induce the best memory state towards that immunogen. In some instances it is necessary to use a living culture of the infective agent in which case 'attenuated' strains of the infective agent are used. An attenuated microorganism is one which has changed or lost its ability to cause a particular disease, often as a result of repeated culture in artificial media rather than in a living cell. BCG (Bacille Calmette–Guérin) vaccination for tuberculosis is an example of an attenuated bacterium, while the polio vaccine is an attenuated form of the virus which causes poliomyelitis. Neutralized preparations of microbial toxins, known as 'toxoids', are used in immunization procedures to protect against particular diseases, e.g. tetanus.

CELLS AND TISSUES OF THE IMMUNE RESPONSE (Barett, 1983)

Lymphocytes

The lymphocytes are the major group of cells

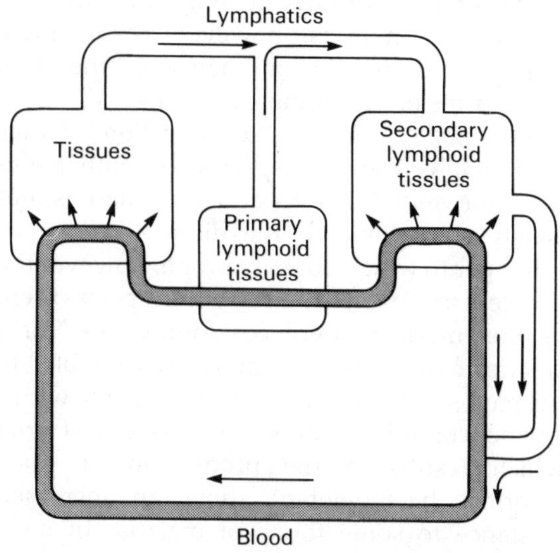

Fig. 5.4 Lymphatic circulation. The lymphatic system drains fluid from the tissues, filtering it in the lymph nodes and returning it to the blood at the thoracic duct. Lymphocytes arising from the primary lymphoid tissues are carried in the lymph to the secondary lymphoid tissues and subsequently enter the vascular circulation. They can pass from the blood into the tissues and again recirculate via the lymphatics.

involved in establishing an immune state; they are primarily associated with the lymphoid tissues of the body, often called the 'reticuloendothelial system' (Fig. 5.2). The lymphatic circulatory system links all the lymphoid tissues and drains fluid from almost all tissues of the body as the 'lymph fluid'. The main immunological functions of the lymphatic system are to filter particles which gain access to, or are formed in, the tissues and to trap them in the filtering structures known as the lymph glands. There is considerable movement of the lymphocyte population between tissues, and the system is responsible for this circulation of cells (Fig. 5.4). As well as providing a means of transport for lymphocytes, the lymph also carries throughout the body tissues the products of the immune response. The lymphatic tissues can be divided into two types. The 'primary' lymphoid organs, the bone marrow and the thymus are responsible for the production and development of the lymphocytes, while the 'secondary' lymphoid organs are populated with lymphocytes from the primary lymphoid organs.

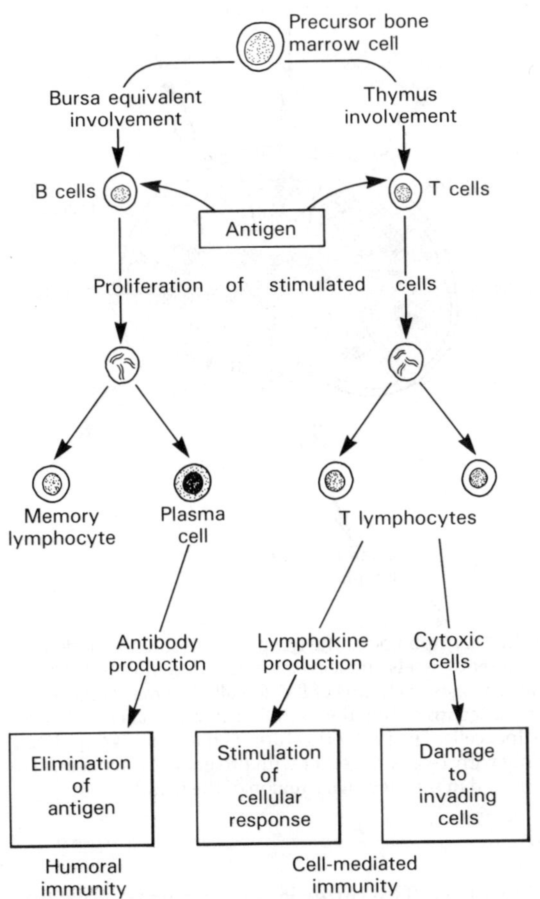

Fig. 5.5 Cellular processes of the immune response. A simplified summary of the sequence of events in both the humoral and the cell-mediated responses to an immunogen.

Types of lymphocytes

Experiments involving the removal of various lymphoid tissues have indicated that there are two different aspects to the immune response. The removal of the thymus impairs the ability of a young animal to reject skin transplants, but does not affect to the same extent its ability to produce antibodies. This aspect of the immune response is known as cell-mediated immunity, and is due to a sub-population of lymphocytes called T-lymphocytes (thymus-derived). Work with fowls demonstrated that the removal of a nodule of lymphoid tissue in the gut known as the bursa of Fabricius resulted in a reduced ability to produce antibodies but did not greatly alter the response to skin grafts. As a consequence of these and similar experiments, the production of antibodies, humoral immunity, is considered to be associated with another sub-population of lymphocytes known as B-lymphocytes (bursa-derived). Although the equivalent of the bursa of Fabricius has not been positively identified in man, it is most likely that the bone marrow acts as the source of B-lymphocytes.

Mechanisms of lymphocyte function

The detailed mechanisms of the immune response are not fully understood but certain major features of the process are generally accepted (Fig. 5.5). The introduction of an immunogen into the tissues of a susceptible animal results initially in the increased proliferation of lymphocytes in the tissues of the reticuloendothelial system, particularly the lymph nodes and the spleen. Subsequently, increased numbers of antibody-producing cells known as plasma cells (see Fig. 5.1) can be seen. These are cells derived from B-lymphocytes and are the direct mediators of humoral immunity. Stimulation of the T-lymphocytes by an immunogen similarly results in rapid proliferation of the cells and the production of two major groups of immunologically active cells. One of these groups, the cytotoxic cells (T_c), is capable of binding to the target or immunogen cell and causing irreversible lytic damage to the cell membrane. The other group of T-lymphocytes (T_d) are capable of releasing soluble substances known as lymphokines; some of these can damage the invading cells and others can further stimulate the immune system of the host. The T-lymphocytes are mainly circulating cells, while the B-lymphocytes tend to be sessile cells in the lymphatic tissue. Apart from the plasma cells, T- and B-cells are morphologically indistinguishable but can be differentiated using immunofluorescent techniques.

Any individual lymphocyte, T or B, is capable of being stimulated by only a limited number of immunogens and recognition is achieved by means of specific receptors on the cell membrane. In the case of B-lymphocytes, receptors are composed of the immunoglobulin which they can produce. Binding of the immunogen by a receptor stimulates the cell to replicate and to differentiate into an 'effector' cell, which is the name given to a cell capable of performing its immunologic function. A plasma cell, being the antibody-secreting cell, is the effector cell derived from a B-lymphocyte. The large numbers of identical cells (clones) which result from this initial immunogenic stimulus are now capable of having a significant effect.

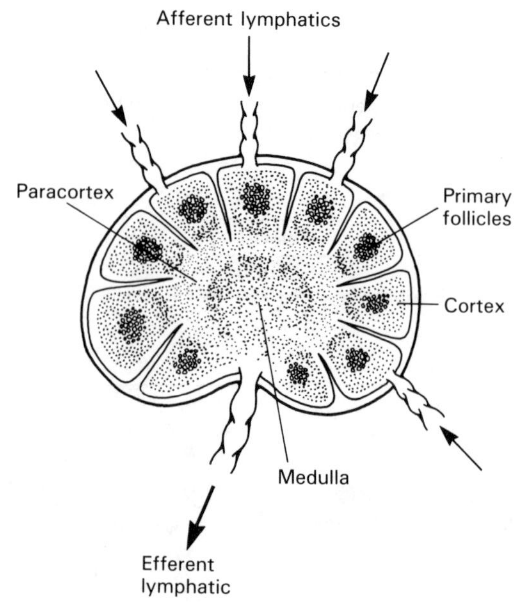

Fig. 5.6 Lymph node. The lymph drains into the node via the afferent vessels and leaves via the efferent vessel. The cortex consists of clumps of B-cells called primary follicles or germinal centres. Together with B-cells are small numbers of T-helper cells. The paracortical area of the nodes is populated mainly with T-cells, together with phagocytic cells which are also found in the medullary region of the gland.

Other cells involved in the immune response

The mechanisms by which the immunogen is recognized are far from clear, but the process does involve several other cells. The macrophage is a large motile cell 15–20 μ in diameter and is found mainly in the lymphoid tissues. Blood monocytes are juvenile forms of these cells in transit to the tissues. Macrophages are actively phagocytic and their cytoplasm is filled with large numbers of lysosomes. Particles that are ingested by the cell are degraded by the lysosomal enzymes and the immunogens subsequently appear on the cell membrane, either in their original form or modified in some way. When a lymphocyte with the appropriate membrane receptor binds to this membrane-bound immunogen, the process of activation can occur. For most immunogens this process will also require the co-operation of another cell, a helper cell (T_h cell) which is a T-lymphocyte and also carries the same or similar receptors for the immunogen. Hence for an immune response to occur, three cells are usually required: a macrophage with bound immunogen, a T-helper cell, and the lymphocyte to be stimulated (B- or T-cell).

Tissues of the immune response

The cellular events of the immune response occur mainly in the secondary lymphoid tissues, particularly the lymph nodes and the spleen. The lymph nodes (Fig. 5.6) are small, well-organized tissues through which the lymphatic fluid drains. The outer layer, or cortex, contains large numbers of lymphocytes concentrated into clumps know as primary follicles. These primary follicles consist mainly of B-cells, whilst the surrounding lymphocytes in the paracortical area of the node are primarily T-cells. A fibrous network throughout the lymph node supports large phagocytes, macrophages and non-phagocytic reticular cells. Lymph-borne immunogens enter the node and are trapped by the macrophages and reticular cells as the first step in an immune response. The primary follicles rapidly show increased cellular proliferation and soon plasma cells can be seen and subsequently immunoglobulin can be detected in the efferent lymph.

The spleen

The spleen is important not only as a lymphoid

organ but also as a site for red blood cell destruction, and in some circumstances for red blood cell production. The red pulp consists mainly of red blood cells and a smaller number of lymphoid cells, while the white pulp is comprised of large numbers of lymphocytes forming a sheath of T-cells around the small blood vessels of the spleen. Larger clumps of lymphocytes on this sheath are primary follicles of B-cells. These lymphocytes, in contrast to the lymph node based cells, will encounter blood-borne immunogens before the lymph node.

The lymph nodes

Immunogens gaining access to the tissues are normally cleared in the lymph and presented to lymphocytes in the local lymph nodes, whereas those entering via the upper respiratory and gastrointestinal tracts are trapped in either the local lymph nodes or the tonsils, adenoids, Peyer's patches in the intestine or the appendix. Blood-borne immunogens may be trapped by macrophages in the liver and the lungs, but the immune response against them is based in the spleen.

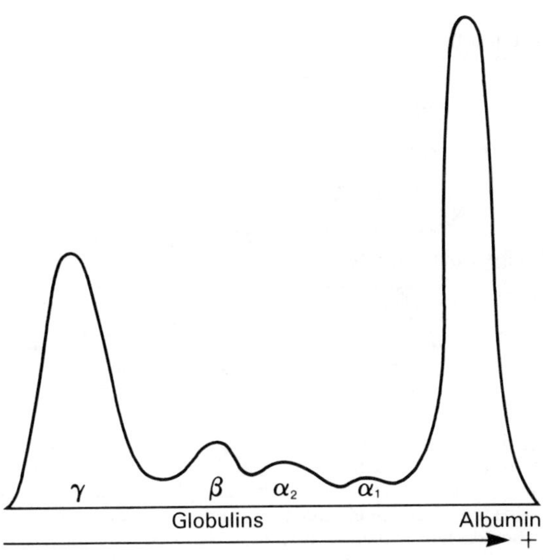

Fig. 5.7 Antibody fraction of human blood serum. A large amount of antibody may be produced in response to an acute infection. This can be demonstrated as an increase in the gammaglobulin fraction after electrophoresis of the serum proteins. The electrophoretic pattern shows a significant increase in this fraction compared with a normal pattern.

ANTIBODIES (Glynn & Steward, 1981)

Antibodies are members of a group of proteins known collectively as immunoglobulins. The name is derived from observations that during electrophoresis of blood plasma, the proteins associated with antibody activity migrate mainly with the gamma globulin fraction (Fig. 5.7). Immunoelectrophoretic studies have shown that the immunoglobulins can be divided into five major sub-classes (Table 5.5) based on their antigenic nature and hence presumably on their overall structure and amino acid sequence.

Structure of antibodies

Porter, working with a purified rabbit immunoglobulin, proposed a four-chain

Table 5.5 Immunoglobulins (Ig)

Ig	Relative molecular mass (daltons)	Serum content (%)	Number of basic immunoglobulin units involved	Number of antigen molecules bound by antibody
IgG	1.5×10^5	80	1	2
IgA	3.2×10^5	13	2	4
IgM	9.0×10^5	6	5	10(?)
IgD	1.8×10^5	1	1	2
IgE	2.0×10^5	1	1	2

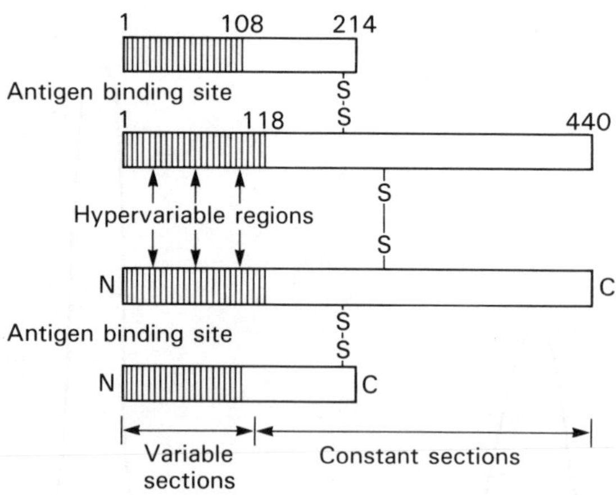

Fig. 5.8 Basic structure of an IgG molecule. Two heavy chains (440 amino acid residues) and two light chains (214 amino acid residues) are joined by disulphide bonds and each chain shows a relatively constant amino acid sequence in one section (C-terminal end) and a variable section (N-terminal end). The variable sections of both heavy and light chains are involved in the formation of the antigen-binding site.

structure involving two 'heavy' chains and two 'light' chains (Fig. 5.8) (Cohen & Porter, 1964). He used proteolytic enzymes to break the immunoglobulin molecules into smaller fragments, separating them using either gel permeation or ion-exchange chromatography. He demonstrated that the basic immunoglobulin molecule could be split into three distinct sections. Two of these seemed to be identical and were capable of binding the antigen. He called these the Fab (antigen-binding) section of the molecule. The remaining section could be crystallized (a feature actually unique to rabbit antibody) and he called this the Fc section. Attempts to study the sequence of amino acids in immunoglobulin molecules is complicated by the fact that extremely large numbers of different antibodies are present in serum. The problem was partly resolved by studying the amino acid sequence of different myeloma proteins and comparing them with one another. Myeloma proteins are produced in large amounts by individuals suffering from the disease known as multiple myelomatosis, in which there is an uncontrolled replication of an antibody cell resulting in a clone of cells all producing the same immunoglobulin.

Comparison of the amino acid sequence of the heavy chains of a particular class of immunoglobulin reveals that approximately three-quarters of each chain shows very similar sequences (the constant section), whereas the remaining quarter of the chain shows considerable variation in the amino acid sequence (the variable section). A similar pattern exists in the light chains except that the variable and constant parts of the chain are approximately equal in size. This means that the variable sections of the heavy and light chains are roughly equal in size and these together comprise the antigen-binding part (Fab section) of the immunoglobulin.

While the simple diagram representing the four-chain structure of an immunoglobulin is very convenient, it does not give any indication of the three-dimensional structure of the molecule. The individual chains show a considerable degree of intertwining in order to give the molecule its characteristic ability to bind specifically with an antigen.

Classes of immunoglobulins

Immunological studies have revealed that the difference between the five classes of immunoglobulins — IgA, IgG, IgM, IgD, IgE — lie in the heavy chains which, although of approximately the same size for all classes, vary in the amino acid sequence of their constant regions. These chains are called alpha, gamma, mu, delta and epsilon chains, respectively. Only two main types of light chain are demonstrable, known as the kappa and the lambda chains. The basic structure of immunoglobulins involves two heavy and two light chains, but although there are five alternative forms of heavy chain and two alternative forms of light chain, any one immunoglobulin can only consist of one type of each polypeptide chain. Mixed immunoglobulins do not occur.

Role of immunoglobulins

IgG

IgG comprises some 80% of the total immunoglobulin in plasma and because it is relatively small it is capable of crossing membranes and diffusing into the extravascular body spaces. It can cross the placental membrane and the presence of maternal IgG provides the major immune defence (passive immunity) during the first few weeks of life, until the immune mechanism of the infant becomes effective.

IgM

IgM is a large molecule composed of five units, each one similar in structure to an IgG molecule with the major exception that mu heavy chains are involved rather than the gamma chains of IgG. The tetramer contains an additional polypeptide, the J chain (relative molecular mass 15 000 Daltons), which appears to be important in stabilizing the pentamer and facilitating its secretion by the cell. It is an effective agglutinating and precipitating agent because of its size and its capability of binding multiple antigen molecules. Although it is potentially capable of binding ten antigen molecules, it usually only binds five (pentavalent) probably because the size of the antigens prevents combination with the full number. Because it is a large molecule it does not cross membranes easily and is largely restricted to the blood stream.

IgA

IgA is associated mainly with seromucosal secretions such as saliva, tears, nasal fluids and gastric secretions and is secreted as a dimer in association with a J chain, as with IgM. In addition, a peptide known as a secretor piece (relative molecular mass 70 000 Daltons) is also involved, apparently to prevent damage to the immunoglobulin by proteolytic enzymes also present in the secretions. Its major role appears to be the protection of mucous membranes and its presence in the blood, mainly as the monomer, may be as a result of the absorption of the degraded dimer through the membrane.

IgE

IgE is also known as a cytophilic immunoglobulin because of its ability to bind to the membrane of certain cells, a factor which may account for its low concentration in body fluids. When IgE which is bound to a mast cell reacts with an antigen, it causes degranulation of the mast cell with the release of vasoactive amines such as histamine. This process may well be helpful in initiating the inflammatory response, but in allergic individuals the reaction is excessive and leads to a hypersensitive or overreactive state.

IgD

IgD has as yet no clearly defined role, but there are suggestions that it may be involved mainly with specific receptor sites on immunocompetent cells to aid in the selection and stimulation of specific cells by an antigen.

DIVERSITY OF THE IMMUNE RESPONSE (Munro, 1975)

It would appear that man can produce an infinite number of different antibodies against immunogens. However, this is not completely true because a large number of substances are not immunogenic: it is generally quoted that man can produce about a million different antibodies. A major problem lies in understanding the genetic basis of this variety.

The molecular events in protein synthesis are well described and any explanation for the diversity in immunoglobulin structures must conform to this sequence of events. The essential genetic information for all cell processes, including protein synthesis, resides in the sequence of nucleotide bases in the DNA molecule. This information is passed on unchanged from one cell to the daughter cell through the process of cell division, mitosis. In a comparable manner, a hybrid of DNA inherited from each parent provides the total amount of genetic information for the development, growth and maintenance of all the cellular processes in the child. If all the information for every antibody that could possibly be produced is acquired in this manner, and knowing that only the lymphocytes can use this information, it would imply that all other cells carry a large amount of unusable genetic information.

There have been a variety of theories which attempt to explain the source of this diversity and they fall into two main categories.

Instructive theories

These suggest that the immunogen is essential for the formation of the antibody molecule and in the simplest form could act as a template for its synthesis. It has been suggested that a flexible unfolded immunoglobulin chain could be moulded around an antigen and then stabilized by disulphide bonds. The fact that the immunogen does not appear to be present in those cells which are actively synthesizing antibody, the plasma cells, is against this theory. In addition, the biochemical evidence that the specificity of an antibody lies in the amino acid sequence of the protein, particularly the variable sections, means that the differences between antibodies lie in the differences in the DNA coding for those proteins.

Selective theories

These suggest that the ability to produce a specific antibody is already available to a lymphocyte and the function of the immunogen is to select that cell and in the process stimulate it to produce greater amounts of the antibody. Initially suggested by Ehrlich in 1900, it has been modified by others, particularly Burnet (1959) into the clonal selection theory. It is this theory which is most widely held at the moment.

Clonal selection theory

The clonal selection theory suggests that an individual can produce a large number of different antibodies because his/her total lymphocyte population is composed of a correspondingly large number of different classes of cells, each able to synthesize immunoglobulin of only one specificity. Each immunogen-sensitive cell is capable of producing a particular antibody, some molecules of which are bound to the cell membrane and can act as receptors. The binding of an immunogen by a receptor results in the stimulation of the cell to proliferate and produce a clone of identical daughter cells, each also capable of producing that specific antibody.

Germ line theory

The basic idea of clonal selection does not explain the source of the immune diversity. The *germ line* theory of clonal selection suggests that all the genetic information is inherited in the normal manner through the germinal cells. Because of the basic structure of an immunoglobulin, the genetic information for all the variable parts must be inherited, but a saving can be made by inheriting only the information for each type of constant part of the chains. At some stage of the development of the cell, one 'variable' gene combines with a 'constant' gene, producing a functional gene.

Somatic mutation. It is also suggested that a process of *somatic mutation* may occur. It is known that the immune system is particularly sensitive to a range of stimuli early in fetal development. It is suggested that a limited amount of information is inherited through the germinal cells, as outlined above. The resulting somatic cells undergo random mutation during this period of fetal development, giving a wider range of variations.

REGULATION OF THE IMMUNE REPONSE (Snyderman, 1984)

The cellular events so far described are related to the activation of immune system cells and the production of antibodies, but it is also necessary to 'switch off' or suppress an immune response at some stage. An additional class of T-cell is known to exist which inhibits antigen-specific T_h cells, and as a result prevents the production of plasma cells and T_c and T_d cells. The mode of action of these suppressor cells (T_s cells) is not understood, but they appear to be able both to act directly on other cells and to secrete suppressor proteins. They appear later in the sequence of events in the immune response than the effector cells (T_h, T_c, T_d and plasma cells) and seem to be induced by T_h cells in a manner similar to the other cells. They are antigen-specific, as with other cells, and as they increase in numbers so that particular specific immune response is suppressed.

The lack of reaction against certain antigens, especially self antigens, is known as tolerance and the role of T_s cells would appear to be crucial both in maintaining this tolerant state and in switching off or slowing down normal responses to antigens. The overall control of the immune response is a complex interaction of activating and suppressing cells and soluble products of cells.

The immunogenic differences between cells from different donors are due to the presence of different membrane markers on the cells. The nature of these markers provides the basis for the recognition of 'self' and 'non-self' and they are known as the histocompatibility antigens. These antigens are derived from a large number of genes known as the major histocompatibility complex (MHC) and are inherited in a normal Mendelian manner. There are three major classes of MHC genes, the first two of which are particularly important in the immune response. Class I genes are primarily responsible for graft rejection and are expressed as membrane markers on practically every nucleated cell. It is the class I genes which are characteristic of the individual — self antigens. Class II genes include a group known as the Ir genes (immune response) which are responsible for the production of membrane markers called Ia antigens (immune reponse associated). These are only found on cells involved in the immune response, particularly the macrophages and T- and B-lymphocytes.

In the discussion on the cellular events of the immune response, it was stated that for an immune response to occur, the co-operation of three cells is usually required; a macrophage, a helper T-cell and the lymphocyte to be stimulated, either a T- or a B-cell. The membrane antigens expressed as a result of the MHC are important in the process of recognition and co-operation. The macrophage takes up the immunogen by various means and presents it on its membrane to be recognized by the T- or B-cell

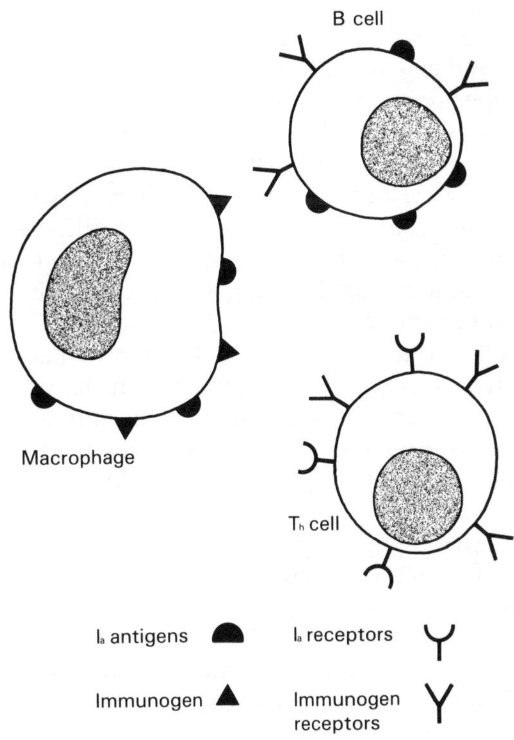

Fig. 5.9 Cellular co-operation. In the majority of cases an immune response, whether it is humoral or cell-mediated, can only be initiated as a result of the concerted action of three different cells. T- or B-cell must bind the immunogen, often presented by a macrophage or similar cell, and be assisted by a T-helper cell which must recognize the immunogen as well as recognizing Ia antigens on the membranes of both cells.

which carries specific receptors for that immunogen. The process of stimulation cannot normally occur without the assistance of the T_h cell which must also carry the same specific receptor and be capable of recognizing the immunogen. However, in addition the T_h cell will only stimulate an immune response if both of the other cells express membrane-bound Ia antigens for which the T_h cell has receptors (Fig. 5.9). A T_h cell will only assist cells which carry Ia antigens and, more specifically, only those cells which carry self Ia antigens, i.e. are from the same individual as the T_h cell itself.

The action of the T_c cell is controlled by the presence on its membrane of receptors for class I MHC antigens. In this way it can bind to macrophages and other lymphocytes in the process of initiating an immune response but subsequently, in its activity as a cytotoxic cell, can bind and destroy only cells which carry both the specific immunogen and the same MHC 'self' antigens as itself. Hence the action of T_c cells are directed primarily against 'self' cells which also exhibit some foreign immunogen characteristics. This might be as a result of a virus infecting and replicating within a cell, or as a result of significant metabolic changes in a cell such as occur in tumour cells.

Both of these examples illustrate what is known as 'associated recognition', which means that in order for an immunogen to initiate an immune response it must be recognized in association with an antigen from the MHC.

The fact that T_c cells function by recognizing 'self' MHC antigens poses problems in attempting to explain how non-self (allografts) transplanted cells, which express 'non-self' antigens, are rejected by the host. It is likely that allografts, although different, do show some MHC antigens which are common, and these common features of MHC could be recognized as 'self' while other antigens of the MHC could act as the foreign immunogen. This would still satisfy the need for associated recognition and yet result in the rejection of the allograft.

EFFECTOR MECHANISMS (Wells et al, 1984)

Antibody effects

Antigen-antibody complex

The ability of an antibody to combine with its antigen is the basis of a range of biological and physical effects. The harmful effects of substances such as toxins can be neutralized as a result of the antibody masking a particular site on the antigen which is normally responsible for initiating its noxious effects. The majority of small antigens are complexed in this manner and the ability of the IgM immunoglobulin to bind at least five molecules or sites makes it particularly effective. Owing to the ability of an antibody to bind to at least two antigen molecules, the interaction of an antibody and an antigen often results in a complex lattice structure being formed which, if it is large enough, may precipitate out of solution. If the antigen is a cell, this effect is known as agglutination and the large aggregates of complexed cells form a sediment. These two effects are usually restricted to in vitro observations and normally do not occur in the tissues because of cellular mechanisms to prevent such potentially harmful aggregation.

Phagocytosis. The in vivo effects of anti-gen-antibody complex formation are extremely important. The binding of antibody to the membrane of a cell enhances phagocytosis by the macrophages present in the blood and the tissues, a process known as 'opsonization'. This enhanced phagocytosis stems from the fact that the macrophages have membrane receptor sites for the Fc regions of IgG and IgM immunoglobulins, resulting in the macrophage and the antibody-coated antigen being brought into close membrane contact. During phagocytosis by polymorphonuclear leucocytes, these cells release substances which lead to the formation of the prostaglandins and leukotrienes which are vaso-active substances and are involved in the inflammatory response.

Activation of complement. An additional and important effect of antigen-antibody reactions is the activation of the complement system in the blood, which results in the lytic damage of cell membranes. Complement is the collective name given to a group of plasma proteins (some 10 or 11) which are present in low concentration and are very labile (unstable). In their normal circulating form they are inactive proteins, but once activated become enzymes reacting in a sequence which results in the formation of a phospholipase. It is this enzyme which causes damage to the cell membranes. The proteins are activated in a cascade sequence, in which one protein molecule once activated can catalyse the activation of many molecules of the protein which is next in the sequence. These secondary proteins also act in a similar manner and the whole cascade results in a dramatic amplification of the initial stimulus and the rapid production of large amounts of the final product.

The process of activation of a complement protein in many instances results in the release

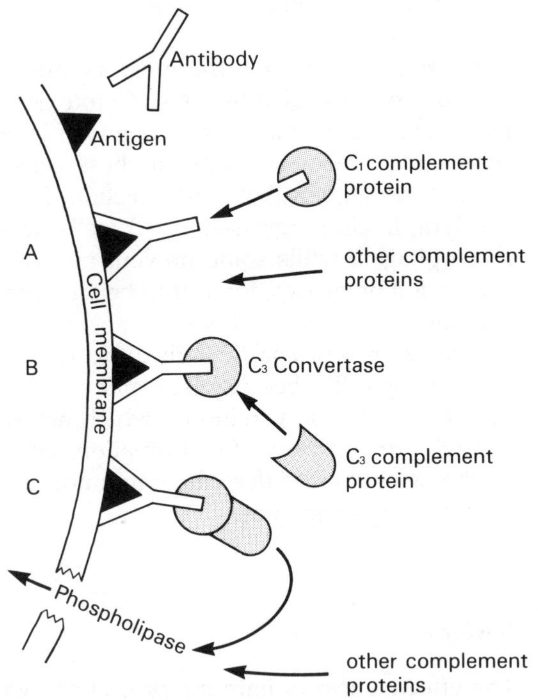

Fig. 5.10 Complement activation. (A) The first stage involves the combination of an antibody with an antigen and the binding of the first of the complement proteins to the Fc portion of the immunoglobulin. Together with the involvement of other complement proteins, a membrane-bound catalytically active complex is formed, C_3 convertase (B). This is capable of activating many molecules of the C_3 complement protein, which together with other complement proteins result in the formation of a membrane-bound phospholipase (C). This is capable of causing damage to the cell membrane which will result in cell lysis.

of specific fragments of the original protein which have biological effects other than the production of the phospholipase. These effects are mainly associated with the inflammatory response, by enhancing chemotaxis of phagocytic cells or by stimulating the release of histamine and similar substances by mast cells.

The initial activation of the first component of the complement sequence demands the presence of an antibody complexed with an antigen. Any antibody so complexed appears to undergo some change in its three-dimensional structure which results in a particular part of the Fc section being available to specifically bind the complement protein. IgM is the most effective activator of complement, but IgG can do so provided there are two molecules suitably complexed and close to each other. Figure 5.10 outlines the sequence of events resulting finally in the formation of the phospholipase. This enzyme, because it is only active for a short time, can usually only damage a cell membrane if it has actually been produced there. However, if there is excessive complement activation, possibly due to the presence of antigen-antibody complexes in the tissues, innocent cells in close proximity may be damaged. This phenomenon is known as 'reactive lysis' and can be significant in certain disease states.

Cell mediated effects

Recognition of, and binding to, an antigen-bearing cell by a cytotoxic T_c cell results in lysis of the target cell. This process can be repeatedly performed by the T_c cell and a number of target cells destroyed. The T_c cell does not undergo any significant changes during the process and must have all the information for recognition and the products necessary for destroying the target cell prior to encountering the cell. The precise mechanisms are not known but membrane to membrane contact is necessary and complement is not involved in the process.

In addition to the action of T_c cells, there are cells of the macrophage type which are not phagocytic which are known as 'killer cells'. These cells have receptors for the Fc section of immunoglobulins and acquire membrane-bound antibodies by an entirely passive process. If these membrane-bound antibodies complex with a target cell, the killer cell is capable of destroying it. This is referred to as 'antibody dependent cell-mediated cytotoxicity' (ADCM cytotoxicity).

Some T-cells, known as T_d cells, release substances known as lymphokines when specifically stimulated by cell-bound antigens. Lymphokines are a group of proteins which show a range of different effects which are not specific to a particular antigen but affect any cells within proximity. Their effects are varied but can be divided into two major categories. Aggressive effects enhance the reaction against the antigen, usually by stimulating or recruiting macro-

Table 5.6 Lymphokines

Lymphokine	Property
Macrophage directed effects	
Chemotactic factor	Attracts macrophages
Migration inhibition	Inhibits macrophage movement
Arming factor	Enhances phagocytic activity in macrophages
Lymphocyte directed effects:	
Lymphocyte activating factor	Induces DNA synthesis in lymphocytes
Lymphotoxin	Slow cytotoxin that spares lymphocytes
Interferon	Prevents viral replication Activates macrophages

phages, whilst other effects are mainly directed towards stimulating the production of more lymphocytes. Table 5.6 lists some of the known effects of lymphokines.

IMMUNE RESPONSE TO INFECTION (Roitt, 1986a)

Viruses

Non-immune phagocytosis

Innate immune mechanisms involving the phagocytic cells, particularly the macrophages, provide a defense against viruses. Tissue-based macrophages in the lungs are active against air-borne viruses whilst those macrophages of the liver, spleen and bone marrow are more effective against blood-borne viruses.

Antibodies

Antibodies produced against viruses mainly restrict the spread of viruses within the tissue fluids, particularly from infected cells. IgA may be particularly important in the protection of seromucosal membranes. The binding of antibodies enhances phagocytosis as well as, in some instances, inhibiting the replication of the virus.

Cell-mediated immunity

This aspect is probably the most significant in the control of viral infections. Cytotoxic cells, raised against the modified antigens of infected cells, cause the destruction of these cells and disrupt the sequence of viral infection. Some of the lymphokines released by T_d cells activate macrophages, while some prevent intracellular replication of viruses, interferon being a specific example.

Viruses present a particularly difficult problem immunologically because so many of them undergo antigenic variations, which are slight enough to prevent the formation of new antibodies but are different enough not to react with existing antibodies.

Bacteria

The effectiveness of immune protection against bacteria depends mainly upon the general mechanism of infection and in particular on whether intracellular growth is a feature of the infection.

Antibodies

Enhancement of phagocytosis is a major feature in the role of antibodies against bacteria, together with the lytic effect of complement activation against Gram negative bacteria in particular. Antibodies are important as neutralizing agents against toxins produced by many bacteria.

Cell-mediated immunity

Cell-mediated immune responses are of major importance against those organisms which infect cells and continue to grow within the cell. Tuberculosis is a classic example, along with other infections such as brucellosis, typhoid and syphilis. The immune mechanisms are very similar to those directed against viral infections, namely lytic damage of infected cells followed by phagocytosis enhanced by either antibody binding or lymphokine activation.

Parasites

As with viruses, a major difficulty in mounting an immune response against parasitic infections lies in the fact that the parasites change their immunogenic characteristics during their life cycles. In addition, they often shed large amounts of surface antigens during their life cycle and these tend to block or neutralize significant amounts of antibody. In some instances the parasite acquires a 'coat' of host antigens, a feature which reduces the effectiveness of the 'non-self' recognition process. In general, immune mechanisms are not always very effective against parasitic infections.

Antibodies

These act mainly against the blood-borne parasites such as malaria and trypanosomiasis. In many parasitic infections, particularly the tissue-based infections, e.g. helminths such as hookworm, there is a significant increase in IgE levels. It has been suggested that the histamine released because of the action of IgE bound to mast cells, in some way aids the expulsion of the parasite from the tissue by means of its action of stimulating smooth muscle.

Cell-mediated immunity

Cytotoxic cells are more effective against tissue-based parasites than are antibodies.

Cancer

Tumour cells exhibit membrane antigens which are not present on normal cells and as a result may be recognized as foreign, despite the fact that they also exhibit 'self' MHC antigens. This feature may be the significant factor in the normal mechanisms for the recognition of altered self cells by the cell-mediated immune processes. There is some debate as to the relative importance of immune protection and non-immune protection against cancer.

Antibodies

The activation of complement (immune lysis) may well be an important mechanism of control, but sometimes the presence of membrane-bound antibody can protect a cell against the action of cytotoxic T-cells.

Cell-mediated immunity

The fact that cancer cells exhibit 'self' MHC as well as new or foreign antigens render them susceptible to specific T_c cells. It is probable that this is an important cancer control mechanism.

Antibody dependent cell-mediated cytotoxicity

The arming of non-specific killer cells by passively bound antibodies directed against foreign antigens on cancer cells is thought by many to be an important mechanism of surveillance and control against cancer cells.

IMMUNOPATHOLOGY

The word immunity was originally intended to describe the resistance to infection but the process can also react against many non-infective agents. It was also assumed to be an entirely beneficial process, but it is now recognized that the immune response can also have adverse effects on the individual. Abnormalities of the immune response can be divided into two main groups, depending upon whether the response to an antigen is exaggerated and excessive (the hypersensitivity group of diseases) or whether the response is reduced or absent (immuno-deficiency diseases).

HYPERSENSITIVE OR ALLERGIC REACTIONS (Roitt, 1986b)

Under certain conditions the development of an immune reaction may be excessive and, for a variety of reasons, may cause damage to the cells or tissues of the person involved. The damage may vary from a mild, local reaction as seen in a skin rash resulting from wearing a metal watch strap, to a violent, systematic shock to the whole vascular system which can, if not controlled, be fatal due to a dramatic fall in blood pressure. One way in which such a reaction may be induced is by the intravenous injection of an antiserum to which the individual is sensitive due to previous injections.

The various reactions are difficult to classify but show a spectrum of effects varying from reactions which occur within minutes of the stimulus (immediate reactions) to those taking hours or days to develop (delayed reactions). In general terms, immediate reactions are associated with humoral immune effects (antibody related) and delayed reactions with cell-mediated immunity.

Type I — immediate hypersensitivity

This is probably the most common form of hypersensitive reaction and is often called an allergic reaction, classical examples being hay fever and asthma.

For some unknown reason, some individuals, in mounting an immune response to certain antigens, produce increased amounts of specific antibodies of the IgE class of immunoglobulin, rather than the usual IgG. Upon a subsequent challenge with the same antigen, an allergic or anaphylactic reaction can occur which involves contraction of smooth muscles and an increased permeability of membranes, resulting in the movement of fluid from the blood vessels into the tissues. If the reaction is systemic, this loss of fluid will cause a fall in the blood pressure. Otherwise, local, limited oedema may develop or secretion of fluid may occur, as in the running eyes and nose of hay fever sufferers. All of these effects are initiated by the release of histamine and related substances, such as 5-hydroxytryptamine, from the mast cells of the tissues by the combined effects of IgE and the specific antigen.

The symptoms of an allergic reaction stem from the fact that IgE immunoglobulins bind very avidly to receptor sites for the Fc section of the immunoglobulin protein, which are found on the membranes of mast cells. Bound in this way to the cell membrane, IgE can still bind to its specific antigen and when this occurs the cell is stimulated to release its lysosomal contents, a process known as degranulation. The lysosomes of mast cells are particularly rich in the vasoactive amines mentioned above.

The natural protective mechanisms against these effects of IgE immunoglobulins involve the blood eosinophils which are attracted to the area and are capable of secreting enzymes which can degrade or neutralize these vasoactive amines. In a comparable manner, artificial relief of symptoms can be given to some extent by antihistamine drugs. Artificial protection can also be attempted by desensitization, a process of immunization against the antigen in which an attempt is made to produce specific antibodies of the IgG class, rather than IgE, with the intention that the circulating IgG will remove the invading antigen before it reaches the IgE antibodies on the mast cells. Alternatively, the stability of the mast cell can be enhanced by the use of drugs which prevent the breakdown of cyclic adenosine mono-phosphate within the cell, a biochemical change associated with the process of degranulation.

Localized allergic reactions involve mast cells in the particular tissues. In food allergies, the reaction of the antigen with IgE bound to mast cells in the upper gastrointestinal tract results in vomiting, while if the process occurs in the lower part of the tract then intestinal cramp and diarrhoea are the major symptoms. Respiratory allergies include hay fever, an allergy associated with the upper respiratory tract, and asthma which involves the bronchi and bronchioles. Systematic allergies result from the degranulation of the blood basophils (mast cells) by blood-borne allergens, for instance bee venom, and the histamine released results in peripheral vasodilatation.

Type IV — delayed hypersensitivity

Whereas Type I hypersensitivity is essentially a feature of humoral immunity, Type IV is primarily a cell-mediated effect. The causative antigen either binds to or modifies some of the patient's own cells and an immune response is initiated, with cytotoxic cells being produced against the antigen but, in the process of reacting against the antigen, they cause damage to the host cells involved. The damage is caused directly by lymphokines released by the T_d cells and, depending upon the severity of the reaction, symptoms will develop which range from simple erythema and swelling to haemorrhage and necrosis of the tissues.

A local skin rash or eczema can develop in sensitized individuals when the offending antigen (allergen) comes into contact with the skin. Contact hypersensitivity, as it is called, develops in about 48 hours and is most frequently caused by certain metals (chromium and nickel), various chemicals present in plastics and synthetic rubbers, and some plant extracts. The allergen is absorbed through the skin and when complexed with tissue proteins can stimulate a cellular response. The consequent infiltration by T-cells results in tissue damage and the symptoms of a local inflammatory response.

Many chronic microbial infections induce a delayed hypersensitive state due to the continuing presence of the antigen in the tissues. The phagocytic cells are not always very efficient at eliminating certain infective agents such as mycobacteria, protozoa and fungi, and the persistence of these microbial antigens stimulates a cellular response which damages not only the infected cells but also antigenically innocent cells. In some instances the process results in the formation of a granuloma in the tissues which becomes necrotic due to the effects of the released lymphokines.

While contact sensitivity can be extremely disconcerting it does not present a major hazard to health. However, the granulomatous type of delayed hypersensitivity causes many pathological effects in a range of serious diseases. In tuberculosis and leprosy, both of which are caused by microorganisms of the mycobacterium class, protection depends almost entirely upon cell-mediated immunity and both diseases show granulomatous delayed hypersensitive reactions which can be extremely serious. In tuberculosis the granulomatous reaction in the lungs leads to cavitation and destruction of the pulmonary tissue, while in leprosy the effects are found mainly in the soft tissues with damage to the nervous and vascular systems.

Other types of hypersensitive reactions

At least three other classes of reaction have been described which are a combination of humoral and cell-mediated effects. In most cases the effects of antibodies, either binding to cells or precipitating as complexes with the antigen, initiate processes which non-specifically damage involved or adjacent cells. Blood transfusion reactions and haemolytic disease of the newborn (Rhesus disease) are examples of hypersensitive reaction in which the cellular damage is directly mediated by specific antibodies. Other reactions are caused by the precipitation in the tissues of antigen-antibody complexes. These complexes initiate an inflammatory reaction and activate the complement system, causing damage to the cells. Deposition of complexes in the glomerulus, for instance, results in damage to the nephron and development of nephritis.

IMMUNODEFICIENCY (Ammann, 1984)

Resistance to infection depends upon both the non-specific and the specific aspects of immunity, and failure in any stage is often reflected in recurrent infections of one type or another. Because of the complexity of immune processes, immunodeficiency diseases are difficult to classify, but they can usually be listed under one of four headings.

Deficiencies in non-specific immunity

The removal of foreign particles and microorganisms by phagocytic cells is itself a complex process, and a variety of abnormalities have been described involving particularly the polymorphonuclear cells of the blood. These abnormalities are all inherited diseases and patients are usually very susceptible to pyogenic infections, with a high mortality rate in early childhood.

Several defects have been described. These

range from the failure of these cells to migrate chemotactically to the site of an infection, to the production of defective lysosomal bodies within the cells which seem to be ineffective at combining with ingested particles and, hence, are unable to destroy invading bacteria.

The cytolytic action of complement is an important non-specific mechanism for the destruction of microorganisms and several hereditary deficiencies of various complement proteins are known. In all cases, patients show reduced resistance to bacterial infections but they may also show an increased incidence of hypersensitivity diseases.

Deficiencies in humoral immunity

The complete lack of antibodies in the blood is known as agammaglobulinaemia, while the reduced production of antibodies is known as hypogammaglobulinaemia.

In the inherited, congenital condition of agammaglobulinaemia (Bruton's disease) there is a complete lack of B-cells and hence of the immunoglobulin that they should produce. As a result the lymphoid tissues which are usually populated by B-cells are depleted of lymphocytes; this is particularly noticeable in the lymph nodes and the spleen. Because the disease is congenital the infected infant shows the symptoms of susceptibility to bacterial infections at about six months of age, when the maternal antibodies have disappeared. The cell-mediated aspects of the immune response are normal, a fact which can be demonstrated by the reaction to BCG vaccination.

Some patients show a congenital condition known as selective dysgammaglobulinaemia in which there is a deficiency of a particular class of immunoglobulin such as IgM, IgG or IgA. Deficiencies of IgM or IgG are usually associated with susceptibility to bacterial infections, while IgA deficiency is associated with gastrointestinal tract disorders.

There are several types of acquired B-cell deficiencies which may result in either agamma- or hypogammaglobulinaemia. In some cases the B-cell population is apparently normal but fails to differentiate into plasma cells. There is some evidence that the abnormality may well reside in the control exerted by either the T-suppressor cells being hyperactive or the T-helper cells being ineffective.

Deficiencies in cell-mediated immunity

There are several congenital defects (not usually inherited) which result in either a lack of T-cells or the inactivity of T-cells. Several abnormalities of thymic development can result in significantly reduced numbers of T-cells and a severely impaired cell-mediated response. Some heritable conditions result in T-cells which lack the ability to synthesize certain enzymes essential for one aspect of nucleic acid metabolism and, as a consequence, are unable to replicate effectively.

The acquired immunodeficiency syndrome (AIDS) is of fairly recent description and has stimulated a considerable amount of concern. The defect lies primarily in the T_h cells, with the levels of circulating lymphocytes being reduced but with a considerable increase in the ratio of suppressor cells compared to the normal state. All aspects of cell-mediated immunity are appreciably impaired, but humoral immunity as reflected in antibody levels may be only slightly reduced.

The direct cause of AIDS is almost certainly a virus known as Human T-cell Lymphotrophic Virus Type III (HTLV III).

However, many who have been infected with the HTL virus do not develop the immunodeficiency. The incubation period is long (periods up to five years have been quoted) and the symptoms are fairly characteristic. As with all immunodeficiency diseases, a wide range of opportunistic infections are common, but particularly frequent is pneumonia caused by infection with *Pneumocystis carinii* which occurs in about 60% of patients. In addition, a significant proportion (about 30%) develop an unusual form of skin cancer known as Kaposi's sarcoma. However, many other types of opportunistic infections are also presented.

At present there is no treatment capable of reversing the immunodeficiency and the disease is usually fatal in about two years, with the direct cause of death often being the pneumonia.

Deficiencies secondary to other diseases or therapy

Any disease or therapy that results in an accumulation of immunosuppressive products may potentially result in immunodeficiency. Renal disease and viral infections generally tend to cause depression of immune responses, a fact which the body can normally compensate for and recover from.

Any malignant disease of the immune cells will obviously seriously impair the immune processes. Patients suffering from Hodgkin's disease, a cancer of the lymph node macrophages, acquire an immunodeficiency because the high concentration of macrophage products blocks membrane receptors on T-cells, preventing their normal stimulation. A disease of the adrenal cortex, Cushing's syndrome, results in the excessive production of cortisol which normally acts as an anti-inflammatory agent but in high concentrations causes the lysis of both T- and B-lymphocytes and inhibits the production of blood monocytes.

There are a variety of situations in which the therapy given to combat a particular disease can also cause a different disease. Such secondary diseases are called iatrogenic diseases. Impairment of the immune response is one such example and can occur as a result of the treatment of cancer by either X-ray therapy or chemotherapy, both of which have an extremely inhibitory effect on the process of cell division which is a vital aspect of both humoral and cell-mediated immunity. In transplantation surgery, therapy is used to directly suppress the immune response in order to prevent tissue rejection. It is very obvious therefore that in both of these situations the prevention of opportunistic infections is a vital aspect of treatment and control.

AUTOIMMUNITY (Smith & Steinberg, 1983)

It was originally thought that it was impossible for the body to produce antibodies against itself — Erhlich called it 'horror autotoxicus' — but the list of diseases known to be caused by either the production of specific antibodies or T_c cells reacting against self antigens grows longer each year.

Theories of autoimmunity

All of the various theories which attempt to explain the wide diversity in the immune response suggest at least some degree of random mutation and it is necessary to explain how, under normal circumstances, cells which are capable of reacting against self are eliminated or suppressed. It has been suggested that, during the development of the immune system in the fetus, contact with high concentrations of self antigens results in the death of the reactive cells, but the increasing recognition of autoimmune disease supports the view that such self-reacting cells are not eliminated but held in a suppressed or tolerant state. It is then a failure of the tolerant state which results in an autoimmune disease. There are various theories proposed which attempt to explain the generation of an autoimmune disease but it appears that no one factor or cause can be identified. Each disease probably results from a variety of factors including such things as immunological variations, genetic and hormonal changes and viral infections, all potentially involved along with other less well-defined features of immunity.

Antigens for one reason or another may evade the normal mechanisms of tolerance. Some antigens are hidden from immune cells within particular tissues and, as a consequence, a tolerant state does not develop. If the tissue is damaged for some reason when the immune system has been fully developed, the escaping antigen will be regarded as 'foreign' and will stimulate an immune response. It is suggested that antibodies which sometimes develop against sperm after a vasectomy or after an attack of mumps, and against heart muscle after a myocardial infarct, do so in this manner. In rather a similar way, existing self antigens may be altered or exposed by the action of drugs. Methyldopa, for instance, is a drug used in the treatment of hypertension and can occasionally result in the production of an autoimmune reaction against red blood cells or

Table 5.7 Autoimmune diseases

Disease	Autoantigen	Lesion
Thyrotoxicosis (Graves' disease)	Thyroid surface antigen	Stimulates thyroid cells
Hashimoto's disease	Thyroglobulin	Reduced production of thyroid hormones
Myasthenia gravis	Acetylcholine receptors	Progressive muscular weakness
Insulin resistant diabetes	Insulin	Cells unresponsive to insulin
Juvenile onset diabetes	Pancreatic islet cells	Decreased insulin production
Addison's disease	Adrenal cells	Adrenocortical failure
Hypoparathyroidism	Parathyroid cells	Parathyroid failure
Haemolytic anaemia	Red blood cells	Lysis of red blood cells
Neutropenia	Blood neutrophils	Lysis of blood neutrophils
Thrombocytopenia	Blood platelets	Lysis of blood platelets
Systemic lupus erythematosus	Cell nuclei	Muliple, e.g. renal and skin lesions

blood platelets. Some microorganisms can stimulate the production of antibodies against themselves in the normal manner but subsequently these antibodies cross-react against host antigens which show similar antigenic features. This sometimes occurs with streptococcal infections, producing antibodies which cross-react against heart muscle protein resulting in the condition known as rheumatic fever.

The normal mechanisms of tolerance may be at fault for a variety of reasons. It is possible that suppressor T-cell function may be generally depressed or that certain specific T_s cells are absent, permitting the spontaneous appearance of the corresponding autoantibodies. Alternatively the B-cells themselves may be less responsive to suppressor messages.

A range of substances known as polyclonal B-cell activators are known to be produced by bacteria and viruses and these are capable of the non-specific activation of B-cells. It is possible that such a process in some situations may also result in the stimulation of B-cells which were previously suppressed.

There is an undoubted genetic connection in the development of autoimmune diseases, with an inherited tendency and an apparent association between certain autoimmune diseases and particular MHC determinants. In addition, there is also a predilection for females in the ratio of approximately 12 to 1.

Autoimmune diseases

The wide variety of autoimmune diseases (Table 5.7) are often divided under two main headings, 'organ specific' and 'non-organ specific' diseases. However there is a considerable degree of overlap and more than one autoimmune condition tends to occur in the same individual. Often autoimmune diseases are associated with proliferative diseases of the lymphoid tissues and also with immunodeficiency disorders. Sometimes autoantibodies develop as part of the ageing process.

Damage to cells and tissues in autoimmune disease can be identified as resulting from three major mechanisms, the relative significance of each varying from one disease to another. The development of autoantibodies against self antigens is a major feature of all autoimmune diseases, but their significance as the prime cause of the symptoms varies. Antibodies directed against cells cause damage by the normal mechanisms of the immune system, that is by activation of complement and the subsequent cytolytic and inflammatory effects and also by antibody-dependent cell-mediated cytotoxicity. Haemolytic anaemia, in which the host red blood cells are destroyed, is a classical example of this type of damage.

Alternatively, antibodies may be directed against specific membrane receptor proteins and as a result can inhibit some specific functions of the cell. Antibodies directed against the acetylcholine receptors at neuromuscular junctions in myasthenia gravis result in a progressive disease with symptoms of muscular weakness and fatigue. Conversely, the binding of antibody to a receptor may stimulate the cell rather than inhibit it. In Graves' disease (hyperthyroidism) the antibody acts in a manner comparable to the normal stimulator for the thyroid gland, thyroid-stimulating hormone (TSH), and results in the thyroid cells secreting excessive amounts of thyroid hormone.

Antibodies reacting against smaller, soluble antigens will result in the formation of complexes which will circulate in the body fluids and finally be deposited in the tissues. Such complexes initiate the general inflammatory processes, including complement activation and phagocytosis, and this will result in damage to the tissue in which the complexes are deposited. Many autoimmune conditions show symptoms as a consequence of immune complex formation but it is particularly characteristic of those described as non-organ specific. Rheumatoid arthritis is an autoimmune disease in which antibodies reacting against IgG immunoglobulins produce complexes which, when deposited in the joints, initiate inflammatory processes causing damage to both cartilage and bone.

The development of self-reactive T-cells is a third aspect of most autoimmune conditions and damage is caused primarily by the release of lymphokines from the T_d cells. Addison's disease (adrenal insufficiency) and juvenile-onset diabetes show significant aspects of cell-mediated immunity.

The diagnosis of an autoimmune condition, often complicated by the diversity of the symptoms, can be assisted by laboratory investigations of the immune processes. There is often an increased level of serum immunoglobulins and, because of the effect of antibody-antigen complexes, there is usually a depletion of the blood complement levels. The most conclusive evidence is the demonstration of the deposition of immunoglobulins in the target tissues, a feature often paralleled by the invasion of the tissue by lymphocytes or plasma cells.

CONCLUSION

From the early days of research into immunity, it has been postulated that the process is essentially a defensive mechanism and that under normal conditions an animal will not react against its own constituents.

It is often assumed that immune protection is directed against foreign, invasive agents, but it is also extremely important in the elimination of 'self' components that have been altered as a result of either an external infective agent or somatic genetic variations. The aspect of immune surveillance against aberrant or cancerous cells would appear to be an extremely important feature of immune responsiveness.

In several important aspects of the immune response, and particularly in immune surveillance, it is an essential feature that the immune cells specifically recognize certain 'self' characteristics of an antigen before they will react against it. Thus the concept that an animal normally fails to react against itself is not due to an inability to recognize or react. There must be an elaborate control mechanism to prevent self-damage rather than prevent self-recognition.

Research into the mechanisms of the immune processes is essential if progress is to be made in many areas of preventative and therapeutic medicine. Enhancement of protective procedures against ineffective agents and the reversal or control of those diseases which result from inadequate immune responsiveness or from the failure of mechanisms for suppression or control, are two different, major areas of clinical science. An understanding of immune control will aid the development of organ and tissue transplantation procedures by enabling less hazardous methods of artificial immunosuppression to be developed.

Acknowledgement

The Editors and Publishers gratefully acknowledge the material submitted by Ms Zonia Argue, Senior Nurse Educator (Clinical Instructor Co-ordinator), Western Australian School of Nursing, Perth, Western Australia.

REFERENCES AND BIBLIOGRAPHY

Ammann A J 1984 Immunodeficiency diseases. In: Stites D P, Stobo J D, Fudenberg H H, Wells J V (eds) Basic and clinical immunology. Lange Medical, Los Altos, California

Barett J T 1983 Textbook of immunology. C V Mosby, St Louis

Burnett F M 1959 The clonal selection theory of acquired immunity. Vanderbilt University Press, Nashville

Cohen S, Porter R R 1964 Structure and biologic activity of immunoglobulins. Advances in Immunology 4: 287–349

Drutz D J, Mills J 1984 Immunity and infection. In: Stites D P, Stobo J D, Fudenberg H H, Wells J V (eds) Basic and clinical immunology. Lange Medical, Los Altos, California

Glynn L E, Steward M W 1981 Structure and function of antibodies. Wiley, Chichester

Mims C A 1980 Pathogenesis of infectious diseases. Academic Press, New York

Munro A J 1975 The genes for antibodies and the origin of diversity. In: Gell P G H, Coombs R R A, Lachmann P J (eds) Clinical aspects of immunology. Blackwell Scientific, Oxford

Richards G K 1976 Resistance to infection. In: Freedman S O, Gold P (eds) Clinical immunology. Harper and Row, London

Roitt I 1986a Immunity to infection. In: Essential immunology. Blackwell Scientific, Oxford

Roitt I 1986b Hypersensitivity. In: Essential immunology. Blackwell Scientific, Oxford

Smith H R, Steinberg A D 1983 Autoimmunity — a perspective. Annual Review of Immunology 1: 175–210

Snyderman R 1984 Regulation of leucocyte function. In: Contemporary topics in immunobiology 14. Plenum Press, New York

Wells J V, Henney C S, Herberman R B 1984 Immune mechanisms in tissue damage. In: Stites D P, Stobo J D, Fudenberg H H, Wells J V (eds) Basic and clinical immunology. Lange Medical, Los Altos, California

6

Degenerative and neoplastic processes

INTRODUCTION

Every cell of the human body may be considered as a small, discrete, membranous package filled with a concentrated solution of many chemicals. All cells share common biologic elements. Each one contains an identical set of genes yet, through the process of differentiation, cells differ considerably from each other in terms of size, shape and function. In man, more than 200 distinct cell types are readily identifiable. The individual characteristics of any one cell type are also influenced by its surroundings. Changes in the external environment of a cell, e.g. through disease processes, will be reflected in alterations in cell structure and function as it grows and strives to maintain a balance between internal and external environments.

Despite its ability to adapt to adverse conditions every cell will eventually die. For an organism to maintain the integrity of its organs and systems its constituent tissues must gain cells at a rate sufficient to replace those it loses. It may be seen then that, in health, the various cell populations contained within an organism are in a steady state.The numbers of cells within individual cell populations remain relatively constant and cell proliferation and cell loss are balanced.

CELL GROWTH AND PROLIFERATION

Cells are replaced in one of two ways. First, a

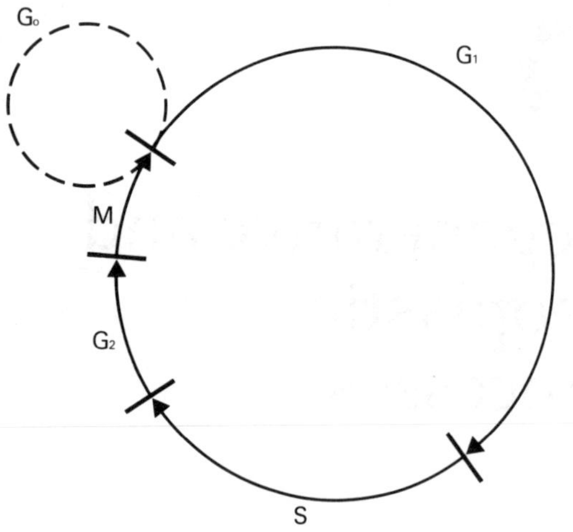

Fig. 6.1 The cell cycle

precursor population migrates from one site in the body to another where differentiation and/or division take place, e.g. precursor cells of the lymphoid series migrate from the bone marrow to the thymus where they undergo differentiation to form mature T-lymphocytes, which will enter the peripheral circulatory system. The second method of cell replacement occurs when a self-maintaining steady-state population reproduces itself to cope with the physiological rate of cell removal, e.g. bone marrow stem cells maintain their numbers although there is continuous migration to other tissues.

Two features central to the maintenance of a steady state population are therefore cell growth and cell division. The majority of the lifetime of the cell is spent during the growth phase, known as interphase. During this time a typical cell doubles its mass and duplicates all of its contents in preparation for cell division which occurs in the mitotic phase.

The events occurring between one mitotic phase and the next span the period of one cell cycle.

The cell cycle is classically divided into four phases of varying duration which are denoted: G1 (growth), S (DNA synthesis), G2 (growth) and M (mitosis) (Fig. 6.1). Cells normally make a choice between proliferation (division) and quiescence (non-division) when they reach G2. It has been proposed that quiescent cells withdraw from the cell cycle into a qualitatively distinct G0 state. Alternatively, quiescent cells may slowly traverse the cell cycle with a greatly extended G1 period. It is the G1 phase of the cell cycle which shows most variation in duration from one cell type to another, the time taken for a cell to pass through the S, G2 and M phases being relatively constant. Once a cell has passed out of G1 it is committed to completing S, G2 and M, there being a 'point of no return', (called a restriction point), late in G1. It is thought that cells need to be 'triggered' by a specific protein or growth factor to enable them to pass the restriction point. The rate of cell division is therefore regulated by certain proteins which may also exert an inhibitory influence on cell division. This is known as feedback control and it ensures that new cells are produced only when required (Pardee et al, 1978).

In multicellular organisms, individual cell types proliferate at a rate that is optimal for survival of the organism as a whole. Some cells, therefore, divide much less frequently than do others. Neurons and red blood cells do not divide at all once they are mature. Other cells divide continuously throughout the life of the organism, e.g. skin cells and epithelial cells lining the gut must continue to divide rapidly to offset cell loss from external and internal surfaces of the body. Overall, the average time taken by a human cell to traverse one complete cell cycle ranges from 8 hours to more than 100 days.

The rate of cell proliferation is also influenced by such external factors as cell-cell contact and interaction. Cells, in culture, grow only to confluence, i.e. once the surface of the culture flask is covered by a monolayer of cells they will not grow over each other, the phenomenon of contact inhibition halting further proliferation. In vivo, a tissue retains its normal shape, size and function by striking a balance between division and differentiation. Differentiation is the process by which cells acquire specific characteristics allowing them to function as one particular cell type only. This requires expression of only those genes within the total genome necessary for the functioning of that cell. The micro-environment in which a developing cell

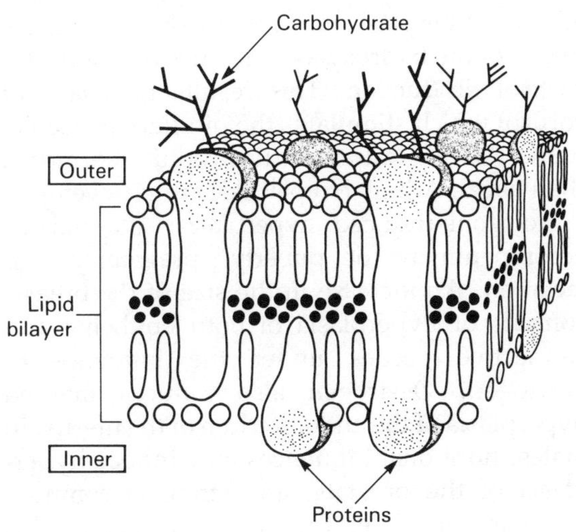

Fig. 6.2 The cell membrane

finds itself can influence the way it differentiates. Populations of somatic cells expressing the same characteristics of structure and function become arranged into tissues, tissues are arranged as organs, and organs comprise the systems of the entire organism.

CELLULAR INTERACTION

In order for specialized groups of cells to function as collaborative units in tissues, and the more highly ordered structure of organs, communication between cells is necessary. This may occur through chemicals, e.g. hormones, produced by one cell, or group of cells, to be recognized by other cells. Such chemicals may be transported in the bloodstream from their site of synthesis to target organ(s) where they are recognized by specific surface receptors embedded in the plasma membrane of responsive cells. Cellular interaction may also occur via direct contact, again mediated by the plasma membrane. Plasma membranes are lipid bilayers into which proteins are inserted (Fig. 6.2). Such proteins may extend right across the lipid bilayer or, alternatively, may protrude from one side only. Proteins extending from the outer surface into the extracellular environment function as receptors for chemicals and as a means by which a cell may be identified. Many proteins functioning in cellular recognition are conjugated to sugar molecules and are known as glycoproteins. Thus, many different protein and glycoprotein cell surface patterns are possible. Molecules by which cells are distinguished are known as surface antigens. Antibodies specific for these antigens would be produced if the cell were introduced into a foreign organism. The antigenic characteristics of a single cell may, however, change. During the course of maturation and differentiation many antigens are lost and others gained. When a virus infects a cell integrating its DNA into that of the host's genome the host cell may express viral antigens. Antigenic variation may occur when antibodies to a particular antigen induce expression of a slightly different molecular determinant. In addition antigens expressed during the embryonic state may disappear only to be re-expressed in old age. The failure of those systems controlling cell growth, division and maturation is associated with a variety of pathological conditions. The sequelae of such events include excessive increases in cell number (hyperplasia), or in cell size (hypertrophy) together with cell shrinkage and net loss (atrophy or degeneration). In this section the pathological conditions responsible for and/or resulting from alterations in cell size and division frequency will be discussed.

HYPERPLASIA

Hyperplasia is the term used to describe the increase in bulk of organ tissue resulting from an increase in the number of individual cells constituting it. The term may be applied to growth of existing body structures or to the appearance of new growths (neoplasia).

Any increase in the number of cellular units characteristic of a tissue must be accompanied by an increase in the total functional capacity of that organ. This is most readily observable in the endocrine system. The congenital absence of a necessary enzyme may inhibit hormone production or secretion by a particular gland. This

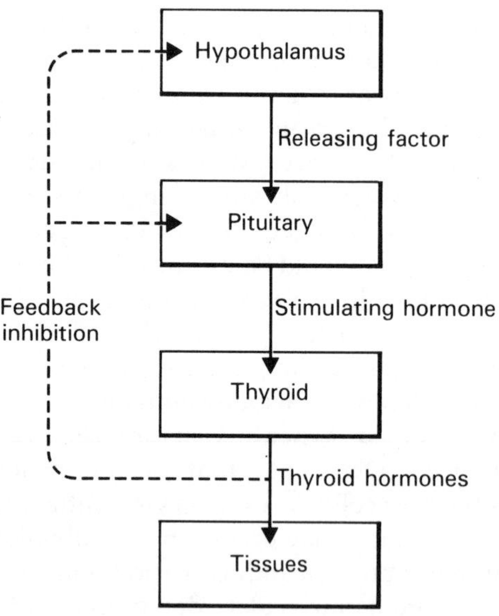

Fig. 6.3 Control of thyroid gland secretions

usually causes hyperplasia of the gland as the body tries to compensate for low hormone levels. Secretion of TSH (thyroid stimulating hormone) induces production of thyroid hormones, the levels of which control the function of the thyroid gland by a feedback mechanism (Fig. 6.3). Inadequate production of thyroid hormones due to a dietary lack of iodine or impaired enzyme activity, secondary to genetic defects or goitrogenic substances, results in excessive TSH secretion. Hyperplasia of the gland ensues. This compensatory mechanism increases thyroid hormone production so as to prevent hypothyroidism.Hyperthyroidism accompanied by enlargement of the gland may be autoimmune in origin as in Graves' disease. Anti-thyroid autoantibodies combine with the TSH receptor on the thyroid gland stimulating hyperplasia and increased hormone production. Thyroid hyperplasia may also be prompted by drugs such as thiouracil or carbimazole which block the synthesis of thyroid hormone. Feedback inhibition of TSH production is therefore released and hyperplasia occurs. The patient is, however, clinically euthyroid as these drugs prevent over-production of the hormones (De Groot & Stanbury, 1975). Similarly, congenital adrenal hyperplasia may ensue from a deficiency in one of the hydroxylase enzymes necessary for cortisol production. This results in a lack of cortisol which stimulates the pituitary to secrete more ACTH (adrenocorticotrophic hormone) than usual. Adrenal hyperplasia thus develops.

Hormone-induced hyperplasia is a normal accompaniment of puberty, pregnancy and lactation. An increase in the size of the breasts consists of hyperplasia of both epithelial and connective tissues under the influence of oestrogen. Oestrogen also induces marked hyperplasia of the endometrium of the uterus. In males, hormonal influences may induce hyperplasia of the prostate, an extremely common event in men over the age of 60 years. This hyperplastic enlargement is thought to be related to hormonal changes occurring as reproductive activity decreases (Purtilo, 1978). Testosterone levels decline, the oestrogen produced in the adrenals then stimulate the prostatic epithelium to grow and undergo hyperplasia. Enlargement of the prostate gland then obstructs the flow of urine through the urethra. Urinary tract infections due to the resultant partial retention of urine are a frequent complication of the disease.

Hyperplasia of the skin, mouth, alimentary and respiratory tract occurs when exposed to any persistent irritating agent. Simple trauma may constitute an irritating agent as when the constant rubbing of ill-fitting shoes causes a corn to develop. Epidermal hyperplasia may also be associated with the presence of inflammatory intradermal lesions e.g. insect bites. The resultant epidermal thickening may often be quite marked.

Hyperplasia may also occur as a result of increased demand placed upon the organ. This can be seen in athletes and also as a compensatory mechanism in cardiac failure (see Ch.22).

NEOPLASIA

Neoplasia concerns the growth of neoplasms, masses of cells that proliferate without normal control to form tumours which do not have any useful function. Neoplastic cells can develop in any tissue of the body that contains cells capable of dividing.

PHYSICAL CHARACTERISTICS OF NEOPLASTIC CELLS

A neoplasm may be either benign or malignant. There is no sharp distinction between the two, although benign tumours generally grow slowly, rarely recur after removal, are composed of cells that look normal and do not metastasize (i.e. do not initiate tumours at a distance from the primary growth). Benign tumours may become life-threatening if they press on nerves or blood vessels or if they secrete biologically active substances, such as hormones, which alter the homeostatic balance of the body. Malignant neoplasms, on the other hand, are invasive, usually grow rapidly, may recur after removal, cause death if growth is not controlled and arrested, are composed of cells of abnormal appearance which are less well differentiated than normal tissue and frequently metastasize via lymphatic channels or blood vessels to lymph nodes and other tissues in the body. (Purtilo, 1978). The presence in the body of malignant growth is usually referred to as cancer.

On examination of cells obtained by surgery, swabbing, washing or secretion of a tissue suspected to contain cancer, a number of observations allow the pathologist to suspect, pending further diagnostic procedures, that cancer is present. The high rate of cell division is manifested by the large number of cells undergoing mitosis at any one time. A 20-fold increase in the number of dividing cells in malignant, relative to benign or normal tissue, would not be an uncommon finding. Among these dividing tissues abnormal mitoses may also be present. These include giant cells containing large, variably-shaped or multiple nuclei. The nuclei of cancer cells often contain very apparent chromatin with prominent large nucleoli.

Chromosomal aberrations

Many malignant tumours contain chromosomal aberrations. The first specific chromosomal change to be associated with malignancy was the discovery in the early 1960s that chronic myelogenous leukaemia is correlated with loss of substance from one of the G-group chromosomes (Nowell & Hungerford, 1960). This results in what has become known as the Philadelphia chromosome (Ph^1). The development of chromosome banding techniques has enabled this change to be defined as a translocation of chromosomal material from chromosome number 22 to chromosome 9. In exceptional cases chromosomes other than number 9 receive the translocated material from chromosome 22 (e.g. numbers 2,3,4,6,11, 13,16,17,19 and 21). It therefore seems probable that the loss of material from number 22 is the significant change associated with the malignancy. The (9;22) translocation is also involved in certain cases of acute lymphocytic and non-lymphocytic leukaemias. The break point in chromosome 22 is very similar in all three diseases (Forman & Rowley, 1982). Deletions involving chromosome 22 have also been found to be associated with many meningiomas and carcinomas (Levan et al, 1977). This suggests that aberrations in the same chromosome region are responsible for the initiation of the malignant transformation, and that different types of malignancies develop depending upon the location and type of the affected cell.

Chromosomal aberrations are almost the rule in haematological malignancies with greater than 90% of all forms of acute leukaemia exhibiting clearly identifiable defects. Distinct patterns have emerged with the aberrations usually only involving a limited number of chromosomes. In acute myeloid leukaemia, while the disease is not associated with a single specific change, there is a strongly preferential involvement of chromosomes 5,7,8,15,17 and 21. Furthermore specific segments of these chromosomes are usually involved in the aberrations (e.g. bands q33–36 on chromosome 7) (Forman & Rowley, 1982).

Most patients suffering from Burkitt's lymphoma have a specific chromosome abnormality involving a translocation of chromosomal material from the long arm of chromosome 8 (band q24) to the long arm of chromosome 14 (band q32) (Manolova et al, 1979). In a minority of Burkitt's lymphoma cases the material from chromosome 8 translocates onto the short arm of chromosome 2 (band p13) or onto the long arm of chromosome 22 (band q11) (Sandberg, 1981). In sixteen out of nineteen cases of follicular-cell lymphoma, it was observed that a translocation had occurred from chromosome 18 to chromosome 14 (also band q32, as in Burkitt's lymphoma).

While it is not always possible to associate specific chromosomal abnormalities with specific tumour types, evidence is growing that only a certain few chromosomes are involved in neoplasia. The nature of the relationship between chromosomal aberrations and neoplasia has been the subject of much debate. The question has been asked about whether chromosomal changes are a causative factor in neoplasia, the result of neoplasia or a side effect of a fundamental factor causing neoplasia. It can be argued that since many tumours do not display chromosomal changes, at least in their early stages, any aberrations observed merely reflect the genetic changes that are possible in a malignant cell without loss of viability. This argument, however, does not account for the finding that certain specific chromosomal abnormalities appear to predispose affected individuals to particular neoplasms or neoplasms in general. An example is provided by Down's syndrome where affected children have at least a 10-fold higher incidence of leukaemia than do normal children (Knudson, 1975).

The association of certain human neoplasms with specific cytogenetic abnormalities and the fact that many human tumours contain detectable, if non-specific, chromosomal changes argues in favour of alterations to the genetic material being a significant factor in the carcinogenic process. Not all changes in the genetic material of the cell are detectable, however, using currently available cytogenetic techniques. Minute base changes in the nuclear DNA of the cell may result in a mutant cell with stably altered properties which would appear unchanged in terms of its gross chromosomal morphology.

The concept that tumours may result from somatic cell mutations (in addition to major chromosomal aberrations) has arisen from experimental findings that the daughter cells of a tumour maintain their neoplastic properties and that there is an almost unlimited variety of tumour types. This mutational theory of cancer is supported by the finding that approximately 90% of known carcinogens (i.e. agents capable of inducing malignant tumours) are also mutagenic (i.e. capable of inducing gene mutations) (McCann et al, 1975). Further support for a mutational origin of tumours has come from the growing evidence that the majority, if not all tumours, have a single cell origin.

The mutation theory of cancer has been further boosted by the finding that in cells taken from a bladder carcinoma, there is a gene which differs from its naturally occurring form in the simplest possible way — one specific nucleotide in the DNA is replaced by another (a guanine-cytosine to thymine-adenine transversion) (Reddy et al, 1982). The resulting protein differs from its normal form (known as p21) again in the most simple way – the twelfth amino acid from the end carrying a free amino group is changed (glycine to valine). That such a minute change could have such profound consequences is perhaps not totally surprising when one considers, for example, that a similar single amino acid substitution in the β-haemoglobin chain results in the normal adult haemoglobin molecule taking on the sickle cell form.

Although there is overwhelming evidence that cancer is a genetic disease, it does not follow axiomatically that it is hereditary. Mutations occurring in the somatic cells are confined to those cells and are not transmitted to future offspring. Only when a mutation occurs in the germ cells which produce the gametes is it possible for the mutation to be transmitted to future offspring. Nevertheless, there are examples of inherited disorders (both dominant and recessive) rendering affected individuals more susceptible to cancer. Three recessively inherited disorders — xeroderma pigmentosum, ataxia telangiectasia, and Fanconi's anaemia — all predispose the individual to cancer through their specific defects in the ability to repair certain kinds of chemical or physical damage to the nuclear DNA of the cell. These disorders provide direct evidence that DNA damage can be carcinogenic and add further strength to the concept that tumours have a mutational origin. Several dominant mutations in humans predispose affected individuals to tissue specific tumours. Virtually all known cancers include a subset of cases that arise due to the affected individuals having inherited a dominant germinal mutation. The most widely quoted example is polyposis of the colon. The gene responsible expresses polyposis of the colon, which is non-malignant, by early adulthood. This is followed by adenocarcinoma of the colon by the age of 50 years in all instances, causing death on average at approximately 40 years (Neel, 1971). Other examples of dominantly inherited mutations predisposing affected individuals to cancer include hereditary adenocarcinoma of the colon (the cancer family syndrome), basal cell naevus syndrome, hereditary retinoblastoma, and hereditary neuroblastoma (McKenna, 1983)

Malignant transformation

There is obviously strong evidence to support the theory that gene mutations (and chromosomal aberrations) are involved in the transformation of normal cells to malignant ones. This concept of the carcinogenic process is not however without its difficulties. There are in fact two main criticisms, namely the observation that 10% of known carcinogens are not mutagenic (McCann et al, 1975), and the finding that some cancer cells are able to revert to 'normality'. Mintz & Illmensee (1975) took cells from a malignant mouse teratocarcinoma and injected them into normal embryos at the blastocyst stage of development. Mice were produced that were cellular-genetic mosaics. Each mosaic mouse had several developmentally unrelated tissues containing tumour-derived cells without any indiction of malignancy. These results show that the transformation of the teratocarcinoma cells genome was not of a mutational nature.

Even the finding described earlier, that a single nucleotide change in bladder cells can result in malignant transformation (Reddy et al, 1982), is not without its contradictions. It is possible to make normal cells malignant by infecting them with DNA of the normal p21 gene to which has been attached pieces of viral DNA necessary for the functioning of the RNA tumour viruses. This results in increased amounts of the p21 protein being produced, suggesting that either a small amount of abnormal p21 or a large amount of normal p21 has similar consequences for the cell, namely malignancy. It must be concluded that a theory of carcinogenesis based solely on gene mutational events does not embrace the experimental evidence thus far obtained (McKenna, 1983).

Stages in carcinogenesis

The clear evidence in favour of both mutational and non-mutational factors being involved in the transformation of a normal cell into a cancer cell has resulted in carcinogenesis being considered, at least in some cases, as a two (or more) step process. This is supported by the finding that if mouse skin is exposed to some mutagens, tumours will appear if a particular non-carcinogen such as croton oil is applied months, or even years, later (Trosko & Chang, 1978).

The two steps in carcinogenesis have been referred to as 'initiation' and 'promotion'. Initiation is regarded as a process which occurs either spontaneously or after a normal cell is subjected to a sub-carcinogenic treatment with a chemical or physical agent. Promotion, which is the second step, involves repeated application of a promoting agent (Fig. 6.4).

Integrative theory of carcinogenesis

The integrative theory put forward by Trosko & Chang (1978) assumes that, in a normal cell, the genes responsible for malignancy (oncogenes) are repressed (i.e. switched off) by the products of certain specific regulatory genes. For carcinogenesis to occur, it is essential that the regulatory genes are defective or repressed and that the oncogenes are in a transcribable

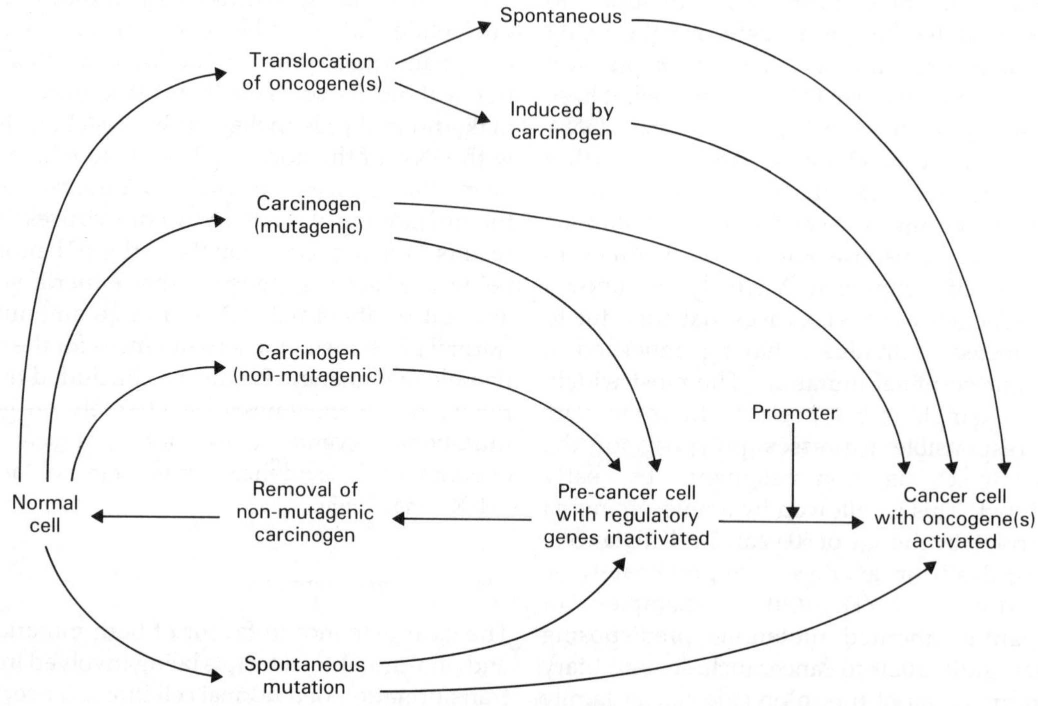

Fig. 6.4 Integrative theory of carcinogenesis (after McKenna, 1983)

condition. The defect in the regulatory genes may be caused by spontaneous somatic mutation, by physical or chemical carcinogens, or by a combination of somatic and germ line mutations (McKenna, 1983). Once the regulatory genes are no longer functioning, carcinogenesis may take place if the oncogenes are in a transcribable condition. The next step therefore is for the oncogenes to become depressed. This 'switching on' may be achieved by tissue specific promoters, e.g. hormones, or by non- tissue specific promoters such as phorbolesters (McKenna, 1983).

The integrative theory of carcinogenesis, therefore, accounts for the finding that not all carcinogens (initiators) are mutagenic by assuming that such carcinogens inactivate the regulatory genes responsible for the repression of oncogenes, but do not alter the DNA base sequence. If the cancer cell subsequently becomes no longer exposed to the non-mutagenic carcinogens, it could revert to normality if the regulatory genes begin to function again. This accounts for the reversion of malignant cells to normality in a changed environment. Promoters, on the other hand, merely assist in the derepression of oncogenes after the regulatory genes have been inactivated. Promoters are not therefore carcinogenic to a normal cell in which the regulatory genes normally responsible for the repression of malignancy are functioning properly (McKenna, 1983).

The concept that the regulation of activity of oncogenes can be a critical factor in carcinogenesis has received support from the recent findings that the genes coding for immunoglobulin heavy chains are contained in the chromosome 14 break-point associated with Burkitt's and non-Burkitt's lymphomas (Kirsch et al, 1982). It can be assumed that one oncogene is located on chromosome 8 and another on chromosome 18. It is believed that these oncogenes are normally repressed or transcribed for protein at a low level. A translocation of either oncogene to chromosome 14 in lymphocytes brings it to a region of high genetic activity so that the oncogene is either derepressed or has its rate of transcription greatly enhanced. It is noteworthy that, in the rare variants of Burkitt's lymphoma where the terminal end of chromosome 8 is translocated onto the short arm of chromosome 2 or onto the long arm of chromosome 22, these are the respective sites of the genes that code for kappa and lambda light immunoglobulin chains (McKenna, 1983). Over a dozen vertebrate oncogenes have now been described.

The model in Figure 6.4 is compatible with these findings, in that it assumes that the translocation of an oncogene to a region of high genetic activity can lead to malignancy. The model also assumes that a direct mutation in an oncogene (e.g. the p21 gene of the bladder carcinoma) might lead to malignancy by the gene then failing to recognize the repressor from the regulatory genes. Tumorigenic RNA viruses can also cause cancer in vertebrates through their regulatory effect on oncogenes. This can occur in at least two ways (McKenna, 1983). The virus can bring an oncogene into the cell and, since the oncogene is under the control of the viral promoter of transcription, it will be transcribed at too high a level. Alternatively, the virus may not contain an oncogene but may by chance become integrated beside one of the cell oncogenes thus bringing about derepression of the oncogene. Present evidence indicates however that human cancer is seldom induced by viruses. What are the normal functions of oncogenes? It is obvious that their normal function is sufficiently important so as not to have been selected out during vertebrate evolution. Evidence is growing that oncogenes may normally be involved in growth regulation during cellular differentiation.

Thus there is overwhelming evidence that cancer is a genetic disease. It does not follow, however, that it is hereditary. Only a few disorders have been shown to predispose affected individuals to cancer and these constitute only a small proportion of cancer sufferers. In other words, the great majority of tumours arise from disturbances of the genetic material after, and not before, conception.

Cellular changes

Following transformation, cancer cells are less subject to most of the feedback mechanisms that control normal cell division. This may be demonstrated in the laboratory where it can be seen that cancer cells in culture will usually continue to divide and proliferate, piling up on top of each other beyond the point at which normal cell division is stopped by contact inhibition (Alberts et al, 1983). The rapid growth of cancer cells is also facilitated by the fact that they require fewer growth factors than normal cells and that they may potentiate their own growth by actually producing growth factors, a phenomenon known as autostimulation (Ruddon, 1981).

Cell cycle counter

Normal cells seems to have an inherent cell cycle 'counter' or 'memory' allowing them to undergo only a certain number of cell divisions in their lifetime. The cancer cell lacks this restraint and can continue to proliferate ad infinitum (Mehlman & Hanson, 1974). Because the balance between cell division and differentiation is impaired following transformation, the function of a tumour may bear no relation to the function of the tissue from which it originally derived. It may assume the function of an entirely different tissue at another site in the body. This may be seen when a tumour functions as a site of ectopic hormone production, high levels of the hormone not being diminished by the normal feedback control mechanisms. For example, an ectopic ACTH-producing lung cancer may continue to produce ACTH even though circulating levels of adrenocortical steroids are sufficient to cause Cushing's syndrome.

Cell differentiation

Malignant tumour cells tend to be 'anaplastic' or less well differentiated than the tissue from which they arose, a process known as dedifferentiation (Ruddon, 1981). Although this term implies that the differentiation process is actually reversed following transformation, this is not so. Rather, the initial cancer cell was one in which the normal differentiation process was blocked. 'Undifferentiated' tumours are those which bear only very little resemblance, either structurally or functionally, to their tissue of origin.

Cell antigens

The antigenic determinants of a cell may be altered following transformation. While this may reflect the expression of viral or of embryonic antigens, the existence of tumour-specific transplantation antigen has been the subject of a large amount of research. To date, however, no specific malignancy associated antigen has been found. Several have been proposed but all have subsequently been demonstrated to be borne by other normal or embryonic cells (Ashall et al, 1982; McGee et al, 1982). The altered antigenic expression of cancer cells suggests expression (i.e. switching on) of those genes coding for specific proteins. This theory is supported by the increased production by tumour cells of several other proteins, e.g. growth factors, and of surface receptors for such molecules. One protein produced in large quantities by virally transformed cells in vitro has been shown to be structurally similar to another protein, platelet-derived growth factor (PDGF), normally produced in large quantities only following haemorrhage (Waterfield et al, 1983). This PDGF could, in theory, cause rapid growth and proliferation of responsive cells, as transformed cells are also known to bear an increased density of surface receptors.

Immune response

Under normal circumstances damaged cells or cells expressing non-self antigens are destroyed by the immune system. It has been proposed, therefore, that the immune response of people in whom malignant tumours develop must be impaired (Kirchner, 1984). Such an impairment has not, however, been positively identified.

Much of the evidence for the contribution of a defective immune system to the development of neoplasms stems from recent evidence suggesting that transplant patients undergoing immunosuppressive therapy have an increased incidence of malignancies both at the site of the transplantation and in other parts of the body (Penn, 1984). Kirchner (1984) does, however, concede that any augmentation in the development of the tumours may be due to a direct carcinogenic effect on the patient by the drugs administered.

The mass of evidence to date suggests that tumours proliferate and metastasize in the face of an intact immune response, any suppression of immunity being a secondary effect promoted by the presence in the body of tumours, by radiation and by chemotherapy. Tumours may also have mechanisms by which to evade the immune system. Tumour cells may shed their antigens into the surrounding extra-cellular fluid, and increased levels of sialic acid, a glycoprotein constituent of surface antigens, have been detected in the sera of patients bearing tumours. Transformed cells may also secrete blocking factors which bind to their antigens, 'hiding' them from potentially destructive antibodies or phagocytic macrophages. Macrophages are known to produce several anti-tumour agents, the best-known of which is tumour necrosis factor (TNF). However, the function of this molecule is not entirely understood. (Playfair et al, 1984).

On activation of the cellular immune system, T-lymphocytes produce a range of protein factors, called lymphokines, some of which may have anti–tumour effects (Roitt, 1977). One group among these, the interferons, has anti-viral properties preventing the spread of virus particles from an infected cell to those surrounding it. Interferons are produced in very small quantities and clinical trials of interferon therapy have not demonstrated conclusively any significant potential in its use to halt the progression of malignancy.

Biochemical changes in the cancer cell

In the early 20th century it was postulated that defective respiration of the tumour cell was the reason for malignancy and was, moreover, the basic difference between normal and cancer cells. This hypothesis was based on the observation that, under aerobic conditions, various tumours produced lactate as a result of glycolysis; normal cells show lactate production only in the absence of oxygen. However, defective respiration in cancer cells has never been established. Lactate production is probably secondary to the loss of growth control reflecting the increased percentage of dividing cells in malignant tissues, rather than having a role in the initiation of malignant transformation (McElroy & Glass, 1958).

Further studies on intracellular enzymes and isoenzymes failed to identify a specific transformation-related pattern common to all neoplasms. Where malignant cells have altered enzyme profiles, such changes are usually elevations in the activities of enzymes of nucleic acid synthetic pathways, consistent with the increased rate of cell replication and therefore unlikely to have initiated the transformation process.

In general, the enzyme complement of a well-differentiated, transformed cell is similar to that of the cell from which it originated. Undifferentiated, highly malignant cells resemble one another and fetal tissues more than their normal adult counterpart. Highly invasive neoplasms appear to release increased amounts of proteases and their activating agents (Ruddon, 1981). For example, large amounts of plasmin produced by the activity of high levels of plasminogen activator increase the fibrinolytic capacity of tumour cells. This release of proteases may be a response to DNA damage, a type of suicide response potentially initiated by DNA-attacking agents, e.g. UV light, Mitomycin C and alkylating agents. Several peptide fragments resulting from proteolytic cleavage uncommon in normal individuals have been observed in serum from cancer patients. These include fragments of the complement component C_3 and a polypeptide derived from fibronectin.

Intracellular cyclic nucleotides, cGMP and cAMP, in conjunction with Ca^{2+} ions, appear to function in the control of DNA synthesis in transformed cells (Jungmann et al, 1983). A transient elevation in cAMP levels is necessary for DNA synthesis, while persistence of these levels inhibits DNA synthesis (Wang et al, 1978). cGMP may function in a similar manner while cAMP may also influence the expression and maintenance of differentiated functions of cells in culture, perhaps by influencing mRNA synthesis. While cAMP levels in transformed cells in vitro are lower than those of normal cells, it is not clear whether this may be responsible for the occurrence of transformation.

THE EFFECT OF TUMOURS ON THE HOST

Tumour detection

The initial early detection of malignant tumours depends on where the tissue involved is situated in the body. The survival rates and curability of specific cancer types reflect this (Purtilo, 1978). Skin carcinoma (cancer of epithelial cells) has a 90–98% cure rate which drops to 30–40% for cancers of hollow organs, e.g. stomach. Because the detection of sarcoma (cancer of mesenchymal cells) relies on the development of obstruction and bleeding, symptoms characteristic of large advanced tumours, its cure rate is only 0–30%.

The earliest detectable malignancies are small tumours, called 'in situ' cancers, localized in particular tissues. They lack a vascular supply so the resultant deprivation of oxygen and nutrients contributes to the slow growth of tumours at this stage. This period of relative dormancy may last for several years, after which the tumour may enter a stage of rapid growth with increased potential for tissue invasion and metastatic growth (Fig. 6.5). The trigger which brings about such changes in the development of the cancer is obscure, although the acquisition of a vascular supply by the malignant growth usually occurs at this time and may contribute to the increased malignancy of the tumour. A factor, tumour angiogenesis factor (TAF), secreted by transformed cells may aid in the establishment of such a vascular supply (Ruddon, 1981).

Tumour growth and spread

As the tumour grows it compresses the surrounding tissue, invading it and metastasizing. The potential for metastatic growth varies between different tumour types. While tumour cells proliferate some cell death occurs,

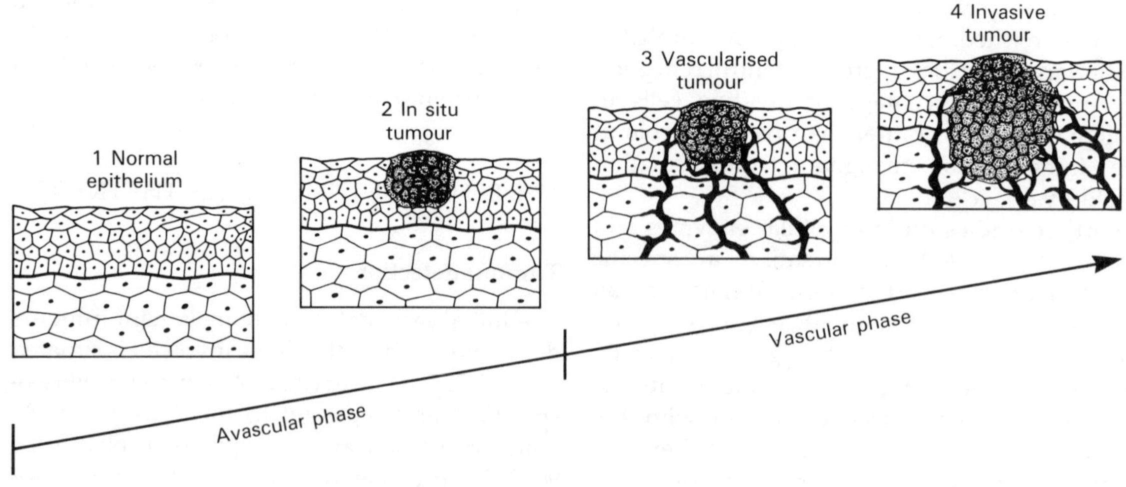

Fig. 6.5 Growth phases of a tumour (carcinoma)

particularly in the centres of large tumours where the vascular supply is limited and cells exist in an essentially anaerobic environment. Death of the patient due to cancer occurs at varying lengths of time after the onset of the rapid growth phase, depending on the tissue involved. Brain tumours, for example, rapidly become lethal because of damage to this vital organ. Acute lymphocytic leukaemia may be lethal within 6–12 months if untreated. Metastatic growth occurs by the penetration of tumour cells into blood or lymph vessels in which they travel to establish secondary growths in tissues at a distance from the primary tumour. It is relatively easy for such cells to penetrate into capillaries, venules and lymph vessels due to the 'spaces' between the epithelial cells in their walls. Arteries and veins have more firmly structured walls and, therefore, are not thought to permit invasion by tumour cells. The secretion of proteolytic enzymes following transformation may also facilitate metastatic growth, increasing the potential of the tumour cell to penetrate into the vascular system and to invade tissue. Tumour cells entering the lymphatic system travel to regional lymph nodes where they may be trapped to form metastatic growths. In general, it is cells from carcinomas which travel in the lymph system, while sarcoma cells are confined to blood vessels. Due to the free communication between the blood and lymph systems this is not, however, always true. During their circulation, tumour cells interact with such cell types as platelets, neutrophils, lymphocytes and macrophages. The result of these interactions may be the formation of an embolus with the capacity to adhere to capillary endothelium. This favours the development of metastases and demonstrates the capacity of the tumour to exploit tumour-directed, cell-mediated, immune responses. Tumours may also spread by the direct shedding of cells into body cavities, e.g. lung cancer may enter the pleural cavity.

The frequency of metastatic growth varies between different organs due in part to differences in vascularization. The lungs and liver, for instance, have a substantial blood supply and are the most frequent sites of visceral metastatic growth. Various other properties of individual host tissues also influence the growth of secondary tumours. Lung cancers frequently metastasize to the brain, carcinomas of the prostate often spread to the spinal vertebrae, and stomach carcinomas are often observed to establish secondaries in the lungs, liver, bone and the remainder of the peritoneal cavity. Overall it may be concluded that metastases do not occur randomly.

The effect on the patient

The growth of cancer in a patient may produce fever, wasting, loss of appetite, infection, anaemia and many other symptoms, depending on the individual tumour. Some of these symptoms may appear in organs where metastases are not apparent and are termed paraneoplastic symptoms. Paraneoplasia may be induced, for example, by a tumour producing a hormone which then induces changes in uninvolved tissues.

Pain associated with malignancy is often one of the greatest problems for the patient, the patient's family and for health care personnel. Pain may be caused by pressure of the growing tumour on surrounding tissue, e.g. brain tumours within the restricted space of the cranial cavity. Pressure on a cranial nerve may induce referred pain in the tissue served by that nerve. Tumours may also cause pain by stretching or obstruction of a hollow organ or by causing infection or inflammation. Cancer-induced pain may also be related to the production of prostaglandins by transformed cells, a function which has also been implicated in the depression of cell-mediated immunity and susceptibility to infection seen in cancer patients (Ziegler, 1982). Infection with herpes zoster virus is also facilitated and can cause nerve pain.

Malnutrition and muscle wasting, seen in almost all cancer patients, have been attributed to the anorexia induced by tumour-released factors and by therapy, to dysfunctions of digestive processes and to the metabolic demands of the tumour (Groer & Shekleton, 1979). Transformed cells utilize nutrients inefficiently because of their high rate of anaerobic glycolysis and their rapid cell growth and division. The persistence of a chronic illness such as cancer places large demands on the bone marrow which must generate vast numbers of the rapidly turning-over cells of the immune system as it strives to cope with the constant invasion. Anaemia may ensue from nutritional deprivation and from the further demands on the bone marrow for erythrocytes to replace those lost due to haemorrhage following tumour-induced damage to blood vessels and haemolysis. An autoimmune, haemolytic anaemia is often associated with certain cancers, usually those of the lymphatic and reticuloendothelial systems (Ruddon, 1981). The reasons for this are not known. Iron deficiency anaemia may also occur in cancer patients. Leucopenia, a depressed white blood cell count, may also be evident due to radiation or drug therapies which depress bone-marrow function. Leucocytosis, an elevated white blood cell count, while a usual result of leukaemia (the malignant proliferation of leucocytes) may, for some unknown reason, be present in other metastatic cancers. This effect may be secondary to infection. Bleeding causes thrombocytopenia, (depression of platelet numbers) aggravated by bone-marrow deficiencies inhibiting megakaryocyte development. Mechanisms contributing to the rare cancer-associated occurrence of thrombocytosis are not understood.

Some of the indirect effects of tumours may be more life-threatening than the cancer itself. One of these is the elevation of plasma calcium levels (hypercalcaemia). This affects the CNS, gastrointestinal tract, kidneys and the cardiovascular system. Calcium may be released when tumours invade bone tissue, although about 15% of patients with hypercalcaemia have no evidence of bony metastases. Theories proposed to explain this phenomenon include the production of parathyroid hormone by tumours and the release of prostaglandins which have osteoclastic activities.

RECENT ADVANCES IN TREATMENT

Recent advances in many areas of medical science are currently being exploited in efforts to prevent and to destroy tumours. While chemotherapeutic and radiation treatment regimes continue to increase the survival rates of cancer patients, such therapies indiscriminately destroy both tumorous and normal cells. Tumour-specific therapies therefore hold the greatest potential for future advancement. Modulation of the immune system to enhance anti-tumour responses is hampered by the complexities of immune control mechanisms. The failure, to date, to identify a tumour–specific

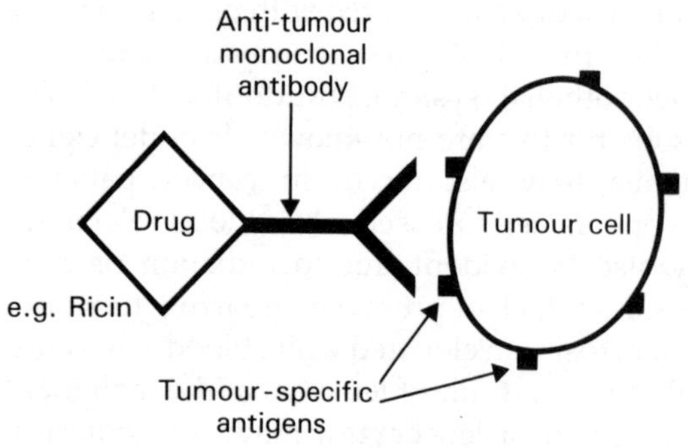

Fig. 6.6 Monoclonal antibody—drug conjugate

antigen has partially overshadowed the development of monoclonal antibody technology, which potentially enables the physician to detect and destroy transformed cells at a very early stage of development without risking damage to healthy tissues (Kohler & Milstein, 1975). Conjugation of a tumour-specific, monoclonal antibody to a potent cytotoxic drug, e.g. the plant-derived chemical Ricin, would greatly facilitate tumour cell killing (Fig. 6.6). Studies on such drug-targeting regimes are currently proceeding in many cancer research centres (Sikora et al, 1984; Dillman & Royston, 1984).

HYPERTROPHY

Hypertrophy occurs when a cell adapts to a sublethal injurious change in its environment by increasing its size without undergoing cell division. This increase in size results from increased synthesis of macromolecules including protein, lipid and nucleic acids. Such a response may be compensatory, resulting from an increased workload placed on the cell, or it may reflect changes in circulating hormone levels.

As a cell increases in size its volume increases relatively faster than its surface area. The cell membrane is the channel through which gases, nutrients and wastes must be transported into and out of the cell. Once cellular volume reaches a critical size, therefore, the flow through the membrane is no longer sufficient to meet the cell's increased requirements, and nutrients and wastes must traverse greater intracellular distances between the plasma membrane and the organelles. In addition, the nucleus may not be sufficient to control this larger unit. The net result of such events is that once cells grow beyond a certain critical level they diminish in efficiency and, under normal circumstances, cell division would then occur giving rise to two smaller and therefore more efficient units.

TISSUE AND ORGAN HYPERTROPHY

Once a tissue has attained its fully differentiated state it loses the capacity to divide and thereafter must grow by hypertrophy. Some tissues never attain such a state and undergo cell division and differentiation throughout the lifetime of the individual. The commitment of a tissue or organ to undergo either hypertrophy or hyperplasia must then depend on the ability of constituent cells to enlarge or to increase in number, or both. Hypertrophy without accompanying hyperplasia occurs only in muscle and may be induced by a number of factors. Obstruction to the outflow of the contents of any hollow organ will cause hypertrophy of the wall muscle. This may occur following inflammatory swellings, or be due to the presence of a hyperplastic growth. The walls of the bladder become hypertrophic in the presence of a urethral stricture, while stomach muscles hypertrophy when thickening of the muscle forming the pyloric valve is caused by congenital hypertrophic pyloric stenosis.

Thickening of the tunica media of arteries may ensue from hypertension which also leads to hypertrophy of muscle fibres of the affected heart chambers, usually the left ventricle, the muscular contractions of which must pump blood around all parts of the body in the face of increased peripheral vascular resistance. Increased workloads may also be applied to cardiac muscle by raised end diastolic volume as a result of aortic regurgitation or hypertrophic cardiomyopathy, or by organic obstruction to outflow by aortic, mitral or pulmonary stenosis. Ventricular hypertrophy makes the myocardium more susceptible to ischaemia as the blood supply does not increase to the same degree as does muscle mass. Congestive heart failure occurs when the heart can no longer pump against the increased resistance. Angina pectoris, the characteristic pain resulting from cardiac ischaemia, may occur. A further example of hypertrophy is that which occurs in the remaining kidney when one kidney is removed or malfunctions due to disease.

Increased workloads may be applied to skeletal muscles by regular exercise. The subsequent increase in muscle mass is due to increases in the number of filaments in the sarcomeres, in the number of mitochondria and in the amount of sarcoplasm. Hypertrophy is accompanied by an increase in strength, because the amount of force a muscle can exert depends on the number of filaments it contains. Once the increased demand ceases, however, the hypertrophic muscle fibres return to their original size.

Muscular hypertrophy induced by hormonal influences is seen during pregnancy when myometrial cells of the walls of the uterus may increase to one hundred times their size during the non-pregnant resting state. This is a response to the increased production of oestrogenic hormones.

HYPERTROPHY AND HYPERPLASIA IN ADIPOSE TISSUE

Adipose tissue, composed of adipocytes, predominates in subcutaneous tissues and mesentery, although it occurs throughout the body. This tissue responds, as an organ would, to stimuli from hormones, the nervous system and changes in the concentrations of blood components. The adipose tissue acts as a storage area for excess ingested calories and its size can increase either by hypertrophy or by hyperplasia. Hypertrophic adipocytes become full of lipids, and hyperplasia occurs during specific periods in the development of adipose tissue. These periods are not yet well-defined although most tend to occur during childhood and adolescence. It is known, however, that the stimulus to hyperplasia is excessive food intake. This hyperplasia is irreversible and is conducive to obesity in adult life. Childhood hyperplasia is mediated by a functioning pituitary gland. In the obese adult excess calories promote hypertrophy of existing adipocytes. Hypertrophic adipocytes appear as large droplets of triglycerides surrounded by a cell membrane. There is, however, a limit to the amount of fat a cell can contain. The degree of obesity in adulthood is thus conditioned by the extent of childhood hyperplasia. There are some exceptions which allow hyperplasia in later life. Adipocyte hyperplasia may occur during pregnancy, so it appears that this event is subject to hormonal control.

CELLULAR DEGENERATION

Cellular degeneration encompasses a variety of morphological changes compatible with cell survival (Gilbert & Huntington, 1978).

The first response of a cell to injury is a reversible increase in intracellular water, termed cloudy swelling. This type of degeneration occurs in many organs but is most frequent in the proximal tubular cells of the kidney. An increase in the size of cytoplasmic vacuoles, vacuolar degeneration, causes the cell to swell further. More severe cellular injury results in fatty degeneration, the reversible accumulation of abnormal amounts of intracellular fat.

In ischaemia the reduced supplies of oxygen, glucose and other essential substrates may precipitate the appearance of cloudy swelling and fatty degeneration in individual cells or groups of cells. Cell death may ensue if the ischaemia persists. Chronic ischaemia in the heart gives it a speckled appearance due to patchy cell death. Fibrosis then occurs in these areas. This loss of cells may alter organ function, causing abnormalities in cardiac electrical behaviour and subsequent dysrhythmias. Fatty degeneration in the liver is thought to be related to nutritional deficiencies, often as a result of alcoholism. Glycogenic degeneration in liver, heart and muscle cells may be promoted by metabolic disorders such as diabetes mellitus or glycogen storage diseases. The latter disorders are of genetic origin. The heritable deficiency of a specific enzyme brings about accumulation of abnormal amounts of glycogen. Coagulation or denaturation of cytoplasmic proteins occurs in the hyaline degeneration characteristic of the muscle fibres of patients with typhoid or diphtheria.

ATROPHY AND DEGENERATION

Causes of atrophy and degeneration

Cells may adapt to an adverse environment by loss or shrinkage of cell substance. This is referred to as atrophy. Decreased size of cells consequently decreases the size of the affected organ. In its early stages atrophy constitutes a decrease in cell size alone whereas in later stages cell loss may also occur. Atrophy occurs in response to a decreased workload, disuse, a diminished blood supply, the loss of nerve supply, decreased hormonal stimulation or malnutrition. On proper restimulation the tissues should return to normal size or undergo hypertrophy.

Atrophy of muscle cells may be caused by the immobilization of muscles (in a cast for example) or by injury to a nerve that supplies a muscle. There is a reduction in the number of filaments and mitochondria and in the amount of sarcoplasmic reticulum. These events may be prevented or retarded by frequent mild electrical stimulation of the muscles. Atrophy due to decreased use is directly related to the principle that catabolic and anabolic processes balance each other. A reduction in catabolic processes leads to a reduction in anabolic processes and thus to a reduction in cell size and available cellular energy. Atrophy and eventual destruction of muscle cells may be brought about by diseases such as muscular dystrophy. Several forms of muscular dystrophy are recognized, all are inherited. The most common is Duchenne muscular dystrophy which is usually diagnosed in young males. Muscular degeneration begins in the area of the pelvic girdle spreading to the legs, abdomen and spine and resulting in death in early adulthood. Other less debilitating forms of the disease are diagnosed in adolescence or adulthood. The mechanism of the cell degeneration caused by the inherited genetic defect is unknown. It is suspected that the fault may lie in the absence or impaired functioning of one or more enzymes. Microscopic examination reveals that the dystrophic muscle tissue degenerates and is replaced by fat and connective tissue.

Atrophy and involution of many structures are general characteristics of ageing. After adolescence, cell division persists in most parts of the body to maintain the tissues and organs in a steady state as regards numbers. With the onset of the ageing process, cell division fails to keep up with cell death and a phase of negative growth begins (Sinclair, 1978).

Cellular changes

At the cellular level degenerative changes are more apparent in permanent cells, i.e. cells from highly specialized tissue; nerve cells, myocardium and sensory cells. These cells do not undergo cell division. The changes essentially involve an alteration in size, shape and number of cellular components with age.

Accumulation of lipofuscin

The most widely observed cellular change associated with the ageing process is the progressive accumulation of lipofuscin granules in certain cells of the body (Wilcox, 1959). These brown granules, which have also been called age pigment or 'wear and tear' pigment (Brody & Vijayashankar, 1977), are autofluorescent and increase with ageing. They are found in a variety of both dividing and non-dividing cells: myocardial cells, spleen cells, liver cells, adrenal glands, seminal vesicles, corpus luteum, prostate, interstitial cells of testes and nerve cells (Brody & Vijayashankar, 1977). Because of the apparent universal occurrence of lipofuscin in phylogeny (Timiras, 1972) and its progressive and irreversible accumulation in postmitotic cells, this process has been proposed as a 'basic law' of cellular ageing.

No single histochemical technique has yet been found to identify this pigment, indicating the heterogeneity of its chemical makeup. It has been observed, however, that ageing pigment contains lipid, carbohydrate and protein with the amino acids arginine, tryptophan, histidine, lysine, cysteine and cystine being present.

Many of the cytoplasmic organelles have been implicated as the originators of lipofuscin. These include lysosomes, mitochondria, endoplasmic reticulum and Golgi apparatus (Brody & Vijayashankar, 1977). Pallis et al (1967), in their study of diffuse lipofuscinosis of the central nervous system, observed the lipofuscin pigments to be the sites of acid phosphatase activity thus providing strong evidence of a lysosomal origin. This is further supported by the work of Brunk & Ericsson (1972) on neurons in rat cerebral cortex. On balance the evidence accumulated thus far appears to support a lysosomal origin for lipofuscin (Brody & Vijayashankar, 1977).

The biological implications of lipofuscin have not yet been resolved, as it is not known whether the pigment is a causative factor in ageing or the result of ageing. The fact that lipofuscin granules can be experimentally induced and modified by drugs, antioxidants, hormones and immunoregulation, suggests that the pigment may represent a harmless by-product of cellular metabolism (Kormendy & Bender, 1971). Zeman (1971) has produced evidence to indicate that the presence of lipofuscin in residual bodies does not impair the function of the cell unless it is present in enormous proportions. In effect it is not currently known what, if any, effect lipofuscin has on the cell, only that it tends to accumulate with age (Brody & Vijayashankar, 1977).

Genetic changes

Degenerative cytogenetic changes also take place with age. Jacobs et al (1961) examined peripheral leucocyte cultures from individuals aged 1–82 years. They found a significant increase in both hyperdiploidy (more than 46 chromosomes per cell) and hypodiploidy (less than 46 chromosomes) as a function of increasing age. The percentage of hypodiploid cells increased from 3.02% in the 5–14 age group to 9.54% in those aged 65 years or more.

The concept that ageing may be a result of the accumulation of somatic mutations has been prevalent among geneticists for a long time. This is supported by the clear association between mutation and cancer described earlier. The occurrence of cancer increases logarithmically with age in man and laboratory animals. If somatic mutations can account for the age associated increase in the incidence of this disease, a relationship between somatic mutation and ageing itself seems logical.

The genetic material (DNA) of most somatic cells is not under constant renewal. If one excludes cells in the digestive tract, the skin, spermatogonial cells and haemopoietic tissue, the DNA of somatic cells is replicated rarely, if at all. As examples, liver cells only divide in response to stress, whereas neurons cannot divide after development in youth. Thus, by far the greater part of a person's DNA is as old as the individual and has time equivalent to the person's age in which to suffer and accumulate damage, some of which will inevitably result in mutations. This is in contrast with the intracellular constituents, most of which are constantly being renewed. Ribosomes, for example, are replaced in the mouse over 100 times during the average lifespan (Hirsch, 1979). Most proteins (including enzymes) are constantly being resynthesized to form new materials, therefore protein damage is unlikely to have lasting effects.

Somatic mutation theory of ageing. The somatic mutation theory of ageing is supported by the observations of Curtis (1966) that there is an increase in the frequency of chromosomal aberrations in liver tissue with age. The increase is linear, with the frequency of cells bearing aberrations reaching about 20% by the end of the lifespan in mammalian species. The rate of increase is slower in long-lived as compared to short-lived species.

Curtis (1966) suggests that mutations in 'fixed' cells with little or no cell division are likely to be much more significant in the ageing process than mutations in cells which are continually proliferating. Wherever there is a rapid turnover of cells, mutants, which are usually less efficient than normal cells, will be selected against and eventually eliminated. As an example there is an exceedingly low frequency of carcinoma of the small intestine, where the lining epithelial cells are constantly renewed. The same is true of the erythroid cell line. Burnet (1974) points out, however, that in both of the above cases the mature functional cell has lost the capacity to divide. The situation is different when epithelial cells exposed to the environment are themselves constantly replacing dead cells and repairing damaged regions. It is in such situations that carcinomas are most likely to arise as in, for example, bronchial mucosa, exposed areas of skin, and in the large bowel and rectum.

Tissue culture studies have also tended to support the somatic mutational theory of ageing. Hayflick (1965) reported on the serial culture of fibroblasts from human embryo lungs. Using optimal culture conditions, these cells continue to proliferate during successive transfers to new medium, and retain the normal diploid chromosome number of 46 chromosomes. However, as the cultures tend towards 50 cell generations (doublings) from the time of their establishment, mitosis becomes irregular and proliferation ceases. Why does mitosis fail? The most widely accepted explanation has its origin in Orgel's concept of error catastrophe (Orgel, 1963). Orgel's model predicts that senescence occurs as a result of mistakes in transcription of DNA into RNA or translation of RNA into protein, or both. The processes of DNA replication and transcription and translation of the 'genetic message' into protein are genetically controlled. The genes in question obviously control the enzymes that ensure accurate synthesis of DNA and the messenger RNA which carries the genetic message from the DNA to the protein synthesizing machinery of the cell. One can readily imagine that, with age, an increasing proportion of the cells of the body will carry a mutation in their DNA. Occasionally the mutation will involve a gene responsible for accurate DNA replication or protein synthesis. This in turn will lead to more mutations. This process of error producing more errors will go on until it cascades into a lethal error catastrophe (Burnet, 1980). At this point so many enzymes are either inactive or faulty that the cell to which they belong is no longer viable. One can readily imagine that such a process occurring in a living person will lead to the death of that individual through the progressive inefficiency and degeneration of the body systems in general and, perhaps, the immune system in particular.

Changes in the immune system

Tissue degeneration may be induced by changes in the body's immune system leading to autoimmunity. The precise sequence of events preceding the production of self-reactive immune effector cells and antibodies is not fully understood. Autoimmunity may reflect a decrease in immune suppressive pathways or the activation of immune responsiveness. (Hallgren et al, 1978). On the other hand, autoimmunity may reflect an inability of the immune system to recognize 'self' antigens due to alteration of the genetic determinants on tissue cells. This alteration might be brought about by a virus. In multiple sclerosis, for example, the myelin sheath is gradually destroyed and replaced by sclerotic plaques which block the transmission of nervous impulses. Rheumatoid arthritis may also be an autoimmune disease in which antibodies are synthesized against an antigen of unknown origin. Antigen–antibody complexes are then deposited in joints and inflammatory processes ensue. The incidence of autoimmune disease increases with age and is common in immuno-deficient individuals.

Central nervous system

Negative growth first shows itself in the progressive cell loss in the central nervous system. This becomes apparent in early middle age although it begins much earlier (hearing ability reaches a peak at the age of 10). The other special senses also deteriorate with age, e.g. the senses of smell and vision. Speech slows down and memory deteriorates, particularly with regard to recently acquired knowledge. This is accompanied by a gradual reduction in the size of the brain with deeper and wider fissuring, so that in old age the brain may weigh up to 10% less than in youth.

After the age of 30 years there is a progressive decrease in the number of fibres in the dorsal roots of the spinal nerves and increasing atrophy in the spinal cord and posterior root ganglia. There is also a deterioration in the peripheral nervous system with age, though not so pronounced as in the central nervous system. There is, for example, a decrease in the maximum speed of nerve conduction in large trunks such as the median and musculocutaneous nerves (Sinclair, 1978).

Connective tissue

Another feature of ageing is an increase in atrophy and wrinkling of the skin and liability to fracture at the hip. These arise from a reduction in the quality and amount of connective tissue. Connective tissue is composed of cellular and extracellular phases and functions as a support for the whole body in the form of fibrous tissue and, as appropriate, in the form of tendons and joint ligaments. Connective tissue is predominantly made up of two tough proteins, namely collagen and elastin. Both of these proteins are synthesized by fibroblasts which also form them into fibres. Collagen and elastin are similar in amino acid composition in that they both contain about one-third glycine and 11–18% proline residues. Collagen is, however, the more abundant of the two and more is known about how it changes with age.

Collagen is the most abundant protein in the body, constituting 25– 33% of the total protein and therefore about 6% of total body weight (White et al, 1978). At least four unique forms of collagen are normally found in specific body tissues, differing from one another in the amino acid content of the constituent chains (called tropocollagen). Type I collagen is made up of two different chains called $\alpha I(I)$ and $\alpha 2$, and its subunit structure is $[\alpha I(I)_2\alpha 2]$. The other three forms of collagen each contain three identical chains, designated $\alpha I(II)$, $\alpha I(III)$, and $\alpha I(IV)$. In all the five types of chains glycine is found at every third residue, except near the NH_2 and COOH terminal ends.

The constituent chains of collagen are synthesized as a higher molecular weight precursor called procollagen. Five enzymatic processes are needed to make the preliminary procollagen and three more to complete fibre formation with cross-linking and hydrogen bonding between the chains. Many additional processes are involved in ensuring that the fibres are laid down properly in order to cope with local stresses, and this must involve movement and proliferation of collagen–producing fibroblasts (Burnet, 1980).

When collagen fibres from old individuals are compared with those from younger members of the population, it can be seen that there is an increase in the frequency of covalent cross-links between the tropocollagen chains in the aged, resulting in increased 'crystallinity' and greater contraction on heating. As stated earlier, the formation of a certain number of cross–links during the period of fibre formation is a normal process. As the individual ages it is continued either spontaneously or under the influence of certain products of metabolism, e.g. aldehydes and free radicals. It is chiefly the increase in these cross-links that is responsible for the inactivation of collagen (Balazs, 1977). In addition to cross-links, characteristic changes occurring in the structure of collagen include an increase in the hydroxyproline ratio and calcification of fibres. There is also a change in the ratio between protein and mucopolysaccharide components. Due to structural changes in collagen there are increases in collagen solubility, in its swelling properties and in its elasticity. Subsequently the fibres become stronger and the replacement procedures correspondingly decrease (Hall, 1978).

The elastic elements of connective tissue are the so-called elastic fibres, which contain the macromolecular complex, elastin. Elastin also shows changes with ageing that are somewhat similar to those found in collagen. Elastic fibres that have been produced during embryonic or early postnatal life undergo chemical alterations later in life. The most significant change is in the formation of cross-links. Up to 30 out of 47 lysine residues per 1000 amino acid residues undergo changes during maturation. The exact

Table 6.1 Physiological changes with age (after McKenna, 1982).

Function	Function at 80 years of age in males (% of function at age 30 years)
Cardiac output	65
Basal metabolic rate	85
Nervous conduction velocity	90
Renal plasma flow	45
Blood pressure	
systolic	115
diastolic	104
Handgrip strength	65
Creatinine excretion (mg/24h)	65

Table 6.2 Changes in serum chemistry with age (after McKenna, 1982)

Substance	% change (↓ lowered, ↑ raised) between ages 20–29 and 60–69 years in males
Albumin concentration	↓ 10
Urea nitrogen concentration	↑ 16 – 22
Creatinine concentration	↑ 4 – 7
Fasting glucose	↑ 5 – 9
Blood potassium	↑ 3.3 – 10.0
Total blood protein	↓ 3.6 – 3.8
Alkaline phosphatase	↑ 8 – 14
Lactate dehydrogenase	↑ 9

mechanism of these changes is not yet clear (Balazs, 1977). Gallop et al (1974) suggest that ome oxidation–reduction carrier systems may play a major role.

Physiological processes

The degenerative cellular and tissue changes associated with the ageing process are reflected in changes in many of the physiological processes necessary for life. Table 6.1 lists some of the changes which occur between the ages of 30 and 80. These are average figures and some 80 year olds have physiological functionality close to that of much younger men.

Changes in serum chemistry also occur as people grow older. Some observed changes are listed in Table 6.2. It can be seen that some serum substances increase in concentration while others decline. Although creatinine blood levels show a small but significant increase with age, creatinine clearance values decline with age (22% between the ages 25–34 and 65–74) (Rowe et al, 1976). Mean cholesterol levels in the blood show more than a 35% increase in American males between the ages of 20 and 60, although there is a small decline in concentration after the age of 60 (McKenna, 1982).

The relative quantities of body constituents also change (Bakerman, 1969). Body water content decreases with age. At birth, water makes up about 75% of total body weight. This value drops by the end of the first year to 65%. At age 25, water accounts for about 61% of body weight (Brozek, 1954) and falls further to 53% by age 70 (Fryer, 1962). The decrease in the proportion of body weight taken up by water is accounted for in part by the increase in the percentage of fat in the body from 14% at age 25 (Brozek, 1954) to 30% at age 70 (Fryer, 1962). Corresponding with the increase in fat concentration is a decrease in lean body mass with age.

Perhaps the most significant age-associated change in the relative composition of the body is that of cell solids, which decrease from a value of 19% total body weight at 25 (Brozek, 1954) to 12% at 70 (Fryer, 1962). Protein is the main component of cell solids, and the age-associated change in protein can be partially explained by the decrease in muscle mass, as muscle accounts for over 16% of body protein (Bakerman, 1969).

CONCLUSION

In conclusion, it may be seen that any damage or alteration in the elegant structural and functional arrangement of the human cell may be fundamental to the genesis of complex and often poorly-understood disease and ageing processes in the body as a whole.

REFERENCES

Alberts B, Bray D, Lewis J, Ralf M, Roberts K, Watson J D 1983 Molecular biology of the cell. Garland Publishing, New York

Ashall F, Bramwell M E, Harris H 1982 A new marker for human cancer cells. 1. The Ca antigen and the Ca 1 antibody. Lancet 8288: 1–6

Bakerman S 1969 Ageing life processes. Thomas, Springfield

Balazs E A 1977 Intercellular matrix of connective tissue. In: Finch C E, Hayflick, L (eds) Handbook of the biology of ageing. Van Nostrand Reinhold, New York

Brody H, Vijayashankar N 1977 Anatomical changes in the nervous system. In: Finch C. E. Hayflick, L (eds) Handbook of ageing. Van Nostrand Reinhold, New York

Brozek J 1954 Measurement of body components in nutritional research. Department of the Army, Office Quartermaster General

Brunk U, Ericsson J L E 1972 Electron microscopical studies on the rat brain neurons. Localization of acid phosphatase and mode of formation of lipofuscin bodies. Journal of Ultrastructural Research 38: 1–15

Burnet F M 1974 Intrinsic mutagenesis: a genetic approach to ageing. MTP Press, Lancaster

Burnet F M 1980 Endurance of life: the implications of genetics for human life. Cambridge University Press, Cambridge

Curtis H J 1966 Biological mechanisms of ageing. Thomas, Springfield

De Groot L J, Stanbury J B 1975 The thyroid and its diseases. Wiley, New York

Dillman R O, Royston I 1984 Applications of monoclonal antibodies in cancer therapy. British Medical Bulletin 40: 240–246

Forman D, Rowley J 1982 Chromosomes and cancer. Nature 300: 403–404

Fryer, J H 1962 Study of body composition in men aged 60 and over. In: Shock N W (ed) Biological aspects of aging. Columbia University Press, New York

Gallop P M, Paz M A, Pereyera B, Blumenfeld O O 1974 The maturation of connective tissue proteins. Israel Journal of Chemistry 12: 305–307

Gilbert E F, Huntington R W 1978 An introduction to pathology. Oxford University Press, New York

Groer M E, Shekleton M E 1979 Basic pathophysiology — a conceptual approach. C V Mosby, St Louis

Hall D 1978 Metabolic and structural aspects of aging. In: Brocklehurst J C (ed) Textbook of geriatric medicine and gerontology. Churchill Livingstone, Edinburgh

Hallgren H M, Kersey J H, Dubey D P, Yunis E J 1978 Lymphocyte subsets and integrated immune function in ageing humans. Clinical Immunology and Immunopathology 10: 65–78

Hayflick L 1965 The limited in vitro lifetime of human diploid cell strains. Experimental Cell Research 37: 614–636

Hirsch G P 1979 Somatic mutations and aging. In: Schneider E (ed) The genetics of aging. Plenum Press, New York

Jacobs P A, Court Brown W M, Doll R 1961 Distribution of human chromosome counts in relation to age. Nature 191: 1178–1180

Jungmann R A, Kelley D C, Miles M F, Milkowski D M 1983 Cyclic AMP regulation of lactate dehydrogenase. Journal of Biological Chemistry 258: 5312–5318

Kirchner H 1984 Immunologic surveillance and human papillomaviruses. Immunology Today 5: 272–276

Kirsch I R, Morton C C, Nakahara K, Leder P 1982 Human immunoglobulin heavy chain genes map to a region of translocations in malignant B lymphocytes. Science 216: 301–303

Knudson A G 1975 Genetics of human cancer. Genetics 79 (suppl): 305– 316

Kohler G, Milstein C S 1975 Continuous cultures of fused cells secreting antibody of predefined specificity. Nature 256: 495–497

Kormendy C G, Bender A D 1971 Chemical interference with ageing. Gerontologia 77: 52–64

Levan A, Levan G, Mitelman F 1977 Chromosomes and cancer. Hereditas 86: 15–29

Manolova Y, Manolov G, Kieler J, Levan A, Klein G 1979 Genesis of the 149+ marker in Burkitt's lymphoma. Hereditas 90: 5–10

McElroy W D, Glass B (eds) 1958 The chemical basis of development. Johns Hopkins University Press, Baltimore

McCann J, Choi E, Yamasaki E, Ames B N 1975 Detection of carcinogens as mutagens in the salmonella/microsome test: assay of 300 chemicals. Proceedings of the National Academy of Sciences (USA) 72: 5135–5139

McGee J O'D, Woods J C, Ashall F, Bramwell M E, Harris H 1982 A new marker for human cancer cells. 2. Immunohistochemical detection of the Ca antigen in human tissues with the Ca l antibody. Lancet 8288: 7–10

McKenna P G 1982 The biology of ageing. 1. A gradual process. Nursing Mirror 155(1): 20–22

McKenna P G 1983 Genetics and cancer — a review. Irish Medical Journal 76: 359–363

Mehlman M, Hanson R (eds) 1974 Control processes in neoplasia. Academic Press, New York

Mintz B, Illmensee K 1975 Normal genetically mosaic mice produced from malignant teratocarcinoma cells. Proceedings of the National Academy of Sciences (USA) 73: 3585–3589

Neel J V 1971 Familial factors in adenocarcinoma of the colon. Cancer 28: 46–50

Nowell P C, Hungerford D A 1960 A minute chromosome in human CML. Science 132: 1497

Orgel L E 1963 The maintenance of the accuracy of protein synthesis and its relevance to ageing. Proceedings of the National Academy of Sciences (USA) 49: 517–521

Pallis C A, Duckett S, Pearse A G E 1967 Diffuse lipofuscinosis of the central nervous system. Neurology 17: 381–394

Pardee A B, Dubrow R, Hamlin J L Kletzien R F 1978 Animal cell cycle. Annual Review of Biochemistry 47: 715–750

Penn I 1984 Depressed immunity and skin cancer. Immunology Today 5:291–293

Playfair J H L, Taverne J, Matthews N 1984 What is tumour necrosis factor really for? Immunology Today 5: 165–167

Purtilo D T 1978 A survey of human diseases. Addison-Wesley, California

Reddy E P, Reynolds R K, Santos E, Barbacid M 1982 A point mutation is responsible for the acquisition of transforming properties by the T24 human bladder carcinoma oncogene. Nature 300: 149–152

Roitt I 1977 Essential immunology, 3rd edn. Blackwell Scientific, Oxford

Rowe J W, Andres R, Tobin J D, Norris A H, Shock N W 1976 The effect of age on creatinine clearance in man: a cross-sectional and longitudinal study. Journal of Gerontology. 31: 155–163

Ruddon R W 1981 Cancer biology. Oxford University Press, Oxford

Sandberg A A 1981 Chromosome changes in the lymphomas. Human Pathology 12:531–540

Sikora K, Smedley H, Thorpe P 1984 Tumour imaging and drug targeting. British Medical Bulletin 40: 233–239

Sikora K, Smedley H, Thorpe P 1984 Tumour imaging and drug targeting. British Medical Bulletin 40: 233–239
Sinclair D 1978 Human growth after birth. Oxford University Press, Oxford
Timiras P S 1972 Degenerative changes in cells. In: Timiras P S (ed) Developmental physiology and ageing. Macmillan, London
Trosko J E, Chang C C 1978 Environmental carcinogenesis. Quarterly Review of Biology 53: 115–141
Wang T, Sheppard J R, Foker J E 1978 Rise and fall of cyclic AMP required for onset of lymphocyte DNA synthesis. Science 201: 155–157
Waterfield M D, Scrace G T, Whittle N, Stroobant P, Johnsson A, Wateson et al 1983 Platelet-derived growth factor is structurally related to the putative transforming protein p 28 515 of simian sarcoma virus. Nature 304: 35–39
White A, Handler P, Smith E L, Hill R L, Lehmann I R 1978 Principles of biochemistry. McGraw–Hill, New York
Wilcox H H 1959 Structural changes in the nervous system related to the process of ageing. In: Birren H E, Imus H A, Windle W F (eds) The process of ageing in the nervous system. Thomas, Springfield
Zeman W 1971 The neuronal ceroid lipofuscinosis – Batten–Vogt syndrome. In: Strehler B H (ed) Advances in gerontological research, vol 3. Academic Press, New York
Ziegler J L 1982 Cancer and the prostaglandins. Current concepts. A Scope publication, Upjohn Ltd, UK

7

The nature and meaning of signs and symptoms

INTRODUCTION

What is it about signs and symptoms within a textbook on nursing the physically ill adult which indicates that we are not dealing with a simple or straightforward set of issues? Health professionals on the whole work on the assumption that when one is sick, one goes and seeks medical advice. But patients have a very different notion, and this relates to their understanding of what constitutes sickness. As the following three sections show, the complexity of ideas about signs and symptoms in relation to health and illness requires separate treatment: a physiological approach, a psychological approach, and finally a sociological approach. Notwithstanding this chapter's analytical separateness, we recognize that real life is less exacting, demonstrating continuous divergence and overlap between the contents of the three sections.

Although signs and symptoms are taken as the first indication of disease before they are actually diagnosed as illnesses, they have to be imbued with meaning to warrant consultation with a doctor. It is not usual to refer all signs and symptoms for medical consideration as Koos' (1954) early study on *The Health of Regionville* clearly shows. Many of the respondents claimed some signs and symptoms of disease which were not considered sufficient to seek expert (medical) advice. Before advice is sought, signs and symptoms have to become invested with types of experience which dictate the taking of a different direction, normally a visit to a doctor or other type of health professional. On the basis of his research Zola (1973) suggests that there is a pattern pinpointing when people will finally make a decision to see a doctor. People will seek medical aid when their persona is no longer able to function in the way that they have taken for granted, in the way that they believe their body and their mind should function. Zola summarized a set of 'non-physiological triggers' which is responsible for a qualitative change in the existing signs and symptoms which lead us to seek medical advice. These are:

- the occurrence of an interpersonal crisis
- perceived interference with social or personal relations
- sanctioning
- perceived interference with vocational or physical activity
- a kind of temporalizing of symptomatology.

On the basis of his study, Zola claims that these particular trigger devices can be related to ethnic groups. While methodological problems suggest that this finding be treated with caution the study nevertheless points to the fact that what eventually persuades people to consult a doctor is not so much a physical deterioration but rather perceived implications of symptoms.

As was pointed out earlier, the analytical separation of these three approaches to treatment is in strong contrast to what actually happens in the real world, and so we would hope that they are not read and digested in isolation from one another. It is worthy of note to consider that irrespective of whether we are dealing with acute or chronic diseases, their signs and symptoms vary not only from type to type but also from period to period. Although we speak of patterns of behaviour, they are not rigid and the same patient might disregard at one time what was differently considered another time. It is really up to the nurse's sensibility and sensitivity to become well-versed and competent in the phenomenon of being ill (Kestenbaum, 1982), and to be able to comprehend and subsequently guide a patient's understanding of his or her own meaning of sickness.

A PHYSIOLOGICAL PERSPECTIVE

When there is a disturbance of normal physiological functioning in the body, the individual generally manifests some abnormal signs and symptoms. Signs and symptoms are simply the terms used to describe the structural and functional changes that accompany disease. A sign is regarded as some objective evidence or physical manifestation of physical (or mental) disturbance which leads to complaints of symptoms on the part of the patient. As such, a symptom is usually a subjective state (e.g. pain, feeling unwell). Thus a sign is what an observer can see for him/herself, whereas a symptom is what the individual subjectively experiences and expresses (Fowler, 1974).

It is not usually possible to observe directly a failing heart or kidney, but signs and symptoms may appear. It follows therefore that signs and symptoms must in some way be a consequence of the underlying pathology or disturbance of function. It is often the presentation of these signs and symptoms that leads to an awareness of illness in the first instance and causes the individual to seek medical attention. Some signs and symptoms such as malaise or nausea are vague in character and, although of significance, give very little information about the precise nature of the illness, for they can be features of many disorders. On the other hand, signs and symptoms may be more specific, e.g. the characteristic nature and distribution of the rash of shingles (*Herpes zoster*) or jaundice associated with liver disease or excessive haemolysis.

Just as the relevance of a particular sign or symptom can be initially obscure, the relationship between signs and symptoms and the underlying pathology is not always obvious. Examples of this include shoulder tip pain with gall bladder disease, or lack of vitamin B_{12} resulting in peripheral neuropathy and presenting as numbness and disordered sensation.

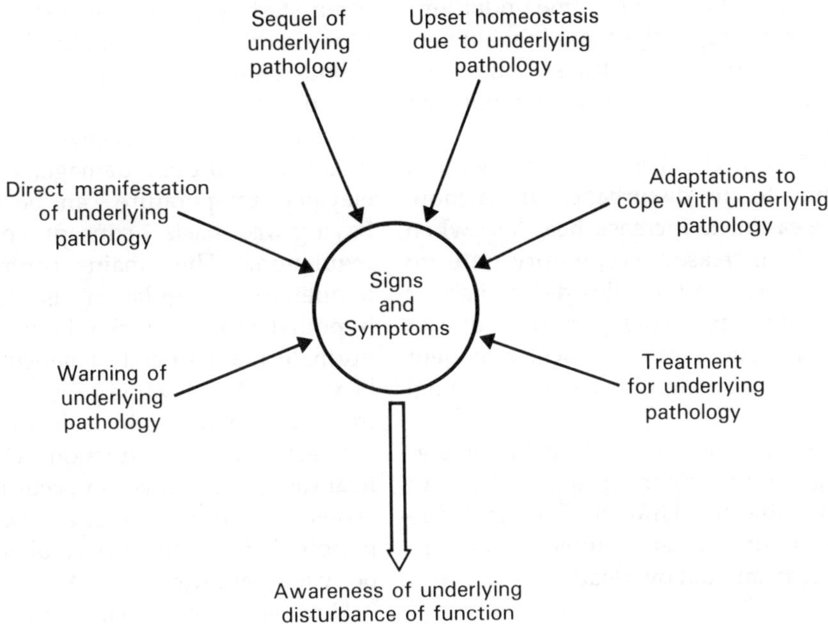

Fig. 7.1 Possible relationships between the signs and symptoms and the underlying disturbance of function (i.e. the pathology).

Although most diseases or illnesses precipitate some form of signs and/or symptoms that make individuals aware of a problem, there are a few disorders that do not. Perhaps the classic example is hypertension. The hypertensive state is defined by statistical norms for age, and is recognized initially only by measurement of blood pressure. At first there are few if any symptoms. Hypertensive retinopathy or left ventricular hypertrophy are complications which in general are indications that the blood pressure has been elevated for some time.

It should also be added that some bodily changes, which in some circumstances are pathological in origin, in other situations are a normal physiological response to some form of activity. An elevated body temperature and sweating are normal responses to exercise, just as constipation is a normal consequence of a diet lacking in fibre and coughing a normal response to the inhalation of irritant gas — smoking!

TYPES OF SIGNS AND SYMPTOMS

As already discussed, the relationship between signs and symptoms and the underlying pathology is not a simple matter of cause and effect. The following groups indicate some of the varying physiological relationships between signs/symptoms and the underlying disturbance (Fig. 7.1):

- a direct manifestation of the disturbance, e.g. a fit in an epileptic, pain in the right iliac fossa with appendicitis, a typical rash of an infectious disease
- the sequel or consequence of the disease process or disturbance of function, e.g. haematemesis and melaena after an upper gastrointestinal bleed, dependent oedema resulting from congestive cardiac failure, fatty stools due to malabsorption disease
- a disturbed homeostatic mechanism, e.g.

an elevated temperature due to an infection, giddiness in postural hypotension
- a warning or indicator of some underlying disturbance, e.g. weight loss in malignant disease, morning stiffness in early rheumatoid arthritis, thirst and polyuria in diabetes
- the body's mechanism for coping with or adapting to the disturbance of function, e.g. sweating to increase heat loss when pyrexial, increased respiratory rate to exhale excess carbon dioxide in diabetic ketoacidosis, pale cold periphery due to vasoconstriction in a shocked patient thereby conserving blood supply to vital organs
- a result of a complication of treatment, e.g. pyrexia and rigor caused by an incompatible blood transfusion, a rash due to sensitivity to an antibiotic, breathlessness from fluid overload.

These categories are by no means mutually exclusive and a particular sign or symptom can often be placed appropriately in several of the categories. However, the categories demonstrate the diversity of the origin of signs and symptoms.

Specific examples

The significance of signs and symptoms lies not in themselves as such, but in the underlying pathophysiology that resulted in the manifestation of the signs and symptoms in the first instance. Thus, it is more important to have a knowledge and understanding of the disease processes that produce the signs and symptoms than to memorize lists of signs and symptoms associated with a particular disease. It is not appropriate to discuss here the numerous signs and symptoms found in different diseases, but it is interesting to consider the possible aetiologies of some of the common signs and symptoms in more detail. As will be shown, the same sign or symptom can be a feature of very different disorders and shows the interactions of body systems in response to disease.

Pyrexia (see also Ch.27)

As indicated earlier, signs and symptoms are often starting points for further investigations. One sign that is commonly observed in hospital is body temperature. An elevated temperature is found in such diverse disease states as thyrotoxicosis, post-myocardial infarction, infections and brain damage. The reason for an elevated temperature can be understood by having a basic concept of temperature regulation. The main control centre for temperature regulation is located in the hypothalamus and the body temperature is normally maintained by balancing heat gain with heat loss. An elevated temperature may result from an increase in cell metabolism, thus increasing heat production without adequate heat dissipation: this can occur in hyperthyroid states or after exercise. Damage to the hypothalamus can also result in an abnormal body temperature.

However, the main cause of a high temperature is infection. Fever does not appear until the infecting organisms have caused an acute inflammatory reaction and cellular necrosis has occurred (hence the link with myocardial infarction). The development of fever is not completely understood, but it is believed that bacterial pyrogens (possibly endotoxin) and/or leucocyte pyrogen produced by dying cells are liberated into the blood stream and eventually reach the temperature regulating centre in the hypothalamus. The pyrogens then 'reset' the internal thermostat so that the set point for the body's core temperature increases above the normal 37°C (Groer & Shekleton, 1979).

Vomiting

Another example to consider is vomiting. The act of vomiting is brought about by a forcible contraction of abdominal muscles, expiration against a closed glottis, a reverse peristaltic wave which originates in the pyloric antrum and relaxation of the cardiac sphincter. The end result is the expulsion of the gastric contents out through the mouth. An increased heart rate, salivation, sweating, faintness and other signs of

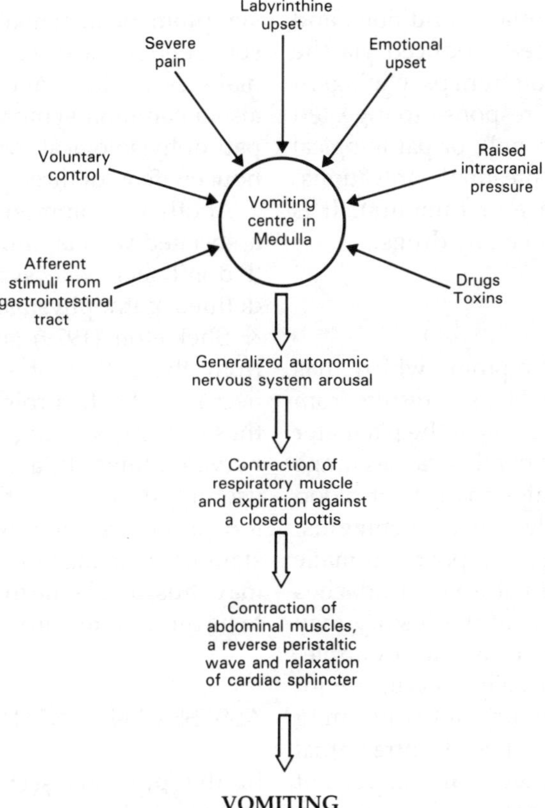

Fig. 7.2 The vomiting reflex.

generalized autonomic nervous system arousal are often associated with vomiting. These events are co-ordinated by the vomiting centre in the medulla of the brain.

As the result is the emptying of the stomach, it is logical that initiation of the vomiting reflex can occur via afferent fibres from the gastrointestinal tract itself, for example, the indulgence in rich and abundant food or ingestion of staphylococcal toxins would set up the vomiting reflex. In these instances the individual would benefit from expulsion of the gastric contents. However, other disorders unconnected with the gastrointestinal tract also result in vomiting. Severe pain, some forms of motion or travel, stimulating receptors in the labyrinth in the inner ear, some cortical and psychic stimuli (emotional upsets, 'nauseating' smells, 'sickening' sights), a raised intracranial pressure and some drugs can all produce the symptoms of nausea and vomiting (Fig. 7.2).

Thus, the initiation of the vomiting reflex occurs by stimulation of the vomiting centre, either directly from afferents from the gastrointestinal tract or via nerve pathways from other areas of the brain, such as the hypothalamus or cerebral cortex. Vomiting could be placed into several of the categories used to describe signs and symptoms.

Diarrhoea

Diarrhoea is another example of a symptom primarily associated with the gastrointestinal tract, and like nausea and vomiting it can have various precipitating factors. The term diarrhoea is usually applied to a condition characterized by the frequent excretion of loose, runny stools. The basic mechanisms underlying the development of diarrhoea are impaired absorption or increased secretion, or a combination of both, within the gastrointestinal tract. The motility of the gut may alter under certain conditions and lead to diarrhoea. Diarrhoea produced via the above mechanisms can result from psychological disturbance (e.g. anxiety), response to ingested irritants (e.g. curry and alcohol), or pathological conditions (e.g. gastrointestinal infections, inflammatory bowel disease or tumours). It is also a common side-effect of many drugs.

Headache

Headache is another symptom which has different aetiologies. The ache itself results from irritation of the sensory endings in the pia mater and the blood vessels. Precipitating causes range from tension, functional disturbances of blood vessels (migraine), hypoglycaemia, meningitis, subarachnoid haemorrhage and post–traumatic concussion. However, the nature of headaches varies, and specific features of the history may give an indication as to the cause, for example, unilateral headaches usually occur with migraine, and headaches worse in the morning are often associated with raised intracranial pressure. This demonstrates an important point — that the precise nature of the sign or symptom does vary and can help define the underlying disturbance of function.

Pain (see also Ch. 9)

The symptom of pain is a common indicator of pathological change where the nature of the pain (e.g. acute, stabbing, nagging, intermittent) and the site of it can be crucial in identifying causation. The classic example is cardiac pain which is typically described as crushing and, after a myocardial infarction, can radiate up into the neck and jaw and down the inner aspect of the left arm (referred pain).

General malaise and lassitude

General malaise and lassitude are non-specific but frequently described symptoms. Lassitude or tiredness is a common presenting symptom in chronic diseases, for example in tuberculosis or malignant neoplasms where it often precedes localized signs and symptoms. It is a cardinal symptom of anaemia and is typically seen in some endocrine diseases including myxoedema, diabetes mellitus and Addison's disease. It is also a common symptom of disturbances not of pathophysiological origin, for example, in a housewife with three young children!

Another common complaint frequently associated with lassitude is general malaise, the 'I don't feel well' syndrome. It has not been defined pathophysiologically. However, Groer & Shekleton (1979) suggest that it may result from the action of substances released from necrotic cells disturbing organs in the body and these changes being detected by the visceral nerve endings. In a sense malaise may serve a useful purpose, as the individual is usually forced to rest, not having the inclination or stamina to engage in normal daily routine. Rest may thus enable the individual's defence system to be directed towards combating the disease.

ASSESSMENT AND INTERPRETATION

In the previous section the physiological or pathological meaning of a few signs and symptoms was considered. The interpretation of the signs and symptoms depends on the nature and characteristics of each sign and symptom, and also the assessment of any associated signs and symptoms.

Observations taken in isolation mean little and can be misleading. A compilation of signs and symptoms that are characteristic of a specific disease state are sometimes grouped together as a syndrome, e.g. Turner's syndrome, Down's syndrome, Stevens–Johnson syndrome.

The significance of signs or symptoms may be different for the patient, the nurse and the doctor (see Fig. 7.3). As already discussed, the presentation of signs and symptoms may be the first indicator to the individual that there is some underlying disturbance of function and may cause them to seek medical attention.

The patient's viewpoint

The patients may be concerned with the intrinsic nastiness (e.g. pain, nausea) or inferred

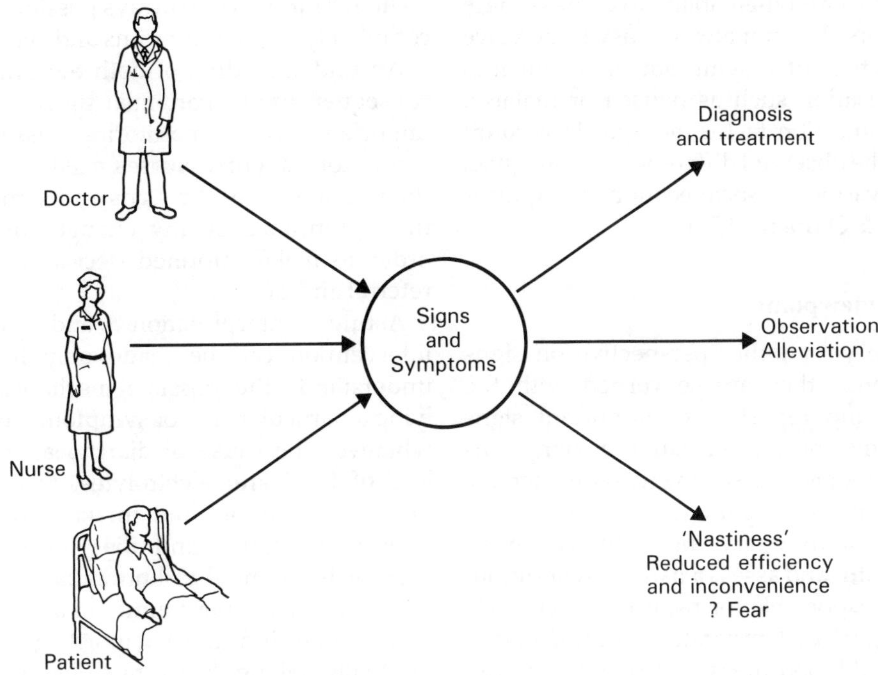

Fig. 7.3 Diagram emphasizing the significance that doctors, nurses and patients may infer from the signs and symptoms

nastiness or threat (e.g. lump in breast or blood in urine) of the symptom. On the other hand, he or she may be more concerned with the inconvenience or reduced efficiency the sign or symptom produces, for instance, breathlessness limiting exercise, back pain preventing lifting. A patient's own interpretation of the significance of a particular sign or symptom is also affected by his or her idea of what is normal or abnormal. An oft-repeated example is that of elderly people who complain of being constipated when they do not have their bowels open every day. Personal experience of illness and that of friends and relatives also modifies an individual's response to a symptom. Symptoms are also influenced by the state of mind of the individual. If he or she is unduly anxious a symptom may be exaggerated, or such symptoms be interpreted as being indicative of life-threatening illness as in the case of a person who considers that his or her 'tension' headaches are due to a brain tumour. The role of anxiety cannot be ignored.

The doctor's viewpoint

On the other hand, doctors are concerned with the interpretation of signs and symptoms in making a diagnosis of the underlying conditon, which then enables them to prescribe the appropriate treatment. Clinical observations, history taking (which includes defining the precise nature and occurrence of signs and symptoms) in combination with laboratory and other special investigations will often lead to the identification of the underlying pathology.

Assessment of clinical signs as observable indicators of disease is relatively more straightforward than interpretation of symptoms which, as has been shown, vary with the individual's perception of the problem. As the nature of any symptom must be communicated by the patient to the doctor or nurse, the wholeness and accuracy of the picture obtained by the doctor or nurse is dependent on a number of factors related to the patient's ability to identify the nature of the sensation, the meaning they attach to it and their ability to express these ideas to others. It is not always easy to perceive the exact nature of a symptom or to put into words a sensation such as nausea or malaise. This communication factor may partly account for some of the observed differences in care given to the various socio-economic groups (Cartwright & O'Brien, 1976).

The nurse's viewpoint

Nurses have yet another perspective on signs and symptoms: they are concerned with the observation and reporting of important signs and symptoms and the alleviation of symptoms whenever possible. Nurses spend a considerable amount of time with patients and so are in a unique position to observe signs, thus enabling them to monitor and assess a patient's condition. Nurses are responsible for recording accurately the 'vital signs' of temperature, pulse, respiratory rate and blood pressure (some would call blood pressure a measurement rather than a sign). In addition, nurses observe the appearance of skin, urinary output, nature of bowel action, amount and character of sputum and any other relevant signs such as neurological observations.

Nurses are also concerned with symptoms expressed by patients and frequently ask 'How are you feeling today?'. Organization of nursing care so that patients are allocated to a particular nurse (as compared with a task allocation system) facilitates more perceptive observation of the signs or symptoms experienced by a particular individual. This must improve the quality of care given.

It is also a primary responsibility of a nurse to try to alleviate unpleasant signs or symptoms whenever possible and to decrease any associated anxiety. Even if it is not possible to treat the cause of the problem it is often possible to alleviate the unpleasant sign or symptom itself (as in administering analgesia for pain relief). The underlying pathophysiology of pain is to some degree understood and this aids the process of treatment or alleviation. In contrast, the patho-physiology of malaise is not understood and there is no real treatment for this feeling. Thus it is not always possible to alleviate completely unpleasant signs and symptoms.

An understanding of both the causation and consequences of a particular sign or symptom is important when monitoring, assessing and caring for patients. Nurses need to understand the importance of the signs and symptoms and the significance of any changes observed, in order to make informed decisions concerning referral and care.

Astute interpretation and appropriate intervention can be made only if the nurse understands the possible mechanisms underlying a particular sign or symptom. For instance, whatever the cause of diarrhoea, the result is loss of fluid and electrolytes, thus the nurse needs to monitor fluid intake and encourage appropriate fluids and diet for replacement. Also, it is essential to know that a rising heart rate of 100 beats per minute in a post-operative patient may indicate haemorrhage, whereas a gradually falling heart rate together with an increasing blood pressure in a patient who has received a head injury are likely signs of rising intracranial pressure.

With an understanding of the relevant pathophysiology, a nurse is more likely to be able to deduce whether a particular symptom or sign is important and routine observations are likely to be more carefully performed if the nurse can interpret their relevance.

Understanding the problems the patient is experiencing also helps the nurse to explain what is happening, and that can be one of the most constructive ways to reassure a patient.

A PSYCHOLOGICAL PERSPECTIVE

A person should not be viewed simply as a biological mechanism with certain body parts to restore. The object and subject of the nurse's concern is a total person, a complex whole, one likely to display both physical and mental experiences. He or she ought to be seen as a self-defining and active individual participating in the complex social relationships involved in an illness situation, in spite of the reality of a biological taxonomy behind physical illness and disease which is often, but not always, evident. By the very nature of total care, the nurse can and should be aware of the possible psychological instigators of physical illness, psychological consequences resulting from physical illness and the extremely close and complex relationship between the physical and psychological aspects of signs and symptoms.

NATURE OF PSYCHOLOGY

Psychology itself is not a unified discipline, nor does it offer a unified model of a person. It has evolved various small-scale conceptual schemes, each of which will determine a framework in which to study the individual.

The purpose of this section is to concentrate mainly on the meanings of signs and symptoms using selective and relevant psychological models. Emphasis will be placed on such models as theories of personality, intelligence and social-psychological approaches. Because of the complexity involved, some detailed information will inevitably be omitted; the reader is therefore advised to refer to the sources of psychological literature recommended throughout this section.

Personality

A brief overview of particular theories of personality will be explored together with some relevant applied research. Psychologists have put forward various definitions of personality. Wright & Taylor (1970) define personality as 'those relatively stable and enduring aspects of the individual which may distinguish him/her from others and which form the basis of our predictions concerning individual behaviour'.

Freudian theory of personality

The intention is to begin with a cursory review of the Freudian theory of personality simply because, regardless of the success or failure of the actual theory, it has had notable influence upon our everyday language and culture, and some of the terms have infiltrated daily discourse. The Freudian theory of personality assumes a connection between aspects of behaviour and repressed material exposed in analysis. Briefly, the mind is held to be comprised of three main parts, id, ego and superego. The id is the biological source of all psychological energy and functions in accordance with the pleasure principle. Because the environment cannot provide instant gratification, the ego develops to optimize the realisation of the id's desires. The ego grows directly from the id but operates independently; it works in order to form a compromise between the id within and the world without (Peck & Whitlow, 1975). In turn, the superego develops from the ego and represents the standards and ethical values which are learned through interaction with others in society. This superego is seen as a 'perfectionist', setting unrealistic standards, and so the ego tempers it (Tomlinson, 1981).

According to Freud, the major personality characteristics originate in early childhood and remain fixed throughout life. Freud was a determinist in both mental and physical aspects of personality, and held that the unconscious mind consisted of desires and wishes which derived their energy from primary physical instincts. Often the unconscious and the conscious mind, the latter being concerned with the external world, are in conflict. This may lead to anxiety. If the anxiety cannot be resolved, the conflict is repressed within the unconscious. According to Freud, repression is one of the important mental defense mechanisms, and psychiatrists, clinical psychologists and others often use it to explain particular aspects of mental disease.

In relation to physical signs and symptoms, interpretations of a person's response to illness may be offered within a Freudian framework. Gyllensköld (1982) for example, in her study of women with breast cancer, identified that women who repressed their knowledge of the lump in their breast delayed going to the doctor. This denial has the potential therefore of seriously affecting the outcome of treatment. Also using the concepts of Freud, Roberts (1976) suggests that denial of the seriousness of myocardial infarction results in patients being overactive, whereas another defence mechanism — regression — is demonstrated by expressed dependence and helplessness.

Although Freud's approach appears to offer some kind of explanation relating to individuals' response to, or apparent interpretation of, signs and symptoms, the notion of mental defence mechanisms remains vague and ill-defined.

The behaviourist view

This view will be discussed briefly, because in one sense it seems to oppose a Freudian analysis. Early behaviourists stressed that habits, rather than being generalized responses with stable and fixed Freudian properties, are learned. The approach, which is utilized within health care systems, emphasizes objective and observable events rather than introspective accounts. The intervening mechanism between the stimulus and response is totally ignored. The behaviourist approach may be appropriate for some types of treatment or particular learning strategies, and relates to social learning theories of personality.

An illness may be stressful, and the response to this experience can be conditioned by the underlying personality. For example, behavioural principles such as reinforcement may well help the individual to moderate and perhaps control chronic pain behaviour.

Trait approaches

Hans Eysenck (1953) supports a 'trait' approach for explanations of personality. According to Eysenck, personality consists of permanent or semi-permanent modes of behaviour which characterize the individual and make him or her different from others (Kristal, 1981). Eysenck calls these individual differences 'traits', and much research has gone into measuring a wide range of traits using questionnaires, self-ratings and observations. Particular personality traits usually correlate with others, giving rise in turn to higher order personality types. Persons can be thought to occupy certain positions along a particular personality type dimension. Eysenck used a statistical procedure, factor analysis, to develop his own type dimensions, one being the extroversion/introversion dimension and the other being an unrelated dimension of emotionality, neuroticism and stability. The extrovert is said to be characterized by traits such as sociability, impulsiveness, venturesomeness, physical activity and talkativeness, whereas introverts seem to display the opposite traits. The Eysenck Personality Inventory (abbreviated to EPI) is often used as an instrument for measuring personality traits in relation to a person's response to illness. Research has indicated that higher scores in neuroticism demonstrate that individuals may have delayed or complicated recovery from surgery (Mathews & Ridgeway, 1981). Further, anti-social behaviour has been seen to be associated more frequently with extroverts, while neurotic behaviour tends to be identified with introverts. However, these generalizations must be treated with caution; behaviour may be more complex than is supposed by trait theorists such as Eysenck.

Measures on the EPI only give an indication or part explanation of the different responses to illness at a given time. Wilson-Barnett (1976) administered EPIs to 202 patients in two hospitals and found that neuroticism was closely related to daily scores of anxiety and depression suffered by patients within a hospital environment. Coleman (1977) cites Bond & Pearson (1969) on individuals' reactions to the symptom of pain. It was found that extroverts had a higher threshold of pain than introverts, and tended to communicate their feelings more readily. These findings may indicate that individuals with particular personality types have different responses towards particular symptoms.

Coping strategies

A hospital is a complex setting in which to study personality, and it is important to bear in mind that staff policy and treatment approaches differ. Likewise, within the wider social situation many external influences interact with personality differences, one such aspect being the individual's coping style. The use of the term 'coping style' relates again to personality types and implies that individuals are thought to have typical ways of managing potentially distressing situations. This may well be relevant to experiences of illness. A classification system has been developed which divides individuals into those preferring vigilant defences and those employing avoidance strategies. Avoiders are thought to have a more benign appraisal of threatening events, and their responses to ambiguous self-reported questions are expected to be more neutral, whereas vigilant subjects are thought to perceive ambiguous stimuli as more threatening (Mathews & Ridgeway, 1981).

Cognitive approaches

It is important to consider not only underlying traits, but also a more cognitive approach to personality. According to Kelly (1963) individuals develop personal constructs: 'These are said to be habitual ways of construing the world based upon hypothesis rather than facts, and which function to help persons categorize and to make sense of their lives'. In other words, Kelly sees the person as a sort of 'proto-scientist'. No two individuals are the same because their construction of the same event will differ, and such constructs are often based upon their own subjective past experiences.

According to Kelly, cognitive processes are involved in thinking, problem-solving and predicting events, and these play an important part in personality development. Each person will view the world through the patterns of constructs, and this relates closely to perceptions of illness and the meaning of signs and symptoms for the person. Kelly developed this repertory grid (Repgrid) technique for measuring these individual constructs.

The application of the Repgrid technique can be useful in understanding how persons construe such bipolar terms as pain/no pain, illness/health, etc. Although constructs cannot be objectively validated they may, in part, indicate to the caring profession how individuals perceive their situation and physical and mental problems.

Psychological theories vary considerably in relation to personality variables, but the point of emphasis lies in the fact that these personality theories can be useful tools in understanding individual differences. Some psychologists have developed sophisticated tests and measuring techniques in order to be more explicit about the differences between persons.

Intelligence

This section attempts a very sketchy overview of aspects of intelligence in relation to signs and symptoms. 'Intelligence' is a concept about which there is much controversy. It can be seen to be both a distinct and a reciprocal aspect of personality. It has been claimed by Eysenck (1953) and others that traits, types and abilities such as intelligence are strongly determined by genetic factors. Eysenck suggests that many people possess specialized verbal, perceptual and spatial abilities which can be measured. Similarly, he held that intelligence is commonly understood to mean a general mental ability which is also measurable. Psychometricians devise tests to measure intelligence, and the rationale behind such action can be traced back to Darwin and Galton who emphasized natural variation and the inheritance of both psychological and physical characteristics. To speak of intelligence as being either genetically or environmentally determined is problematic, not only because such claims are difficult to validate, but because the underlying psychological aspects are complex and interactive. In practice, it may be impossible to distinguish between the effects of nature or nurture on intelligence since the realization of the potential of the genes depends upon the environment in which they operate.

The main concern of this section lies in determining what kind of information about intelligence can be considered useful for understanding people's responses to signs and symptoms. It is obvious that some cognitive ability is necessary for the individual to be able to understand illness and, in turn, to have control over his or her own behaviour and responses. The Wechsler's Adult Intelligence test (Wechsler, 1958) was devised to distinguish between intellectual functions which endure with increasing age and those that do not. Further, psychologists make a distinction between 'fluid' and 'crystallized' mental abilities; the former reflect the inborn potential, and the latter the extent to which experiences and education shape a person's abilities.

It may also be useful and interesting to consider intelligence from a developmental point of view. Piaget's theory of cognitive development makes it clear that a child's understanding of concepts such as illness and health is likely to be different from that of an adult's. The concepts of cause and effect are very complicated in medicine, and it may not be until the age of 9–10 years that the child can understand these ideas and their implications. For example, children may consider illness as some kind of punishment. According to some psychologists, native intelligence (nature) begins to level off at 13 years and is completed by adolescence. The gifted person reaches output peak in the early 30s and steadily declines after this period. Psychometric surveys indicate that from the early 20s there is a steady impairment of functions such as productive thinking, mental speed, attention and memory (Coleman, 1977). It would seem, then, that mental abilities and intelligence deteriorate with age, However, particular experiences (nurture), such as an occupation, may stimulate and develop individual abilities to the extent that they are maintained throughout life, regardless of age. In other words, cognitive changes are not universally related to ageing. The elderly person in hospital can understand the illness and the related signs and symptoms. Impairment to fundamental sensory and perceptual skills does not imply impairment to cognitive functioning. Cognitive disturbance may show increasing incidence with age, but it may be a symptom of physical disease rather than a sign of mental deterioration as such, as dementia due to impaired cerebral circulation is frequently associated with the elderly.

SOCIAL-PSYCHOLOGICAL APPROACHES

Perceptions of illness

Given the fact that there exist wide variations between social–psychological viewpoints, the intention here is to provide a somewhat global review of the perception of illness. For present purposes, the point of interest lies in establishing links between the individual's perceptions, both of social situations and of illness and subsequent response and behaviour, while recognizing that the establishment of causality is indeed problematic.

Social influences encourage individuals to disregard or attend to evidence presented by the senses. As some emphasis is placed upon diversity and similarity between individuals, particular psychological interpretations should not be taken as predictive. Signs and symptoms may be direct manifestations of physical disturbances which in turn involve complex internal analysis by the individual. A person's own theory of illness can be influenced by bodily experiences and information from internal and external sources.

Important consideration lies, then, with the information that the person receives, processes and interprets. When interpretation proves particularly difficult for the person, a search is made for possibilities that are likely to reduce uncertainty (Robinson, 1971). The experience of having symptoms of illness is an example of this tendency. Symptoms may be ambiguous and entail underlying threats to health and life style. Evidence suggests that the difficulty in interpreting symptoms is an important cause of delay in seeking help or medical advice (Kent & Dalgleish, 1983).

Current aspects of research give increasing attention to the interrelationship between social, psychological and physiological determinants of illness. Particular symptoms may have relevance and, as Mechanic (1962) remarks, vague and complex symptoms such as abdominal pain are considered more important than the obvious localized and visible symptoms. It appears that if the former cannot be explained by the person then medical advice is usually sought. Lipowski (1975) also points out that the nature and type of a particular symptom will influence an individual either to ignore it or attend to it. In this case adequate attention may not be forthcoming. Imboden

(1972) indicates that people often deny the onset of invidious or general illness or of impairment, e.g. cognitive impairment or impairment associated with psychiatric disturbances. Cases are also reported where others may recognize changes long before the individual notices alterations. Although certain specific sensations — e.g. bleeding, dyspnoea, or severe pain — will demand our attention, other less serious or non-specific symptoms can be ignored.

In attending to, or interpreting, those sensations, individuals rely heavily on past experiences. Signs and symptoms have meaning therefore only in so far as they fit into a larger context in which past experience plays an important part.

In the absence of specific relevant past experiences, uncertainty can result. Comaroff (1982) observes also how complex aspects of personality and culture are involved in both interpretations and meaning. When Robinson (1971) asked mothers to record the signs and symptoms of illness and the reactions and interpretations of such within the family, the results indicated a considerable degree of uncertainty about the meaning of such events. Mothers themselves adopted a strategy of 'wait and see'. A child might therefore have been feeling quite ill for several days or wet the bed on numerous occasions before a decision was made to visit the doctor. It is only when the signs and symptoms are construed as indications of illness that action is taken. Other research on this aspect relates to patients' perceptions at the time of a myocardial infarction. The results of the interviews showed that, on the whole, alternative explanations of the pain were considered first, and only when the pain had worsened was action taken appropriate to the recognition of myocardial infarction (Kent & Dalgleish, 1983).

Closely related to the importance of interpretation are studies concerned with 'perceived' health. These refer to symptoms held to be serious by the doctor but not necessarily perceived as serious by the patient or other members of the public, or vice versa. For example, Kent & Dalgleish (1983) report how, in one research study, one in five elderly people deemed themselves to be in poor health. The doctors on the other hand perceived their health as perfectly satisfactory. Conversely, two out of three elderly people who were rated by their doctors as not being well gave themselves good reports. Kent & Dalgleish cite a study by Shepherd et al (1966) reporting that only when patients failed to respond to medication and continued to complain, did doctors begin to suspect psychological difficulties. While this may indicate that initially doctors only concern themselves with organic pathologies, it may also suggest a doctor's inclination to believe in stereotypes where failure to respond to medication, coupled with a continuation of complaint, necessarily points to a psychological problem. It has been estimated that approximately 40% of consultations between doctors and patients are based upon a patient presenting physical symptoms as a means of talking to the doctor about more personal matters. The above illustrates individuality and variation between people and the nature of the mediation between symptoms and action by physical, psychological and social factors. The important point lies in understanding that the presentation of symptoms should be seen against the total background of a person's life and relationship with others.

Effect on individuals

Psychologists taking a social psychological perspective emphasize the importance of interpersonal relationships and stress their influence on individual perception. If, for instance, the signs and symptoms affect the 'normal' behaviour of the person, psychological discomfort is evident and the individual may seek medical help. Likewise, help will be sought if signs and symptoms affect 'normal' physical functioning and/or cause any level of disfigurement, in turn affecting the person's self-image. When interviewing people with long-standing physical problems, Zola (1973) noted that they were attending hospital out-patient departments only when their symptoms were beginning to interfere with their 'normal' activities. He claims that people often adjust to their difficulties. Only when coping fails is action taken.

Relationship between physiological disturbance and psychological distress

It is well known that particular illnesses appear to have an intricate relationship with both physiological disturbance and psychological distress. Castelnuovo-Tedescu (1961) noted that certain illnesses with their attendant signs and symptoms were likely to produce emotional reactions, e.g. ulcerative colitis is said to be related to depression. Brown (1950) also pointed out that chronic illnesses can produce feelings of indifference and apathy, particularly in relation to intractable pain. Rogers et al (1979) observe that the release of stress hormones such as corticosteroids can suppress immune responses and therefore increase a person's susceptibility to disease.

All aspects of a person's life can cause stressful situations, ranging from a very demanding occupation to 'crisis' life events (Parkes, 1985). Stress can be described in terms of mechanisms that intervene between the stimulus and response. That is to say, what is considered as stressful for an individual depends on the nature of the intervening mechanism coupled with his or her perception of the social situation. Some factors viewed as a source of stress are conflicts, threats, or challenges. The important point lies in the observation that signs and symptoms experienced by the individual can induce a stressful situation, irrespective of whether stress is caused by 'external' sources, such as family, occupation or illness, or by 'internal' factors such as anxiety, fear or paranoia. Because stress affects both mental and physical health, individual perceptions are important and need to be taken very seriously.

Swift (1962) argues that emotional factors are involved in our perception. He suggests they fall into the following categories: the nature and severity of illness (which includes signs and symptoms), the age of the person, personality, previous experiences, environmental and social factors. Clearly, the perception of illness is complex and the influences upon the individual's interpretation and meanings embrace social-psychological dimensions. One of the central debates in recent years focuses on whether individual behaviour in different situations is more closely tied to personality or more dependent upon the social context.

Essentially, nurses ought to be concerned with making qualitative rather than quantitative assessments, taking into account the physical, psychological and social aspects of the person. What makes us human is individuality; the way each person selects, perceives and interprets information in order to deal with his or her own life. To study this uniqueness, in order to understand the individual person's perception of signs and symptoms of illness and their subsequent responses, is the appropriate focus for the health care professional. Hopefully, psychological knowledge can develop insight, awareness and understanding and hence facilitate better patient care.

A SOCIOLOGICAL PERSPECTIVE

When the nurse meets a patient for the first time, a diagnosis of disease has usually been made by a doctor. It is on the basis of this diagnosis that the patient's ongoing treatment and care is planned. A discussion of the meaning of signs and symptoms to patient, family and health professionals must therefore acknowledge the dominance of medicine in constructing the disease picture and subsequent plan of treatment. It is proposed, therefore, to examine the medical model of disease as a series of dichotomies between signs and symptoms, mind and body. It is suggested that these dichotomies are analagous to the distinction made between disease and illness in the sociological literature and are of relevance to nurses in alerting them to assumptions implicit in how they view the patient and plan nursing care.

It is proposed to examine the way in which meaning will affect response to the presence of signs and symptoms. Since meaning and response are intimately linked, it is suggested that the factors which affect meaning will also affect response. These factors include age, class and gender in differing historical, cultural and social contexts in which the illness episode takes place.

Although the nursing process will not be discussed at length, it is relevant to the present discussion in the following ways. At best, the nursing process not only provides a means of integrating lay and professional meaning in the sign/symptom, disease/illness dichotomy, but also facilitates a departure from a rigid adherence to the medical model. When taking the nursing history, the nurse asks the patient about his or her daily living activities and how they have been affected by illness. In this way, patients' needs and problems may be defined in their own terms, rather than translating them first into a list of medical signs and symptoms. A section in the nursing history about perceptions and expectations of health and the current illness should be used by the nurse to explore with patients the meaning they attach to their present condition.

The nursing process therefore asks nurses to break with at least a semantic dependence on medical definitions, and to beware of substituting for them a new nursing language or jargon. The process should also permit patients to have an opportunity for planning and evaluating their own care, based on how they are experiencing and describing the illness and its treatment (Kratz, 1979).

It is proposed therefore that the ongoing discussion of the meanings of and responses to signs and symptoms for doctors and nurses on the one hand, and patients and their social networks on the other, is fundamental to a more sensitive and effective use of the nursing process in the delivery of care which is truly patient-centred.

THE SOCIAL CONSTRUCTION OF DISEASE AND ILLNESS: MEDICAL AND LAY MODELS

Health professionals (viz. doctors and nurses for the purposes of this discussion) learn as students to recognize disease as an immutable list of signs and symptoms. In this way, diseases such as rheumatoid arthritis or multiple sclerosis, with their attendant treatment and nursing care, become meaningful to the professional. These disease terms, however, also 'implicate a host of social and psychological factors' (Fabrega, 1975) which do not form part of the conventional disease picture. That the patient does have some input into constructing this picture is acknowledged by the traditional dichotomy between signs and symptoms. Signs are what the health professional elicits by observation, clinical examination and investigations such as noting pallor, high blood pressure or abnormal X-ray readings. Symptoms are what the patient complains of, e.g. fatigue, headache or sleeplessness.

Mind-body dichotomy

A further dichotomy in the disease picture is that of mind and body, i.e. physical and psychological signs, symptoms and disease. Wing (1978) considers the distinction to be artificial and 'created by the belief that symptoms should be defined in non-social terms'. He sees no reason why both physical and psychological symptoms should not interact, since all illness behaviour is to a greater or lesser extent learned. Coronary heart disease is given as an example. The cardinal symptom of this disease is chest pain which radiates down the left arm. The doctor, therefore, reaches an initial diagnosis based on the subjective experience of an individual complaining of a primarily psychological symptom, namely that of pain.

It is interesting to note the source of these dichotomies in medicine. The origin of the body-mind dichotomy is Descartes' treatise which 'legitimated the study of the body as mechanism by the science of physiology and preserved the soul as the domain of theology' (Eisenberg, 1977). The development of medical science and technology since the middle of the 19th century has strengthened this dichotomy even further and is similarly reflected in the sign/symptom dichotomy. Foucault (1973) notes that prior to this period 'the sign was not by nature different from the symptoms'. In current medical practice, however, symptoms only become part of the disease picture if they are accompanied by demonstrable physical and biochemical changes. Alternatively, Eisenberg (1977) draws attention to the fact that some signs, such as raised blood pressure, may be detected by a doctor but are of little significance to the individual unless they lead to incapacitating symptoms, such as the breathlessness of heart failure or the paralysis of cerebrovascular accident.

Disease-illness dichotomy

These dichotomies are analagous to the distinction made between disease and illness in the sociological literature. Hence, in this literature the professional is described as viewing signs and symptoms as the biological disturbances, evident during clinical examination, X-rays and laboratory tests, which together constitute a disease. Illness on the other hand, as defined in the sociological literature, is concerned with the patient's own feelings about signs and symptoms as well as how 'his family and his social network perceive, label, explain, valuate and respond to disease' (Kleinman, 1978).

Causality of illness

Developing this theme further, it is apparent from studies carried out in both sociology and anthropology that lay and professional perceptions of health and disease co-exist (Blumhagen, 1980; Illsley, 1980; Taussig, 1980). One important and fundamental difference in perception that is often cited originates from Evans-Pritchard's (1968) study of the Azande. He observed that individuals are preoccupied with why disease affects them at that particular point in time rather than others. The health professional is able to explain the 'how' of the disease, i.e. why changes in the organism produce certain signs and symptoms but not 'why' it has happened to that particular person. It is partly this search for explanation that imbues disease with meaning and transforms it into a significant event for the person and family concerned.

Health professionals need to be aware therefore that the clinical meanings they attach to signs and symptoms are not always synonymous with those of their patients in relation to causality. Comaroff & Maguire (1981) in a study of children with leukaemia described the concern of parents in looking for reasons other than medical explanations for the onset of the disease. The parents focused on a variety of psycho-social causes related to their own biographies and belief systems: 10% of them looked upon their child's leukaemia as 'a punishment for something we've done'.

Interpretation of information

Interpretation of lay meaning, that is, the information supplied by patients and their families, should not be underestimated by health professionals. Parents of handicapped children, for example, often have difficulty in co-operating and communicating with professionals because both parties are interested in different things. The goals of the participating parties may be at variance in that the parents are seeking a cure whereas the professionals, knowing that one does not exist, look for other forms of care.

In the majority of health care settings, information is collected routinely by taking a medical or nursing history through the medium of the interview. Although most medical and nursing courses may teach students how to interview, the training is often limited. Greater emphasis is put on clinical observation and examination, especially for doctors. It is interesting to compare this situation with the development of social research methods where the question of meaning is a key issue. This is particularly important in causal enquiry where the meaning attached to social phenomena by both researchers and subjects needs to be considered when interpreting the data (Menzel, 1978; Brown, 1974). Brown & Harris's work (1975) on depression in women is an example of this. A complex system of interviewing and rating scales was developed to measure the emotional significance which life events had for the respondents, and their subsequent effects in the aetiology and outcome of depressive illness.

FACTORS AFFECTING MEANING AND RESPONSE TO SIGNS AND SYMPTOMS

Cultural and social factors

In discussing this section of the chapter, the paper by Taussig (1980) referred to above is a useful starting point. Signs and symptoms are viewed as 'social as well as physical and biological facts' in relation to their meaning over time and in different cultural and social settings. Health professionals are thus asked to reconsider disease in the light of individual patient differences and social change.

Gender

Figlio (1978), in an historical review of disease in 19th century Britain, claims that not only did the demarcation between physical and psychological illness become apparent, but also that certain disease pictures that have since disappeared reached peak prevalence during this period. Such an example is chlorosis, a form of anaemia described as 'a common feminine disease of adolescence'. The disease seems to have disappeared from the medical literature after 1925. Figlio rejects the possibility that this was a simple case of changing its name.

He introduces another factor, that of gender, into the meaning of and response to signs and symptoms by suggesting that chlorosis reflected the popular view of women at that time as 'naturally frail and prone to disorder'. Anorexia nervosa may be taken as a comparative example which, although it did exist in early medical literature, only became commonly reported during the 1970s (Palmer, 1980). These two examples of predominantly female disorders illustrate the interplay of disease categories constructed by doctors in response to the prevailing social attitudes of each period towards women.

The women's movement has also highlighted the fact that disease pictures are usually constructed by doctors, i.e. members of a male–dominated profession which frequently projects stereotypical female attributes on to how diseases and their attendant signs and symptoms are described and interpreted. Indeed, Ehrenreich & English (1979) state: 'For decades into the twentieth century doctors would continue to view menstruation, pregnancy and menopause as physical diseases and intellectual liabilities. Adolescent girls would still be advised to study less and mature women would be treated indiscriminately to hysterectomies, the modern substitute for ovariotomies'.

Class, position, age

The patients' class, position and age, vis-à-vis the health professionals', are additional factors influencing the meaning of and response to signs and symptoms. The influence of both class and age in affecting meaning and response was demonstrated during interviews recorded by Blaxter & Paterson (1982) in Aberdeen. Two generations of women from social classes IV and V, 'the product of a very disadvantaged social and medical history', considered themselves healthy as long as they could carry on their everyday routines and go to work. They also did not regard as 'illness' those illnesses which they considered occurred as an 'inevitable' ingredient of the life cycle from childhood to senescence. By way of contrast, Herzlich's (1973) study in the 1960s of middle–class Parisians showed that many respondents saw illness not as 'inevitable' but as a reaction to a stressful lifestyle generated by urban living, which they could do something about.

Seeking medical advice

It is important to note that not all people with symptoms seek medical advice. This phenomenon, referred to as the 'iceberg' syndrome, is frequently described in health surveys. For example, a study in a London borough found that during the two weeks prior to interview only 5% of a sample of 2153 respondents were symptom–free. The majority complained of one or more disease symptoms. However, only 32% of those who complained had consulted a doctor (not always in the two weeks prior to interview) and 19% had done nothing at all about their complaints (Wadsworth et al, 1971).

Lay referral

Indeed, the factors influencing people's decisions to visit their doctor are many and complex. The lay referral network of family and friends is often an important determinant in this respect. A study by Suchman (1965) of people in Washington Heights showed that three-quarters of those seeking care had previously discussed their symptoms with others.

Perception of normal

Related factors influencing an individual's decision to seek medical advice include class, culture, age, gender and marital status. Zola (1966), for example, discusses how working-class women regard low-back ache as normal and Mexican-Americans perceive diarrhoea, sweating and coughing as common daily experiences.

It is also well documented that many elderly people do not report ill-health until they are severely incapacitated (Johnson, 1972; Williamson et al, 1978). Part of the reason for this is their belief that growing old is inevitably linked to a decline in health, for which nothing can be done. Their eventual decision to seek medical advice is often based on the degree to which that incapacity interferes with their normal functions, particularly those related to the maintenance of independence.

Lay-professional encounter

Once the potential patient has decided to seek help, the subsequent lay-professional encounter is also influenced by the characteristics of the participants. Most of the sociological literature relates to doctor-patient relationships and little empirical work has been undertaken relating to patient-nurse contact. However, Cartwright's (1976) findings compare with Friedson's (1961) that working-class patients were more likely than middle-class patients to consult nurses during a stay in hospital. However, only a small percentage of the sample (11%) had received their main source of information from nurses and it is possible that most patients, regardless of class, did not consider nurses to be 'appropriate' for this purpose. Cartwright also found that the middle-class patient was more critical of nurses' behaviour than the working-class patient.

In a later study, Cartwright & O'Brien (1976) documented that consultations with doctors took, on average, two minutes longer for a middle-class than a working-class patient. This may reflect the findings in the earlier study that the higher the class the more likely the individual was to 'ask about things rather than being told'.

A similar finding is noted in Comaroff & Maguire's (1981) study referred to above, where doctors are described as being 'explicitly self-critical' about their more frequent use of 'reductions' in the quality and quantity of information given to ' "less-educated" working class families'. As Comaroff & Maguire go on to point out, 'the conceptual structure of medical knowledge translates more readily into terms of everyday middle-class communication'.

AN EXAMPLE — PAIN

By taking the complex symptom of pain, manifest in many disease conditions and originating from a variety of causes, it is possible to examine the interplay of these factors more closely. If no pathological cause can be found, the pain may be termed 'functional' or 'psychosomatic'. Doubt may be thrown on the justification of the individual to be ill at all.

Although it is well documented that different cultural and racial groups respond to pain in different ways (Zborowski; 1952, Zola, 1966), studies of subjective pain experience are few (Fairhurst, 1977). Taussig's (1980) patient, a 49-year-old white working-class woman with a history of multiple admissions over the past 8 years with a diagnosis of polymyositis, voices how she experienced the doctor's response to her pain: 'They don't feel the pain. They give an order what to do but they don't feel the pain. So they really don't know the type of hazard you're going through'.

Hayward's study of pain experienced by hospital patients recounts similar opinions but focuses primarily on nurses (Hayward, 1975). He also examines both lay and nursing attitudes towards the control of pain. By drawing attention to the complex communication patterns within hospitals, he shows how these may actually militate against the patient's meaning of pain. Since analgesia cannot be administered without a doctor's prescription, patients are frequently dependent on nurses for transmitting their need for pain relief. This may result in long delays. One patient who had waited many hours commented, 'I felt angry at being treated in such an off-hand manner when I was in real pain like they thought I was putting it on'. Hayward also observes that drug regimes for pain control often 'deny individual differences between patients' since they are 'routinized'. He further suggests that patients may not admit they are in pain nor nurses offer analgesia, because of the 'fears and misconceptions' that such drugs induce dependence and addiction. Here we have an example of how signs and symptoms can take on contradictory meanings and affect response to the detriment of the patient.

CONCLUSION

In conclusion, signs and symptoms are seen to have different meanings for professional and lay people. Hence these meanings will affect the way in which both professional and lay persons will respond to them and to each other. For the professional, meaning is related to a set of models based on the sign/symptom, mind/body dichotomies. In this way an 'objective' disease picture is constructed seemingly immune from the dynamics of individual patient differences and social change. A corresponding model for treatment and care is developed, based on how the professional views the disease rather than on the person suffering from it. That lay people may have their own meaning which does not correspond to that of the professional is often not acknowledged within medical and nursing circles. The development and use of the nursing process is suggested as a way of integrating lay and professional meanings, at least at the level of planning and evaluating nursing care. By broadening the disease model to include notions of illness, the professional may begin to acknowledge why the symptom is of prime importance to the lay person, irrespective of the presence or absence of the sign. Furthermore, the professional may learn to recognize that the dichotomies inherent in the medical model are socially constructed.

REFERENCES

Blaxter M, Paterson E 1982 Mothers and daughters; a three-dimensional study of health attitudes and behaviour (SSRC – DHSS Studies in deprivation and disadvantages. Ser: 5. Heinemann, London. Also in: Illsley R 1980 Professional or public health. The Nuffield Provincial Hospital Trust, London

Blumhagen D 1980 Hyper-tension — a folk illness with a medical name. Culture Medicine and Psychiatry 4(3): 197–227

Bond M R, Pearson I B 1969 Psychological aspects of pain in women with advanced cancer of the cervix. Journal of Psychosomatic Research 13: 13–19

Brown G W 1974 Sociological research — how seriously do we take it? Inaugural Lecture Bedford College, University of London

Brown G W, Harris T 1975 Social origins of depression. Tavistock, London

Brown J R 1950 Symposium on psychiatry and the general practitioner: the holistic treatment of neurologic diseases. Medical Clinics of North America 34: 1019–1028

Cartwright A 1976 Social class variation in health care and in the nature of general practitioner consultations. Institute for Social Studies in Medical Care (Mimeo), London

Cartwright A, O'Brien M 1976 Social class variations in health care and the nature of general practitioner consultations. In: Stacey M (ed) The sociology of the NHS. Sociological Review Monograph 22. Keele

Castelnuovo-Tedescu P 1961 Depression in patients with physical diseases. Cranbury, Wallace Labs: New Jersey

Coleman C (ed) 1977 Introductory psychology. Textbook for health students. Routledge & Kegan Paul, London

Comaroff H, Maguire P 1981 Ambiguity and the search for meaning — childhood leukaemia in the modern clinical context. Social Science in Medicine 15B: 115–123

Comaroff J 1982 Medicine, symbol and ideology. In: Wright P, Treacher A (eds) The problem of medical knowledge. Edinburgh University Press, Edinburgh

Ehrenreich B, English D 1979 For her own good, 150 years of the experts' advice to women. Pluto Press, London

Eisenberg L 1977 Disease and illness. Culture Medicine and Psychiatry 1: 9–23

Evans–Pritchard E E 1968 Witchcraft, oracles and magic among the Azande. Clarendon, Oxford

Eysenck H J 1953 The structure of human personality. Methuen, London

Fabrega H 1975 The need for an ethnomedical science. Science 189: 969–975

Fairhurst E 1977 On being a patient in an orthopaedic ward –

some thoughts on the definition of the situation. In: Davis A, Horobin G (eds) Medical encounters. Croom Helm, London, p. 159–174

Figlio K 1978 Chlorosis and chronic disease in 19th century Britain — the social constitution of somatic illness in a capitalist society. International Journal of Health Services 8(4): 589–617

Foucault M 1973 The birth of the clinic. Tavistock, London

Fowler P B S 1974 Common symptoms of disease. Blackwell Scientific, Oxford

Freidson E 1961 Patients' views of medical practice. In: Cartwright A 1964 Human relations and hospital care. Routledge & Kegan Paul, London

Groer M E, Shekleton M E 1979 Basic patho–physiology, a conceptual approach. Mosby, St Louis

Gyllensköold K 1982 Breast cancer: the psychological effects of the disease and its treatment. Tavistock, London

Hayward J 1975 Information — a prescription against pain. RCN, London

Herzlich C 1973 Health and illness. Academic Press, London

Illsley R 1980 Health beliefs and health and illness behaviour. In: Professional or public health, Nuffield Provincial Hospital Trust, London

Imboden J B 1972 Psychosocial determinants of recovery. Advances in Psychosomatic Medicine 8: 142–155

Johnson M L 1972 Self–perception of need amongst the elderly: an analysis of illness behaviour. Sociological Review 20: 521–531

Kelly G A 1963 A theory of personality. Norton, New York

Kent G, Dalgleish M 1983 Psychology and medical care. Reinhold, Wokingham

Kestenbaum V 1982 The humanity of the ill. The University of Tennessee Press, Knoxville

Kleinman A 1978 Concepts and a model for the comparison of medical systems as cultural systems. Social Science and Medicine 12: 85–93

Koos E L 1954 The health of Regionville. Columbia University Press, New York

Kratz C R (ed) 1979 The nursing process. Baillière Tindall, London

Kristal L 1981 The ABC of psychology. Pelican, Harmondsworth

Lipowski J 1975 Physical illness, the patient and his environment. Psychosocial foundations of medicine. American Handbook of Psychiatry 4: 1–42

Mathews A, Ridgeway T 1981 Personality and surgical recovery. A review. British Journal of Clinical Psychology 20: 243–260

Mechanic D 1962 The concept of illness behaviour. Journal of Chronic Diseases 15: 189–194

Menzel H 1978 Meaning — who needs it? In: Brenner et al (eds) The social contexts of methods. Croom Helm, London

Palmer R L 1980 Anorexia nervosa, a guide for sufferers and their families. Penguin, Harmondsworth

Parkes K R 1985 Stressful episodes reported by 1st year student nurses. Social Science and Medicine 210(9): 945–953

Peck D, Whitlow D 1975 Approaches to personality theory. Methuen, London

Roberts S L 1976 Behavioural concepts and the critically ill patient. Prentice Hall, Englewood Cliffs

Robinson D 1971 The process of becoming ill. Routledge & Kegan Paul, London

Rogers M P, Dudley D, Reich P 1979 The influence of the psyche and the brain on immunity and disease susceptibility. A critical review. Psychosomatic Medicine 41: 147–164

Shepherd M, Cooper B, Brown A, Kallton J 1966 Psychiatric nursing in general practice. Oxford University Press, London

Suchman E A 1965 Stages of illness and medical care. Journal of Health and Human Behaviour 6: 114–128

Swift N I 1962 Psychological reactions to illness. Psychotherapy 48: 172

Taussig M T 1980 Reification and the consciousness of the patient. Social Science and Medicine 14B: 3–13

Tomlinson P 1981 Understanding teaching — the interactive approach to educational psychology. McGraw–Hill, New York

Wadsworth M E J, Butterfield W J H, Blaney R 1971 Health and sickness: the choice of treatment. Tavistock, London

Wechsler D 1958 The measurement and appraisal of adult intelligence. 4th edn. Baillière, Tindall & Cox, London

Williamson J et al 1978 Old people at home: their unreported needs. In: Carver V, Liddiard P (eds) An ageing population. Hodder and Stoughton, London

Wilson–Barnett J 1976 Patient's emotional reactions to hospitalisation. An exploratory study. Journal of Advanced Nursing 3: 221–229

Wing J K 1978 Reasoning about madness. Oxford University Press, Oxford

Wright D S, Taylor A 1970 Introducing psychology: An experimental approach. Penguin, Harmondsworth

Zborowski M 1952 Cultural components in responses to pain. Journal of Social Issues 8: 16–30

Zola I K 1966 Culture and symptoms — an analysis of patients presenting complaints. In: Cox C, Mead A (eds) 1975 A sociology of medical practice. Collier–Macmillan, London

Zola I K 1973 Pathway to the doctor — from person to patient. Social Science and Medicine 7: 677–689

8

The nature of stress and its relationship with physical illness

INTRODUCTION

There can be little doubt that the development, in this century, of the concept of stress has contributed significantly to current understanding of health and disease. It is now widely recognized (Hinkle, 1973) not only that stress can be a major contributory factor in the aetiology of disease, but also that it can adversely affect the course and outcome of an illness. Cox (1978) has stated that 'stress is a threat to the quality of life and to physical and psychological well-being.'

This chapter discusses the nature of stress and its relationship with physical illness, focusing on theoretical material which has important implications for nursing practice.Chapter 12 examines the alleviation of stress.

As nurses have prolonged day-to-day contact with physically sick people, they are perhaps the best placed of all health care workers to take action which will reduce the likelihood of unnecessary suffering and a prolonged, complicated course to an illness, by preventing or alleviating their patients' experience of stress. Conversely, nurses who lack understanding can unwittingly increase stress levels in their patients. In addition, because of the very nature of the job they do, nurses may themselves become stressed. For these reasons nurses should have a clear understanding of stress and its relationship not only with ill health, but also with everyday life. They require the background knowledge and skills to enable them to accurately assess their patients' experience of stress, plan and carry out appropriate nursing interventions and evaluate the effectiveness of their patient care. Understanding stress is the basis for preventing and alleviating it, and the importance of this aspect of the nurse's role cannot be overemphasized.

APPROACHES TO STRESS

In a general context the word 'stress' is used frequently in relation to human experience, for example, one often hears phrases such as 'he is under stress', or 'this is stressful'. However, difficulties often arise when, in order to enable the term to be used precisely in a scientific and clinical sense, one attempts to define it. The Concise Oxford Dictionary (Sykes, 1982) contains five definitions. The word is derived from the Latin 'strictus', 'to draw tightly together' and, in Middle English, was a shortened form of the word 'distress'. According to the first two definitions in this dictionary, stress is 'a constraining or impelling force', or 'effort and demand on mental energy'. There is also reference to the idea that stress causes disease.

Three main ways of viewing stress emerge from a study of the literature.

STRESS AS A STIMULUS

The word 'stress' is sometimes used to describe a stimulus which gives rise to a stress reaction, or strain, in an object, animal or person. This is the way in which the word is often used in everyday language, for example, 'the stress of overwork'.

The use of the word in this way is a misinterpretation of its precise use in physics and engineering (mechanics), where stress is defined as 'the force per unit area which tends to distort an object'.

The major problem associated with thinking of stress as some force or stimulus outside ourselves lies in the identification of stimuli which are stressful. Man is an animal capable of complex mental activity and behaviour and so there are many variables which can affect whether a stimulus is stressful to an individual. For example, the extent to which identical experiences of exposure to a hot climate, restricted periods of sleep, disco noise or aircraft flight are stressful to different individuals is likely to vary according to their age, physiological constitution, personality and past experience.

As a result of this limitation, the concept of stress as a stimulus is rarely used by biological and social scientists. Despite this, a great deal of research has been carried out in an attempt to identify situations which can reliably be described as stressful. This research will be discussed in a later section since much of it relates to man's cognitive ability to consciously appraise a situation.

STRESS AS A RESPONSE

According to this school of thought, stress can be understood in terms of an animal's or person's response to an environmental demand for adaptation. The presence of stress is, therefore, dependent on a stimulus or stressor. The stress response has physiological and psychological manifestations.

The response based approach has been particularly important in the development of biological concepts of stress. The work of the Canadian doctor and physiologist, Hans Selye is probably the first and major example of such an approach to the study of stress. He published his first major work on the subject in the form of a book entitled *The Stress of Life* in 1956 (a second edition of this book was published in 1976). Selye's biological concept of stress is founded in the work of the French physiologist, Claude Bernard and grew in parallel with that of the American physiologist Walter B. Cannon.

In the latter half of the nineteenth century, Bernard (1927) taught the fundamental physiological principle that one of the most characteristic features of living things is their ability to maintain the constancy of their internal environment, despite changes in their external surroundings. He realized that the extracellular fluid provided the cells of a higher animal with a thermostatically controlled and chemically stable 'milieu intérnale' (internal environment) in which they can function optimally.

Cannon (1932) first referred to the process by which an organism attempts to maintain the constancy of the fluid part of its internal environment as 'homeostasis'. A basic feature of his concept of homeostasis was the recognition that the composition of the internal environment is repeatedly disturbed as a result of the metabolic activities of the animal. The term homeostasis refers to the continual tendency of the internal fluid environment to return towards a steady state after each disturbance. Cannon and other physiologists showed this phenomenon to be due to a complex system of feedback mechanisms and buffers which are an integral part of living organisms.

Cannon (1929 and 1935) also carried out detailed experiments on the reaction of the adrenal medulla and sympathetic nervous system in laboratory animals and humans exposed to conditions such as cold, lack of oxygen and loss of blood. He documented the 'fight and flight' reaction and described his subjects as being 'under stress'.

Against this background, Hans Selye's early work and concept of stress developed.

Hans Selye's stress theory

In 1926, as a young medical student, Selye wondered about the mechanisms which might underlie what he has since called 'the syndrome of just being sick'. The collection of signs and symptoms making up this syndrome include the diagnostically unimportant ones of feeling and looking ill, a coated tongue, fatigue and diffuse aches and pains in the joints. In other words, 'non-specific' features not characteristic of any one disease.

General Adaptation Syndrome

Ten years later, Selye was working as a research assistant on the identification and functions of

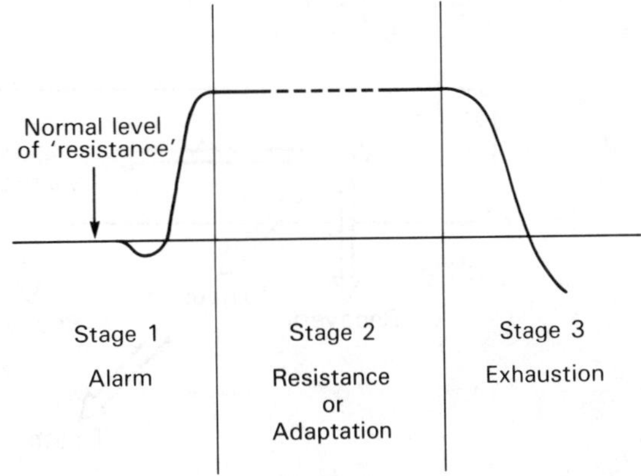

Fig. 8.1 The three phases of the General Adaptation Syndrome (GAS) (Selye, 1956).

ovarian hormones. This research involved injecting rats with extracts of glands of varying degrees of purity. On later postmortem examination he found the following changes, irrespective of the tissue or hormone content he had injected:

- enlargement and hyperactivity of the adrenal cortex
- atrophy (wasting) of the thymus and lymph nodes
- bleeding ulcers in the stomach and duodenum.

The physiological mechanisms associated with these changes are discussed in detail in the section on the physiological response to stress.

Selye then discovered that this syndrome, which he called the General Adaptation Syndrome (Fig. 8.1) could be elicited consistently by many other stimuli; heat, cold, infection, trauma, haemorrhage and even injections of formalin. In fact, he found that the syndrome was produced by any noxious agent he tried. It seemed to be a pattern of response to the fact of injury and perhaps an experimental replica of the clinical syndrome of 'just being sick'.

Stages of the general adaptation syndrome. Selye also found that it was possible to divide the physiological response of his experimental animals to those noxious stimuli into three distinct phases occurring over time. He called the initial response the alarm reaction. In this stage he noticed that stores of hormone in the

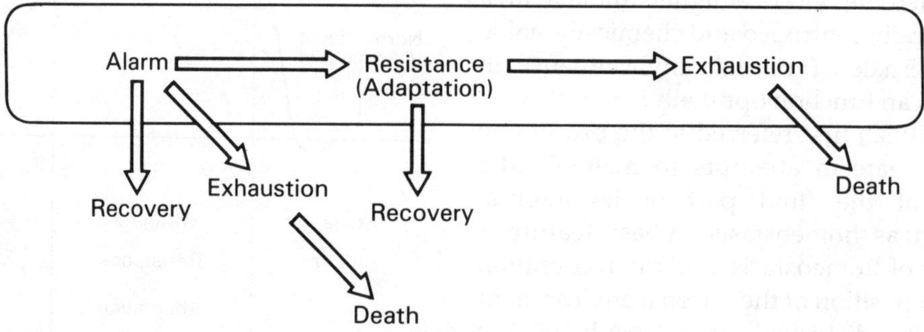

Fig. 8.2 The General Adaptation Syndrome and alternative routes of the response to stress

adrenal cortex were depleted by secretion into the blood. Other features were loss of weight and increased concentration of the blood. No animal could remain in this state for long. Selye viewed it as the expression of a generalized 'call to arms' of the defensive forces in the body. Depending on the intensity of the stressor, the animal either recovered, passed into the second stage, that of resistance or adaptation, or died. The characteristics of the second stage were quite different from those of the first, in that the adrenal cortex accumulated a reserve of hormone and haemodilution and a return to normal body weight occurred. The animal successfully adapted to the effects of the agent to which it was exposed. However, if the effects of the agent were not removed or greatly diminished, the animal eventually entered the third phase, that of exhaustion. The symptoms of this phase were essentially similar to those of the alarm reaction and the animal eventually died. Figure 8.2 illustrates the alternative outcomes.

Meaning of general adaptation syndrome. Selye called the entire response the General Adaptation Syndrome (GAS). He called it 'general' because it was produced only by agents which have a general effect on large portions of the body; 'adaptive' because it stimulated defence and helped in the acquisition and maintenance of a state of habituation; and 'syndrome' because the individual manifestations were co-ordinated and inter-dependent. He postulated that the syndrome was produced by 'non-specific stress' (Selye, 1946). He later (Selye, 1976) defined stress as 'the state manifested by a specific syndrome which consists of all non-specifically induced changes within a biologic system'. Selye emphasized that the state of stress is manifested only by the appearance of this specific syndrome.

By 'non-specifically induced changes', Selye means changes that can be produced by many or all agents, as opposed to specifically caused changes that can be elicited by only one, or a few, agents. For example, a specific effect of infection by the measles virus is the characteristic and diagnostic skin rash, whereas a non-specific effect is simple inflammation which is also produced by any irritant that enters the body.

Selye views the response to stress as the adaptive response of the body to any demand made upon it. He has described (Selye, 1976) it as 'the rate of wear and tear of life'. As such it is part of life itself and cannot be avoided. The effect of a stressor depends on the intensity of the demand it makes on the adaptive capacity of the body. Selye (1976) introduced the term 'eustress' to mean the amount of stress necessary for an active, healthy life and has stated that unpleasant and potentially damaging stress would be more accurately termed 'excessive stress' or 'distress'.

Local adaptation and stress

The three stages of the General Adaptation Syndrome (GAS) reflect the physiological response of the body to stress over time. It is important to distinguish local inflammation (Local Adaptation Syndromes (LAS) Selye, 1956) from the GAS. The defensive inflammatory response of tissue to irritation, for example by local infection by *Staphylococcus aureus* (a boil), represents a local adaptation syndrome. When muscle becomes exhausted after exercise and eyes strained after prolonged reading these are final stages of local adaptation syndromes. If several local adaptation syndromes occur simultaneously, in various parts of the body, they may activate the GAS, which is produced only by agents which have a general effect on large portions of the body.

Diseases of adaptation

Selye (1956) was one of the first research workers to claim that inappropriate stress responses can produce physical diseases. He called these 'diseases of adaptation' and during his years of research has named many disorders, including all psychosomatic disease and conditions of inflammatory and immunological origin as falling into this category.

Later Selye (1974) developed his concept of stress beyond biology and medicine to discuss and propose a code for living. He summarized this code in a short jingle: 'Fight for the highest attainable aim, but do not put up resistance in vain'. According to Selye (1965), the art is to learn how to live a full life with a minimum amount of wear and tear. The secret is not to live less intensely, but more intelligently. Each individual must find his innate stress level and live accordingly.

Alternative views

Selye's very broad concept of stress has been extremely influential and is still used by both biological and behavioural scientists. However, there is now evidence, contrary to Selye's theory, that some noxious physical conditions, for example, heat, fasting and exercise, do not always produce the general adaptation syndrome (Mason, 1971).

There is also evidence that the response to stress does not always have the stereotyped and phylogenetically old pattern described by Selye. The components of the response can vary with the characteristics of the stressor, between species and between individuals. For example, human individuals tend to exhibit characteristic and possibly familial patterns of response to stress. In one person, for example, changes in heart rate and blood pressure may be the predominant features of stress, while in another person changes in breathing pattern may be the most obvious sign of stress (Smith, 1967).

Selye's discussion of the effect of 'conditioning factors' (Selye, 1976) goes some way towards making this evidence compatible with his theory. The reaction of tissues to various stressor agents, he suggests, is affected by conditioning factors. These factors can be internal or external to the body. Internal conditioning factors are those which have become part of the body through heredity and past experiences, particularly those of coping with the stressor. External conditioning factors include the effects of diet, climate and concurrent psychological and social events.

However, in concentrating on the body's physiological response to stressors, Selye has largely ignored the role of psychological processes in stress. There is now a strong movement towards viewing stress as an interactive process in which the physiological response is not directly determined by the actual presence of the stressor, but by its psychological impact on the person.

STRESS AS AN INTERACTION

This essentially psychological approach to understanding stress arose largely because of the limitations of stimulus-response models. It overcomes these limitations in that it enables one to view the person experiencing stress as an active rather than passive entity and as an individual different from any other. This

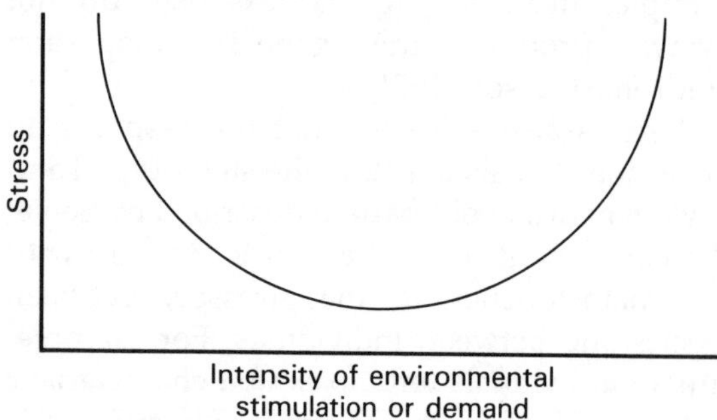

Fig. 8.3 The relationship between the intensity of environmental demand and stress.

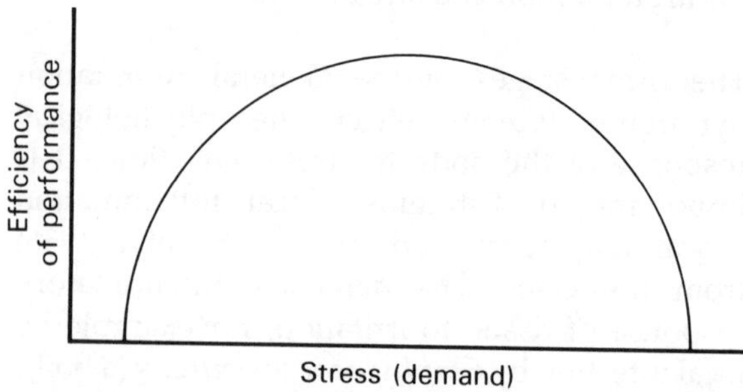

Fig. 8.4 The relationship between stress and efficiency of performance

approach views stress as the reflection of imbalance between the demands of the environment on an individual and that individual's perceived ability to cope with, or adapt to, those demands. Lazarus (1971) pointed out that while both the environmental stimulus and reacting individual are vital elements in stress, it is the nature of the relationship between the two which is crucial. A person's reaction to environmental demand depends on how that person interprets or appraises (consciously or unconsciously) its significance for him. The appraisal of threat is based on a wide range of past and current experiences and expectations and change in any one of these can radically alter perceived interpretation. For example, a man may ignore his chronic smoker's cough, although he has read about the health risks of smoking, until he hears that a friend of his, who also smokes, has been diagnosed as having lung cancer.

This interactive viewpoint allows individual variations in type and level of stress to be attributed to characteristics of the individual. Appley & Trumbull (1967) have described a 'vulnerability profile' made up of such factors as constitution, personality, past experience and motivation.

The concept of environmental demand

Welford (1973) suggested that stress occurs whenever the demand for adaptation made on an organism departs from a moderate level. This idea is important because it illustrates that low levels of demand on an individual can be as stressful as high levels of demand (Fig. 8.3). For example, monotonous production line work in a factory may be as stressful as the highly pressured work of a business executive, and it can be just as stressful for a patient to be isolated in a hospital cubicle as to be in a busy, noisy ward. Clearly, this will depend on each individual's perception of their situation.

It seems too that most organisms, including man, have evolved to produce optimum adaptive performance under conditions of moderate demand (Fig. 8.4). The Yerkes-Dodson Law (Hilgard et al, 1983) states that:

> The optimum level of aversive stimulation in the control of learning is at some moderate intensity, lower and higher values being less effective; the optimum level decreases as task complexity increases.

This general law is an expression of the relationship between demand and performance demonstrated by learning. This concept has many applications in nursing and it is helpful for the nurse to be able to assess whether a patient's or colleague's 'poor' performance is due to their perception of either too little or too much demand on their ability to cope. For example, a newly-diagnosed diabetic may have difficulty in learning how to give him/herself injections of insulin either because he/she has been told that the community nurse could be available to do this (too little demand), or because he/she has not yet sufficiently recovered from the shock of the diagnosis and its implications or has had unpleasant past experience of injections (too much demand).

Situations likely to be stressful

As already mentioned a great deal of research has attempted to identify situations which can reliably be described as stressful to man. Such situations can be viewed in terms of a person's perception of the demand being made on the person by his/her environment. Weitz (1970), Lazarus (1966, 1976) and Frankenhauser (1975a, 1975b) have identified various situations as likely to be stressful. A modified list of these is presented below:

- extremes of environmental stimuli, for example, heat, cold, noise
- disrupted physiological function due, for example, to starvation, disease, injury, drugs, sleep loss
- sensory deprivation, for example, isolation, confinement, underwork
- sensory overload, for example, crowding, overwork
- perceived threat, for example to one's physical survival, sense of identity, values and goals, community life, or resulting from group pressure
- goal frustration
- lack of control over events
- loss, for example of loved ones, or symbolic loss, for example of life expectations when a serious illness is diagnosed
- the need to respond to information being given too rapidly.

Life events. The first systematic attempt to quantify the degree of stress associated with life events was made by Holmes & Rahe (1967). They constructed a scale of 43 life events after asking a sample of 400 people to rate each event according to the length of time and amount of effort involved in adjusting to it. Death of a spouse was consistently rated highest and was given a value (score) of 100. All other events were given proportional values based on this value. For example, retirement ranks tenth and has a proportional value of 45. This scale is known as the Social Readjustment Rating Scale (SRRS) and its use has shown that individuals in the United States, Western Europe and Japan tend to rate life events in almost exactly the same way (Rahe, 1969; Rahe et al, 1971). It should be mentioned, though, that retesting with SRRS has not always produced the same results. One explanation for this is that the events allow too much room for interpretation by the subjects and that subjects' perceptions change with the passage of time.

The SRRS has had some success in establishing a relationship between certain life events and physical ill-health. High scores are associated with a greater risk of illness (Wyler et al, 1971; Rahe, 1969).

Transactional model of stress

Developing the interactionist approach, Cox & Mackay (1976) suggested that stress can best be described as part of a complex system of interaction between man and his environment.

The transactional model of stress proposed by Cox (Fig. 8.5) to some extent meets the requirements that previous models cannot accommodate. His model embodies a mixture of characteristics which are central to an understanding of the concept of stress. Generally, Cox's model describes the dynamic process by which people experience and respond to problems and difficulties encountered.

Stress itself is viewed as an individual phenomenon and is the result of a transaction between the person and his situation (Cox, 1978). The process of transaction refers to the active and adaptive nature of the process.

The basis for Cox's model is the relationship between the individual and the environment. The external environment supplies a certain proportion of the demands and constraints placed upon the individual. The individual's personal resources and capabilities are largely directed towards internal needs according to a personal system of values. These components interact to form a balance or an imbalance within the person.

One of the major characteristics that Cox attempts to explain is the notion of demands made upon the individual by the situation he/she is in and, in turn, his/her ability to meet those demands. The notion of demands relates to satisfaction of needs, where the individual

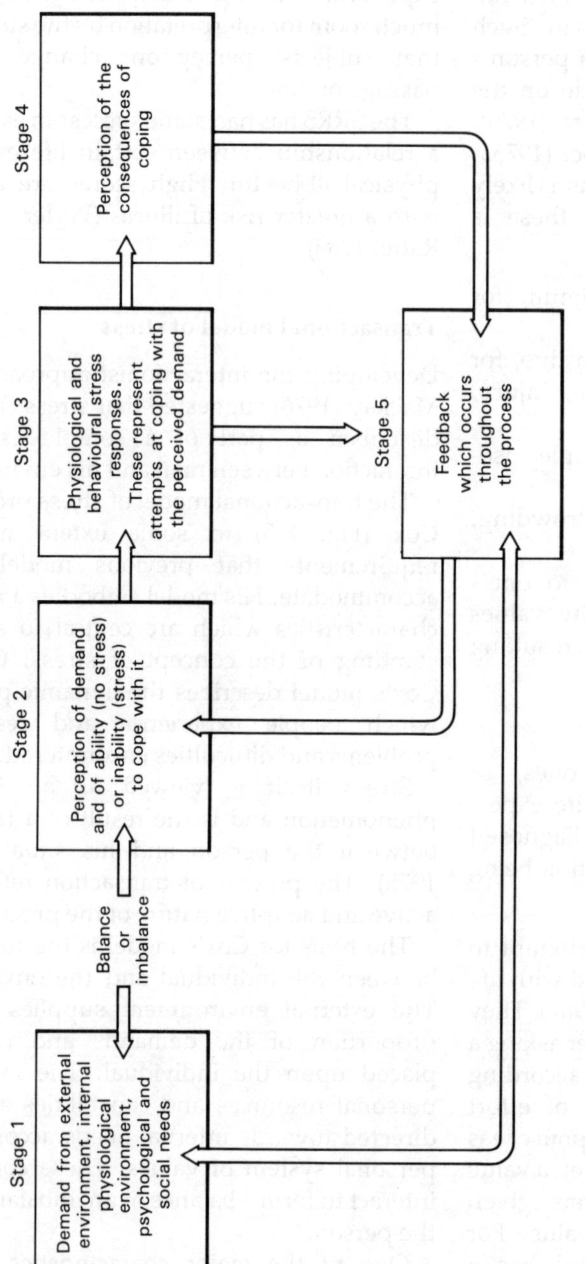
Stage 1
Demand from external environment, internal physiological environment, psychological and social needs
Balance or imbalance
Stage 2
Perception of demand and of ability (no stress) or inability (stress) to cope with it
Stage 3
Physiological and behavioural stress responses. These represent attempts at coping with the perceived demand
Stage 4
Perception of the consequences of coping
Stage 5
Feedback which occurs throughout the process

Fig. 8.5 Diagrammatic representation of stress as part of a complex system of interaction (Cox & Mackay, 1976).

within a given environment may or may not be provided with the opportunity to satisfy those needs. According to Cox the needs are viewed as internally generated demands.

'Demand' in this context denotes the requirement for physical or mental action on the part of the individual, and implies constraints with respect to the time allowed. Cox & Mackay (1976) remark that the perception of time alters with the experiencing of stress and this can affect the balance between perceived demand and perceived capabilities. The person may make use of the rate of change over time of the variables involved in order to evaluate the given situation.

Cox's 'personal resources or capabilities of the person' include not only those skills that relate to dealing with 'demands' but also the general characteristics of personality and learnt behavioural patterns of the individual. Constraints are placed upon the person by his/her situation or by his/her own value system and support given by others.

An integral part of Cox's transactional model are the interactions within and between its different levels and stages. Each of these interactions relies upon the concept of feedback mechanisms which are concerned with returning the individual to a state of balance. Cox refers to coping strategies which involve the use of an individual's psychological resources. The first stage of the coping process is concerned with the selection of appropriate responses and the second stage with the individual's uncertainty concerning his/her decision. It is perhaps the uncertainty which may have unwanted results such as anxiety or panic. It is therefore obvious that the selection and subsequent implementation of coping responses represent skills in themselves. Initiation of coping strategies, and their effect upon the demands, leads to a process of secondary appraisal where imbalance may have been reduced, remained the same or increased.

Cox's model not only emphasizes the individual's experiences; the interactive approach is also clearly emphasized. The transactional model reflects a phenomenological basis in that the agent, i.e. the person, influences both him/herself and the environment, and in turn the environment influences the individual. Stress itself is viewed as an individual phenomenon reflecting idiosyncratic viewpoints in the way persons interpret their world and their situations. It is a model that fits well with the nursing viewpoint of individual assessment and care, and therefore is extremely useful for understanding a person's possible predisposition towards stress when experiencing an illness serious enough to confine him or her to a hospital environment.

Cox (1978) produced the following working definition:

> Stress, it is argued, can only sensibly be defined as a perceptual phenomenon arising from a comparison between the demand on a person and his ability to cope. An imbalance in this mechanism, when coping is important, gives rise to the experience of stress and to the stress response. The latter represents attempts at coping with the source of stress. Coping is both psychological (involving cognitive and behavioural strategies) and physiological. If normal coping is ineffective, stress is prolonged and abnormal responses may occur. The occurrence of these and prolonged exposure to stress, per se, may give rise to functional and structural damage. The progress of these events is subject to great individual variation.

UNDERSTANDING STRESS

Each of these approaches to understanding stress has areas of overlap with the others and useful applications. Appreciation of the existence of all three can only aid the attainment of a clear understanding of the uses of the term 'stress'.

In the remainder of this chapter, stress is considered essentially from the transactional viewpoint of Cox but also taking into account Selye's model of stress. Selye's work, and that of others, clarifies the physiological stress response and its effects as identified in Cox's model.

THE PHYSIOLOGICAL RESPONSE TO STRESS

CONTROL MECHANISMS

The physiological stress response is regulated by

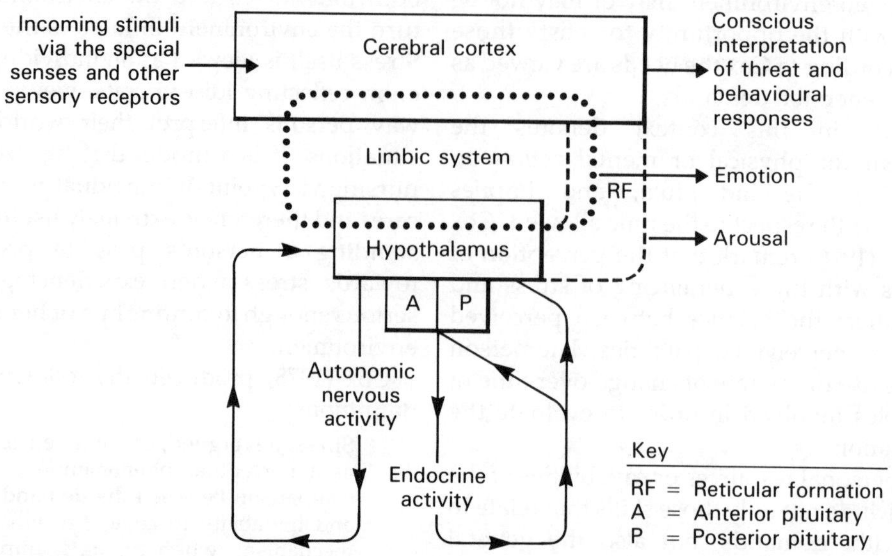

Fig. 8.6 Diagrammatic summary of the major control mechanisms of the stress response.

the hypothalamus, which is a small area of the brain lying, as its name suggests, below the thalamus in the floor of the third ventricle. The hypothalamus controls autonomic nervous activity and, as a result, a number of homeostatic mechanisms, for example temperature regulation. It also contains centres which control hunger, thirst and sex drive. Through its nervous and vascular connections with the pituitary gland, which lies just below it, it plays a major role in the control of endocrine secretion.

The hypothalamus forms part of the limbic system of the brain. The limbic system is a rim of cortical tissue surrounding the hilum of the cerebral cortex and some associated deep structures. As well as the hypothalamus, these include the amygdala, hippocampus and septal nuclei (Ganong, 1985). The limbic system is the area of the brain involved in the interpretation of emotion (Hilton, 1981) and also has nervous connections with the reticular formation, which controls the level of arousal.

The hypothalamus has many nervous connections within the limbic system. There are also established pathways between the limbic system and the cerebral cortex. These pathways are probably the ones by which life events, perceived by the cerebral cortex, influence physiological function, i.e. these nervous pathways form the biological basis to the long recognized phenomenon of the mental state influencing the body. Stimulation of the limbic system can lead to the experience of emotions such as anger, fear and anxiety and, via the hypothalamus, to physiological responses to stress. For example, a patient who sees another patient have an epileptic fit may experience both acute anxiety and a physiological stress response. Figure 8.6 diagrammatically summarizes the major control mechanisms of the stress response. Feedback to the hypothalamus occurs by a number of routes, depending on the nature of the stressor. In certain situations the hypothalamus may override medullary homeostatic reflexes and so, temporarily, abolish mechanisms which usually operate to maintain the constancy of the internal environment (Hilton, 1981).

ACUTE STRESS

The physiological and emotional changes that characterize the alarm stage of the GAS are short

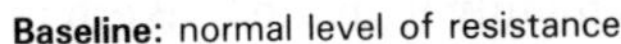

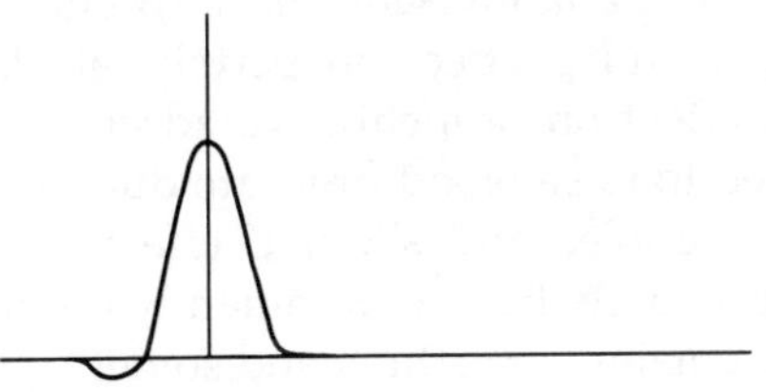

Acute stress
Alarm followed by return to normal level of resistance on removal of stressor

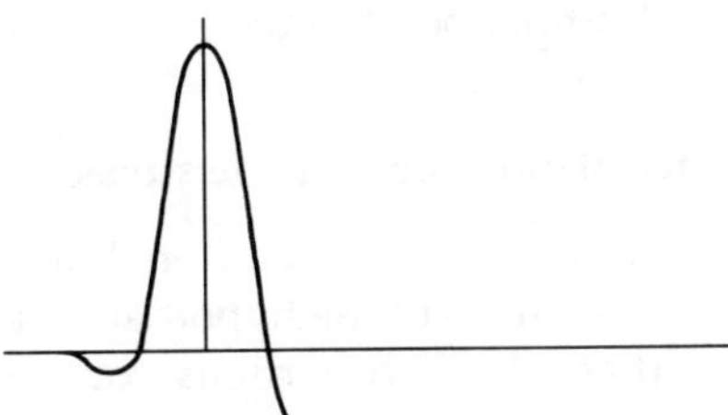

Very intense acute stress
Extreme alarm reaction. Exhaustion and death occur before stressor removed

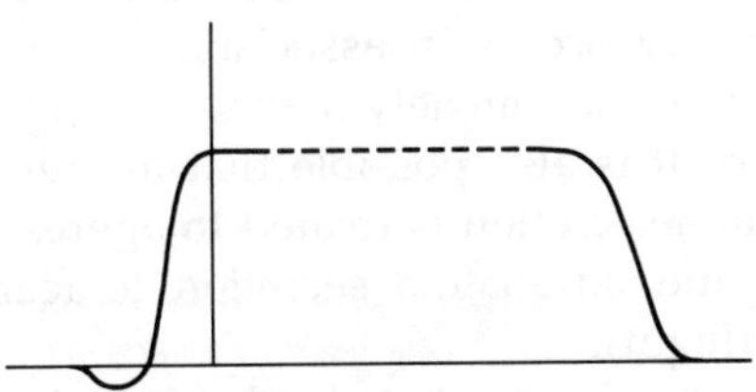

Long-term (chronic) stress
Alarm, followed by adaptation and return to normal level of resistance on removal of stressor

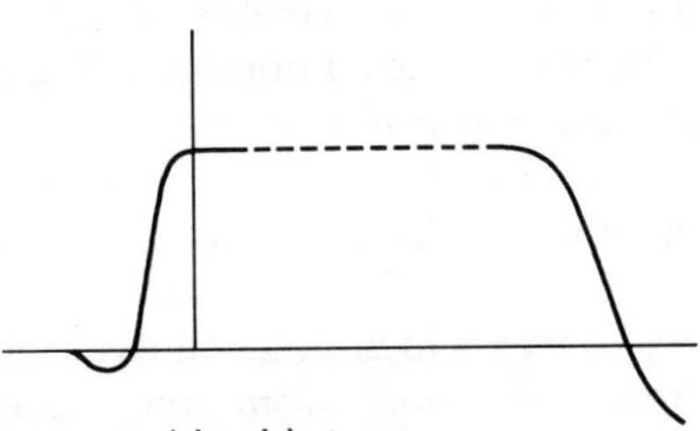

Long-term (chronic) stress
Alarm and adaptation, eventually followed by exhaustion and death, i.e. the complete general adaptation syndrome

Fig. 8.7 Stages of the physiological stress response.

term responses, to cope with acute stress. These responses occur mainly as a result of increased sympathetic nervous activity, although increased secretion of glucocorticoid hormones from the adrenal cortex also begins. There may also be increased secretion of hormones such as antidiuretic hormone, aldosterone, thyroxine and glucagon.

This state of arousal cannot be maintained for long because the physiological changes associated with it upset homeostasis and, in the long term, are not compatible with life. If the demand for adaptation is intense and the stressor not removed the affected person will become 'exhausted' and die (Fig. 8.7). For example, the physiological stress response to a sudden severe haemorrhage functions to preserve sufficient blood supply to prevent damage to vital organs such as the heart and brain. This occurs at the expense of organs such as the kidneys and gastrointestinal tract. If the response has to be maintained for long, the latter organs can suffer irreversible damage from hypoxia. Rapid replacement of the blood loss is therefore essential and serves to reduce the physiological stress experienced.

The function of the sympathetic nervous system in stress

The sympathetic nervous system has an important role in the alarm stage of the stress response, and the majority of the physical signs and symptoms of acute stress, as well as the experience of emotion, are the result of sympathetic arousal. The sympathetic nervous system is part of the autonomic or involuntary nervous system which controls the activity of smooth muscle, cardiac muscle and the secretion of exocrine glands, for example digestive glands and sweat glands. Activation of the sympathetic nervous system via the hypothalamus brings about physiological changes which are adaptive insofar as they lead to preservation of the animal in a situation which requires physical activity and may involve physical injury. These were described by Cannon (1929) and have become known as the 'fight or flight' response.

Sympathetic nervous activity produces most of these changes quickly and specifically. Most postganglionic sympathetic fibres are adrenergic, that is, they produce noradrenaline (norepinephrine) as the chemical transmitter at tissue receptor sites. Exceptions are the sympathetic neurons supplying sweat glands and also those which end on blood vessels in skeletal muscle. These are cholinergic (produce acetylcholine as the chemical transmitter at receptor sites). These cholinergic postganglionic sympathetic fibres produce vasodilatation when stimulated and are known as sympathetic vasodilator nerves (Ganong, 1985).

The adrenal medulla is supplied by a long, cholinergic, preganglionic fibre from the sympathetic nervous system. Activation of this fibre stimulates the adrenal medulla to secrete its hormones into the bloodstream. In man this secretion consists mainly of adrenaline (epinephrine) and small amounts of noradrenaline. These hormones produce a more widespread and longer lasting effect than sympathetic nervous activity, also by combining with tissue-based receptors.

Tissue-based adrenergic receptors have been classified according to their function and termed alpha (α) and beta (β) receptors (Ganong, 1985). α receptors are localized in smooth muscle, mainly in the walls of blood vessels in the skin, viscera and in the eye. Stimulation of these receptors causes contraction of smooth muscle and hence vasoconstriction in the skin and viscera and dilation of the pupil in the eye (due to contraction of the radial muscle of the iris).

β_1 receptors occur in cardiac muscle. Stimulation of these causes increased conduction velocity and decreased refractory period and hence increased contractility of cardiac muscle fibres. The rate of firing of the sinoatrial node is also increased.

β_2 receptors occur in smooth muscle in the walls of blood vessels supplying skeletal muscle (Laurence, 1980) and the walls of the bronchi, bladder and uterus. Stimulation of these receptors causes relaxation of smooth muscle and so dilatation of skeletal muscle blood vessels, dilatation of the bronchi and relaxation of the bladder and uterus.

Adrenaline combines with both α and β receptors, whereas noradrenaline has predominantly α effects. These effects explain the therapeutic uses of adrenergic substances. Adrenaline is used mainly in asthma (β effect on bronchi) and in anaphylactic shock (β effect on the heart, α and β effect on peripheral blood vessels, β effect on bronchi). Noradrenaline is mainly used to raise blood pressure due to its α effect on arterioles and slight β effect on the heart. Isoprenaline has predominantly β effects and is used mainly in asthma and sometimes in heart block, because of its powerful β effect on cardiac conduction tissue (Laurence, 1980). The changes of acute stress mediated through the adrenal medullary hormones develop rapidly and last for a short period of time.

The experience of emotion in acute stress

Blood-borne adrenaline and noradrenaline may stimulate different areas of the hypothalamus. It is possible that the proportions of these substances secreted in stress may partly explain whether the associated emotional experience is one of anger or fear. Funkenstein (1955) introduced evidence that marginally higher adrenal activity occurs in association with the emotions of fear and anxiety than when anger is experienced. It is also possible that in animals noradrenaline secretion is related to aggressive behaviour and adrenaline secretion to fearful behaviour (flight).

For example, the adrenal glands of predatory animals such as lions contain more noradrenaline than adrenaline. This situation is reversed in prey animals such as rabbits. The human adrenal medulla secretes about four times as much adrenaline as noradrenaline and this may suggest that primitive man's primary behavioural response to threat was of 'flight' rather than 'fight'. Today, however, many factors may modify the behavioural and emotional responses which occur in association with hormone secretion from the adrenal medulla.

Physical signs and symptoms in acute stress

The majority of physical signs and symptoms that occur in acute stress are the result of sympathetic arousal. Clinical signs are those which may be observed by others. Symptoms are experienced by the person and may be communicated verbally to nursing and medical personnel.

As well as appreciating the situations which are likely to produce stress in physically ill people, the nurse can recognize and assess the presence of acute stress in patients by monitoring the physiological signs and symptoms which may be associated with it. These are summarized in Table 8.1.

Clinical and research measurement of acute stress, as indicated by sympathetic arousal

Catecholamine release. Until the early 1970s most research evidence of catecholamine release in stressful situations in man was based on measurement of levels of the hormones excreted in the urine. This method was largely unsatisfactory as only 5% of the hormone secreted by the adrenal medulla is excreted in urine, and urine samples consist of urine secreted over a period of at least one hour. Plasma levels are now being measured with increasing accuracy (Hilton, 1981) and the use of indwelling venous catheters for blood sampling reduces the stressor effect of venesection on the secretion of adrenaline and noradrenaline.

Substantial and rapid increases in the secretion of both adrenaline and noradrenaline have been found in students prior to examinations and patients before operation, as well as with general excitement (Hilton, 1981).

Galvanic Skin Response (GSR). This is a measurement of the skin's resistance to electric current. The response is associated with the sweating of the palms which occurs with sympathetic arousal but it is not due simply to increased activity of the sweat gland membranes.

Palmar Sweat Index (PSI). This is also dependent upon sympathetic sweating. This index was used by Munday (1973) in her study entitled *Physiological Measures of Anxiety in Hospital Patients* because its use was feasible on the ward.

Other indices of acute stress. Other indices employed as objective measures of stress include blood pressure estimations and monitoring heart rate and pulse volume. However, practical problems due to extraneous variables have been encountered when using these clinically (Munday, 1973).

The use of the polygraph, an instrument which simultaneously records as many as twenty physiological stress parameters (and is used in lie detection) has produced further research information on people's reactions to various stressors (Smith, 1967).

LONG TERM STRESS

If the demand is less severe but prolonged, the person is able to adapt and passes into the stage of resistance or adaptation. The physiological responses to such long term, or chronic, stress are mainly the result of increased glucocorticoid secretion from the adrenal cortex, although again it is likely that the secretion of many other hormones is altered (Mason, 1968). The length of time for which resistance can be maintained depends on several factors. These include the intensity of the stressor, the ability of the individual to adapt and the nature of the feedback which occurs between the two. Eventually though, if the stressor is not removed, exhaustion occurs (see Fig. 8.7) as the adrenal cortex can no longer maintain its increased secretion of hormone.

Selye (1956) used the term 'adaptation energy' to describe the energy consumed during stress and postulated that this is inherited and finite and that when it is used up, exhaustion and death follow. The 'stress theory of ageing' has developed from this idea and is discussed on page 180.

The physiological changes that occur in chronic stress can cause disease and therefore may be viewed as maladaptive (Raab, 1971; Levi, 1971; Selye, 1976). The concept of the adaptive/maladaptive nature of the response to stress is discussed on pages 170–175.

The function of the adrenal cortex in stress

Despite their anatomical proximity, the adrenal cortex is histologically and functionally distinct

Table 8.1 Physical signs (including common clinical measurements) and symptoms which may occur in acute stress

Site	Physiological basis	Physical signs and common clinical measurements	Physical symptoms
Cardiovascular system	Increased cardiac rate and output	Tachycardia Pulse of full volume Raised blood pressure	Pounding heart Palpitations Chest pain Headache
Respiratory system	CNS arousal If the hyperventilation is not in response to physiological need, low pp CO_2 results and leads to vasodilatation, fall in blood pressure and, in extreme cases, tetany	Increased rate and depth of ventilation Tetany in extreme cases	Dizziness, faintness, panic (in extreme cases) Tingling in the extremities Muscle spasm (in extreme cases)
Gastrointestinal system	Reduced blood supply to and reduced secretion in gastro-intestinal tract		Dry mouth Indigestion/dyspepsia
	Decreased or increased mobility of tract	Vomiting Diarrhoea Constipation Anorexia or overeating	Nausea Diarrhoea (often frequent) Constipation Anorexia or overeating
Skin	Contraction of pilomotor muscles Cholinergic sweating Reduced blood supply	Erection of hair Sweating Pallor	Clammy palms
Eye	Contraction of radial muscle	Dilated pupils	Blurred vision
Muscle	CNS arousal	Muscle tension, tremor Muscle spasm in severe cases Lack of coordination	Headache Muscle tension, tremor, twitching Lack of coordination Backpain
General	CNS arousal	Insomnia Restlessness	Insomnia Restlessness Fatigue/weakness
	Increased metabolic rate	Low grade pyrexia	Feeling hot or cold

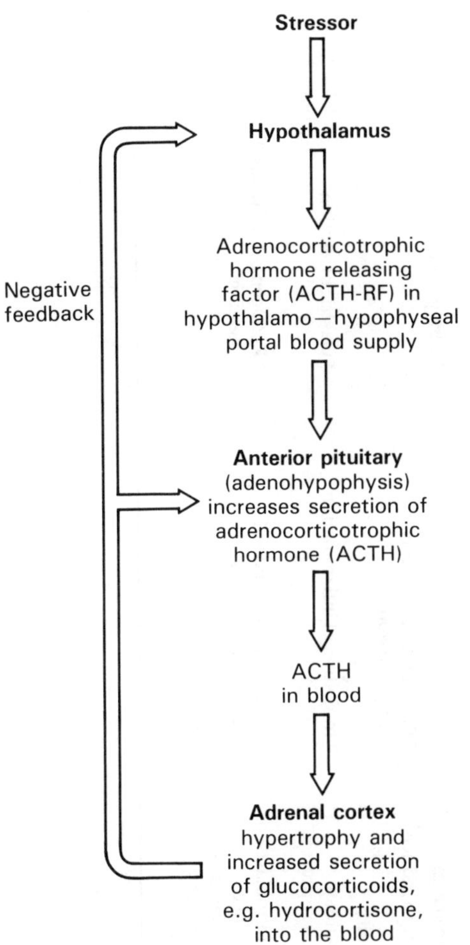

Fig. 8.8 Control of glucocorticoid secretion.

from the adrenal medulla. It is not controlled by direct innervation but by the action of other hormones and variations in plasma concentration of certain substances. The adrenal cortex secretes steroid hormones which are divided into three groups according to their principal effects, glucocorticoids, mineralocorticoids and sex hormones. The first two groups are C-21 steroids (having 21 carbon atoms in their lipid soluble molecule). All C-21 steroids from the adrenal cortex have some mineralo- (control salt and water balance) and some gluco- (regulate general metabolism) activity.

The major glucocorticoid hormone in humans is cortisol (hydrocortisone) and for many physiologists increased secretion of this hormone is synonymous with stress (Vander et al, 1985). The physiological changes of the General Adaptation Syndrome described by Selye (1976) included and are the result of the increased adrenocortical activity which occurs in acute and chronic stress.

Control of glucocorticoid secretion (Fig. 8.8)

Stimulation of the hypothalamus by stressors leads to hypothalamic secretion of adrenocorticotrophic hormone releasing factor (ACTH-RF) into the portal capillary blood supply to the anterior pituitary gland. ACTH-RF stimulates increased production and secretion of adrenocorticotrophic hormone (ACTH) from the anterior pituitary into the blood. On reaching the adrenal cortex, ACTH stimulates increased activity of the cells of the gland and increased secretion of glucocorticoid hormones into the blood.

The level of glucocorticoids in the blood regulates the secretion of ACTH (and hence glucocorticoids themselves) by negative feedback to the anterior pituitary and hypothalamus. However, the stimulating effect of the stressor may overcome this negative feedback mechanism. In addition, animal studies have suggested that, in long term stress, the feedback loop may function at a higher 'set point' so that a greater than usual steroid level is necessary before negative feedback occurs (Ramsey, 1982).

The physiological effects of glucocorticoid secretion

The physiological effects of glucocorticoid secretion are summarized in Table 8.2. The major physiological effect of cortisol is on carbohydrate metabolism, stimulating the production of glucose, and this is closely linked with its effects on protein and fat metabolism.

When large quantities of circulating cortisol are present, further effects become apparent and some of these have clinical value. Cortisol's action in blocking all stages of the inflammatory response means that the hormone can be used therapeutically in many inflammatory conditions, such as rheumatoid arthritis. Its

Table 8.2 Physiological effects of glucocorticoid (cortisol) secretion in acute and chronic stress

Body function or site	Glucocorticoid effect	Short-term physiological effects	Additional long-term physiological effects
Carbohydrate metabolism	Stimulates hepatic gluconeogenesis Enhances elevation of blood glucose produced by other hormones e.g., adrenaline, glucagon Inhibits uptake of glucose by most tissues (not brain) by antagonizing peripheral effects of insulin Inhibits activity of glycolytic enzyme hexokinase	Increased plasma glucose * Glycosuria (if renal threshold exceeded) (Steroid diabetes)	
Protein metabolism	Stimulates breakdown of body protein and depresses protein synthesis Stimulates hepatic deamination of amino acids	Increased plasma levels of amino acids Increased nitrogen content of urine Negative nitrogen balance	* Muscle wasting * Thinning of the skin * Loss of hair * Depression of the immune response
Lipid metabolism	Promotes lipolysis	Increased plasma levels of fatty acids and cholesterol Increased ketone body production and ketonuria	* Redistribution of adipose tissue from periphery to head and trunk
Calcium metabolism	* Antagonizes vitamin D metabolites and so reduces calcium absorption from the gut Increases renal excretion of calcium		* Osteoporosis Kidney stones
Vascular reactivity	Permissive for noradrenaline to induce vasoconstriction Reduces capillary permeability	* Prevents stress-induced hypotension	
Inflammatory response	* Stabilizes membranes of cellular lysosomes (inhibiting their rupture) * Suppresses phagocytosis * Reduces multiplication of fibroblasts in connective tissue and hence decreases production of collagen fibres * Inhibits formation and release of histamine and bradykinin	* Inhibition of inflammation * Decreased formation of granulation tissue * Reduced allergic response	* Gastric ulceration * Reduced rate of wound healing

Table 8.2 continued

Body function or site	Glucocorticoid effect	Short-term physiological effects	Additional long-term physiological effects
Immune response	* Reduced immunoglobulin synthesis * Decreased levels of lymphocytes, basophils and eosinophils * Atrophy of lymphoid tissue	* Decreased white blood cell count * Immunosuppression and decreased resistance to infection	
Water and electrolyte balance	Enhances sodium ion and water reabsorption in distal tubules and collecting ducts of renal nephrons Reciprocal potassium and hydrogen ion excretion (mineralocorticoid effect)	Increased extracellular fluid volume	
Blood	* Enhances coagulability * Reduces levels of lymphocytes basophils and eosinophils * Increases levels of erythrocytes, platelets and neutrophils	* Reduced blood clotting time * Decreased white blood cell count * Haemoconcentration (increased viscosity)	
Central nervous system	* Emotional changes (in excess or deficiency) May facilitate learning and memory (Levine 1971) (ACTH may, independently facilitate learning and memory)	* Emotional changes Increased rate of learning Enhanced learning	

* These physiological effects occur only when high plasma levels of glucocorticoids, similar to those found during steroid therapy, are present.

immunosuppressive effect allows it to be used clinically to reduce rejection of foreign tissue in transplant and graft operations. However, it must be remembered that these same effects suppress wound healing and reduce resistance to infection in patients receiving steroid therapy.

Pathologically increased secretion of ACTH and cortisol has now been replaced by therapeutic use of these hormones and their derivatives as the most common cause of very high plasma levels of these hormones. The physiological effects which result, collectively known as Cushing's syndrome, are now often referred to as 'the pharmacological effects of cortisol'. There is now evidence that approximate doubling of normal plasma cortisol levels and ACTH levels as high as those found in patients with Cushing's disease occur in severely stressed people. For example, people in anxiety states, patients during the first week after thoracotomy and medical students after oral examination, have been found to have such increases in plasma cortisol levels. It seems that the pituitary-adrenocortical system is very sensitive to distress and arousal (Hilton, 1981).

Glucocorticoid hormones are metabolized in the liver. Here they are conjugated, usually with glucuronic acid, and approximately 90% are excreted, as 17-hydroxycorticoids, in the urine.

Clinical and research measurement of stress as indicated by glucocorticoid secretion

In man, glucocorticoid secretion can be accurately assessed by measuring plasma and urinary 17-hydroxycorticoid levels. The major advantages and disadvantages of these methods are similar to those discussed for the estimation of catecholamines.

Urinary hormone levels were successfully used as stress indices by Boore (1978) when she was assessing the effect of pre-operative preparation on the level of stress experienced by patients postoperatively.

Boore (1978) used the sodium/potassium ratio in urine as a further stress index. This ratio reduces in stress because of the mineralocorticoid action of cortisol. The biochemical estimation is a relatively quick and simple one to perform. Boore found that this indicator did not distinguish between the experimental and control groups in her study, although it had been used successfully in investigations of stress in patients who had not undergone surgery (Gentry et al, 1973; Foster, 1974). It may be that in Boore's study the effect of the stressor (anxiety) due to 'lack of pre-operative information', was masked by the greater physical stressor of the operation itself. However, a consistent negative correlation was found between sodium/potassium ratio and amount of steroid hormone excreted and this indicates that the ratio is a valid measure of stress.

The secretion of other hormones in stress

As illustrated in Figure 8.6, a stressor can, via the hypothalamus, influence the secretion of most hormones and research evidence suggests that the secretion of almost every hormone is changed in stress (Mason, 1968; Vander et al, 1985).

Table 8.3 summarizes the secretion and major effects of hormones, other than the catecholamines and cortisol, in stress. Plasma levels of catecholamines, cortisol, growth hormone, glucagon and thyroxine increase in acute stress. All these hormones have a predominantly catabolic effect on the body and there are many examples of interactions between them, both in facilitating secretion and reinforcing metabolic effect. Some of these interactions are noted in Table 8.3.

IMPLICATIONS OF THE PHYSIOLOGICAL RESPONSE TO STRESS

The adaptive nature of the response

The physiological changes that occur in acute stress are adaptive insofar as they facilitate effective coping and survival in situations requiring physical activity or in which physical injury may occur. They represent the mobilization of resources in response to signals of dangerous situations. Anatomical and physiological evidence shows that the apparatus and

Table 8.3 The secretion and effects of other hormones in stress

Hormone	Endocrine gland of origin	Physiological functions	Effect of stressor on secretion	Physiological effects in stress
Somatostatin	Hypothalamus	Inhibits secretion of growth hormone and thyroid stimulating hormone Suppresses output of insulin and glucagon	Inhibited	Secretion of growth hormone and thyroid stimulating hormone facilitated Secretion of insulin and glucagon increased
Antidiuretic hormone	Hypothalamus and posterior pituitary	Increased water reabsorption from the distal tubule and collecting duct of renal nephrons May also influence learning by direct action on the brain	Increased	Increased extracellular fluid volume Enhanced learning
Growth hormone	Anterior pituitary	Reinforces carbohydrate and lipid mobilizing effects and insulin antagonism of catecholamines and cortisol May stimulate uptake of amino acids by injured tissue, but unable to counteract catabolic effect of cortisol on body protein	Increased in acute stress Cortisol suppresses release, so decreased in chronic stress	Promotes gluconeogenesis and elevation in blood glucose Facilitates tissue growth and repair Retarded growth in chronic stress
Thyroid stimulating hormone Thyroxine and Tri-iodothyronine	Anterior pituitary Thyroid	Raised metabolic rate Acts synergistically with catecholamines	Increased in acute stress but secretion suppressed by cortisol in chronic stress	Potentiation of catecholamine effects in acute stress
Aldosterone	Adrenal cortex	Increased sodium ion reabsorption from distal tubule and collecting duct of nephron	Increased	Increased extracellular fluid volume

Table 8.3 continued.

Hormone	Endocrine gland of origin	Physiological functions	Effect of stressor on secretion	Physiological effects in stress
Glucagon	Pancreas (α-cells)	Promotes glycolysis and gluconeogenesis Presence of cortisol permissive for these actions	Hypoglycaemia is major stimulus for secretion but large increases in secretion also occur in response to other stressors, such as cold exposure, exercise and acute anxiety	Raised plasma glucose
Insulin	Pancreas (β-cells)	Promotes entry of glucose into most body cells Anabolic effect on lipid and protein metabolism	Catecholamines suppress release Cortisol and Growth hormone antagonize peripheral effects	Actions inhibited
Gonadotrophins (Follicle stimulating and luteinizing hormones)	Anterior pituitary	Secretion of gonadal steroids reduced	Inhibited	Irregularity or cessation of menstrual cycle Failure of ovulation Infertility

mechanisms which result in the response to stress became specialized early in vertebrate evolution (Hilton, 1981) and the response varies very little between species.

The contents of Tables 8.1, 2 and 3 summarize the nervously and humorally induced changes which produce this physiological 'state of readiness'. Central nervous arousal occurs and skeletal muscles tense. The pupils of the eye dilate, enlarging the field of vision. Erection of hair increases the apparent size of the animal. This latter response is of little or no significance in man but is an important defensive reaction for many furry mammals. Freezing and 'playing dead' defensive behaviour seen in some species, including man, is a manifestation of extreme muscle tension.

Nutrients are mobilized for use during a period of physical activity and fasting and are directed in increased quantities via the bloodstream to organs such as the heart and skeletal muscle, whose efficient activity is essential during fight or flight. Meanwhile, metabolic activity which is non-essential in the short term emergency, for example, gastrointestinal activity, is reduced.

Amino acids become available for tissue repair and blood coagulability increases, as does extracellular fluid volume. These latter responses would be adaptive if blood loss occurred. The occurrence of inflammation and its concomitant symptoms may reduce ability to cope with a stressor and this is a possible explanation for the suppression of inflammation that occurs in severe stress.

In animal and primitive human societies, this emergency response to physical threat must often have had survival value and it is not surprising that its efficient production has become established during evolution. Even in modern industrial societies there are many instances in which the physiological stress response is adaptive and many of these occur in association with physical injury and surgery.

In the short term the response establishes a new physiological equilibrium which aids survival. Indeed, it may be that in critically ill people, therapeutic efforts to restore physiological parameters such as heart rate and blood pressure to 'normal' values may not be appropriate, since values above or below the 'normal range' may be more conducive to recovery. This concept, which is clearly of importance in intensive care, is further discussed by Bland et al (1978).

The new 'stress equilibrium' is only made possible by the interruption of normal homeostatic mechanisms and prolonged reactions are therefore potentially harmful. Prompt relief of physiological stress minimizes the risk of tissue damage.

Animals and humans who for some reason are unable to produce an efficient stress response are less able to survive disease and trauma. Complete loss of adrenomedullary function is not incompatible with life, as sympathetic nervous activity is able to parallel most of the functions of circulating catecholamines. However, complete loss of adrenocortical function is quite rapidly fatal unless treated. Death usually occurs as a result of hypotension, hypoglycaemia and resultant brain dysfunction.

Both animals and man suffering from undersecretion of glucocorticoids (Addison's disease) have a greatly enhanced susceptibility to stressors. Patients suffering from this disorder may succumb to what may seem relatively trivial stressors, for example, dental extraction, unless given appropriate hormone cover.

Similarly, people taking glucocorticoids therapeutically have their normal mechanisms of glucocorticoid secretion suppressed because of their artificially high plasma levels of the hormone. Such individuals require increased doses of hormone if they are successfully to resist stressors such as injury or surgery.

The maladaptive nature of the response

Human stressors are frequently of psychosocial origin. Via the hypothalamus, these stressors can also trigger the physiological response to stress. However, in these circumstances, although the reactions of our internal organs persist, we have learnt more or less successfully to inhibit our movements of 'flight or fight', since these are not appropriate behavioural responses (Hilton, 1981). In the absence of physical injury and/or exercise, physiological responses to stress are inappropriate and potentially harmful, both in the short and long term, because the 'mobilized resources' are not utilized.

In sick people, the effects of psycho-social stressors are often superimposed on the stressor effect of their physical illness itself, unnecessarily increasing the intensity of the physiological response beyond an adaptive level.

In this situation sympathetic arousal produces unpleasant mental and physical symptoms (see Table 8.1) and, in the longer term, physiological responses to stress can cause tissue damage and disease as well as hindering recovery from illness.

In severe prolonged stress, the effects of increased glucocorticoid secretion may result in the manifestation of signs and symptoms of Cushing's syndrome. Wound healing may be delayed and resistance to infection reduced. Boore (1978) found, in her sample of surgical patients, that those who developed post-operative infections had higher levels of stress, as indicated by 17-hydroxycorticosteroid excretion, than those who did not, but the difference between the two groups was not statistically significant. These manifestations of the physiological response to stress have obvious adverse implications for a sick person's recovery.

Adrenal reserve of glucocorticoids varies considerably, both between individuals and at different times in the same individual. If someone is confronted with stressors over a period of time without relief, these reserves become greatly diminished and may become exhausted. Signs and symptoms of diminished glucocorticoid reserve include feelings of weakness, fatigue, irritability, gastrointestinal disturbances, hypotension, hypoglycaemia and abnormal sensitivity to change in environmental temperature. This situation is unusual in people with normal adrenocortical function. However, it can and does occur in severe and prolonged stress and nurses should be aware of this. This is the condition represented by Selye's 'stage of exhaustion' in the general adaptation syndrome. Clearly the best therapeutic action is to relieve the stress experienced before glucocorticoid exhaustion occurs. However, once a person experiences these symptoms, rest and relief from avoidable stress are essential in order to restore normal adrenocorticoid function. Artificial glucocorticoid cover may be necessary if stress avoidance is impossible. Otherwise irreversible tissue damage and death will eventually occur.

Large amounts of cortisol may accelerate the development of atherosclerosis, hypertension, gastric ulcers and interfere with the menstrual cycle (Vander et al, 1985). The physiological changes that occur in stress have been implicated in the aetiology of many 'diseases of civilization' since there are similarities between the pharmacological effects of catecholamines and cortisol and other hormones secreted in stress and the pathological changes associated with these diseases. It is known that plasma levels of cortisol in severe stress can be as high as those found in Cushing's syndrome (Hilton, 1981). However, it is not yet clear whether or not the lesser elevations of cortisol associated with more moderate stress also cause disease if continued over a long period of time.

Stress relief

Physiological responses to stress of psycho-social origin are unnecessary and should, as far as possible, be prevented or controlled, not only to relieve mental distress but also to minimize tissue damage. Methods of preventing or alleviating stress are described in Chapter 12.

Stress can be relieved either by altering the situation itself so that it becomes less threatening, or by increasing the individual's perceived ability to cope, for example, by education and counselling.

Learning a technique such as tension control (muscle relaxation) or meditation can be beneficial. Use of these techniques produces a mental and physical state which seems to be the antipathy of sympathetic arousal and the physiological response to stress may, therefore, be controlled effectively (Wallace & Benson, 1972; Macdonald Wallace, 1980). Many healthy people relieve their symptoms of stress by taking exercise, for example, a vigorous game of squash. Such exercise can relieve stress by channelling the associated physiological response appropriately.

The use of alcohol, tobacco and medically prescribed tranquillizing drugs relieves stress by temporarily suppressing the person's perception of the problem and hence reducing the unpleasant symptoms of stress. Although these methods fail to affect the actual cause of the stress and carry other health risks, they can be useful in helping the person to cope until either the problem resolves or more effective methods of coping can be found and learned.

PSYCHO-SOCIAL RESPONSES IN STRESS

MOOD CHANGE

Mood change is probably the most commonly recognized symptom of stress. Usually the emotion experienced is negatively toned or unpleasant (Cox, 1978) and is associated with sympathetic arousal.

The emotion most commonly associated with stress in the literature is anxiety. Feeling anxious must be an almost universally recognized experience. Spielberger (1972) defines it as a 'transitory emotional state or condition characterized by feelings of tension and apprehension and heightened autonomic nervous system activity'. It generally occurs in relation to an event in the future or in response to something which is unknown.

It is essential when describing a person as 'anxious' to distinguish between 'trait' and 'state' anxiety. In the former the tendency to be anxious forms part of the individual's personality. In other words, the person is characteristically more anxious than average. In the latter the 'state' of anxiety has occurred in response to a particular, stressful situation. The two are often interrelated, but the difference between them is now reflected in the design of various scales for measuring anxiety, for example, the Institute for Personality and Ability Testing (IPAT) self-analysis form (Cattell, 1963). Anxiety scales are usually standardized questionnaires requiring yes/no or multiple choice type answers. The pattern of answers given is often significant, as well as the total score.

Depression is another mood commonly encountered in stress. In depression there tends to be a much reduced level of behaviour characterized by withdrawal and lethargy. The person may experience feelings of guilt and worthlessness. Anxiety may accompany depression and, as with anxiety, the distinction between 'trait' and 'state' is important when assessing the presence of depression.

Anger, fear, grief, jealousy and shame are further emotions which may be experienced in association with stress. Emotional lability is also common. Just as individuals vary in what they perceive as stressful, so their emotional responses are likely to vary.

It is not possible to directly observe a person's experience of emotion. Sometimes a patient will say, 'I feel anxious/depressed/angry/frightened', either spontaneously or in response to enquiry. More frequently though, the emotion is expressed in behaviour, for example tearfulness, short temper or irritability. In addition, the nurse may observe the associated physiological signs of increased sympathetic nervous activity. These are summarized in Table 8.1.

CHANGES IN BEHAVIOUR

Emotion affects a person's thought processes and this is reflected in his/her behaviour. Through informed observation of patients, the nurse may recognize behavioural cues which indicate the presence of stress. Examples of these behavioural cues are:

- intolerance of noise and other disturbing stimuli
- overreacting to apparently minor events
- impulsive behaviour
- poor memory
- difficulty in judging a situation, making decisions and planning ahead
- reduced willpower, inability to concentrate and to finish tasks that have been started.

All these are common reactions and most readers will recognize the occurrence of at least some of these behavioural symptoms of stress in their own everyday life.

Some people suffering from these disturbing symptoms will understandably take steps to avoid them or to minimize their effect. A nurse might notice that a person occupies his or her time in mundane trivial activities, which do not require concentration, even when there are more pressing calls on the person's time. For example, a stressed senior nurse in charge of a busy ward might spend long periods of time unnecessarily tidying cupboards and organizing the ward office instead of planning patient care priorities in the ward.

Activity may be reduced because the person perceives that the quality of his/her performance is reduced, for example, a stressed person may spend long periods staring into space. Such behaviour often serves only to increase the stress as the person perceives his lack of performance and this, in itself, becomes a stressor and forms a vicious circle.

Reduced activity is often accompanied by muscle tension, one of the manifestations of sympathetic arousal in stress. This may be observed in rigid body position, clenched hands showing white knuckles and gritted teeth. These responses also occur when someone is in pain, a stressor in itself. If the pain is aggravated by movement, reduced physical activity is an appropriate coping strategy, but muscle relaxation rather than tension usually serves to relieve pain.

A stressed person unconsciously may spend his/her time in aimless, non-productive activities such as pacing the floor (the classical occupation of the expectant father), repetitive tapping of fingers and feet, frequent blinking and the hand-wringing of the grief stricken. These and other hyperkinetic activities probably serve to relieve muscle tension.

PSYCHOLOGICAL COPING STRATEGIES

These are discussed in detail in Chapter 12.

STRESS AND PHYSICAL ILLNESS

Stress may be involved in physical illness both as a contributing cause to the onset of illness and resulting from physical illness.

THE ROLE OF STRESS IN THE ONSET OF PHYSICAL ILLNESS

As mentioned earlier, the physiological changes that occur in excessive or inappropriate stress have been implicated in the aetiology of many diseases. This idea originated in Selye's (1956) work and the role of stress, particularly that of psycho-social origin, in the aetiology of organic disease is still an important area of research and speculation. The term 'psychosomatic' is applied to diseases in which the physical manifestations are caused by, or significantly influenced by, the emotional state of the patient.

It is possible to argue that the very nature of stress means that it must be implicated in the onset of every illness. It would follow from this that research should be concerned not with which diseases are caused by stress, but with the mechanisms by which each disease is caused. However, this is a fairly extreme view and, to date, most clinical observation and research has been concerned with identifying illnesses in which stress has an aetiological role.

Physical symptoms which are the direct result of the stress response were given in Table 8.1. Many of these are unpleasant and often cause affected individuals to consult health workers in order to obtain relief. Some of these symptoms of underlying disorder, for example, headache due to prolonged contraction of the muscles of the head and neck (tension headache), are instances of illnesses in which the aetiological role of stress is clear.

However, for the large majority of illnesses the contribution of stress to their onset is not nearly so clear-cut. In many cases the bulk of the evidence is based on clinical observation of affected people. It may have been consistently noticed that people affected by the disease seem to be more tense, nervous, or highly strung than the general population, or that they display a particular personality trait. Examples of diseases to which such observations apply are hyperthyroidism and ulcerative colitis. It has also been observed that the onset of disease often follows a period of stress, for example gastric ulceration, diabetes mellitus, multiple sclerosis; or that signs and symptoms are aggravated by emotional stress, for example bronchial asthma, eczema and hypertension.

For some diseases, notably those which are major causes of morbidity and mortality in industrial societies, for example coronary heart disease, cancer and diabetes mellitus, more formal research has been performed. However, such research is fraught with methodological problems which have limited the design and usefulness of the findings of many of the investigations that have been performed. Some of these problems are discussed below. They should always be taken into account when assessing research on the relationship between stress and the onset of physical illness.

Problems associated with research

One of the first problems encountered involves the conceptualization, definition and standardization of terms and criteria, such as 'stress'. Variation in this between projects makes it difficult to compare findings and, when conceptualization is poor, findings may be invalidated.

A further problem lies in the fact that it is neither ethical nor practical to manipulate artificially the variable of psycho-social stress in human subjects in order to see if this affects the occurrence of disease. If animals are used manipulation is more feasible, but problems of extrapolating findings to humans are encountered. There are, therefore, two major alternative strategies for human research in this area.

The first is to look for evidence of stress in the past lives of people who are already suffering from the disease under study. This retrospective course is the one that has been followed most frequently. It has several disadvantages.

Probably the most fundamental of these is that the research relies on the memory of subjects and/or their relatives for incidents in their lives previous to the onset of the disease and how they felt about them. Memory in such instances is not always reliable and may be coloured by current emotion associated with the presence of disease. Retrospective studies also have difficulty in obtaining appropriate control groups.

The second strategy (a prospective study) is to wait for stressful events to occur naturally during the lives of the study population and assess their effect on the occurrence of disease. Stress levels and disease incidence are assessed at intervals after the start of the study. The major disadvantage of a prospective research design is the time involved from commencement to completion. It is often many years before results become available.

The demonstration of a link between the occurrence of psycho-social stress and the development of illness does not mean that the link is necessarily causal. The likelihood of the link being causal increases with the quality of the controls placed on other variables. The ideal requirement is for a control group identical to the experimental group except for the variable of stress. This is usually attempted either by using pairs of people matched for the variables considered important, or by using large populations of people identified by broad criteria such as age or type of work. Neither of these alternatives is wholly satisfactory as there may be unknown factors operating. Once a link between two variables has been established, the search for possible mechanisms to explain that link can begin.

Few of the illnesses studied have exact, identifiable points of onset and most have pre-symptomatic periods of development. This means that there are often difficulties in dating the onset of illness in relation to the occurrence of stress. It also raises the possibility that early symptoms of the illness could have contributed to the occurrence of the stress, for example, if someone loses his/her job and shortly afterwards develops renal failure, one might question whether or not the pre-diagnostic symptoms of kidney disease contributed to the loss of employment.

Stress as an aetiological factor in disease

Despite the retrospective nature and lack of

Table 8.4 Physical illnesses which have had psycho-social stress implicated in their aetiology

Disturbed body function	Physical illness	Postulated mechanisms by which stress contributes to pathology
Control and co-ordination:		
Nerve function	Multiple sclerosis	Possibly autoimmune — see below
Endocrine function	Diabetes mellitus	Stress regarded as factor precipitating symptoms of dormant condition rather than as a direct causal factor In pre-diabetic, stress response may exhaust already vulnerable pancreatic cells. Glucocorticoid secretion in stress results in increased blood glucose and ketosis — this may precipitate diabetes (Cox, 1978) Autoimmune mechanism has been postulated for juvenile onset diabetes mellitus
	Hyperthyroidism	Hypothalamic effect on pituitary regulation of thyroid hormone secretion Possibly autoimmune — see below
	Reproductive disorders	Hypothalamic inhibition of gonadotrophin secretion. Disturbed autonomic regulation of smooth muscle in the reproductive tract, for example, in the Fallopian (uterine) tubes
	Growth retardation	Hypothalamic inhibition of growth hormone secretion in chronic stress (Gardener, 1972)
Internal transport:		
Cardiovascular function	Coronary heart disease (atheroma, coronary thrombosis and myocardial infarction)	Sympathetic nervous activity and glucocorticoid secretion leads to breakdown of adipose tissue Free fatty acids are converted to triglycerides and these and cholesterol are available for incorporation into atheroma (Carruthers, 1969) Presence of atheroma reduces potential oxygen supply to myocardium. Sympathetic nervous activity increases cardiac work and oxygen demand (Raab, 1971) Raised blood viscosity and reduced clotting time increases risk of intravascular thrombosis Sustained, raised blood levels of adrenaline may be toxic to cardiac muscle by depleting high energy phosphates in cells (Ramsey, 1982) Glucocorticoid activity results in sodium retention and potassium and magnesium loss by the body. This may lead to changes in electrolyte balance at myocardial cell membranes and cause abnormal cell function (Raab, 1971)
	Hypertension	Sympathetic nervous activity and catecholamines are powerful vasoconstrictors, raising total peripheral resistance and blood pressure: habitual increase in activity leads to development of essential hypertension: glucocorticoids permissive for noradrenaline to induce vasoconstriction; they also raise blood viscosity and cause retention of sodium and water which increases blood volume and contributes to hypertension Receptors in hypothalamus and brain stem are activated by brain noradrenaline and stimulate hypertensive response. (Ramsey, 1982)

Table 8.4 continued

Disturbed body function	Physical illness	Postulated mechanisms by which stress contributes to pathology
	Cerebrovascular accident	Hypertension increases risk of cerebral haemorrhage Presence of atheroma, raised blood viscosity and reduced clotting time increase risk of cerebral thrombosis and embolus
	Migraine	Vasoconstriction of cranial vessels during periods of mental stress is followed by marked vasodilatation which causes throbbing pain
Acquisition of nutrients and removal of waste:		
Respiratory function	Bronchial asthma	Wheeze, produced by narrowing of lumen of bronchi and trachea, can be induced voluntarily, indicating central nervous system involvement. Postulated that changes in respiratory physiology which produces wheeze are centrally controlled and a response to psycho-social stress (Groen, 1971) Allergy theory more orthodox and widely accepted
Gastrointestinal function	Gastric and duodenal ulceration	Three factors must exist for stress ulcers to occur: presence of gastric acid; agents that increase H^+permeability through mucosal cells, for example, regurgitated bile salts, aspirin, alcohol; and the occurrence of a period of decreased mucosal blood flow such as that which may occur in acute stress Decreased mucosal blood flow results in cellular hypoxia and damage which is aggravated by acid and pepsin (Groer & Shekleton, 1983) Secretion of gastric acid and pepsinogen are increased in association with emotions of anger, anxiety and fear Raised glucocorticoid levels in chronic stress inhibit the normal protective, inflammatory response in gastric mucosa: this allows gastric acid and pepsin to attack mucosa
	Ulcerative colitis	Autonomic nervous activity, associated with the experience of emotion, produces increased mobility, hyperaemia and congestion of colon wall Possibly autoimmune — see below
	Spastic colon	Autonomically mediated hypermotility and cramping
Mobility and support:		
Musculoskeletal function	Rheumatoid arthritis	Autoimmune — see below
Protection and survival:		
Skin	Eczema and dermatitis	Allergic responses — see below
Immune function	Cancer Autoimmune disease Allergies Susceptibility to infection	Raised glucocorticoid levels in stress suppress normal immune responses: this results in impaired surveillance mechanisms, ie, recognition of self and non-self and increased susceptibility to cancer, autoimmune disease, allergic responses and infection

controls in many of the investigations performed, there is now sufficient evidence available for there to be little doubt that the experience of stress contributes to the aetiology in coronary heart disease and gastrointestinal conditions such as dyspepsia and ulcers (Cox, 1978; Hurst et al, 1976). However, the evidence remains inconclusive for a large number of other conditions. There is a great need for long-term, prospective investigations, with carefully defined and selected controls, and also for more research which investigates the mechanisms by which stress causes disease.

Table 8.4 summarizes some of the physical illnesses which have had stress of psycho-social origin implicated in their aetiology, and the postulated mechanisms by which stress may exert its pathological effect.

A reciprocal relationship exists between stress and disease, in that disease acts as a stressor and stress may promote disease. It is therefore at best artificial to separate the effects of a specific disease producing agent on a person from the effects of the state of stress existing in the person at the time.

It is also important to note that the emotions experienced in psycho-social stress frequently leads to changes in behaviour which may themselves constitute health risks and cause pathological change. For example, sleep may be lost, eating and exercise habits may change and smoking, alcohol intake and drug consumption may increase. This can create a positive feedback loop, or vicious circle, and hence increase still more the direct and indirect contribution of psycho-social stress to eventual tissue damage.

Thus, the progressive breakdown of homeostasis which leads to disease is far more likely to be caused by a number of different stressors, reinforcing each other over time, than by a single stressor.

The stress theory of ageing

This theory stands beside others which attempt to explain the pathogenesis of ageing and death, such as programmed theory, mutation theory and autoimmune theory.

Stress theory holds that ageing is due to the accumulated effects of stress on the body and originates in Selye's (1976) work. He postulated that each individual possesses a finite amount of 'adaptation energy', determined by genetic make-up and used up during life by the 'wear and tear' of stress. Tissues whose cells undergo a rapid turnover are least affected by wear and tear while those with low turnover, such as connective tissue, muscle and nerve are most affected and eventually indirectly damage other tissues. At the end of the life span, the stage of exhaustion of the general adaptation syndrome is reached.

An important aspect of this theory is that exposure to stressors accelerates ageing and this has been shown for certain stressors, for example prolonged exposure to cold, high altitude, radiation and mentally stressful events. Accumulation of the 'old-age' pigment, lipofuschin, is also associated with stress.

Aged people generally secrete glucocorticoids efficiently, but it may be that target tissues are relatively unresponsive because membrane receptors no longer bind as effectively. Theoretically this would reduce ability to 'resist' a stressor and hasten 'exhaustion'. This mechanism of deterioration of endocrine function has also been suggested for other hormones such as adrenaline, insulin and thyroid hormone and may, in part, explain the occurrence of certain diseases in old age, such as diabetes, hypertension and osteoporosis.

Evidence for the role of stress in the ageing process is, as yet, inconclusive. However, the proposition that genetically programmed events can be influenced by life experience of stress seems both logical and feasible.

STRESS RESULTING FROM PHYSICAL ILLNESS

Physical illness or injury, and sometimes the mode of treatment, are in themselves some of the most powerful stressors recognized. Every step should, therefore, be taken to minimize their occurrence and severity and hence to prevent unnecessary stress and its potentially harmful physiological sequelae. The ways in which this can be done obviously vary with the situation and range through primary, secondary and tertiary preventive measures.

For example, the prevention of stress resulting from injury involving haemorrhage in a road traffic accident can be considered as :

- primary prevention: injury is minimized if the individual is wearing a seat belt
- secondary prevention: prompt and appropriate first aid measures at the scene of the accident
- tertiary prevention: medical treatment involving transfusion to restore extracellular fluid volume and minimize shock (a manifestation of the stress response) and its potential sequelae, for example acute renal failure resulting from renal hypoxia following the constriction of renal blood vessels which occurs in shock.

As well as being a stressor in itself, physical ill-health invariably brings with it events of psychological significance which can trigger the physiological responses to stress already discussed. Perceived inability to cope is invariably associated with the experience of emotion, such as anxiety, fear, depression, grief or anger. The experience of emotion and the behavioural changes which may accompany it are further manifestations of the response to stress. However, the experience of emotion may itself act as a stressor, thus potentiating the stress response and creating a vicious circle. For example: a patient who is about to undergo an operation may perceive this as a threat to survival and may feel that he/she has little control over the events taking place. Little information may have been given about what is happening and why. These circumstances act as stressors, he or she experiences stress and manifests a stress response. One of the components of this response is the emotion of anxiety. Anxiety is an unpleasant subjective sensation and may be recognized by the patient as further evidence of inability to cope with the situation. The anxiety itself then acts as a stressor and potentiates the stress response.

Situations causing stress

Types of situations likely to evoke stress were listed previously, and many of these may be associated with physical illness. For example, a person who is ill already has disrupted physiological function, he/she may be experiencing pain and losing sleep. Particularly if admitted to hospital, he/she may experience loss of identity in a strange environment and with the assumption of the patient role. The illness may frustrate plans already made and disrupt family and social life. Such situations are likely to be stressful to most people, but it must be remembered that each individual interprets events occurring in his or her life against a wide range of variables, and so responses to illness and its concomitant events vary considerably.

Most research into emotional responses to illness is hospital-based. It therefore records the effects of more serious illnesses and probably, as a result, the more severe emotional and behavioural reactions which can occur. Wilson-Barnett (1979) has reviewed some of the research literature on patients' psychological reactions to illness and health care, and this text forms a useful introduction to more detailed study of primary as well as more recent sources.

Hospital care

Several studies have focused on specific events associated with a stay in hospital which might be expected to be stressful, and some of these are summarized below.

Hospital admission, associated events and care. Findings from studies of patients' reactions to admission to hospital indicate that this can be a particularly stressful event (Hugh-Jones et al, 1964; Franklin, 1974; Wilson-Barnett & Carrigy, 1978). Franklin (1974) attempted to determine if there was a relationship between patient anxiety on admission to hospital and quality of nursing care. She used a sample of 160 patients admitted to surgical wards in four London hospitals: 31 of these patients stated that they were 'very worried' on admission , 59 were 'worried' and 70 'were not worried'. 'Worry' is an affective state closely allied with anxiety.

Replies to the question: 'What have you been mainly worried about?' were as follows:

- 32% did not know what to expect
- 31% the operation
- 18% anaesthesia
- 11% family
- 8% general dislike of hospitals.

Wilson-Barnett (1976) undertook an interview study with 200 patients on medical wards in two hospitals to determine which hospital events were most commonly liked and disliked. Questions were asked on 60 aspects of hospital life and items ranked according to the subjects' responses. Far more items elicited positive responses than negative ones. However, certain items elicited predominantly negative responses from patients. These were:

- using a bedpan
- anticipating a treatment or procedure which is likely to be painful
- seeing another patient who is very ill
- leaving your usual 'work' while you are in hospital
- being away from the family
- your own illness or condition.

The main findings of this study are in agreement with those of other studies (Wilson-Barnett, 1979) and imply that patients generally have positive feelings and attitudes towards ward events.

Many people undergo medical investigations both as in-patients and out-patients and there is evidence that these are also stressful occurrences (Wilson-Barnett, 1976). Studies have also produced evidence that giving patients prior information and explanation about the investigation reduces their experience of distress during the procedure and increases their ability to tolerate it without sedation (Johnson, Morrissey & Leventhal, 1973; Wilson-Barnett, 1978). The latter experimental study aimed to measure patients' emotional responses to the procedures of barium meal and barium enema and assess the effect on these responses of giving prior information about the procedure. Current emotional state was measured using a standardized mood adjective check list and the Eysenck Personality Inventory was employed to assess 'trait' emotionality. The main findings were that barium enema was associated with higher levels of anxiety than was barium meal. Barium enema patients who had received structured explanation prior to the procedure were significantly less anxious during the procedure than those patients who had not received explanation. There was a similar, though non-significant, trend for barium meal. A positive correlation existed between trait and state anxiety scores at each stage of the experiment.

Wilson-Barnett & Carrigy (1978) reported on their longitudinal interview study in which they aimed to assess how personality, medical and personal factors affect reactions to events in hospital. Their findings indicated that particular types of patients report most anxiety and depression during their stay in hospital. For example, patients who were generally prone to feelings of anxiety and depression, as indicated by their high scores on the Eysenck Personality Inventory, were most likely to report strong negative emotion and to make negative comments about their stay in hospital. In addition, female patients under forty years of age admitted for investigations and those suffering from neoplastic, infective or unknown disorders all reported relatively higher levels of anxiety or depression during their stay in hospital. Findings such as these could contribute to the development of methods of assessing which patients may be particularly 'at risk' of experiencing distress in hospital.

Hospital discharge. Findings from the Wilson-Barnett & Carrigy (1978) study also indicated that discharge from hospital may be quite stressful for some patients. The researchers had anticipated that anxiety and depression, as measured daily by a mood adjective check list, would be less on day of discharge than during their hospital stay. However, this was not always the case. Some patients were generally dissatisfied with the arrangements for their discharge, for example short notice had been given or they were worried about the arrangements for the journey or how they would cope at home.

Few studies have assessed how people feel about their discharge from hospital (Wilson-Barnett, 1979) but several have described patients' unpleasant experiences after discharge, for example, Skeet (1970) and Roberts (1975).

Surgical patients. There is now considerable research evidence that patients awaiting a surgical operation experience stress as indicated by emotions such as anxiety, and studies have related the psychological state of the physically ill person to their postoperative course. Janis (1958) undertook a study of anxiety in surgical patients viewed from a psychoanalytical perspective. One of the most significant findings from his qualitative analysis of the data was that patients who display moderate pre-operative anxiety show less emotional evidence of stress during recovery. Patients who display high or low pre-operative anxiety, however, had significantly more symptoms, such as acute anxiety states, hostility and depression during their recovery. Janis considered that the patients exhibiting moderate pre-operative anxiety were basically emotionally stable and able to form a rational assessment of their situation. High anxiety patients were assessed as having a neurotic personality disposition, whereas the denial mechanism appeared to be operating in those patients showing less pre-operative anxiety. These findings clearly fit with the concept of the relationship between demand and performance discussed earlier.

Johnson, Dabbs & Leventhal (1970) studied 62 patients who were due to have either a cholecystectomy or hysterectomy. They used trait and state emotionality measures and found that their trait measures were good predictors of pre- and postoperative state anxiety scores. Individual levels of anxiety recorded pre and postoperatively were similar and Janis' (1958) findings were not confirmed, in that moderate pre-operative anxiety did not reliably predict best postoperative recovery.

Experimental studies. A number of experimental projects have assessed the effects of giving information to patients pre-operatively. Egbert et al (1964) found that length of postoperative hospital stay was shorter and less analgesics were required by a group of patients who had received a pre-operative explanatory visit from an anaesthetist.

Hayward's (1975) work assumed that pain is a combination of physiological and psychological factors and that pain and anxiety are closely related phenomena. His major experimental hypothesis, that giving relevant pre-operative information would reduce postoperative pain and anxiety, was upheld for his samples of patients in two hospitals. Informed patients required fewer analgesics postoperatively.

In a similar study Boore (1978) examined the relationship between giving pre-operative explanation to patients and their postoperative levels of stress. Physiological and biochemical measures of stress were used as well as patients' subjective ratings of their physical and mental state. Boore also measured recovery rates and postoperative complications as potential indices of stress. Her data was collected on a sample of 80 patients undergoing either cholecystectomy or herniorraphy/appendicectomy. She found that 17-hydroxycorticosteroid excretion was significantly lower in the experimental (informed) group of patients on the second and third postoperative days, indicating that the pre-operative explanation was associated with reduced stress. There was also a lower incidence of postoperative infections in the experimental group and this difference was significant for wound infection. Patients who developed infections were found to have higher levels of stress, as indicated by 17-hydroxycorticosteroid excretion, than those who did not, but the difference was not significant.

There are, therefore, strong indications from recent nursing research that giving structured pre-operative explanation to patients reduces stress and/or anxiety and has a beneficial effect on recovery. A great deal of research in a variety of areas has demonstrated patients' expressed needs for relevant information which helps them anticipate and prepare for their experiences of their illness and its treatment. The effective communication of such information is an important aspect of the nurse's role. Information giving, as a method of preventing and alleviating stress, is discussed in Chapter 12.

The research findings summarized in this

section relate to patients in general medical and surgical wards. In addition to these findings, there is strong evidence that high percentages of seriously ill patients requiring intensive care in specialist units suffer psychological changes which can be extreme. These are probably related both to the organic effects of their disease and to features of the 'intensive care environment' (Hackett et al, 1968; Baxter, 1975; Neary, 1976; Ashworth, 1980). Relevant too, here, are discussions of the stressful nature of working in these units, both for nurses and other health care staff, such as those by Roger (1975) and Melia (1977).

All these findings provide nurses with useful pointers to common sources of distress amongst physically ill people and to potential psychological and physiological benefits of reducing such distress. They also indicate areas where further research is required to confirm or extend the findings of earlier studies, but it is already clear that nurses and other health professionals should be developing their expertise in stress prevention and alleviation.

REFERENCES

Appley M H, Trumbull R 1967 Psychological stress. Appleton, New York

Ashworth P M 1980 Care to communicate: An investigation into problems of communication between patients and nurses in intensive therapy units. Royal College of Nursing, London

Baxter S 1975 Psychological problems of intensive care. Nursing Times 71:22–23 and 63–65

Bernard C 1927 Introduction to the study of experimental medicine. Translation by H C Green. Macmillan, New York

Bland R, Shoemaker W, Shabot M 1978 Physiologic monitoring goals for the critically ill patient. Surgery Gynaecology and Obstetrics 147:833–841

Boore J R P 1978 Prescription for recovery: the effect of pre-operative preparation of surgical patients on post-operative stress, recovery and infection. Royal College of Nursing, London

Cannon W B 1929 Bodily changes in pain, hunger, fear and rage, 2nd edn. Appleton, New York

Cannon W B 1932 The wisdom of the body. Appleton, New York

Cannon W B 1935 Stresses and strains of homeostasis. American Journal of Medical Science 189:1

Carruthers M A 1969 Aggression and atheroma. Lancet 2:1170

Cattell R B 1963 IPAT — self-analysis form. Institute for Personality and Ability Testing. Champaign, Illinois

Cox T 1978 Stress. Macmillan, London

Cox T, Mackay C J 1976 A psychological model of occupational stress. A paper presented to the Medical Research Council meeting Mental Health in Industry, November, London

Egbert L D, Battit G E, Welch C E, Bartlett M K 1964 Reduction of postoperative pain by encouragement and instruction of patients. New England Journal of Medicine 170:825–827

Foster S B 1974 An adrenal measure for evaluating nursing effectiveness. Nursing Research 23:118–124

Frankenhauser M 1975a Experimental approaches to the study of catecholamines and emotion. In: Levi L (ed) Emotions: their parameters and measurement. Raven Press, New York

Frankenhauser M 1975b Sympathetic—adrenomedullary activity, behaviour and the psychosocial environment. In: Venables PH Christie M J (eds) Research in Psychophysiology. Wiley, New York

Franklin B L 1974 Patient anxiety on admission to hospital. Royal College of Nursing, London

Funkenstein D H 1955 The physiology of fear and anger. Scientific American 192:74–80

Ganong W F 1985 Review of medical physiology, 12th edn. Lange Medical Publications, Los Altos, California

Gardener L I 1972 Deprivation dwarfism. In: Readings from the Scientific American 1976 Human Physiology and the Environment in Health and Disease, Part IV Responses to Psychosocial Stress. W H Freeman, San Francisco

Gentry W D, Musante G J, Haney T 1973 Anxiety and urinary sodium/potassium as stress indicators on admissions to a coronary care unit. Heart and Lung: The Journal of Critical Care 2:875–877

Groen J J 1971 Psychosocial influences in bronchial asthma. In: Levi L (ed) Society, stress and disease, vol 1. Oxford University Press, London

Groer M E, Shekleton M E 1983 Basic pathophysiology, a conceptual approach, 2nd edn. C V Mosby, London

Hackett T P, Cassem N H, Wishnie H A 1968 The coronary care unit, an appraisal of its psychological hazards. New England Journal of Medicine 278:1365

Hayward J 1975 Information — a prescription against pain. Royal College of Nursing, London

Hilgard E R, Atkinson R C, Atkinson R L 1983 Introduction to psychology, 8th edn. Harcourt Brace Jovanovich, New York

Hilton S M 1981 The physiology of stress — emotion. In: Edholm O G, Weiner J S (eds) The principles and practice of human physiology. Academic Press, London

Hinkle L E 1973 The concept of stress in the biological and social sciences. Science, Medicine and Man 1:31–48

Holmes T H, Rahe R H 1967 The social readjustment rating scale. Journal of Psychosomatic Research 11:213–218

Hugh-Jones P, Tanser A R, Whitby C 1964 Patients' views of admission to a London teaching hospital. British Medical Journal 2:660–664

Hurst M W, Jenkins C D, Rose R M 1976 The relation of psychological stress to the onset of medical illness. In: Garfield CA (ed) 1979 Stress and survival: the emotional realities of life-threatening illness. C V Mosby, St Louis

Janis I L 1958 Psychological stress. Wiley, New York

Johnson J E, Dabbs J M, Leventhal H 1970 Psychosocial factors in the welfare of surgical patients. Nursing Research 24:404–410

Johnson J E, Morrissey J F, Leventhal H 1973 Psychological

preparation for endoscopic examination. Gastrointestinal Endoscopy 19:180–182

Laurence D R 1980 Clinical pharmacology, 5th edn. Churchill Livingstone, Edinburgh

Lazarus R S 1966 Psychological stress and the coping process. McGraw–Hill, New York

Lazarus R S 1971 The concepts of stress and disease. In: Levi L (ed) Society, stress and disease, vol 1. Oxford University Press, London

Lazarus R S 1976 Patterns of adjustment, 3rd edn. McGraw–Hill, New York

Levi L (ed) 1971 Society, stress and disease, vol 1. The psychosocial environment and psychosomatic disease. Oxford University Press, London

Levine L 1971 Stress and behaviour. In: Readings from the Scientific American 1976 Human physiology and the environment in health and disease, Part IV, Response to psychosocial stress. W.H. Freeman, San Francisco

Macdonald Wallace J 1980 Stress and tension control. Nursing (Oxford) 1st series, 10:451–454

Mason J W 1968 A review of psychoendocrine research on the pituitary adrenocortical system. Psychosomatic Medicine 30:567– 607

Mason J W 1971 A re-evaluation of the concept of 'non-specificity' in stress theory. Journal of Psychiatric Research 8:323

Melia K M 1977 The intensive care unit — a stress situation. Nursing Times 73:17–20

Munday A 1973 Physiological measures of anxiety in hospital patients. Royal College of Nursing, London

Neary D 1976 Neuropsychiatric sequelae of renal failure. British Medical Journal 1:122–130

Raab W 1971 Cardiotoxic biochemical effects of emotional—environmental stressors — fundamentals of psychocardiology. In: Levi L (ed) Society, stress and disease vol 1. Oxford University Press, London

Rahe R H 1969 Life crisis and health change. In: May P R, Whittenborn R (ed) Psychotropic drug responses: Advances in prediction. Thomas, Springfield, Illinois

Rahe R H, Lundberg U, Theorell T, Bennett L K 1971 The social readjustment rating scale: A comparative study of Swedes and Americans. Journal of Psychosomatic Research 15:241–249

Ramsey J M 1982 Basic pathophysiology, modern stress and the disease process. Addison-Wesley, London

Roberts I 1975 Discharged from hospital. Royal College of Nursing, London

Roger B 1975 The role of the psychiatrist in the renal dialysis unit. In: Pasnau R O (ed) Consultation — liaison psychiatry. Grune and Stratton, New York

Selye H 1946 The general adaptation syndrome and the diseases of adaptation. Journal of Clinical Endocrinology 6:117

Selye H 1956 The stress of life. McGraw-Hill, New York

Selye H 1965 The stress syndrome. American Journal of Nursing 65:97–99

Selye H 1974 Stress without distress. Hodder and Stoughton, New York

Selye H 1976 The stress of life, 2nd edn. McGraw-Hill, New York

Skeet M 1970 Home from hospital. The Dan Mason Nursing Research Committee, London

Smith B M 1967 The polygraph. Scientific American 216:25–31

Spielberger C D (ed) 1972 Anxiety: current trends in theory and research, vol 1. Academic Press, London

Sykes J B (ed) 1982 The concise Oxford dictionary of current English, 7th edn. Oxford University Press, London

Vander A J, Sherman J H, Luciano D S 1985 Human physiology: the mechanisms of body function, 4th edn. McGraw–Hill, London

Wallace R K, Benson H B 1972 The physiology of meditation. In: Readings from the Scientific American 1976 Human physiology and the environment in health and disease, Part IV, Responses to psychosocial stress. W H Freeman, San Francisco

Weitz J 1970 Psychological research needs on the problems of human stress. In: McGrath J E (ed) Social and psychological factors in stress. Holt Rinehart and Winston, New York

Welford A T 1973 Stress and performance. Ergonomics 16:567

Wilson-Barnett J 1976 Patients' emotional reactions to hospitalisation: an exploratory study. Journal of Advanced Nursing 1:351–358

Wilson-Barnett J 1978 Patients' emotional responses to barium X-rays. Journal of Advanced Nursing 3:37–46

Wilson-Barnett J 1979 Stress in hospital — patients' psychological reactions to illness and health care. Churchill Livingstone, London

Wilson-Barnett J, Carrigy A 1978 Factors affecting patients' responses to hospitalisation. Journal of Advanced Nursing 3: 221–228

Wyler A R, Holmes T H, Masuda M 1971 Magnitude of life events and seriousness of illness. Psychosomatic Medicine 33:115–122

(See Appendix (p. 895) for a discussion of the biological basis of pain and its management.)

9

Pain: helping to meet the challenge from a nursing point of view

It is not expected of nurses to do something about pain but it should be. (A teacher of nurses, 1985)

INTRODUCTION

The management of pain is receiving increasing attention within the health caring professions. Many advances have been made in recent years through contributions by both the biological and behavioural sciences yet, despite many available therapies, the complex phenomenon of pain continues to present a challenge to health carers. For nurses in particular there is an exceptional challenge because we, more than any other health professionals, have frequent contact with ill people. There are many opportunities for us to help relieve pain and suffering. Unfortunately, however, these opportunities may sometimes be overlooked through deficiencies of communication among staff or between staff and patients, or because of deficiencies within the educational system of the nursing and medical professions resulting in a lack of up to date knowledge.

This chapter is an attempt to encourage nurses to be more aware of their responsibilities in relieving pain. The practical aspects of management related to nursing care are emphasized. Theoretical information from the biological sciences is included in the Appendix (p. 895) and the reader is strongly urged to read this in conjunction with this chapter. The already extensive bibliography on pain is growing all the time and it would be quite impossible in this one chapter to cover all the relevant available material.

SOME DEFINITIONS OF PAIN

It is difficult to define pain. Pain cannot simply be reduced to a physiological phenomenon. It is a subjective experience, the expression of which has social and cultural determinants. Some attempts to define pain allow for its subjective nature. For example, 'pain is a complex phenomenon, a signal of tissue damage threat, an integrated defence reaction and a private experience of hurt' (Sternbach, 1968). The International Association for the Study of Pain Subcommittee on Taxonomy (1979) stated that 'Pain is an unpleasant sensory and emotional experience associated with actual or potential tissue damage or described in terms of such damage'. Wall (1977), in The Encyclopaedia of Ignorance, simply stated 'Pain is'.

As nurses, we are faced daily with many different types of behaviour in patients with similar medical diagnoses. Consequently we must try to understand pain expression on an individual basis. For us, therefore, an appropriate and valuable definition of pain is an operational one — 'Pain is what a person says it is and hurts when he says it does' (after McCaffery, 1983).

ETHICS AND PAIN MANAGEMENT

There are general, humanistic, ethical principles which give a person the right to be free from pain (Edwards, 1984). Consequently, we have certain moral obligations to a patient, the first being not to inflict additional pain and suffering beyond that required to make a diagnosis, and the second being to do all that is possible within available knowledge and resources to relieve as much suffering and pain as possible. Edwards also reminds us that whereas, as far as inflicting additional pain is concerned, there are occasional carers who may be careless, the duty to relieve pain as much as possible is one that is widely infringed.

There is abundant evidence to substantiate this claim. Serious deficiencies in clinical practice have been shown to occur. These include: stereotyping of patients by nurses on surgical wards and subsequent treatment according to the prejudices of nursing staff (Wiener, 1975); differences of knowledge, belief and experience among health professionals resulting in wide variation in staff's perceptions of patients' pain and subsequent decisions regarding relief (Charap, 1978; Jacox, 1979); differences between patients' and nurses' perceptions of patients' pain (Hunt et al, 1977); and fewer postoperative analgesia administrations being received by patients than are allowed for within the prescriptional framework (Cohen, 1980).

CURRENT TRENDS IN UNDERSTANDING AND TREATING PAIN

In the early and mid-twentieth century it was thought that pain was simply a sensory experience and that relief could be achieved through the modification of sensory processes. Now it is acknowledged that, although sensory processes play a part, social, psychological and cultural factors also contribute to the pain experience. The recognition that pain is complex and multidimensional has led to the formulation of many theories in different disciplines. However, the search still continues for a theory of pain that will be acceptable in all fields of scientific endeavour. For information about theories of pain the reader is referred to the Appendix and to Melzack & Wall (1982).

PAIN ENTITIES

Acute pain and chronic pain are different entities and are treated differently. In the treatment of chronic pain there is a difference also between the management of protracted pain not associated with terminal illness, and that of protracted pain that is associated with terminal illness.

ACCOUNTABILITY, COMMUNICATION AND ASSESSMENT

ACCOUNTABILITY

Usually the management of pain takes place within an organizational setting such as a hospital, nursing home or hospice. It has been noted that the setting has an effect on the character of the interactions taking place between those in pain and the health care team, and that these interactions in turn affect pain management (Fagerhaugh & Strauss, 1977).

Sometimes, it may be that staff take for granted the day to day work and routines and are unaware of important personal interactions that relate to the management of pain and involve nurse accountability. It is important, for example, that we realize the onus is very often on us to monitor the efficacy of a particular therapy. There may be a tendency to forget that, even though the doctor has prescribed a medication, this is not the end of the story since he/she may not be on hand to assess the result. It is all too easy to assume, just because a medication has been prescribed and administered, that it is bound to be effective. It is the responsibility of the nurse to check and to request review of a therapy if the result is not satisfactory.

Being accountable also involves continuity of care. This may be partially achieved through improved documentation of pain relief, and there is certainly plenty of scope for this. For example, it was found, through scanning records of approximately 450 patients who had undergone surgery, that only three comments had been recorded by nurses relating to pain (Sofaer, 1984). It is usual practice for nurses to record when an analgesic is administered to a patient but it would be valuable also to record its effect. This would help new shifts of nurses coming on duty to be alert to any problems, it would assist medical colleagues in making decisions about changing prescriptions and it should therefore be of ultimate benefit to the patient.

COMMUNICATION

One factor contributing to poor pain management is poor communication. The essential ingredients of good communication are trust, respect and empathy. These dynamics should involve patients, nurses and doctors as well as other members of the health care team. However, nurses have a special role to play as they are often bridges between the patients and the doctors. Porritt (1984) has noted that, as nurses, we will increase effectiveness in communication with others if we become aware of how much we are able to influence colleagues and patients. The implementation of good communication skills by nurses is therefore imperative for the management of patients with either acute or chronic pain.

The following anecdote illustrates a problem of communication in pain management. During a teaching session on drug administration with a student of nursing, a teacher came to the bedside of a female patient. The patient had undergone surgery the previous day following a compound fracture of one leg. The patient looked as if she was in pain. She had not been offered medication by the nursing staff nor had she requested any relief since the last drug around six hours earlier. The prescription was for paracetamol tablets 1–2, 4–6 hourly prn. The teacher asked how effective the medication had been, to which the patient replied 'It doesn't touch me'. The teacher approached the staff nurse in charge of the ward and asked if it would be possible for the nurse to request the doctor to review the prescription. The nurse refused, saying, 'I cannot argue with the doctor'. The teacher assured the nurse that it was not a question of arguing with colleagues and that it was perfectly reasonable to make this request on behalf of the patient. The nurse again refused to take any action but invited the teacher to approach the doctor herself. Since the teacher was a guest on the ward she felt a little uncomfortable at this suggestion but nevertheless agreed to do so.

The teacher approached the doctor, introduced herself and explained that the patient was not feeling relief from the prescribed analgesic. 'These patients are never satisfied,' said the doctor. It was then put to the doctor that other people cannot feel what the patient is feeling, so the best that could be done in the situation was to believe the patient. At the same time the teacher pressed the patient's chart into the doctor's hands, smiled and, while maintaining eye to eye contact, said, 'I am sure we all want to help the patient. I would be most grateful if you could review the prescription and consider a stronger medication.' The doctor took the chart and prescribed a different analgesic. The teacher returned to the patient and instructed her to report the effect of the new analgesic to the staff. She also reported the outcome of her conversation with the doctor to the staff nurse.

In this situation, poor communication already existed in the health care team. Were it not for the teacher's intervention, improved pain control may not have been implemented. The question of whether or not the patient could have been successful in requesting a change of medication raises the issue of patient versus staff responsibility. However it seems that, given the situation as it was (unaware nurse who was unwilling to take the initiative), the patient's chances were not good.

The models shown in Figure 9.1 are intended as food for thought when considering communication with medical colleagues and with patients. Figure 9.1A simply depicts potential communication between a patient in pain, a nurse and a doctor (broken lines). Figure 9.1B shows the patient 'not speaking' of her need for relief, the nurse 'not seeing' and the doctor 'not hearing'. In Figure 9.1C, the patient is pain-free and smiling because of successful communication between the three participants (unbroken lines).

A further point we should always keep in mind is the need for nurses and doctors to explain, in terms that can be understood by patients, the physiological or pathological basis for pain. This may contribute to a patient's peace of mind. Nevertheless, sometimes health carers use technical jargon when talking to patients. Furthermore, Dangott et al (1978) suggested that we may give information in a 'controlling way' when communicating with patients. For

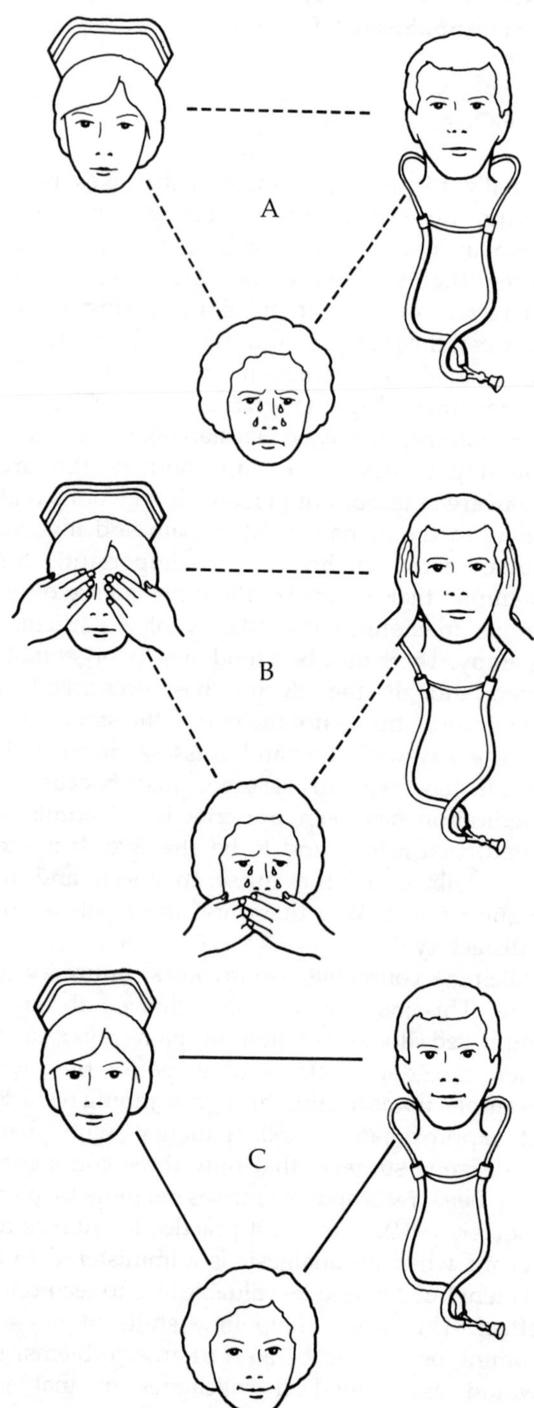

Fig. 9.1 Models of communication between nurse, doctor and patient in pain: (A) potential communication; (B) non-communication; and (C) successful communication.

example, rather than actually telling a person what he will feel during a procedure it would be more valuable to allow him expression of his own feelings openly and in an atmosphere of trust.

PAIN ASSESSMENT

The idea of pain assessment is related to that of communication. With assessment, it is easier to initiate effective treatment. Since we cannot feel what the patient is feeling we must somehow bridge the gap between his experience and relief. One way to do this is to assess pain using some sort of tool with the patient. In postoperative care this should present no difficulty. As we note the general condition of each patient on a regular basis, a simple assessment chart could accompany any other documentation. In a study where four teams of nurses were encouraged to use pain assessment charts in caring for patients postoperatively, the author found a significant reduction in pain assessed compared with pain not assessed. It was evident that the use of an assessment chart was helpful to the nurses when requesting review of patients' medication by medical staff.

One night nurse was concerned about the pain of an elderly patient following cholecystectomy. The nursing staff felt that perhaps the dose of medication prescribed was too small and administration too infrequent, but a young doctor had refused to increase the dose. The night nurse was experienced in dealing with such matters and was an exceptionally compassionate nurse. She approached the doctor. 'Could you please help us? Mrs ... has now suffered for two nights in considerable pain and has not slept. Please come to the ward as soon as you can and suggest some changes in the medication.' This approach did not offend the doctor, and the assessment chart that had been used was valuable in showing up the inefficacy of the medication prescribed.

Assessment of pain may involve both quantitative and qualitative measurements. The simplest assessment instruments have been found to be preferred by patients (Sriwatanakul et al, 1983) and to be more reliable than other clinical measures of pain. An example of a simple quantitative tool is the visual analogue scale (after Scott & Huskisson, 1976) as shown below.

No pain ├──────────────┤ Pain as bad as it can be

It may be helpful to give a patient a scale such as this and to ask him to place a mark on the line indicating the intensity of pain experienced. There are no firm guidelines as to how often a patient should use such a scale. However, postoperatively, it may be appropriate to use this form of assessment every two or three hours initially, gradually increasing the time between assessments according to the patient's requirements. Obviously, if a medication is found to be unsatisfactory, the nurse will want to keep a closer eye on the situation. The same type of scale could be adapted to assess relief as a result of treatment. In this case, 'complete relief' could be written at one end of the scale and 'no relief' at the other. Such scales could be used several times a day and a profile drawn up to show if treatment has been effective. This involves superimposing a scale of the same length broken into ten equal subdivisions, reading off the corresponding score and transferring this to a plot of pain score against time (Fig. 9.2). The use of scales may be particularly helpful in assessing acute pain and its relief.

Alternatively, patients may use category ratings such as 'slight pain' (or relief), 'pain' and 'a lot of pain'. In assessing pain of multifocal distribution, perhaps with terminally ill patients, an observation chart with a body diagram may be helpful in locating the pain and recording this information (Twycross & Lack, 1983). A detailed discussion of assessment tools can be found in McCaffery (1983) and pain measurement in clinical research has recently been reviewed by Chapman et al (1985). However, the most important part of the assessment process is that we accept the patient's statement about his pain, since different patients have different ways of

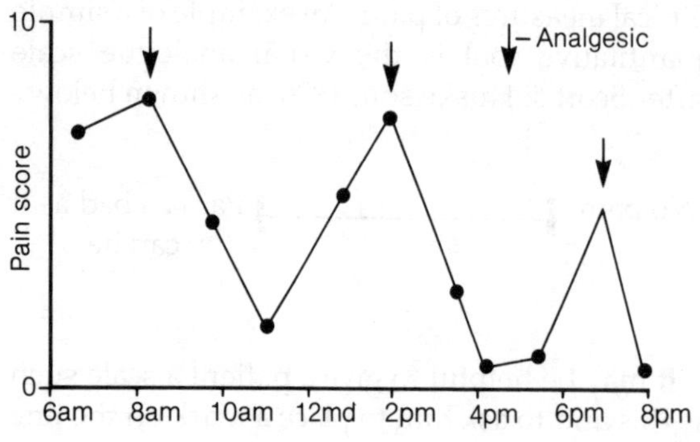

Fig. 9.2 A pain profile showing the effect of a medication on pain score. The arrows indicate times at which analgesia was administered.

coping with the same condition. Furthermore, patients may be reluctant to tell staff about their own coping strategy. Lastly, it should always be remembered that lack of pain expression does not mean lack of pain since, for some people, expression of pain is an embarrassing event.

ACUTE PAIN

Acute pain is pain of sudden onset and foreseeable end. It tends to get better. Even so, we are still responsible for assisting a patient by controlling acute pain with whatever means are at our disposal. We encounter patients suffering acute pain mainly in hospital surroundings: in emergency rooms, intensive care units, postoperative recovery areas and surgical wards. Most patients in acute pain therefore do not have control over their environment and are subject to the customs and practices of their particular ward and the traditional behaviour patterns of the staff. These may vary from routines based on convenience, such as the four-hourly drug round, to practices based on myth, such as the withholding of narcotic medications for fear of addiction.

In relation to drug rounds, it is common for patients to be offered analgesics at these times but the variation in patient requirements may not be accommodated by this routine. It has been demonstrated (Sofaer, 1984) that where nurses in surgical wards broke with this tradition and administered analgesics according to individual requirements, pain intensity and duration were reduced, the patients were more satisfied with their care and the staff more confident in their management of pain. As far as the fear of addiction is concerned, this is completely unfounded in the short term treatment required for acute pain. In fact, undertreatment of pain can result in 'clockwatching', the anxious wait for the next pain relief treatment, with consequent psychological distress. The resulting negative feelings related to unrelieved pain may delay recovery and rehabilitation. A patient may feel resentful and/or angry about the staff and so view future hospitalization with trepidation. Sometimes, people even apologize to staff for their behaviour while in pain, leading to a lowering of their self esteem (Sofaer, 1985).

TREATMENT OF ACUTE PAIN

Although a number of treatments must be prescribed by doctors, several others can be implemented on a nurse's own initiative. The appropriate type of therapy depends on the nature of the pain. Combinations of therapies may also be useful. Distraction techniques, for example, are valuable in preventing peaks of pain while waiting for an analgesic medication to take effect. Table 9.1 lists some common treatments for acute pain.

Table 9.1 Some common treatments for acute pain.

Comfort	Sleep and rest
Drugs	Analgesics
Central modulation	Explanation Distraction Relaxation Hypnosis
Peripheral modulation	Transcutaneous electric nerve stimulation (TENS)
Nerve interruption	Pharmacological — local analgesia Sympathetic nerve blocks

Sleep and rest

An important therapy seldom given priority in the literature on pain is sleep and rest. It is mentioned here to emphasize that nurses can be more instrumental in pain relief than they might imagine, simply by allowing people in pain to have some peace and sleep. During a recent visit to a relative in hospital the author was told, 'You know, the nurses are very nice here, but they don't give you a moment's peace!' 'So why don't you ask them to leave you to sleep awhile?' 'I can't, they have so much to do and besides, they are *so* nice.' This patient went on to say that standard issue to patients undergoing surgery should be ear plugs and a black mask, as issued to some long distance air travellers, to keep out the light.

On one occasion a patient who had not slept for several nights because of uncontrolled pain was having an afternoon nap. Pain is very fatiguing and so the nurses were happy at last to have found a method of pain control for this patient that allowed her to rest. Visiting relatives waited outside the patient's door, but a medical professor entered the room and woke the patient to examine her. When a nurse teacher was approached by the staff and asked for suggestions as to how they might prevent this kind of thing happening, they were asked why they had simply not explained the situation to the professor and requested him to return a little later. 'But he is a *professor*', they said 'besides, we have a little problem with him! He would not have listened to us.' It was recommended that the staff discuss the situation with him openly, honestly and in the spirit of colleagueship for the benefit of the patient. It was also suggested that a 'Please do not disturb' notice might be tried out on the doors of patients' rooms when appropriate.

Analgesics

The rationale for using a particular medication for pain relief is a complicated subject, so only general guidelines are offered to the reader. Analgesic drugs should be viewed as part of an overall approach to the patient's pain and emphasis should be placed on assessing the efficacy of the medication. Since the medical staff are responsible for prescription policy, nursing responsibility is defined by certain limits. Nevertheless, the following suggestions may prove useful:

- a patient has a right to pain relief
- the duty of the nurse is to respond to the needs of a patient
- the responsibility of the nurse is to communicate these to medical colleagues where appropriate
- the nurse must implement a prescribed treatment if it is within her ability and legally acceptable
- the nurse should assess the effect of the treatment
- the nurse should report the results of treatment to colleagues.

Where practicable, the nurse should assess with a patient his response to a particular therapy and discuss possible adjustments with him. The most important criterion in administering analgesics is safety, but the use of all drugs carries risks.

In combating severe pain, narcotic analgesics such as morphine usually provide the only effective treatment. These drugs are subject to national and local regulations regarding their use and have to be prescribed by a medical or dental practitioner. The duration of action of morphine given intramuscularly or subcutaneously is usually considered to be about four hours. However, this should not be taken for granted because there is individual variation. The major side effect is dose-related respiratory depression. Particular care is therefore required in its use for patients who have pulmonary disease. An overdose of morphine can cause death through respiratory suppression, but its depressant effect on the respiratory system can be counteracted by the specific morphine antagonist, naloxone. If naloxone is used, care must be taken not to counteract all the analgesic effect afforded by the morphine. The duration of action of naloxone may be as short as 30 minutes whereas the depressant effects of morphine may last longer.

Repeated doses of naloxone may therefore be required.

As a general rule, it is safe to give a patient enough narcotic to relieve the pain. Yet, unfortunately, many people suffer unrelieved pain through underprescription and inadequate administration. For initial treatment, the intramuscular or intravenous routes may be used, changing to oral, sublingual or rectal routes as the intensity subsides. New preparations for the treatment of pain are constantly appearing on the market and there are many non-narcotic drugs now available. These drugs are helpful in the control of mild to moderate pain and may be useful as the intensity of acute pain subsides further. Aspirin, paracetamol, diflunisal, mefenamic acid and ibuprofen are a few of the more commonly used non-narcotic analgesics. The drugs buprenorphine and pentazocine have narcotic properties but are not classed as narcotics. Detailed information on analgesics can be found in pharmacology texts. For their use in the treatment of different types of pain the student is referred to McCaffery (1983) and the Appendix.

Current ideas on the management of acute pain are aimed at prevention rather than treatment. One approach is known as patient controlled analgesic therapy. A purpose built, preprogrammed drug injector is connected to a venous cannula in the patient's arm or hand. A preset dose of analgesic can then be delivered over a predetermined time when the patient feels the need for it. When this method is used postoperatively, patients may experience better pain relief than would have occurred with more conventional methods (Keeri-Szanto & Heaman, 1972; Tamsen et al, 1979).

Explanation

As mentioned earlier, different people respond differently to the experience of pain. Some factors influencing the response are social background, cultural beliefs, motivation and personality. As far as acute pain is concerned, it has been suggested that there is a relationship between the level of anxiety and degree of pain experienced (Parbrook et al, 1973). However, as nurses we are faced with the actual behaviour of the patient and do not usually have the tools or the skills to assess all these variables. We do not, for example, use 'psychological tools' to assess personality although we know that this may be important in a patient's response to pain. Petrie (1967) described three types of subject in relation to their response to pain: reducers, who decreased what they perceived; augmenters, who increased what they perceived; and moderates, who neither decreased nor increased their perceptions. If we were able to have this kind of information about a patient we might be more understanding about his pain response. Nevertheless we can ask each patient how he normally copes with pain.

There is some conflict in the literature regarding the possible beneficial effects of 'information giving'. Preparing a surgical patient by giving information has been advocated by some authors as a way to decrease pain postoperatively (Egbert et al, 1964; Johnson, 1973). Others have suggested that imparting knowledge can be detrimental (Andrew, 1970; Langer et al, 1975). More recent research (Scott & Clum, 1984) found that information- giving alone was not sufficient for reducing distress associated with surgery. However, when information was given together with a brief training in relaxation techniques, patients who were overtly anxious (sensitizers) found it beneficial. Those who were not anxious about their operation, or who refused to think about it, were better off without the information and training. These findings have implications for nurses who are faced daily with preparing people for surgery. Deciding what to explain, when to tell it and whom to tell it to may present some difficulties. The best we can do is to ask the patient what he would like to know and to go along with his wishes. In a sample of 87 patients, Sofaer (1984) found that 94% interviewed following major surgery felt it would be a good idea for nurses to discuss pain relief with patients prior to surgery.

Previous experience of pain may contribute to coping style. As Wise et al (1982) noted, patients' responses to surgical pain may differ between those who have experienced chronic pain and those who have not. A patient who was mobile the day after major abdominal surgery was giving psychological support to others on the ward. She requested no pain relief. 'I have had so much pain in my lifetime, this is nothing', she said. Another, very elderly, patient underwent major surgery on her foot. She declined all offers of analgesics from nurses, saying 'My dears, I have been through two world wars. This is the first time in my life I have been in hospital and it is nothing by comparison. I know exactly what I have to do'. On the other hand, a third patient, who had suffered chronic pain for several years, was terrified when faced with surgery and afraid to mobilize post-operatively. 'I have had so much pain, but this is something else', she said. 'I can't take any more'. Thus, as nurses caring for patients with a wide variety of responses to pain, we must be able to individualize our care.

Distraction

Distraction may be developed with a patient or initiated by a nurse without telling the patient first. Often patients develop their own method without telling staff for fear of ridicule. What may be appropriate for one person may not suit another, and so assessment of the interests of a patient is important before planning how to proceed. Generally speaking, distraction will result in pain being less bothersome to a patient, but it should be noted that there are limitations to what can be achieved by this technique.

When a person has severe pain, distraction is not likely to be the best method of relief. However, it may be helpful for short periods of time. The most effective distraction techniques are usually developed in consultation with the patient, using the senses of hearing, sight and touch. The idea is to concentrate on positive stimuli inimical to the experience of pain. On a very hot day, a nurse and a patient worked on the following distraction involving visual imagery while waiting for an analgesic drug to take effect. The nurse drew the patient into a casual conversation about a picture that was hanging on the wall. The scene was a wintry one. Snow covered the ground, the trees were bare and the sky clear. Blue smoke poured from the chimney of a little cottage. A bird sat on a fence. Two people were walking in the snow, holding hands. As they talked, the patient and the nurse became these two people. They imagined what they could hear, see and smell. They held hands as the soft snow crunched under their feet. When they had finished, the patient said, 'I feel calm now. As we walked together and you held my hand I forgot about the pain.' This patient was subsequently successful in using her own imagination to distract herself during further bouts of pain. At a later stage, the nurse taught her how to distract herself using, as a tool, a set of coloured bangles.

A nurse can use all sorts of ways to initiate distraction. Encouraging a person to talk about himself and being an interested listener can be of great help. McCaffery (1983) has some further suggestions, including one where a patient stares at a particular spot and, at the same time, massages an area of skin slowly and rhythmically.

Relaxation

Relaxation can be regarded as mental and physical freedom from tension and stress. People have to *learn* relaxation techniques. There are many of these, including meditation, biofeedback, progressive relaxation exercises and self hypnosis. Relaxation tends to reduce anxiety, enhance the effect of different types of pain relief and facilitate sleep. Most techniques are best carried out in a quiet environment with the patient in a comfortable position. McCaffery (1983) gives excellent guidelines for the use of relaxation techniques by nurses. One short exercise that can be carried out, for example prior to or during a procedure or at the scene of an accident, is as follows:

- breathe in deeply and clench your fists
- breathe out and go limp as a rag doll
- start yawning.

These instructions can be repeated as often as

necessary. Step 1 should be followed by step 2, while steps 2 and 3 can be repeated alone at intervals. Slow rhythmic breathing can also be effective. Prior to teaching a patient, the nurse should have some instruction and practice. It may be helpful to a patient if instructions are recorded on a tape recorder with some imagery.

Hypnosis

Hypnosis induces an altered state of reality, in a trusting relationship, and can be used to modify the perception of pain. Hypnotic techniques are numerous but special training and supervision are required.

Transcutaneous electric nerve stimulation (TENS)

Peripheral modulation of pain may sometimes be achieved by the use of TENS, where a mild electric current is applied to the skin via electrodes. A TENS unit consists of two or four electrodes connected by wires to a battery-powered stimulator which is about the size of a bar of soap. The mechanism whereby TENS results in pain relief is not fully understood, although some researchers feel that it activates peripheral nerve endings in the same way as rubbing or the application of heat or cold (Loeser & Black, 1977). TENS may be useful in treating acute pain such as postoperative pain and that associated with trauma such as sprains. Following surgery, the electrodes may be placed near the wound using sterile pre-gelled electrodes. The use of TENS is not widespread, but favourable results have been achieved with 20–30 minutes of stimulation twice a day (Hymes et al, 1974).

Nerve interruption

Nerve blocks may be carried out by doctors to relieve acute pain. Those most commonly used are epidural and intercostal blocks. The role of the nurse during these procedures is to offer support to the patient, to position the patient during and after the procedure according to the instructions of the doctor and to be aware of possible complications, such as urinary retention following an epidural block. Maintaining eye contact and holding a hand if necessary may help a patient to relax.

PAINFUL PROCEDURES

Honesty can be a useful therapy. It is often valuable for a patient to know what is being done. Pain may sometimes be avoided during potentially painful procedures by the administration of Entonox, a 50/50 mixture of nitrous oxide and oxygen.

THE ENVIRONMENT AND PAIN

Wainwright (1985) suggested that privacy, appropriate lighting, heating, ventilation and toileting arrangements are aspects of the environment that make an impact directly or indirectly on the patient in pain. Bryan-Brown (1986) has argued that the environment in intensive care units is conducive to the development of stress which in turn may lead to greater anxiety and greater pain.

CHRONIC PAIN

Chronic pain is considered to be pain that has lasted at least six months, although it may have been present for several decades (Finer, 1982). It is therefore more of a situation than an event. Patients who suffer chronic pain may have developed a ‘pain career’, seeking treatment from many doctors. Because treatment may not have been successful and the patient may not be believed, there is frequently a loss of self-esteem, increasing depression and a lessening of freedom to enjoy life. Chronic pain is seldom life-threatening, but it can be death-threatening. Patients worn down by unremitting pain may be driven to (thoughts of) suicide.

Chronic pain may be associated with disorders

of the spine, arthritis, post-traumatic injuries, postoperative complications, neuralgias and (migraine) headaches. Often a patient suffering chronic pain is seen by a physician who is a specialist in the patient's underlying condition. Unfortunately, progressive disability from pain may not be recognized before it is too late. The patient then becomes a chronic pain patient and develops problems associated with the pain rather than the disease. This may have serious implications for his quality of life. In recent years, pain clinics of a multidisciplinary nature have been developed to try and help these patients, and chronic pain has come to be regarded as an illness in its own right rather than a symptom of disease. Volumes have been written on the medical management of chronic pain and there are many therapies available.

Table 9.2 Some treatments for chronic pain

Comfort	Sleep and rest
Drugs	Analgesics Psychotropics Tranquillisers
Central modulation	Explanation Distraction Relaxation, imagery, hypnosis Social remodelling Family therapy
Peripheral/central modulation	Heat, cold Vibrotherapy, massage TENS Acupuncture
Nerve/tract interruption	Surgical, e.g. cordotomy Pharmacological – sympathetic nerve blocks Heat – radio frequency diathermy Cold – cryoprobe
Other	Physiotherapy Mud baths Hydrotherapy

TREATMENT OF CHRONIC PAIN

Therapies used in the management of chronic pain that fall within the province of the nurse have already been mentioned in connection with acute pain. However, their use in the treatment of chronic pain is rather different. It may be, for example, that a nurse will teach a patient to use a TENS unit, after which he can use it according to his own needs at home. Psychological strategies employed in the treatment of acute pain are often used as adjunct therapies in the management of chronic pain, in combination with other treatments such as medications. Behaviour therapy can sometimes be applied to change habits to more healthy patterns of behaviour. In using drugs for the management of pain not associated with malignancy, drugs that do not have a potential for abuse are chosen, since the treatment of chronic pain is long-term. Psychotropic drugs such as antidepressants and phenothiazines are sometimes found to be helpful. Medication may consist, for example, of an antidepressant, a medium strength analgesic and a tranquillizer three times a day. Some treatments for chronic pain are listed in Table 9.2.

It is astounding to consider that, in the United States alone, 50 million people are partially or totally disabled by pain for periods of up to months or years at a time. For many it is the pain and not the underlying cause that impairs their normal way of life (Chapman, 1984). These patients therefore require psychological and social management as well as medical attention. Yet, even though various combinations of therapies may be tried, often there is only partial success and patients go from doctor to doctor seeking a miracle. Unfortunately, many doctors do not know how to help a person manage chronic pain because they are used to thinking of pain as a symptom of underlying pathology. Such patients often feel isolated, depressed and angry with the world. Specialized pain clinics try to help these patients, and the literature on management is steadily growing. However, although the doctor's role in the management of different pain syndromes – such as orofacial pain and low back pain – has received considerable attention, little is available regarding the nurse's role in the management of chronic pain.

One point to remember is that many chronic pain patients are hospitalized from time to time and, because these are short-term stays, the chronicity of their pain may not be recognized by nursing staff. The possibility that nurses may play an important role in the *prevention* rather than the management of chronic pain is also worthy of attention, and it is up to us to develop this further. Finer (1986) has suggested that once the first medication has been found to be unsuccessful in relieving pain, there is a chance that the patient could become a chronic pain patient. This may be an appropriate time to use group therapy to educate and encourage potential chronic pain sufferers. This could be multidisciplinary in nature and include a nurse, physiotherapist, social worker and occupational therapist. It is hoped that these ideas will be developed further and findings published at a future stage.

SPECIAL OPPORTUNITIES

While caring for a patient who is suffering chronic pain either at home or in hospital, the nurse may have a special opportunity to influence progress. There *are* aspects of a patient's life where we may be able to offer support and advice.

The patient could be asked about the areas in which he would welcome help. If he is not ready to identify these we may need to offer encouragement for him to do so. All this may be easier if the nurse has training in counselling skills and, fortunately, this type of training is becoming more readily available to the nursing profession. Sometimes sound common sense and intuition are all that is required. At other times more specific information may be needed as to what therapies are available. We should also be able to direct the patient to some relevant literature. Two books currently available for patients are by Sternbach (1983) and Lipton (1984). The type of problem with which the nurse may be confronted is illustrated below.

I was once asked to help a young woman (age 32) who had sustained multiple injuries to the lower half of her body in a road traffic accident three years earlier. She had a young family, one child having been delivered by caesarean section three months before the accident. Together we identified four areas of her life for discussion with a view to improvement: restoration of feelings related to her femininity, reintegration into society, motivation to work and reduction in the use of medication.

Her feelings of loss in relation to femininity had much to do with the extensive scarring on her body. She was encouraged to assess her own appearance from head to toe and together we suggested potential improvements. The discussion was open and frank and the tone neither intrusive nor offensive. The patient achieved an attractive outcome, there being a marked difference in the appearance of her hair, face and hands. This pleased her. She even began to like herself a little. Her facial expression changed from being rather sad to pleasant. Some relaxation and imagery enhanced her positive feelings. The concern over body scarring decreased as we thought of imaginative ways to cover the unsightly areas. We talked of the perceptions of other people as they look at you. It seemed a natural and sensible idea to pursue restoration of femininity with this young patient. Most nurses would be helpful in this respect and well able to encourage these ideas with patients.

Turning to the question of improving social contacts, we simply used a diagram to summarize her present pattern of relationships. Since these were mostly with members of her immediate family, we explored possible ways of extending her social contacts, for example, in collecting a child from school there would be the chance to meet other parents. In discussing goals related to work, the patient had a realistic idea based on her own preferences and strengths. The possibility of reducing medication was discussed but she felt the need to continue. Decreasing the dose by half a tablet every other day was encouraged, with a view to decreasing further at a later stage under medical supervision.

The patient recalled how she used to go waterskiing and was fond of sports. Now she walked with a stick. Frequently, people who suffer chronic pain suffer a degree of disability and there is always the danger that they will slide into invalidism and rely on others for income because they have developed a low opinion of themselves. In this particular instance there was motivation to earn and my role was simply to encourage it.

Not all patients will seek advice in a direct way as did the patient discussed, but many may benefit from guidance at an early stage in their 'pain career'. As nurses, we are in a position to try and identify potential chronic pain sufferers and initiate strategies which could prevent pitfalls later. Consultations and group discussions with our fellow health carers, using a team approach during initial hospitalization, might be one way. Occupational therapists, physiotherapists, social workers and physicians all have an important role to play. It is essential not only to identify present problems but to help patients plan realistically for the future. This prevents the development of a negative identity and feelings of uselesness.

GUIDELINES IN ASSISTING PEOPLE NOT TO BECOME CHRONIC PAIN PATIENTS

Try to identify with a patient key areas of life which might be encroached upon as a result of injury or illness. Discuss with him realistic goals to be met in overcoming difficulties so that he has hope for the future. Help him plan. Give information when appropriate and offer sound common sense advice. Help him to be specific about activities. If a person will be unable to work at his old trade or profession, help to develop ideas about new possibilities. Maintain body image as much as possible during hospitalization. Encourage family and social contacts. Discuss personal issues if you think this would be of help, but always in a non-intrusive way. Allow privacy, so that feelings of sexuality and tenderness are preserved. This is essential, especially during long periods of hospitalization, so that the interacting and loving part of a person is maintained as intact as possible. Logistically this may be a little difficult to achieve in large, open wards, but it is always possible to draw curtains around the bed so that a modicum of privacy is provided in an otherwise public place. Encourage fun and humour as these are powerful distractions. Share ideas and thoughts with professional colleagues and encourage each other.

Encouraging pleasant feelings

One aspect of care seldom addressed by nurses is how to help a person have fun. We try to help a patient in pain over a hump but he also may need to maintain the ability or even relearn how to enjoy life a little. An elderly retired miner once told a nurse how he had forgotten the joys in life through years of suffering pain. 'Nobody believed my pain, but you do,' he said. He wept in his despair and, when he said goodbye to her later they shook hands and he kissed her cheek. 'I need more of that in my life,' he said.

Several patients have mentioned the need for help in reshaping relationships eroded through the experience of pain. Sometimes requests are met by avoidance on the part of doctors and nurses. Encouragement given in an open manner for partners to talk over difficulties with each other, and referral for professional help where appropriate, may be steps in the right direction.

Occasionally, difficulties in someone's personal and/or sexual relationship manifest themselves as pain. This may have been a contributory factor in the following example. A female patient (age 48) reported headaches for the past two years. Medical investigation failed to reveal an underlying cause, so the patient was referred to a pain clinic. She was offered a number of therapies, including analgesics and acupuncture, but they all proved unsuccessful and, after several months, the patient was referred for counselling. She was invited to talk about herself and made the following statement. 'I can't understand it. I go to bed at night, give my husband a kiss and wake up the next morning with a headache.' Standard counselling techniques were used to feed back to the patient what she had said. She found it helpful to talk openly and frankly. It subsequently occurred to her that she was not satisfied with only a kiss!

She returned only once more to the pain clinic, to report a decrease in her headaches.

Encouraging appreciation of music, literature and art, together with involvement in hobbies such as gardening, needlework or woodwork, is all part and parcel of working towards the enhancement of pleasant feelings in life.

THE PAIN OF TERMINAL ILLNESS

Pain and terminal malignant disease do not necessarily go hand in hand, the incidence of pain varying according to the primary site of cancer (Twycross & Lack, 1983). However, when pain does occur it may be continuous and may get worse over time. Nevertheless, there are ways to relieve it. For a person who is dying, the most important aspect of care is the trust that develops between him and the caring team. Most people who are dying know when they are nearing the end of their life. There is security for these patients in honesty and we have to prepare ourselves to deal with this. Pain relief is also part of providing security. Once it is realized that a person is suffering a terminal illness there is no reason to withhold medication. Likewise, there is no reason to wait until a person is 'really dying' before using narcotic analgesics. There are a number of useful therapies we can draw on to help the patient, for example oral morphine, sustained release morphine, nerve blocks and non-pharmacological methods such as relaxation and imagery.

Cancer pain may be caused by the cancer itself or by other factors, for example by various forms of treatment. Associated pains may also occur, caused by bed sores or constipation, but these can be dealt with. Severe pain is fatiguing and should be avoided by the optimal use of analgesics (and co-analgesics where appropriate) administered in regular doses and in sufficient quantity. The exhaustion resulting from unrelieved severe pain can lead to distrust of nursing and medical staff.

The hospice movement has been instrumental in advocating symptom control in the care of the terminally ill. The pain of dying is 'total pain', that is not only physical pain but psychological and spiritual pain as well. People who are dying should be allowed to die the way they want to. It is valuable if they can be cared for by those who have deep understanding of human life, and who know something of pain and suffering, separation and loss.

SOME GUIDELINES FOR CONTROLLING TERMINAL PAIN

Believe what the patient says. Identify when analgesics are too weak and communicate this to medical colleagues. Abandon fears of addiction. Don't wait until almost the end before encouraging the use of morphine. Many people with cancer lead useful and fulfilling lives while taking narcotic medication. Use non-pharmacological measures where appropriate. Provide information and emotional support for the patient and his family. Don't shy away from open discussion with a patient when he needs your companionship. Encourage participation of the family in the patient's care if the patient welcomes this.

OPEN DISCUSSION

Open discussions between nurses and terminally ill patients should not be avoided. The following story may be helpful in illustrating the value of such discussions. A student and I were bedbathing a woman (age 52) who had undergone abdominal surgery for advanced cancer. The nurse left the room for a few moments during which time the patient said to me: 'I have inoperable cancer. The staff will not discuss the situation with me. The only person I can communicate with is the young nurse. She cannot be with me all the time, of course, but she is the *only* one who gives me courage. She gives me spiritual strength. You know, she even prays with me.' When the nurse returned I taught the patient some relaxation and imagery. As the nurse held her hand, I suggested that she experience that feeling very strongly and that she concentrate on the face of the nurse so that then she would be able to recall the nurse's presence whenever she wished to and so not feel alone. She appreciated this.

She then expressed her fear that decreasing mobility would soon prevent her from taking her evening walks round the harbour town where she lived. Again using imagery, and with encouragement, she was able to recall the sensations as these walks took place – the smells, sights and sounds. She asked for some suggestions as to what work she might do to keep herself productive. We suggested needlework and she liked the idea. As I was leaving the room the patient said, 'I want to live to see my only child celebrate her 21st birthday (in three months time). Do you think I will?' I replied, 'One cannot predict anything, but I encourage you to make it one of your goals.' 'I'll do that,' she responded.

I did not meet the patient again as my teaching commitment on that ward came to an end. Some weeks later, I bumped into the student. She reported that the patient had taught her husband and daughter the imagery about the harbour so that when she herself become too weak they could recite it to her. The nurse had accompanied the patient to a hospice and had been able to make contact there with a nursing colleague who promised to continue the spiritual companionship and pray with the patient.

Several months later, I had a chance conversation with a medical colleague who worked in the hospice. I asked if he remembered this patient. 'Yes,' he said, 'a matter of fact I remember her very well. She arrived with a thick file of notes. For years she had reported abdominal pain but nobody had believed her. In her professional life she had been a medical secretary and doctors thought the pains were 'psychogenic', so she had been referred for psychiatric care. She was transferred to the hospice from hospital with a letter and a phone call indicating that she was 'difficult to deal with' and 'demanding' of the staff'. 'How did you find her,' I asked. 'Well, to tell you the truth, we saw her as a very courageous woman. We felt the medication prescribed in hospital was probably not adequate. She encouraged other patients and was an example in her activity. She worked on embroidery and derived much pleasure from the visits of her husband and mentally handicapped daughter. You know, we even threw a little party for her daughter's 21st birthday and she was in fine form. Yes, I remember the patient well. Two days after the birthday she asked me to sit down next to her. 'Doctor,' she said, 'I am now ready to die.' She did so 24 hours later. I felt she had peace of mind at last.'

Helping a patient achieve peace of mind is most important in terminal care. The situation of a male patient in his early 60s illustrates this point too. He asked to be taught relaxation at home. Very open discussions about his approaching death had taken place between him and his wife. 'I know I am dying', he said. 'I have cancer of the pancreas. It is not nice to die, but it is happening. Probably I have three months to live. More or less, I have accomplished all the goals I set myself, but I need some encouragement to prepare my wife for afterwards. The pain killers are not adequate but I want at least to have the strength and courage to maintain self-respect and self-esteem in front of relatives.' He was taught relaxation as he requested and the ideas of courage which he wished to achieve were suggested to him. Afterwards, he smiled a gentle wry smile and said, 'Thank you, now I feel more calm and have more peace of mind.' He died a week later.

Support of family and friends is also part of relieving pain for patients. There are fears and anxieties around separation, and we must offer people the opportunity to express these. Furthermore, support for each other and for our medical colleagues is necessary when caring for patients who are terminally ill.

SPECIAL PATIENT GROUPS

The discussion in this chapter has focused on the different pain entities and some general approaches to management by nurses. However, there are certain groups whose pain may present particular difficulties of management to health carers. One such group is the elderly. Assessment can be a problem because sometimes there are difficulties of communication due to impaired bodily function and, in some instances, confusion. Increased awareness by staff and relatives of changes in behaviour with age, and special skills and patience, are all required. One experienced geriatrician commented, 'It is sometimes so hard to tell if an elderly, confused, deaf person is in pain.' A student nurse recalled how a patient was prescribed an analgesic for abdominal pain but, when constipation was relieved, the patient's personality and behaviour were quite transformed. Overcoming difficulties caused by language, dysphagia and deafness are all avenues which need to be explored in caring for elderly people in pain. Managing the pain of someone who has an existing physical handicap presents a challenge too, while pain detection in the mentally handicapped has received little or no attention in the literature (Fraser & Ozols, 1980).

Nursing the patient who has sustained severe burns is also worthy of special mention because the pain and suffering may be considerable. In addition to dealing with the pain, the patient has to cope with the emotional stress related to body disfigurement. Nurses who learn imagery and relaxation may find these techniques of great value when trying to relieve the pain of burns patients.

THE CHALLENGE AND THE PRIVILEGE

Effective caring by nurses begins with intuition: offering a hand to hold when it seems right, maintaining eye to eye contact when words are meaningless and talking too strenuous for the sufferer, listening at times when the patient needs to talk. All this means sharing the negative, but also the positive, using the moments of freedom from pain to share a thought, an idea or laugh with the patient but also sharing these things with the patient's relatives and friends, and our own colleagues too. Pain for a patient is pain for his family. Sometimes there is also the pain of failure for us and our medical colleagues. It is no good saying that a patient is 'comfortable' when in truth he is rather uncomfortable but receiving the best care we can give. In such situations, consultation with patients and relatives is particularly important. 'Is there anything you could suggest that might be more helpful in relieving the pain?' Sometimes patients and relatives are reluctant to offer suggestions for fear of offending staff. This is perhaps understandable because suggestions are not always well received.

A colleague was with her husband postoperatively. He was suffering a lot of pain. She asked the nurse for pain relief for her husband and was met with the response, 'I am in charge of the ward.' On another occasion, a doctor who was very experienced in the care of terminally ill patients requested a narcotic for himself the night before surgery on his back. 'I was in terrible pain,' he said. 'I asked for a narcotic so that I could get some relief. The staff (both doctors and nurses) told me that I was only asking for a narcotic because I knew what a narcotic was! They gave me paracetamol. Of course, it did not relieve the pain. Following surgery I was offered morphine but they would have spared me unnecessary pain if they had given it when I needed it.'

Generally speaking, incidents like these are on the decrease. Nurses are becoming more aware of their potential in relieving pain and of the importance of believing the patient. A combination of empathetic skills, good communication and up-to-date knowledge about treatment options goes a long way in facing the challenge of managing pain with patients. It is our privilege to offer what ability we have to ease the suffering and pain of our fellow human beings. These efforts cut across language and culture, across politics and power struggles. Sometimes we face failure, sometimes we have a measure of success. Our efforts, given in a spirit of trust and respect for our patients and colleagues, will be received in the same light.

It is hoped that this short chapter, inadequate as it stands in the context of so much literature on pain and its treatment, will offer some encouragement to students of nursing, and strength and confidence to colleagues who have been in practice for some time.

REFERENCES

Andrew J M 1970 Recovery from surgery, with and without preparation instruction for three coping styles. Journal of Personality and Social Psychology 15:223–226

Bryan-Brown C W 1986 Development of pain management in critical care. In:Cousins M, Phillips G D (eds) Acute pain management. Churchill Livingstone, Edinburgh

Chapman C R 1984 New directions in the understanding and management of pain. Social Science and Medicine 19:1261–1277

Chapman C R, Casey K L, Dubner R, Foley K M, Gracely R H, Reading A E 1985 Pain measurement: an overview. Pain 22:1–31

Charap A D 1978 The knowledge, attitudes and experience of medical personnel treating pain in the terminally ill. Mt Sinai Journal of Medicine 45:561–580

Cohen F L 1980 Post-surgical pain relief: patients' status and nurses' medication choices. Pain 9:262–274

Dangott L, Thornton D C, Page P 1978 Communication and pain. Journal of Communication 28:30–35

Edwards R B 1984 Pain and the ethics of pain management. Social Science and Medicine 18:515–523

Egbert L D, Battit G E, Welch C E, Bartlett M D 1964 Reduction of postoperative pain by encouragement and instruction of patients. New England Journal of Medicine 270:825–827

Fagerhaugh S Y, Strauss A 1977 Politics of pain management: staff—patient interaction. Addison-Wesley, Menlo Park, California

Finer B 1982 Treatment in an interdisciplinary pain clinic. In: Barber , Adrian C (eds) Psychological approaches to the management of pain. Brunner-Maazal, New York

Finer B 1986 Personal communication

Fraser W, Ozols D 1980 Cries in pain and distress in the severely mentally handicapped. In: Mittler P (ed) Proceedings of the 5th Congress of the International Association for the Scientific Study of Mental Deficiency, Jerusalem

Hunt J M, Stollar T D, Littlejohns D W, Twycross R G, Vere D W 1977 Patients with protracted pain: a survey conducted at the London Hospital. Journal of Medical Ethics 3:61–73

Hymes A C, Raab D E, Yonehiro E G, Nelson G D, Printy A L 1974 Acute pain control by electro-stimulation: a preliminary report. Advances in Neurology 4:761–767

International Association for the Study of Pain Subcommittee on Taxonomy 1979 Pain terms: a list with definitions and notes on usage. Pain 6:249–252

Jacox A 1979 Assessing pain. American Journal of Nursing 79: 895–900

Johnson J E 1973 Effects of accurate expectations about sensations on the sensory and distress components of pain. Journal of Personality and Social Psychology 27:261–275

Keeri-Szanto M, Heaman S 1972 Postoperative demand analesia. Surgery Gynecology and Obstetrics 134:647–651

Langer E J, Janis I L, Wolfer J 1975 Reduction of psychological stress in surgical patients. Journal of Experimental Social Psychology 11:155–165

Lipton S 1984 Conquering pain. Martin Dunitz, London

Loeser J D, Black R G 1977 Electrical stimulation for pain relief. In: Management of pain, circuit course (syllabus). University of Washington (Seattle), Continuing Medical Education

McCaffery M 1983 Nursing the patient in pain. (Adapted by Sofaer B) Harper and Row, London

Melzack R, Wall P 1982 The challenge of pain. Penguin, Harmondsworth

Parbrook G D, Steel D F, Dalrymple D G 1973 Factors predisposing to postoperative pain and pulmonary complications. A study of male patients undergoing elective gastric surgery. British Journal of Anaesthesia 45:21–33.

Petrie A 1967 Individuality in pain and suffering. University of Chicago Press, Chicago

Porritt L 1984 Communication:choices for nurses. Churchill Livingstone, Edinburgh

Scott J, Huskisson E C 1976 Graphic representation of pain. Pain 2:175–184

Scott L E, Clum G A 1984 Examining the interaction effects of coping style and brief interventions in the treatment of postsurgical pain. Pain 20:279–291

Sofaer B 1984 The effect of focused education for nursing teams on postoperative pain of patients. Unpublished PhD thesis, University of Edinburgh

Sofaer B 1985 Pain: a handbook for nurses. Harper and Row, London

Sriwatanakul K, Kelvie W, Lasagna L, Calimlin J F, Weis O F, Mehta G 1983 Studies with different types of visual analogue scale for measurement of pain. Clinical Pharmacology and Therapeutics 34:234–239

Sternbach R A 1968 Pain:a psychophysiological analysis. Academic Press, New York

Sternbach R A 1983 How can I learn to live with pain when it hurts so much? Pain Treatment Center, Scripps Clinic and Research Foundation, La Jolla, California

Tamsen A, Hartvig P, Dahlstrom B, Lindstrom B, Holmdahl M 1979 Patient controlled analgesic therapy in the early postoperative period. Acta Anaesthesiologica Scandinavica 23:462–470

Twycross R G, Lack S A 1983 Symptom control in far advanced cancer: pain relief. Pitman, London

Wall P D 1977 Why do we not understand pain? In: Ducan R, Weston-Smith M (eds) The encyclopaedia of ignorance. Pergamon Press, Oxford

Wainwright P 1985 Impact of hospital architecture on the patient in pain. In: Copp L A (ed) Perspectives in pain. Recent Advances in Nursing. Churchill Livingstone, Edinburgh

Wiener C L 1975 Pain assessment on an orthopaedic ward. Nursing Outlook 23:508–516

Wise T N, Hall W A, Wong O 1982 Factors determining acute pain response. In: Hendler N H, Long D M, Wise T N (eds) Diagnosis and treatment of chronic pain. Wright, Bristol

FURTHER READING

Brena S F, Chapman S L (eds) 1985 Chronic pain: management principles. Clinics in Anaesthesiology. Saunders, London.

Copp L A (ed) 1985 Perspectives on pain. Recent Advances in Nursing. Churchill Livingstone, Edinburgh

Cousins M, Phillips G (eds) 1986 Acute pain management. Churchill Livingstone, Edinburgh

Fagerhaugh S Y, Strauss A 1977 Politics of pain management: staff—patient interaction. Addison-Wesley, Menlo Park, California

Kotarba J A 1983 Chronic pain. Its social dimensions. Sage Publications, Beverley Hills

Melzack R, Wall P 1982 The challenge of pain. Penguin, Harmondsworth

Menges L J (ed) 1984 Chronic pain. Social Science and medicine 19:No 12 (special issue)

McCaffery M 1983 Nursing the patient in pain. (Adapted by Sofaer B) Harper and Row, London

Sofaer B 1985 Pain: a handbook for nurses. Harper and Row, London

Twycross R G, Lack S A 1984 Symptom control in far advanced cancer: pain relief. Pitman, London

10

Shock

INTRODUCTION

The syndrome of shock can arise from a number of different causes, but it is always imperative that treatment is started promptly. Awareness of factors predisposing to shock, early detection if it occurs, and prompt and effective treatment may make the difference between a relatively rapid and complete recovery, and increasing organ damage leading to death. It can also be a very stressful experience for any patient, and one in which nursing can make a considerable contribution to the support he/she receives as a suffering person.

Shock is a state in which tissue perfusion is inadequate either to maintain the necessary supply of oxygen and nutrients for normal cell function or to remove the waste products of metabolism. This results from 'pump failure' (inadequate cardiac function) or real or apparent reduction in circulating blood volume; that is, fluid is actually lost from the intravascular space, or excessive vasodilation increases the volume of space so that the circulating fluid is inadequate for effective circulation. Figure 10.1 indicates physiological factors affecting blood pressure.

Different kinds of shock originate at different points in the system, e.g. cardiogenic shock may result from changes in cardiac contractility/rate/ rhythm, hypovolaemic shock from loss of circulating volume. In anaphylactic shock changes in vessel size/resistance are the main feature, while septic shock is much more complex.

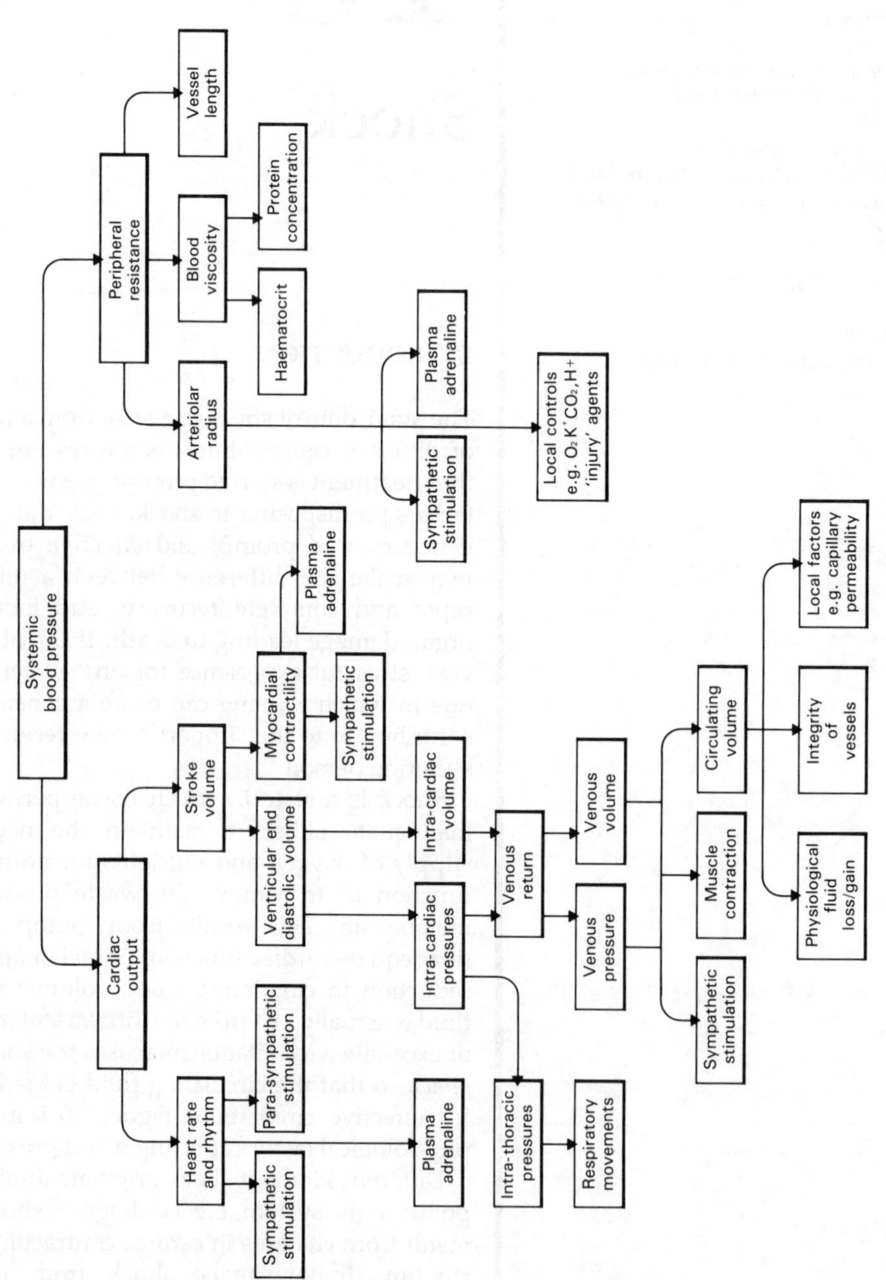

Fig. 10.1 Physiological factors affecting blood pressure

SIGNS AND SYMPTOMS OF SHOCK

Whatever the cause, the signs and symptoms of shock usually include hypotension (i.e. low compared with the patient's usual blood pressure), tachycardia (though bradycardia may occur), hyperventilation, oliguria or anuria, anxiety or clouding of consciousness, and a low PCO_2 and PO_2 (partial pressure of carbon dioxide and oxygen). Frequently the skin is cold, pale and moist, but in early bacteraemic or endotoxic shock there may be vasodilation, so that the skin is pink and warm though hypotension still occurs. In this situation the cardiac output may be high rather than low, the so-called hyper-dynamic shock syndrome. What causes these signs and symptoms? Effective nursing care and co-operation in medical treatment requires understanding of this so that the care can be planned intelligently, the effects constantly observed, and modifications made as necessary.

MAINTENANCE OF EFFECTIVE CIRCULATION

To understand the pathophysiology of the main types of shock, the signs, symptoms and effects, it is necessary to review briefly the major physiological mechanisms for maintaining effective circulation (Vander & Sherman, 1985). The maintenance of good peripheral perfusion depends on adequate systemic arterial pressure, which in turn depends on an adequate cardiac output in relation to the peripheral resistance. The cardiac output varies according to the heart rate and stroke volume (volume of blood pumped out by the ventricle with each contraction). Left ventricular contractility and venous return of blood to the heart together largely determine stroke volume. Variation in either the rate of contraction or the stroke volume will alter the cardiac output unless other factors alter at the same time. Similarly, changes in venous return to the heart will affect the cardiac output unless other mechanisms compensate for the change. The venous return may be increased or decreased according to the circulating blood volume and the amount of blood pooling in the peripheral and major vessels. The peripheral resistance depends on the degree of peripheral vasoconstriction or vasodilation, and to some extent on the viscosity of circulating blood.

The interaction of the autonomic nervous system, the vasomotor centre and feedback mechanisms such as the baroceptors in the aortic arch and the carotid sinuses, and the chemoreceptors in the aortic carotid bodies, control the balance of cardiac output (rate and contractility) and peripheral resistance (degree of vasoconstriction/dilatation) to maintain adequate arterial pressure and perfusion of the tissues. The main humoral factors affecting circulation are the release of adrenaline and noradrenaline (epinephrine and norepinephrine), both vasoconstrictors from sympathetic nerves and the adrenal medulla; aldosterone (increasing renal absorption of sodium and water) from the adrenal cortex, which increases the circulating fluid volume; and angiotensin which both stimulates the release of aldosterone and is a powerful vasoconstrictor.

Local factors also play a major part in controlling tissue perfusion by regulating the opening or closing of the pre-capillary sphincters, thus increasing the flow of blood through the capillaries or causing some or all of it to be shunted through small bypass vessels from the arterioles to the venules. The main factors affecting the sphincters are the tissue oxygen demand and carbon dioxide level, a low oxygen or high carbon dioxide level causing opening of the sphincters; but the complex mechanisms which may affect vascular tone and capillary permeability include such factors as potassium, hydrogen ions, adenosine triphosphate (ATP), histamine and less well-known factors such as kinins and lysozymes (Ledingham & Routh, 1979). It should not be forgotten that emotion, by its effect on the hypothalamus which controls the autonomic system, may exert considerable influence on the circulation. This is readily seen when, for example, a person becomes flushed when angry, or pale with a rapid heart rate when anxious. While harmless for the healthy person, such reactions may be damaging to an individual whose physiological function is already severely disturbed. This has considerable implications for nursing and is discussed later.

TYPES OF SHOCK

All authorities seem to agree that, in shock syndromes, general tissue perfusion fails to maintain an adequate supply of oxygen and removal of carbon dioxide and other metabolites, with the consequence that cell function progressively deteriorates. However there are various ways of classifying the different types of shock. For example Ledingham & Routh (1979) describe hypovolaemic, cardiogenic and septic shock, while Jones (1978) dislikes the term septic shock since in his experience the blood may be sterile when septic shock is diagnosed by some people. He prefers to use the terms hypovolaemic shock, pump failure, and neurogenic shock. Holloway (1979) describes the major types of shock according to physiological mechanisms. First, cardiogenic shock due to failure of cardiac function; second, vasogenic shock, with decreased arterial resistance and/or increased venous capacitance, either of which decreases venous return unless there is compensation by other physiological mechanisms (examples are anaphylaxis, intense pain, and sometimes sepsis); third, hypovolaemic shock, in which blood volume is depleted.

In order to explain the main factors leading to shock syndromes, it is proposed here to discuss four types in order of prevalence:

- hypovolaemic
- cardiogenic
- septic, bacteraemic or endotoxic
- neurogenic and anaphylactic shock.

HYPOVOLAEMIC SHOCK

Any condition which depletes the circulating fluid volume may lead to this if it is severe enough; examples are haemorrhage, diarrhoea and/or vomiting, dehydration due to inadequate fluid intake, or burns. Fluid need not actually leave the body for circulation to be depleted. Collection of several litres of electrolyte-rich fluid in the stomach or gut (as may occur in paralytic ileus and/or acute dilatation of the stomach or obstruction) may quite rapidly lead to the signs and symptoms of shock. Furthermore, the abdominal distension may exacerbate these by pushing upwards on the diaphragm and impeding cardiac and respiratory function. As the circulating fluid decreases, adequate circulation to the vital organs, brain, kidneys, liver and heart may at first be maintained by vasoconstriction and an increased heart rate. But sooner or later this mechanism fails, not least because the tachycardia increases myocardial work and oxygen demand while decreasing the diastolic period during which most circulation through the coronary system occurs, thus limiting oxygen transport to the myocardium. At the same time peripheral tissues, deprived of adequate perfusion by the vasoconstriction, produce more lactic acid due to the change to anaerobic metabolism necessitated by inadequate oxygen supply. As this accumulates in the blood and metabolic acidosis develops, this further decreases myocardial function and reduces cardiac output.

This situation is compounded by failure of the kidneys to maintain their usual function in maintaining acid-base balance by excreting excess hydrogen ions (urine output ceases from even a previously healthy kidney when the arterial pressure falls below about 50 mmHg). Myocardial depressant factor (MDF) produced by hypoxic pancreatic cells may decrease myocardial function still further (Ledingham & Routh, 1979). Hyperventilation, stimulated by hypoxic tissues, may at first increase oxygen intake but cannot compensate for inadequate oxygen transport, and the extra muscular effort further increases oxygen demand. Circulation to the brain is maintained as long as possible, the cerebral vessels dilating as lactic acid accumulates and the plasma PCO_2 (partial pressure of carbon dioxide) rises. But as cerebral circulation decreases and hypoxia increases, the patient's anxiety, often associated with the increased circulating catecholamines, is replaced by clouding of consciousness and eventually coma. It can be seen that simple fluid depletion, if severe enough, may lead to a downward spiral of tissue hypoxia, myocardial failure, acidosis and multiple organ failure ending in death, unless the process is reversed before it becomes irreversible.

CARDIOGENIC SHOCK

In this condition the downward spiral is similar to that seen in hypovolaemic shock, but the cycle of events begins with 'pump failure' (failure of the heart to maintain adequate output to perfuse the body tissues), and far from being depleted the circulating blood volume may be increased. There are several possible mechanisms, each of which impedes cardiac function in a different way. In acute myocardial infarction, some kinds of poisoning, or endotoxaemia, the myocardial muscle is damaged and fails to contract adequately. When massive pulmonary embolism occurs, resistance to the outflow from the right ventricle is greatly increased. In addition, there is a decrease in blood flow through the left side of the heart and, thus, in coronary perfusion and myocardial oxygenation. Cardiac tamponade (when fluid in the closed sac of pericardium round the heart impedes cardiac filling by compression, preventing expansion of the heart chambers) is comparatively rare. It may be seen, however, after cardiac surgery or stab wounds to the chest. It is perhaps less rare to see conditions such as acute asthma or tension pneumothorax, when raised intrathoracic pressure reduces venous return of blood to the right atrium. The raised intrathoracic pressure reduces the 'thoracic pump' effect, which normally increases venous return during inspiration when intrathoracic pressure is decreased. Cardiac dysrhythmias such as persistent severe tachycardia or bradycardia may similarly cause the signs of shock, particularly when the myocardium is already damaged and thus more susceptible to the resulting deficiency in myocardial circulation.

Whatever the mechanism, as cardiac output decreases, hypotension and vasoconstriction occur, tissue oxygenation fails and lactic acid accumulates and the cycle continues downwards as previously described. But it seems that some of the physiological reactions which may initially be protective in hypovolaemic shock may actually be counterproductive in cardiogenic failure. Vasoconstriction increases resistance to the outflow of blood from the heart and therefore increases the workload of the left ventricle, thus extra demands are made on an already failing pump. Similarly the hormonal response is likely to include increased release of aldosterone from the adrenal cortex, stimulated by activation of the renin-angiotensin system which, in turn, is caused by poor blood flow to the kidneys. Aldosterone causes increased reabsorption of sodium and water thus increasing the circulating volume, but this does little to help the failing heart. The increased retention of sodium may not, however, be obvious on measuring the serum sodium, since cell damage due to hypoxia may reduce the efficiency of the 'sodium pump' which, normally, actively keeps sodium out of the cells. Cell membrane function is impaired by the reduced availability of ATP, increased lactate and acidosis, and other such effects of hypoxia. Thus sodium and water leak into the cells while potassium leaks out — the 'sick cell syndrome'.

Despite modern treatment, the mortality rate for patients with severe cardiogenic shock is still high, around 60% (Forrester & Waters, 1978).

SEPTIC, BACTERAEMIC OR ENDOTOXIC SHOCK

This is most likely to occur where there are local infections in the gut, respiratory or urinary tracts, or obstruction or intervention of some kind such as operation, instrumentation or artificial ventilation. Gram negative infection seems to be associated with rapid onset of a fairly typical picture of the shock syndrome, with hypotension and tachycardia, vasoconstriction and cold peripheries, oliguria and impaired cerebral function, and tachypnoea or hyperpnoea. However, in other infections the picture may be deceptive, with hypotension and tachycardia associated with vasodilation and warm pink peripheries, a good urine output and a respiratory alkalosis. Mortality in bacteraemic shock is around 50% or more (Wardle, 1979) and, although it is lower for those patients with 'warm hypotension', this too may progress to the typical picture of impaired blood flow and multi-organ failure. In septic shock the patient is liable to feel cold and shivery, show pyrexia or hypothermia and there may be diarrhoea and vomiting and possibly jaundice (10%).

Cell damage and increased capillary permeability lead to loss of fluid from the circulation, while endothelial damage increases susceptibility to disseminated intravascular coagulation (DIC). Increased capillary permeability may be due to bacterial toxins (Wardle, 1979) or to bradykinin, which is also an extremely potent vasodilator and is a vasoactive polypeptide. Such polypeptides are released by powerful enzymes which in turn are released by the lysosomes of damaged or dying cells as the cells break down (Wilson, 1976). Although endotoxins are usually inactivated by the Kupffer cells in the liver, when there is a brisk endotoxaemia these are paralysed and the resulting systemic endotoxaemia is thought to be the cause of 'shock lung' or 'shock kidney' which are common complications of endotoxic shock.

NEUROGENIC AND ANAPHYLACTIC SHOCK

Examples of neurogenic causes of shock include intense pain and damage to the central nervous system mechanisms concerned with the maintenance of circulation. Anaphylactic shock is an extreme example of allergic response which may be provoked by many antigens such as bee-stings, injection of drugs (especially those such as penicillin) or other chemicals. The onset is rapid and the typical symptoms of shock may be accompanied by urticaria, localized tissue swelling and laryngeal oedema or bronchospasm. The histamine and other substances released dilate and increase the permeability of venules and capillaries, thus causing fluid loss from the circulation and pooling of blood in the vessels, thus reducing venous return. Because of the accompanying respiratory embarrassment, the urgency to treat anaphylaxis is even greater than in other kinds of shock. Treatment recommended is a subcutaneous injection of adrenaline 0.3–0.5 ml of 1:1000 accompanied by an antihistamine, or sublingual isoprenaline and an antihistamine (Holt, 1979), or adrenaline injection BP 1 ml intramuscularly, promethazine hydrochloride 50 mg intravenously, and hydrocortisone 100 mg intravenously (Jones, 1978). Patients who have previously had an anaphylactic reaction may carry drugs with them, having been taught how to use them.

COMPLICATIONS OF SHOCK

Since the shock syndrome has such a widespread effect throughout the body there are a number of possible complications, including paralytic ileus, stress ulcers and gastric bleeding, venous thrombosis and embolism. Liver failure may occur with septic shock or hypovolaemia, though necrosis is rare if the hypotension lasts less than 10 hours (Ledingham & Routh, 1979).

However, three of the most common and potentially fatal complications are renal failure, disseminated intravascular coagulation (DIC), and 'shock lung' or adult respiratory distress syndrome (ARDS). It is important to consider complications along with the main shock syndrome, since continuous assessment of the patient's condition must include vigilance to ensure that early treatment is instituted as soon as signs of complications appear. As Harken (1974) has said, to some extent 'We see what we look for and we look for what we know'. Furthermore, some of the treatment of shock is ordered with the prevention of complications in mind.

RENAL FAILURE — 'SHOCK KIDNEY'

This is particularly liable to occur where there is crush injury or sepsis, or where there is pre-existing kidney function deficiency. However, it may occur after any period of prolonged severe hypotension. Normally the kidneys receive up to 25% of the cardiac output and if the blood pressure drops sufficiently (at about 50 mmHg systolic) urine output ceases. One of the aims of treatment in shock is to maintain circulation to the kidneys, as demonstrated by a flow of urine, and in this respect some of the more recent inotropic drugs (which increase cardiac contractility) such as dobutamine (dopamine) are useful in that they selectively increase renal circulation. If there are no other complications, this kind of renal failure is often reversible and kidney function may return to normal if the patient can be maintained meantime by haemodialysis. However, if the recovery is to be as complete and rapid as possible it is essential that it should be detected and treated early, before excessive overhydration occurs. Therefore, if the urinary output remains below 30 ml per hour when the arterial pressure and circulating volume are adequate, and despite the administration of diuretics, renal failure should be suspected and fluid balance carefully controlled according to the medical regime ordered. Peritoneal or haemodialysis may be required in addition to this.

DISSEMINATED INTRAVASCULAR COAGULATION (DIC)

In this condition, due to vasoconstriction and sluggish peripheral circulation, cell dysfunction and damage to the vascular endothelium and other factors, diffuse clotting of blood and formation of microemboli occurs. Thus the clotting factors in the blood become used up, as demonstrated by the low platelet count and fibrinogen level, the prolonged thrombin and prothrombin time, and the increased fibrinogen degradation products found in the blood. Only if the mechanism of this syndrome is understood does it make sense when heparin is ordered for a patient who oozes blood from every skin puncture or trauma site, and may show profuse bleeding from the gastrointestinal or genitourinary tract.

ADULT RESPIRATORY DISTRESS SYNDROME (ARDS) — 'SHOCK LUNG'

This condition is now more often termed ARDS, since it may be associated not only with the shock syndrome but also with factors such as massive transfusion and/or overhydration, fat embolism, non-thoracic trauma, disseminated intravascular coagulation, central nervous system hypoxia, metabolic disorders, oxygen toxicity, or aspiration of gastric contents or other fluids. Sepsis is a very important factor, and other aetiological factors seem to include prolonged hypoperfusion of the lungs, pulmonary microemboli and circulating vasoactive material such as histamine or other enzymes due to the breakdown of damaged cells.

Beyer (1979) suggests that there are four phases:

Phase	Characteristics	Clinical features
• First	Shock Resuscitation Haemodynamic stabilization	Hyperventilation Respiratory alkalosis Metabolic alkalosis Hypoxaemia Normal chest X-ray
• Second	Respiratory distress	Marked hypoxaemia Respiratory alkalosis Chest X-ray shows interstitial pulmonary oedema
• Third	Refractory pulmonary failure	
• Fourth	Hypoxic cardiac arrest	

The picture is often one of a patient who appears to be improving in some ways after the initial episode of shock, but shows increasing respiratory distress. He works harder to breathe thus increasing oxygen demand; the lungs become stiff with poor compliance (alterations in the lung surfactant, which normally lowers surface tension and keeps the alveoli open, leads to areas of collapse); imbalance develops between the ventilation and blood flow through lung tissue which leads to a physiological right to left shunt (some blood passes through the lungs without being oxygenated) and the pulmonary hypertension and oedema increase the strain on the right ventricle. The rapid respiratory rate does not increase ventilation as might be expected, since for each breath there is the 150 ml or more of air in the dead space which does not take part in gas exchange, so that rapid relatively shallow respiration may actually decrease the gas exchange while increasing respiratory effort and oxygen demand. Thus the patient becomes increasingly hypoxic and will eventually become hypercapnoeic also, with complete respiratory failure.

Management

Early artificial ventilation is instituted when hypoxia begins to develop and increase, with a high fixed inspired oxygen concentration (FIO_2), and positive end expiratory pressure (PEEP) (Aspinall & Tanner, 1982) to maintain or increase patency of the alveoli. Even so, the mortality rate is high if this syndrome reaches the later stages. One of the difficulties is that lung perfusion is as important as ventilation. PEEP, by maintaining a constantly raised intrathoracic pressure, may decrease lung perfusion and also increase the workload on the right ventricle. Early detection is essential so that treatment can be started, thus increasing the chances of success. The presence of risk factors such as sepsis and/or trauma should make staff particularly alert to early signs of respiratory distress.

MANAGEMENT OF THE PATIENT IN SHOCK

The overview given indicates the complex nature of changes in physiological mechanisms which may be associated with the shock syndrome and its consequences, and their potentially fatal nature. Good nursing care is vital to patients with this syndrome to increase their chance of survival, or if this is not possible, to provide the care and support they (and their family or significant others) so much need. There are three main components to the nursing care:

- initial and continuing assessment of the patient's condition in order to provide a rational basis for and evaluation of treatment and care
- assisting medical staff and giving the treatment ordered
- providing the essential care needed by any human being in this stressful situation, including physical, psychological, social and spiritual care.

These three components will be discussed in the order stated because, although the last is at least as important as the other two, some of the care needed derives from the measures used in assessment and treatment. If nursing care is to be as effective, efficient and individualized as possible, then these three components are provided within the framework of the nursing process, with assessment, planning, implementation and evaluation proceeding in a systematic and cyclical way, though often these may overlap or take place almost simultaneously in the care of an acutely ill person.

ASSESSMENT

This should have begun with awareness of risk factors even before any signs of shock are evident. These risk factors may relate to the physical disease, medical regimes or organization of care, or to characteristics such as age, sex and psychosocial factors. For example, pre-existing disease of the cardiovascular system, lungs or kidneys will make the patient more susceptible to the effects of any of the causes and sequelae of shock stated, such as hypovolaemia or sepsis. Medical treatment regimes such as steroid therapy reduce resistance to infection and may therefore increase the likelihood of septic shock, for example after operation. The damaged cardiovascular system and ischaemic myocardium may be unable to tolerate and compensate for a period of dehydration or hypoxia which could be coped with quite adequately by someone without these deficiencies.

The organization of care and the speed with which treatment is instituted — whether in the community where the patient suffers trauma, a coronary occlusion and/or cardiac dysrhythmia, or in hospital — may make the difference as to whether or not he or she develops the shock syndrome, its severity, and the likelihood of complications.

Factors such as age are also relevant, for example a higher proportion of the infant or child's body is fluid (Beland & Passos, 1975) and it may very quickly become dehydrated whatever the provoking factor. Both the very young and the very old often lack the ability to compensate adequately when physiological functions are grossly disturbed by, for example, fluid depletion or electrolyte imbalance.

Emotional factors may make a difference by their effects on the circulation via the hypothalamus and humoral controls. Intellectual ability and capacity to co-operate in treatment measures in illness may influence whether factors leading to the shock syndrome develop. The anxious independent man with myocardial infarction who is unable to comprehend the need for rest may exert himself excessively, leading to increased heart rate and oxygen demand, myocardial hypoxia and possibly dysrhythmias resulting in cardiogenic shock.

All the activities of daily living are likely to be affected in the patient with shock syndrome, and these will mostly be considered in the section on basic nursing care and support. Circulation and breathing are, in the short-term, most vital to life and therefore usually most urgently treated. Careful and constant assessment of circulation and oxygenation are therefore vital in the care of patients with shock, since without adequate tissue perfusion and oxygenation all other functions will eventually inevitably fail.

Assessment of circulation

The circulation can be assessed directly by invasive methods or, as is more commonly the case, by simpler clinical methods. All the measurements and observations made can only be properly interpreted when considered in relation to each other, and to the trends of repeated observations recorded on accurately completed charts. This will become obvious as individual measurements are discussed. If used intelligently, such records of even the more simple observations can provide a good basis for treatment and evaluation. Assessment of the circulatory state usually includes evaluation of the following parameters.

Arterial pressure

This may be measured by sphygmomanometer, in which case it is essential that the cuff should be of the right size, since too small a cuff produces a falsely high recording and too big a cuff a low one. Holloway (1979) recommends a cuff with a bladder 20% wider than the diameter of the patient's limb and long enough to go halfway round the limb, i.e. 12–14 cm wide for the average adult's arm. However, when the arterial pressure falls to less than 50 mmHg systolic, the cuff pressure tends to read lower than arterial pressure as measured directly via an intra-arterial catheter and pressure transducer (Fig. 10.2) which is more accurate. If a transducer and electronic monitor are used then it is essential, as with all such systems, to make sure that the lines are patent with a minimal flow of heparinised solution via a pressurised system, that they are not kinked and contain no bubbles, and that the machines are correctly calibrated so that readings are accurate. Also, the patient must be protected from such hazards as infection via catheter and tap systems (Walrath, 1979), air embolism (though this is more likely in an intravenous system), loss of a broken catheter fragment into the blood vessel, or blood loss through leaks in the system. Blood can be lost rapidly through a disconnected arterial catheter, and the external end should, for this reason, always be kept visible if possible, or observed frequently. These hazards are present with any intravenous or intra-arterial catheter, though modern design has reduced the danger of broken catheters. If the medial artery is cannulated, movement of the hand should be checked regularly as nerve damage can occur.

A systolic arterial pressure of 80–90 mmHg or less in an adult is usually considered to represent hypotension and to be a cause for concern. However, a systolic pressure of 100 mmHg when the patient shows considerable vasoconstriction and tachycardia may be equally or more worrying, since it may show that all possible compensatory mechanisms are active and collapse is likely to occur suddenly when these fail. Furthermore a systolic arterial pressure of 100 mmHg for a person whose system is used to working on a pressure of 160/100 may be very inadequate. It is the total patient state and trend, rather than just the pressure recorded which is important.

Central venous pressure (CVP)

The catheter is inserted into a main vein such as

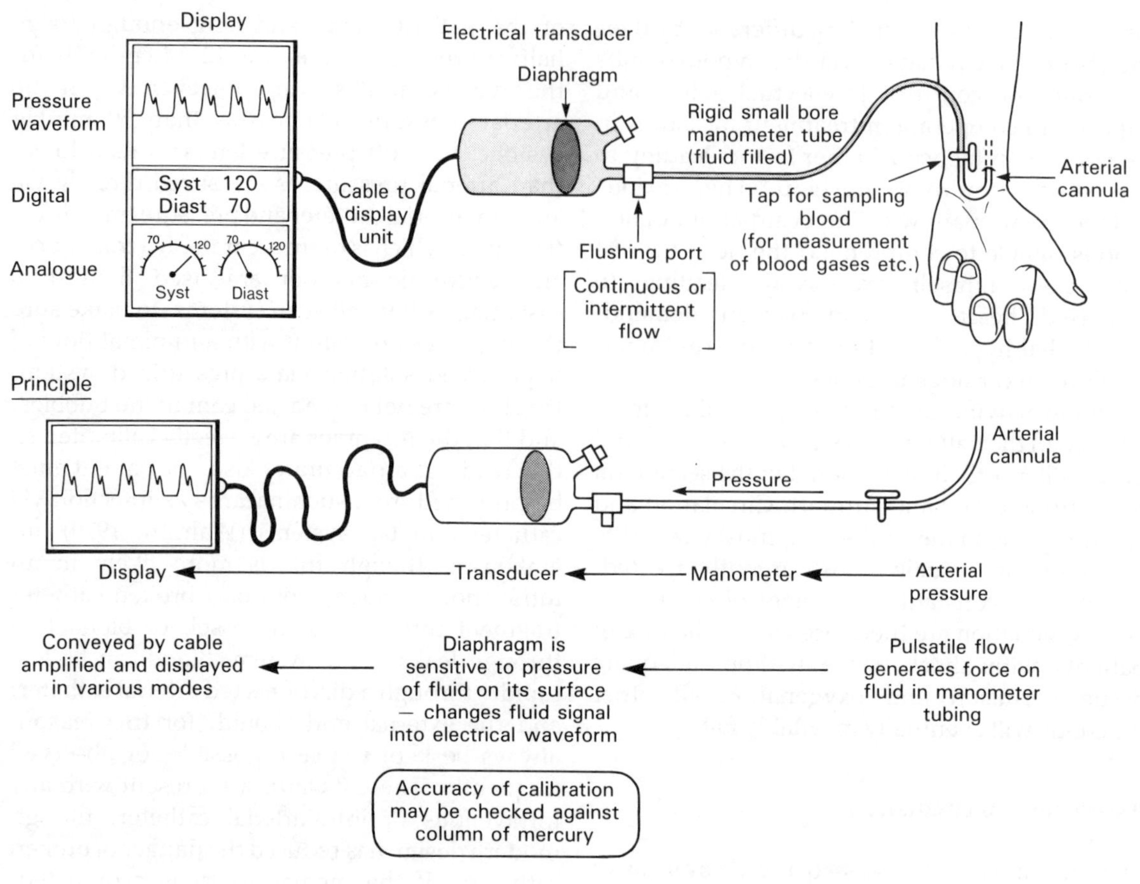

Fig. 10.2 Arterial pressure monitoring.

the subclavian or the superior vena cava (via an arm vein, Fig. 10.3A). It may be connected to a pressure transducer or to an intravenous system with a side arm attached to a ruler or other measuring device. Whichever is used, the pressure transducer or zero point should be levelled with a fixed point each time, usually the sternal notch, a point halfway from front to back of the chest at the level of the 5th intercostal space (mid axillary line), or some other point near the right atrium (Fig. 10.3B & C). The patient should be in the same position each time, or else the fact that he is not must be considered in interpreting the reading since it may be altered (though this is not always so for either central venous or pulmonary artery pressures) (Woods & Mansfield, 1976). Figure 10.4 illustrates the sequence of events for the measurement of CVP.

Central venous or right atrial pressure is usually around 2–6 mmHg (multiply by 1.34 to convert mmHg to cm H_20). It rises in conditions such as heart failure or fluid overload and falls when the circulating volume is depleted. It reflects changes in pressure in the venous system and right heart, but may not reflect changes in the left ventricular and diastolic pressure (caused for example by left ventricular failure or myocardial infarction) if the lungs and heart valves are normal to begin with. It is not always, therefore, an accurate guide to fluid replacement.

Pulse rate, rhythm and pressure

Pulse rate normally varies according to such factors as activity, emotional factors and age. However, in shock the pulse rate is usually

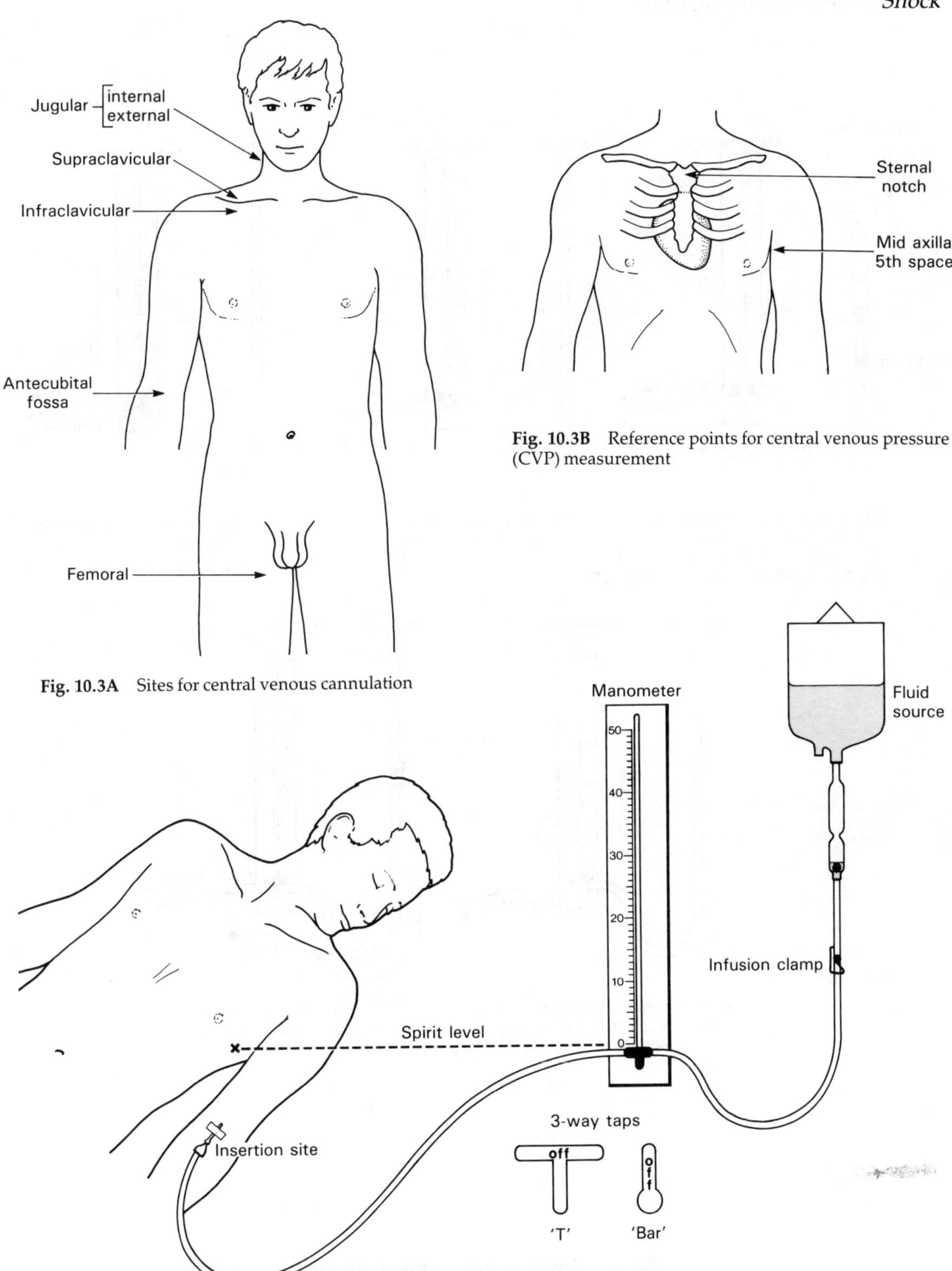

Fig. 10.3A Sites for central venous cannulation

Fig. 10.3B Reference points for central venous pressure (CVP) measurement

Fig. 10.3C Setting zero using mid-axilla reference point

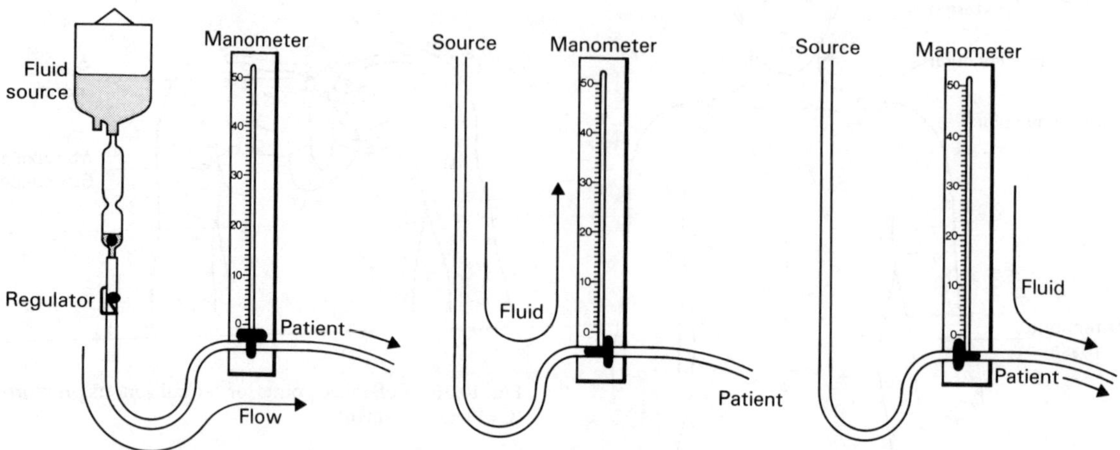

1 Fluid flows from source to patient. Tap 'Off' to manometer. Set zero on manometer with fixed reference point as illustrated, Fig. 10.3C

2 Fluid fills manometer. Tap 'Off' to patient.

3 Fluid flows from manometer to patient. Tap 'Off' to fluid source.

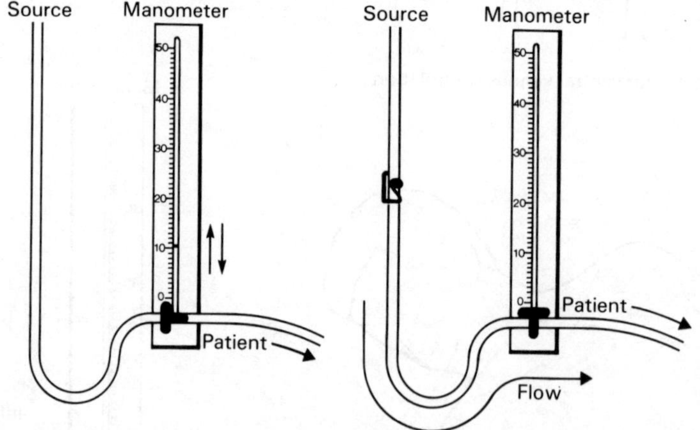

4 Fluid level in manometer settles. Some oscillations with respirations noticeable (0 – 1 cm H_2O). Read mean value as CVP.

5 Tap 'Off' to manometer. Regulate flow as prescribed.

Fig. 10.4 Measuring CVP — sequence of events

rapid, though it may be excessively slow, and an irregular rhythm may be contributing to the circulatory deficiency. For this reason a cardiac monitor is often used. The pulse pressure is the difference between the systolic and diastolic arterial pressure, and a decreased pulse pressure usually only occurs when the stroke volume is decreased, peripheral vascular resistance is increased, or with valve disease such as aortic stenosis. This can be quite a useful measure of improvement or deterioration in the patient's condition when sophisticated monitoring is not in use.

Peripheral temperature and skin colour

Cold and pale or cyanosed peripheral tissues are a sign of vasoconstriction, and sluggish circulation may be confirmed by applying finger pressure and watching the slow return of colour to the area. But temperature felt by the hand depends partly on the temperature of the hand itself, as well as that of the object felt. A cold limb may not feel as cold to a cool hand as to a warm one. Therefore peripheral temperature may be measured by attaching a thermister to the big toe or lower leg and comparing temperature recordings with the central temperature as measured in the ear or oesophagus (rectal monitoring is now thought to increase infection risks [Stoddart, 1975]). Unless the legs are exposed to a colder atmosphere than the body, more than about 2°C difference in temperature at the two sites usually indicates some decrease in peripheral circulation.

Urine output

Since the kidneys are dependent on adequate perfusion for function, urine output is a useful indication of renal perfusion. In the absence of severe dehydration the urine output should be at least 30 ml per hour from an adult. The importance of knowing the urine output makes it essential to have a patent catheter in situ despite the risks of infection, though all possible precautions, such as maintaining a closed drainage system to a urimeter or special bag, should be taken to prevent infection of this critically ill and susceptible patient (such systems permit frequent measurement of small amounts of urine without opening the system and risking infection). Usually urine output is diminished or absent in shock, but in the so-called 'warm hypotension' of some septic shock, the output may at first be normal or even increased.

Cerebral function

In the early stages of shock the patient may be alert and anxious, possibly partly both cause and effect of the increased circulating catecholamines. But as hypoxia increases and eventually cerebral circulation decreases he becomes less alert, less aware and oriented to surroundings, and eventually comatose. Some units use a measure such as the Glasgow coma scale (Teasdale & Jennett, 1974) to assess consciousness (Fig. 10.5). However, as in any person lapsing into unconsciousness, hearing may persist longer than is obvious. A number of recovered patients have subsequently described what happened while they were apparently unconscious, sometimes to the chagrin of the staff!

Haemodynamic monitoring by Swan-Ganz catheter

The measures described so far are likely to be used to assess the circulation of patients in any hospital setting. However, in specialized units one of the methods of haemodynamic monitoring which is used increasingly is measurement of the pulmonary artery pressure, the pulmonary artery wedge pressure (PAWP), and sometimes the cardiac output by means of a balloon-tipped catheter such as the Swan-Ganz (Fig. 10.6). This is a thermal dilution catheter which is inserted via a main vein (e.g. the antecubital) and floated into place via the right atrium, ventricle and pulmonary artery. Usually a 4-lumen catheter is used.

One lumen leads to a 1 ml capacity balloon near the tip of the catheter. Distal to this is the opening from the second lumen which measures pulmonary artery pressure while the balloon is deflated, but pulmonary artery wedge pressure

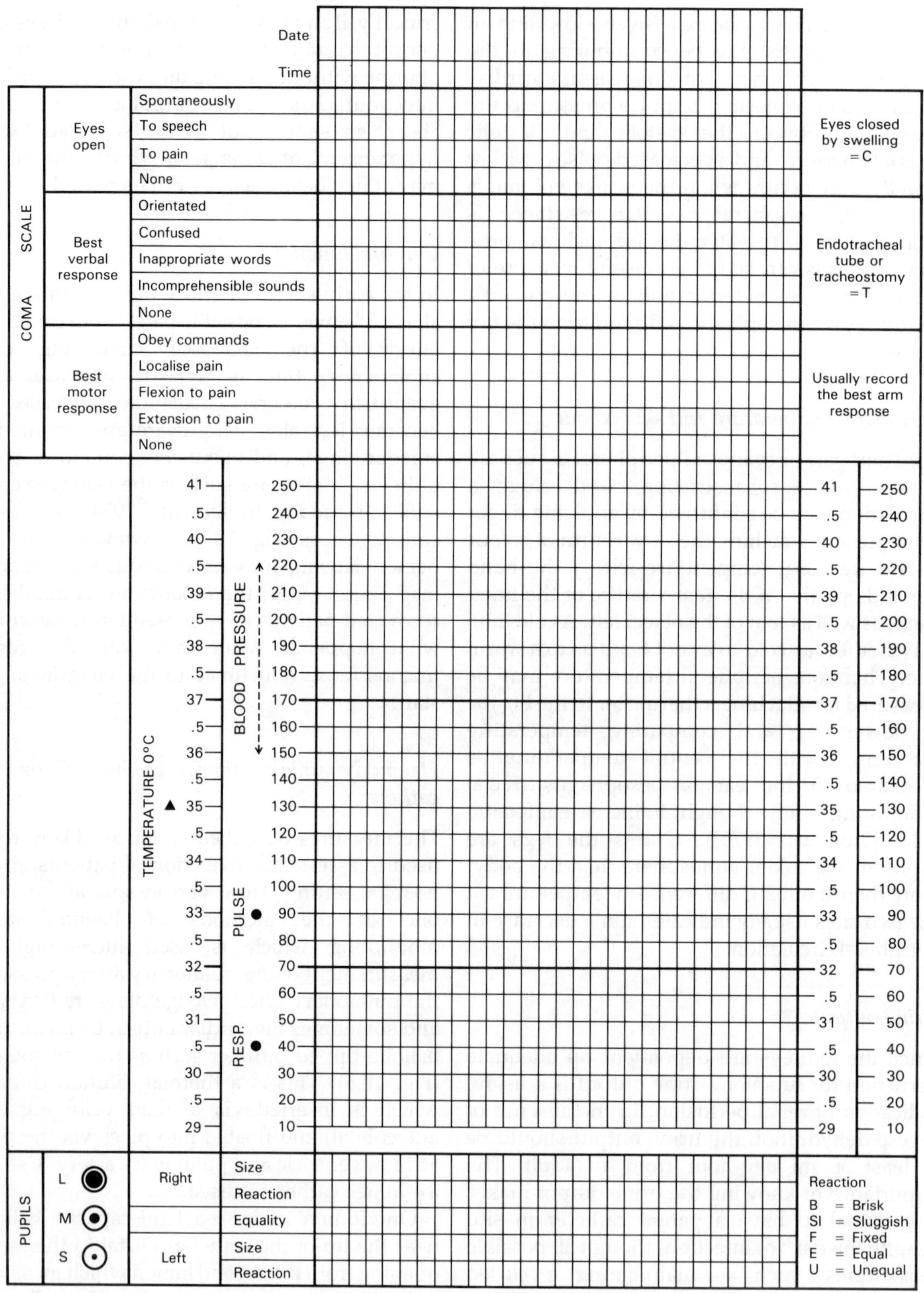

Fig. 10.5 Glasgow coma scale

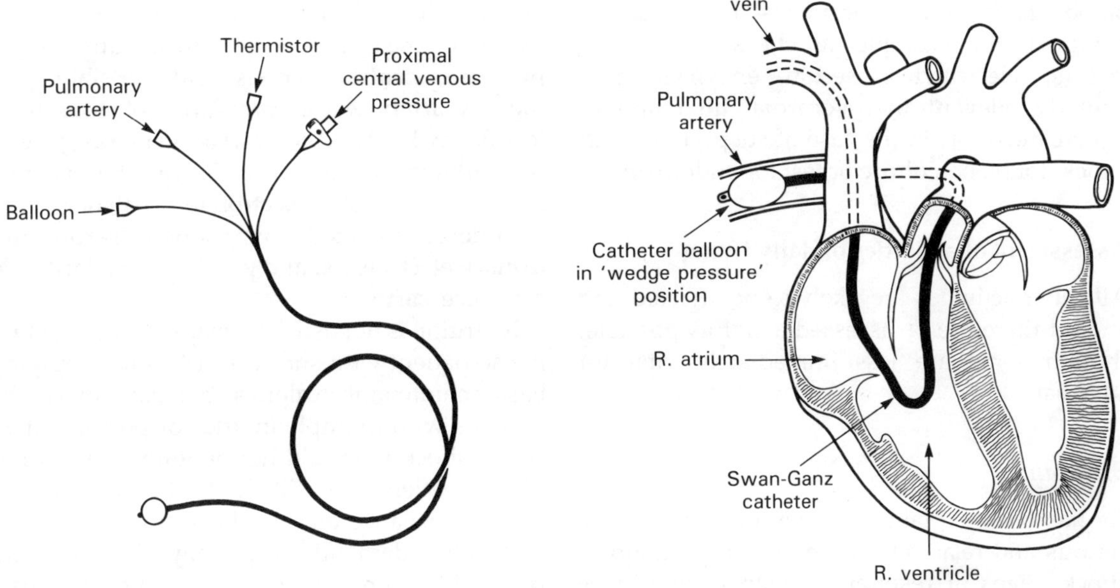

Fig. 10.6 Swan-Ganz catheter with four lamina (left), shown in situ in 'wedge' position (right)

when the balloon is inflated and wedged in a small branch of the pulmonary artery. This reflects left atrial and left ventricular filling pressure (rather than right ventricular pressure as reflected by the central venous pressure) and is therefore a useful measure of cardiac function.

The third lumen is used to connect the electronic unit to a carefully calibrated thermister in the catheter tip, used for measuring the cardiac output by the thermodilution technique. The electronic unit, which is used to store the baseline temperature, gives a signal for the injection via the fourth lumen (which lies in the right atrium or superior vena cava) of a small volume (usually 10 ml) of fluid at known temperature, and as the temperature again reaches the baseline records the cardiac output in litres per minute. This takes only 20–30 seconds and so can be recorded as required. This can be useful in determining the 'optimal filling pressure', which in critically ill patients is usually that at which cardiac output is greatest (unless there is pulmonary oedema). This is determined by giving aliquots of 50–100 ml fluid intravenously followed by cardiac output and PAWP measurement, and repeating the process until either the cardiac output begins to fall or the PAWP reaches 18 mmHg. The curve plotted from serial measurements is sometimes known as a Starling Curve, since it makes use of Starling's law of the heart indicating that within physiologic limits the heart pumps all the blood that comes into it.

It is important that the balloon is not left inflated or it may cause infarction, and that the nurse is alert for this or other complications (Walinsky, 1977). Left atrial pressure may be monitored directly, but such a line is only put in at operation so will only be seen after cardiac surgery.

Blood gases

While these do not directly assess circulatory efficiency, they do reflect it. A fall in the PO_2 and PCO_2 and an increase in the arterio-venous difference in PO_2 are often early signs of shock. Usually there is an increasing metabolic acidosis due to anaerobic metabolism in the tissues and excessive production of lactic acid. However, in patients with septic shock there may be metabolic alkalosis, possibly due to the inhibition of anaerobic metabolism (Holloway, 1979).

While blood is being obtained to measure blood gases other specimens may also be obtained, for example to check on clotting factors, electrolytes, serum enzymes (particularly relevant in myocardial infarction or pancreatitis), or, in the case of suspected septic shock, for blood culture or test for endotoxins.

Assessment of activities of daily living

All other activities are likely to be affected and should therefore be assessed as far as possible, though some are less immediately vital for survival.

Breathing

As has been explained, respiratory failure is a serious and relatively common complication of shock. Signs of respiratory distress should be noted carefully so that progress over time can be assessed. It is important to be constantly aware that rapid, shallow breathing is relatively inefficient and often means that the patient is, or will shortly become, very hypoxic. Looking for cyanosis is not a very reliable way of detecting hypoxia, since whether it is seen depends partly on the lighting, and a very anaemic patient will not become cyanosed (since cyanosis only occurs when there is at least 5g deoxygenated haemoglobin per 100ml blood). However, cyanosis should be noted, including whether it is central or peripheral. It should also be noted whether there are any factors impeding respiration, e.g. a distended abdomen, position, or in the injured person a chest dressing or non-functioning intercostal tube which should be relieving pneumothorax or haemothorax.

Eating and drinking

Usually the patient will not wish to eat while suffering from shock. Since normal gastro-intestinal function is likely to be decreased and paralytic ileus may occur, it is important to know whether bowel sounds are present before even fluids are given orally. The necessary fluids and, if the state is prolonged, nutrients are usually supplied intravenously until gastro-intestinal function improves. Fluid requirements are usually calculated according to haemodynamic measures, e.g. pulse rate, blood pressure, central venous and possibly pulmonary artery wedge pressures, obvious fluid loss of any kind and clinical signs such as general or pulmonary oedema. Since the normal mechanisms of electrolyte balance are disordered repeated estimations of serum and urinary electrolytes, and possibly osmolarity are also necessary.

Nutrition is not usually a major concern at first in the patient with shock, apart from supplying basic maintenance calories, but particularly for patients with multiple injuries or postoperative septic shock it should not be ignored for long. These patients are likely to be in negative nitrogen balance and are likely to have a high metabolic demand, especially if they are pyrexial. Serum proteins play an important part in maintaining the balance between the hydrostatic pressure and the plasma osmotic pressure in the peripheral circulation and thus preventing oedema. Also protein deficiency is likely to increase susceptibility to infection. Hyperglycaemia is a feature of traumatic shock due to catecholamine-induced hepatic glycogenolysis and depressed insulin secretion (Shatney & Lillehei, 1976), so the blood sugar is usually estimated at intervals. A combination of little fluid given orally, possible mouth-breathing, and the patient's inability to maintain self-care makes it likely that the mouth will need extra attention, so assessment should include this.

Stress ulcers are always a possibility with the combination of stressful conditions and an empty stomach, and with the shock syndrome there is the added risk of disseminated intravascular coagulation (DIC). It is therefore important to note and report any signs of gastrointestinal bleeding, since this may become severe.

Elimination

It has already been explained that oliguria or anuria are likely to occur and that urine output is a useful indicator of renal perfusion. Defaecation is unimportant during the acute stages of shock except when diarrhoea occurs. In this case the frequency and amount should be estimated to assess fluid loss, and the appearance should be noted since this may indicate, for example, blood loss.

Movement and protection from hazards

The patient is frequently unable to move himself and thus is liable to all the complications of immobility and, in particular, pressure damage to tissues which are already deficient in circulation. Discomfort or even damage from lying in unnatural body positions may occur, particularly when the patient has various bits of equipment attached with limbs, perhaps purposely, immobilized. Some of the various hazards of infection, bleeding or air embolism via various lines or tubes have been mentioned, and electrical hazards are added when electronic equipment is in use. Awareness of such hazards and the need for protection even in the midst of crisis situations is necessary, but becomes part of the mental equipment of nurses only when deliberately developed during less stressful times.

Rest and sleep

It may require all the nurse's skills in planning, giving care and treatment, and negotiating with other staff to ensure that the patient is allowed to rest at times. It is all too easy for staff constantly to disturb the patient every 15–30 minutes, or even more often, when this could be avoided with a little thought and organization. Indeed, Lynch (1978) describes observation periods of 4–5 hours before a curarized patient in a shock unit was undisturbed for even 7 minutes.

Even though shock is usually a fairly short-term condition this point is not irrelevant since constant discomfort and disturbance is an additional stressor affecting this critically ill person.

Seeking stimulation and reward, maintaining self-concept and relating to others

These functions are all very much altered for the patient in shock. There are people who would maintain that these are no longer important in a crisis situation and that 'maintaining life' is the essential focus of interest. However, that view seems misguided for several reasons. It is well-recognized now that emotions may have considerable physiological effects mediated by the hypothalamus-endocrine links and autonomic nervous system (Vander & Sherman, 1985), and in the critically ill person these may be important. In a crisis situation the patient's whole personal world, support systems and ways of coping may be disrupted, adding to the various physical stressors already taxing his resources. Some patients will be in a state of irreversible shock and will therefore spend their last hours in this situation, which could be made more tolerable by good nursing. Probably there will be only too much available stimulation of an abnormal kind, uncomfortable or even painful procedures, strange noises and people talking about strange and perhaps anxiety-provoking things. It is difficult to maintain one's self-concept as an adult human being when deprived of normal functions, invaded by various tubes, surrounded by people who handle one's body, yet may pay a lot of attention to the various bits of equipment and little to the person whose body it is. It is difficult to relate to others when communication is impeded by oxygen mask or endotracheal tube, inability to move, and diminished cerebral function which make it difficult to think clearly and make sense of the environment.

Assessment must therefore include what is conveyed by the patient verbally and non-verbally, the frightened face and eyes, the clutching hand or other signs. The nurse, since she can to some extent control the environment while the patient cannot, must assess and seek to avoid those stimuli which may be disturbing and provide those which appear helpful. There is evidence from studies in a shock unit (Lynch, 1978) as well as personal observation that critically ill and apparently unresponsive patients can be affected by stimuli such as human touch, perhaps perceived as a recognizable and comforting stimulus amongst all the unfamiliar sights, sounds and sensations For example, when a nurse quietly took the pulse of a critically injured woman who had been in a coma for two days, her pulse rate slowed by almost 20 beats; a similar change was observed in another severely injured man when a nurse held his hand.

Additional areas of assessment

Observation and ongoing assessment should include two other aspects:

- Coagulation and control of bleeding. Are there signs of clotting deficiencies and DIC, such as persistent oozing from skin puncture sites or wounds, or excessive bruising, or any other bleeding?
- Temperature regulation. The measurement of core and peripheral temperature difference to estimate peripheral blood flow has already been mentioned under circulation. However, control of the total body temperature is also relevant in assessment.

The patient in septic shock may become very pyrexial, or shock may result in hypothermia. Excessive exposure of the body, which sometimes occurs when many procedures and examinations are taking place, may lead to considerable cooling of the body surface as well as distressing the patient. Cold blood transfused quickly may also cause the temperature to fall. For many years it has been recognized that active warming of the body surface may be undesirable for patients with the shock syndrome since it may divert circulation from the vital organs. However, excessive vasoconstriction caused by cooling may also be undesirable if the circulating volume is adequate, since it increases the afterload on the heart (i.e. provides increased resistance).

It is helpful in planning individualized care to have knowledge of the patient as a person and of his normal life and ways of maintaining his integrity, and if the patient has been in hospital for a while this may already be available. If not, since he is too ill to talk much, any information from the patient's visitors which can help to build up a picture of the person, his lifestyle and his reaction to illness forms part of the nursing assessment. Information about any religious affiliation and spiritual beliefs and practices is essential, for in a crisis these are likely to become an even more important part of life and indeed may be the main source of support.

TREATMENT OF SHOCK

The overall aim of this is to restore adequate tissue perfusion for normal physiological requirements. As may be concluded from the description of the pathophysiology of shock, the treatment is mainly:

- to restore and maintain circulating fluid which is adequate in volume, oxygen-carrying capacity and plasma osmotic pressure
- to achieve cardiac function which is as effective and as efficient as possible, in balance with peripheral resistance
- to minimize and if possible correct the physiological effects of shock such as hypoxia and metabolic abnormalities, and to minimize or prevent complications such as renal, respiratory or other failure, or DIC
- to give appropriate treatment for any specific cause of shock such as bleeding, cardiac pathology, sepsis, anaphylaxis or pancreatitis.

Which of these takes priority depends on the presenting problems, but they will be discussed in the order listed.

Restoring circulating fluid

As an immediate measure to counteract hypotension the patient may be put in the Trendelenberg position with the bed foot raised about a metre. This drains blood from the legs increasing the circulating volume by 400–800 ml, but is undesirable when there is raised intracranial pressure, cardiogenic failure of circulation, or bleeding from the upper part of the body. It may also impede respiration, though this problem may be diminished by using the 'jack-knife' position with the upper half of the body raised a little as well as the legs. It has been suggested that the sudden rise in arterial pressure may stimulate the baroceptors and cause vasodilation and cardiac deceleration and that, if the Trendelenberg position is used, pillows should be put under the head to prevent this by raising intracranial arterial resistance and increasing venous drainage (Sun, 1971). Medical anti-shock trousers (MAST) may be put on and inflated, thus squeezing some 500–1000 ml of the patient's blood into his central circulation (Budassi, 1981). When the circulating volume has been restored and the MAST is to be deflated, this must be done slowly to avoid hypotension as the peripheral resistance falls.

An intravenous infusion is necessary to control fluid intake and provide a route for drug administration. Usually a separate intravenous cannula is inserted into a central vein for pressure measurements, and clear fluids such as dextrose or electrolyte solutions are given through this. It is often considered undesirable to use it for purposes such as giving blood or drugs because of the dangers of blocking or infecting it. While crystalloid fluids may be given, these stay within the circulation for a relatively short period and therefore colloids such as low molecular weight dextran, 5% albumen solution, blood or degraded gelatin, which Jones (1978) suggests is an excellent plasma substitute with no side-effects, may be administered. Dextran 70 has several advantages: it decreases blood viscosity and rouleau formation, improves microcirculatory flow and attracts fluid from the interstitial fluid. Blood should be taken for cross-matching if it is likely to be required, before giving dextran, since some dextrans interfere with cross-matching. If large quantities of blood are to be given quickly a blood warmer must be used to bring the blood nearer to body temperature, or excessive cooling of the heart may occur. It should also be remembered that stored blood may be quite rich in potassium, and the citrate content (used to prevent coagulation during storage) of large quantities of blood may be sufficient to cause hypocalcaemia. Because of these factors, amongst others, a monitor displaying cardiac rhythm is useful even if shock is not of cardiogenic origin. The fluid given needs to be carefully titrated against the patient's needs, particularly if cardiac function is deficient or suspect. In the early stages of treatment the CVP, arterial pressure and heart rate and, if available, the pulmonary wedge pressure may need to be recorded every 15 minutes; alternatively, in some units these are checked after every 200–500 ml of fluid. Most authorities recommend continuing rapid infusion until the CVP reaches 15–18 cm H_2O and the PAWP 18 mmHg if necessary to achieve adequate arterial pressure and tissue perfusion (as demonstrated by urine output, skin colour and temperature and heart rate), but the levels permitted depend partly on whether venous and pulmonary artery pressures were previously high due to cardiac abnormalities. Continued vasoconstriction with a high CVP and PAWP usually indicate pump failure, and pulmonary oedema may occur if rapid infusion is continued. As the skin-core temperature difference nears around 2°C and the skin feels warm and dry, urine output remains over 30 ml per hour (for an adult), arterial pressure and heart rate stabilize near the patient's pre-shock levels, and cerebral function improves, the rate of infusion can usually be decreased (unless loss continues) to maintain the current PAWP and/or CVP. Since several intravascular lines may be present it is important to keep a careful check on fluid going through each, so that accidental overloading does not occur.

Improving cardiac function

Drug therapy

Various drugs may be used for this purpose. Vasoconstrictors such as noradrenaline and metaraminol are now rarely used since they may raise the arterial pressure, but at the expense of reducing peripheral perfusion and increasing cardiac work. More commonly used are the beta receptor stimulators such as isoprenaline or dopamine (Inotropin) which increase cardiac impulse formation and are inotropic (increase myocardial contractility), and decrease peripheral resistance. These drugs are usually given via a carefully regulated infusion pump since the required dose is small and must be given accurately. For example isoprenaline dosage is usually 1–4 micrograms (μg) per minute, according to the blood pressure, and effects such as tachycardia or dysrhythmias are likely if this is exceeded. With dopamine, a natural precursor of noradrenaline, a low dosage (below 30 micrograms/kilogram body weight/minute) causes moderate vasoconstriction in the skin and muscles but vasodilation in the renal, mesenteric and splanchnic circulation, as well as being inotropic. But it is an alpha as well as a beta stimulator, and at doses higher than 30–40 μg/kg/min, the alpha effects predominate, leading to vasoconstriction in the vital areas such as the kidneys and the skin, and ventricular dysrhythmias may occur. A cardiac monitor is therefore necessary.

Digoxin may also be ordered to increase myocardial contractility, starting with 0.5 mg i.v. and continuing with doses of 0.25–0.125 mg, remembering that hypokalaemia will increase and hyperkalaemia decrease the effects.

When peripheral resistance is so high as to decrease cardiac output drugs may be used to reduce this by peripheral vasodilation, thus decreasing the workload of the left ventricle. Some of those commonly used are i.v. chlorpromazine 5–10 mg (diluted 1 in 10) at intervals of 10 minutes, phenoxybenzamine 5 mg every 10 minutes up to 4 times, or thymoxamine 5 mg then 30 mg over 4–6 hours, but the choice of drug and to some extent the dosage vary according to medical staff choice. Whenever vasodilators are given it is essential to make sure that the circulating volume is sufficient, and be prepared to increase it as necessary to fill the increased vascular space, monitoring the arterial pressure, PAWP and/or CVP at frequent intervals as vasodilation occurs.

While some doctors do not find them useful, glucocorticosteroids have been shown to have effects likely to be beneficial in shock, notably restoration of vascular membrane integrity, stabilization of lysosomal membranes, increase in visceral organ blood flow and lactic acid metabolism, decrease in sympathetic nerve transmission, arteriolar and venular resistance, platelet and leucocyte viscosity, kinin production and extravascular lung water, and pulmonary arterio-venous shunting amongst others. Shatney & Lillehei (1976) suggest that 30 mg/kg methylprednisolone sodium succinate given intravenously over 10 minutes, repeated once or twice in the first 12–24 hours then stopped, provides the benefits without the disadvantages of more prolonged dosage and that it is particularly beneficial in improving the haemodynamic and metabolic state of patients with septic shock.

Glucagon may be ordered for its effects in increasing cardiac output and stroke volume, lowering peripheral resistance, stimulating hepatic conversion of lactic acid to glucose and possibly increasing ATP production. It appears to be effective in cardiogenic shock with peak action after 10 minutes and duration of 30 minutes, and it appears most effective when used with isoprenaline (Seal, 1980).

When cardiac dysrhythmias are a major cause of shock, drugs such as atropine (for bradycardia), or xylocaine or procainamide may be used to control them, though hypotension may be made worse by either of the latter two. Other measures such as a cardiac pacemaker for heart-block, or cardioversion for rapid dysrhythmias may also be used.

Mechanical methods

Several mechanical means of augmenting cardiac function in cardiogenic shock have been developed. One non-invasive aid is the external counterpulsation unit. The legs are placed in two rigid tapered sleeves. A waterbag wrapped round each leg fills the intervening space, and pressure is applied during diastole, triggered by the attached electrocardiogram, thus forcing venous blood back and also producing counterpulsation in the arterial system. However, while this increases diastolic pressure, therefore increasing coronary circulation, it does not decrease and may increase cardiac work and increases myocardial oxygen consumption. It also is very uncomfortable for the patient. It has therefore been shown to be less effective in reducing cardiogenic shock than invasive counterpulsation, i.e. intra-aortic balloon pumping, probably the most widely used method of cardiac assistance used outside the operating theatre. There are various kinds of balloon catheters with 1–3 balloons, but in each case the basic principle is the same. The catheter is inserted, via a Dacron sleeve graft attached to the femoral artery after a 'cut-down', and the balloon positioned in the aorta just distal to the left subclavian junction, checked by X-ray. The catheter is then attached to a unit which causes the balloon to be inflated by helium during diastole (triggered by the ECG) thus raising aortic pressure proximal to the balloon, and deflated early in systole thus decreasing aortic pressure and resistance to outflow from the left ventricle. Thus coronary blood flow is increased when the balloon is inflated and left ventricular workload decreased with deflation of the balloon.

If hypoxic cardiac arrest occurs, then of course the immediate procedure for cardiopulmonary resuscitation consists of external cardiac compression and artificial maintenance of ventilation as in any similar situation, followed by continued definitive treatment as before.

Reducing the physiological effects of shock and minimizing complications

Oxygen supply

Oxygen supply to the tissues is vital if normal cell function is to be regained and the patient is to recover. Therefore oxygen — 5–6 litres per minute by mask or nasal cannulae — is usually started immediately and the concentrations then adjusted according to the PO_2 as soon as blood gases have been estimated. Hypoxia is usually so evident that the danger of removing the hypoxic respiratory drive of people with chronic respiratory disease is not relevant. However, artificial ventilation via an endotracheal tube may become necessary to achieve adequate oxygenation to relieve the hypoxia, or it may be necessary in severe shock when the PCO_2 eventually begins to rise with respiratory failure. Positive end expiratory pressure (PEEP) and a high FIO_2 (fixed inspired oxygen concentration) may be necessary, but a careful check on haemodynamic parameters is important as the persistently raised intrathoracic pressure may impede venous return and diminish cardiac output. Early and adequate artificial maintenance of ventilation and oxygenation, together with controlling fluid intake to avoid overload, offer the best chance of avoiding ARDS or the 'shock lung' syndrome.

Acid-base balance

The restoration of normal acid-base balance is also essential to normal cell function but is complex because of the various factors which may be affecting it — increased lactic acid production, disturbed electrolyte balance, increased CO_2 removal via the lungs, decreased kidney function, and the administration of large amounts of blood (which may initially cause acidosis followed by alkalosis), to name a few. Therefore arterial blood specimens are usually taken quite frequently for estimation of blood gases and acid-base balance, and also serum and if possible urine electrolytes are measured. Since there is frequently a metabolic acidosis, intravenous sodium bicarbonate is likely to be needed, usually given as a bolus since it tends to precipitate when mixed with other drugs. Electrolyte intake intravenously will need to be adjusted according to the serum levels and losses. Intravenous infusion of glucose and insulin is often ordered to maintain glucose metabolism and to cause potassium to re-enter the cells in the 'sick cell' syndrome.

Renal function

Renal function can be protected to some extent by maintaining a flow of urine throughout the period of shock. Mannitol 100 ml 20% i.v. will usually produce a diuresis of 30–60 ml even in the presence of dehydration, but in many units frusemide (Lasix) is now preferred. This may initially be given in doses of 20–40 mg i.v., but if this is unsuccessful 100–500 mg may be given. A patent catheter to the bladder, maintained aseptically, is essential.

Disseminated intravascular coagulation

If disseminated intravascular coagulation is to be successfully treated it must be treated early. Any signs of excessive bleeding, bruising or abnormality in blood clotting factors may be a warning sign. The treatment is intravenous heparin, and possibly replacement of clotting agents such as platelets and fibrinogen as well as blood where there is severe bleeding, with control by repeated estimation of clotting factors. In some units every patient at risk of stress ulceration, e.g. those likely to need very intensive therapy for more than 48 hours, is given an alkali such as magnesium trisilicate 10 ml alternating with aluminium hydroxide 10 ml every 2 hours to reduce the risk of gastric haemorrhage (Stoddart, 1975) or an intravenous infusion of cimetidene, an H_2 receptor blocker (Wardle, 1979) is given.

Treating the cause of shock

The traumatic or pathological causes of shock, and therefore the specific treatments, are very varied. In anaphylaxis the immediate administration of adrenaline and an antihistamine is top priority, along with the maintenance of an airway. Similarly, external bleeding must be controlled initially by pressure, followed if necessary by surgery or other measures. Severe gastrointestinal haemorrhage may necessitate early operation, but sometimes this can be postponed to become an elective measure, or avoided by fibreoptic endoscopy and electrocoagulation or application of local styptics. Gastric cooling and freezing seem to have lost favour due to the dangers and likelihood of further bleeding later (Eiseman & Norton, 1977). Oesophageal balloon tamponade, as with a Sengstaken tube, may be useful in controlling bleeding from oesophageal varices.

Antibiotics used to combat infection in septic shock vary according to the proven or suspected causative organism, and the preference of the medical staff, since many of the drugs do carry some risks. Some examples of antibiotics in use are intravenous clindamycin and gentamicin, metronidazole for anaerobic infections, and carbenicillin which is weaker than polymyxin for neutralizing toxins but is less toxic. Often drug dosage is controlled by estimating serum levels, since the response may be unusual if, for example, there is kidney failure.

In cardiogenic shock, specific measures such as insertion of a cardiac pacemaker for heart block, operative relief of cardiac tamponade or correction of abnormalities such as ruptured chordae tendinae, may occasionally be needed. Pulmonary embolectomy now seems to be less in favour as rapid cardiopulmonary bypass is required. Fibrinolytics such as streptokinase or urokinase sometimes prove successful in breaking up large emboli, particularly if given through a catheter into the pulmonary artery. However careful control is required. Other possible treatments include anticoagulant therapy and, if embolization persists, insertion of an umbrella-like device in the inferior vena cava to catch the emboli before they reach the lungs. When pancreatitis is the cause of shock one of the main treatments may be the administration of the enzyme inhibitor aprotinin (Trasylol) to inhibit the deleterious effects of trypsin, chymotrypsin and kallikrein released into the peritoneal cavity. Possible dosage may be 300 000 units then 600 000 units 12-hourly for 5 days (Jones, 1978).

NURSING CARE OF THE INDIVIDUAL IN SHOCK

Maintenance of physiological integrity

One of the overall functions of nursing is to promote and maintain the integrity of the individual patient, and this is by no means easy with a patient in shock. Promoting physiological integrity includes all the necessary measures so far described, but also others such as prevention of the complications of immobility and deficient local circulation, and avoidance of the possible hazards of treatment. If the patient must be kept flat then the heels and sacrum are likely to be most at risk of pressure damage. This may sound a relatively trivial and mundane concern in a crisis situation, but relief of pressure every 1–2 hours or the use of aids such as sheepskin pads may avoid weeks of discomfort or even prolonged time in hospital for the patient who recovers. Careful re-positioning at 2-hourly intervals and gentle movement of limbs if there is no contra-indication may increase comfort, decrease stasis of the circulation, and improve respiratory function. If skilfully done it need not cause deterioration in even critically ill patients. The patient who has a distended abdomen and/ or dyspnoea may benefit from having his head and shoulders raised on pillows to about 30°, if necessary with the legs raised to increase venous return (the 'jack-knife' position).

The various necessary monitoring and treatment measures involve a number of hazards, ranging from bleeding from disconnected intra-vascular lines, infection via the various catheters into the body, electrical hazards from inadequately earthed equipment, and pressure damage due to tightly strapped or dragging tubes, taps or other equipment, to the dangers of inadvertently allowing fluid overload, or injecting drugs through the arterial instead of the venous line. The patient's physical safety depends on all staff being aware of these hazards and taking measures to avoid them.

Psychological care

The patient's psychological safety depends on staff remembering that he is a suffering human being, who may be aware of the surroundings even if this is not obvious, and not just a set of disordered systems. Explanations and orientation to time and environmental stimuli should be given, and staff working under pressure in a familiar environment need to be careful what they say in the presence of patients and their visitors. Light-hearted chat or irritable remarks may be a release of staff tension but are usually better kept outside patient areas. The patient needs human support, whether by staff or his family (or both). It has been shown that human touch does appear to have physiological effects such as changes in heart-rate, even when the patient is curarised (Lynch, 1978) and this fits with the comments of many people who have been critically ill that it meant a lot to them to have someone sympathetic just to 'be there'.

Care must be planned to try to provide periods of rest, and in this respect electronic monitoring and arterial and venous lines are useful since they may permit observation of physiological function and the obtaining of blood specimens without disturbing the patient. When procedures must be carried out, whether technical procedures or basic care such as changing the bed clothes when there is faecal incontinence (diarrhoea is sometimes a feature of septic shock, or melaena may occur), despite the need to be careful of the various tubes and wires it is essential to remember that such things may be distressing, particularly to an adult, even if they are not painful. Even critically ill patients may be conscious of loss of dignity and personal identity. These, like fear, may all be added psychological stressors. The benefits of simple comfort measures and cleanliness should not be underestimated. One woman, asked several days after open-heart surgery what she had found helpful, said 'Oh, that lovely wash now and again', while others have been distressed by unchanged stained linen.

Control of pain

Adequate control of pain and discomfort contribute to both physiological and psychological well-being. Sometimes there is reluctance to give analgesics in case they cause increased hypotension. In practice the blood pressure may rise when pain and the accompanying anxiety are relieved, since these may be contributory causes of hypotension. However, multiple relatively minor discomforts which may be causing distress can be alleviated relatively simply with a little thought. Patients could often tell much more than they have opportunity to, about the discomforts of such things as awkwardly placed and stiff limbs (usually those with intravascular lines in place), glaring lights, unfeeling manipulation of equipment or patient, or badly strapped nasogastric tubes.

Support of family and others

Care of those who support the patient is part of patient care, since they can only provide support most effectively if they receive it. It is often particularly difficult for the family or friends when a lot of active treatment is going on, since they know that the patient is critically ill yet they must remain away from him in the visitors' room for long periods. They can be greatly helped by ensuring that their physical needs are met, such as hot drinks, meals and toilet facilities, being kept well informed, and given the opportunity to express their feelings. The frequency and duration of time spent with the patient must depend on such factors as the effect of their presence on him, their ability to tolerate necessary activities while they are there, and the space available when staff must work around the bedside. One or sometimes two visitors sitting quietly with the patient even for quite long periods can sometimes be of great comfort, while not impeding the staff's work or becoming too distressed. But this requires that they be properly prepared beforehand with explanations of the patient's appearance, condition and ongoing procedures and attached equipment, and feel accepted by the staff. Visits by the chaplain or other religious adviser may require privacy, within the limits of good treatment, and he too may need help and advice from the staff if he is unused to such acute hospital situations. Again the attitude to and acceptance by staff of such visits, and of small objects of religious significance to the patient, are often important to him. For example, a religious medal attached with care somewhere may be safer than pinned to a gown liable to be sent off to the laundry, or some other symbol may be kept within view, or disturbance reduced for a few moments while someone reads or prays with him. What the patient believes is important, whether or not the nurse shares his faith, yet such things may easily be forgotten in the bustle of activity and effort to reduce the clutter round the bed in the cause of efficiency.

Communication

Sometimes, when shock reaches the irreversible stage, there are difficult decisions to be made about what is appropriate treatment, questions as to what is a justifiable balance of suffering versus benefit. Should all possible measures be used to support physiological function? At such times the good interdisciplinary communication which is essential for effective care becomes even more essential if patients, relatives, and indeed staff, are to be protected from unnecessary harm. The death of a patient in an acute illness such as this can be an extremely traumatic, or a tolerable, or even in some ways a good experience for all concerned, depending on how it is managed.

Recovery

Despite the persistently high mortality rate associated with the fully developed shock syndrome (especially the cardiogenic and bacteraemic varieties), many patients do recover from it with early and effective treatment. As recovery begins, thoughtful planning is required to ensure that gradual, increasing independence in the activities of daily living is encouraged, with the recognition that energy and endurance will be limited after such a severe illness. Generally those who have suffered cardiogenic or bacteraemic shock will be slower to recover. But other factors such as age, previous activity and fitness level, concurrent diseases, or temperamental adaptability are also relevant, so care needs to be planned and performed according to individual needs.

EVALUATION

Evaluation of the care given and patient responses to it should be both intermittent, in that it occurs at preplanned intervals, and also continuous in that relevant changes and responses are noted at any time. In this way care and treatment can be modified as necessary at any time in response to the information obtained, but less obvious changes will be observed even if only at the times planned for evaluation. When the patient is conscious, calm and comfortable, with pink, warm, dry skin, stable vital signs within his normal limits, a good urinary output, effortless breathing, and no signs of bleeding then he appears well on the way to total recovery from shock. But in the acute stage of shock, obviously great and vital changes in the patient's condition may occur within a few minutes. As recovery begins they may be much less obvious, and it may be some hours or days before it can be said with reasonable certainty that recovery of the various normal functions is satisfactory.

CONCLUSION

To summarize, successful recovery from shock is most likely to occur when there is early detection of the warning signs, prompt and effective treatment responsive to the results of careful and continued assessment and, throughout all this, awareness and care of the person suffering the syndrome. In all of this the nurse plays a vital role which requires knowledge, skill, constant awareness, conscientiousness and compassion, as well as the ability to co-operate with other people.

Acknowledgement

We are grateful to Addison-Wesley Publishing Company Inc. for permission to include in this chapter Figure 10.2 from Holloway N 1979 Nursing the Critically Ill Adult (copyright 1979).

REFERENCES

Aspinall M J, Tanner C A 1982 Decision making for patient care. Applying the nursing process. Appleton-Century-Crofts, New York
Beland I, Passos J 1975 Clinical Nursing: pathophysiological and psychosocial approaches, 3rd edn. Macmillan, New York
Beyer A 1979 Shock lung. British Journal of Hospital Medicine 21(3):248,253, 256–258
Budassi S A 1981 Giving an autotransfusion with MAST. Nursing 81 11(10):50
Eiseman B, Norton L 1977 Massive upper gastro-intestinal haemorrhage. In:Ledingham I McA (ed) Recent advances in intensive therapy. Churchill Livingstone, Edinburgh
Forrester J S, Waters D D 1978 Hospital treatment of congestive cardiac failure. Management according to hemdynamic profile. American Journal of Medicine 65:173–180
Harken D 1974 Post-operative care following heart surgery. Heart and Lung 3:893–902
Holloway N M 1979 Nursing the critically ill adult. Addison-Wesley, Menlo Park, California
Holt D 1979 Anaphylactic shock. A shock that's easy to see. Nursing Mirror 148:32–34
Jones E S 1978 Essential intensive care. MTP Press, Lancaster
Ledingham I McA, Routh G S 1979 The pathophysiology of shock. British Journal of Hospital Medicine 22:472,476, 478–480
Lynch J J 1978 The simple act of touching. Nursing (Horsham) 78(8):32–36
Seal A L 1980 Cardiogenic shock. Appleton-Century- Crofts, New York
Shatney C H, Lillehei R C 1976 Pathophysiology and treatment of circulatoryshock. In: Zschoche E (ed) Comprehensive review of critical care. Mosby, St Louis
Stoddart J C 1975 Intensive therapy. Blackwell Scientific, Oxford
Sun R 1971 Trendelenburg's position in hypovolaemic shock. American Journal of Nursing 71:1758–1759
Teasdale G, Jennett B 1974 Assessment of coma and impaired consciousness. Lancet ii:81–84
Vander A J, Sherman J H 1985 Human physiology, 2nd edn. McGraw-Hill, New York
Walinsky P 1977 Acute haemodynamic monitoring. Heart and Lung 6:838–844
Walrath T M 1979 Stopcock: bacterial contamination in invasive monitoring systems. Heart and Lung 8:100–104
Wardle N 1979 Bacteraemic and endotoxic shock. British Journal of Hospital Medicine 21:223–225, 229–231
Wilson R F 1976 The diagnosis and management of severe sepsis and septic shock.Heart and Lung 5:422–429
Woods S L, Mansfield L W 1976 Effect of body position upon pulmonary artery and pulmonary capillary wedge pressures in non–critically ill patients. Heart and Lung 5:83–90

FURTHER READING

Barrow J J 1982 Shock demands drugs — but which one's best for your patient? Nursing (Horsham) 82(12):34–41
Brantigan C O 1982 Haemodynamic monitoring: interpreting values. American Journal of Nursing 82:86–89
Crumlish C M 1981 Cardiogenic shock: catch it early! Nursing (Horsham) 81(11):34–41
Hancock H 1984 Monitoring vascular pressures. Nursing (Oxford) 2(26): 755–760
Hudson-Civetta J, Carruthers-Banner T E 1983 Intravascular catheters: current guidelines for maintenance and care. Heart and Lung 12(5):466–476
Jenner E 1983 Infused with safety. Nursing Mirror 156(14): 23–27
Kaye W 1983 Invasive monitoring techniques: arterial cannulation, bedside pulmonary artery catheterisation, and arterial puncture. Heart and Lung 12(4):395–427
Kennedy G T, Bryant A, Crawford M H 1984 The effects of lateral body positioning on measurements of pulmonary artery and pulmonary wedge pressures. Heart and Lung 13(2):155–158
Kitchen I 1984 Congestive heart failure and cardiogenic shock – drug therapy. Nursing (Oxford) 2(25):743–745
Lamb L S 1982 Think you know septic shock? Read this.

Nursing (Horsham) 82(12):34–43
McCulloch J 1983 The pulmonary artery catheter. Nursing Times 79(13):27–30
Pyles S H 1983 Role of critical care nurses in the early detection and prevention of cardiogenic shock: discovery of the weak link. Heart and Lung 12(4):429–430
Rasie S M 1980 Meeting families' needs helps you meet ICU patients' needs. Nursing (Horsham) 80(10):32–35
Runkel R, Burke L 1983 Trouble-shooting Swan-Ganz catheters. Heart and Lung 12(6):591–597
Sumner S M, Grau P A 1981 To defeat hypovolaemic shock, anticipate and act swiftly. Nursing (Horsham) 81(11):46–51
Townsend A 1983 The intra-aortic balloon pump in the coronary care unit. Nursing Times 79(13):24–26
Wroblewski SS 1981 Toxic shock syndrome. American Journal of Nursing 81:82–85

SECTION TWO

Diagnosis and therapy

This section examines the nursing implications of diagnostic and treatment methods. The first chapter looks at the process of medical diagnosis. It concerns itself with the implications for patients of this process and an exploration of methods used in obtaining diagnostic labels.

Methods of treatment and management are then considered, beginning with those that could be seen to be more within the realm of nursing decision-making, followed by those that are clearly the province of the doctor. In reality any patient will experience a wide variety of treatment modalities. For example, a person undergoing surgery will need support and teaching (socio-psychological therapy), will need to alter his or her level of activity (physical therapy), and will require drugs to alleviate pain (drug therapy). The nurse is in the unique position to collate her knowledge and skills to integrate appropriate therapeutic modes in the act of caring for the person before, during and after treatment partially initiated and given by medical and paramedical staff.

Socio-psychological approaches are vital tools available to nurses to promote patient well-being. Physical and dietary therapy in a highly specialized sense are the province of paramedical staff. Nursing's unique and large contribution in these areas lies in the prevention of further problems by supporting persons receiving specialized therapy, and in activities to optimise the health of those in their care. Though drugs are prescribed by doctors, their administration is mainly effected by nurses who are also responsible for educating patients about their drug therapy and monitoring the effects of treatment.

Clearly, all these forms of therapy have considerable implications for nursing observation and care. For example, both radiotherapy and surgery are prescribed and carried out by medical staff and/or other specialists. Radiotherapy can result in effects on the patient which can be modified by nursing intervention, while the final results of surgery can be greatly influenced by the pre- and post-operative nursing management of the patient.

11

Medical diagnosis and the implications for nursing

INTRODUCTION

THE NEED FOR A DIAGNOSIS AND THE NATURE OF MEDICAL DIAGNOSIS

The process of diagnosing a disease provides medical meaning to a patient's illness, from which a chain of consequences ensue in relation to investigations, treatment and care. The provision of a diagnosis usually implies understanding by doctors of the disease state and the cause of pathology involved. In reality, however, this is often just a label for a recognized cluster of signs and symptoms. Nevertheless the process of making a diagnosis is deemed necessary by physicians, providing the basis both for prognosis and management.

The search for definitions of any one diagnosis and the level of sophistication of knowledge considered necessary to provide a diagnostic label have occupied many authors. The range of definitions varies because of disagreement on the level of sophistication and knowledge held to be necessary before accepting that an illness is recognized as different from all others, yet consistent in its presentation. At its crudest level the process involves providing a label (for economy of words) for a recognized pattern of signs and symptoms. However, Kendall (1975) asserts that any definition of disease that boils down to what people complain of or what doctors treat or some combination of the two is almost worse than no definition at all. Others concede that it is necessary to describe patients' illness at this level in order to systematize observations and aid comprehension, and clearly recognize this process as that of diagnosis. For instance, Taylor (1979) believes that:

> The diagnosis of illness is described in the language of medicine. Illness is diagnosed by description of the phenomena in the language of medicine and comparison with existing descriptions. The language of medicine consists of labels, which are intended to promote brevity and precision.

Most authors accept that the final aim is to diagnose a disease which is differentiated from others and which has an identified cause and, hopefully, a clearly indicated course of treatment. However, in many instances this is not possible, partly because of the constantly developing or mutating disease patterns and also because of other factors which influence symptoms, pathology and the patient's response to them. As Kraupl Taylor (1979) suggests:

> Most diseases which are acknowledged in medicine today are certainly not monogenic disease entities. Yet the final hope and aim of medical science is the establishment of monogenic disease entities and that means the detection of pathological onsets and their causal consequences. Such detection is not only a task for practical investigations, it also requires a scrutiny of the principles of causality so that the various problems which can arise in causal analysis may be understood.

Diagnosis, or medically acceptable diagnosis, is therefore a complex task. First, from the initial interview and examination there may be several possible diagnoses. Secondly there may also be many disease processes in one patient, increasingly so with an ageing population. Thirdly, patients vary in their presentation of any one disease and often complain of symptoms for which there are either too many possible underlying causes, or none readily apparent. These three aspects contribute to the problem of diagnosis. If the doctor were to consider each patient's illness as novel and treat symptoms without knowledge of the underlying cause he would be abandoning a sizeable body of knowledge, and treatment would be a matter of trial and error. Most doctors, therefore, work on the basis of comparing the 'individual' with the 'general' in terms of finding the 'best fit' of signs and symptoms. Thus, most doctors utilize a scientific and disease-oriented approach to medicine.

It is helpful to maintain a distinct terminology. 'Disease processes' are medically recognized with a diagnostic label. 'Illness' is the patient's experience of what may or may not be associated with a recognized disease. Because of the patients' different perceptions of illness, the doctor's role, and of cultural and family expectations of health care (see Ch. 7), it is necessary to broaden professional views beyond the disease model.

This model is concerned primarily with physical causation, pathological disturbances, physical methods of treatment, and the determination of progress. There is increasing evidence of the interrelationship between the sociological, the psychological and the physiological aspects of health/illness (see Chapters 2, 7 and 8). To help patients, therefore, it is often not enough to think only of the disease model of illness, or to cure or treat their physical symptoms. Patients who are ill experience certain problems or symptoms for which they may or may not seek medical aid. These symptoms can be associated with a disease process, but are frequently affected by other factors such as stress, lack of support, a need to abdicate responsibility or to avoid an undesirable situation. In order to help it is necessary to understand the multiplicity of such influences.

Nurses, in particular, should understand not only the aims of medical diagnosis for a patient, but also the role of other contributory factors. There is thus growing support for a more patient-centred view of illness and a problem (and symptom) oriented approach to care by doctors and nurses. This has probably developed in opposition to Parsons' (1966) concept of the 'medical model' and 'the sick role'. The disease oriented approach is epitomized by this concept, in which the patient abdicates other roles and ceases to be responsible for his or her own welfare. The doctor takes over the care of the patient (hence the patient is *under* the doctor's care); the patient then accepts the doctor's judgements and adheres to the doctor's prescriptions until he or she is deemed fit. This model is therefore clearly inappropriate for those who wish to continue to manage their lives as best they can during illness. It also negates the concept of the patient as an active partner in his or her own care, understanding and participating in the decisions about treatment and management and actually concerned with all aspects of care and rehabilitation.

Further research on the 'sick role' by Mechanic (1962) demonstrated how various factors influence both visits to the doctor and individuals' response to illness. In one study students' attendance at a health centre was recorded and related to their perceived levels of stress. Cultural background was also found by Zborowski (1952) to affect the way people responded to symptoms. For instance, Italians suffering from pain would respond with considerable emotion and primarily seek relief from pain, while 'Old Americans' were more stoical and concerned about the meaning and significance of the pain. Jews on the other hand were both very emotional in the expression of pain and concerned to find meaning and significance in the pain experience. Differences in presentation, therefore, may confuse diagnosis and require a different sort of medical attention.

THE HEALTH CARE PROFESSIONALS' RESPONSE TO THE DIAGNOSTIC LABEL

Medical diagnosis thus can be seen to fail in providing an explanation for variation in individuals' responses. For instance, difficulties arise when behaviour during illness is deemed disproportionate to the severity of the disease, as judged by staff. This is particularly problematic when organic pathology is not detected yet the patient remains ill. Doctors used to dealing with physically detectable disease often conclude that the patient is 'faking' or that they cannot help because the illness has 'psychological' causes. This is seen to be an unsatisfactory or incomprehensible reason for illness by those trained in the disease oriented discipline of medical science. Patients become labelled as 'a psychosomatic problem' or 'hysterical' and are referred for a psychiatric opinion.

Discrepancy between the doctor and the patient in judging the illness has led to different approaches in caring for patients' problems, and obviates the use of a simplistic dichotomy between organic and psychological causes of illness. Pilowsky (1975) has discussed instances in which doctors are unable to identify disease and fail to understand why a patient is ill. Patients are said to be manifesting 'abnormal illness behaviour'. He advises that a more holistic approach at both initial assessment and later care provides a better picture of the various contributory factors. Discussion of needs, concerns and problems as well as physical and psychological symptoms will, he says, enable more continuous and rational care. This view thus moves towards the multiple causation of illness and away from the monogenic diagnosis of disease processes.

Nurses and other health workers have traditionally accepted the disease oriented framework, and this has unfortunate implications for those patients whose illness does not fit a disease hypothesis. The separation of general and psychiatric nurse training further demarcates those diseases which are appropriate to each setting, and delays understanding about the interaction of social, psychological and physical processes. Stockwell's (1972) study showed how patients with a psychiatric diagnosis were 'unpopular' on general wards. Robinson (1976) also discussed the low priority given to psychological care by students only skilled in acute and technical forms of care.

The clinical setting, or the suitability of this in relation to the condition of the patient admitted, tends to influence the response to diagnosis. For instance, a young person's attempt at suicide may be seen as a tragic event requiring expert intervention if admitted to an acute psychiatric clinic. In a general ward opinions may be very different, particularly if several other critically ill 'medical' patients require attention. The immediate aim is for rapid psychiatric referral and discharge from hospital. A psychiatric label often acts as a barrier to empathetic treatment in a general ward. Simplistic and pejorative terms such as 'nutter' are often heard in this setting, and even appear in ward reports. This tends to reduce nurse-patient contact and penalizes patients with this type of unfavourable label.

It is not, however, only those who acquire a 'psychiatric' label whose diagnosis will influence the approach to care by health professionals. In Stockwell's (1972) study the chronic long stay patient was also found to be 'unpopular'. Traditionally both the status and the financing of the geriatric, psychiatric and mental handicap wards and units have been low. The 'young chronic sick' are still found in some geriatric wards on the basis that physical dependency is a more important determinant of need than psychosocial environment. The chronic sick and elderly will therefore be seen as 'illegitimate' within the context of a care situation dominated by the disease/medical model, in spite of the physical nature of their disease.

There is a a third group of patients whose diagnostic label — malignancy — has a particular connotation for staff. A diagnosis of 'cancer' or 'leukaemia' appears to move the patient into a different category of being. The continuing debate relating to 'should the patient be told', and the large number of hospices recently opened and partially financed outside the state system of provision, demonstrate the im-plications of the disease/medical model for this group.

Clearly, therefore, the diagnostic label is of considerable significance to health care professionals beyond the simple diagnosis — treatment link.

THE PATIENT'S RESPONSE TO DIAGNOSIS

Patients as well as doctors accept that a diagnosis is a necessary part of the medical process. It tends to serve as a reassurance for them. As Lipowski (1975) pointed out, individuals need an explanation for any symptom or health problem. Although patients may not understand the diagnostic label, it helps them by implying that the illness is 'bona fide'. Further, they can now take on the 'patient role' and can abdicate their responsibility for their welfare to their doctor. Occasionally doctors may use this effect to legitimize a patient's sickness. He may diagnose a 'coryza' rather than a cold so that a busy, tired mother is given 2 days in bed while the family look after themselves and her for a change!

Beyond the initial impact, further meanings and consequences accrue from a diagnosis. Certain types of disease will certainly be unpopular and threatening. Having to alter one's lifestyle, food intake, cigarette smoking and drinking will obviously be a nuisance, but the greatest threat or underlying fear for a majority of patients is malignancy. This fear was previously associated with tuberculosis, but now 'cancer' is seen as the 'worst' diagnosis — 'intractable and capricious — that is, a disease not understood.' (Sontag, 1979).

Whereas patients' tolerance for recurrent chest infections or long-term arthritis is often remarkable, an unexplained symptom or change in body function is frequently the source of considerable anxiety. This anxiety may result in rapid medical consultation, but may alternatively lead to denial of the problem, the threat being too great to face. As Aitken-Swan & Paterson (1955) found, 45% of early symptomatic patients tended to delay seeking advice. During the first out-patient visit, patients with a malignant breast lump were found to be highly anxious, expressing this as a fear of a fatal disease (Maguire 1978). For such patients, doctors and other staff have adopted 'softer', more generalized labels, such as 'ulcer' or 'growth', to avoid the use of emotive diagnostic terms (Bond, 1978).

CONCLUSION TO THE INTRODUCTION

Patients and doctors both accept that diagnosis is a necessity prior to the treatment of illness. Initially, doctors may list tentative diagnoses before any further confirmation is available, and occasionally they may withhold treating the symptoms before a final diagnosis is reached. Patients may be less likely to understand that several diagnoses are possible, and lack an appreciation that sophisticated tools are sometimes required to confirm a diagnosis. They may also be relieved when they are given an incomplete diagnosis, such as 'anaemia', not understanding the full implications that a cause, which may be more sinister, has to be established. It is therefore not surprising that the process of diagnosis is itself often bewildering, the complexity and medical sophistication seemingly incomprehensible and, therefore, beyond their control.

THE PROCESS OF DIAGNOSIS AND NEED FOR DIAGNOSTIC TESTS

The process of diagnosis for all patients will initially involve taking a clinical history and carrying out physical examination. These will not necessarily indicate a diagnosis, or alternatively they may indicate too many. All the symptoms, the sequence in which they occurred, the conditions which surrounded them, the family history and every piece of information offered by the patient must be noted during the history. Each piece may offer a vital clue.

These clues are picked up in the context of the physical examination. On the basis of this information, certain diagnoses will not then be considered further. A list of tentative diagnoses will be postulated, then a series of tests may be planned. The more probable diagnoses will be more thoroughly tested. Some tests, or combinations of tests, are considered to be 'diagnostic' for certain diseases, i.e. a positive finding will be strongly indicative of that specific disease. Thus by a process of elimination and deduction, a diagnosis (or diagnoses) is reached. This initial diagnosis, or 'hypothesis', may then be confirmed by further testing. This disciplined approach avoids making snap judgements based on a few clues which seem to fit the puzzle. Perhaps the biggest challenge for a specialist is admitting that he is unable to explain an illness in terms of a disease and so has to ask for another's opinion. This referral may lead to a different and more useful perspective, but it also frequently leads to more tests being requested, and a greater delay for the patient before (what he may see as) useful action.

Diagnosis for the practising physician is thought to depend on a blend of clinical skills and scientific evidence. When there is doubt, a full survey of diagnostic tests may be ordered. Although this is an extravagant and often tiring procedure for the patient, it is undertaken during preventative screening and prior to major surgery to eliminate complicating, previously undetected, pathology. A single abnormal test result seldom provides a diagnosis. For example, a high blood urea may indicate cardiac, liver, kidney or nutritional abnormalities; however in conjunction with other results, such as albuminuria and a raised erythrocyte sedimentation rate, an infection of the kidney would seem likely.

THE NATURE OF DIAGNOSTIC INVESTIGATIONS

The nature of diagnostic investigations is inevitably diverse due to the widespread and diverse nature of disease. Theoretically, it would be helpful if every organ, tissue or fluid in the body could be examined both macroscopically and microscopically, and every cell, organ or system tested functionally. In reality this is clearly impossible. Most organs are essential for survival one way or another, so investigations are limited to those tests that do not disturb that function too much. Assumptions and generalizations therefore have to be made from the examination of part of a structure or an aspect of function. Thus, a sample of blood or urine or a fragment of tissue gained by biopsy may be considered as indicative of the state of the whole. Similarly, function may be estimated by the rapidity with which an organ deals with a selected chemical.

Clearly, such indicators are subject to questions both of reliability and validity. A series of samples may be taken or a group of different tests performed in order to increase the reliance that can be placed on results. While this may be readily apparent to medical staff, the need for a test to be repeated or for several different tests to be performed is often not so clear to the patient, who not only has to tolerate the physical deprivations and discomforts, but whose future plans may depend on the outcome.

In addition to the problem of sampling, some structures in the body are particularly inaccessible or do not process chemicals that are specific or known. The brain is such an organ and is notoriously difficult to investigate, much of our knowledge being gained from autopsy rather than in vitro investigation. In this situation, patients may undergo extensive and prolonged investigation only to find that the outcome is the acceptance of a disability state of unknown causation.

A third problem is that of individual variation. This is overcome to a certain extent by defining a range of 'normal' values, these being theoretically derived from large samples of the population. In practice however, large numbers of 'normal' individuals do not make themselves available for the physical discomforts of numerous tests. The definition of 'normal' for any one test is therefore likely to change value from time to time, as new evidence beomes available. Similarly when a new test or technique is developed, 'normal' has to be identified and standardized. Epidemiological and cross-cultural studies are helpful in identifying what can be considered 'normal' in a given population. It must be pointed out, however, that 'normal' is not to be confused with either 'healthy' or 'desirable'. For example, the fact that the majority of the population of the UK will have carbon deposits in their lungs cannot be considered desirable, although it is quite normal.

Within the diagnostic context investigations are carried out with a number of aims in mind:

- to establish the nature of the disorder, i.e. to fix the appropriate label to the signs and symptoms presented
- to establish the causative factors relevant to that individual
- to establish the extent of the disease.

This latter point is important not only as an indicator of prognosis but also of treatment. Radical operative therapy is unlikely to be undertaken if disease is widespread, or if vital organs or vessels are infiltrated; a single small dose of an orally administered antibiotic is unlikely to be effective in fulminating pneumonia.

IMPLICATIONS OF THE MEDICAL DIAGNOSTIC PROCESS FOR NURSING

Patients are particularly vulnerable to psychological distress (Wilson-Barnett & Carrigy, 1978) during the process of diagnosis. When this is protracted and requires hospitalization, there are many reasons for their distress, including the fear of what the diagnosis might be, the feeling that staff suspect they are frauds because test results are normal, and their lack of contact and attention from staff who are tending those who are obviously ill. Nurses have an important role in helping such patients through this difficult period. This may be considered in relation to four areas:-

- providing psychological comfort and informed reassurance
- co-ordination of tests and communication of results and further plans to patients
- preparing patients physically and providing physical comfort during and after tests
- arranging necessary equipment or facilities, to promote a smooth procedure with minimal interruptions or delays.

Although these patients are frequently independent, they clearly have special needs for nursing care. Uncertainty about the future is one of the most unpleasant and energy-consuming responses to any situation. As well as empathising, getting to know and showing understanding of how the patient feels about his or her situation, the nurse must be able to provide sufficient knowledge of what is happening through contact with medical and other staff involved in caring for the patient. Nursing will involve giving the patients plenty of opportunities to ask questions, talking with them and providing some form of enjoyable and constructive diversional therapy. The very fact that staff care enough to try to think of odd trips outside the hospital or to spend days at home is reassuring to patients.

Where the process of diagnosis is undertaken in the out-patient department or through general practice liaison with the hospitals, the waiting period may involve uncertainty and worry. This is often relieved by the presence of family members, and the usual daily activities also act as distractions. During any stressful or threatening period the presence of others, particularly those significant to the individuals concerned, acts as a mediating or buffering force. Nuckalls et al (1972) found that support from the spouse reduced complications and stress reactions during the important and potentially stressful event of childbirth. The implication of this for nursing is clearly that staff should encourage contact between family and patient, and promote the formation of meaningful and supportive relationships between nurses and patients.

It is important to note that all aspects of the diagnostic process, i.e. clinical history, physical examination and diagnostic testing, contribute not only to the labelling of the disorder but also to the identification of the extent and aetiology of the pathological process. This information not only forms the basis for treatment but may also give an indication of prognosis.

For some patients the process of diagnosis is extremely rapid. For example, a person at home may wake with severe, crushing chest pain and a feeling of impending death (see Ch. 22). The family practitioner, when called, observes a severely shocked patient (see Ch. 10) who continues to complain of severe chest pain. He makes a tentative diagnosis of myocardial infarction, which is subsequently confirmed by the changes in the electrical potential of the heart muscle demonstrated in an ECG (undertaken in the home or in hospital). At this time, blood is also taken for examination of enzymes released into the blood stream from damaged myocardial tissue (see Ch. 22). When these results are available, they act as additional confirmation of the diagnosis and are indicative of the amount of tissue damage.

The process of diagnosis for other patients may be a more prolonged affair. For example, a person may experience 'indigestion' for some days and treat himself with proprietary antacids before going to his family doctor. After taking a history and examining the patient, a diagnosis of gastric ulceration may be reached. The doctor prescribes a more sophisticated antacid and advises the patient about diet and smoking. If the problem persists the family doctor is likely to refer the patient for specialist advice. In the out-patient department of the hospital, investigations such as barium meal and gastroscopy will be arranged. These may or may not result in hospital admission for treatment.

Some problems are resistant to diagnosis. Pyrexia of unknown origin is, by definition, one of these problems, and is discussed in Chapter 27. In some instances the cause of abdominal pain is very difficult to establish. Other problems of this type include some metabolic and endocrine disorders, collagen diseases and allergic disorders.

If diagnosis evades the resources of the general practitioner, it may well be necessary to refer the patient for specialist advice. Out-patient appointments would then be made for consultations, and diagnostic tests might be carried out before or after this visit.

The traditional organization of out-patient departments gives rise to very brief contacts between individual patients and staff, and makes it unrealistic for nurses to seriously develop their supportive and counselling roles.

In addition, the practice of doctors in informing patients of test results (whether performed as in-patients or out-patients) within a clinic setting, and without a nurse being present, further detracts from the nurse's ability to support patients when necessary. That means that it is crucial to encourage the presence of a close friend or relative and to make every effort to be friendly and informative. Close liaison with the family practitioner is also essential.

INVESTIGATIONS FOR OTHER PURPOSES

Some people also have various investigations performed outside the narrow diagnostic context. These people fall into three main groups:

- Individuals presumed to be healthy who are undergoing some form of health screening. This may be in relation to occupation, age/sex, or insurance, or they may be self-referred for general or specific screening.
- Those patients with a known diagnosis who are undergoing routine physical examination and 'routine' tests, such as urine testing, full blood count, serum urea and electrolytes and chest X-ray. This includes patients admitted for surgical treatment and antenatal women. The specific tests used will vary in different patient groups.
- Those people with a known disorder which may or may not be treated but whose condition needs to be intermittently monitored.

In all three of these situations, while patients may be happy to undergo physical examination, they may be less willing to undergo potentially painful or embarrassing procedures, such as venepuncture or check cystoscopy. In these circumstances it is important that the nurse ensures that the patient fully understands the rationale for the proposed investigation.

THE ROLE OF THE NURSE DURING DIAGNOSTIC INVESTIGATIONS

The nurse's prime responsibility in caring for patients during diagnostic investigations is her direct support of the patient. Satisfying their physical and psychological needs involves attending the patient prior to, during and after the test. If the test is undertaken on the ward it is also conventional that nurses collect and prepare necessary equipment. However, as doctors usually perform the test it is wise if they help with this, ensuring that everything needed is readily available, to avoid unnecessary delay and discomfort for the patient. Whether the doctor also assists in disposal of this equipment tends to depend on personal charm and charity of both the nurse and the doctor! This is actually less arduous when 90% of the equipment is disposable. Clearing away together has the distinct advantage of allowing staff to discuss the significance of the test for the patient's progress, and to clarify any special precautions or care that may be required as a consequence of the test. This should only be done after the patient is made comfortable and any questions he or she may have been dealt with.

If patients are taken to special departments for investigation, it is the responsibility either of the accompanying ward nurse or the departmental nurse specialist to ensure that patients are inconvenienced as little as possible. Clear instructions about where and when to wait, what they can or cannot do, completion of the test and follow-up arrangements should be given.

PATIENTS' RESPONSES TO DIAGNOSTIC TESTS

Patients' responses to the process of diagnostic tests are very variable, the same procedure evoking very different reactions. However, despite this overall variability a few objective individual factors provide some indication of those who are most emotionally and physically vulnerable. On the whole the major emotional dimension involved is anxiety, which tends to be specifically related to what will happen during the test. Patients fear pain, discomfort and embarrassment or indignity.

Anxiety

Studies of patients' emotional responses to investigations reveal that anxiety is frequently experienced, often at extreme levels. However, Hawkins (1979) and Wilson-Barnett & Carrigy (1978) found that older patients tend to be less anxious than others, possibly explained by the fact that they tend to expect illness and to be more philosophical about the procedures that this entails. They also seem to accept a passive role more easily, abdicating responsibility for decisions about their care and complaining or making negative comments less frequently than others (Wilson-Barnett, 1977). Their capacity to adjust to life in hospital is also greater than that of younger patients (i.e. those under 40 years). The study by De Wolfe et al in a TB sanatorium also found that educated young people were more highly dissatisfied and unhappy than other groups of patients (De Wolfe et al, 1966).

Nurses should not be deceived by patients' stoical attitudes. Despite much anxiety, most patients go through some very unpleasant tests without complaint or request for rest or analgesia. This should not reduce the efforts of staff to provide optimum support, tailored to individual needs. As yet, research only gives general guidelines for practice which have been validated by the results of several studies.

Patients who will need most support, who are likely to suffer extreme anxiety over tests, are those with a predisposition towards emotionality. In a study by Johnson et al (1973), this was demonstrated by measuring patients' trait, or predisposition towards anxiety, and correlating this with reports and observations during gastroscopy. Although most patients are likely to feel some anxiety, whatever their trait, it was also shown during barium X-rays (Wilson-Barnett, 1979) that those with high scores on a trait test were highly likely to experience high level anxiety. Reasons for this response tend to be in terms of 'fear of the unknown', fear of pain, complications and what they might find. Hawkins (1979) also found that, although two-thirds of patients who had experienced a range of tests would agree to a repeat test, the remainder would be unwilling or would only agree reluctantly to having the test repeated.

Physical illness and incapacity

Physical illness and incapacity will also affect how patients respond to tests. Many investigations involve lying in one position, or alternatively moving from side to side or from a lying to sitting position on hard X-ray tables or theatre trolleys. For example, over half the patients who have a barium enema are over 60 years of age, and Wilson-Barnett (1979) found they were very distressed by the physical effort required for this procedure, particularly by the bowel preparation the night before which usually caused abdominal pain and repeated trips to the lavatory.

Invasiveness

The physical invasiveness of the test may well be thought to influence patients' responses. Although to some extent the medical procedures such as lumbar puncture and bone marrow biopsy are invasive and do evoke much anxiety, this is anticipated and staff tend to be reassuring. Cardiac catheterization is an extremely 'invasive', uncomfortable and sometimes lengthy procedure, but many staff are around the patient throughout and they usually provide ongoing information, reassurance and at least one dose of intramuscular analgesia in addition to the pre-medication. Patients are therefore surprisingly calm about this procedure (Hawkins, 1979). For more routine tests, less attention or time is devoted to preparing patients. It appears that the presence of another person is a factor that helps them to cope, and therefore when this support is not available the patient feels more alone and unsupported.

Coping with investigation

In general, those patients who have better coping mechanisms, intellectual and social resources, as well as a positive, questioning and confident attitude are likely to be less anxious in the anticipation and experience of stressful episodes such as tests or surgery. The reasons for this are thought to relate to their use of information in preparing for a novel experience. Those who are too reticent, withdrawn and ill to ask for or understand any explanation are in a more vulnerable position. Several research studies have demonstrated how information giving can reduce anxiety at the time of tests, although the way this is achieved is still open to question. Johnson et al (1973) showed how detailed explanation before a gastroscopy had a significant association with lowered anxiety levels and a reduced need for sedation. Wilson-Barnett (1979) also demonstrated significantly lower anxiety levels for experimentally informed patients during barium enema, and there was a suggestion that this also reduced anxiety immediately prior to the X-ray. Johnson et al also showed that the type of information given to the patients was important. Descriptions of the likely sensations, sights, sounds and degree of pain (if any) was significantly more helpful in reducing anxiety than procedural details. They hypothesized that the more accurately the information describes the patient's experience, the more useful it is as a preparation. They suggest that the opportunity to think about the procedure helps the patient anticipate and plan how they will cope with and react to events. Without explanation or previous experience the patient faces the unknown and at each step may expect something more painful or uncomfortable, imagining the worst.

IMPLICATIONS FOR NURSING

Preparation of patients

Findings from this growing body of research should encourage practitioners to provide explanations which are relevant to their patients. Lack of explanation prior to tests is frequently reported (Reynolds, 1978; Hawkins, 1979). Although nurse educators stress the importance of explanation, the wide range of tests and related information is increasing so rapidly that nurses have to be highly motivated and conscientious to satisfy all their patients' needs. It is also difficult for staff to witness and learn about each and every investigation. More time is needed for nurses to talk with and observe patients' during and after such tests. The information gleaned could then be used for the benefit of future patients. Aspects of this psychological preparation may be considered under the headings below.

Purpose. The way in which any procedure aids diagnosis should be explained, always in everyday, non-technical language. For instance, an electrocardiogram, or ECG, may be explained as a tracing on paper illustrating how nervous impulses pass through the heart activating the muscle, indicating how the heart is functioning. An intravenous pyelogram could be described as an X-ray of the kidney, which is made possible by injecting a dye concentrated by the kidney and passed into the urine and which can be seen draining down into the bladder on X-ray. Any interruption or abnormalities in flow can then be seen.

How and where is it done? Nurses are usually in a position to say where a procedure will be undertaken. As an example, biopsies may be undertaken on the ward or in the X-ray department, where visualization of the organ is possible. This may need to be clarified with those who are to do this test so that the patient can prepare for it realistically. A department such as 'nuclear medicine' may worry a patient simply because of its name. Radiation hazard signs such as 'Danger do not enter' in departments such as X-ray may also be interpreted as indicating harm to the patient. Unless clearly told, patients may not realize that many procedures undertaken in these departments are non-invasive in the normal sense of the word, except for the administration of dyes or radioactive isotopes. However, with increasing public awareness of the dangers of radiation, many patients may also be worried about the insidious or long term effects of the investigation.

The equipment involved, particularly in such procedures as scans, may be overwhelming without adequate preparation. In some instances it may be useful for the patient to see the equipment beforehand and/or be accompanied by a nurse familiar to the individual concerned.

Preparation for the procedure. If preparation is required prior to a test, such as a period of fasting or bowel cleansing, it is important that both the need for it, and what is involved are explained. Patients find the preparation as stressful as the investigation itself and need time to adjust to this expectation. If, as sometimes happens, wards differ in their preparation routine, some fasting and others not, nurses should initiate discussion on this with the appropriate personnel and not accept variation which unnecessarily inconveniences patients.

The timing of explanation about the investigation is related to how much preparation is required. The preparation for major investigation such as special X-ray or a biopsy may take 24 hours or more, and the explanation should therefore be given prior to physical preparation commencing. Without research evidence on the efficiency of the timing it is impossible to prescribe in detail. Intuitively, there should be enough time to prepare but not too long to forget. A blood test, rarely a novel experience, is usually not explained beforehand, but as it is such a rapid procedure a short preparatory sentence just before it would normally be adequate. In general, the longer the procedure, the longer the time required for preparation.

Delay or variation in the procedure. One of the most difficult problems in a large institution is the co-ordination of events such as tests and preparations. Ideally, patients should spend a minimum amount of time in the investigatory department, as lengthy waiting inevitably creates anxiety. In addition, waiting patients are often on trolleys or in wheelchairs sometimes in draughty corridors. This is uncomfortable and tiring and may be detrimental both physically and psychologically. Close liaison between ward and departmental staff may prevent undue delay. Awareness of the departmental requirements in terms of patients' notes, X-rays and escort will also reduce delay.

When waiting time is usual and unavoidable, for instance between stages of a test, patients should be prepared and advised on how to cope with this, e.g. to take a blanket, newspaper and foam ring to sit on.

Where variations may occur for patients having the same test, the possibilities should be mentioned. If extra procedures occur patients will be prepared; if not, so much the better.

The sensations involved. As mentioned, this is a key area of information giving, gleaned from others who have experienced the test. If these reports mention a 'sharp pain', staff should prepare patients for the fact that it may be painful, say how long this lasts and provide prophylactic analgesia beforehand if possible. After local anaesthetic, always used prior to tissue biopsy, the sensation tends to be one of pressure rather than pain. In the particular examples of a sternal marrow puncture or lumbar puncture, the amount of pressure which has to be applied for penetration not only surprises the patients, but also staff. Likewise, it is important to mention muscular reflex contractions where this is relevant. For example, in order to introduce speculae per vaginum or rectum, patients often get frightened that initial contraction will persist so that the instrument will have to be introduced under pressure. It is reassuring for them to know that this spasm is usually momentary. In many procedures where discomfort and anxiety, rather than pain, are expected, such as endoscopies or cardiac catheterization, sedatives such as diazepam are often used. Apart from creating relaxation (general and smooth muscle) this also diminishes the memory of an unpleasant experience. It is a false kindness in explanations to patients to minimize the degree of discomfort 'usually' experienced. From empirical observation, every one of us has seen how the majority resent a falsehood and are shocked and resentful after experiencing unexpected or negated discomfort. Once warned about this and 'psyched up', most people cope with much less distress. The effectiveness of adequate preparation for potentially distressing experiences has been well documented and justified by work in the field of childbirth and surgical care.

The length of the procedure. It is also important to tell patients how long a procedure, and any related discomfort, will last. For instance, during barium X-rays bowel distension from barium and gas becomes extremely uncomfortable towards the end of the procedure (after about 20–25 minutes), and remains for about 10 minutes before patients are escorted to the lavatory with resultant relief.

Similarly with an IVP, the pressure pads only remain tied to the abdomen during screening for about 10 minutes.

If patients mention ways that they were able to alleviate discomfort, for instance by certain adjustments in breathing or leg exercises when lying still on a bed or table, these should be remembered by staff for their successive patients.

Who will be there? When the nurse from the ward will be accompanying the patient or helping with the procedure this should be mentioned. Many studies, originally done with animals (e.g. Liddell, 1950), have shown that at a time of stress the effects can be alleviated by the presence of another. Every step possible should be taken to accompany a patient who is to go for a special test, especially when they are particularly nervous or frail. In some instances the presence of an informed, supportive relative should be considered.

After effects. Once more, by using the reports of other patients' experiences any likely after effects can be described and steps taken to prevent them when possible. Tiredness is to be expected in anyone who is unwell, but more specific effects must also be described. These include, for example, headache for about 24 hours after lumbar puncture; ache or soreness for one or two days after biopsy, cardiac catheterization or angiography; constipation and indigestion after tests requiring previous bowel clearance; stiffness and backache after lengthy X-rays and possibly a sore throat after a general anaesthetic.

Giving information and psychological support

Giving information which is understood and retained is a complex task which requires training. Staff may look for interest, recognition or perplexity in their patient, and need to provide plenty of opportunity for questions before, during and after the session. A few patients may appear not to want this explanation. Where this is the case, it is probably wise to give a brief insight into what is involved prior to procedures that are invasive, lengthy or risky, and to provide company and continuous support to avoid adverse reactions from such an unprepared, vulnerable patient.

It is difficult to predict what will be considered as intrusive, painful or embarrassing by individual patients. The problems created by radiation have already been mentioned. For some patients a series of searching questions may be seen as more threatening than physical procedures or examination.

Staff should be aware of the possible implications for patients' responses throughout the diagnostic process. Not only is a disease being revealed, but patients are experiencing novel events where taboo, 'private' functions have to be discussed, observed and analyzed. During diagnosis, patients are subject to a process whereby questions are asked and they feel obliged to comply to strange requests and accept what is done 'for their own good'. If they are unable to do what is required of them, such as producing a stool or swallowing a Ryle's tube, it is upsetting and frustrating.

In this vulnerable state some patients are expected to assess whether they should accept risks which, although small in statistical terms, may in the event affect them. For procedures where some risk is involved, as in cardiac catheterization, written consent is obtained. The problem for the staff is how best to explain the risk involved, and this clearly raises ethical issues. Figures are not available or sufficiently meaningful to present the information realistically. Death from fatal arrhythmias does sometimes occur, and arrhythmias are certainly common. However, this procedure is only undertaken when thought to be absolutely necessary for diagnostic purposes prior to treatment.

Research which has examined preparation of patients for diagnostic tests does have clear implications for practice. However, more knowledge is required in a number of areas. First, there is relatively little knowledge about the ways in which different patient characteristics affect the response to investigatory procedures and therefore influence their specific requirements for preparation. Secondly, more information is needed on the patient's perception of the experience of tests and of helpful/unhelpful nursing and other support and interventions.

There is no research to show that information about tests produces an overall drop in anxiety levels in groups of patients, but this requires further evaluation in the clinical field. It is also clearly established that patients report a lack of sufficient helpful information for preparation before tests.

SPECIFIC TESTS

While this chapter has been concerned with medical diagnostic tests, it is important to

Table 11.1 Diagnostic tests: What is being investigated

What is being investigated	What is being looked at	Means of investigation	What can be identified
A Structure			
Cells, Tissues	Macroscopic and Microscopic appearance	Physical and digital examination Endoscopy Laparotomy Histological examination Microbiological examination Haematological examination	Basic pathophysiological changes — inflammatory degnerative neoplastic
Organs, Vessels	Arrangement of structures Size and patency	Physical and digital examination Straight and serial X-rays Contrast medium X-rays Endoscopy Laparotomy	Congenital and acquired malformations Ulceration, aneurysms, leakage Obstruction, strictures, stenosis Irregular surfaces Enlargement or contraction
B Function			
Organ, System	Levels of substances Ability of organ to process substance Nature of flow of fluid Electrical activity	Biochemical examination Radioactive isotope studies Pressure and sound recordings Electrical recordings Thermal recordings	Quality of function

recognize that nursing is less concerned with the medical diagnostic process than with assisting the patient to cope with his experiences. However, understanding both the diagnostic process and the implications for the patient of the diagnostic label is essential for the nurse to plan effective physical and psychological care.

Making sense of the numerous diagnostic tests is a daunting task. In the section that follows three questions are asked:

- What is being investigated?
- By what means is the investigation carried out?
- What tests are carried out on specific body fluids, tissues or systems?

In answering these three questions some specific implications for patient and/or nurse are identified, the more general implications having already been discussed. For ease of reference much of the material has been tabulated.

What is being investigated?

Within the context of identifying the nature and extent of the disease process diagnostic investigations are concerned with examining either the structure or the function of cells, tissues, organs or systems. Table 11.1 outlines these in more detail. In terms of preparation it is clear that if structure is to be looked at, that structure has to be made as readily available as possible and without attendant debris. Thus, organs to be infiltrated with a contrast medium must first be empty; radio-opaque ornaments or fastenings must be removed prior to X-ray; the patient must be positioned appropriately for various physical or digital examinations. If function is to be investigated, that function must be understood so that it will not be interfered with during the test. For example, if uptake of a substance by an organ is the principle upon which the test is based, then it is important that the substance is not given in natural form for a known amount of time prior to the test — e.g., no fish prior to ^{131}I uptake tests, fasting prior to glucose tolerance.

By what means is the investigation carried out?

As already mentioned, ideally each organ or tissue should be available for direct examination.

Table 11.2 The means by which diagnostic investigations are carried out

Types and means of examination		What can be identified	Examples
A. Direct examination of the gross structure of organs, tissues or cavities			
General physical examination		Condition and appearance of skin Body masses	'Routine' physical
Digital		Size of cavity Position of organs Texture, tension, masses	Rectum, vagina
Direct vision through natural orifice*		Condition and appearance of epithelium	Nose, ear, retina, mouth
with speculum		Size of cavity, vessels	Oesophagus, stomach, duodenum, colon, rectum
with endoscope	— rigid with or without light	Constrictions, state of valves and sphincters	Bile duct Larynx, trachea, bronchi
	— fibreoptic	Fluids present or being produced Reaction of organ to presence of instrument	Vagina, Urethra, bladder
Direct vision via a fibreoptoscope* inserted through a small incision		Structures in a body cavity	Abdominal cavity Mediastinum Amniotic sac
Direct vision through a major incision*		Structures in a body cavity	Abdominal cavity

* It is important to note: (1) that these examinations are often carried out when the patient is sedated or under local or general anaethesia
(2) that the direct gross examination is combined with specimens being taken for laboratory investigation or other measures being taken for indirect examination of structures or function

Types and means of examination		What can be identified	Examples
B. Indirect examination of the gross structure or function of organs, tissues, or cavities			
Radiographic	Single X-rays	Radio-opaque structures such as bone or fluid for size, relationship to other structures, radio-opacity	Chest Abdomen
	Serial X-rays Tomograms Computerized axial tomography (CAT scan)	Radio-opaque structures such as bone or fluid for size, relationship to other structures, radio-opacity	Chest Skull Abdominal organs
	Using radio-opaque dyes	Outline of cavity of vessel, tube or organ	Gastrointestinal tract — barium studies Biliary system Blood vessels — angiography Heart chambers Spinal cord and cerebral ventricles
Pressure recordings		Pressure of fluid within a vessel or organ	Blood pressure CSF Pressure of blood within heart chambers
Sound recordings			
Auscultation		Sounds within body	Heart sounds Breathing Peristalsis
Ultrasound (reflection back of high frequency waves)		Density of tissue	Fetus and placenta Liver
Thermography		Differential temperatures of body tissue	Breast

Table 11.2 continued

Types and means of examination	What can be identified	Examples
Electrical activity	Changes in action potentials of nerve or muscle	Electrocardiogram (ECG) Electroencephalogram (EEG) Electromyogram (EMG)
Radioactive isotope studies	Uptake and/or excretion pattern of elements often normal to function of tissue being studied, given in radioactive form	Thyroid — ^{131}I Liver Deep vein thrombosis — radio-actively-labelled fibrinogen
C. Laboratory examination of body fluids or tissues		
Biochemical	Levels of chemicals normally present Levels of toxins	Blood, e.g. urea and electrolytes Urine CSF
Haematological	Level and appearance of blood constituents	Blood — red blood cells, Hb White cells, platelets
Histological	Cell and tissue abnormality — microscopic structure	Tissue biopsy
Microbiological	Presence of infective organisms including parasites Antibiotic sensitivity	Urine Sputum Pus Blood
Immunological	Presence and level of antibodies Immune response tests	Blood Skin

While this is still not possible in many instances, the scope of direct examination has been increased enormously with the development of flexible fibre-optoscopes. Other technological advances are similarly likely to expand and refine the techniques available for diagnostic testing. Table 11.2 outlines the various methods currently in common use. It is important to note that some investigations that a patient will undergo use more than one method of investigation — e.g. lumbar puncture is used to measure pressure of the CSF within the spinal column, to obtain samples of CSF for bacteriology and biochemistry and to inject air or a radio-opaque dye for indirect examination of structure.

What tests are carried out on specific body fluids, tissues or systems

This is the classification scheme most commonly used in standard texts on investigations. It is not intended here to give a comprehensive or detailed account, simply an indication of the variety of common tests available. For detailed aspects of care the reader is referred to texts such as Pagana & Pagana (1982), Evans (1978) or Bomford et al (1975). It is important to note here, however, that where specimens are being collected it is vital that the appropriate containers are used and that the containers are clearly labelled with the patient's details, the nature of the specimen and the time and date at which it was collected. Different tests require different additives or none at all and samples are easily confused or mislaid. Any inaccuracies of this nature are likely to prolong the diagnostic process. Table 11.3 indicates common tests on specific body fluids, tissues or systems. Fuller explanation of tests in relation to systems structure and function are included within the subsequent chapters on disturbances of function. One general point, while most tests are reasonably specific to a particular system,

Table 11.3 Notes on some common tests

Type of test	What is being identified	Nursing notes
A. Tests on specific body fluids		
1. *Blood*		
Venous blood (Venepuncture)	Number and characteristics of red and white blood cells, platelets.	Variations in some levels due to circadian rhythm, pyrexia, food intake
	Urea and electrolytes Blood glucose	
	Hormone and enzyme levels Plasma proteins, antibodies Drug levels Presence of infective organism	Risk of bruising. As needle removed apply direct pressure over swab until oozing stopped.
Arterial blood (Arterial puncture)	PCO_2 PO_2	May relate to controlled O_2 intake or artificial ventilation Very painful Risk of bleeding and extensive bruising As needle removed, press firmly over swab for 5 minutes or until oozing has stopped
Capillary blood (finger prick)	Blood glucose	Used regularly for monitoring diabetes control. Rotate sites
Glucose tolerance test	Measures pattern of blood glucose level and urinary excretion of glucose after administration of known (50 g) amount of glucose after a period of fasting	Overnight fast except for water Fasting blood sugar, bladder emptied, specimen discarded. Administer 50g glucose. ½ hrly blood sugars for 3–6 hours. Urinary sugars at same time as blood sugars
2. *Urine*		
Single specimen		
Freshly voided urine	pH and constituents	'Routine' ward testing
Clean Midstream Catheter	Bacteria	
Early morning		
Over period of time e.g. 3 h, 6h 24h	17–hydroxycorticosteroids Other hormones	Patient to void immediately prior to collection commencing — this specimen discarded. All specimens from that time then collected. Patient to void at time collection due to be completed — this specimen is the final specimen of the collection. Note times on bottle.
	Creatinine clearance	Blood sample to be taken within the 24 hours of the urine collection
	^{131}I excretion	Radioactive precautions
B. Tests for specific purposes		
3. *Tests for infective organisms*		
Swab of exudate from wounds, rectum, vagina, throat Samples of CSF, saliva, faeces, fluid from sinuses and wounds, pleural aspirate, blood, urine, sputum	a. Bacteria and bacterial sensitivity to antibiotics	Clean dry swabs or container required Samples to laboratory immediately or put into refrigerator
	b. Viruses	
	c. Parasites	Usually only faeces — whole very fresh specimen to laboratory immediately
4. *Tests for biochemical analysis*		
Blood, urine, CSF, faeces	CSF — sugar, proteins Faeces — fat content	See Section C for notes on lumbar puncture 5 day collection

Table 11.3 continued

Type of test	What is being identified	Nursing notes
5. *Tests for cell changes*		
CSF, pleural aspirate Ascites fluid, bone marrow Biopsy of any tissue including liver, kidney pleura, skin, lymph nodes, mucosa of bronchi, stomach, rectum, cervix, etc. Undertaken via puncture with or without direct vision, endoscoscopy open operation	Malignant changes Degenerative changes Inflammatory changes	Usually an invasive procedure, therefore performed under sedation, local or general anaesthesia Except for some endoscopies, involves invasion into sterile cavity See Section C for further nursing notes
6. *Tests for changes in gross structure*		
Undertaken via endoscopy Contrast medium X-rays	Obstructions and constrictions Enlargement	Cavity being investigated must be empty
C. Specific notes on procedures undertaken in ward and requiring skin puncture		
7. *General points*		Problems common to all procedures 1. Pain/discomfort from puncture Local anaesthetic Post-procedure analgesia 2. Potential infection Strict asepsis Skin antiseptic used — sometimes iodine — needs skin patch test 24h before procedure Puncture site sealed with e.g. OpSite, collodion dressing 3. Potential leakage of fluid or haemorrhage Rest — probably in bed — for 24h Direct pressure if appropriate Nurse on affected side to observe problem quickly Problems and potential problems specific to each procedure listed below
8. *Lumbar puncture*		
Subarachnoid space at L2/3 in adults Lumbar spine flexed	CSF — pressure — constituents — infection Instillation of antibiotics Instillation of cytotoxic agents	Headache — keep flat if present Pressure on vital centres leading to respiratory arrest due to reduced intrathecal pressure drawing brain-stem into foramen magnum
9. *Pleural tap*		
Between visceral and parietal pleura at point where fluid present Ribs separated at entry point	Pleural fluid — constituents — infection Instillation of cytotoxic agents Withdrawal of fluid	Puncture of visceral pleura Air into pleural space — pneumothorax — prevent by taking care with three way tap during procedure. Treat by inserting pleural drain and attaching to water seal drainage
10. *Abdominal paracentesis*		
Peritoneal cavity Bladder empty Patient semiprone	Peritoneal fluid — constituents — infection Instillation of antibiotics Instillation of cytotoxic agents Withdrawal of fluid	Rapid reduction in abdominal pressure causing shock. Prevent by slow fluid withdrawal or application of pressure to abdomen by abdominal binder Trauma to bladder
11. *Liver or renal biopsy*	Cell change	Haemorrhage
12. *Bone marrow puncture*		
Sternum or iliac crest	Cell change	Bone pain

'indicators' within blood and urine may relate to the function of a system apart from the reticuloendothelial and renal systems; for example, PCo_2 relates to respiratory function while ^{131}I secretion in the urine is a measure of thyroid function.

REFERENCES

Aitken-Swan S J, Paterson R 1955 The cancer patient delay in seeking advice. British Medical Journal 1:623

Bomford R, Mason S, Swash M 1975 Hutchinson's clinical methods. Baillière Tindall, London

Bond S 1978 Routinization of nurses' communication with cancer patients. PhD thesis, Edinburgh University

De Wolfe A S, Barrell R P, Cummings J W 1966 Patient variables in emotional response to hospitalization for physical illness. Journal of Consulting Psychology 30(1):68–72

Evans D M D 1978 Special tests and their meanings. Faber & Faber, London

Hawkins C 1979 Patients' reactions to their investigations: a study of 504 patients. British Medical Journal 2:638–640

Johnson J E, Morrisey J F, Leventhal H 1973 Psychological preparation for an endoscopic examination. Gastrointestinal Endoscopy 19(4):180–182.

Kendall R E 1975 The role of diagnosis in psychiatry. Blackwell Scientific, Oxford

Krauple Taylor F 1979 The concepts of illness, disease and morbus. Cambridge University Press, London

Liddell H 1950 Some specific factors that modify tolerance for environmental stress. In: Wolff, Wolff, Hare (eds) Life stress and bodily diseases. Williams & Wilkins, Baltimore.

Lipowski S J 1975 Physical illness, the patient and his environment: psychosocial foundations of medicine. American Handbook of Psychiatry 4:1–42

Maguire G P 1978 The psychological effects of cancers and their treatments. In: Tiffiny R (ed) Oncology for Nurses, vol. 2. Allen & Unwin, London

Mechanic D 1962 The concept of illness behaviour. Journal of Chronic Diseases 15:189–194

Nuckalls L B, Cassel J, Kaplan B H 1972 Psychological assets, life crises and the prognosis of pregnancy. American Journal of Epidemiology 95:431–444

Pagana K D, Pagana T J 1982 Diagnostic testing and nursing implications. Mosby, St Louis

Parsons, Talcott 1966 On Becoming a Patient. In: Folta J R, Deck E (eds) A Sociological framework for patient care. Wiley, New York

Pilowsky I 1975 Dimensions of abnormal illness behaviour. Australian and New Zealand Journal of Psychiatry 9:141–147

Reynolds M 1978 No news is bad news: patients' views about communication in hospital. British Medical Journal 1:1673–1676

Robinson L 1976 Psychological aspects of the care of hospitalized patients. 3rd edn. Davis, Philadelphia, Pennsylvania

Sontag S 1979 Illness as metaphor. Penguin, Harmondsworth

Stockwell F 1972 The unpopular patient. Royal College of Nursing, London

Taylor D C 1979 The components of sickness: diseases, illness and predicaments. Lancet 2:1008–1010

Wilson–Barnett J 1977 Patients' emotional reactions to hospitalization. PhD Thesis, University of London

Wilson-Barnett J 1979 Stress in hospital: patients' psychological reactions to illness and health care. Churchill Livingstone, Edinburgh

Wilson-Barnett J, Carrigy A 1978 Factors affecting patients' responses to hospitalization. Journal of Advanced Nursing 3 (2):221–228

Zborowski M 1952 Cultural components in response to pain. Journal of Social Issues 8:16–30

12

Psychological therapies and the alleviation of stress

INTRODUCTION

The role of the autonomic nervous system in the alarm stage of the stress reaction has already been discussed in Chapter 8. Physiological changes mediated by the autonomic nervous system are vital in coping with physical threat. These changes may also occur when the threat is not physical, but of a purely psychological nature. A physiological response to a psychological threat may be inappropriate and useless and can even be quite harmful. How is this?

In order to emphasize the way in which such a response may be harmful, it might be useful again to state the components of the immediate physiological response to threat:

- increased heart rate and cardiac output
- increased blood pressure and muscular tension
- redistribution of blood from skin and the gastrointestinal tract to muscle
- increased metabolic rate and oxygen consumption
- increased blood glucose levels
- increased blood clotting
- increased levels of serum free fatty acids leading to raised serum lipid and cholesterol levels
- increased central nervous system arousal mediated through the reticular activating system to give alertness and prevent sleep.

Physiology books often include a description of reduction in peristalsis and tightening of sphincter muscles as part of this response, but in practice there may be urination and defaecation brought about by interference with parasympathetic function.

Control systems involved in the response to threat include the pituitary and adrenal glands, the limbic system, the hypothalamus, the cerebrum, the reticular activating system. However, the precise role of these and the way in which they interact together are not known.

Enhanced sympathetic activity has been detected in people just before driving a car, when taking an examination, on being admitted to hospital, and during repetitive industrial work, office work, and among supermarket checkout personnel during a busy period. These activities are all relatively sedentary in nature, but stimulation by the sympathetic nervous system prepares the body for 'flight' or 'fight', i.e.for rapid muscular activity. However, behavioural responses shown by animals during intense fear may include a pattern of 'freezing' with extreme muscular tension, muteness, piloerection and defaecation. Such a behavioural pattern is not usually accounted for in accounts of neurophysiology although it is activated by the sympathetic nervous system (Gray, 1971).

Under normal circumstances, the 'fight', 'flight' or 'freezing' response is relaxed or reversed after the threat has ceased. It has been suggested that in response to psychological threat, elements of the physiological response may persist long after the threat has ceased. This constitutes a long-term alteration in physiological function. It has also been suggested that alteration in physiological function over a long period of time may result in structural change resulting in disease. It follows that any modification or prevention of the stress response to psychological threat may prevent disease.

The autonomic component of the stress response has been emphasized here, not because the corticosteroid response is less important but because autonomic responses are amenable to some control by behavioural methods, especially those accompanying the experience of negative emotion. Some of these behavioural methods of control are described in this chapter. At the moment we do not know how to influence the corticosteroid response although psychological methods may have a secondary or indirect effect upon the endocrine glands.

Given that it is an individual's perception of an event which determines whether or not it is a stressor for that person, it follows that there are large individual differences in the type of sitution which an individual treats as threatening. These individual differences are largely a function of past experience and social learning.

When an individual is presented with a threat, a part of the general physiological response may occur rather than the 'full- blown' response. This partial response may be characteristic of the person. For example, one person may respond to threat by tensing muscles, particularly those of the neck and face, whilst another might respond with an increase in blood pressure. In this way individuals, or even families, may be vulnerable to the development of a particular pattern of response which over time may lead to a characteristic type of illness.

It has been claimed that a number of illnesses may be caused by stress. Among them are coronary artery disease, hypertension, asthma, back pain, tension headache, ulcerative colitis, dyspepsia, peptic ulcer. Some authorities also attribute the onset of diabetes mellitus (maturity type) to the effects of stress (Ch. 8).

The conceptualization of the person's perception of threat as the important determinant of the response, together with a knowledge of the possible pattern of response has led to the development of methods of helping people both to cope with threat and to prevent or curtail the stress response. These methods include:

- altering the situation in some way so that it is actually no longer threatening, e.g. a patient having investigation of a lump in the breast is told that it is benign, following biopsy
- altering the person's perception of the situation so that it is no longer seen as threatening, e.g. a patient who had a bad experience of an anaesthetic as a child is

brought to understand the improvement in technique and safety in administration of anaesthetics that has taken place
- supporting and helping a person so he/she no longer feels he/she has to cope with a threatening situation alone, e.g. admitting an elderly person to hospital for 2 weeks in every 4 to allow the single daughter a period of rest
- a person is given full information before a frightening event takes place so that he/she can rehearse the events, gain a measure of familiarity with them and plan methods of coping. This helps him/her to feel in control of the situation, e.g. explaining in the pre-operative period the use of chest drains postoperatively
- teaching a person various methods by which he/she can cut short or reverse the physiological effects of stress
- prescribing drugs which will help to reduce unpleasant emotions experienced as a component of a stress response.

A number of these methods are available for nurses to use to help patients and their relatives as a part of professional practice, and a fuller discussion of these will be found later in this chapter. The next section is concerned with some of the methods which can be used to prevent or at least curtail aspects of the stress response.

RELAXATION OR TENSION CONTROL

One common component of the response to threat is a tensing of the muscles. If this is prolonged it can not only lead to tiredness but also to pain, as when headache results from clenching the jaw or tensing neck muscles. It is also a common experience that tension in muscles prevents sleep. Loss of sleep or pain adds to the initial problem. Ideas about muscular tension and relaxation have become part of our everyday language. We say of someone that they 'got very uptight', that we felt all 'wound up', and that music helps us to 'unwind'. We even say that we feel 'tense'.

The principle behind relaxation or tension control is that by teaching the individual to relax tense muscles, pain, tiredness and insomnia can be prevented. The individual begins to feel that he/she has some control over the situation and this allows a reappraisal of the threat. Some authorities claim that muscle relaxation is actually incompatible with a feeling of threat and can be used to prevent or curtail stress. Other functions of relaxation include the slowing down of mental and physical activity, the promotion of sleep, and a calming effect on autonomic function by lowering the heart rate and blood pressure.

RELAXATION THERAPY

The objective of relaxation therapy is to train clients in the ability either to relax specific muscles and/or to relax the whole body. In the latter case a number of different activities may be involved, such as exercise of muscles, diaphragmatic breathing, massage and conscious relaxation of the body.

The client needs to understand that much of the problem posed by the threat may be his/her own response to it and that given certain conditions responses can be modified and controlled. One of the important components of training is getting the individual to recognize and to perceive his/her own bodily responses, because we often fail to perceive that there is tension in our own muscles.

Method

The client is first instructed to tense his/her muscles, then to perceive how this feels, and then to relax them. In this way what is understood to have been taught is to distinguish between the sensations arising from tensed muscles and those associated with their relaxation.

This learning uses proprioceptive information from muscles. Learning can be enhanced through the sensory modality of touch. The client is asked to palpate tense muscles using the finger tips. It is possible to recognize muscle tension in another person by this means. This is a skill which a nurse can develop.

When a person is upset, changes in respiration take place. These changes include gasps, catching of breath, panting or laboured breath. Overbreathing may occur through increased activity of the intercostal muscles. This washes carbon dioxide out of the lungs and leads to changes in blood carbon dioxide and hydrogen ion levels. In turn this may cause dizziness, fainting, tingling and numbness, symptoms which are distressing if they are not understood. Relaxation training includes learning slow, steady diaphragmatic breathing. Once the client has learned this skill it can be used in stressful circumstances, preventing the ill effects mentioned above. During relaxation training, concentrated attention on breathing may lead to easy and natural relaxation. It is worth noting that diaphragmatic breathing forms a part of meditation and yoga regimes.

Massage helps muscles to relax. It also stimulates the flow of blood to the muscle and this helps to remove potentially painful waste products of metabolism. The repetitive stimulation of massage helps to relax the whole individual as well as the specific muscles concerned.

A nurse who can help a patient to get a good night's sleep helps him/her cope with the stress of illness. We know that a person is best able to sleep when in a completely relaxed physical state and a calm mental state. Complete relaxation occurs when all muscles are relaxed and the attention is prevented from focusing on worries.

Helping patients to achieve that state requires planning and a knowledge both of the factors which induce sleep and those which prevent sleep. Warmth helps to induce sleep whilst feeling too cold or hot prevents it. A high ambient temperature causes vasodilatation with overactivity of the cardiovascular system.

Evidence from a survey carried out for the Royal Commission on the Health Service (Gregory, 1979) showed that patients who had difficulty in sleeping complained of the hotness and sweating caused by plastic drawsheets. Potentially vasoactive food substances should be avoided late at night as they can also lead to overactivity of the cardiovascular system. These include chocolate, cheese, alcohol, coffee, tea, and indeed rich meals of any kind. Comfort promotes sleep whilst pain and discomfort prevent it. Timing the administration of analgesic drugs carefully so that they begin to have their maximum effect at bed time as well as utilising nursing methods of promoting comfort can facilitate sleep.

Environmental stimulation causes arousal and prevents sleep. Noise and light should be avoided when patients are being settled for the night. Above all, anxiety prevents sleep. Patients can be helped by allowing them to talk over their anxieties in the day time and by keeping them fully informed of investigations and treatments as well as their progress throughout their illness. Teaching the patient relaxation skills may help to promote sleep at night.

AUTOGENIC TRAINING

Schultz & Luthe (1959) noticed that 'good' hypnotic subjects often reported a feeling of heaviness throughout the body and warmth in the limbs before a successful therapeutic session of hypnosis. He began to teach the patients to put themselves into a state of physiological quietness by silently repeating phrases associated with heaviness and warmth. This gave general relaxation. He found that in this generally relaxed state subjects were able to instruct themselves to produce bodily changes. An example was the ability to raise the temperature of one or both hands. There was an objectively recorded 10°F rise in one subject but the average rise was 3-4°F. Such instruction can be aimed specifically to modify physiological dysfunction suffered by the subject. The example mentioned of raising the temperature of the hands has been shown to prevent migraine and even to curtail an attack. Migraine is associated with dilatation of extracerebral arteries of the dura mater and scalp. Some data from the Soviet Union indicates that vasodilatation of the scalp is generally associated with vasoconstriction in the hands. It is assumed that the vasodilatation which occurs in the hands when an individual succeeds in raising the temperature of the hands prevents or reverses any dilatation of vessels in the dura and scalp.

Autogenic training is more usually used to bring about general bodily relaxation. During the training period the individual is asked to practise in a quiet environment where there is little visual stimulation and under the supervision of a qualified practitioner. Learning includes repeating phrases such as 'my arms are heavy'. During the session individuals put themselves in a state of relaxation and warmth. Subjects report feelings of wellbeing and peace, but occasionally report tension release with accompanying emotion such as laughter or tearfulness.

Though autogenic training has been reported to reduce the frequency of asthmatic attacks and tension headaches as well as generally helping people to cope with or prevent stress, its application is not without its own problems. An individual's past, the strength and depth of experience and learning will shape his or her response to stress situations. The likely success of any autogenic training will have to take account of deep-seated stress-inducing events.

AUTOGENIC TRAINING COMBINED WITH FEEDBACK

Feedback is concerned with helping the person to recognize tension within muscles by producing a visual display of the tension on a meter or monitor. This may be combined with the autogenic training to help the individual to gain rapid control over muscle tension. Using this technique it is possible to teach some migraine sufferers to raise the temperature of their hands more rapidly and effectively.

BIOFEEDBACK

The ability to relax or tense at will those muscles which are normally under our conscious control can be readily understood. However, it has been shown over the past two decades that it is also possible for the individual to gain control over physiological functions which are wholly or partially within the domain of the autonomic nervous system.

Two lines of research have contributed to this development. One is the work mentioned above, since blood vessels implicated in changes of temperature in the hands are innervated by sympathetic nerves. The second line of research is with animals. It has been found that animals which have been paralysed with curare can be taught to raise or lower their heart rates by means of positive reinforcement (a pleasant sensation delivered to the brain). From this was developed the concept of biofeedback, which involves the individual in learning to control 'unconscious' physiological processes such as heart rate, the regularity of the heart beat, blood pressure, brain wave activity and skin temperature.

The principle is similar to that already explained in the section on autogenic training with feedback. A person is taught to recognize first what is happening to one physiological function within his own body and then to recognize a desirable change in that function and then to be able to bring it about. Recognition is aided by the amplification of physiological signals obtained through a transducer attached to the body. The amplified signal is then displayed to the patient by means of a visual or auditory signal. Thus information which is normally transmitted through visceral sensory pathways to the brain stem is being transmitted through extero-perceptual sensory pathways to the cerebrum. Eventually the patient is able to recognize the visceral sensory pathways without the use of the amplified signal and can bring a symptom under control at will.

One of the theoretical difficulties involved in this method is whether the apparent control of visceral activity is a side-effect of voluntary muscular control or a result of the relaxation brought about by concentrating the attention upon one particular function and thus lowering arousal.

One of the physiological changes which can be brought about by the use of biofeedback is a change in brain wave activity which can be detected by the use of an EEG. During the rested relaxed state prior to sleep, alpha waves become apparent on the EEG record. Individuals can be trained to relax through the display of the waves produced by the relaxation.

MEDITATION

People in trance states and during meditation also exhibit alpha waves on EEG. It is claimed that those who are extremely well practised in going into a trance-like state can also control the feeling of pain and even stop bleeding during such a state, showing that they have control over internal visceral function.

Meditation techniques usually involve the subject sitting quietly with the eyes closed for 15–20 minutes twice a day. They focus on a special thought or sound in a special way without effort. Physiological changes during meditation have been documented and include a marked reduction in oxygen consumption, arterial carbon dioxide and lactate concentration; a decrease in heart rate, respiratory rate and metabolic rate; an excess of base in the plasma; a rise in basal skin resistance. The EEG shows alpha wave activity with occasional frontal theta wave activity. The subject appears wakeful. People practising meditation over a long period of time show lowered plasma cortisol levels and decreased levels of the excretory metabolites of catecholamines. There is evidence that people who are regular meditators are less susceptible to stress from psychological causes than non-meditators, and report fewer minor complaints such as headaches, colds and insomnia. Wallace & Benson (1972) suggest that transcendental meditation activates an innate physiological response which is antagonistic to the activity of the sympathetic nervous system. This has been called the 'relaxation response' or the 'hypometabolic' state. It is remarkably similar to the trophotropic state said to be induced by autogenic training, which is also incompatible with the actions of the sympathetic nervous system.

BEHAVIOUR THERAPY IN THE TREATMENT OF PHOBIA

A development based on psychological experiments in the classical conditioning of responses is the use of desensitization in the treatment of phobia. Patients who develop a phobia suffer extreme anxiety and fear in the presence of the object or situation causing the phobic response. One could say that the object or situation acts as an extreme stressor for the patient, although to the majority of people an identical object or situation is accepted as perfectly normal. Examples of objects and situations arousing such responses include snakes, heights, enclosed spaces, open spaces, and objects thought to have been contaminated with germs. Sometimes phobic conditions are extremely incapacitating, not only for the patient but for his family.

In 1920 Watson & Rayner induced a fear response to a white rat in an 11-month-old child by conditioning. Whilst the conditioning model cannot explain the acquisition of all phobic reactions, counter-conditioning is one of the elements in the treatment of phobias by systematic desensitization as developed by Wolpe (1958).

The use of counter-conditioning in overcoming fear of specific objects was shown by Jones (1924). The patient was a child who was frightened of a rabbit. Treatment involved feeding the child in the presence of the rabbit which was initially placed at a considerable distance from the child. Gradually in subsequent counter-conditioning sessions the rabbit was brought nearer and nearer the child until he was able to touch the rabbit without fear. The usual response to food came to be attached to the sight of the rabbit by conditioning. This was incompatible with the previous response (fear) evoked by the rabbit.

Wolpe's method of systematic desensitization developed in 1958 consists of three elements:

- training in muscle relaxation
- construction of the fear hierarchy
- counter conditioning.

Muscle relaxation is taught so it can be used as a response to be associated with the object or situation which evokes the fear response and in turn replaces the fear response. The second stage is to construct a fear hierarchy from the event/object causing the patient the slightest unease up to the event/object causing the greatest fear. A case Rardin (1969) often quoted to illustrate the point is an appropriate one to quote here. The client was an 18-year-old student nurse. She had been fearful of blood and generally squeamish for several years, but this was of no great importance until she took up nursing, and she found that she felt nauseous and dizzy watching films in the classroom and sometimes had to leave the room. The staff were beginning to question her suitability for nursing.

The hierarchy which was constructed consisted of the following items:

1. bleeding from nose and mouth due to internal injury.
2. a sucking chest wound.
3. seeing a blood sample drawn.
4. blood foaming from the mouth.
5. waters breaking for childbirth.
6. baby's head emerging and its effect on mother.
7. blood flowing after birth.
8. delivery of placenta.
9. stitching after delivery.
10. scraped elbow.
11. a torn hangnail.
12. squeezing out one drop of blood.
13. a cut in the sole of the foot.
14. a compound fracture of the leg.
15. needle in the skin for a stitch.
16. gash in the arm with blood.

After training in muscle relaxation and a few sessions of counter-conditioning in a clinic, she practised imagining the scenes while relaxing at home. At the end of 6 weeks she succeeded in feeling relaxed whilst imagining the most severe of these situations (number 1 above). She also attempted to attend a birth in the hospital, although she felt dizzy and left. However, she observed the next delivery satisfactorily. After a year she was able to cope with all real life events in which blood was involved.

An important element in such treatment is that the hierarchy is developed individually for each client and is based on personal fears. As the treatment proceeds if the client shows or feels any signs of fear then treatment returns to the preceding item in the hierarchy so that the session ends with the client feeling calm and relaxed. An interesting aspect is that the response of calm to the imaginary situation generalizes to the real one.

It must be pointed out at this stage that though behaviourism and its many different schools are immensely appealing, nevertheless their argument can be said to be fallacious. As a technology of behaviour based on 'operant conditioning' the judicious use of reinforcement is no doubt a highly effective technique for shaping and controlling behaviour. But the ability to control responses and thereby to predict them in no way guarantees that they can be predicted in other less controlled circumstances. As a method which does not recognize a relationship beween introspection and behaviour, behaviourism in no way helps our understanding about the determination of the casual status of consciousness or the need to study the relations between introspection and behaviour. At another level an indiscriminate use and application of behaviourism is also morally suspect because of its manipulative aspects, and it should only be used with the informed consent of the client.

STRESS INNOCULATION

Imagery may also be used as part of a technique known as stress innoculation. Haggard (1949) stated that 'A person is able to act realistically and effectively in a stressful situation only if he knows what to do and is able to do it'. Obviously one thing which not only allows one to know what to do but also to know that one can cope, are previous experiences of the stressful situation. Thus one can learn to deal with stressful circumstances through prior experiences. It is also suggested that mastery of situations which produce 'manageable units' of stress provides 'innoculation' against future stressors and that exposure to a mildly stressful stimulus allows tolerance of similar stimuli of a greater intensity.

The idea of stress-innoculation training involves the client in understanding his/her own responses when confronted with stressors, learning possible strategies and practising strategies in role play.

The technique can best be illustrated by describing stress innoculation as carried out by Meichenbaum & Novaco (1978) with police officers.

First the officers learned the functions and determinants of anger, the properties of aggressive sequences and the importance of cognitive factors in the self-instruction of behaviour. Next, they participated in group discussions where coping processes were suggested and reviewed. Finally, they were involved in a graduated series of role plays in which the officers were provoked into anger and learned to control it. Training included learning a number of statements with which the individual could instruct himself during a confrontation.

Examples include the following:

'This could be a rough situation but I know how to deal with it. I can work out a plan to handle this. As long as I keep my cool I am in control of the situation. There is no point in getting mad. Look for the positive, and don't jump to conclusions. Muscles are getting tight. Relax and slow things down. Time to take a deep breath.'

Trainees were also taught phrases to provide subsequent analysis and reflection after the conflict, such as 'Forget about the aggravation. Thinking about it only makes you upset. Remember relaxation, it's a lot better than anger', or 'I handled that well. My pride can get me into trouble but I'm doing better at this all the time.'

Thus the elements which are important are:

- understanding and recognizing one's own responses
- learning a range of new coping skills as alternatives to self-destructive stress responses
- gaining confidence in one's ability to cope.

PSYCHOTHERAPY

Psychotherapy, a well-established method in therapy, lies at the other end of the continuum of therapy from the behaviourist approach. It is subjective, interpretive and is a theory about meaning. During treatment, when the client is encouraged to develop a relationship with the therapist, the focus of the therapy is on the meaning of the client's experiences. Problems for which this may be a useful method include those which involve interpersonal relationships and particularly those resulting from low self-esteem.

Therapists belonging to the more specialized psychoanalytical school of psychotherapy based on Freud's work may ask the client to reflect back on his childhood. In childhood there is conflict between instinctual behaviour (the id) and the curbs imposed during socialization which are internalized (the super-ego and ego). The function of the socialization process encompasses the initiation of children into their appropriate family and cultural adult group. Guilt responses evoked in circumstances of pleasure in adult life are said to reflect unresolved childhood conflicts. Similarly, it is claimed that so-called immaturity in relationships in adult life may reflect earlier subconscious conflicts with parents. Clients are supposedly helped to work through old conflicts with the therapist as a substitute for other people, in a safe and controlled environment.

Therapists who do not belong to the psychoanalytical school feel it is by no means always necessary to refer back to the past, but prefer to analyze the current situation in terms of the dynamics which are operating and causing it to be stressful. A relative newcomer in the growing field of new methods of psychotherapy is Transactional Analysis (TA for short), which is well discussed by Harris & Harris (1985). This originated in California and became generally known in the 1960s. It claims that in each of us is a Child, a Parent and an Adult. The Child is our experience as a child, the Parent is our history of contact with our parents (or substitute) during the first 5 years and the Adult is that part of ourselves which reasons, thinks and predicts. Any transaction involves two people; someone saying and doing something to another, and the other saying and doing something back. TA determines which of the three parts of a person initiated the transaction and which part of the three parts of the other responded.

Group psychotherapy is increasingly popular. Here, clients discover 'fellow feeling' with others who have problems and learn to understand the implicit, covert and even symbolic meaning of words and actions. They can then look at their problems in this way, as well as having the help of the group in analysis. Sometimes coping with interaction within the group brings to light characteristic but non-functional habits of interaction of which the client is unaware. When they are pointed out, new interaction skills can be learned which provide more satisfying outcomes.

Whichever form of therapy is used the outcome should be a restructuring of the perception of self and relationships, together with the acquisition of new skills to bring about more satisfying and therefore less stresssful relationships.

Merely talking about one's problems may in itself help by catharsis, to bring about relief of tension and therefore induce calmness and relaxation. Repressed emotion is examined and released. The aim is to relieve the symptoms of anxiety and depression brought about by pent-up emotion such as anger. Talking about problems often brings insight since the client begins to see how the problems might appear to others and thus begins to develop a new perception.

Therapists vary in the amount to which they engage in interpretation of clients' problems. Some use only a technique of elaborating and clarifying what the client himself said. This is called 'reflecting'.

Psychotherapy has been described as designed to modify behaviour which is personally or socially painful. The therapist helps the patient to gain further knowledge of his/her behaviour, an understanding of its possible origins, forms, functions and goals. The therapist will also point out the options available and the restrictions and costs. A therapist does not attempt to plan or enforce a way of life for the client, but to counsel and clarify. As a professional he/she must recognize and deal with the expression of anxiety in interpersonal situations (Will, 1977).

As with all other attempts at relieving stress, psychotherapies in their various forms are not without their problems. On the one hand they can foster unacceptable levels of dependency between the client and the therapist or the client and the group. On the other hand, psychoanalysis is not only considered suspect as a science, it has also little demonstrable proof of effectiveness. It is evident that rarely is psychotherapy successful for the black single mother of two living in overcrowded housing in Brixton, London, for example. It is aimed on the whole at members of the largely well-to-do middle-class, and is criticized (TA in particular) as it does not deal with the strength of unconscious motives and defences, and only covers surface tension.

SOCIAL SKILLS TRAINING

Some psychologists state that stress may be caused by difficulty in forming and maintaining interpersonal relationships. A recent approach to helping people has been developed from work on social skills by social psychologists such as Argyle. The skill performance involved in social interaction has only been analyzed in a useful way by psychologists over the past two decades. Argyle (1969) states:

> 'For many years very little was known about the process of social interaction, there were no concepts to describe it or methods to study it.'

From this analysis has emerged the realization that whilst social interaction skills are learned in childhood, some people fail to learn adequately or have inadequate models from whom to learn, with disastrous consequences upon their relationships with others. This in turn has deleterious consequences for their health and happiness. Training in social skills forms part of the range of treatments offered by many clinical psychologists. The development of skill in social interaction allows people to develop more satisfying interpersonal relationships.

While it is also the fact that conditions of illness affect the best learned and acquired skills, the therapist's ability lies in the recognition of the nature of an illness's interference with what were originally perfectly adequate skills, so that the focus of therapy can be directed appropriately. There is also a danger associated with the notion of 'adequate social skills'. It defines people by what they cannot do, rather than by what they can or might. This focus on a definition of incapacity has a tendency to preclude the identification of the areas in which people might be helped to adjust the demands of their lives to their capacities, and to start emphasizing what they can do instead of what they cannot. This would constitute a recognition of continuity within oneself, rather than having to face an alienating process of discontinuities in the learning of new skills.

FORMS OF DRUGS — AS AN AID TO COPING

Many people use alcohol and tobacco to help them to cope with stressors. Unlike some of the methods mentioned earlier, they usually only suppress the problem for the duration of the action of the drug. Alcohol works by changing the person's perception of the problem and smoking helps to boost the confidence. Sometimes the problem resolves itself, which then reinforces the use of alcohol or tobacco.

One of the main difficulties of using these substances to aid coping is that the drinker or smoker habituates and needs more of the drug to gain the same effect. Heavy use of alcohol can lead to cirrhosis of the liver, whilst habitual use of tobacco, especially in the form of cigarettes can lead to lung and heart disease. The use of alcohol in particular may increase a person's problem due to the behaviour manifested whilst 'under the influence'.

Medically prescribed drugs for the alleviation of severe anxiety or depression due to stress also suppress symptoms whilst failing to affect the cause of the stress. They may however enable the patient to cope until more permanent skills of coping can be learned.

There are two major groups of drugs which may be prescribed. These are the tranquillizer or anxiolytic drugs and the antidepressants. They all come under the general classification of psychoactive drugs.

Tranquillizer or anxiolytic drugs are used to combat insomnia, induce muscle relaxation and reduce psychological aspects of stress. Within this group of drugs are included barbiturates, propanediols, and benzodiazepines.

Barbiturates have a sedative effect upon the central nervous system and they suppress paradoxical sleep. They are the most likely drugs of the group to induce physiological and psychological dependence. Propanediols also have a sedative effect upon the central nervous system and suppress paradoxical sleep. They have the useful effect of causing relaxation of skeletal muscle. The benzodiazepine group also relax skeletal muscle. They are reported not to suppress paradoxical sleep. They depress the limbic system to a greater extent than the other types of drug and this is an important effect in reducing anxiety.

There are major groups of antidepressant drugs: the monoamine oxidase inhibitors (MAOIs) and the tricyclics.

Depression appears to be associated with a relative lack of three closely related neurotransmitters: dopamine, 5-hydroxytryptamine and noradrenaline. These are amongst the substances collectively called catecho-lamines. Monoamine oxidase inhibiting drugs work by blocking the breakdown of catecholamines. These are normally broken into less active substances by the enzyme monoamine oxidase. MAOIs prolong the action of the amine neurotransmitters. Most nurses will realize that patients taking MAOI drugs should avoid foods and drinks containing the amino acid tyramine or other amines. Tyramine has a chemical structure similar to catecholamines and can be dangerous when the action of monoamine oxidase is depressed. Patients receiving these drugs should be given a detailed list of the foods to be avoided. These include cheese, yoghurt, chocolate, broad beans, yeast and meat extracts such as Marmite and Bovril, wines and beers. Drugs containing phenylephrine such as nose drops and cold cure should also be avoided. Patients who are taking MAOI drugs and come into hospital for physical treatment may need to have their blood pressure monitored, especially if the drugs are withdrawn.

The other group of antidepressant drugs is the tricyclics. These work by blocking the neuronal uptake of 5-hydroxytryptamine and noradrenaline into the pre-synaptic vesicle. This also has the effect of prolonging the action of the transmitter upon the post-synaptic membrane. These drugs have the disadvantage that they take several days to work and may take up to 3 weeks. Patients should be warned about this. Tricyclics may cause potentially dangerous side-effects such as the induction of glaucoma, jaundice, purpura, paralytic ileus, and urinary retention. They may also induce cardiovascular symptoms such as tachycardia, arrhythmias, faintness and postural hypotension. Care should be taken in their use for patients who have a heart condition.

Anxiolytic drugs are prescribed more frequently than any other group of therapeutic agents (Rogers et al, 1981). Yet undoubtedly they are unsatisfactory as a treatment for anxiety. They are often prescribed inappropriately for interpersonal problems which are better treated by some of the other methods mentioned earlier.

A report in *The Observer* of 19 April 1981 by Peter Durisch states, 'General practitioners who readily prescribe tranquillizers for patients under stress are being blamed by hospital specialists for a worrying growth in the number of people taking overdoses. The increase is particularly alarming in women aged 15–24 among whom the rate has risen more than ten times over the past 20 years. Dr Norman Kreitman, Director of the Medical Research Council psychiatric unit at the Royal Edinburgh Hospital said last week that drug overdoses are now the commonest single cause of acute medical admissions to hospitals.'

The ease with which tranquillizers and other drugs are prescribed is also seen as a major reason for the burgeoning problem by Dr Colin Berry, a consultant psychiatrist at Walsgrave Hospital, Coventry. 'I'm certain that many GPs prescribe them because they are under pressure. Often these doctors are faced with patients who want to be treated as sick people rather than people with problems.'

This ends the section on some possible therapeutic methods of helping people to cope with stressors and stress. There are several common themes in the methods reviewed. There is an emphasis on learning skills which may help the individual to cope directly with the stressful situation and so change it to a non- stressful one. There is an emphasis on learning skills which should help the person to modify his/her responses to stressors. Actions which can be learned to bring about this modified response are:

- muscle relaxation
- knowledge and understanding, and recognition of bodily reactions
- the use of self-instruction
- the use of imagery
- learning responses which are incompatible with the activity of the sympathetic nervous system.

While there are problems with each one of the therapies mentioned, the choice as to which one to deploy and which ones to discard depends in the final analysis on the research evidence available as to the efficacy of individual therapies, on an intelligent assessment of a client's situation, and on the voluntary co-operation of a patient who understands his/her own situation and can therefore be involved in decisions affecting his/her own person.

THE NURSE'S CONTRIBUTION TO THE PREVENTION AND ALLEVIATION OF STRESS

For many reasons there has been a good deal of recent interest in the social nature and significance of the act of nursing. At a superficial level this may be surprising when much of nursing is seen as no more than a physical task carried out for a patient by a nurse who engages in no verbal exchange at all. Therein lies what is now regarded as a fallacy. It is precisely within the exchange between the patient and the nurse during these multitudinous nursing tasks that relationships between a nurse and a patient are established. Whether these exchanges occur at a conscious verbal or at a nonverbal level is immaterial to the fact that a relationship is involved. The level of exchange and its quality may be absolutely crucial to the positive or negative nature of the relationship.

That the relationship is also affected by the entire organization within which nursing care takes place is shown by research, of which Isobel Menzies' (1961) study is the classical example. It is now recognized that nurses themselves can ill afford to overlook the development of their own competence in social skills.

It is therefore now becoming apparent to nurses themselves that teaching nurses social skills based on Argyle's (1969) work has much to offer the nursing profession, not merely those engaged in psychiatric care but also those in the care of patients with physical disorders.

Whilst it has been recognized for a long time that psychiatric nurses work through the relationship they form with the patient, it is only recently that it has been recognized that the therapeutic role of general nurses is also dependent to a large extent upon the relationship they form with their patients. It must be noted, however, that in a study by Altschul (1972) of nurse/patient interaction in four psychiatric wards she failed to show that relationships formed between nurses and patients were in any way therapeutic. Interactions which occurred were based on intuitive action on the part of the nurses rather than through conscious planning based on treatment ideology.

Many research studies have described general nursing in terms of tasks (e.g. Goddard, 1953; Pembrey, 1975), perhaps because general ward work has usually been organized in the form of task assignment. Task assignment means that each nurse is delegated a specific task to perform for all those patients who require it. One nurse may be instructed to record blood pressures, for example. The nurse then interacts with one patient only long enough to record the blood pressure before passing to the next patient. Under such circumstances it is difficult to form a helpful relationship with the patient. Indeed Menzies (1961) suggested that nursing was organized in this way to avoid forming deep relationships with patients, preventing the anxiety that the nurse might experience as a result of such a relationship.

Many of the subject areas which a patient may wish to discuss are to do with sickness and death. The latter particularly is a taboo subject in our society. In growing up, people no longer learn how to discuss death or how to comfort someone who is grieving. Instead avoidance is practised, a form of behaviour in which many nurses and doctors participate as was shown in the study by McIntosh (1977). This is none too surprising because doctors and nurses like any other members of their society share its values and belief systems.

From what has been said earlier in this chapter, it is suggested that stress may increase if patients are prevented from talking about their anxieties and concerns.

COMMUNICATION

Increasing evidence of the importance of communication between patients and nurses and doctors has been documented.

Several investigators (McGhee, 1961; Cartwright, 1964; Ley & Spelman, 1967) have shown that between 54–65% of patients surveyed up to one month after discharge from hospital were dissatisfied with communication during their hospital stay. This was in spite of the fact that they reported high levels of satisfaction with other aspects of care. Patients at any rate recognize the importance of communication between hospital staff and themselves.

Communication with patients is important not only because it promotes satisfaction with care. Work first carried out in the USA and then developed by nurse researchers in this country has shown the importance of communication with general hospital patients in promoting more rapid and complication-free recovery (Johnson et al, 1978). One argument against giving patients information has always been that it would frighten and worry them. One of the earliest workers in this area, Janis (1958), investigated the relationship between pre-operative fear and recovery. He found that patients who displayed a moderate amount of fear prior to operation coped much better in the recovery period than those who had suffered excess fear, or those who appeared to suffer none. He suggested that the latter had denied their fear only to be overwhelmed by the effects of the surgery in the postoperative period. He suggested that patients needed a certain level of fear before the event in order to develop and rehearse coping strategies for the postoperative period. He talked about the 'work of worrying'. However, this finding by Janis has rarely been replicated by other workers (Newman, 1984).

Cohen & Lazarus (1973) studied coping in surgical patients. Amongst their subjects they found a group of patients whom they categorized as relying on 'vigilance' as a coping mechanism. This group actively sought out information about their medical condition. They were doing this in an irrational and rather neurotic way, voicing worries about extreme and unlikely outcomes. The vigilant group showed the poorest recovery in terms of the number of days in hospital, the frequency of minor complications and negative psychological reactions.

Burstein & Meichenbaum (1976) showed in a group of 20 children aged 4–9 years about to undergo surgery that those who denied worrying manifested the greatest postoperative distress.

Egbert et al (1974) in an experimental study found that patients given detailed pre-operative information required less morphine and were discharged earlier after operation than a group of patients who were not given such information. Hayward (1975) and Boore (1978) have carried out similar studies in this country which tend to support Egbert's results. In her study Boore more clearly linked giving information with the prevention of stress in her study by using biochemical measures of glucocorticosteroid secretion, whilst Hayward used anxiety measures.

Most workers have concentrated their investigations upon patients undergoing surgery. This is perhaps because it provides a clearly identifiable period of stress rather than the more diffuse stress of disease and medical treatment. Wilson-Barnett & Carrigy (1978), using anxiety measures showed, the importance of giving patients in a medical ward information before they underwent a barium enema. Franklin (1974) explored the relationship between the admission procedure and anxiety in hospital patients.

Based on these studies and others, the interest in nurse-patient communication has grown, together with a more widespread recognition of the importance of such communication in helping patients to cope with stress.

Information giving alone, however, has proved not to be entirely unproblematic. What is equally important is a consideration of the nature of the information, its timing, its frequency, its form of repetition (which at times may reinforce or negate its actual message), the manner in which it is given, and the language used. In particular, information must be specifically tailored to the needs of the individual patient and his/her potential experience. The point to be made about communication is that at one level the earlier researchers had a point when they argued that information giving can induce fear or worry. Clearly inappropriate or badly given information can do just this. To focus on information giving as a social skill without understanding the social nature of an individual is one-sided and unlikely to produce the relaxation hoped for by both the client and the nurse.

The link between stress and the development of disease has been discussed in Chapter 8. However, one of the most powerful physiological stressors we know is to be seriously ill. A person who is ill will experience anxiety about diagnosis, prognosis, future life and circumstances. Lazarus (1966) classified and grouped the underlying factors in stress-producing circumstances. His list was as follows:

- uncertainty about physical survival
- threat to one's sense of identity
- loss of loved ones
- lack of ability to control one's environment
- disruption of community life
- pain and privation.

A person who is ill is not only uncertain about physical survival, but loses control over his environment, suffers disruption of community life and may also suffer pain and privation. While a major element of the nursing role is to help the patient to cope with unavoidable stress, it is also to prevent additional stressors from affecting the patient whenever possible. Chapman & Cox (1977) carried out a study of anxiety in surgical patients which shows the effect of stress over and above that caused by the surgery itself. They found that a sub-group of the patients they studied entered surgery already stressed. This group of patients showed greater postoperative pain and anxiety than those patients who were not already stressed when having surgery.

Helping patients to cope with unavoidable stress can be carried out by the means mentioned earlier in this chapter:

- by attempting to alter the situation so it is no longer threatening
- by attempting to alter the patient's perception of the situation so he/she no longer sees it as threatening
- giving the patient support and help so he/she no longer feels he/she has to cope alone. This includes physical nursing care and medical treatment as a means of giving support and help
- by giving the patient full information before any treatment so he/she can rehearse the events, gain a measure of familiarity with them and plan methods of coping
- teaching a patient methods by which physiological effects of stress can be cut short or reversed
- administering drugs at appropriate timing prescribed by the doctor to reduce unpleasant emotions and pain.

Taking those elements of Lazarus's classification of stressors which are relevant to patients, it is possible to see how nursing care may help to minimize the effect of these. This is particularly relevant to care in hospital since the process of hospitalization potentially creates a more stressful situation for patients than being cared for at home. Yet care at home may also be associated with stress. At home, where presumably reign love, tolerance and understanding, the nervous patient will miss the apparent security of high technology and the constant availability of highly trained staff. Stress is likely to be present in most ill people, and one needs to weigh up very carefully the type of stressor and how much can be tolerated before making an irreversible decision about the ideal place for being nursed.

Loss of ability to control one's environment

For a patient, coming into hospital means not only losing control over his/her environment, but also entering one which is strange and can at times be frightening. Probably, this new environment will be shared with several strangers whose own environmental needs may clash with this patient's requirements for sleep and rest. In any case, it is an environment controlled by nursing and other staff for whom it is a place of work.

Under such circumstances there are two main strategies open for the patient to use. One is to give up all attempts at any control and to become a passive recipient of care, trusting the staff to make all decisions and to adjust the environment to his/her needs and in his/her interests. Such a patient will be completely compliant in hospital.

The other strategy is to attempt to gain as much control as possible, by asking questions and altering the environment within the limits of the possible to his/her own requirements.

The first of these strategies will be favoured by many staff because the patient appears co-operative and no trouble. However, this may not be a very adaptive strategy in the long term. First, because the patient may be repressing emotions such as anger and self-assertion. Second, there will come a point at which the patient needs to become active and independent in order to get better and to become a member of the wider society again, functioning to his own optimum level.

A middle course, which is better than either strategy considered above, is for nurses to help patients to gain as much control over their environment as possible, or at least to gain sufficient information so that he/she can infer what might happen next. This can be done by showing the patient around the ward, or, if this is not possible, by providing as much information about it as is available. Rules of behaviour such as smoking restrictions, watching TV, listening to the radio, having lights on and certain behaviour expected of patients during consultants' rounds can be given. Of particular importance is the need to initiate patients into ward patterns of the patient's day. In this way, though it is recognized that a patient's freedom to wash, eat and sleep at his/her normal time is being curtailed, such events can reasonably be expected at given times and the rest of the day structured around them. Likely treatments and investigations (of which see details later) require the fullest information so patients know the reason for each procedure, as well as what is expected of them before, during and after such procedures.

On the whole, patients new to hospital life and new to the whole array of medical investigative procedures cannot be expected to assess their own likely reactions to them. While it is of course difficult for nurses to envisage how patients might feel before, during and after investigations, nurses' powers of observation and their eventual accumulation of data of how patients feel should be of immense benefit to the unsuspecting or overwrought patient. For successful patient outcomes from medical therapy, both doctors and nurses require a patient's active co-operation, and this includes any information which the patient may have and which may or may not directly relate to the investigation under discussion. While there is no way patients can report on what they don't know about, the significance of what is reported can be measured only by the medical expert. On the other hand, experiential aspects may be understood only by a patient.

Threat to one's sense of identity

The maintenance of the patient's identity as an individual is emphasized a good deal in nursing textbooks and lectures. It is important not only on humanitarian grounds, however, but also, according to Lazarus (1966), in preventing stress. Means by which the patient's sense of identity can be expressed, preserved or even enhanced include: addressing patients by name; knowing their occupation; learning about friends, families and hobbies; discussing current events. While all these things may be dismissed as 'social chit-chat' they are immensely important in building a relationship between a nurse and a patient, as well as in preserving the patient's own sense of identity. Respect for the patient as an individual has to permeate all nursing care. This includes involving the patient in decisions whenever possible; helping him/her preserve dignity in the face of invasive procedures such as catherization, enemas and others; and helping him/her to maintain appearances and to save face. Contacts with friends and relatives must be encouraged as much as possible and provided for within the busy time-table of any hospital ward.

Uncertainty about physical survival

It is not normally part of the nurse's role to give information to patients about their medical diagnosis and prognosis. However, the patient's knowledge or suspicions about diagnosis and prognosis form the context within which nursing interactions take place. In the final analysis, it is only the patient who will be able to assess whether and to what extent doubts, anger, fear and frustrations are reasonable concomitants of the nature of being ill. Many a doctor and/or a nurse's somewhat facile understanding of what really moves a patient to despair undermines many of the best thought out therapies. Doctors and nurses work in an environment which, because of the very nature of its pressures in depth and over time, has a tendency to blunt their sensitivity, and that is why it may indeed be very uncomfortable for a nurse merely to sit and to listen. What comfort can be given by sitting and listening? How can the nurse cope with his/her own feeling of despair, fear and impotence? These problems, complex though they are, should be explored in the development of social skills of a kind which allows patients to talk and express their feelings freely and may thereby ease momentarily or over a longer period problems which appear to be insurmountable.

Talking over problems with an empathetic listener serves to release emotion, sharing the burden so that the patient no longer feels he/she must cope alone, and brings to light unrealistic fears so that they can be dealt with. For example, part of the fear of death is the fear of pain. Patients can be kept pain free (Twycross, 1975) and so can be reassured about this.

Recent research (Faulkner, 1980; Gott, 1982; Macleod Clark, 1982) has shown that nurses communicate in an inhibitory and authoritarian way. An example is a nurse who goes up to a patient and says 'Hello Mr Jones. I'm just going to take your blood pressure, all right? Give me your arm'. Such communication gives the patient no chance to answer, let alone suggest that he might prefer not to have his blood pressure taken right there and then.

The type of therapeutic communication which allows the patients to talk over their fears requires a high degree of skill, including the ability to appear relaxed and to have plenty of time. Non-verbal techniques can encourage the patient to talk, as can the ability to ask questions which encourage the recognition of feelings. Some of the skills used in psychiatric nursing within a therapeutic relationship are needed. The technique of 'reflection', reiterating in different words what the patient said and questioning its meaning, may be useful, opening avenues of insight not previously thought about. Above all, sensitivity to verbal and non-verbal cues that the patient may want to talk is an essential quality. Patients, like many other human beings, rarely say directly that they are frightened and wish to talk. Most of us speak indirectly, employing a series of metaphors. An example comes from a patient who was dying: 'I think I am ready for the scrap heap'; another, also from a dying patient: 'My wife's very worried about me'. Unfortunately, in both instances the nurse took the remark at its face value and missed a valuable opportunity to ease the patient's own acute discomfort.

Giving patients information

Janis (1965) has said, 'The ability to cope with an impending stressful situation requires:

- preparatory communication regarding the sensations to be experienced and the probable change
- reassuring statements indicating how the changes will be kept under control or mitigated
- recommendations of what can be done to protect the individual or reduce the damaging impact of the potential change
- the belief or expectation that those recommendations will be effective in reducing the threat.'

It can easily be seen how pre-operative information can fulfil these criteria, but information about any procedure or treatment can contain these elements.

Research carried out by Ley and his associates (1967) into patients' recall of medical information and instructions has given us valuable knowledge which can help nurses to structure the information they give patients.

Bradshaw et al (1975) analyzed X-ray leaflets and diet instructions for ease of reading using the Flesch formula. He found that the easier the material was to read the greater the amount which was recalled by his subjects. Whilst this study used written material the results can be generalized to spoken information, suggesting that the simpler the language is, in terms of short words and short sentences, the more likely it is to be recalled.

Ley (1974) himself carried out work which demonstrated that the number of statements which are forgotten increases with the number of statements which a patient is told. The implication of this is that one should give information rather slowly, and preferably write it down as well so that patients can refer to it later.

Ley (1972) also found that patients recall best the statements which are made first. However, he also found that patients recall best the statements which they consider the most important. It is likely that the patient assumes that a doctor states the most important thing first when giving information and instructions. In practice, they often do not. Nurses can use this finding, however, not only to structure information so that the most important statements are made first, but also to gain attention by saying 'Now, this is important...'.

Structuring and clustering of information in a logical way was found by Ley to improve recall, especially if patients were told what the structure was. This is similar to the way teachers are told to introduce a lecture by saying first what it is they are going to cover in the lectures.

In terms of giving advice or instructions, Bradshaw et al (1975) found that specific advice was recalled better than general advice. For example, 'You must lose half a stone in weight' was recalled better than 'You must lose weight'. Applying this to nursing it suggests that a patient would recall better if told the number of cupsful of tea and glasses full of water he should drink a day, rather than just being told to drink plenty. A finding of Ley & Spelman's (1967) which is particularly relevant to the topic of this chapter is that volunteer subjects who were very high in anxiety recalled less information than volunteers who had a moderate amount of anxiety. This suggests that in giving information to patients who are already anxious we should be particularly careful to give it in a way which can be understood, remembered and acted upon.

It is important for nurses that patients do recall information given them since we wish them to use it to help themselves in anticipatory and realistic coping when stressful events occur.

CONCLUSION

When considering the acquisition of social skills of one type or another, it is equally important to recognize that, in spite of the bridging between theory and practice, gaps do exist and are likely to remain in spite of the best laid out therapies. Social encounters of any sort, especially within large organizations such as hospitals, which because of the nature of their business easily claim solutions to difficult and intractable problems, are subject to an enormous number of variables which are difficult to control. It is therefore all the more important that nurses are well versed and competent in the deployment of social skills and in recognizing complex human responses as well as in understanding the effects of the nature of organization on social encounters.

REFERENCES

Altschul A T 1972 Patient-nurse interaction. Churchill Livingstone, Edinburgh

Argyle M 1969 Social interaction. Tavistock Publications, London

Boore J R P 1978 Prescription for recovery. RCN, London

Bradshaw P W, Kincey J A, Ley P, Bradshaw J 1975 Recall of medical advice, comprehensibility and specificity. British Journal of Social and Clinical Psychology 14(1):55–62

Burstein S, Meichenbaum D 1976 The work of worrying in children undergoing surgery. Unpublished, University of Waterloo. Quoted in Bakal D A 1979 Psychology and medicine. Tavistock Publications, London

Cartwright A 1964 Human relations and hospital care. Institute of Community Studies, Routledge and Kegan Paul, London

Chapman C R, Cox G B 1977 Determinants of anxiety in elective surgery patients. In: Spielberger C, Sarason I G (eds) Stress and anxiety, vol 4. Wiley, New York

Cohen F, Lazarus R S 1973 Active coping processes, coping dispositions and recovery from surgery. Psychosomatic Medicine 35:375–389

Egbert L D, Battit G E, Welch C E, Bartlet M K 1974 Reduction of post-op pain by encouragement and instruction of patients. New England Journal of Medicine 270:825–827

Faulkner A 1980 The student nurse's role in giving patients information. Thesis submitted for the degree of MSc, University of Aberdeen

Franklin B L 1974 Patient anxiety on admission to hospital. RCN, London

Goddard H A 1953 The work of nurses in hospital wards. Nuffield Provincial Hospitals Trust, Oxford

Gott M 1982 Learning nursing: A study of the effectiveness and relevance of teaching provided during student nurse introductory courses. Thesis submitted for the degree of PhD, University of Hull

Gray J 1971 The psychology of fear and stress. Weidenfeld and Nicholson, London

Gregory J 1979 Patients' attitudes to hospital services. HMSO, London

Haggard E 1949 Psychological causes and results of stress. In: Lindsley D (ed) Human factors in undersea warfare. NRC Press, Washington

Harris A B, Harris T H A 1985 Staying OK. Cape, London

Hayward J 1975 Information, a prescription against pain. RCN, London

Janis I 1958 Psychological stress. Academic Press, New York

Janis I L 1965 Psychodynamic aspects of stress tolerance. In: Klausner S (ed) The quest for self-control. Free Press, New York

Johnson J E, Rice V H, Fuller S S, Endress M P 1978 Sensory information, instruction in coping strategy and recovery from surgery. Research in Nursing and Health 1:4–17

Jones M C 1924 The elimination of children's fears. Journal of Experimental Psychology 7:382–390

Lazarus R S 1966 Psychological stress and the coping process. McGraw-Hill, New York

Ley P, Spelman M 1967 Communicating with the patient.

Staples Press, St Albans
Ley P 1972 Primacy, rated importance and recall of medical information. Journal of Health and Social Behaviour 13 : 311–317
Ley P 1974 Communication in the clinical setting. British Journal of Orthodontics 1:173–177
Macleod Clark J 1982 Nurse-patient verbal interaction: An analysis of recorded conversations on medical wards. Thesis submitted for degree of PhD, University of London
McGhee A 1961 The patients' attitude to nursing care. Livingstone, Edinburgh
McIntosh J 1977 Communication and awareness in a cancer ward. Croom Helm, London
Meichenbaum D, Novaco R 1978 Stress innoculation: a preventive approach. In: Spielberger C, Sarason I G (eds) Stress and anxiety, vol 5. Wiley, New York
Menzies I E P 1961 The functioning of social systems as a defence against anxiety. Centre for Applied Social Research, Tavistock Institute of Human Relations, London
Newman S C 1984 Anxiety, hospitalization and surgery. In: Fitzpatrick R, Hinlon J, Newman S, Scambler S (eds) The experience of illness. Tavistock, London
Pembrey S C 1975 From work routines to patient assignment. Nursing Times 71(45):1768–1772
Rardin M 1969 Treatment of a phobia by partial self-desensitization. Journal of Consulting and Clinical Psychology 33:125–126
Rogers J H, Spector R G, Trounce J R 1981 A textbook of clinical pharmacology. Hodder and Stoughton, Sevenoaks
Schultz J H, Luthe W 1959 Autogenic training: a psycho-physiologic approach in psychotherapy. Grune and Stratton, New York
Twycross R G 1975 Relief of terminal pain. British Medical Journal 4:212–214
Wallace R K, Benson H 1972 The physiology of meditation. Scientific American 226:84–90
Watson J B, Rayner R 1920 Conditioned emotional reactions. Journal of Experimental Psychology 3:1–16
Will O A 1977 The future of the therapeutic relationship as an agent of change. In: McCabe O L (ed) Changing human behaviour. Grune and Stratton, New York
Wilson-Barnett J, Carrigy A 1978 Factors affecting patients' responses to hospitalization. Journal of Advanced Nursing 3:221– 228
Wolpe J 1958 Psychotherapy by reciprocal inhibition. Stanford University Press, Stanford

13 Physical methods of therapy

INTRODUCTION

Physical methods of therapy are non-invasive therapies, achieving their end result by the external manipulation of parts of the body by a skilled therapist. The effectiveness of the treatment lies with the skill and resources of the therapist, the use of aids and appliances and his or her rapport with the patient. The basis of all physical methods of therapy rests on a sound understanding of body mechanics, knowledge of correct posture and the effect of degrees of inactivity and exercise on the body. Built upon this framework is an understanding of physical dysfunction, caused by pathological change or congenital abnormality, coupled with the expertise of knowing how to help an individual to compensate for such physical defects.

Manipulation and touch are integral parts of the therapist's skill repertoire, in addition to the use of a range of external treatments and appliances including cold and heat treatments such as ice packs or wax baths, the use of pulleys, weights and exercise machines, and the use of common pieces of equipment to achieve maximum mobility.

WHO ARE THE THERAPISTS?

At one level, knowledge relating to correct body posture, movement and exercise ought to be part of each person's regimen for healthy living. Knowing how to stand correctly, how to lift heavy objects and how to choose well-designed and appropriate house furnishings are ways in which mobility and posture problems can be avoided. Knowledge of basic body mechanics is necessary in caring for a disabled or dependent person at home. Statistics show that the majority of elderly disabled and physically handicapped people are cared for in their own homes (Harris, 1971; Townsend, 1979), thus underlining the need for lay carers to be made aware of techniques related to positioning, moving and exercising relatively immobile people at home.

Providing information on the basic rules of body mechanics related to correct posture, how to position oneself before moving or lifting a heavy load and how to minimize fatigue or muscle strain ensures that the lay carers are more adequately equipped to provide supportive care.

The nurse's knowledge of physical therapies is linked with his/her role in helping patients to manage their activities of daily living and guiding them towards optimal self-care and independence. The patient's level of mobility is an activity which may have been disrupted during a period of illness or injury. It is the nurse's responsibility to ensure that during any period of immobility or controlled mobility the patient comes to no harm and that no complications develop due to lack of exercise or inactivity.

Professionals specializing in mobility problems include physiotherapists, occupational therapists and medical practitioners with an interest in physical therapies and rehabilitation. This group of specialists is concerned with the particular problems of patients suffering mobility limitations caused by congenital defects such as spina bifida, spasticity, or caused by pathological change and injury including paralysis following a cerebrovascular accident, spinal cord damage, motor neurone disease, rheumatoid or osteoarthritis. Such specialists require a range of specific skills to plan and evaluate therapeutic regimens, the aims of which are to restore function as far as possible in the light of the disability.

'ROUTINE' VERSUS 'SPECIALIST' PHYSICAL THERAPIES

The main distinction between the activities of the nurse and that of other workers, such as physiotherapists and occupational therapists, in the area of physical therapies can be illustrated by using the term 'routine' therapies to describe the nurse's function and that of 'specialist' therapies to describe the work of the other groups. 'Routine' therapies include those activities which go toward maintaining the patient's present level of function and the prevention of further deterioration. 'Specialist' therapies, on the other hand, comprise those activities which relate to the evaluation and restoration of function and the adaptation of aids and appliances to optimize mobility. Achieving the goals of specialist therapy is impossible without the execution of successful routine physical therapies.

Maintenance of the patient's actual level of function and the prevention of further deterioration, when related to mobility, involves an understanding of the effects of activity and rest on the body, both in terms of the normal limits and of the effect of illness or incapacity. It also involves a knowledge of the body's need for exercise, knowing how much and what sort of activity to initiate. Finally, successful routine physical therapy requires a knowledge of the use of aids and appliances such as beds, chairs, clothing, walking aids and, perhaps most importantly, the skill of helping the patient relax.

Before discussing the nurse's role in the provision of 'routine' physical therapy a brief mention will be made of the physical agents utilized in 'specialist' physical therapy.

SPECIALIST PHYSICAL THERAPY

The use of physical agents in the treatment of patients involves the application of various types of physical energies to the body tissues. Types of energy included are the thermal, electrical, radiated and mechanical.

Some of the principles underlying the application of these energies are now described.

HEAT

When heat is used as a treatment modality the type of heat, its intensity and its duration need to be carefully planned. Certain safety precautions should always be taken before heat is applied. Some patients may have reduced sensitivity to heat and there is then a serious danger of a burn. Patients with nerve lesions, and certain pathological conditions associated with sensory impairment or vascular deficiencies, are particularly at risk. Heat should not therefore be used as a panacea, but, like other medical prescriptions, the precautions and contra-indications must be observed.

Conduction

Methods of heat production in tissues depending on conduction all rely on the contact of some heated object with the body tissues. Common examples are the use of wax, hot packs, or even placing part of the body in hot water. The initial effect of such applications is to heat the area of skin involved, and the heat so generated is carried away to other parts of the body by convection in body fluids such as blood and lymph. This dispersion of heat is quite rapid and heating by conduction, unless excessive and over a wide area, only significantly alters the temperature of the area of skin involved and, to a lesser extent, the more superficial underlying tissues. Any signs of tissue damage (burns) should be reported immediately, but if the precautions already mentioned have been strictly observed such accidents should not occur.

Radiation

Heating by radiation depends on rays of the electromagnetic spectrum of specific wavelengths.

Infrared

These wavelengths are from 7700 – 4 000 000 angstrom units (Å). (There are 10 million angstrom units in 1 millimetre.) This waveband produces heat when absorbed by the tissues. The deepest penetration occurs at between 10000 – 12000Å. Infrared lamps used in hospital departments are a common source of therapeutic infrared rays. The precautions and contra-indications are generally as for other heat treatments. Infrared forms a useful source of heat for some types of open wounds, as the source of heat does not come into contact with the exposed damaged tissue. The deeper penetrating rays are also useful for relieving superficial pain and muscle spasm, and increasing the local blood supply.

Microwave

Microwave treatment units emit rays of 12.5 cm, which is considerably longer than the infrared rays. Microwaves are absorbed by the deeper tissues which contain relatively large amounts of water, and the majority of heat production occurs specifically in highly vascular tissues such as muscle. Higher temperatures can therefore be achieved more safely in deep muscle than could be achieved using conduction or superficial radiation. Safety of microwave applications has been a matter of some public concern and the reader can check literature for further details (Health and Equipment Information, 1980).

Short wave diathermy

The detailed physical principles underlying this treatment are complex, and outside the scope of this book. Briefly, the patient's tissues form the dialectric of an electrical condenser. An alternating potential is applied to the plates of the condenser at a frequency of approximately 27 million cycles per second. Tissue forming this dialectric becomes heated by the particular behaviours of ions and molecules of which the tissues are composed. The principal difference in effect between short wave and microwave is that short wave tends to heat relatively more of the fatty tissues. If circulation is impaired during treatment (for example by pressure) the heat formed cannot be conducted away and there will be a serious danger of a burn. Complaints of heat or discomfort during or after treatment should always be investigated. Excessive reddening or any blistering of the skin should be reported immediately.

Short wave treatments can be pulsed, producing specific curative and regenerative effects which are not yet fully understood (Oliver, 1984; Barclay et al, 1983).

THE USE OF COLD IN THERAPY

Cold is not a form of energy. It is, quite simply, the absence of heat energy. The physiological and therapeutic effects of cold are well documented and it has become a treatment of choice for many therapists, particularly in dealing with recent injuries and muscle spasm.

The usual methods of application are by means of cold packs, ice cubes, immersion in cold water, or ethyl chloride spray. Cold therapy should not be used on patients with coronary heart disease or other circulatory disorders. Caution must always be exercised in cold applications to ensure that irreversible tissue damage does not occur. The common skin reaction is a vasoconstriction followed by vasodilatation, and experience is necessary in order to judge whether or not the observed response is normal. Techniques of application and therapeutic effects have been documented (Lee & Warren, 1974; Lee et al, 1978; Lee, 1978).

ULTRASONIC THERAPY

Ultrasonic therapy does not involve the passage of electricity through the patient's tissues. The treatment head of the machine vibrates at about a million cycles per second and this vibratory massaging effect is transmitted to the patient's tissues. The results are analgesic and, if sufficiently intense, cause heating and vasodilatation. It is useful in pain relief, reducing oedema due to recent trauma, reducing muscle spasm, and mobilizing collagen tissue.

Particular care must be taken when treating organs of special senses, regions close to the reproductive organs, and areas of neoplasm, infection or impaired circulation, especially in haemophiliacs.

Ultrasonic therapy can also lower blood sugar levels and trigger cardiac reflexes, and therefore diabetic patients require close observation during and following treatment (Sumner & Patrick, 1964).

ULTRAVIOLET RADIATION

Ultraviolet rays are also part of the electromagnetic spectrum, consisting of a band from 1849 to 3900 Å in wavelength.

These rays are absorbed in the superficial skin layers, and produce a variety of effects specific to different parts of the ultraviolet band. It is important to appreciate that there is no immediate sensory stimulation from ultraviolet rays. Unlike infrared rays, they do not result in a sensation of warmth. The physiological effects are delayed, and include:

- various degrees of erythema (sunburn)
- thickening of the epidermis
- desquamation (peeling)
- pigmentation (tanning)
- abiotic effects (used in treating infected wounds)
- vitamin D formation.

Any ultraviolet source capable of producing these effects at practicable therapeutic levels is also capable of producing dangerous overdoses, and considerable technical knowledge and skill is necessary in order to provide a treatment which is both safe and effective.

In planning a treatment programme with ultraviolet irradiation the therapist will consider:

- the pathological condition to be treated
- the patient's sensitivity to ultraviolet rays
- the size of the area to be treated
- the distance of the lamp from the skin surface
- the duration of the treatment
- the type of lamp to use.

Failure to take any of the above into account may result in a dangerous treatment.

A variety of conditions benefit from radiation by ultra violet rays. Pressure sores and ulcers are two examples with which the ward nurse may be familiar. Other common examples are psoriasis and acne.

Patients vary considerably in their individual sensitivity to ultraviolet rays and certain drugs can increase this sensitivity. Ultraviolet is contraindicated in certain pathological conditions, such as TB and eczema, and also in patients undergoing deep X-ray therapy.

The nurse should report immediately any excessive reaction to ultraviolet treatment, as the hazards of an overdose can sometimes be reduced if caught in time. Infrared radiation is one way of reducing the effects of an overdose of ultraviolet.

More detailed information on the technical aspects of ultraviolet irradiation can be obtained from standard texts such as Forster & Palastanga (1985).

LOW FREQUENCY ELECTRICAL CURRENTS

Probably the most important physiological effect of low frequency electrical currents is their ability to stimulate motor nerves to muscles, thus producing a muscle contraction. The low frequency pulses are up to 1 millisecond (ms) in duration, and occur at a frequency of 50 pulses/second. Such currents are usually varying in intensity in order to produce rhythmic contraction and relaxation similar to normal muscle function. This type of current is sometimes referred to as Faradic. Such a current is useful in the re-education of muscles which have lost their full function as a result of trauma, denervation, or immobility in plaster.

During the 1960s, when many therapists were questioning the value of the Faradic current because of lack of scientific evidence, Melzack and Wall discovered another important effect of low frequency pulses. They can relieve pain by closing the 'pain-gate' in the spinal cord (Melzack & Wall, 1965). This discovery led to the development of a new treatment modality in electrotherapy known as Transcutaneous Electrical Nerve Stimulation (TENS). TENS has proved to be a highly effective means of relieving certain types of pain which have proved resistant to other methods of pain relief (Wall, 1985; Lundeberg, 1984).

Muscle-stimulating currents can be used very effectively in an area of treatment known as biofeedback. Biofeedback increases the amount of information available to the patient about his/her bodily functions. It is sometimes possible for the patient to use this information in order to function more efficiently. Use of electrical equipment such as electromyography (EMG) recording and muscle stimulating currents can be used to good effect in re-education of voluntary muscle function, particularly in patients with neurological disorders (Harvey, 1978; De Weerdt & Harrison, 1985; Danskin & Crow, 1981).

The main limitation to intensity of low frequency current applications is the sensory effect. Some patients find these currents particularly difficult to tolerate. This problem can be overcome by using 'interference' currents or 'interferential'. Briefly, two separate currents of about 4000 cycles/second are applied to the affected area, the two currents differing in frequency by up to one hundred cycles/second. In the region where the currents cross in the tissues, a current frequency of the difference between the two original currents is produced. This results in effects similar to standard low frequency currents, but much higher intensities can be tolerated, since the skin is far less sensitive to the 4000 cycles/second applied at individual electrodes. The benefits to muscles and other soft tissues can be considerably greater than with traditional low frequency currents (Willie, 1969; Savage, 1984).

ROUTINE THERAPIES — THE NURSE'S FUNCTION

The nurse's therapeutic role in providing physical therapies is linked to the performance of 'routine' therapies. More specifically, her* role is seen in terms of protecting the patient from the dangers of prolonged immobilization and bed rest, maintaining proper body posture and alignment, and meeting the patient's need for regular and sustained exercise. Finally, the nurse's contribution to physical therapies also

* Throughout the rest of this chapter, the patient will be referred to as 'he', the nurse or carer as 'she'.

involves her awareness of the use of touch as a therapeutic treatment. Nursing expertise may therefore be seen to encompass the following areas:

- understanding and supplying the patient's need for rest and relaxation
- understanding and supplying the patient's need for activity and exercise
- understanding and supplying the patient's need for contact through touch and massage.

The nurse's activity in each of these areas is seen as complementary to and supportive of the more specialized action of the physiotherapist, occupational therapist or other remedial therapist. Crucial to the success of any physical therapy treatment is the preparatory and maintenance treatment performed by nursing personnel.

UNDERSTANDING AND SUPPLYING THE PATIENT'S NEED FOR REST AND RELAXATION

Bed rest as a treatment regimen

The concept of rest, and specifically bed rest, as a therapeutic measure was first introduced in a series of lectures by John Hilton, a surgeon at Guy's Hospital (1860–1862). According to Browse (1965), Hilton's words were misinterpreted and bed rest came to be viewed as a cure for every ailment and consequently became the treatment for many illnesses without specific evidence that it was helpful. More interest has been shown in recent years in trying to assess the effect of bed rest on the recovery rate of patients suffering from illnesses.

Studies (Chalmers, 1969; Repsher et al, 1969) have shown that for patients suffering from TB, hepatitis and myocardial infarction, prolonged total bed rest has been ineffective in altering the course of the disease. Harper et al (1971), in a study of patients with myocardial infarctions, found that patients who were out of bed after seven days fared no worse than those patients who were kept in bed for twenty days. Similarly, Boyle et al (1972) found that post myocardial infarct patients classified 'not at risk' tolerated discharge from hospital within ten days and had less incidence of deep venous thrombosis, postural hypotension and cardiac neurosis than those kept in bed for longer periods.

In a study of patients suffering from rheumatoid arthritis, Mills et al (1971) reported no significant difference in improvement of the acute attack for patients randomly assigned to a group treated with ten weeks intensive bed rest and a group in which ambulation was encouraged as the patients desired. Browse (1965) cites findings where 200 patients with the diagnosis of TB were on drug therapy: 100 patients were ambulatory, and the other 100 were placed on bed rest. The X-ray results showed that both groups had the same rate of recovery. Similar recovery rates for ambulatory and bedfast patients have also been found in studies of persons with gastric ulcers and respiratory infections.

It would seem therefore that bed rest per se does not increase recovery rate. Indeed, current practice is geared more toward early ambulation of patients after illness or surgery with only short periods of bed rest. However, restricted mobility (i.e. bed rest) is acceptable in cases of paralysis, pain, in conditions of physical weakness caused by ageing, neuromotor disease, anaemia or other nutritional problems. Bed rest can relieve pain resulting from surgery, sprains, trauma or disease by taking undue weight and pressure off the affected part. Wounds can also be immobilized by enforced bed rest as in the case of fractures or after cataract extraction.

In cases where the individual is suffering from cardiac overload or shortness of breath, bed rest in an *upright position* can serve a therapeutic purpose by aiding cardiac output and venous return. Bed rest can also provide support when there is too little strength to fight the pull of gravity. By reducing this effect conditions such as oedema, varicosities, venous ulcers, hernias and a prolapsed rectum can be helped and treated.

In deciding the extent of immobilization or bed rest required by any patient, it is always important to balance the physiological advantages against the disadvantages. If one part of the body requires resting and results in the patient being put to bed, it means that the rest of the body is immobilized, regardless of whether such immobilization is either necessary or helpful. Reasons for the immobilization of a particular patient should always be clearly articulated so that those parts of the body which do not require immobilization as treatment are put through a range of movements and muscular exercise.

Adverse effects of bed rest/enforced immobilization

Knowledge of the adverse effects of bed rest ensures that the decision to keep a patient in bed for prolonged periods is not taken lightly. Bed rest affects the normal functioning of most of the main systems in the body.

Cardiovascular system. Coe (1954) studied the effect of imposed rest on the cardiac system and found that when a patient lies *flat* in bed his pulse rate drops from an average of 90 beats to around 60 beats per minute, his blood pressure remains the same, whilst the distribution of blood alters in the body. Blood leaves the legs and 11% extra goes to the thorax, thus increasing the blood volume of the heart and hence increasing the heart's workload. Coe also found that turning in bed and getting on and off a bedpan also increase cardiac workload. The increased strain on the heart from moving and using the bedpan is related to the complex of movements termed the Valsalva manoeuvre used to perform either task. During the Valsalva manoeuvre, a person takes a deep breath and, holding his breath with his chest fixed, the air pushes against the closed glottis leading to an increase in intrathoracic pressure, the individual either turns or gets on or off the bedpan. When the person exhales suddenly (usually after the task has been completed), there is a sudden increase in venous return to the heart causing tachycardia. In order to minimize the effect of this on the cardiac system, cardiac patients are encouraged to breathe through their mouths when turning in bed and are given commodes rather than bed pans.

Patients confined to bed may also suffer from orthostatic hypotension. Due to the decreased effect of gravity, the patient experiences a generalized vasodilatation and increased venous return, cardiac output and blood volume. When the patient first sits up or changes from a lying to a vertical position, the resulting change in pressure may cause dizziness and nausea, signs of orthostatic hypotension. This phenomenon was studied by Taylor et al (1949) who found that when healthy individuals, who were kept in bed for 21 days, were given work requiring moderate exercise, their heart rates on average increased to about 40 extra beats per minute compared to their heart rates before bed rest. Taylor also noted that it took 5–10 weeks for heart rates during work to return to rates prior to the period of rest. This knowledge has implications for the preparation and advice health personnel give to convalescent patients.

Respiratory system. Bed rest also interferes with the function of the respiratory system, reducing the potential for chest expansion, decreasing the movement of secretions and contributing generally to a decrease in ventilation. It is important that compensatory measures are activated, such as encouraging deep breathing exercises and coughing.

Bones, renal system and skin. Demineralization of bones also takes place with a resultant change in the chemistry, strength, size and general appearance of the bone. Bone demineralization may also affect kidney function, the excess calcium predisposing to calculus formation. Changes in urine composition, particularly the increase in the concentration of calcium, also affect bladder sensitivity, with incontinence and urinary tract infections not uncommon occurrences in patients who have been confined to bed for prolonged periods. Skin breakdown is also a danger in prolonged bed rest, particularly at sites such as the heels, sacrum, elbows, shoulders and pinnae of the ears — areas where the skin covers a bony prominence and where prolonged pressure can predispose to tissue breakdown and necrosis (see Ch. 20).

Muscular system. It is also estimated that muscle weakness and atrophy begin from the 3rd to 7th day in bed, most noticeably affecting the antigravity muscles of the limbs used for standing and walking. When motion is reduced or absent, connective tissues surrounding bone joints and muscles also tend to become dense — a condition known as fibrosis. This has been known to cause a loss of motion within a few days which in turn results in contractures (shortening and thickening of connective tissue). Contractures can occur very rapidly in people immobilized from a cerebrovascular accident. Stryker (1977) reports that as many as 60% of stroke victims develop shoulder contractures, and 30% develop ankle contractures. Whilst it may take only a matter of days before connective tissue becomes fibrosed and contractures begin to develop, it may take weeks and sometimes months to reverse fibrosis. Perkins (1953) outlined the length of time needed to regain full range of motion following shoulder dislocation with varying periods of immobilization. Even when the length of immobilization was less than 24 h, Perkins found that it took up to 18 days to recover complete range of motion for the shoulder joint. Where patients were immobilized for a period of 21 days, range of shoulder movements did not recover fully until almost one year later.

Therapeutic bed rest

Before the nurse can act in a positive way, she must know why the patient has been prescribed a period of bed rest as part of his treatment regimen. The clearly articulated treatment plan will help the nurse identify specific organs or tissues which are being intentionally immobilized. Having established which systems are to be kept relatively inactive, the nurse can then initiate a regimen of movement to ensure that complications do not occur. It is the nurse's duty also to ensure that enforced bed rest, or any period of rest, is as beneficial as possible to the patient. Therapeutic rest is linked with the patient's ability to relax. There is generally a false assumption made that when a person is lying in bed, he is resting. This is not necessarily the case — indeed, to be motionless in bed all day is not relaxing for a normally active person. Adequate rest depends on the degree of muscular relaxation that is present as well as relief from mental stress.

Relaxation. Ideally the nurse should see teaching and encouraging patients to relax as part of her therapeutic role. She could do this by first of all ensuring that the patient is in a posture favouring relaxation. This relates to positioning the patient in bed in a way which he finds most comfortable. By attempting to allay or relieve emotional tensions the nurse may also be able to induce a more relaxed state in the patient. According to Kraus (1963), emotional tensions manifest themselves through the striated musculature of the body. If such irritations recur daily and establish similar patterns of response, then an habitual pattern of muscular reaction is formed resulting in such symptoms as sleeplessness, hyperirritability, backache or headache. Jacobson (1964) has shown that by teaching a person how to relax, such tensions can be alleviated.

Rest and relaxation may be best induced by planning a routine of exercise during the day. Baekeland & Lasky (1966) found that exercises in the afternoon increased the amount of sound sleep athletes experienced, whereas exercise and complex mental activity before bedtime had an adverse effect on sleep. Again, it is part of the nurse's therapeutic function to provide treatment plans which will reduce muscle tensions, alleviate any mental or emotional anxieties which may be causing muscle tension and provide some sort of activity which will help relax patients.

Ensuring that the patient is in a posture favouring relaxation. Two main considerations are involved in ensuring that the patient is in a posture favouring relaxation. The first requires that the nurse has knowledge of the range of basic positioning techniques; the second, that she can apply these techniques to the particular requirements of the patient.

Before the nurse comes to position or move a patient in bed, it is important that she knows how to position herself. Before attempting to lift or move any object she ought to give herself as broad a base of support as possible by keeping her feet apart, one slightly in front of the other.

She should make maximum use of her centre of gravity by moving close to or holding objects close to her own body. Leg muscles should always be used to move and lift objects, and the back can be further protected by never twisting it when lifting. Abdominal and gluteal muscles should be contracted to stabilize the pelvic floor prior to moving the object. This protects both the ligaments and joints from strain. If the object to be lifted is too heavy or awkward for one nurse, then either mechanical help in the form of hoists or lifts, or additional manpower, should be employed. The nurse's knowledge of body movement and lifting techniques will help to reduce fatigue and muscle strain and conserve energy. It will also help to minimize the danger of injury by preserving muscle tone and joint mobility.

Once the nurse has acquired the basic skills of positioning herself correctly in relation to the patient, she is ready to assess the most beneficial position for the patient in bed. The correct bed position ought to reproduce the normal erect posture, that is, one in which the feet are together, the toes and knees are facing forward, arms are relaxed and at the side, the trunk straight and the head high (Fig. 13.1A&B). This vertical stance can be reproduced on a horizontal plane by ensuring that the patient has a firm bed, one flat pillow underneath his head rather than a stack of pillows, with his knees straight and toes and knees pointing to the ceiling (Fig. 13.1C). A firm mattress is an important prerequisite for all patients when attempting to achieve correct body alignment in bed, particularly in maintaining the straight line of the hips in relation to the upper and lower limbs. Stryker (1977) notes that if the patient's hips sag from between 2–5 inches, forming an angle of about 120° at the hip joint, the result can be a hip contracture. When the patient is put in the semi-Fowler's position, an angle of approximately 110° is formed at the hips, which again may result in a hip contracture if used continuously. Prolonged use of this position can cause the same problem as poor mattresses or poor positioning (Fig. 13.2). With correct positioning on a firm mattress, where the hip joint angle is 150° the possibility of hip contractures is diminished.

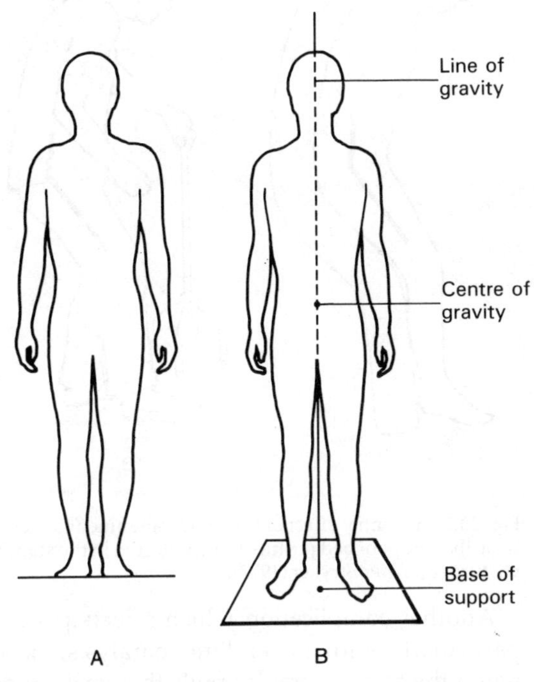

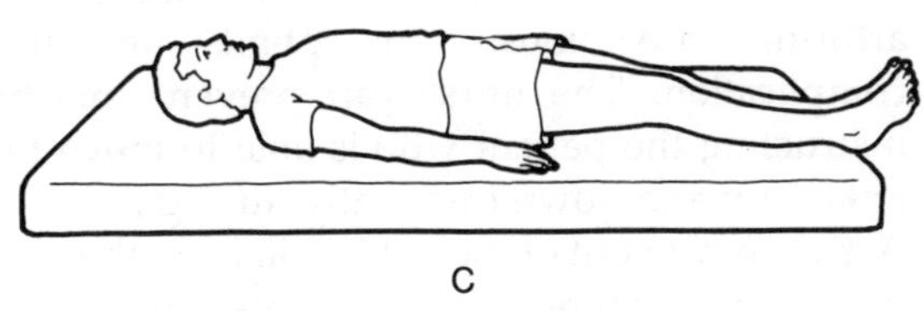

Fig. 13.1 Correct body alignment, standing and supine. (A) Standing figure correctly aligned. (B) Standing figure showing base of support, line of gravity and centre of gravity. (C) Supine figure correctly aligned. Note that there is no pillow, or one flat pillow, under the head, legs are straight, knees together, arms are straight and at the sides. Note also the space above head and below feet. After Stryker (1977).

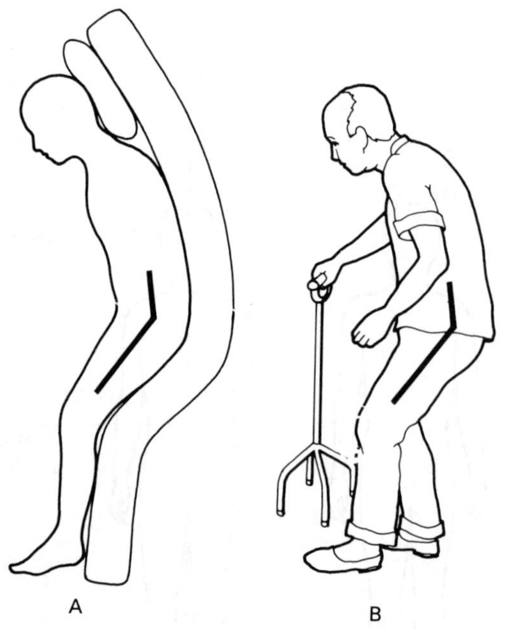

Fig. 13.2 Potential effect of poor body alignment in bed. Note that the poor bed posture (A) is reflected in the standing posture (B). After Stryker (1977).

Another complication which affects patients, particularly with lower limb paralysis, occurs when the force of gravity pulls the weakened or paralysed foot into a 'foot drop' position, that is, where the calf muscles and heel tendons shorten in response to prolonged hyperextension of the ankle joint. Patients who suffer from foot drop are unable to put their heel to the ground with the result that walking is impaired. Those suffering from strokes, Parkinson's disease and arthritis are most susceptible to this complication. The nurse can prevent this by instructing the patient who is able to move his ankles up and down frequently during the day. Active movement of the ankle will keep the heel tendon from tightening and will also strengthen the ankle muscle. If the patient is unable to do this the nurse is responsible for ensuring that passive movements of the ankles are carried out. Bedclothing should also be kept loose over patients' feet, or bed cradles used, to ensure that the extra pressure of tight bedclothes does not accentuate the problem.

The nurse should also be aware of the danger of using too many pillows to support and position the patient. The use of pillows under the patient's knees leading to continued elevation of the knee joint can produce contractures and increase the extent of hip contractures. Multiple pillows under the patient's head and shoulders can lead to a rounding of the back and can push the head forward.

Body posture — assessment and planning for care. Thus, in trying to ensure that the body is in a position favouring relaxation, it is imperative that the nurse work out a position plan for each patient. This will take into consideration such factors as the patient's level of consciousness, comprehension, pain sensation, muscle function, presence of oedema, skin integrity, body type, bowel and bladder control, the patient's ability to assist in his own positioning and whether contractures have developed. When each of these areas has been assessed, the nurse selects a range of positions most appropriate for the patient and takes on the responsibility for ensuring that the plan is carried out.

The importance of the nurse's assessment of the patient's position plan is well illustrated in a study by Lamb (1979) who assessed the postoperative comfort levels of patients who had fractured hips. Lamb found that there was a range of opinions about the most appropriate way of positioning such patients: Larson & Gould (1974) noted that patients with fractured hips may be turned onto the affected side, the bed acting as a type of splint, to provide comfort and to promote gravity drainage for the wound, whilst Bradley (1970) suggested that patients would be more comfortable lying on the unaffected side. Lamb found that up to 50% of the patients in the study sample preferred lying on the operative side, commenting that they found this position more comfortable. These results would suggest that postoperative positioning to achieve optimal comfort is linked more to patients' individual preferences than any pre-set pattern.

Nurses also need to be aware of the physiological effect of moving and repositioning patients suffering from certain pathological conditions. Mitchell et al (1981) studied the effect of position change on patients' intracranial pressure and found a significant increase in ventricular fluid pressure (VFP) following several of the movements, both immediately after the movement and one hour later. Turning in all directions (supine to right lateral; right lateral to supine; supine to left lateral and left lateral to supine) was found to produce more variability in VFP than either passive range of movements or head rotations. Whilst the increase in VFP was not seen to be harmful in the majority of patients, the researchers underline the importance of monitoring such reactions as a routine nursing procedure, particularly in patients whose VFP is a crucial factor in prognosis and recovery.

Using nursing techniques to relieve emotional and muscle tension

In addition to preventing complications of bed rest and trying to increase patient comfort, the nurse can also help the patient to relax by carrying out certain nursing procedures in a manner which minimizes pain or which actively instils in the patient a feeling of well-being and relaxation.

Intra-muscular injections. In a study of the effect of using different body positions to reduce discomfort from dorsogluteal injection, Rettig & Southby (1982) took a sample of 60 general surgery and gynaecology postoperative patients and asked them to comment on the level of discomfort they experienced when given two injections. One injection was given when the patient's femur was internally rotated (toes pointing inwards) and the other given when the patient's femur was externally rotated (toes pointing outwards). The degree of discomfort experienced when the patient lay in the prone position as opposed to the side-lying position was also tested.

Patients reported significantly more discomfort when they assumed the prone externally rotated position than when they received the dorsogluteal injection in the prone internally rotated position. Similarly, patients complained of more pain from the dorsogluteal injection when it was administered in the side-lying externally rotated position than when it was given in the side-lying internally rotated position. When the prone and side-lying internally rotated results were compared, no significant differences were noted, suggesting that it is the internal rotation position of the limb which induces muscular relaxation, thus reducing pain. Rettig & Southby's results confirmed the findings of Zelman (1961), Pitel & Wemett (1964) and Lang et al (1976), that an injection into a relaxed muscle reduces discomfort.

Bathing. Another nursing activity which can help patients relax is bathing. Whilst the therapeutic effects of bathing are expected to relieve anxieties and increase patient comfort, Barsevick & Llewellyn (1982) argued that very often the choice of the bathing procedure was determined more by the amount of time available to the nursing staff rather than on any assessment of the therapeutic value of the procedure to the patient. Barsevick & Llewellyn thus attempted to compare the effect of a towel bath (a method of bathing a patient in bed using a towel soaked in a warm lubricated solution, where the patient's skin is massaged through the towel and then air dried) and the conventional bed bath on patient anxiety levels. A total of 105 patients were included in the study, divided into two groups: one group had undergone surgery and another group was suffering from unrelieved pain caused by a range of pathological conditions. Anxiety levels were measured using the State-Trait Anxiety Inventory (STAI), the Palmar Sweat Index (PSI) and the Behavioural Cues Index (BCI). Patients in either group were then randomly allocated to the towel bath group or the conventional bed bath group. Both bathing procedures were found to have significant anxiety-reducing effects on both groups of patients. When the baths were compared with each other, the towel bath was found to be more effective in reducing anxiety than the conventional bed bath. Barsevick & Llewellyn attributed this finding to the relaxing effect of heat and massage inherent in the towel bath. Unlike the conventional bed bath, where the patient's body is exposed to the cold, in the towel bath method, the patient is wrapped in a large, solution-soaked warm towel and massaged clean. The towel bath thus reduces heat loss, conserves energy and utilizes a relaxing massage technique shown to reduce anxiety levels, particularly in postoperative patients.

Muscle-relaxant exercises. Wells (1982) reported on a study of the effect of relaxation on postoperative muscle tension and pain, noting that it was a necessary part of the nurse's function to be able to teach patients how to reduce muscle tension by performing a series of muscle relaxant exercises. Results showed that distress caused by painful sensations was lower for patients who learned the relaxation technique.

UNDERSTANDING AND SUPPLYING THE PATIENT'S NEED FOR ACTIVITY/EXERCISE

It is important to remember that the normal healthy person has almost unlimited choice of posture and that his body is constantly moving. Activity is not only linked to movement of voluntary striated muscle in the body; the involuntary or smooth muscles in the viscera also depend indirectly on the tone of voluntary musculature for its effect. Thus, for normal body function, the voluntary muscles must be constantly stimulated. For those patients who find themselves unable to move it is essential that they be given assistance in order to maintain joint and soft tissue mobility. The aim of such exercise is to minimize the effect of inactivity, correct the inefficiency of specific muscles or muscle groups and help the individual maintain or regain a range of joint movements.

Stryker (1977) has identified five reasons why exercise is prescribed:

- to increase or maintain joint and soft tissue mobility
- to improve musculoskeletal co-ordination
- to develop muscular strength
- to develop muscular endurance
- to promote physical rehabilitation.

The nurse is seen to be primarily responsible for the preservation of the patient's present range of movement, thereby preventing deformity and further loss of motion. It is in the maintenance of present function and the prevention of further deterioration that the nurse's responsibility for the provision of routine physical therapies lies.

Therapeutic exercise

Having established the fact that the patient requires routine exercise does not automatically mean that it will be therapeutic. Merely getting a patient to move around and waggle his legs does not constitute therapeutic exercise; rather therapeutic exercise comprises the prescription of bodily movements to correct an impairment, improve musculoskeletal function or maintain a state of well-being (Kottke, 1971). Henderson & Nite (1978) see the main purpose of therapeutic exercise as increasing and maintaining mobility of joints and soft tissue. It can be directed toward the correction of abnormalities, both structural and functional, as well as toward rehabilitation covering physical, social and mental aspects.

In order to appreciate the need for therapeutic exercise, the nurse must be aware that immobile patients require muscle and joint activity from the very beginning of their immobilization in order to prevent further discomfort and disability. The nurse may also have to explain the need for exercise to patients who are uncooperative and refuse to do exercises daily or at prescribed periods, especially if they are trying to deny incapacity. The specific exercises to be performed will vary with the person's treatment goals, which are evaluated by the nurse and therapist together.

In initiating and carrying out a range of motion exercises, it is important that the nurse distinguishes between her responsibility and goals for patient mobility, and those of the physiotherapists. The physiotherapist's primary role concerns evaluation and restoration of function, whilst the nurse's primary responsibility is related to the maintenance of present function and prevention of further deterioration.

Range of motion (ROM) exercising is one of the various nursing skills used as a preventive measure. It helps to prevent contractures and to maintain joint integrity and mobility. Other preventive measures which are used in conjunction with exercising include proper body alignment, change of position, adequate support to various parts of the body and use of equipment to prevent pressure.

Range of motion (ROM) exercises

The most effective way for the nurse to integrate the therapeutic exercise programme is to link range of motion exercises with the performance of patient's activities of living. Before she does this, however, the nurse must decide on the most appropriate type of exercise regimen. There are three main types of ROM exercise: passive, isometric and active. All three are designed to ensure that all joints and muscles in the body are exercised. The degree to which the patient requires help determines whether the ROM is passive, isometric or active. Figure 13.3 shows the normal range of joint motions which are covered by the ROM exercises.

Assessment and planning. Range of motion exercises are planned to meet the individual needs of each patient, the objective being to maintain or achieve the degree of motion necessary to regain independence. Often patients' uninvolved joints can be used as a guide for the normal range of motion which can be achieved in the involved joints. By assessing the patient's range of motion at the beginning of hospitalization, the nurse is then able to devise an exercise routine which will ensure that the patient will receive appropriate activity throughout the day.

A primary consideration in formulating the treatment plan is the patient's medical condition. If there is any evidence of inflamed joints, infection or oedema, then exercise to those areas is contraindicated. Similarly, if the patient suffers from osteoporosis, the nurse needs to handle him gently. The presence of spasticity, contractions or decreased sensation will limit the patient's exercise potential and may require a specific set of ROM to be performed by the nurse after consultation with the physiotherapist. Any voluntary muscle control possessed by the patient should be noted and incorporated into the treatment regimen. The nurse should also be assessing continually those activities which the patient can or cannot do, as well as noting any which can be done with difficulty. The patient's fatigue tolerance during activities and exercise is another important factor which must be identified and considered.

Before starting the exercises, the nurse should position herself correctly in front of the patient, ensuring that she has a broad base of support and is able to exercise the patient without injuring herself. She ought to ensure at this point that the patient is in good body alignment. When handling the patient's extremities, the nurse should hold the limb at the joint if the patient has muscle pain. If joint pain is the problem, then the nurse grasps the patient's limb above and below the joints. The motions should be performed smoothly, slowly and rhythmically.

It is important that the nurse never exceeds the patient's existing range of motion; movements should never be forced and if pain is felt then the movement should stop. Exercises should be integrated as far as possible into the daily self-care routine of each patient.

Passive exercises (Figs 13.4–13.15). When the patient is unable or not allowed to exercise his body, the nurse takes on the responsibility of ensuring that each joint in the body is exercised. Passive ROM is more commonly used as preventive rather than corrective therapy and consequently should be seen as an activity which is initiated and performed by the nurse. The purpose of passive ROM is to increase circulation, maintain joint movement and minimize contractures. Each joint in the body should be put through full ROM five times each and repeated several times a day depending on the patient's condition. Brower & Hicks (1972) suggest that exercises should be performed at least every hour, while Kottke (1971) suggests that a complete ROM should be performed between two to five times daily.

The nurse must also be aware that the body's complete range of movement may not be utilized even though the patient may be able to perform most of his activities of living. It is often the case that upper extremity exercises are neglected when self-care activities such as washing and dressing are performed. The nurse therefore must be able to assess which movements are

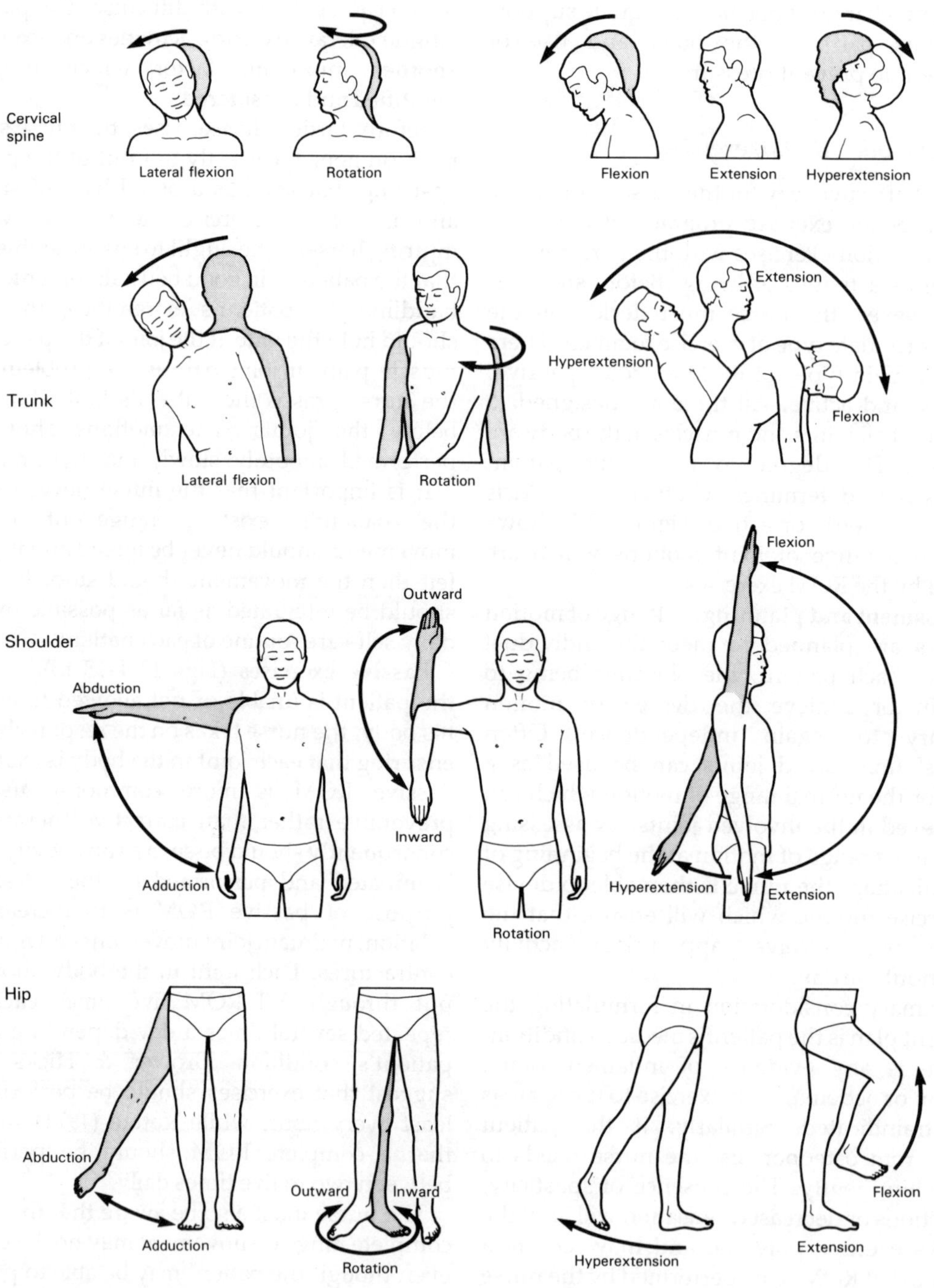

Fig. 13.3 (A & B) Range-of-motion exercises for joints: cervical spine, trunk, shoulder, hip, elbow, knee, wrist, ankle, fingers and toes. After Henderson & Nite (1978).

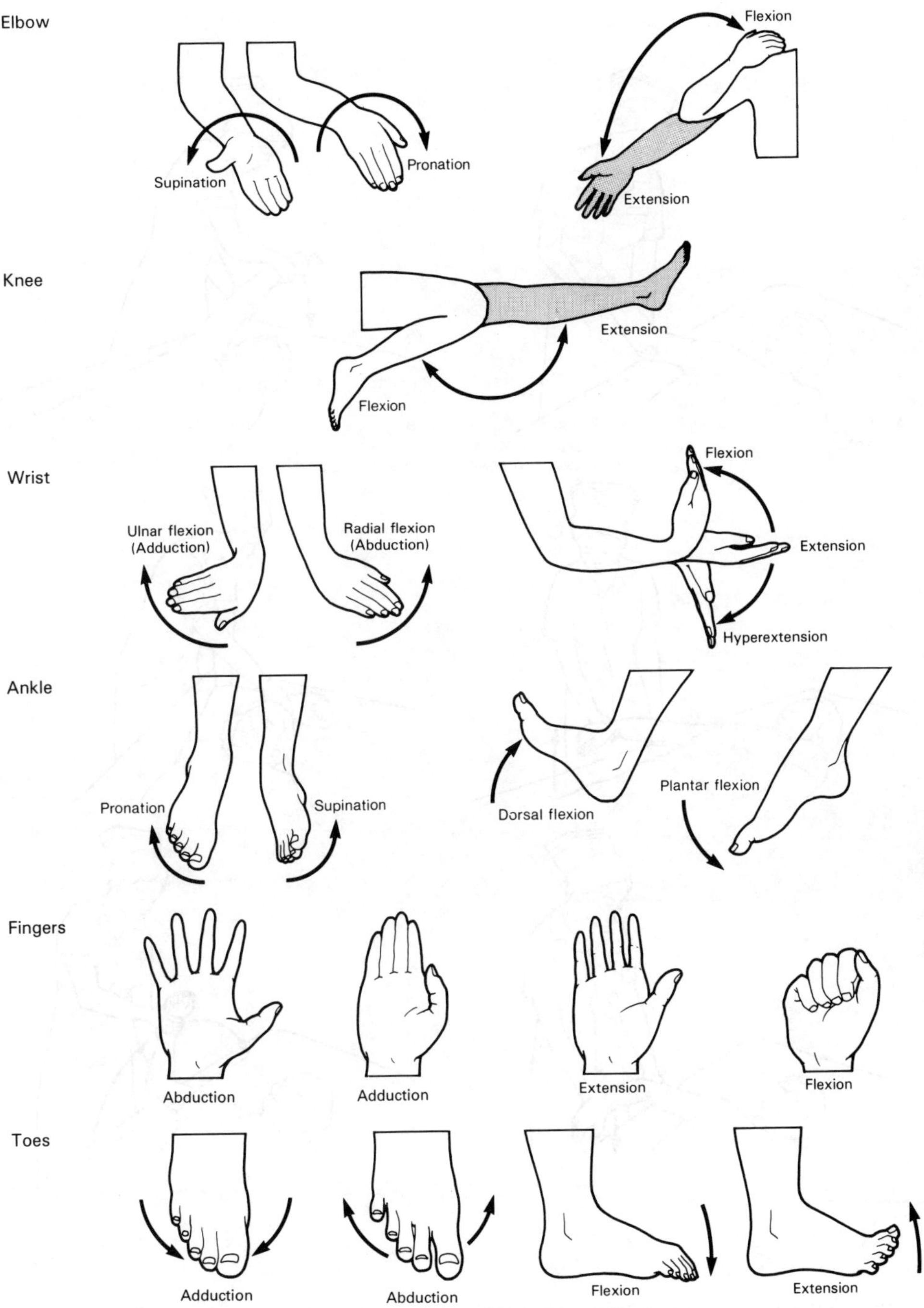
Elbow
Supination
Pronation
Flexion
Extension
Knee
Extension
Flexion
Wrist
Ulnar flexion
(Adduction)
Radial flexion
(Abduction)
Flexion
Extension
Hyperextension
Ankle
Pronation
Supination
Dorsal flexion
Plantar flexion
Fingers
Abduction
Adduction
Extension
Flexion
Toes
Adduction
Abduction
Flexion
Extension

Fig. 13.3 B

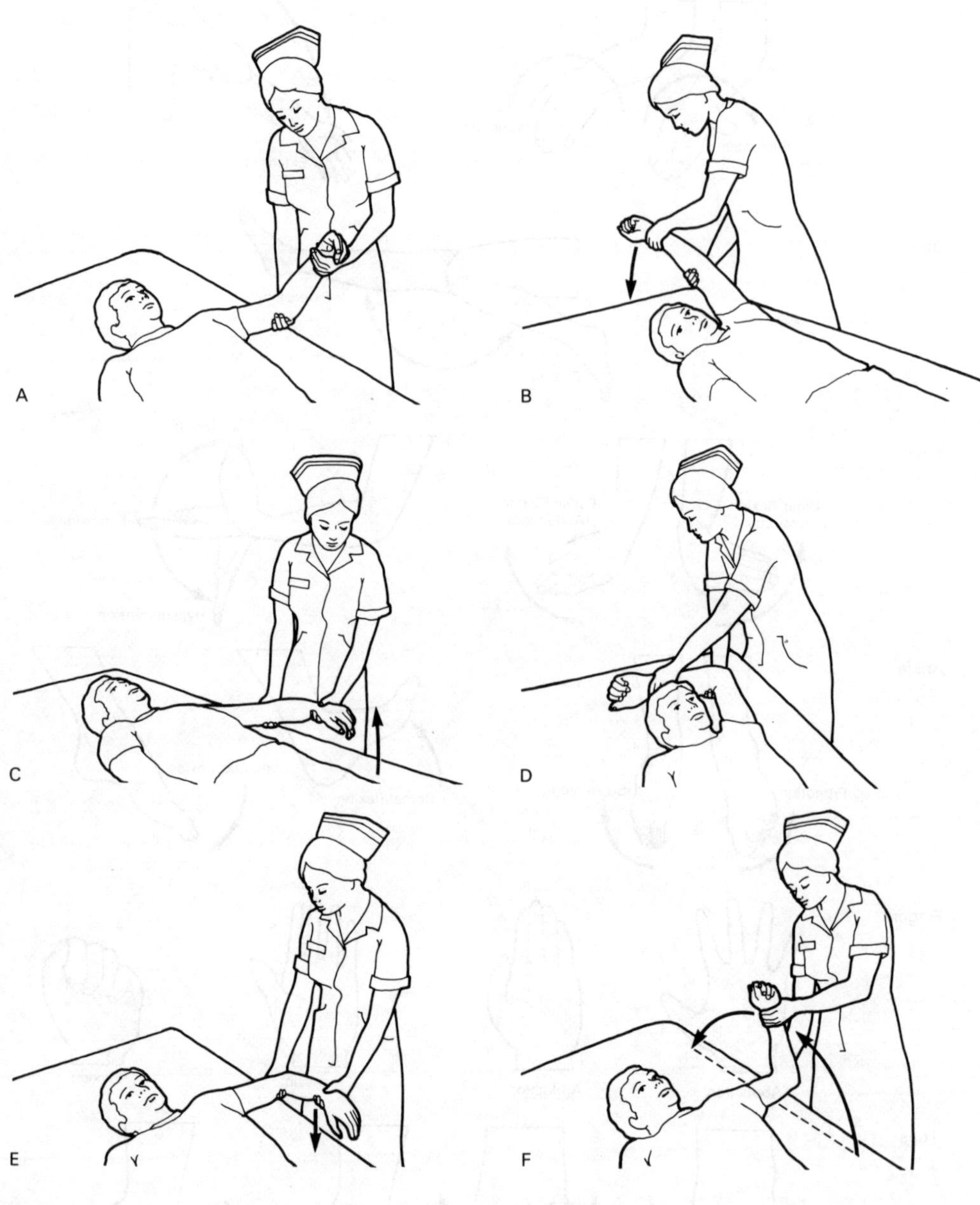

Fig. 13.4 Passive shoulder exercises, patient supine. (A) Lift the arm straight up towards the ceiling, supporting the elbow. (B) Continue the movement towards the patient's head until tightness or pain occurs. Return the arm to the side. (C) Move the arm away from the patient's side, turning the palm up. Continue the motion towards the patient's head. (D) Put one hand on the patient's shoulder if it tends to move up. (E) Place the upper arm to the side, at a right angle to the body. Bend the forearm to form a right angle with the upper arm. Maintaining this position, bring the arm down until the palm touches the bed. (F) Bring the forearm up so that the back of the hand touches the bed. After Stryker (1977).

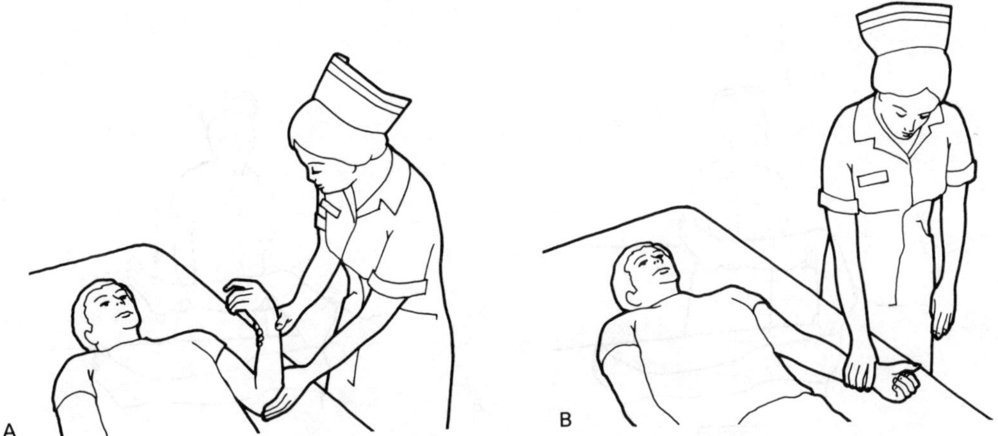

Fig. 13.5 Passive elbow exercise, patient supine. (A) Bend the patient's elbow, keeping the palm turned up (i.e. moving fingers towards shoulder). (B) Then straighten elbow completely.

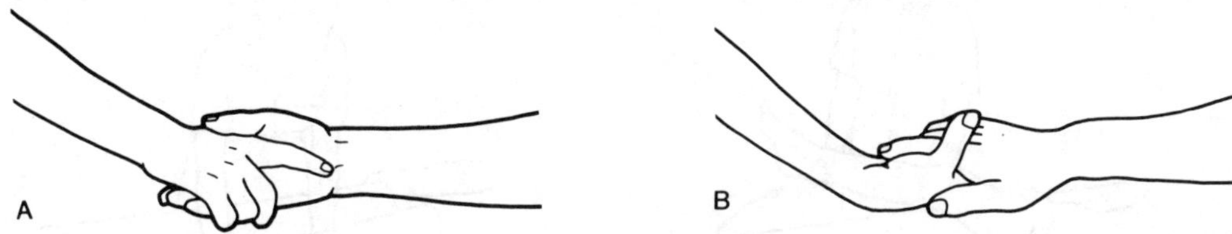

Fig. 13.6 Passive forearm exercise, patient supine. Grasp patient's hand as if to shake hands. Hold the upper arm with the other hand to ensure that the motion takes place in the forearm, not the shoulder. Supporting the wrist, turn the palm up (A) and down (B).

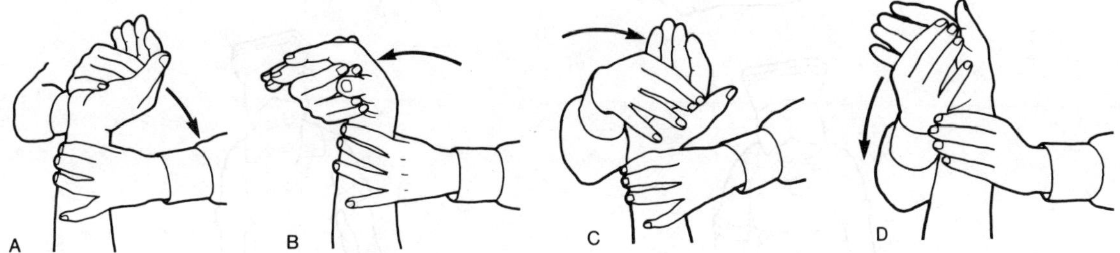

Fig. 13.7 Passive wrist exercise, patient supine. Supporting the forearm, bend the wrist backwards (A) and forwards (B). Straighten, then move the hand toward the thumb side (C) and toward the little finger side (D). Movement (D) can be omitted if the wrist assumes this position when relaxed.

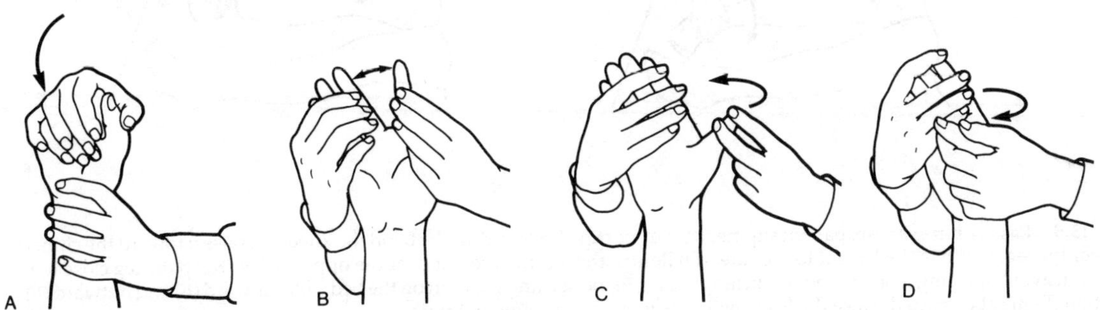

Fig. 13.8 Passive finger and thumb exercise, patient supine. (A) Supporting the wrist, bend and straighten the thumb and fingers at all joints. For the hemiplegic hand, only extend the joints. (B) Move the thumb and each finger, in turn, away from the adjacent finger and then back. (C) Bring the thumb out in a circling motion. (D) End with the thumb toward the little finger.

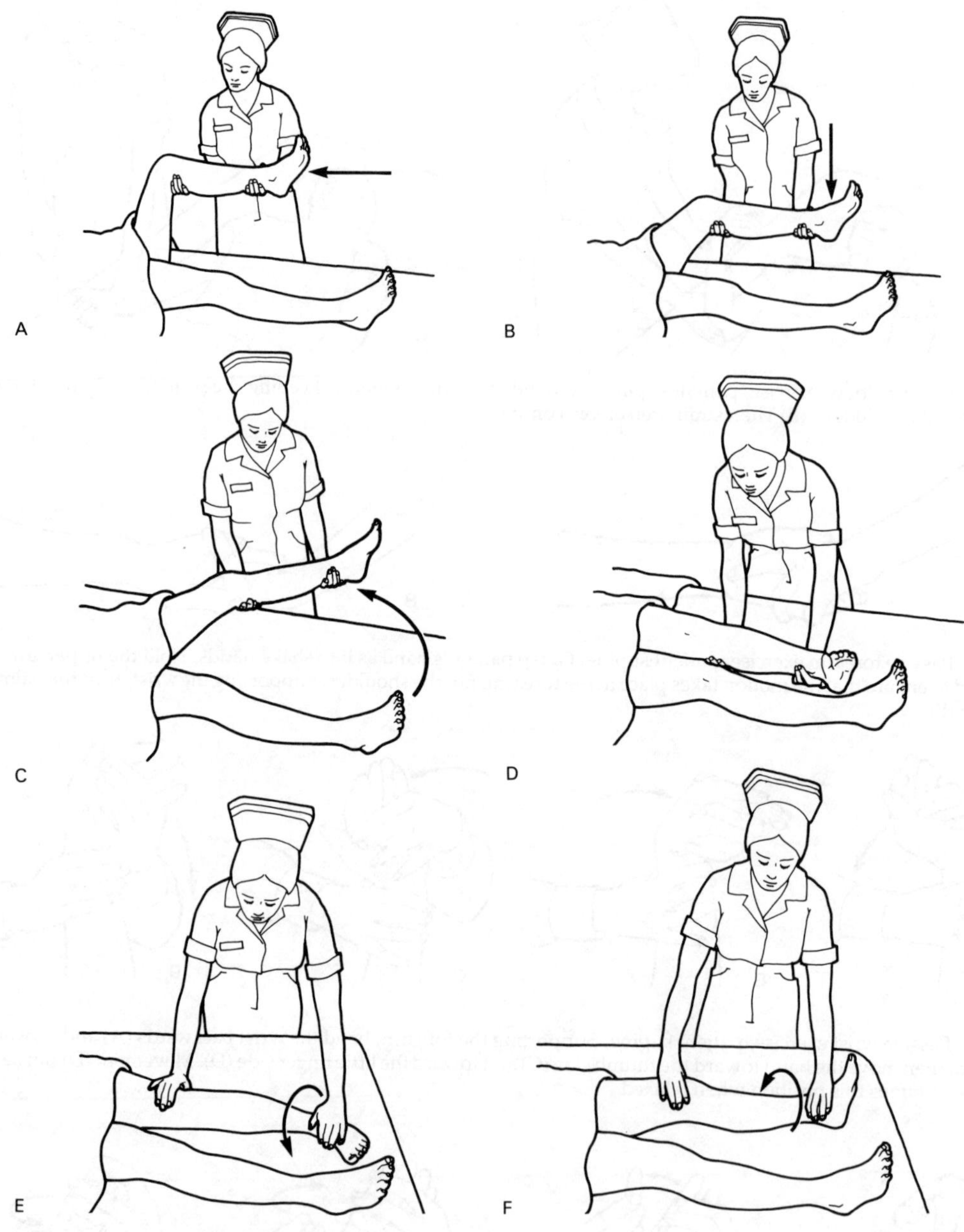

Fig. 13.9 Passive hip exercise, patient supine. (A) Supporting knee and ankle, bend the knee and raise it toward the chin. (B) Lower the leg. (C) Take the leg out to the side. (D) Return the leg and cross it over the opposite leg. Keep the leg close to the bed, but avoid dragging it on the bed. Returning the leg to the starting position on the bed, roll it inward (E) and outward (F). Motion (F) may be omitted, since the leg usually assumes this position naturally.

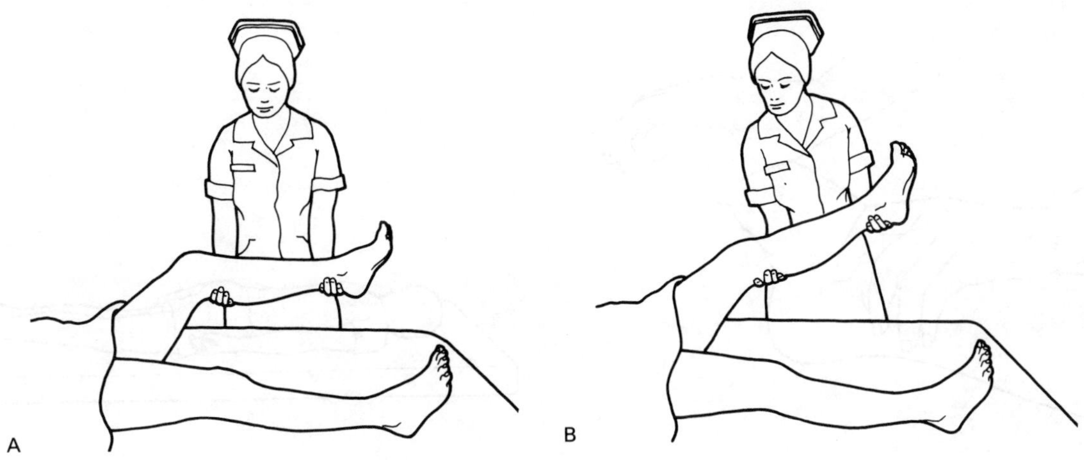

Fig. 13.10 Passive knee exercise, patient supine. Supporting just below the knee and at the ankle, raise the leg and bend at the knee (A), then straighten leg (B).

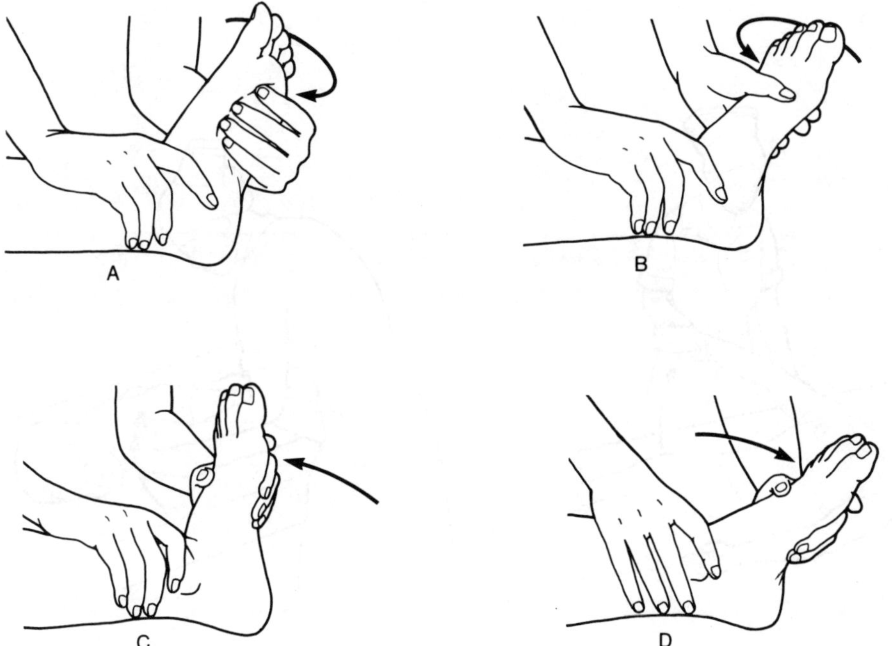

Fig. 13.11 Passive ankle exercise, patient supine. Support the leg and turn the foot outward (A), then inward (B). (C) Bend the foot up and backward. A right angle of the ankle joint is sufficient for standing; a little more range is needed for walking. It is seldom necessary to bend the foot down (D), since gravity and the weight of bedclothes tend to encourage this position.

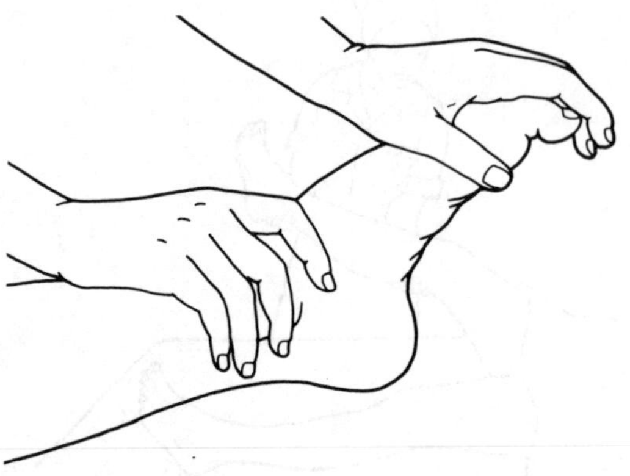

Fig. 13.12 Passive toe motions, patient supine. Supporting the ankle, bend and straighten the toes.

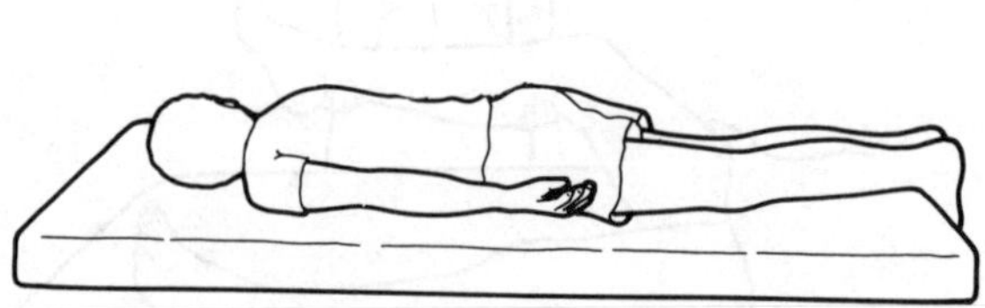

Fig. 13.13 Proper prone position. When the patient is lying prone, the toes should not rest on the mattress, but should extend over the edge. If this is impossible, place a small roll under the ankles to prevent pressure on the toes and feet. If the prone position is medically contraindicated, most of the following exercises can be done with the patient in the side-lying position.

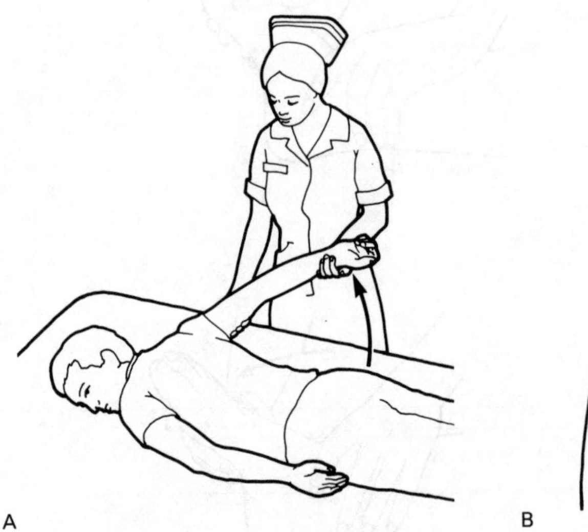

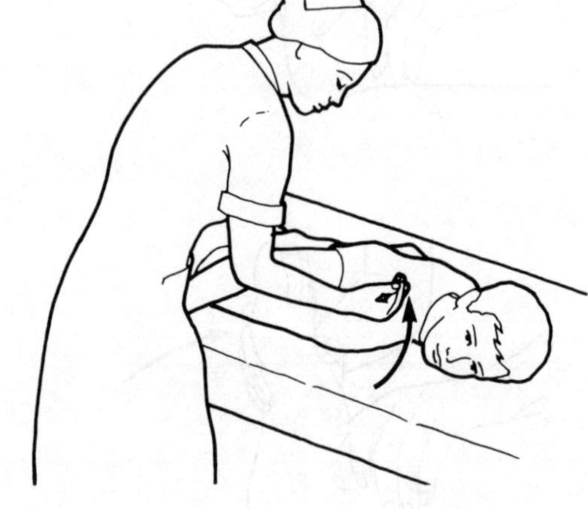

Fig. 13.14 Passive shoulder exercise, patient prone. (A) Bring the arm straight back, not bending at the elbow. (B) With the arm at the side, lift the shoulder off the bed, as if bringing the shoulder blades together.

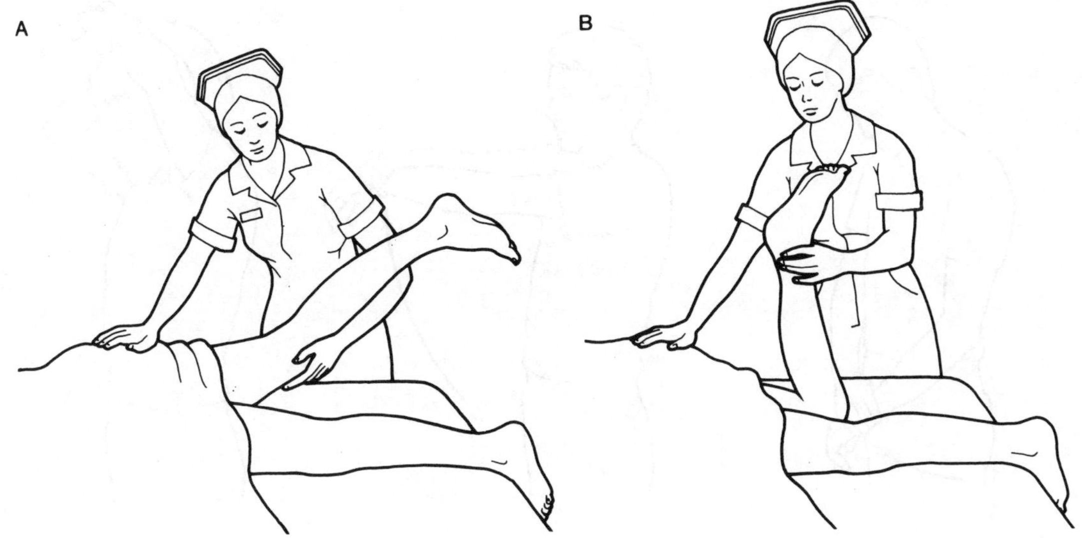

Fig. 13.15 (A) Passive hip exercise, patient prone. Keeping light pressure on the buttocks to prevent the hip from lifting off the bed, raise and lower the leg. This exercise helps to achieve optimal hip mobility.
(B) Passive knee exercise, patient prone. Keeping the hip from rising off the bed, bend the knee, taking the heel toward the buttocks. Stop the exercise at the point of resistance.

being performed so that she can compensate and encourage the patient to perform the additional movements. The most effective way for the nurse to integrate the therapeutic exercise programme is to link ROM with the performance of patients' self-care activities. Thus the nurse may be able to put the patient through a range of motions to ensure that he has performed them during such activities as a bed bath, an ordinary bath, brushing or combing hair, whilst moving the patient in bed, getting him in or out of bed or helping him to sit out on a chair. While the nurse may begin her exercise plan by performing most of the movements for the patient, it is important that as the patient's condition improves, so the nurse teaches and encourages him to perform the exercises unaided. The nurse's role is constantly one of an enabler and support to the patient.

Isometric exercises. Isometric exercises are those in which muscles contract against an immovable outer resistance. The purpose of such activities is to improve the strength of a muscle group. Isometric exercises do not involve joint motion, a change in muscle length or any external muscular movement. They are useful when joint movement is contraindicated and can be done by patients confined to bed rest for long periods. The exercises, also called muscle setting, are performed by contracting and relaxing muscles alternately, without joint movement. Kelly (1966) believes that such setting or isometric exercises are particularly useful for maintaining the tone of the postural muscles of the buttocks, abdomen and thighs. The patient can set these muscles separately, or he may set all of them simultaneously by lying supine with legs extended, hands at his sides, then lifting his buttocks off the bed bearing his weight on his shoulders and heels. The nurse can encourage this type of movement when assisting the patient to move in bed or when performing certain self-care activities, e.g. using a bed pan.

The therapeutic benefit of such exercises has been reported by Müller (1970) who noted that five maximal isometric contractions, each lasting six seconds, with a two-minute rest period between contractions, would prevent loss of muscle strength in the immobilized person.

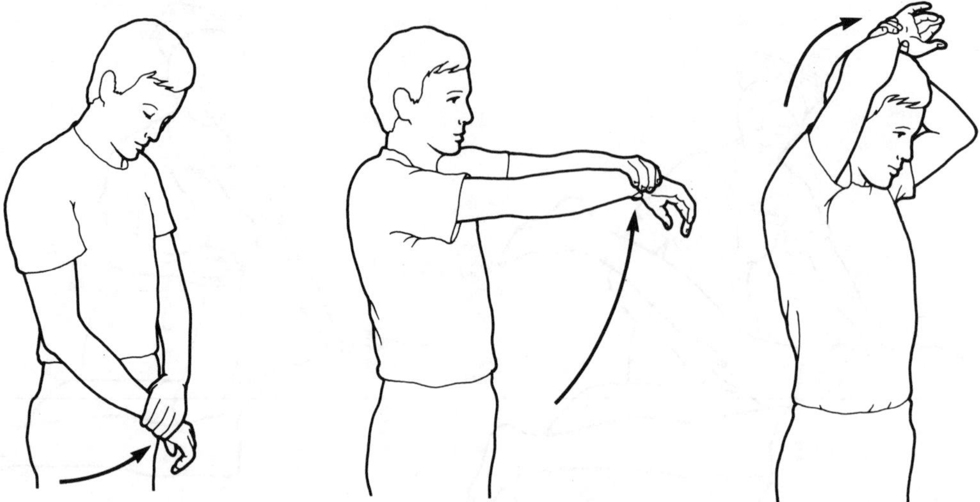

Fig. 13.16 Active self-assistive shoulder exercise — patient supine, sitting or standing. The patient grasps the involved arm at the wrist and performs all the exercises of the shoulder, elbow and wrist. The uninvolved hand extends the fingers and thumb of the involved hand.

Given the fact that when muscles are kept at complete rest, loss of muscle strength occurs at a rate of 10–15% per week of inactivity (Kottke, 1971), it is important that the nurse be aware of simple activities which could prevent such deterioration. A further benefit of isometric exercise is that after appropriate instruction and supervision the average patient is able to carry out these exercises independently. Stryker (1977) notes that isometric exercises place little demand on the cardiovascular system if the breath is not held during contraction. They should not be recommended to persons with cardiovascular disease, however, without a specific medical order. Such exercises are recommended for postsurgical and orthopaedic patients, as well as other inactive persons.

Active exercises (Figs 13.16, 13.17). Active exercises are those in which motions are performed without, or with minimal, assistance. They can be performed either individually or in groups. Huddlestone (1961) has identified five types of active exercise:

- Static active exercise describes a situation where the patient contracts and relaxes muscles alternately without joint motion (isometric exercises).
- Assistive active exercises are those where the patient is helped by the nurse or therapist, or by weights or pulleys, to perform the exercise.
- Resistive exercises refer to situations where patients perform the exercise against resistance offered by the nurse, gravity or weights.
- Progressive-resistive exercises utilize pulleys and weights to provide a resistance load to develop muscle strength.
- Free exercises refer to those carried out by the patient.

Whilst it is the physiotherapist's responsibility to work toward increasing and developing the patient's exercise tolerance, the nurse must be aware of the treatment goals and be able to assess whether the patient is progressing. As patient activity is so closely tied up with the performance of self-care activities, the nurse is in a key position to monitor response to prescribed exercise — the patient's pulse rate before, directly after and several minutes after the activity, his respiratory rate and his temperature. Any muscle soreness or joint stiffness ought also

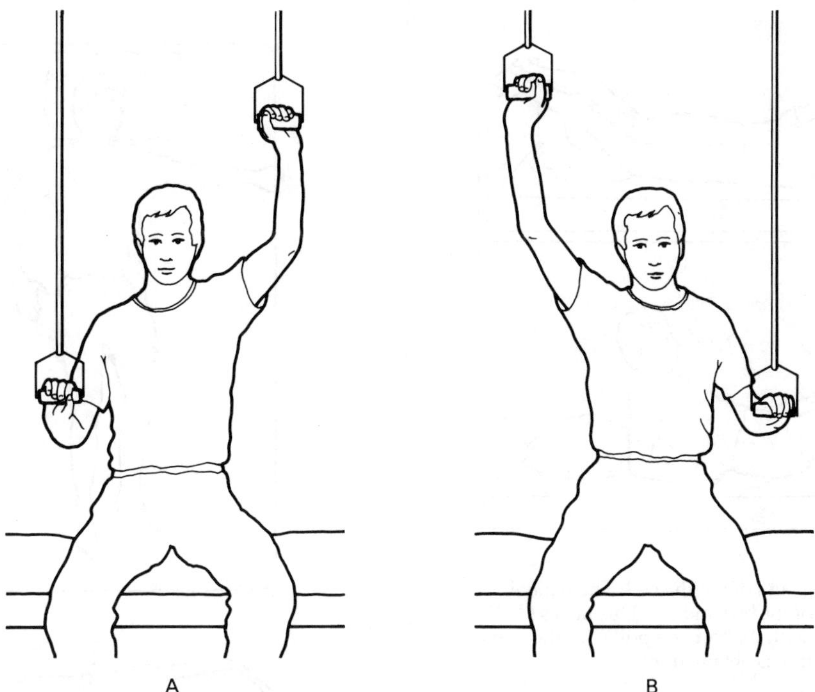

Fig. 13.17 Active self-assistive shoulder exercises using a reciprocal pully. (A) As the patient pulls down with the unaffected hand, the involved hand is brought up over the head. (B) As the unaffected arm raises, the other will automatically return to the side. After Stryker (1977).

to be reported to the physiotherapist.

The nurse is able to encourage all patients to use simple forms of exercise that will keep joints free moving and prevent loss of muscle tone. Such exercises could be performed by a group of patients together. Goldberg & Fitzpatrick (1980) looked at the effect of participation in a movement therapy group on morale and self-esteem in a group of institutionalized elderly people. The residents were divided into a control group who participated in the usual treatment programme whilst the experimental group participated in a series of movement therapy sessions. The movement therapy group members were found to have greater improvement in total morale and attitudes toward their own ageing than those in the control group. It is not impossible to envisage similar exercise classes having beneficial effects on the well-being of postoperative surgical or orthopaedic patients when an active exercise programme could be worked out by the therapist in conjunction with the nurse.

Reduced mobility has also been found to affect the ability of patients to perceive and judge the passage of time. Tompkins (1980) found that when subjects were asked to judge the length of time they had been performing an activity (walking in a circular track), they judged that they had been walking for a much longer time when one limb had been restricted than when they were able to walk freely. When encouraging the disabled or immobilized patient to exercise, it is worth noting that he will not only fatigue more quickly but will also perceive that he has been exercising for a longer period of time than he actually has. The nurse must be able to respond in a sympathetic yet positive way by encouraging the patient to reach certain exercise goals set jointly by the two of them.

Transfer techniques (Figs 13.18–13.23)

The nurse has an important contribution to make in ensuring that patients maintain and practise therapeutic exercises when assisting or directing

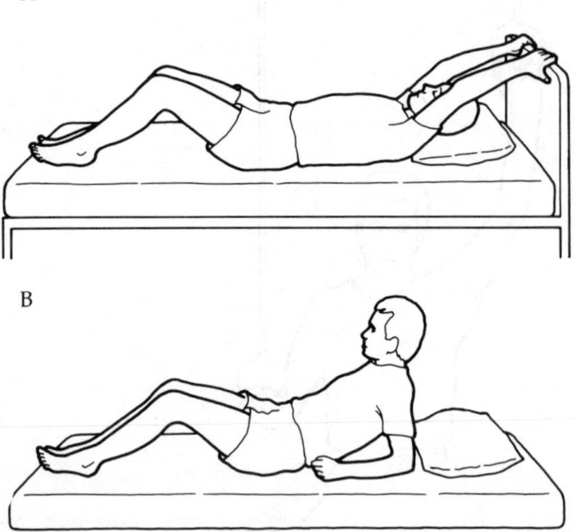

Fig. 13.18 Moving up and down the bed. The patient should grasp the top of the bed and bend his knees (A) then simultaneously push with the feet and pull with the arms, until the desired position is obtained (B).

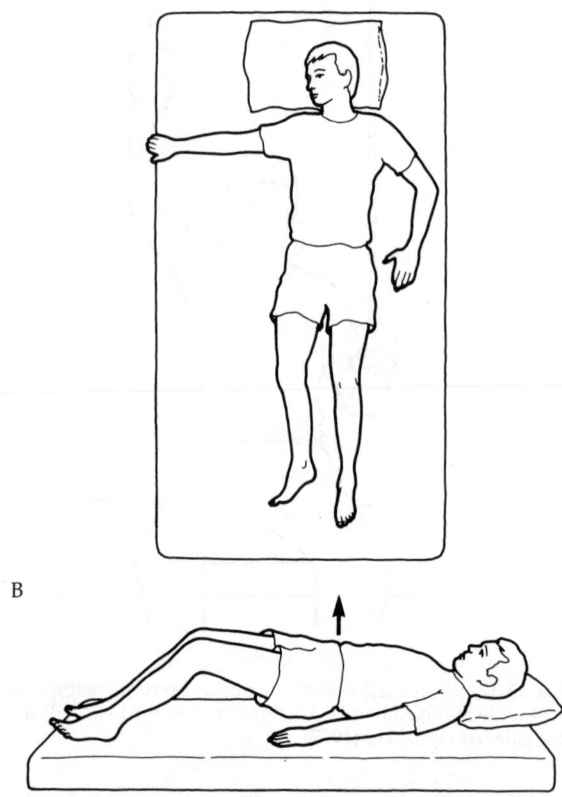

Fig. 13.19 Moving sideways. The patient, lying supine, grasps with his near hand the side of the bed he wishes to move towards (A). Bending his knees and putting his feet flat on the bed, the patient lifts his hips off the bed and moves them sideways (B). He then pulls his shoulders over.

patients in a range of transfer activities. The nurse, with the physiotherapist, is responsible for assisting and teaching the patient how best to move up and down the bed, roll over, assume a sitting position and how to transfer from a bed to a chair. By being aware of the mechanics involved in each of these procedures, the nurse is able to assess the exercise potential of the patient.

Moving up and down the bed (Fig. 13.18). The nurse can use this activity as part of the patient's active ROM exercises. It is important that she position herself correctly, facing the bed which is at the right height for the nurse and flat with the blankets turned down. It is best that the nurse teaches the patient how to move up and down the bed so that he can do it himself.

Lying flat on his back, the patient is asked to reach above his head grasping hold of the top of the bed and to bend his knees and hips. Then the nurse asks him to push with his feet and pull with his arms simultaneously. This movement is repeated until the patient has moved up into position. The nurse could offer assistance to hemiplegic patients by helping to raise the paralysed hip and moving it up the bed, but not by hitching her arm under the patient's arm.

Moving sideways in bed (Fig. 13.19). After preparing the bed and checking the patient's cardiac signs, the nurse asks the patient, who is lying in the supine position, to put one hand on the raised cotside or the side of the bed (Fig. 13.19A) at about his shoulder level. She then gets him to bend his knees and put his feet flat on the bed. The patient is next asked to lift his hips off the bed by pushing on the mattress with his feet and shifting his hips sideways before putting them down on the bed and relaxing (Fig. 13.19B). The nurse then asks the patient to pull his shoulder over.

For hemiplegic patients there may be some difficulty in moving the involved leg in bed. To move it, the patient should be told to place his uninvolved foot under his involved ankle. He then is asked to lift the uninvolved leg just enough to clear the bed and moves the involved leg along with it. Likewise the upper extremity is moved by the uninvolved arm, by grasping it at the wrist. Hemiplegic patients can be helped by the nurse to practise lifting their buttocks off the bed in the following way: the nurse holds the patient's knees and feet in a flexed position and gives him assistance to clear his buttocks off the bed by sliding her hand underneath them. By encouraging the performance of such movements, the nurse is helping to strengthen his hip flexor muscles, his hamstring muscles, his buttock, back and abdominal muscles.

Rolling in bed (Fig. 13.20). Another important activity is teaching the patient how to roll over to one side of the bed. If the patient is being asked to roll to the right hand side, the nurse should position herself on the left hand side of the bed, just off centre. The patient is asked to cross one leg over the other (if the patient is turning to the right,then the left leg goes over the right leg). The left arm is crossed over the chest and grasps the cotside or mattress

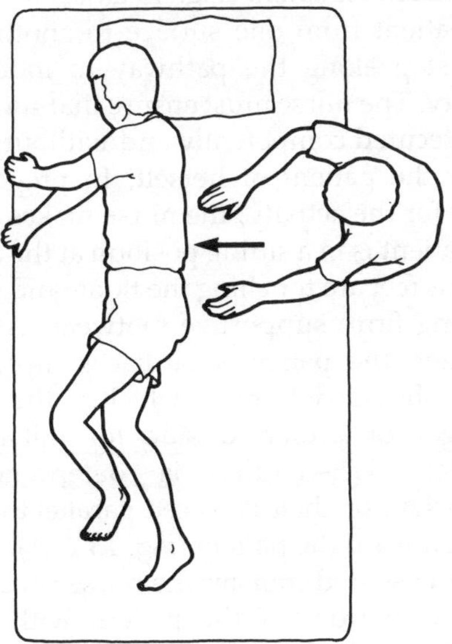

Fig. 13.20 Rolling over in bed. The patient crosses the far leg over the near one, the far arm grasps the near side of the bed. The nurse then helps the patient to pull himself over.

edge. The nurse then helps the patient to pull himself over.

If the patient is hemiplegic, the nurse puts the uninvolved foot under the involved ankle to cross the patient's legs. If the patient cannot roll over by himself the nurse can encourage him to swing his arm or leg across. This will help to create some movement to initiate the roll. The nurse may need to help the patient when he first tries this activity, but as he practises it he ought to be able to manage it independently.

Assuming a sitting position (Fig. 13.21). Before initiating this movement the nurse should check the patient's cardiac symptoms and pulse response. Changing from a prone to an erect position often causes dizziness. The patient can be prepared for sitting up by having to dangle his feet at the bedside for five minutes daily before he gets up to sit. The nurse prepares the scene by putting the bed flat and checking that the patient is wearing shoes and socks. The nurse then puts together the sequence of movements that the patient has already been practising in bed: namely, moving sideways toward the edge of the bed and rolling over in bed (Figs. 13.19 & 13.20). When on his side, the nurse asks the patient to slide his right arm underneath his torso with his elbow in a flexed position. The nurse, who is standing directly in front of the patient, may need to help him get his arm between the mattress and his torso. Then the patient drops his legs off the side of the bed and as his legs move downwards he pushes up with his arms. When his weight is on his right elbow it is shifted to his right hand, all the time the patient is pushing upwards (Fig. 13.21 B,C).

The hemiplegic patient should always roll onto his uninvolved side to sit up. If help is needed, the nurse should be there but ought to encourage him to do as much as he can by himself. Sitting can be a very stressful activity for a debilitated patient and it is important to build up the patient's sitting tolerance from 1–1½ hours per day to anything up to 12–14 hours per day. The nurse can assess this by considering how much time the patient has previously been up, by noting his pulse response and other cardiac symptoms. If the heart beat is over 122 beats per minute on sitting then the activity is too

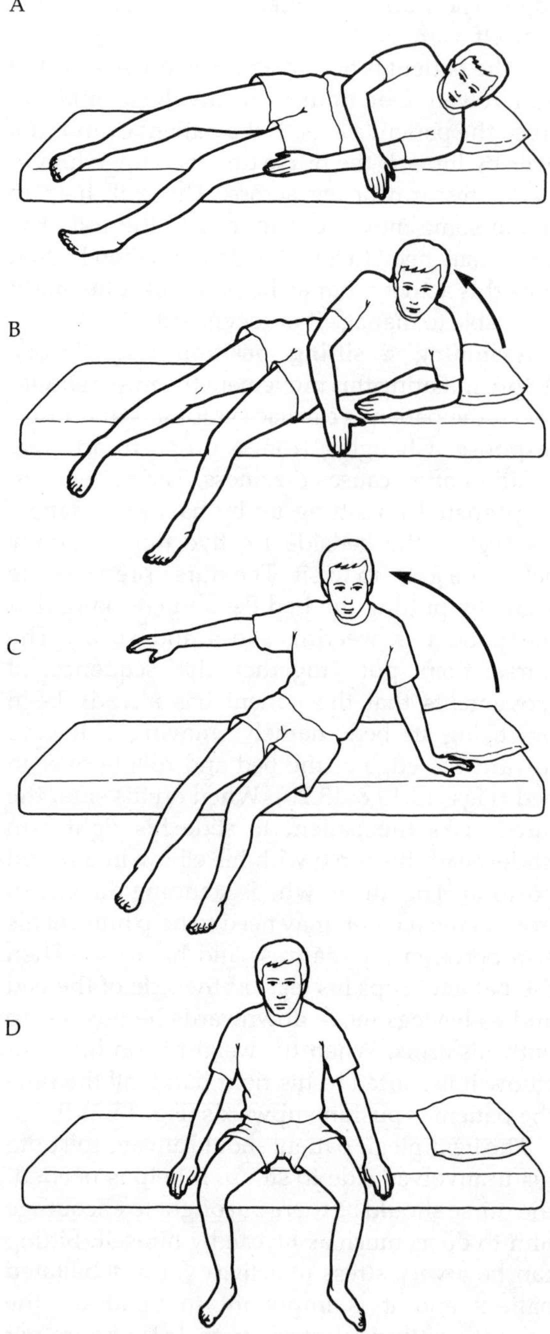

Fig. 13.21 Assuming a sitting position. (A) The patient moves sideways in bed and rolls over (see Figs 13.19 and 13.20). (B) The patient slides his lower arm underneath his torso and raises himself on his elbow. (C) Dropping his legs off the edge of the bed, the patient transfers his weight from his elbow to his hand. (D) The patient should now be sitting on the edge of the bed.

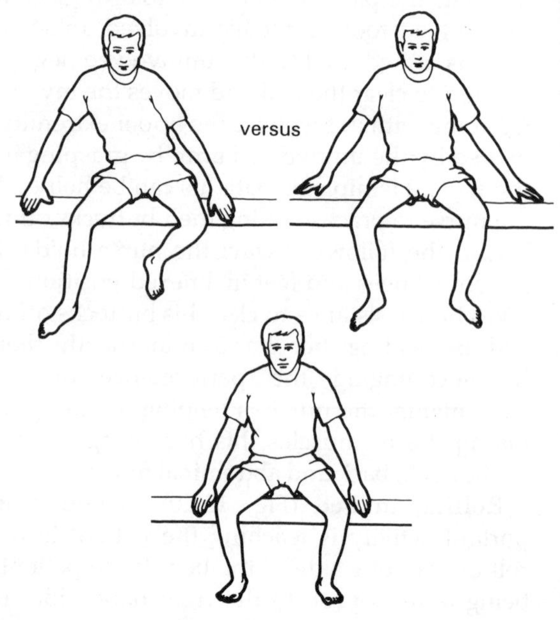

Fig. 13.22 Sitting balance

strenuous. If the pulse rate is 100 beats per minute or less without any other cardiac symptoms then the patient may stay up (Sine et al, 1981) (Fig. 13.22).

Assisted transfers (Fig. 13.23). Transferring the patient from one surface to another is the next step along the pathway to independent activity. The nurse must ensure that such actions are executed competently and without harming either the patient or herself. In preparing the scene for the activity, the nurse makes sure that the patient is in a sitting position at the bed side, that his feet are touching the floor, and that he is wearing firm, supportive footwear. As well as checking the patient's cardiac symptoms, the nurse should determine which is the patient's stronger or preferred side for initiating the transfer. When this is determined, the wheelchair or chair is placed parallel to the bed, facing toward the patient (Fig. 13.23A).

In an assisted transfer the nurse should stand directly in front of the patient with her feet slightly apart. The patient is sitting at the bed side and the nurse bends her hips and knees to the level of the patient and assists him by pulling him up to a standing position by grasping him

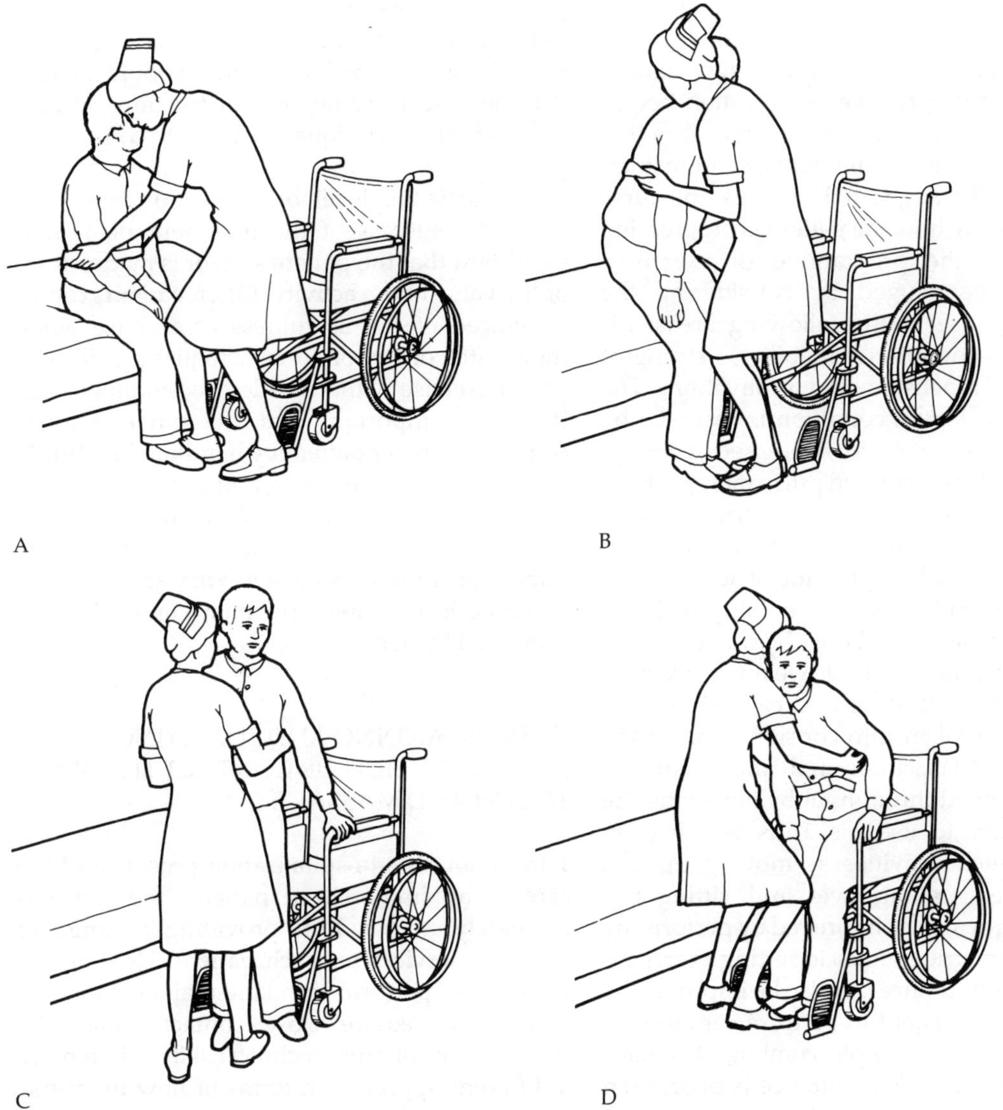

Fig. 13.23 Assisted standing transfer. (A) The assistant bends her knees, putting her hips and knees at the same level as the patient's. Grasping the transfer belt from underneath, she moves the patient to the edge of the bed. (B) The assistant's knees support the patient's knees while the patient comes to a standing position. (C) Still supporting the knees, the assistant pivots the patient around so that his bottom is just above the chair seat. (D) Continuing to brace the patient's knees against her own, the assistant lowers the patient into the chair, still holding the transfer belt for stability.

round the waist (Fig. 13.23B). If the patient has weakness at the knees, the nurse can brace her knee against the patient's weak knee in order to stabilize it. Once in a standing position, the nurse helps the patient to pivot round so that his bottom is poised above the chair seat (Fig. 13.23C,D). He then leans gently forward and lowers himself into the chair, guided and supported by the nurse. As the patient gets stronger, he will require progressively less help. Gradually a time will come where the nurse can stand further away while the activity is being performed. It is important that the nurse only gives assistance when it is required.

Evaluation

In all aspects of patient activity it is important to remember that progressive mobilization begins on the day of admission with a plan of care that comprises preventive, maintenance and restorative measures. Throughout the process the nurse must be assessing how the patient is progressing in relation to the programme of exercises. Success can be gauged by considering the patient's response in the following areas: his physiological condition, mobility, strength, balance, comprehension and motivation. The patient's physiological condition is assessed by his physical reaction to increased activity. Symptoms such as increased pulse rate, postural hypotension, a feeling of nausea, dizziness and fainting would alert the nurse to the need to reassess the planned programme of activity.

The patient's prior level of mobility will also affect the exercise goals set by the nurse, in that any joint limitations or muscle weakness existing before the hospitalization or treatment period will have to be taken into consideration in the setting of goals. Muscle strength and endurance can be determined throughout by observing the patient's ability to use his arms and legs in performing such activities as moving up and down the bed, rolling over and sitting up. Muscle strength may be improved by performing a range of isometric or muscle setting exercises. Strength and endurance can also be improved by encouraging the patient to perform certain self-care activities, for example combing his hair, washing his face. If his endurance is poor, then periods of rest between scheduled activities can be introduced. Balance is of vital importance in helping an immobile patient become independent again. The nurse can help the patient practise balancing while seated at the edge of the bed, standing in front of him to provide support.

The patient's level of comprehension and the clarity and consistency with which exercises and activities are explained are important factors in evaluation of the success of the treatment programme. It is important that the patient is taught a sequence of movements one step at a time. The nurse ought to use short commands only and repeat the same instruction until the patient understands, using gestures and praising the patient when he has achieved something new. All personnel should ensure that they use the same set of instructions and the same transfer techniques so as not to confuse the patient.

The patient's level of motivation may also affect the success of the treatment plan. It is important that the patient sees or is made aware of the value of the activity. Often patients can be convinced of the usefulness of exercise when they watch others or when activities are done as group exercise with an added social dimension. It is also important that the nurse inspires confidence in her patient by handling him firmly and competently, praising and encouraging him and taking time with him, allowing him time to talk out his fears and frustrations. In this way the nurse transforms a set of everyday actions into a therapeutic treatment regimen controlled and evaluated by her.

UNDERSTANDING AND SUPPLYING THE PATIENT'S NEED FOR CONTACT THROUGH TOUCH AND MASSAGE

Throughout the hospitalization process and the care of an immobilized patient, the nurse is intimately involved in providing a range of personal services for each patient. Helping the patient to perform fundamental activities of living will require close contact whilst the performance of more technical skills will require a different approach in terms of how the nurse moves, positions, makes contact with and manipulates the patient. All the time she should be aware of the social and cultural context within which both she and the patient operate, noting that many of the more intimate procedures which she is required to do, are permitted by the patient because of the nature of his incapacity. In order to make these interactions as therapeutic as possible, the nurse must know something about the effect she has on the patient when she comes in contact with him. Touch is a medium through which the nurse constantly communicates and thus it is important to recognize the effect she has and how she can use the interaction to help the patient.

Touch as communication

Touch has been described as the most fundamental means of communication (Barnett, 1972 a&b), delivering the simplest and most straightforward of all messages (Geldard, 1960). In all human cultures the touching of another is evidence of affection and friendliness. Avoidance of touching another indicates the withdrawal of affection or social rejection. Touching has been found to have a positive influence on perceptual and cognitive functions and an environment enriched with sensory stimulation can produce an accompanying and proportional increase in development (Cratty, 1974). Brody (1956) and Casler (1965) found that infants who received an extra 20 minutes of handling each day demonstrated a greater visual attention than those not handled as much.

Whilst it is accepted that touch represents an all-pervasive, all-positive attribute of interaction, it is important that the nurse knows how to evaluate the effect she has on the integrity and well-being of the patient. The meaning a touch will have between a therapist and a patient will be determined by a number of factors: namely, the frequency of the interactions, cultural norms, personality factors and the amount of trust the patient has in the nurse's skills and abilities.

The meaning of touch

Weiss (1979) believes that the meaning of touch or tactile interaction between the nurse and a patient cannot be derived totally from merely the presence or absence of touching. She has outlined six ways touch can be described.

The duration of touch. The duration of a touch refers to the temporal length of the touch, from the initiation of the contact to its cessation. According to Montagu (1971), the length of time in a touch can help the individual develop a greater awareness of his own body. Short durations are likely to occur below the level of self awareness whilst longer contact appears to allow the body time to experience the sensory stimulation provided by another human being. Weiss (1975) found that longer durations of touching have been shown to nurture a knowledge of body detail and body boundaries, and to develop a high level of body esteem.

Location of touch. A second criterion used to judge the effect of touch on the patient is a consideration of location, or the area of the body being stimulated. Weiss (1979) identifies three components in location:

- the threshold or the degree of innervation within the body area and the resulting sensitivity of the body to touch
- the extent or the number of areas of the body being touched in relation to the number of areas available to be touched
- the centripetality or the degree to which the trunk of the body is touched rather than the limbs.

In considering the location of touch, the nurse has to consider cultural norms and sexual connotations related to body contact. Also, if a part of the body carries stigma as a result of a physical defect, e.g. paralysed or contracted limb, the degree of contact with the body part by others can be significantly influenced. For example, Murray (1972) and Watson (1970) found that the more sensitive areas of the body often acquire overtones of disgust or fear in an individual because of the nature or actual lack of physical contact they have received. Patients suffering from paralysis with concomitant incontinence may have to overcome strong feelings of disgust or loss of self-esteem resulting from having to accept continual assistance from the nurse or other carers.

Speed of touch. The way in which the action is carried out may also affect the patient's response. The action can be abrupt or gradual, graded according to the speed or rate of approach to the body. An abrupt approach by the nurse or therapist may cause muscular resistance or a spastic muscle response which determines a different degree of discrimination in neural representation than is found in a more gradual action (Zubeck, 1969). Weiss (1975) found that rapid onset of approach in a touch was highly related to body esteem and perceptions of oneself as an independent, sexual individual.

Intensity of touch. Linked to the way in which the action is carried out is the intensity of the tactile stimulation. Touch can either be described as strong, moderate or weak, depending on whether the degree of skin indentation caused by the touch is deep, shallow or barely perceptible. Geldard (1972) and Weiss (1975) found that moderate intensity of touch was least therapeutic and that variation in the type of intensity, including both strong and weak touching, helped to improve body esteem.

Frequency of touch. The frequency of tactile stimulation refers to the overall amount of touching which an individual experiences in his everyday life. Montagu (1971) linked frequency of touch with changes in the individual's metabolism, intestinal mobility, glandular, biochemical and muscular changes. Frequency of touch has also been found to have positive psychological and emotional value, in that high frequency of touching relates to having a high positive regard and self-esteem (Burnside, 1973; Casler, 1965; Frank, 1957).

Sensation of touch. Finally, the degree of comfort or discomfort experienced by the individual describes the sensation of touch. Sensations in the body can be broadly divided into two groups: those sensations which are designed to warn body tissue of potential harm by effecting somatic discomfort or pain, and those sensations which are concerned with higher discriminative functions related to pleasurable sensations. Shilder (1950) and Tyler (1972) found that when a patient experiences a series of uncomfortable or painful sensations his body image is distorted and his ability to experience pleasurable sensations is diminished. Conversely Brody (1956) and Weiss (1975) found that pleasurable tactile interaction allowed for maximal discrimination and provided vital information for the development of a positive attitude to one's body image.

The therapeutic use of touch in nursing

It is important that the nurse is aware of the different nuances and reactions she may unknowingly evoke in a patient by the way in which she performs a nursing procedure. The following discussion will focus on this notion of the nurse being in a position to affect the patient either in a positive or negative way by the manner in which she initiates or responds to tactile stimulation. Therapeutic touch is seen as that form of tactile interaction which is deliberative and responsive to the clearly identified needs of the patient. It may be seen in terms of helping to build up a more positive body image through acceptance, demonstrated by touching, of a disfigured limb or body part; or conversely therapeutic touch may describe the way a nurse responds to a patient's emotional distress by holding his/her hand. Finally therapeutic touch is seen as a means whereby the nurse can encourage the patient to feel more relaxed by using techniques such as massage or other methods of treatment which induce relaxation.

Deliberative touch

It is part of the nurse's function to have continued and intimate contact with patients. In this position she can increase the physical and emotional adaptation of patients through messages of reassurance and support which she communicates as she performs certain physical procedures. The act may simply be moving a patient in bed, but the way in which the nurse makes contact with the patient, the confidence, authority or hesitancy with which she performs the procedure will be transmitted to the patient, either reinforcing fears about his own well-being or inspiring him with confidence. The nurse must also attempt to understand the patient's own frame of reference in relation to tactile stimulation. Barnett (1972b) found that marked cultural differences exist in the frequency and interpretation of tactile interaction between patient and nurse. It is important therefore that the nurse is aware of the patient's normal tactile pattern. She can do this by observing the degree of physical contact between the patient and his spouse and other members of the family. Some individuals are more demonstrative and touch more frequently; others prefer to communicate their feelings in less overt ways.

The intimate zone. The nurse must also

remember that she has been permitted to enter the patient's 'intimate zone' (Hall, 1966), that space from the patient's body and extending to a distance of 3–4 feet (1–1.3 m) from his person. This zone is normally reserved for close, intimate expressions of emotions such as love, comforting and protecting another individual. Yet by the very nature of her job, the nurse has been allowed relatively free access to the patient's body. Consequently she must take note of the effect her presence has on the patient and consciously work out ways of helping him cope with the situation. Jourard (1964) has identified a further problem for the nurse in attempting to provide a meaningful and therapeutic experience for the patient when he states that 'one of the latent functions of the bedside manner is to reduce the probability that patients will behave in ways that are likely to threaten the nurse'. If this is the case, then again the nurse has to take more seriously the potential effect she may have on the patient when she treats him.

Body integrity. The stage of development and pathological condition of the patient will also affect the way in which the nurse will make contact. In the case of a hemiplegic patient who may be denying the affected side, the nurse may need to concentrate on moving, manipulating and massaging the paralysed side, all the time drawing the patient's attention to the body parts. For a disabled patient or for someone who has undergone radical surgery and finds their altered body image unacceptable and disgusting, the nurse is faced with the difficult task of helping the patient accept or come to terms with the situation. By gently and confidently taking hold of, or feeling, or massaging the body part, the nurse can demonstrate her acceptance of the part, thus encouraging the patient to do likewise. Patients who have undergone surgery which has altered their body image, particularly in terms of their sexual identity (e.g. mastectomy patients or patients with stomas), require sensitive and careful preparation and support. Again it is important that the nurse does not react in a negative way to the patient through such ordinary reactions as a hesitant gesture or a facial expression of fear or disgust. Rather the nurse has to communicate to the patient a sense of their body wholeness and integrity.

Non-necessary touch. That the nurse has a special responsibility to the patient in this area was demonstrated by Barnett (1972b), who studied the utilization of touch by health team personnel with hospitalized patients. She focused on the amount of 'non-necessary' touch utilized by doctors, nurses and other health team personnel and found that nurses touched patients more frequently than any other group of health personnel. Parts of the patient's body which were touched most frequently included the hand, forehead, shoulder and abdomen. In total, Barnett found that 60% of non-necessary touches occurred on the patient's extremities, i.e. there was a low level of centripetality or touching of the trunk. Barnett also found that paediatric wards, labour wards, the intensive care unit and recovery rooms were the clinical areas where most touching occurred, whilst patients in psychiatric wards, surgical and post-natal wards received least touch.

The occurrence of touch in relation to the patient was also found to vary: those patients classified as 'good' or 'fair' received 70% of all occurrences of touch, whilst patients classed as being in a 'serious' or 'critical' condition received 30% of touch. Barnett speculated that this finding may be linked with health workers' fear of death and their inability to provide emotional support necessary for acutely ill patients. Touch was also found to be least frequent with children from the age of 8–17 years and adults between 41–47 years. Infants up to the age of 12 months received most touch. Female patients were touched more frequently than male patients.

From Barnett's study it would seem that nurses respond to patients in a way that few other health team members do. The increase in non-necessary touch may be a direct result of the more intimate relationship between the nurse and patient. Consequently it is important that the nurse perceives such interaction as purposeful, where she in one sense is encouraging self disclosure by increasing the amount of physical contact between herself and the patient (Jourard & Rubin, 1968). If the nurse does see her actions as therapeutic, then she must consider the logistical problem of a number of nurses being involved in caring for the same patient whereby the trust and confidence built up between a nurse and a patient may be undermined by a lack of continuity in the relationship.

A second point from Barnett's work is the observation that tactile interaction seems to be influenced by such factors as the condition of the patient, their age, sex and race. Again, if the nurse perceives herself as acting in a therapeutic way then such factors ought not to determine the duration, frequency and character of the tactile interaction.

Massage

Body massage is thought to have a positive effect on both the physiological function of the body and on the psyche. Massage is described as the rhythmic movement of skin and underlying soft tissues by hand or by a device (Boroch, 1976). Through the reflex effects initiated in the skin by massage, muscles are relaxed and arterioles are either dilatated or constricted; the return flow of blood and lymph is increased by the mechanical effect of massage. General massage causes peripheral vasodilatation with a visible reddening and slight elevation of temperature of the area being manipulated. With the dilatation of capillaries there is increased permeability so that interchange of fluid and solids between the blood stream and tissue is accelerated. With the continued movement of the superficial tissue there is an increase in the number of sensory impulses carried to the spinal cord segments and to the brain from the peripheral nervous system. This facilitation helps in re-establishing the effectiveness of nerve pathways and in the repatterning of reflex arcs.

Massage is useful in loosening and dissolving soft tissue adhesions, in reducing swelling of superficial tissues and in stretching tightened tendons and stiff joints. There are six main types of massage:

- effleurage
- friction
- pressure
- kneading
- vibration
- percussion.

The aim of each of these is to reduce tension and release elasticity of spastic muscles, to relieve pain, promote relaxation and provide non-verbal communication through touching. Massage does not increase muscle tone (Beard & Wood, 1964); its main purposes are to help the patient relax and to promote a feeling of well-being. The nurse may initiate and carry out a range of massage techniques, either incorporating them into certain aspects of her daily routine, for example massaging the patient whilst giving him a towel bath (Barsevick & Llewellyn, 1982), or in conjunction with the physiotherapist, devising a massage regimen most beneficial to the patient.

Thus, in terms of effecting a positive change in the patient's condition through touch or tactile interaction the nurse's activity may be divided into two distinct areas. She may effect a positive change through the use of a well-defined manipulative technique such as massage, whereby rhythmic movement of the skin induces a range of physiological and relaxation inducing responses; she may help her patient to relax by using less well-defined means related to the duration, frequency, location and intensity of her tactile interaction with the patient. By being aware of her effect on the patient through touch, the nurse is able to develop a set of tactile responses which will communicate such emotions as acceptance, warmth, compassion, encouragement and concern. By this means physiological and psychological responses similar to those achieved with massage are obtained, as measured by levels of relaxation (Wells, 1982; Barsevick & Llewellyn, 1982), but they are achieved through less focused activities. Rather, the reduced levels of muscle tension are more a result of the continual interaction and the development of the nurse's therapeutic relationship with the patient. From this perspective, touch is seen as an essential therapeutic tool for nursing staff, not confined to the performance of techniques such as massage but comprising an integral part of the nurse's therapeutic function. This interpretation of the nurse's role in touch as a physical therapy must be distinguished from what has been called therapeutic touch, or the art of interpersonal energy transfer for the purpose of healing (Krieger et al, 1979).

Therapeutic touch

The concept of therapeutic touch has developed beyond the notion of a therapist and patient interacting in a purposeful and deliberate way; further, it has been viewed as a method of healing or positive energy transfer, where the therapist (or nurse) is able to effect a positive change in the patient's well-being. Therapeutic touch, according to Turton (1984), is another name for psychic or faith healing which has been practised over the centuries. The use of therapeutic touch has been linked with nursing by Krieger (1973, 1975, 1976, 1979), whose pioneering work in America has led to a growing interest in the subject.

Research base for therapeutic touch. The justification of therapeutic touch as a treatment modality is based on Krieger's belief that all human beings possess an innate potential to be healers, and that a person's body is surrounded by an energy field which in good health is sufficient, but in bad health is depleted. Therapeutic touch, according to Krieger, is based on the assumption that the healer can act as a channel transferring energy to the patient. The scientific basis of Krieger's assumption and consequent analysis of the effectiveness of therapeutic touch have been questioned (Schlotfeld, 1973, Clark & Clark, 1984).

Krieger (1976) stated that the effect of therapeutic touch could be measured in the patient by recording the increased levels of haemoglobin which occurred after the patient had been treated through therapeutic touch. She used this physiological indicator as a measure of the positive or healing effect the therapist had on the patient, postulating that the healer facilitates a flow of healing energy from his/her body to that of the patient. She also claimed that this energy is bound to oxygen in the blood stream. The haemoglobin level was chosen as an indicator of this energy flow because, according to Krieger (1976), haemoglobin is one of the body's most sensitive indicators of oxygen uptake. Clark & Clark (1984) have questioned this basic premise, commenting that the level of haemoglobin in the body is not a measure of oxygen uptake but rather a measure of oxygen capacity. A more appropriate measure of oxygen uptake, if that was what Krieger had wanted to measure, would have been the oxygen saturation level of the blood.

Clark & Clark (1984) also raised a number of doubts about other assumptions Krieger (1973, 1975, 1978, 1979) made in the development of her study design. Krieger had used the work of Grad (1965, 1967) and Smith (1972) to develop a scientific basis for the study of the effect of a 'faith healer' on the robustness of groups of wounded mice and on the growth of barley and rice seedlings. She justified the use of human haemoglobin as an indicator of therapeutic touch by comparing it to the role of plant chlorophyll, stating that Grad (1965) had found treated seeds to have a greater net weight and significantly more chlorophyll content than non-treated seedlings. Clark & Clark (1984) comment that it is difficult to know how this conclusion was reached, in that the measures Grad (1963) had reported using were the mean number, height and yield of plants. He did not report any measure of the chlorophyll content.

Krieger (1973) had also referred to studies carried out by Smith (1972) who examined the potential effect of a healer and a magnetic field on enzyme activity. Smith hypothesized that cellular metabolism involves specific enzyme activity and supposed that illness could be a result of the absence or dysfunction of enzyme activity. Clark & Clark (1984) report that there was no conclusive evidence to support the hypothesis that a healer can increase the enzyme activity of a solution. Krieger (1976), however, used Smith's study as evidence to support the use of haemoglobin, arguing that Smith's study indicated that enzyme systems responded to laying-on-of-hands.

Clark & Clark (1984) continue their criticism of Krieger's approach by drawing attention to certain methodological weaknesses in her research design. First, she omitted to report the manner in which the experimental and control groups in her study were selected. She also failed to control such independent variables as whether the patients being observed in the experimental and control groups were on medication, a factor which may have affected the haemoglobin level. Other criticisms involve Krieger's apparent lack of utilization of a range of physiological variables such as galvanic skin resistance, pulse, temperature and other indicators of the effect of therapeutic touch on the patient.

Krieger's work was also criticized for omitting to take account of the 'placebo effect'. As the therapeutic touch technique comprised a set of specific actions performed by the nurse on the patient, it could be argued that it was the contact rather than the healing powers or the energy transfer which effected a change in the patient. As Krieger (1973) had not set up a group receiving the action without the 'energy transfer', the results were still ambiguous as to whether it was the contact or the energy transfer which made the difference. Randolph (1984) attempted to separate these two factors by exposing both the control and experimental group to an identical set of tactile stimuli. The treatment of both groups was the placement of practitioners' hands on the subjects' abdomen and back. The experimental group was presumed to have received the hypothesized energy transfer involved in therapeutic touch whilst the control group did not receive any energy transfer. The results of the study showed no difference in the post-treatment measures employed to assess anxiety levels of either group.

Clark & Clark (1984) conclude from these observations that the current research base supporting continued nursing practice of therapeutic touch is at best weak. Results from double blind studies (Randolph, 1984) have shown transient results supporting Krieger's claims of the benefits of therapeutic touch.

Value of touch. Whilst Krieger's claims are somewhat suspect, it is likely that the nurse can still effect a positive change in the patient's level of well-being by knowing how best to communicate and interact with him. Thus it would not be inappropriate for the nurse to possess, as part of her general therapeutic function, the ability to enhance the patient's self-esteem or body image by the way she performs certain activities with and for him. Part of the process would include her knowledge of the effect of tactile stimulation on patient well-being, and her need to communicate at a tactile level in order to transmit such feelings as support, comfort, trust and empathy.

Jourard (1964) believes that people get better because they have faith in the symbols and rituals of the hospital and health team. When the patient has tangible proof that he is a unique and worthy individual and is treated as such by everyone, he experiences a rise in spirit that in some way helps his body to throw off illness. Touch is a basic means of communication and one which is least open to the masking of true feelings. This may be the reason why patients respond most positively to tactile stimulation which is focused and deliberative. Rather than attributing the resulting improvement in the patient's condition to energy transfer, one could explain the change in terms of one human being responding in a positive, empathetic, knowledgeable and therapeutic way to another. It may also be the result of a decrease in the physiological stress response (Ch. 8). In this sense, touch is seen as a basic nursing skill for all practitioners to utilize in a positive and therapeutic way.

CONCLUSION

The focus of this chapter has rested on the singular contribution the nurse has to make in devising, controlling and carrying out physical methods of therapy. The nurse's role in this area is least dramatic in that she must attend to the prevention of complications and guard against any deterioration in the patient's level of mobility, striving to maintain function at its optimal level. In attempting to achieve these goals, the nurse must develop a range of skills and a level of expertise in four main areas.

First, she must be aware of the dangers of

induced immobility, either of the whole body or parts of it; she must have at her disposal a thorough and working knowledge of how to position patients correctly in bed and how to maintain optimal joint mobility. Once these skills have been mastered, the nurse must then be able to assess the individual requirements of each patient according to his or her level of self-care, medical condition and prognosis. A second important nursing skill is to be able to exercise the patient by incorporating a range of motion exercises into daily self-care activities, or by devising group exercise activities.

Finally, the nurse must also be taught how to help patients to relax. This may be achieved through the use of such techniques as massage, or by devising and organizing exercise programmes at certain times of the day. The nurse can also use her normal course of interactions with the patient to help relaxation by ensuring that through touch she is communicating a sense of acceptance, warmth and reassurance as well as professional competence to the patient.

The nurse's action in terms of carrying out a range of physical therapies is not dependent on a range of gadgets or pieces of equipment. Whilst it is in the domain of the physiotherapist to devise exercises which build up muscle strength and tension, the nurse's primary concern is to maintain the body at its optimal level of function throughout the rehabilitation period. As rehabilitation develops and the patient grows stronger, so the nurse's actions will change. In the initial stages of any patient's illness, however, it is the nurse who is the primary physical therapist whose level of knowledge and skill may have a considerable effect on the eventual prognosis and level of recovery of the patient.

REFERENCES

Baekeland F, Lasky R 1966 Exercise and sleep patterns in college athletes. Perceptual and Motor Skills 23:1203

Barclay V, Collier R J, Jones A 1983 Electromagnetic energy. Physiotherapy 69(6):186–188

Barnett K 1972a A theoretical construct of the concepts of touch as they relate to nursing. Nursing Research 21:102–110

Barnett K 1972b A survey of the current utilization of touch by health team personnel with hospitalized patients. International Journal of Nursing Studies 9:195–209

Barsevick A, Llewellyn J 1982 A comparison of the anxiety reducing potential of two techniques of bathing. Nursing Research 31:22-27

Beard G, Wood E 1964 Massage: principles and techniques. W B Saunders, Philadelphia

Boroch R M 1976 Elements of rehabilitation in nursing. C V Mosby, St Louis

Boyle D McC, Barber J M, Walsh M J et al 1972 Early mobilization and discharge of patients with acute myocardial infarction. Lancet 2:57–60

Bradley D 1970 Fractures of the upper end of the femur 2: treatment. Nursing Times 66:1552–1555

Brody S 1956 Patterns of mothering. International Universities Press, New York

Brower P, Hicks D 1972 Maintaining muscle function in patients on bed rest. American Journal of Nursing 72:1250–1253

Browse N L 1965 The physiology and pathology of bed rest. Thomas, Springfield, Illinois

Burnside I M 1973 Caring for the aged: touching is talking. American Journal of Nursing 73:2060–2063

Casler L 1965 Effects of extra tactile stimulation on a group of institutionalized infants. Genetic Psychology Monographs 71:137–175

Chalmers T C 1969 Rest and exercise in hepatitis. New England Journal of Medicine 281:1421–1422

Clark P E, Clark M J 1984 Therapeutic touch: is there a scientific basis for the practice? Nursing Research 33:37–41

Coe W S 1954 Cardiac work and the chair treatment of acute coronary thrombosis. Annals of Internal Medicine 40:42–48

Cratty B J 1974 Motor activity and the education of retardates, 2nd edn. Lea and Febiger, Philadelphia

Danskin D G, Crow M A 1981 Biofeedback. An introduction and guide. Mayfield Publishing Company

De Weerdt W J G, Harrison M A 1985 The use of biofeedback in physiotherapy. Physiotherapy 71(1):9–12

Forster A, Palastanga N 1985 Clayton's electrotherapy. Baillière Tindall, London

Frank L K 1957 Tactile communication. Genetic Psychology Monographs 56:211-251

Geldard F 1960 Some neglected possibilities of communication. Science 131:1583–1588

Geldard F 1972 The human senses, 2nd edn. Wiley, New York

Goldberg W G, Fitzpatrick J J 1980 Movement therapy with the aged. Nursing Research 29:339–346

Grad B 1963 A telekinetic effect on plant growth. International Journal of Parapsychology 5:117–133

Grad B 1965 Some biological effects of the laying-on-of-hands: a review of experiments with animals and plants. Journal of the American Society for Psychical Research 59 : 95–127

Grad B 1967 The laying-on-of-hands: implications for psychotherapy gentling and the placebo effect. Journal of the American Society of Psychical Research 61:286–305

Hall E T 1966 The hidden dimension. Doubleday and Company, New York

Harper J E, Kellett R J, Conner W T et al 1971 Controlled trial of early mobilization and discharge from hospital in uncomplicated myocardial infarction. Lancet 2:1331–1334

Harris A 1971 Handicapped and impaired in Great Britain. HMSO, London
Harvey P G 1978 Biofeedback — trick or treatment? Physiotherapy 64(11):333–335
Health and Equipment Information 1980 77/80 Microwave diathermy is safe in normal use. No. 88, September
Henderson V, Nite G 1978 Principles and practice of nursing, 6th edn. Macmillan, New York
Huddlestone D L 1961 Therapeutic exercises, kinaestherapy. F A Davis, Philadelphia
Jacobson E 1964 Anxiety and tension control: a physiological approach. Lippincott, Philadelphia
Jourard S 1964 The transparent self. Van Nostrand, New York
Jourard S, Rubin J E 1968 Self disclosure and touching; a study of two modes of interpersonal encounter and their inter-relation. Journal of Humanistic Psychology 8:39–48
Kelly M 1966 Exercises for bedfast patients. American Journal of Nursing 66:2209–2213
Kottke F J 1971 Therapeutic exercises. In: Krusen F H et al (eds) Handbook of physical medicine and rehabilitation, 2nd edn. W B Saunders, Philadelphia
Kraus H 1963 Therapeutic exercise, 2nd edn. Thomas, Springfield, Illinois
Krieger D 1973 The relationship of touch with intent to help or heal to subjects' in vivo haemoglobin values: a study in personalized interaction. In: Proceedings of North American Nurses Association. Ninth Nursing Research Conference, San Antonio, Texas, March 21–23
Krieger D 1975 Therapeutic touch: the imprimatur of nursing. American Journal of Nursing 5:784–787
Krieger D 1976 Healing by the 'laying on' of hands as a facilitator of bioenergetic change: the response of in-vivo human haemoglobin. Psychoenergic Systems 1:121–129
Krieger D 1979 Therapeutic touch: how to use your hands to help and heal. Prentice Hall, Englewood Cliffs, New Jersey
Krieger D, Peper E, Ancoli S 1979 Therapeutic touch, searching for evidence of physiological change. American Nurses Association 79:660–662
Lamb K 1979 Effect of positioning of post-operative fractured hip patients as related to comfort. Nursing Research 28:291–294
Lang S H, Zawacki A M, Johnson A E 1976 Reducing discomfort from intra-muscular injections. American Journal of Nursing 76:800–801
Larson C B, Gould M 1974 Orthopaedic nursing, 8th edn. C V Mosby, St Louis
Lee J M 1978 Aids to physiotherapy. Churchill Livingstone, Edinburgh
Lee J M, Warren M P 1974 Ice, relaxation and exercise in reduction of muscle spasticity. Physiotherapy 60(10):296–302
Lee J M, Warren M P, Mason S M 1978 Effects of ice on nerve conduction velocity. Physiotherapy 64(1):2–6
Lundeberg T 1984 Electrical stimulation for the relief of pain. Physiotherapy 70(3):98–100
Melzack R, Wall P D 1965 Pain mechanisms — a new theory. Science 150:971–979
Mills J A, Pinals R S, Ropes M W et al 1971 Value of bed rest in patients with rheumatoid arthritis. New England Journal of Medicine 284:453–458
Mitchell P H, Ozuna J, Lipe H 1981 Moving the patient in bed: effects on intracranial pressure. Nursing Research 30:212–218
Montagu A 1971 Touching: the human significance of the skin. Columbia University Press, New York
Müller E A 1970 Influence of training and of inactivity on muscle strength. Archives of Physical Medicine and Rehabilitation 51:449–462
Murray R 1972 Principles of nursing intervention for the adult patient with body image changes. Nursing Clinics of North America 7:697–707
Oliver D E 1984 Pulser electro-magnetic energy — what is it? Physiotherapy 70(12):458–459
Perkins G 1953 Rest and movement. Journal of Bone and Joint Surgery 35b:521–539
Pitel M, Wemett M 1964 The intramuscular injection. American Journal of Nursing 64:104–109
Randolph G L 1984 Therapeutic and physical touch: physiological response to stressful stimuli. Nursing Research 33:33–36
Repsher L H, Freebern R K 1969 Effects of early and vigorous exercise in recovery from infectious hepatitis. New England Journal of Medicine 281:1393–1396
Rettig F, Southby J 1982 Using different body positions to reduce discomfort for dorsogluteal injection. Nursing Research 31:219–221
Savage B 1984 Interferential therapy. Faber and Faber, London
Schlotfeld R 1973 Critique of the relationship of touch with intent to help or heal to subjects' in vivo hemoglobin values: a study in personalized interaction. Paper presented at the North American Nurses Association. Ninth Nursing Research Conference, San Antonio, Texas, March 21–23
Shilder P 1950 Image and appearance of the human body. International Universities Press, New York
Sine R D, Holcomb J D, Roush R E, Liss S E, Wilson G B 1981 Basic rehabilitation techniques. A self instructional guide, 2nd edn. Rockville Aspen Publications, Rockville
Smith J 1972 Paranormal effects on enzyme activity. Human Dimensions 1:15–19
Stryker R 1977 Rehabilitative aspects of acute and chronic nursing care. W B Saunders, Philadelphia
Sumner W, Patrick M K 1964 Ultrasonic therapy — a textbook for physiotherapists. Elsevier, Amsterdam
Taylor H L, Henschel A, Brozek J, Keys A 1949 Effects of bed rest on cardiovascular function and work performance. Journal of Applied Physiology 2 : 223–239
Tompkins E S 1980 Effect of restricted mobility and dominance on perceived duration. Nursing Research 26:333-338
Townsend P 1979 Disability in Britain. Martin Robertson, Oxford
Turton P 1984 The laying on of hands. Nursing Times 80:47–48
Tyler N 1972 A stereognostic test for screening tactile sensation. American Journal of Occupational Therapy 26:256–260
Wall P D 1985 The discovery of transcutaneous electrical nerve stimulation. Physiotherapy 71(8):348–350
Watson W 1970 Body image and staff-to-resident deportment in a home for the aged. Ageing Human Development 1(4):345–359
Weiss S J 1975 Familial tactile correlates of body image in children. Unpublished doctoral thesis, University of California, San Francisco
Weiss S J 1979 The language of touch. Nursing Research 28:76–80

Wells N 1982 The effect of relaxation on post-operative muscle tension and pain. Nursing Research 31:236–238
Willie C D 1969 Interferential therapy. Physiotherapy 55(12):503–505
Zelman S 1961 Notes on techniques of intramuscular injection. Hospital Topics 39:79–84
Zubeck J P (ed) 1969 Sensory deprivation. 15 years of research. Appleton-Century-Crofts, New York

14

Dietary therapy and nutritional care

INTRODUCTION

The use of diet in the maintenance of health and the treatment of disease began with the ancient Greeks and Romans. Hippocrates (460–370 BC), the 'father of medicine', was a firm believer that diet was the best way to treat disease and Galen (AD 130–200), a Roman physician, recognized that health depended chiefly on the choice of food. Throughout the ages the importance of diet, in both the prevention and cure of disease, has been recognized, but with the move away from crude plants and foods as therapeutic agents came the movement away from diet as a therapeutic entity, and nutrition was considered 'old fashioned' and 'second class'. However, as the science of nutrition has re-emerged and developed, the emphasis of dietary therapy has been placed on the adequate diet, with modifications to specific nutrients as prescribed by the physician and with modifications to the consistency of the food depending on the condition of the patient. Today dietary therapy is still based on modifications of the 'normal' diet and is under the guidance of the dietician.

Nutritional care, however, goes much further than this to include all the services necessary to enable the scientific principles of nutrition to benefit the health of the individual. In simple terms nutrition is the study of food and food components, their ingestion, absorption, utilization and excretion and their effects on life and health. It is also concerned with the social, cultural, economic and psychological implications of both food and eating. Dietetics, on the other hand, involves the use of food as a factor in aiding recovery from illness by relating the science of nutrition to the symptoms and treatment of disease.

THE NURSE AND NUTRITIONAL CARE

But why does nutritional care involve nurses? It is not commonly recognized that Florence Nightingale, the 'mother of nursing', was also the 'mother of dietetics', establishing the first diet kitchens during the Crimean War. Dieticians at first followed her example and came from within the nursing profession, but this gradually became a specialized field of activity. Nurses reduced their involvement with patients' eating behaviour and now have limited knowledge of this area of patient care.

Yet a large part of nursing care involves meeting basic needs common to all persons sick or well. The framework for a systematic approach to identifying and meeting the patient's needs enables, and requires, the nurse to assist him/her in meeting those needs. Basic biological needs include those for oxygen, fluids, food, elimination of body wastes, rest and sleep. The patient may or may not require assistance in meeting these needs but, when this is required, it must be adapted to the individual. For example, the selection of food to meet individual requirements differs in the case of a young child from that of an adult. Modifications or special assistance may be needed due to the patient's pathological problems and the nurse is the person in the best position to judge when specialized help is required. In other words, the provision of care is directed towards meeting the total health needs of the individual which includes adequate nutrition whether or not specialized dietary therapy is required. The dietician comes into her/his own when dietary modificaton is required.

Thus Henderson (1960) states 'There is no more important element in the preparation for nursing than the study of nutrition', as this aspect of patient care cannot be carried out unless the nurse is adequately prepared to do so. This requires an understanding of normal nutrition, the role of food on life and health, its social and cultural implications, the determinants of food choice and the development of food habits, in addition to a knowledge of current nutritional theories.

NORMAL NUTRITION

NUTRITIONAL NEEDS

The physiological need for food actually represents the need for nutrients — the chemicals obtained from food which allow the proper functioning of the body and each of which has one or more of the following functions:

- providing energy for body processes and activity
- providing structural material
- participating in the regulation of body processes.

Some nutrients are simple elements, such as iron; others are complex molecules, such as proteins. As there are many different nutrients, similar ones are grouped together; thus broad nutrient categories include carbohydrate, protein, fat, vitamins, minerals and water. Table 14.1 shows the sources and functions of these major nutrient groups.

There are, in addition, a number of substances present in foods which cannot be considered to be nutrients but which, nonetheless, play important roles in the diet. Non-nutrient components include fibre, caffeine, alcohol and most food additives.

There are many body compounds which are not found in foods but which are synthesized from particular nutrients in the diet. Only when an abnormal condition prevents adequate synthesis of one of these compounds would it become a dietary essential.

The most basic nutrient need is for water which is vital to all body processes. The next priority is for energy as every body cell requires a continuous supply of fuel. Hunger creates the

Table 14.1 Components of food of nutritional importance

Function	Nutrient	Sources
Supply energy	Carbohydrate	Sugars, syrups, sweets, cereals and cereal products, potatoes and starchy vegetables, fruits
	Fat	Butter, dairy products, cooking fats and oils; margarine, meat and meat products; cheese
	Protein	Expensive and wasteful as an energy source
Synthesize, maintain and repair body tissues	Protein — providing amino acids including essential amino acids	Meat, fish, poultry, eggs, milk, pulses and legumes, cereals and cereal products
	Fat — providing complex lipids and essential fatty acids	From sources shown above
	Minerals — particularly calcium	Milk and milk products, vegetables, meat
	— iron	Lean meat, offal/liver, eggs, leafy green vegetables
Regulate body processes	Minerals, Vitamins } as co-enzymes	All foods supply *some* vitamins or minerals
	Protein } as enzymes and hormones	See above
	Fat — complex lipids — essential fatty acids } as enzymes and hormones	See above

need to eat and is satisfied only by nutrients providing energy, i.e. carbohydrate, fat or protein. The amount of energy a food can supply (measured in kilojoules or kilocalories) is still sometimes described by the term 'caloric value'; foods supplying the same number of kilojoules (kJ) or kilocalories (kcal) will supply the same amount of energy. The vehicle which enables the physiological need for nutrients to be met is food but, as foods differ in their nutrient content, no one food can be depended upon to supply all the nutrients required. Hence the need for a varied diet. The term 'nutritional value' refers to the nutrient content of a specific amount of food.

NON-NUTRITIONAL NEEDS

Food meets many other needs in addition to those for nutrients; it fulfils many social and psychological needs. Storing food may satisfy the need for security; cooking or tasting new foods provides opportunities to meet the need for manipulation and exploration. Following traditional or cultural food habits provides many with a sense of belonging to a particular social group, and eating at an expensive restaurant may create a feeling of self-esteem; creating a new dish may meet the need for self-fulfilment.

FOOD HABITS

Food habits are 'characteristic and repetitive acts performed under the impetus of the need to provide nourishment and meet social and emotional goals' (Gifft et al, 1972). Many of the patterns of eating seen in adult life are established during early life when children depend on others for their food supply.

The development of food habits can be seen in terms of socialization which embraces the actions of imparting culturally valued norms and, more specifically, knowledge, values, attitudes and routines adopted by the society in which we live (Tones, 1978). In nutritional terms the strongest influence is likely to be the mother, who prepares and presents food to the child. Transmission of norms and adoption of routines occurs at this time as the child identifies with the parent's behaviour. The processes of reinforcement, modelling and imitation result in the adoption and integration of new behaviour with previous experience. Children tend to learn through a system of reward and denial, and food often takes on an emotional significance which may well override its nutritional value. In particular, sweet foods are often used as treats, gifts and tokens of affection as well as rewards and bribes.

Later, secondary factors influence behaviour. For example, at school the child is exposed to a wider range of influences and to differing values and opinions. Environmental experiences then become important; school meals set important examples and, because they are presented within the educational setting, may be seen as representative of nutritionally acceptable meals. It is, therefore, important that such meals are of a high standard. As adulthood is reached other factors influence food habits. Peer group values, attitudes and behaviours are frequently adopted by individuals. Certain practices are seen as acceptable or unacceptable either in cultural or social terms, whereas others are promoted as desirable, largely through the mass media;

> Advertising persuades us that the right taste for a food results from a particular concept designed by marketing men, created by food techno-logists and produced in factories with sales potential (Hanssen 1980),

irrespective of the nutritional consequences. Thompson (1978) highlights the profit motive behind the majority of food production by drawing attention to the large sums of money spent on market research and advertising designed to alter food habits.

Established values, attitudes and routines can be difficult to change and require a process of resocialization. Nutritionists believe that nutrition education is primarily concerned with persuading people to eat 'properly'. However, what is 'proper' is not always clear and there are dangers in the educators imposing their own values on other groups. This is particularly true of this field as nutrition is a comparatively new science. Many of its concepts must therefore be regarded as subject to modification as knowledge increases. Nutrition education should, there-fore, confine itself to providing current facts so that individuals have a rational basis for their decisions.

NUTRITION AS A DETERMINANT OF HEALTH

The control of communicable disease by improvements in standards of hygiene and sanitation, combined with the ready availability of antibiotics, has led to considerable changes in the pattern of disease in Britain. Similarly, within the developed countries improvements in the supply and distribution of food have helped to eradicate many of the nutritional deficiency problems previously seen, and advances in nutritional knowledge have led to better recognition of the relationship between nutrition and health (Drummond & Wilbraham, 1939). However, although the risks of deficiency diseases have largely been eliminated, nutritional problems do arise. These may be widespread, such as obesity, or confined to a particular section of the population. Dietary imbalance may arise from a conscious desire to adopt an eating pattern which, although not commensurate with long-term health, is suited to the current lifestyle. This has led to the development of a different type of malnutrition, overnutrition, which has been linked to many of the now common degenerative diseases of the Western world, for example, cardiovascular disease, gastrointestinal disorders, dental caries and periodontal disease. As these are believed to result from the considerable changes in lifestyle they have become known as the 'diseases of modern civilization' or 'diseases of affluence'. Aspects of the nutritional state of particular adult groups are discussed briefly below.

NUTRITIONAL STATES DURING ADULT LIFE

Adolescents

The nutritional intake of a child is largely dependent on what is provided by the mother but, as children become older, they assume more responsibility for their own food intake. At this stage dietary patterns may be influenced by social and psychological factors and by economic considerations — an outline of these is provided by Lennon & Fieldhouse (1979).

Obesity is a common problem believed to affect at least 10% of adolescent girls. Even those who are not overweight however may wish to lose weight. If this results in a restricted food intake then there is cause for concern as inappropriate or excessive attempts at weight loss may precipitate anorexia nervosa (see Ch.23).

Selective nutrient deficiency may arise from poorly balanced diets resulting from restricted food preferences, food aversions, religious beliefs or weight-reducing regimes. The concept of dietary balance depends on consumption of an appropriate mixture of foods which will supply the minimum requirements for nutrients. A diet supplying a limited number of foods is less likely to meet these requirements; thus, by ensuring a varied and unrestricted diet, one item rich in a particular nutrient will 'balance' a deficiency in another.

Common nutritional deficits occurring in adolescence are those of iron and calcium. The adolescent growth spurt increases the demand for iron and, in females, extra iron is needed to compensate for menstrual losses (Heald, 1969). A dislike of iron-rich foods — liver, kidney, lean meat — will reduce the dietary intake predisposing the person to iron deficiency anaemia. Wholegrain cereals, egg yolks, vegetables and fruits can be included in the diet to compensate for a failure to eat iron-rich meats.

Pregnant women

The increased nutritional requirements of pregnancy may precipitate nutritional deficiencies reflecting inadequate intakes over the preceding years or associated with an inadequate intake during pregnancy itself. Poor nutritional intakes tend to be associated with the social classes IV and V and with teenage pregnancy (Smithells et al, 1973).

Although severe nutritional deprivation during pregnancy may have serious effects on the developing fetus, many physiological and nutritional adaptations occur so that a wide range of dietary intakes may be compatible with normal fetal growth and development.

The development of the fetus and placenta, together with the increased maternal red cell volume, increases the requirement for iron so that, when the dietary intake is inadequate, the mother can become severely anaemic. In addition, megaloblastic anaemia may arise as a result of folate deficiency. Chanarin (1973) has suggested that its incidence is a sensitive indicator of the nutritional folate status of a population as it reflects the status before pregnancy, exhibits socioeconomic class differences and shows seasonal variations. Vitamin B_{12} deficiency may also result in megaloblastic anaemia, which can lead to severe deficiencies in the infant, but this is less common.

The elderly

In general, nutritional requirements do not differ greatly with age although, if the level of energy expenditure declines, energy needs may decrease. However, many factors come into play in the elderly which may combine to envelop the individual so that their food intake becomes affected and malnutrition develops (Table 14.2).

From a study in 1972, the DHSS concluded that the number of malnourished elderly people was probably small, about 3% of the population over 65. However, as the number of elderly individuals increases it is possible that this percentage may increase. Exton-Smith (1978) suggests that, although frank malnutrition is rare, subclinical nutritional deficiencies are relatively common.

The nutrients most likely to be deficient in the

Table 14.2 Factors contributing to nutritional deficiency in the elderly

Reduced overall intake	Physical/mental disability Reduced ability to obtain, prepare and eat food Impaired appetite — drug therapy — illness
Disturbed balance of nutrient intake	Inadequate dentition Ignorance Social isolation Alcoholism
Increased or modified requirements	Malabsorption Increased cell destruction or excretion of nutrients Drug therapy

diet of the elderly are vitamins C, D, the B complex and iron. Frank signs of scurvy are rare although the blood levels of vitamin C are commonly found to be low, particularly in widowers suddenly finding they are required to feed themselves and relying heavily on processed convenience foods. Subclinical deficiencies of riboflavin (B_2), thiamin (B_1), and pyridoxine (B_6) are relatively common in elderly individuals (Vir & Love, 1979). Signs of folate deficiency may be present in those living alone under poor economic circumstances, although megaloblastic anaemia through dietary inadequacy is uncommon. It is difficult to assess folate status as there are many interacting factors; for example, deficiency of iron or vitamin C may lead to lower serum folate levels, whilst vitamin B_{12} deficiency may have the opposite effect. There is some evidence that a deficiency of folate may result in malabsorption, which may in turn lead to reduced folate levels thus creating a spiral of decreased intake and decreased absorption.

Vitamin D deficiency can arise from a variety of causes including a poor dietary intake, inadequate exposure to sunlight and malabsorption. Calcium absorption is then impaired and the risk of osteoporosis and pathological fractures increased. Osteomalacia may also be seen (see Ch.21).

CURRENT NUTRITIONAL THEORIES

It is outside the scope of this chapter to discuss in detail all the current hypotheses on diet and disease. However, many such theories have come to the attention of the media and therefore to the attention of the public; nurses must be able to answer the inevitable questions. 1983 saw the publication of 'A Discussion Paper on Proposals for Nutritional Guidelines for Health Education in Britain' (National Advisory Committee on Nutrition Education, (NACNE) 1983), an important document presenting the consensus of views, derived primarily from Government and other major bodies, on what dietary changes would be advisable to promote the maintenance of health and the primary prevention of disease in this country. A summary of the recommendations is given in Table 14.3.

Body weight

The problem of obesity (see Ch.23) has been considered in detail by the Royal College of Physicians (RCP)(1983) in their report on obesity. This report concludes that even mild degrees of overweight are, on a public health basis, important and the risks of obesity are no longer believed to be applicable only to the substantially obese. There is a progressive increase in morbidity and mortality with even small increases in body weight. This is of particular importance in those with a familial tendency to diabetes mellitus and cardiovascular disease and in those already suffering from hypertension.

The RCP calls for a fundamental change in nutrition education so that it is made clear that carbohydrates are not peculiarly fattening

Table 14.3 Long-term dietary proposals (NACNE, 1983)

Energy intake	Should be appropriate to maintain optimal weight for height — must be combined with adequate exercise
Fat intake	To represent 30% of the total energy
Saturated fatty acid intake	To comprise 10% of the total energy (i.e. ⅓ of total fat)
Cholesterol	No recommendation
Sucrose intake	Total sucrose should be reduced from 38 to 20 kg/head/year
Dietary fibre	Average intake should be increased from 20 to 30 g/head/day
Salt intake	Should be decreased, on average, by 3 g/head/day
Alcohol intake	Should comprise only 4% of total energy
'Vulnerable' and 'at risk' groups	Separate information required; supplied by separate government reports
Mineral/vitamin intakes	Should match those intakes recommended by the DHSS (1979)

dietary components and every encouragement is given towards a substantial reduction in the dietary fat intake (see later discussion). A reduction in the sugar (sucrose) intake would also be beneficial as this would limit energy consumption whilst maintaining the nutrient intake.

Carbohydrate with particular reference to dietary fibre

NACNE (1983) advocate an increased consumption of carbohydrates, particularly the complex carbohydrates which are higher in fibre. This approach differs totally from all previous nutritional directives in which restriction of carbohydrate was paramount in any weight reduction regime. However, not all carbohydrates should be regarded in the same light and an increased intake of carbohydrates rich in fibre is now considered nutritionally desirable (Royal College of Physicians, 1981).

Dietary fibre is an aspect of health which, until recently, has received little attention. The Royal College of Physicians' Report on the Medical Aspects of Dietary Fibre (1981) highlighted many of the suggested links between a deficiency of fibre and ill-health, particularly with regard to disorders of the large bowel (e.g. irritable bowel syndrome, diverticular disease, constipation and cancer of the colon). Burkitt (1971) was amongst the first to associate such disease with a fibre deficiency, and human metabolic studies have shown that fibre is a dietary constituent having marked effects on faecal weight (bulk), shortening transit time and reducing intraluminal pressure (Painter, 1969). Dilution of the intestinal content may reduce the contact time of potential carcinogens with the intestinal wall.

Vegetarians consuming a dietary fibre intake in excess of 30 g/day have been shown to have a lower incidence of diverticular disease (Gear et al, 1979), and a high fibre intake is now used to beneficial effect in the treatment of both diverticular disease and constipation. On this basis it is recommended that the daily fibre intake should be at least 30 g/day for adults (DHSS, 1979). This is best derived from 'natural' foods rather than those to which fibre has been added, as this will ensure increased intakes of minerals, trace elements and other necessary micronutrients. It has been suggested that fibre may reduce mineral absorption (Royal College of Physicians, 1981) which could exacerbate existing mineral deficiencies.

Sugar and dental caries

This provides an area of intense controversy amongst the different members of the health care team. Many members of the dental profession advocate dramatic reductions in the sugar intake (Sheiham, 1983) whereas others believe this to be of only minor significance when studied in the context of the complex interacting factors which involve the host, the microbial population and the environment. Dental caries, in this context, is regarded as an infectious oral disease which, although related to the intake of fermentable carbohydrate, can be prevented by the use of fluoride in the water supply, toothpaste and mouthwashes together with scrupulous oral hygiene.

It is interesting to note that this food commodity, which is responsible for a great deal of controversy, is one which is a relatively new addition to our diet. The diet of early man was rich in protein, moderate in fat and low in carbohydrate; it was not until the 17th century that sugar first entered the UK when it was considered a luxury. Sugar consumption has risen during the last 100 years, its present value being 38 kg/head/year (Ministry of Agriculture, Fisheries and Food, 1980) although, as most of the sugar currently consumed is present in manufactured food products, it is difficult to obtain an accurate figure for that consumed by an individual. Sugar is an excellent preservative which inhibits the growth of moulds and bacteria and as such is useful to the food industry particularly as its flavour is acceptable, it is cheap and it is not toxic. There is, therefore, intense commercial pressure to maintain sugar intakes at their current level and, due to the scientific controversy, the evidence for a reduced intake is under dispute.

The DHSS (1978) clearly indicates that sugar

intake is the basis for the development of dental caries. Evidence suggests that, in the process of decay, there is first a build up of plaque on the teeth which is composed of protein, carbohydrate, food particles and deposits from saliva and bacteria. Demineralization of hydroxyapatite, present in the enamel, depends on the acid generated in the plaque by the action of bacterial enzymes on the fermentable carbohydrates contained within it. The pH within the plaque can fall as low as 4.5–5.0 within 1–3 minutes and it can take between 10 and 30 minutes for this to approach neutrality. This level of acidity is sufficient to produce a marked increase in the solubility of the tooth enamel.

However, in view of the many factors contributing to the development of dental caries (which include the frequency of the sugar intake, the degree of salivary flow, the 'stickiness' of food, the degree of fluoridation and the care taken over dental hygiene), epidemiological studies have failed to demonstrate a clear causal relationship between sugar and dental caries. Other workers (e.g. Hargreaves, 1980; Burt & Ekland, 1980) have concluded that it is the form and frequency rather than the amount of sugar consumed which is more important and, for this reason, the DHSS (1978) advocates a specific reduction in sugar intake between meals and, therefore, a reduction of sugar in the form of confectionery, soft drinks and snacks.

Sugar and other diseases

In addition to its role in dental caries, sugar has been implicated in the aetiology of other disease states including ischaemic heart disease (IHD) and diabetes mellitus (Trowell, 1972). Yudkin (1972) in his book *Pure, White and Deadly* suggests that, whilst IHD is clearly of multifactorial aetiology, sugar is an important factor as the rise in deaths from the disease closely follows the rise in sugar consumption. Yudkin (1957) also relates the number of individuals dying from diabetes to the amount of sugar and fat consumed some 20 years earlier, finding a high correlation with sugar but not with fat. He was not, however, the first to suggest such a relationship; Stocks (1944) first drew attention to the decline in diabetic mortality during the two world wars, which he linked with a decrease in sugar consumption.

Although many factors, some nutritional, are involved in the aetiology of diseases such as obesity, IHD and diabetes mellitus, sugar clearly plays a part and is a part of the diet which could be omitted without upsetting the nutritional balance or creating any deficiency.

Fats (lipids)

Triglycerides and fatty acids

The term lipids refers to many fat-like and waxy compounds but, as dietary constituents, the triglycerides are of primary importance as the majority of fat in foods is in this form (Holmes, 1983). Each triglyceride comprises three molecules of fatty acid combined with one molecule of glycerol; there are many different fatty acids and it is these which give foods their particular characteristics. The various types of triglyceride result from the combination of different fatty acids with glycerol. There are three types of fatty acids: saturated, monosaturated and polyunsaturated fatty acids (PUFA). When applied to fats the terms saturated and unsaturated refer to the number of hydrogen atoms present and the number of double bonds between adjacent carbon atoms. When there are no double bonds present in the carbon chain, a saturated fatty acid results; one double bond means a monosaturated fatty acid and two or more a polyunsaturated fatty acid. The degree of saturation of a fat determines its physical properties (i.e. whether it is solid or liquid at room temperature); those fats containing predominantly saturated fatty acids are solid while those with predominantly unsaturated fats tend to be liquid at the same temperature.

Fat has the effect of delaying gastric emptying and, therefore, creates a feeling of satiety but, apart from its satiety value, fat has other functions in the diet including making the diet more palatable. Fat has a high energy content (37.6 kJ/g or 9 kcal/g) and is particularly useful in those requiring a high energy intake. It also provides a vehicle for the fat soluble vitamins and the essential fatty acids, thus some fat is necessary to the diet although the amount which is either desirable or necessary has yet to be firmly established.

Fats and disease

It was Keys (1953) who first suggested that fat intakes correlated with the incidence of IHD in various countries, and in 1980 he and others published the findings of the 'Seven Countries Study', which clearly demonstrated a strong correlation between the dietary fat intake and the incidence of IHD. Death rates from this disease in the UK are amongst the highest in the world; the UK also has a poor record in its prevention (DHSS, 1981). The consensus of opinion is that its incidence could be reduced by a decrease in the total fat consumption. The Royal College of Physicians and the British Cardiac Society (1976) recommended that this should represent only about 35% of the total energy; NACNE (1983) have reduced this still further, suggesting that fat should comprise only 30% of the dietary energy and only 10% should come from saturated (animal) fats. If the total fat is reduced to this level, and saturated fat comprises only one-third of this, the polyunsaturated fat intake must of necessity be increased as this combination of recommendations can only be achieved by substituting different oils and fats for the animal fats eliminated.

Cholesterol

There is considerable variation in scientific opinion about dietary cholesterol. Neither the DHSS (1979) nor the Royal College of Physicians & the British Cardiac Society (1976) made any recommendations regarding cholesterol although the Royal College of Physicians did advise that egg consumption be reduced and the WHO Expert Committee (1982) recommended an intake of less than 300 mg dietary cholesterol per day. However, although cholesterol is present in most Western diets (about 500 mg/24 h), it is also synthesized in the body, primarily by the liver. Cholesterol is excreted, unchanged, in the bile or may be oxidized in the liver to form the bile acids; these are the routes of cholesterol loss from the body. Its metabolism is subject to feedback control so that when dietary cholesterol increases, endogenous synthesis is inhibited and breakdown increased. Cholesterol levels in the plasma usually fall when a diet low in cholesterol is consumed, although this reduction does not always persist as the plasma cholesterol levels are also related to the total dietary fat intake. Analyses of this relationship suggest that a fat intake representing 30% of the total energy is needed to reduce the cholesterol levels towards 200 mg/dl (5.2mmol/litre), the level considered appropriate by the World Health Organization Expert Committee (1982). A plasma cholesterol concentration of 160–180 mg/dl (4.1–4.6mmol/l) is associated with a very low risk of IHD (American Heart Foundation, 1979).

Sodium (salt)

Epidemiological studies consistently show hypertension to be a major risk factor in the development of both IHD and cerebrovascular disease. A reduction in hypertension reduces the risk of death from such diseases.

Animal experimentation has shown that high sodium intakes lead to high levels of hypertension and even moderate sodium intakes can lead to hypertension in genetically susceptible animals (Dahl et al, 1962). Human metabolic studies have shown a fall in blood pressure when subjects consume a low sodium diet (Morgan et al, 1978; Macgregor et al, 1982). However, a fall in blood pressure has also been demonstrated when additional potassium is given even on a relatively high sodium intake and it appears that the sodium:potassium ratio may be of more importance than the absolute sodium intake (Meneely & Ball, 1958). In those populations in which hypertension is unknown the dietary potassium intake is high and the sodium low but there are also other common characteristics:

- a lack of obesity
- high levels of physical activity
- diets low in animal fat.

Clearly obesity is related to hypertension and studies have shown that some of the differences between populations can be explained by differences in body mass. Similarly dietary fat, particularly saturated fat, has been related to hypertension through its link with arteriosclerosis. However, fat intake is unlikely to be the sole cause of the international differences in the prevalence of hypertension. For example, in Japan, where hypertension and cerebrovascular disease are common, the incidence of strokes is falling although fat intakes are increasing (Keys et al, 1980).

Nonetheless, the WHO Expert Committee (1982) consider the evidence sufficient to suggest that a high sodium intake may be a cause of hypertension in susceptible individuals, particularly when this is associated with a low potassium intake and, as the proportion of susceptible individuals is unknown, it is considered appropriate to encourage a low salt intake for the whole population. The average salt intake is 12 g/24 h (Bull & Buss, 1980) which is far above that necessary for even physically active individuals. A gradual reduction to 6 g or even 3 g is unlikely to be associated with any danger to health, although this would necessitate considerable changes in food manufacturing techniques. Gleibermann (1973) has calculated that a reduction in salt intake of 3 g/24 h would, in men aged 50–59 years, lead to a reduction in mean systolic blood pressure of 5 mmHg which would substantially lower the prevalence of hypertension and, therefore, the morbidity and mortality arising from the condition.

NUTRITIONAL CARE

NUTRITIONAL STATUS; DEFINITION AND ASSESSMENT

The term nutritional status refers both to the types and amount of nutrients available to the body and to the body's ability to utilize them. Nutritional status may be influenced by many factors and the form of the food eaten may also influence the bioavailability of nutrients, i.e. whether or not the body is able to utilize them. Once absorbed, nutrients work together in physiological processes; these can be influenced by many factors including the psychological state. The interactions of nutrients both with each other and with the individual consuming them are extremely important to the nutritional status. Health cannot be optimal when nutritional status is poor although it is important to realize that if an individual becomes ill it does not of necessity indicate that his/her nutritional status is poor, although this should be considered as a possible contributory factor.

Nutritional status is assessed in four ways, of which two are particularly relevant to nurses:

- dietary history } particularly
- physical examination } relevant to nurses
- biochemical tests
- immunological tests.

Dietary history

Disturbances in nutritional status develop over time and may be due to inadequate nutrient intake. In order to identify areas where modification is advisable the individual's dietary intake must be assessed.

It is difficult to record an individual's dietary intake without influencing it, although the extent of change depends on the person's understanding of the need for such a record. Nonetheless, this may highlight possible areas of deficiency. There are three main methods of assessing the food intake.

24 hour recall

This involves the use of a questionnaire and an interview in which the individual is asked to recall what he has eaten during the previous 24 hours and to estimate the quantity. It is an easy way of gaining an idea of the food intake but contains several possible sources of error, as the memory is not a reliable tool and estimates of quantity are difficult to make. In addition the previous day's intake may not be typical or the individual may not be truthful.

Food frequency questionnaire

This technique may help to overcome some of

Table 14.4 Data included in a dietary history

- Economic data
  - Income: frequency of paycheck
  - Amount of money available for food per week — is this adequate to meet food needs?
  - Social benefit recipient?
- Physical activity
  - Occupation: type, hours/week
  - Exercise: type, frequency (seasonal?)
  - Sleep:hours/day (uninterrupted?)
- Influence on eating habits
  - Ethnic/cultural background
  - Religion
  - Educational level
- Homelife, meal patterns
  - Number in household: who does shopping/cooking?
  - Number of meals per day? Composition?
- Appetite
  - Good, poor, any changes?
  - Factors which may affect appetite
  - Taste and smell perception
  - Allergies, intolerances, food avoidances
  - Foods avoided and reasons
  - Length of time of avoidance
- Eating problems
  - Foods which cannot be eaten. Why?
  - Problems with swallowing, chewing, food 'sticking'
  - Dental/oral health
  - Handicaps — physical/mental
- Gastrointestinal health
  - Problems e.g. 'indigestion', flatulence, diarrhoea, constipation
  - Frequency?
- Chronic disease
  - Treatment: length of treatment
  - Dietary modification: prescribed or self determined?
  - Length of time, compliance
- Medication
  - Type, dosage, frequency: length of time on therapy.
  - Vitamin/mineral supplements: frequency, type, amount, prescribed or self administered

the weaknesses inherent in the recall method and to validate the accuracy of recall by clarifying the real food intake. This provides an indication of the frequency — monthly, weekly, daily, several times daily — with which a particular food is consumed.

Dietary history

A true dietary history is more complete than either of the above methods and incorporates both. It also includes economic data, the level of physical activity, cultural background and normal food patterns together with information on appetite changes, food intolerances or avoidances, the presence of chronic disease and medications currently being taken. Table 14.4 shows the data included in a dietary history and indicates that only minor modifications are required to the nursing assessment of patients admitted to hospital in order to obtain such a history.

Food diary or record

This can be useful but involves more time and a great deal of motivation by the patient and, in most circumstances, is not of value in acute clinical care.

Physical assessment

Physical assessment includes a general clinical examination, which can give a number of clues to the patient's nutritional status, and anthropometric or physical measurements. Table 14.5 indicates some clinical signs of nutritional deficiency.

Anthropometric measurements

Physical measurements may reflect nutritional status over a lifetime; some, such as height or head circumference, reflect past or chronic nutritional status; others reflect present nutritional status and include measurements such as mid-arm muscle circumference and skinfold thickness (Table 14.6). Measurements such as height and weight are of particular value in evaluation of growth and development and are used especially in infants, children, adolescents and pregnant women.

Some of these measurements require practice and care in order to achieve accuracy and are discussed in detail in Moghissi & Boore (1983). The measurements obtained are compared with standard tables (Tables 14.7 & 14.8) and with the patient's previous measurements.

Biochemical assessment

Data regarding the nutritional status can be

Table 14.5 Clinical signs indicating nutritional status (Moghissi & Boore, 1983)

	Normal condition	Clinical disturbance	Possible disorder/deficiency
General appearance and condition	Normal weight for height, age, sex, etc.	Overweight/underweight	Obesity/starvation
			Protein lack/Thiamin deficiency
	Good muscle tone and posture	Muscle wasting/tenderness	Vit. C deficiency
		Skeletal deformities	Vit. D deficiency, calcium lack
	Smooth, pink, elastic skin	Haemorrhage/bruising/dry, rough inflamed skin	Vit. C or K/A or B complex deficiency
	Normal subcutaneous tissue	Oedema	Kwashiorkor
		Fat over/under standard	Obesity/starvation
Face and head	Shiny, not easily plucked hair	Dull, dry, sparse, depigmented hair	Kwashiorkor/marasmus
	Face and neck not swollen	Moon-face/enlarged thyroid	Kwashiorkor/iodine deficiency
	Pink healthy appearance	Nasolabial seborrhoea	Riboflavin deficiency
	Clear, bright eyes with pink moist membranes	Dry, thickened, inflamed cornea or conjunctiva	Vit. A or B complex deficiency
		Fissures at corners of the mouth	
		Corneal arcus, yellow deposits near eyes	Hyperlipidaemia
	Smooth, pink lips	Angular lesions or scars, inflammation	Riboflavin deficiency/B complex deficiency
Mouth	Red, normally rough tongue	Swollen, red, beefy tongue	Vit. B complex deficiency
		Papillary atrophy, smooth appearance	
	Healthy, red gums	Spongy, bleeding, receding gums	Vit. C deficiency
	Bright, pain-free teeth	Mottled enamel/carious teeth	Fluorosis/excessive sugar
Gastrointestinal function	Good appetite and digestion	Anorexia, indigestion,	Niacin deficiency/may lead to multiple deficiencies
	Normal elimination	Constipation, diarrhoea	Inadequate fibre or fluid, inadequate food
	Flat abdomen	Hepatosplenomegaly	Kwashiorkor
Cardiovascular system	Normal heart rhythm/rate	Cardiac enlargement, tachycardia	Thiamin deficiency
	Normal blood pressure	Hypertension	Sodium excess/Potassium deficiency
		Oedema	
Nervous system	Alert, responsive, psychological stability	Listless, apathetic, mental confusion, depression	Vit. B complex deficiency
	Normal reflexes	Psychomotor changes	Kwashiorkor
	Normal sensory and motor nerve function	Sensory loss, paraesthesia	Thiamin deficiency
		Motor weakness, loss of some reflexes	

Table 14.6 Some anthropometric measurements used in nutritional assessment

Measurement	Procedure	Interpretation
1. Weight	Measurement at same time of day, on same scales, in same clothing, after emptying bladder and bowels. Scales regularly checked	Single measurement — no value Rapid loss of 10% of usual weight indicates malnutrition
2. Height	Measurement at same time of day, without shoes	Short stature — may indicate chronic childhood malnutrition
3. Weight/height	Compared with standard weight for height and sex (see Table 14.7)	Indicates under/over nutrition
4. Mid-arm circumference (MAC)	Measured around upper arm at mid-point between acromial process of scapula and olecranon process of ulna. Use same arm each time, non-stretchable tape measure. Compare with standard tables (Table 14.8)	Indicates under-nutrition: no published standards for over nutrition
5. Triceps skin-fold thickness (TSF)	Measured at same level as 4 over triceps muscle. Mark point on skin, use skin-fold calipers, same person (takes practice to obtain proficiency): record average of 3 measurements, compare with standard table (see Table 14.8)	Indicates fat stores of body $<90\%$ of standard — moderate malnutrition $<60\%$ of standard — severe malnutrition
6. Mid-arm muscle circumference (MAMC)	Calculated from 4 & 5 above MAMC = MAC (cm) − (0.134 × TSF (mm)) Compare with standard tables (see Table 14.8)	Indicates muscle mass of body $<90\%$ of standard — moderate malnutrition $<60\%$ of standard — severe malnutrition

Table 14.7 Acceptable weight ranges for men and women*

	Height (without shoes) ft in	cm	Weight (without clothes) lb	kg
Men	5 5	165	121-152	55-69
	5 6	168	124-156	56-71
	5 7	170	128-161	58-73
	5 8	173	132-166	60-75
	5 9	175	136-170	62-77
	5 10	178	140-174	64-79
	5 11	180	144-179	65-80
	6 0	183	148-184	67-83
	6 1	185	152-189	69-86
	6 2	188	156-194	71-88
	6 3	191	160-199	73-90
Women	4 11	150	94-122	43-55
	5 0	152	96-125	44-57
	5 1	155	99-128	45-58
	5 2	157	102-131	46-59
	5 3	160	105-134	48-61
	5 4	163	108-138	49-62
	5 5	165	111-142	51-65
	5 6	168	114-146	52-66
	5 7	170	118-150	53-67
	5 8	173	122-154	55-69
	5 9	175	126-158	58-72
	5 10	178	130-163	59-74

*Prepared from data published in the Royal College of Physicians' Report on Obesity, 1983

Table 14.8 Adult anthropometric standards (Jeliffe, 1966)

	Sex	Standard	90% standard	80% standard	70% standard	60% standard
Mid-arm circumference — adults (cm)	Male	29.3	26.3	23.4	20.5	17.6
	Female	28.5	25.7	22.8	20.0	17.1
Triceps skin-fold thickness (mm)	Male	12.5	11.3	10.0	8.8	7.5
	Female	16.5	14.9	13.2	11.6	9.9
Mid-arm muscle circumference — adults (cm)	Male	25.3	22.8	20.2	17.7	15.2
	Female	23.2	20.9	18.6	16.2	13.9

obtained from examination of urine, plasma, erythrocytes, leucocytes or tissues such as liver, bone or hair. Some accepted tests for the evaluation of specific nutrient status are shown in Table 14.9.

Nitrogen balance studies are carried out by estimating the nitrogen ingested in the form of protein in the diet and measuring the amount of nitrogen lost from the body in urine. The balance is estimated by subtracting the nitrogen excreted from that ingested, and making a number of corrections to allow for other losses from faeces, sweat and other secretions (e.g. wound drainage, vomit) (Moghissi & Boore, 1983). Normally intake and output of nitrogen should be in balance. When someone is in positive balance then protein is being laid down within the body. This is the usual state during growth and in the recovery stage following trauma. Negative nitrogen balance indicates that body protein is being broken down and used as a source of energy. This situation is found in someone who is fasting or whose energy needs are greater than his intake and is the usual situation immediately following surgery or trauma.

Immunological tests

The body's immune response is reduced in malnutrition and certain tests may be useful indicators of the degree of malnutrition. In severe malnutrition, individuals may lose the ability to respond to antigens to which they have previously been exposed and developed immunity. This state of unresponsiveness is known as anergy. Tuberculin, *Candida albicans* and streptokinase antigen are those most commonly used for these tests in the UK. The total lymphocyte count may also be reduced in malnutrition.

Overall nutritional assessment

Nutritional status should be assessed in all patients, but the depth of assessment required will vary. Those requiring parenteral feeding will require a range of methods of assessment, but in most cases a dietary history and physical assessment will be adequate. These can readily be carried out by the nurse, following instruction and practice in anthropometric techniques.

Table 14.9 Some examples of biochemical measurements of nutritional status

Nutrient	More sensitive	Less sensitive
Protein	Plasma amino acids Hair root morphology Serum albumin Urinary creatinine:height index Nitrogen balance studies	Total serum protein
Fats (Lipids)	Serum cholesterol Serum triglycerides Lipoproteins	
Vitamin D	Serum 25-hydroxy vitamin D Serum alkaline phosphatase	Serum calcium Serum phosphorus
Vitamin B_1 (Thiamin)	Urinary thiamin Erythrocyte transketolase activity	Blood pyruvate
Folic acid	Red cell folate	Serum folate Bone marrow aspirate Urinary FIGLU
Vitamin C	Serum and leucocyte ascorbic acid	Urinary ascorbic acid
Iron	Iron deposits in bone marrow Serum iron % saturation of transferrin	Haemoglobin Haematocrit Thin blood film
Zinc	Serum or plasma zinc	Hair zinc

DIETARY PRESCRIPTION

The aim of nutritional assessment is to obtain the information needed to define the type of diet required by the patient. Regardless of the type of diet required, the aim is to supply adequate quantities of nutrients in a form acceptable to the patient. In general this will be based on modifications of the normal diet with alterations to the consistency depending on the condition of the patient.

The normal diet

A 'normal diet' is one supplying all the nutrients necessary for normal body function. It therefore provides protein for growth, maintenance and repair of body tissues, fats and carbohydrates for energy, vitamins and minerals to regulate body processes, and water, which, after oxygen, is the most important substance for the maintenance of life. 'Normal' diet is not to be confused with the person's usual diet, which may or may not supply all the necessary nutrients.

For optimal health the body requires all nutrients in optimum amounts and an adequate supply of energy (calories). In general, the recommended hospital diet provides 8400–10 500 kJ(8.4–10.5 MJ)(2000–2500 kcal) and contains 80–100 g protein, 60–80 g fat and 300–400 g carbohydrate. The task of planning nutritious meals is based on inclusion of all the essential nutrients. There are many ways to plan a diet; to be sure that all needs are met the simplest method involves the use of the 'basic four' food groups (Table 14.10). Whatever method is used, it is essential that the patient is fully involved as successful im-plementation is usually dependent on the patient maintaining the regime.

As the requirements for some essential nutrients, particularly trace elements, has not been clearly established it is essential that a wide variety of foods is consumed to provide for these uncertainties. It must be remembered that any nutrient, even if supplied in the recommended amount, will only be valuable as long as the requirement for all other nutrients is met. A 'balanced diet' is one supplying all necessary nutrients in the correct amount and in the right relationships to each other.

The table of recommended intakes (DHSS, 1979) gives an indication of the average nutritional requirements for different groups of people and should be used as a guide (Table 14.11).

Modifying the normal diet

Modification of the diet is indicated in the

Table 14.10 The 'basic four' food groups

Basic groups	Adult daily needs
Milk group	
Milk including foods made with milk, e.g.cheese, ice-cream and yoghurt	500 ml or more
Meat group	
Eggs,meat, cheese, fish, poultry, pulses,legumes, nuts	2 servings
Bread/cereal group	
Bread; wholegrain or enriched Cereals, rice, pasta	4 or more servings
Fruit/vegetable group	
Include a citrus fruit daily Include a dark green/deep yellow vegetable on at least alternate days Other vegetables and fruit	4 or more servings
In addition	
Other foods as necessary to complete a meal and to provide additional food energy and trace nutrients, e.g. oils, cooking fats, salad dressings and other sauces, flour, sugar.	

Table 14.11 Recommended daily amounts of nutrients for population groups (Department of Health and Social Security, 1979)

Age ranges	Energy		Protein	Calcium	Iron	Vitamin A (retinol equivalent)	Thiamin	Riboflavin	Niacin equivalent	Vitamin C	Vitamin D*
years	MJ	kcal	g	mg	mg	μg	mg	mg	mg	mg	μg
Boys											
under 1	3.25	780	19	600	6	450	0.3	0.4	5	20	7.5
1	5.0	1,200	30	600	7	300	0.5	0.6	7	20	10
2	5.75	1,400	35	600	7	300	0.6	0.7	8	20	10
3-4	6.5	1,560	39	600	8	300	0.6	0.8	9	20	10
5-6	7.25	1,740	43	600	10	300	0.7	0.9	10	20	–
7-8	8.25	1,980	49	600	10	400	0.8	1.0	11	20	–
9-11	9.5	2,280	56	700	12	575	0.9	1.2	14	25	–
12-14	11.0	2,640	66	700	12	725	1.1	1.4	16	25	–
15-17	12.0	2,880	72	600	12	750	1.2	1.7	19	30	–
Girls											
Under 1	3.0	720	18	600	6	450	0.3	0.4	5	20	7.5
1	4.5	1,100	27	600	7	300	0.4	0.6	7	20	10
2	5.5	1,300	32	600	7	300	0.5	0.7	8	20	10
3-4	6.25	1,500	37	600	8	300	0.6	0.8	9	20	10
5-6	7.0	1,680	42	600	10	300	0.7	0.9	10	20	–
7-8	8.0	1,900	48	600	10	400	0.8	1.0	11	20	–
9-11	8.5	2,050	51	700	12**	575	0.8	1.2	14	25	–
12-14	9.0	2,150	53	700	12**	725	0.9	1.4	16	25	–
15-17	9.0	2,150	53	600	12**	750	0.9	1.7	19	30	–
Men											
18-34 Sedentary	10.5	2,510	62	500	10	750	1.0	1.6	18	30	–
18-34 Moderately active	12.0	2,900	72	500	10	750	1.2	1.6	18	30	–
18-34 Very active	14.0	3,350	84	500	10	750	1.3	1.6	18	30	–
35-64 Sedentary	10.0	2,400	60	500	10	750	1.0	1.6	18	30	–
35-64 Moderately active	11.5	2,750	69	500	10	750	1.1	1.6	18	30	–
35-64 Very active	14.0	3,350	84	500	10	750	1.3	1.6	18	30	–
65-74	10.0	2,400	60	500	10	750	1.0	1.6	18	30	–
75 and over	9.0	2,150	54	500	10	750	0.9	1.6	18	30	–
Women											
18-54 Most occupations	9.0	2,150	54	500	12**	750	0.9	1.3	15	30	–
18-54 Very active	10.5	2,500	62	500	12**	750	1.0	1.3	15	30	–
55-74	8.0	1,900	47	500	10	750	0.8	1.3	15	30	–
75 and over	7.0	1.680	42	500	10	750	0.7	1.3	15	30	–
Pregnant	10.0	2,400	60	1,200	13	750	1.0	1.6	18	60	10
Lactating	11.5	2,750	69	1,200	15	1,200	1.1	1.8	21	60	10

* Most people who go out in the sun need no dietary source of vitamin D, but children and adolescents in winter, and housebound adults, are recommended to take 10μg vitamin D daily.

** These iron recommendations may not cover heavy menstrual losses.

treatment of many disease states. Certain general principles of dietary management will enhance the therapeutic effect whatever form of modification is required:

- any therapeutic diet should vary as little as possible from the patient's usual diet, unless this is inadequate
- the food habits and preferences of the patient must be taken into account; religious practices must be upheld
- economic status must be considered when recommending specific foods
- requirements for essential nutrients must be met as closely as the diet will allow.

While the last of these is essential for physiological functioning, the first three reflect an aspect of dietary therapy that distinguishes it from other therapeutic modalities. Unlike the other modalities, e.g. surgery, drug therapy, it requires that the patients themselves take the responsibility for the therapy in a treatment regime which basically modifies an essential aspect of their daily living. The therapy does not consist of something the patients 'do' or 'have done' to them in an active sense. They cannot ask themselves 'have I taken my pill' or even 'have I done my exercises'. It is all intrusive in that it is a continuing part of their daily life. Additionally they cannot look to someone or something else, e.g. the surgeon, the physiotherapist or a cobalt machine, to perform miracles for them. And, as eating and drinking are usually very significant in daily living and social relationships, modification of the diet potentially disrupts the whole way of life. It is not surprising therefore that non-compliance with dietary treatment is very high even within the relatively controlled environment of the hospital (Davies et al, 1975).

Energy requirements

The body requires a source of energy to maintain the normal processes of life. Energy intake is defined as the sum of metabolizable energy provided by the diet from available carbohydrate, fat, protein and alcohol. Available carbohydrates represent those carbohydrates which can be digested and absorbed by the human digestive tract (e.g. glucose, fructose, sucrose, and maltose present in foods). Dietary fibres (e.g. cellulose or lignin) provide examples of unavailable carbohydrates.

Metabolizable energy is calculated by the application of the appropriate energy conversion factors to the amounts of energy provided by constituents of the diet. These are:

- protein 17 kJ/g (4 kcal/g)
- carbohydrate 16 kJ/g (3.75 kcal/g)
- fat 37 kJ/g (9 kcal/g)
- alcohol 29 kJ/g (7.00 kcal/g)

The total energy requirement includes that needed to power all functions and actions. Thus an accurate estimate of total energy needs must allow for support of the following:

- basal metabolism (BMR)
- activity/external work
- the specific dynamic action of food (heat production following food ingestion)
- any increases in metabolism due to disease or trauma

Table 14.11, above, shows the recommended intakes in health, but allowance must still be made for illness states.

Pyrexia increases the energy requirements by 13% for each degree centigrade rise above normal body temperature (Ganong, 1985). The metabolic effects of surgery or trauma result in increased energy needs from about 0.1 MJ/kg/day (25 kcal/kg/day) to demands which may be as high as 0.17–0.21 MJ/kg/day (45–50 kcal/kg/day).

Protein requirements

The body's requirement for protein reflects the need for amino acids necessary to form new tissue and to meet the demand for protein during normal growth and maintenance. However, protein can also be used as a source of energy, particularly when the food intake is inadequate and fails to meet the energy demand. Amino acids are then oxidized to provide energy and the protein requirement for growth and repair may not be met. Under such circumstances this cannot be remedied by an increase only in the dietary protein; the total energy intake must also be raised. Thus, after calculating the daily energy requirement, the protein content of the diet is estimated.

Proteins vary in their usefulness to the body depending on their essential amino acid content (amino acids which cannot be synthesized by the body at a rate commensurate with its needs). Without these, body protein cannot be synthesized or body tissue maintained. For this purpose a mixture of proteins may be more useful than a single protein source, as a deficiency of an amino acid in one protein may be balanced by a high proportion of that amino acid in another. At least one-third of the protein intake should consist of proteins of high biological value. Protein foods of high quality are usually of animal origin; those of fair or low value are usually of grain or vegetable origin. The value of a protein depends also on the availability of the amino acids which are present. Greaves & Tan (1966) have calculated the utilization value of food proteins to be 70%.

Protein needs are often calculated on the basis of nitrogen balance (protein is the major dietary source of nitrogen) the aim being to maintain nitrogen equilibrium although, in disease states, a positive nitrogen balance is desirable.

Sherman (1920) concluded that a protein intake of 45 g/day, or about 0.7 g/kg, is sufficient to maintain nitrogen balance for many weeks provided that it is of good quality. This then is the minimum requirement. However, the recommended intake for an average sized man (65 kg) of middle age (35–65) is 65 g (DHSS, 1979), which takes account of the acceptable composition of the diet and also ensures that the recommended intakes of the trace nutrients are met. The DHSS also recommends that protein should comprise 10% of the total energy intake which, in this case, represents a protein intake of 58.5 g, a figure close to 65 g.

Patients requiring long stays in hospital or who are losing protein (e.g. from burns, exudates or renal disease) may require an increase in this amount.

Carbohydrate and fat

Once the protein content of the diet has been determined the remainder of the energy intake is assigned to either carbohydrate or fat. But how is the correct proportion of these nutrients decided? Exact data on this ratio is scarce but present knowledge in nutrition indicates that too much fat is harmful. NACNE (1983) recommend that less than 35% of the total energy should come from fat, and of this percentage 10% should be saturated fat and 25% polyunsaturated fat. However, Bender (1979) suggests that 10% fat is all that is necessary to maintain health and supply both essential fatty acids and fat soluble vitamins.

Trace nutrients — vitamins and minerals

The diet must also satisfy the requirements for the essential vitamins and minerals.

The vitamins are essential organic compounds required for the normal metabolism of other nutrients as well as for normal growth and maintenance, but which are required in relatively small amounts. They are classified as being soluble either in water (the B vitamins and vitamin C) or in fat (vitamins A, D, E and K). Requirements for vitamins under conditions of stress (such as illness) have not yet been completely determined.

Over 26 minerals and elements are needed for normal body function (Table 14.12). They have

Table 14.12 Essential minerals

Essential at levels of 100 mg/day	Calcium Phosphorus Sulphur Potassium	Chlorine Sodium Magnesium
Essential at no more than a few mg/day	Iron Fluorine Zinc Copper	Cobalt Chromium Iodine
Essential although amounts necessary for humans not estimated at present	Silicon Vanadium Tin Selenium	Molybdenum Nickel Manganese
Minerals present in body: function not yet known	Strontium Bromine Gold Aluminium	Boron Arsenic Silver Bismuth

important metabolic functions through their participation in enzymatic reactions in which they may act as cofactors or as an integral part of an enzyme. Many are present in only small quantities in foods and as mineral requirements have not, in many cases, been precisely determined this emphasizes again the need for a varied diet.

The therapeutic diet

The 'normal diet' may be modified to produce a specific therapeutic diet to help compensate for a specific dysfunction of the body or to meet specific needs induced by disease, stress or trauma. Modifications may affect the quality or the quantity of the diet; a qualitative modification is one adjusting the type(s) of food allowed; a quantitative change is calculated either to increase or decrease the amounts of specific nutrients. Therapeutic diets are required for one or more of the following reasons:

- to maintain or improve nutritional status by relief of nutritional deficiencies — clinical or subclinical
- to maintain, decrease or increase body weight
- to rest certain organs
- to eliminate particular food constituents which the patient is unable to utilize or to which he/she is sensitive
- to adjust the dietary composition to meet the ability of the body to metabolize or excrete certain nutrients or other substances

The diet may also be modified in terms of its consistency to meet specific needs. For example, a soft or liquid diet may be necessary for patients having difficulty in chewing or swallowing. In cases of severe dysphagia, tube feeding or total parenteral nutrition may be required. The choice of feeding method then depends on gastro-intestinal function.

Thus dietary adjustments may include any of the following:

- energy content may be increased or decreased
- specific nutrient content may be increased or decreased
- specific foods may be omitted
- the form in which the nutrients are supplied may be altered.

Such changes are not mutually exclusive and there is no rigid demarcation between them.

Therapeutic diets are named after the type of dietary modification required and only rarely after the name of the disease or its symptoms (such as the diabetic diet). This makes the terminology universal. Nonetheless every diet should be planned on an individual basis which takes account of the patient's preferences and lifestyle as well as his/her individual physiological needs. Each diet prescription should, therefore, be based on the energy requirements (dependent on the individual's weight and level of activity) as well as the needs for protein, fat, carbohydrate, vitamins, minerals and dietary fibre and with due regard to the increased or decreased needs as a result of illness. The prescription is then 'translated' into foods and meals suitable for the individual patient. The need for the diet as a therapeutic measure is discussed fully with the patient as well as specific ideas about how to adjust his/her normal life style. Table 14.13 shows examples of, and indications for, some therapeutic diets.

Changes in energy content

Reducing (restricted energy) diet. Whatever the cause of obesity (see Ch.23) the energy intake must be restricted to the point where the body must draw on its energy reserves to meet energy needs because at this point weight will be lost.

Table 14.14 shows the energy output during various activities. This highlights the variations in requirements which are dependent on the activity level. As a result a businessman may require only half the energy of a manual labourer. This clearly demonstrates one aspect of the individuality required when planning a therapeutic regimen.

Protein in the diet is kept at the maximum amount permitted to maintain nitrogen balance at equilibrium. Usually 0.8 g/kg ideal body

Table 14.13 Examples of, and indications for, some therapeutic diets

	Type of diet	Indications
Fat modification	Low fat	Gallbladder disease, hepatic or pancreatic disease, all forms of hyperlipoproteinaemia
	Fat controlled, low cholesterol	Often used to treat hypercholesterolaemia, occasionally used in atherosclerosis
Protein modification	Low protein	Renal or hepatic disease, hepatic coma, chronic uraemia
	Gluten free	Coeliac disease, nontropical sprue
	Restricted phenylalanine	Phenylketonuria
	High protein	Any condition in which protein deficiency is present, e.g. burns, surgery, trauma, nephrotic syndrome, ulcerative colitis cystic fibrosis and many others
Carbohydrate modification	Controlled carbohydrate	Diabetes mellitus
	Lactose free	Lactose intolerance
Electrolyte	Restricted	Congestive cardiac failure, hypertension, renal failure, eclampsia or toxaemia of pregnancy

Table 14.14 Approximate energy costs of some physical activities

Activity	kJ/min	kcal/min
Sitting quietly	5.0	1.2
Sitting writing	10.9	2.6
Walking	18	4.3
Domestic work	10.5 – 20.5	2.5 – 4.9
Bricklaying	10.5 – 21	2.5 – 5.0
Driving a truck	10.5 – 21	2.5 – 5.0
Golf	18.8 – 25	4.5 – 6.0
Cycling	21 – 31	5.0 – 7.4
Agricultural work (non-mechanized)	23.8 – 31	5.7 – 7.4
Lumber work	> 42	> 10
Running (7 minute/mile)	> 42	> 10

weight/day is sufficient for this purpose (approximately 50 g).

Once the protein content has ben estimated, the remainder of the diet is determined, calories being allocated between carbohydrate and fat. There is, however, some controversy over this aspect of the diet as some workers believe carbohydrate rich foods should be restricted as these are often responsible for the initial development of obesity. However, provided the diet is well balanced and restricted in calories, loss of weight is ensured. A rapid weight loss in the first few days is explained by the loss of water released when body glycogen is depleted. (Each gram of glycogen binds 3.4 g water which is released as glycogen is broken down.) Fat intake is often maintained at 30–35% of the total energy as this helps to eliminate the hunger and fatigue which are commonly associated with reducing diets.

In general carbohydrates should be in the form of complex carbohydrates while simple sugars should be eliminated, particularly sucrose which supplies ‘empty calories’ (i.e. supplies only calories and no other nutrients). The dietary fibre associated with complex carbohydrates is a valuable addition to the diet as it contributes to a feeling of satiety by delaying both gastric emptying time and nutrient absorption. Such a diet should, where possible, be combined with an exercise regime to increase the metabolic rate and, therefore, the efficiency of energy utilization.

High energy content. Patients with particularly high energy requirements such as those who have become severely malnourished or who have suffered trauma and acquired infections will need very high amounts of energy. Manufactured nutrient solutions may be helpful in supplementing the diet. Sometimes their requirements may be so high that they cannot be met through normal oral feeding and nasogastric feeding or parenteral feeding will be necessary.

Alteration of specific nutrient content

Low protein diet. Such a diet is used, for example, in chronic renal failure when the glomerular filtration rate falls and the excretion of nitrogenous waste products is reduced. It then becomes necessary to control the level of the protein intake whilst maintaining a positive nitrogen balance and preventing the loss of lean body mass. Protein restriction is usually initiated when renal function has decreased to about 25% and further restricted as renal function continues to decline. This is measured by renal function tests such as creatinine clearance and blood urea estimations (see Ch.26); when blood urea rises above 39 mmol/l and plasma creatinine above 500 mmol/l, protein is restricted.

However, even on a diet which is devoid of protein but which supplies adequate quantities of energy and other nutrients the body continues to produce nitrogenous metabolites from the breakdown of endogenous protein. Sufficient protein must be given to balance these endogenous losses which correspond to approximately 0.25 g protein/kg body weight/day (approximately 22 g in the average adult).

When protein restriction is commenced, at least 75% of the protein intake must be of high biological value to ensure that the requirements for essential amino acids are met. The body then utilizes its excess nitrogen to synthesize non-essential amino acids thus reducing the amount of nitrogenous waste which must be excreted. Energy intake must be sufficient to prevent protein metabolism for energy and to spare protein for tissue protein synthesis.

Such a diet is tedious for patients as they must not only control their intake of protein but also its quality and they cannot substitute low biological value proteins for high. However, variety and energy may be added by use of low protein or protein-free products, although these may prove expensive and require extra effort in preparation. Nonetheless the patient should be informed about these and given the opportunity to try them.

The diabetic diet is discussed in Chapter 19.

The omission of specific foods

In the past this type of diet was only rarely used in the care of the physically ill adult as, in general, such diets are only used in the treatment of inborn errors of metabolism such as phenylketonuria or galactosaemia which are primarily diseases of childhood. However, the increasing use of hypoallergenic/oligoallergenic diets in the treatment of food allergy means that these are now more commonly found in general nursing practice.

Gluten-sensitive enteropathy (nontropical sprue), the adult form of coeliac disease, perhaps provides the best example of this type of dietary modification. The causation of this condition remains a matter of conjecture although several theories exist.

Whatever the cause, the symptoms remain the same: the patient is unable to tolerate the glutamine rich polypeptide present in the gliadin fraction of gluten (wheat protein) so that this acts as a cytotoxin towards the intestinal epithelium. It interferes with the normal maturation of the epithelium, injuring the mucosa and causing pathological changes (Baker et al, 1964). Treatment includes correction of the malfunction of the small bowel by removing gluten from the diet. This involves elimination of wheat, barley, rye and oats from the diet as these all contain large amounts of gluten. Cereal products which can be substituted include cornflour, cornmeal, rice flour and wheat starch (gluten free). Potato flour is also of value. Such a diet creates considerable problems when shopping for food and means all labels must be carefully scrutinized and ingredients questioned prior to purchase or consumption.

Other common elimination diets include lactose (milk) free diets, egg-free diets and diets which exclude shellfish, nuts, all cereals or preservatives and additives.

Table 14.15 Situations in which 'artifical feeding' may be required

Physiological problem	Clinical disorder	Recommended feed
Difficulty in ingestion of food	Carcinoma of oesophagus or stomach; dental or oral surgery; coma; inflammatory disease of the oesophagus	Liquid: whole food or milk based formula either orally or via tube. Commercially available products can be used
Inability to ingest food	Oesophageal obstruction/surgery	Parenteral nutrition
Inability to digest food	Pancreatitis; enzyme deficiency; disease of biliary tract	Predigested or defined formula either orally or via tube
Reduced absorption	Radiation therapy; sprue; inflammatory bowel disease; short bowel syndrome	Defined formula
Inability to meet normal requirements through normal food	Major surgery, burns, trauma; extended pyrexia; anorexia of chronic illness; anorexia nervosa.	Liquid feeding as oral supplement or via tube Parenteral nutrition

Factors to be considered when selecting a feeding formula:

- Form of nutrient related to absorptive capacity
- Type of carbohydrate used
- Electrolyte content
- Recommended uses of selected formula
- Nutrient density and osmolality

Changes in consistency

Liquid or soft diets needed for the edentulous or dysphagic patient may be prepared by purέeing or liquidizing the food. Apart from this, changes in consistency are rarely required except when 'artificial feeding techniques' must be used (Table 14.15). Liquid feeding, which provides all the nutritional requirements of the individual, is used in the care of patients unable to take solid food. These may be used as sip feeds or, more commonly, as tube feeds (enteral feeding).

Some patients will be unable to deal adequately with food taken into the gastro-intestinal tract. These patients will require parenteral feeding, in which the nutrients in solution are instilled directly into the circulation. The indications for enteral and parenteral feeding are discussed in detail in Moghissi & Boore (1983).

Enteral feeding. Enteral feeding depends on using the normal physiological mechanisms for dealing with the digestion and absorption of food, but bypassing the normal route of entry. The commonest method of administration is via a nasogastric tube, but feeding can also be via a gastrostomy or jejunostomy tube.

The effectiveness of enteral feeding is dependent on the adequacy of the planned nutritional regime and the efficiency of its administration. This method of feeding is usually managed by nursing staff and it must be emphasized that it is a therapeutic regime that should be planned as carefully as any other method of treatment. Jones (1975) found that this task was often left to junior nurses with inadequate knowledge and patients were not obtaining a satisfactory nutritional intake.

Nutritional content of feeds. Tube feeds may be used either when oral intake is not possible or as a supplement when a patient cannot meet his nutritional requirements through oral intake alone. Feeds may be composed from a mixture of foods served in the 'normal' diet, finely homogenized in a blender and strained to ensure passage through the tube, or from combinations of foods planned to meet specific therapeutic needs. Such feeds may have psychological benefits for the patient in that the use of such a mixture may reduce the isolation at mealtimes felt by patients requiring tube feeds. It is, however, more common to use commercially available, defined formula mixtures when tube feeds are required. These have the advantage of being formulated in such a way as to pass through a fine bore feeding tube which is more comfortable for the patient than the previously used wider bore nasogastric tubes. When a feeding formula is being evaluated it is necessary to look at the osmolality, caloric concentration and vitamin and mineral composition.

Osmolality is a measure of the osmotically active particles per kg of the solvent in which the particles are dispersed, which is usually water. The normal osmolality of body fluids is about 275–298 milliosmoles/kg; solutions taken into the body which have an osmolality greater than this are hyperosmolar and cause water to be drawn into the intestine. Most tube feeds are hyperosmolar and will cause gastrointestinal disturbances if given too rapidly. For this reason it is usual to commence with feeds diluted to quarter strength gradually increasing to full strength over 3–5 days to allow tolerance to develop.

Most feeding formulae provide approximately 4.2 J/ml (1 kcal/ ml) when mixed to full strength: thus, to give 4.2 MJ (1000 kcal), 1000 ml must be given. Some formulae have a higher caloric concentration; such calorically dense formulae are specifically designed for severely debilitated patients requiring very high energy and protein intakes.

The protein content may vary between 9 and 24% of the total energy content. It is usually provided by a complete protein (e.g. casein or albumin) which may be partially hydrolyzed into peptide fragments or into individual amino acids for easier digestion.

Fat is added to the feed as it provides a good source of energy yet does not increase the osmolality; it also gives the patient a feeling of satiety. In most commercial formulae fat is supplied through corn, soya or safflower oil; the amount may range from 1–47% of the total energy content.

There are many possible sources of carbohydrate ranging from pureed fruit or vegetables to glucose, fructose, sucrose and lactose. The source depends on the type of feed being used.

The majority of commercially produced liquid diets are fortified with vitamins and minerals to meet the recommended daily intakes (RDI) which are calculated to meet the needs of healthy individuals. Thus additional quantities may have to be added to meet the requirements of an ill person. For some patients electrolytes may also have to be added to replace losses.

Defined formula (elemental) diets are designed for easy digestion and absorption and to leave minimal residue in the bowel. The carbohydrate is present in the form of glucose or dextrins and the protein as amino acids, dipeptides or tripeptides as these are easily absorbed. Very little fat is present — usually only enough to prevent essential fatty acid deficiency. All products are supplemented with vitamins and minerals to meet the RDI.

Such products can be taken orally but are better tolerated when given through a tube as they are somewhat unpalatable due to the presence of the peptides and amino acids. However, when they are to be given orally, they must be offered with a positive attitude and not with a look of disgust! The palatability can be improved by the addition of various flavours and by serving them chilled or in fruit juice.

Administration of feeds. The route of administration will largely determine the type of feed used and how it will be tolerated by the patient. The route may be nasogastric or through an oesophagostomy, gastrostomy or jejunostomy. If feeds are being given via the nasogastric route a fine bore catheter should be used as the risk of oesophagitis and later oesophageal stricture is reduced (Allison, 1981).

Ideally continuous drip administration at a rate of 80–150 ml/h is carried out but this tends to limit the patient's activity (although some will push the drip stand around with them) and, for this reason, bolus feeding is often given. In this case 200–350 ml should be given over a period of at least 10–15 minutes followed by 100 ml water. This is necessary to 'clean the tube' (the protein in the feed tends to coagulate when it comes into contact with the gastric acid) and, more importantly, to prevent hypertonic dehydration from solute overload. The feed should be administered to the patient with the head and thorax elevated and the patient should remain in this position for at least one hour after feeding to prevent the possible aspiration of the feed into the lungs. The stomach contents should be aspirated prior to administration of a feed to ensure that there is only minimal residue from the previous feed. Excess residue may indicate an obstruction or a digestive problem which should be resolved before feeding is continued.

Once such problems have been overcome six feeds of 300–400 ml each at 3 hr intervals will allow administration of 7.56 — 10.08 MJ/day (1800–2400 kcal/day) with an additional 1000 ml water. However, the precise quantity given will depend on individual requirements. It is important to remember that, when dilute formulae are given, the patient's needs for energy and other nutrients are not being met, and further supplementation or extra feeds may be required.

Patients who are being tube fed require a great deal of encouragement to help them adjust to the situation; the nurse can be of help in establishing pleasant associations with the feeding routine. The meal should be attractively presented and, when possible and appropriate, the patient should be encouraged to learn the procedure and to feed himself under supervision.

The monitoring of the patient and of the enteral feeding is discussed in detail in Moghissi & Boore (1983). The possible complications of this method of feeding fall into two groups (Allison, 1981):

- those associated with the equipment
  - displacement of the tube with possible aspiration of nutrients
  - blockage of the tube
  - discomfort/ulceration as a result of the tube
  - oesophagitis and oesphageal stricture.

  These can be minimized by using a fine bore tube, checking the position of the tube and flushing it through with water after each feed.

- those related to nutrient intake and metabolic complications
  - nausea and vomiting
  - diarrhoea
  - hyperosmolar state and osmotic diuresis
  - uraemia
  - deficiency complications.

  These are prevented or dealt with by planning the feeding regime with care to ensure adequate nutrients and adequate fluid, but with a gradual build-up from diluted to full-strength feeds to allow the body to adjust.

Parenteral feeding. This involves the instillation of nutrients directly into the circulation via a central venous line and is discussed in detail by Moghissi & Boore (1983). This form of feeding is medically prescribed but the nurse has an important role in monitoring the effectiveness of the nutritional care and in managing the regime and equipment.

The possible complications associated with the equipment are the same as those which may occur with any central venous line but in addition there are metabolic complications which may occur. These complications fall into three groups:

- those related to the infusion system and technique
  - catheter displacement
  - disturbance of flow of the solution
  - air embolism
  - fracture of the catheter and catheter embolus (now rare)

  These are prevented by care in the insertion of the catheter and continuing care in changing of dressings etc. to reduce the risk of movement, by monitoring the infusion rate and by care when changing the infusion set. Air embolism is a risk whenever the central venous catheter is open to the air because the intrathoracic pressure is subatmospheric. It can be prevented by asking the patient to carry out the Valsalva manoeuvre (the patient tries to breathe out against closed mouth and pinched nose) or by putting the patient into the Trendelenburg position with the head lower than the body whenever any procedure which involves this risk is carried out.

- infective complications – particularly at risk because of compromised immune system.

  These can be minimized by taking particular care when changing the nutrient container, changing the intravenous set etc. The IV set should be changed every 24–48 hours as the risk of infection rises after this period, and the use of a semi-occlusive transparent dressing (e.g. Op-Site) over the entry site allows observation and appears to discourage bacterial growth (Phillips et al, 1976).
- metabolic and deficiency complications are similar to those which can arise with enteral feeding.

NUTRITIONAL PROBLEMS ASSOCIATED WITH HOSPITALIZATION

GENERAL ASPECTS

Even in relatively healthy patients undernutrition can lead to the first steps in the sequence of deterioration.

Patients admitted to hospital often do not eat adequately; perhaps they dislike the type of food provided or find the timing of meals unacceptable. Such a patient will often enjoy food prepared at home and brought into hospital by their family and friends. Institutional food, whilst providing all the necessary nutrients, cannot be cooked to individual specifications; such problems can often be overcome by asking the relatives to bring seasonings or sauces to add to the hospital diet. But there may be other reasons for a failure to eat; the patient may be in pain or one of his medications may be interfering with his appetite (e.g. digoxin), altering his taste sensations (e.g. cyclophosphamide) or causing nausea. Such effects may also cause depression and, with it, anorexia and a marked reluctance to eat.

It is particularly important to be aware of psychological factors which may underlie food refusal. This can create something of a dilemma; the patient requires nutrients to aid recovery but also needs a sense of control over his/her environment. This situation requires a sensitive and supportive approach.

There are other factors which may affect the patient's ability to meet his/her nutritional needs – the 'physician induced factors' (Butterworth, 1974). Patients are often denied sufficient food in order that they may undergo diagnostic tests, they are rarely supplied with additional vitamins or minerals even when these are indicated and they are often provided with inadequate feeding through intravenous lines (e.g. glucose or saline without added amino acids, vitamins or minerals and with inadequate energy). Such factors may significantly delay recovery prolonging the length of the hospital stay, delaying convalescence and thereby increasing the cost of their medical treatment.

If nutritional intake is to be observed and problems identified, then someone clearly has to be present on the ward when patients are eating. Chapman (1983) has clearly shown that as patients' meals are served the nurses disappear! In many hospitals food is distributed by the domestic staff who are untrained and do not recognize the patient's need to be helped to sit up, to have the tray moved closer or the food cut into manageable sized pieces. The same staff remove the trays and the nurse has little opportunity to ascertain either the quality or the quantity of food consumed. In some instances the relatives can play an important role by being present at meal times to help to feed the patient and to encourage him/her to eat.

It can therefore be seen that, although specific dietary therapy may not be needed by all patients, all will need adequate nutritional support throughout their stay in hospital. In the section that follows some aspects of providing this support are explored more fully.

RESPONSIBILITY FOR NUTRITIONAL CARE

As with many other aspects of treatment and care of persons in hospital, the responsibility for adequate nutritional care is shared between a number of health carers. This creates its own difficulties, well illustrated by the disturbing

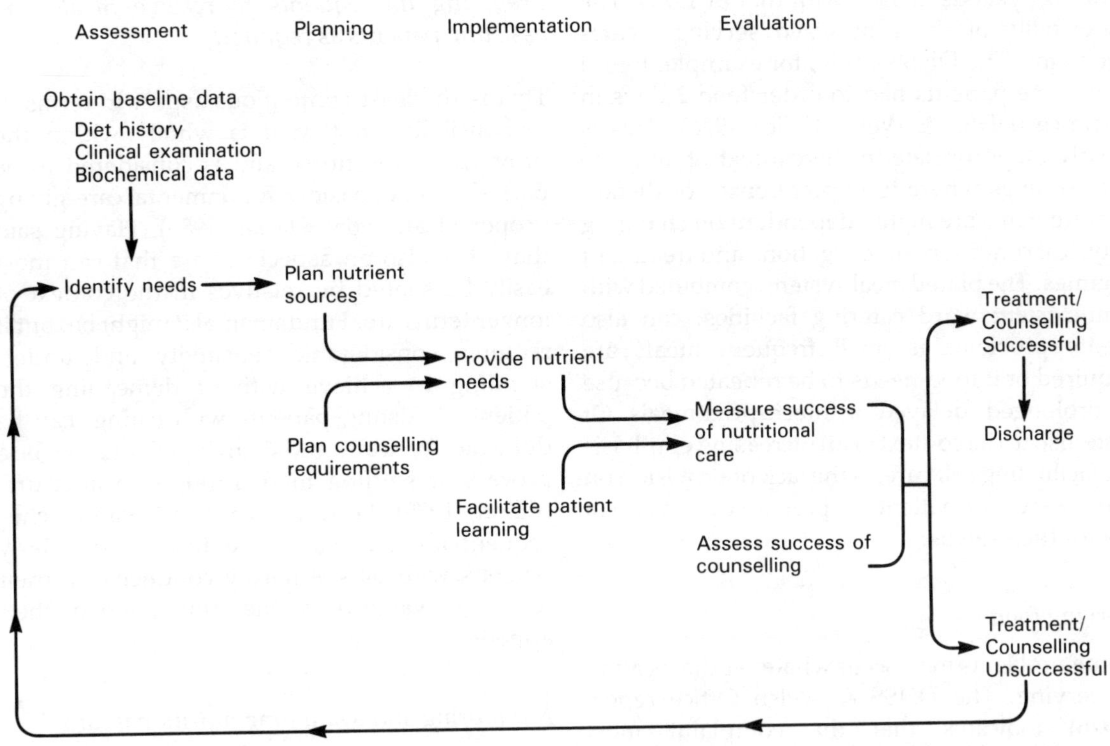

Fig. 14.1 The nutritional care process

findings of studies such as Jones (1975) and Davies et al (1975). Both of these highlight the lack of responsibility taken by any one professional group for ensuring that patients receive the prescribed or the appropriate special diet. Others report the general undernutrition of patients in hospital whether they are undergoing surgery or not (Coates, 1984; Whitehead, 1983). Indeed a small study undertaken by Todd et al (1984), 24% of patients on medical, surgical and orthopaedic wards reported an intake identified as less than predicted for basal metabolic rate and 16% less than required for daily protein requirements.

At each stage of management, the confusion of responsibility exists.

Figure 14.1 diagrammatically represents the nutritional care process irrespective of who takes responsibility for that care.

Assessment and planning

The increasing emphasis on nursing assessment may focus nursing attention once more onto nutrition. Certainly nursing theorists acknowledge nutrition as a fundamental aspect of nursing care (e.g. Roper et al, 1980, Henderson, 1960, Roy, 1980), but there is no evidence that nurses have adequate knowledge. By contrast the dietician has the necessary specialist knowledge but cannot gain access to the patient without medical or nursing referral. Doctors have little nutritional education (Gray 1983) and do not always appreciate the problems.

Preparing food

Preparation of food is now the total responsibility of the catering staff with the same relatively small input from the dietician. Plated meal systems are supplanting plug-in trolleys and ward serving, and ward kitchens equipped for cooking even a light meal are increasingly rare. Nurses are no longer taught 'invalid cookery' in the introductory course (compare the training syllabus of 1959 with that of 1979). The inflexibility of the centralized serving creates problems. The DHSS study, for example, found that some patients had to order food 2 days in advance (DHSS & Welsh Office 1976). This is clearly inappropriate in the context of all acute care settings where food preferences or dietary requirements are highly dependent on changing physical condition, investigations and treatment regimes. The plated meal system, combined with non-existent ward catering facilities, can also create problems if small frequent meals are required or if food needs to be reheated because of prolonged, delayed or interrupted meals. Of note also in the context of an increasing emphasis on facilitating self care, is the lack of provision on most wards for patients to prepare even a cup of tea for themselves.

Serving food

Some problems may occur whatever the location of serving. The DHSS & Welsh Office report (1976) indicates that the complaint most frequently voiced by patients was that of hot food being served cold. Other studies show that choice is an important element, as is the amount of food offered, the latter being generally too much rather than too little (Elliott, 1975; Raphael, 1977). Raphael's study was reassuring in that it showed an improvement in satisfaction with meals since the previous survey in 1971, although she also points out that the level of satisfaction showed no relationship to the catering costs of the hospital.

The responsibility for serving food is again contentious. While a number of reports indicate that it is not, or may not be, the perceived role of the nurse to physically serve the food (non-nursing duties) (Anderson, 1973; Champion, 1979), the nurse is uniformly seen as being responsible for its serving. The DHSS & Welsh Office report (1976) states that it is the fundamental duty of nurses to see that the patients are offered the correct food in appropriate quantities. It is difficult to see how this can be achieved with or without a central plating system if nurses do not actually serve the food to the patient.

Preparing the patients to receive meals and assisting patients as required

This is the least contentious aspect in terms of responsibility in that it is wholly within the province of the nurse and is considered to be part of general, basic or fundamental care-giving (Roper et al, 1985; Clarke, 1983). Having said that, it is also an aspect of care that can most easily be shared by relatives in the context of longer term care. Fundamental it might be, but it requires considerable sensitivity and understanding to achieve without demeaning the patient. Assisting patients with eating 'can be done nicely, neatly and with dignity or it can be a process of stuffing food through an aperture' (Elliott, 1975). Feeding marmalade sandwiches sequentially, a bite at a time, to a row of elderly persons with bibs is hardly conducive to their feeling of value or to the stimulation of their appetite.

Monitoring and evaluating nutritional care

The evidence of studies such as Davies et al (1975), Jones (1975) and Todd et al (1984) would suggest that this is of low priority. Clearing after meals has traditionally been seen as the duty of housekeeping staff. Successful monitoring of food intake by nurses would be difficult to achieve without officiousness unless they themselves are directly involved in serving and clearing meal plates. Systematic recording of food intake may be as important as that of fluid intake or bowel action for some patients, but is seldom undertaken outside of the context of tube feeding or monitoring patients suffering from anorexia nervosa.

Routine, regular weighing of patients is valuable and was a traditional task when the patient's length of stay on medical or surgical wards was longer than a week. This is a crude guide however and will not indicate malnutrition in relation to lack of specific nutrients as opposed to overall adequacy of energy intake. Similarly, anthropometric measurements will indicate body fat, for example, but will not highlight mineral or vitamin deficiencies or short-term protein lack.

Observation and reporting of food intake appears therefore to be the only valid method of estimating nutritional balance, but the problems inherent in gaining reliable data by this method are obvious (Davies et al, 1975). Certainly there is no evidence that any one group of health care professionals takes this aspect of nutritional care at all seriously.

Responsibility of the nurse

There is a strong argument that the nurse should take responsibility for the assessment and planning of nutritional care, for ensuring that care is carried out and for monitoring its effect in those patients for whom there is no requirement for specialist dietary advice. This will promote the development of the role of the practitioner nurse as one whose independent function is to assit patients in those things they would normally do for themselves (Henderson, 1960) or to compensate wholly or partially in self-care activities (Orem, 1971). For those who are identified by the nature of their medical diagnosis (e.g. diabetes mellitus) or from their nursing assessment to have a need for specialist intervention, the dietician and the nurse must share the responsibility, and in certain instances the doctor may also become fully involved. This implies an effective means of communication between them and a mutual understanding of their various roles. This does not occur automatically.

In the section that follows the role outlined above is assumed i.e. that it is the nurse's responsibility to ensure that all patients are offered or have available an appropriate diet (that is, a diet in a form they can ingest, in quantities and nature that will enhance their well-being) and which is presented in a way and within an environment that is conducive to their ingestion and enjoyment of the food.

Three broad aspects of management are considered: firstly, environmental aspects, secondly (and in more detail) specific aspects related to assisting patients, and thirdly, aspects of nutritional education and support.

Environmental aspects

Environmental aspects of nutritional care can be highlighted with the single question — are the surroundings of the patient conducive to the enjoyment of their food? Noxious smells, sights and sounds are sometimes difficult to mask in an open ward setting, and are probably responsible for the periodic emphasis by the ward manager on the use of tables at one end of a ward, the day room or a dining room. However the social significance of sharing a meal may suggest that forcing strangers to sit at a table together will inhibit rather than encourage eating. There is also the very real problem of some patients, by virtue of themselves, their disease or their treatment, creating sights, sounds or smells that will quickly put another person off their food. Where patients eat, therefore, must be subject to individual preference and not bound by institutional rules. For example, a patient may prefer to join another, named person for their meal, rather than eat alone at their own bedside or join a larger group of strangers.

With whom one eats is therefore significant. Relatives or friends may be just what is required to encourage or cajole. However, the trend towards 'open visiting' patterns has created the 'feeding time at the zoo' phenomenon; that is, patients being served with food at their bedside and being expected to eat it when surrounded by visitors. Inevitably a running commentary ensues on the state of the patient's appetite, the problems of eating food sitting on a bed, what they ate yesterday or anticipate tonight and so on. Again, more sensitive and active management by nurses might overcome some of these problems.

Aspects relating to assisting patients

Lack of serious study in this area inevitably results in ideas being suggested based on common sense and experience rather than substantive evidence. It is convenient to consider these aspects under headings modified from a functional framework. Initial students of nursing are also referred to basic nursing texts such as Roper, Logan & Tierney (1985) and Clarke (1983) for further details of practical nursing.

Altered breathing. A patient whose breathing is in any way distressed will find that the effort of chewing and interruption by 'mouth breathing' seriously diminish their ability to consume an adequate diet. For a limited period such patients may replace their normal diet with high nutrient fluids, especially if they require a high fluid intake to compensate for the increased fluid loss inevitable when respirations are rapid and distressed. Foods easily chewed, or able to be swallowed without chewing, are more likely to be acceptable than sliced meat or salad, for example. The effort expended by the patient at mealtimes will be reduced if food is cut into small, 'mouth-sized' pieces if this can be achieved without diminishing the patient's self-esteem.

Effort is also reduced by ensuring that the patient is well supported in an upright position and that conversation is kept to a minimum. For patients receiving continuous oxygen, delivery via nasal cannulae during meals will increase the likelihood of the patient coping with the additional effort required during eating. The inflexibility experienced with some centralized meal systems can create problems if smaller, more frequent meals are indicated or if food becomes cold during the longer time breathless patients require to complete a meal. Crumbly foods may be a hazard if patients are distressed by coughing.

Sensory input. Persons unable to smell or taste food are likely to lose interest in eating and particular efforts should be made to present food that is visually attractive. This includes a large number of the elderly in whom the normal physiological changes associated with ageing may diminish their ability to appreciate flavours.

Patients who have oral pathologies, e.g. infections or carcinoma, experience altered taste which may seriously diminish their desire for or appreciation of food, quite apart from the mechanical problems they may encounter with chewing. Related treatments further contribute to the problem, often resulting in tasteless and/or bitter tasting food. Strohl (1983) suggests that, apart from the general presentation and environment in which food is served, the patient may find mouthwashes immediately prior to food helpful. Some patients may also find artificial saliva helps to lubricate food.

Any patient who has diminished sensation in his/her mouth will be at risk of burning and scalding.

Visual presentation of food can enhance or detract from its enjoyment and those with reduced sight may be helped to enjoy their meal by a description of the food and the location of different items on the plate. Helping the patient to feel items on the tray or table will help him or her to locate things and acquire detailed information about the exact direction and distance the hand has to travel to deliver food to the mouth. Persons whose sight is reduced by injury or operation will need particular sensitivity on the part of the nurse in order for them to continue to feed themselves without feeling hopelessly frustrated by futile attempts to transfer food from the plate to their mouths. The provision of adequate but not demeaning protection for clothes is likely to enhance a person's confidence in coping with the food on his/her own.

Similarly patients who cannot see their food by reason of their position, e.g. if being nursed supine, will need food located for them unless a mirror is appropriately positioned. Such patients may need feeding if they are to maintain an appropriate food intake. Foods which are easily swallowed are preferred in this situation.

Reduced mobility. Patients whose mobility is restricted will not have the same freedom of choice with regard to where and with whom they eat as those without these problems. The social importance of eating has already been noted. Enough here to point out the problems inherent for a disabled or incapacitated person in preparing food or in carrying prepared food from one location to another. In a hospital situation the problem will be more one of the location of served meals. It is often assumed that when the patient is 'getting better', he/she will sit at a table with other patients with varying eating habits — a practice already challenged as being of doubtful rehabilitative value.

Altered movement. Movement is here meant to imply the ability of the individual to move various parts of the body rather than the body as a whole. In terms of eating, the functional parts most essential are those of the arm, hand and mouth, and to a lesser extent the eyes (discussed previously).

The positioning of drinks or of a meal tray in relation to patients who have diminished ability to move themselves generally is an important consideration. Thus it is easier, as well as more therapeutic, to place a bedside cabinet with drink in front of or on the affected side of the person rather than on the unaffected side. He/she will then reach forward or over the body and the hand will be in a natural grasping position. Otherwise the person tries to bend the elbow backwards to reach articles parallel to the body on the unaffected side.

If arm or hand movement is diminished, consideration should also be given to the provision of any of the wide variety of aids available, for example utensils with large grip or long or curved handles, combined knife/forks, anti-slip mats for plates, plate guards. The occupational therapist may be of assistance here. Every effort should be made to enable the person to be self caring in respect of feeding, this often being one of the few areas of care that severely disabled persons, reliant on others for mobility and for meeting their hygiene and elimination needs, can undertake for themselves. Again, ensuring that food is presented in a form requiring minimal additional effort with respect to cutting is important.

A particular problem is created by difficulty in co-ordinating movement or flexibility of hand or arm or uneven chewing. Such patients tend to drop food on the way to or from their mouths, creating stained and unpleasant clothing. The tying of a bib around the necks implies childhood. Substantial plastic-backed serviettes well tucked in might be an acceptable alternative but promoting self care and dignity often exercises a nurse's creative abilities to the full in this situation.

If movement within the mouth is uneven or diminished, or if swallowing is impaired, foods requiring little chewing but definite swallowing are preferable until awareness of control has been learned (see Ch. 18). Such foods tend to be semi-solid such as milk-softened cereals, porridge, milk puddings and desserts. These can be boring and distasteful, as well as nutritionally inadequate, and should be combined with more stimulating foods such as specially prepared pureed casseroles, thick soups, soft or pureed fruit. Persons with a complete absence of the swallowing reflex will need to be fed parenterally or via intragastric tube.

However, the use of tube feeds for the majority of persons who have had a stroke is contentious on two grounds. First, that the tube itself, if left in situ, will decrease the ability to sense the bolus of food for swallowing, thus diminishing their ability to learn to swallow. Secondly, the early re-establishment of swallowing is more likely to result in rapid and complete recovery. Appropriate semi-solid/soft food can be swallowed without danger by the vast majority of stroke patients. Liquids are less controllable and dry, crumbly foods can easily be inhaled accidentally, while foods which require much chewing are tiring.

Consideration should also be given to the needs of those with few or no teeth and who choose not to wear dentures. A single piece of beef can last a long time!

Altered position. The normal position enabling food to be safely passed into the upper gastro-intestinal tract is upright with the chin at right angles to the body. Most people lean forward slightly as they deliver food to their mouth to reduce the likelihood of dropping food or dripping food onto their clothing.

In Western society, tables are approximately at waist height to the sitting person. Sitting on a chair with the legs down or on the floor with crossed legs are the most natural positions to adopt if the upper thorax is to maintain an upright or slightly forward leaning position. Sitting with the legs up but not crossed, as in patients who are confined to bed, creates a strain on the muscles of back and thighs when the thorax is held upright for any length of time. Leaning back slightly supported on pillows reduces this strain but then creates more difficulties in delivering food to the mouth without spillage. Some patients have to eat in very unnatural and sometimes potentially dangerous positions such as supine. In this situation the patient needs to be warned of the additional control he/she will have to exert over swallowing food and of the problems that are likely to be experienced when eating dry or crumbly food such as biscuits. Initially moist foods with real substance requiring chewing or definite swallowing are advised until the person has adjusted.

Altered elimination, pain, discomfort. These elements have been combined, as it is usually the pain/discomfort aspects associated with altered problems of elimination that create nutritional problems rather than the altered patterns per se. Symptoms such as gastric pain, 'indigestion', associated with peptic ulceration, feeling bloated following vagotomy, colic or abdominal cramping associated with diverticulitis or colitis, or distension associated with excess flatulence or constipation, will lead to disinclination to eat foods associated with these discomforts. In the short term this is not a problem, but in the long term, dietary management may become a major issue as the patient may reduce the amount or balance of the nutritional intake below that which is commensurate with physiological need. Where disorders of the mid or lower gastrointestinal tract are concerned severe diarrhoea with associated nutrient, electrolyte and fluid loss creates additional problems.

Changes in our understanding of physiological responses and disease causation have dramatically changed nutritional management in this respect. For example, in the management of a patient with peptic ulceration, the bland 'gastric' diet has been replaced by a more normal one (see Ch.23). Also, the low residue diet for patients with any lower intestinal problems given in order to 'rest' the gut has given way to high fibre diets which decrease the amount of time food remains in the gut (Burkitt, 1971; Painter, 1969).

In negotiating diets of adequate nutritional value with persons in great distress over their gastro-intestinal function great patience, understanding and sensitivity is required on the part of the nurse. The demoralising and excruciating pain associated with abnormal intestinal function should never be underestimated and every effort should be made to link appropriate palliative drugs with mealtimes or nutrient fluid intake.

Safety aspects. A further note in relation to assisting patients with their food concerns safety. Some points have already been made, for example, potential problems of choking when ability to swallow is diminished, or of scalding when sensation is altered. Another major aspect is that of prevention of cross infection. Norms of hygiene require that handwashing takes place after dealing with excrement and before handling food. This is a fundamental and simple principle but requires that nurses remember and make provision for handwashing for those persons not able to provide this for themselves.

Another potential source of infection is the utensils and crockery used — chipped glazing on cups or plates allows micro-organisms to invade the crockery, and dried on food on cutlery can also harbour bacteria. Patients with diseases or undergoing treatment that render them particularly vulnerable to infection or particularly liable to infect others may have crockery and cutlery for their specific use.

Chipped or cracked crockery or glasses not only create risk of infection but also of cutting the user's mouth. Oversharp knives or pointed forks create similar risks, although the value of the plastic varieties of these in any situation is dubious.

General note. Assisting patients with eating, and feeding them when necessary, requires considerable imagination and sensitivity and a lot of thoughtful common sense. 'Problem-solving' should be active and continuous, however dependent the patient has become: active involvement in choosing the meal, indicating preference for mixed or unmixed mouthfuls of food, preference for the utensil to be used, order and pace of delivery, can make the meal an enjoyable, sociable and enhancing occasion.

Aspects related to nutritional education and support

Nutritional education is required by many patients and provides a means of helping the individual to maintain or improve his/her health. Although the dietician is the person best qualified to provide such help, her/his time is limited and is focused on those requiring special diets. The other members of the health care team have, therefore, an important role to play in promoting healthy eating patterns in all patients, whether or not a special diet is involved. Many patients are willing to use a period of hospitalization as a learning experience and are motivated to change their eating practices; this provides the nurse with the opportunity to assist the patient in adopting healthy eating habits.

The way an individual behaves with regard to food is unique as it relates specifically to his/her past experiences and his/her perceptions of particular situations. Changing deep seated food habits is a slow process and, as habits may have emotional connotations, they are often particularly resistant to change; resentment is a common reaction to attempts to force change. The social meanings of food are less emotive and changes in the social environment, such as those produced by illness and hospitalisation, may be accompanied by concurrent changes in the perceived social role of food. Food practices which are deleterious to health and which are motivated primarily by social concerns are, therefore, more amenable to alteration provided that adequate explanation is offered. However, it must be remembered that alteration to any aspect of the environment — be this physical, physiological, psychological or social in origin — can of itself motivate change particularly if the individual can see that this will be of benefit to him or her.

Thus, in attempting to instigate change — whether this be to meet the requirements of a therapeutic diet or to instigate the adoption of healthy eating practices — the potential benefits must be realistically presented. Good health (or its recovery) is not guaranteed by the 'proper' choice of foods, although this does mitigate in its favour. It is often necessary first to correct faulty or misguided beliefs before new learning can be initiated. This must, however, be approached with care as, if the belief has strong emotional roots, arguing against it may close the mind to further teaching. When faulty information is merely misguided, and has no emotional connotations, providing accurate facts may act as a stimulus to further learning. It is the patient's motivation which provides the key to his/her willingness to learn; thus the nurse must first work at motivating the patient whilst, at the same time, establishing needs, wants and worries as these may be central to the learning process. Teaching will not be successful unless the patient accepts the value of it and is prepared to put in the necessary effort.

Progress is often slow when attempting to change food habits as the future gains are obscured by the immediate benefits of not changing and of maintaining the present life-style. For education to be successful the gains must be clearly identified and the educator must help to interpret the facts and identify possible courses of action based upon these. Nurses, whether in hospital or in the community, have many opportunities to talk to the patient and can use these to teach good food habits within the context of personal health behaviour.

Patients in hospital are under stress; the stress of illness and that of an unfamiliar and threatening environment. Some may have a superficial knowledge of nutrition or believe in the value of certain foods or a 'fad' diet in the recovery of health; many believe hospital food is 'bad' and that doctors and nurses know little about nutrition. They know that they will not get well unless they have the 'right' food; they are naturally worried and distressed and they don't feel secure that the doctor will take note of their nutritional problems.

The responsibilities of the nurse are clear. First, she/he must be supportive and find ways by which to reinforce the patient's confidence in the caring team. Secondly, she/he must be aware of her/his own limitations and realize that, in many instances, the best help which can be given is referral of the patient to the dietician or nurse-nutritionist. The nurse's role then becomes one of helping the patient to understand the advice given, to 'translate' terms and to explain, interpret and offer suggestions as to how the advice given might be implemented. Counselling of this sort is supplementary to, and supportive of, the actions of the medical team and the dietician.

Nutrition is now considered to be one of the

important medical sciences and has a vital place in health care today. It is critical in both the attainment and maintenance of good health as well as in the treatment of disease. The study of nutrition provides knowledge applicable to nurses in their personal lives as well as in their professional practice. It is the nurse's responsibility to consider the application of its principles to her/his own life as well as to the patients in her/his care, for, as Florence Nightingale (1859) said: 'The nutritional nursing care of the patient is one of the most important duties of the nurse.'

REFERENCES

Allison S P 1981 Fine bore tube feeding. Second European Congress of Parenteral and Enteral Nutrition, September 1980. Acta Chirurgica Scandinavica (suppl. 507)

American Heart Foundation 1979 Conference on the health effects of blood lipids: optimal distributions for populations. Preventive Medicine 8 : 621–678

Anderson E 1973 The role of the nurse. Royal College of Nursing,London

Baker H, Frank O, Sobotka H 1964 Mechanisms of folic acid deficiency. Journal of the American Medical Association 187:119–121

Bender A E 1979 The pocket guide to calories and nutrition. Mitchell Beazley, London

Bull N L, Buss D H 1980 Contribution of foods to sodium intake. Proceedings of the Nutrition Society 39(2) : 30A

Burkitt D P, 1971 Epidemiology of cancer of the colon and rectum. Cancer 28 : 3–13

Burt B A, Ekland S A 1980 Sugar consumption and dental caries;some epidemiological patterns in the US. Fourth Annual Conference on Foods, Nutrition and Dental Health. Report of the American Dental Association

Butterworth C E 1974 The skeleton in the hospital closet. Nutrition Today, March/April : 4–8

Champion R 1979 The administration of patient care. Unpublished MSc Thesis, University of Wales

Chanarin I 1973 In : Howard A N (ed) Nutritional deficiencies in modern society. Newman, London

Chapman J 1983 Nutritional status of hospitalised elderly patients : nursing implications. In : Proceedings of nutritional care of the elderly : a nursing responsibility. Conference held at Northwick Park Hospital, June 1983

Clarke M 1983 Practical nursing. Nurses Aids Series, Baillière Tindall, London

Coates V 1984 Inadequate intake in hospital. Nursing Mirror 158 (4) : 21–22

Dahl L K, Heine M, Tassinari L 1962 Effects of chronic excess salt consumption : evidence that genetic factors play an important role in susceptibility to experimental hypertension. Journal of Experimental Medicine 115 : 1173—1190

Davies G J, Evans E, Stock A, Yudkin J 1975 Special diets in hospitals : discrepancy between what is prescribed and what is eaten. British Medical Journal 1:200–204

Department of Health and Social Security 1972 Report on public health and medical subjects No. 3. HMSO, London

Department of Health and Social Security 1978 Prevention and health; eating for health. HMSO, London

Department of Health and Social Security 1979 Recommended daily amounts of food energy and nutrients for groups of people in the UK. Report on health and social subjects No. 15. HMSO, London

Department of Health and Social Security 1981 Prevention and health; avoiding heart attacks. HMSO, London

Department of Health and Social Security and Welsh Office, Central Health Services Council 1976 The organisation of the in-patient's day. HMSO, London

Drummond W C, Wilbraham A 1939 The Englishman's food. Jonathan Cape, London

Elliott J R 1975 Living in hospital. King Edward's Hospital Fund for London, London

Exton-Smith A N 1978 Nutrition and the elderly. In : Dickerson J W T, Lee H A (eds) Nutrition in the clinical management of disease. Edward Arnold, London

Ganong W F 1985 Review of medical physiology, 12th edn. Lange Medical Publications, Los Altos, California

Gear J S S, Fursdon P, Nolan D J, Ware A, Mann J L, Brodribb A J M, Vessey M P 1979 Symptomless diverticular disease and intake of dietary fibre. Lancet 1 : 511–514

Gifft H H, Washbon M B, Harrison G G 1972 Nutrition, behaviour and change. Prentice Hall, New Jersey

Gleibermann L 1973 Blood pressure and dietary salt in human populations. Ecology, Food and Nutrition 2 : 143–156

Gray J 1983 Nutrition in medical education : report of the British Nutrition Foundation's task force on clinical nutrition. The British Nutrition Foundation, London

Greaves J P, Tan J 1966 The amino acid pattern of the British diet. Nutrition 20 : 112–115

Hargreaves J A 1980 Sucrose and total sugar intake and dental caries of Ontario children. Kellogg Nutrition Symposium, Toronto, Canada

Heald F P 1969 Adolescent nutrition and growth. Butterworth, London

Henderson V 1960 Basic principles of nursing care. International Council of Nurses, Geneva

Holmes S 1983 A vital power supply. Nursing Mirror 156 : 39–41

Jeliffe D B 1966 The assessment of nutritional status in the community. WHO Monograph 53, Geneva

Jones D 1975 Food for thought. Royal College of Nursing, London

Keys A 1953 Prediction and possible prevention of coronary disease. American Journal of Public Health 43 1399–1407

Keys A, Aravanis C, Blackburn H, Van Buchem F S P, Buzina R, Djordjevic B S, Dontas A S, Fidanza F, Karvonen M J, Kimura N, Menotti A, Puddu V, Punsar S, Taylor H I 1980 Seven countries :A multivariate analysis of death and coronary heart disease. Harvard University Press, Cambridge, Massachusetts

Lennon D, Fieldhouse P 1979 Community dietetics. Forbes Publications, London

Macgregor G A, Markandu N, Best F, Elder D, Cam J, Sagnelli G A, Squires M 1982 Double blind randomised crossover trial of moderate sodium restriction in essential hypertension. Lancet 1 : 351–355

Meneely G R, Ball C O T 1958 Experimental epidemiology of chronic sodium chloride toxicity and protective effect of potassium chloride. American Journal of Medicine 25 : 713–725

Ministry of Agriculture, Fisheries and Food 1980 Household food consumption and expenditure. HMSO, London

Moghissi K, Boore J 1983 Parenteral and Enteral Nutrition for Nurses. Heinemann, London

Morgan T, Gillies A, Morgan G, Adam W, Wilson M, Carney S 1978 Hypertension treated by salt restriction. Lancet 1 : 227–230

National Advisory Committee on Nutrition Education (NACNE) 1983 Proposals for nutritional guidelines for health education in Britain. Health Education Council, London

Nightingale F 1859 (republished 1974) Notes on nursing. Blackie, London

Orem D E 1971 Nursing concepts of practice. McGraw Hill, New York

Painter N S 1969 Diverticulosis of the colon and diet. British Medical Journal 1 : 764–765

Phillips I, Meers P D, D'Arcy P F (eds) 1976 Microbiological hazards of infusion therapy. M T P Press, Lancaster

Raphael W 1977 Patients and their hospitals. King Edward's Hospital Fund for London, London

Roper N, Logan W W, Tierney A J 1985 The elements of nursing, 2nd edn. Churchill Livingstone, Edinburgh

Roy C 1980 The Roy adaptation model. In : Riehl J P, Roy C (eds) Conceptual models for nursing practice, 2nd edn. Appleton-Century-Crofts, New York

Royal College of Physicians 1981 Report on the medical aspects of dietary fibre. Pitman Medical, Tunbridge Wells

Royal College of Physicians 1983 Obesity. Journal of the Royal College of Physicians 17 : 3–58

Royal College of Physicians and the British Cardiac Society 1976 Prevention of coronary heart disease. Journal of the Royal College of Physicians 10 : 213–275

Sheiham A 1983 Sugars and dental decay. Lancet 1 : 282–284

Sherman H C 1920 Protein requirements of maintenance in man and nutritive value of bread protein. Journal of Biological Chemistry 41 : 97–109

Smithells R W, Ankers C, Carver M E, Lennon D, Scorah C J, Sheppard S 1973 Maternal nutrition in early pregnancy. British Journal of Nutrition 38 : 497–506

Stocks P 1944 Diabetes mortality in 1861–1942 and some of the factors affecting it. Journal of Hygiene, 43 : 242–247

Strohl R A 1983 Nursing management of the patient with cancer experiencing taste changes. Cancer Nursing 6 (5) : 353–359

Thompson A M 1978 Problems and politics in nutritional surveillance. Proceedings of the Nutrition Society 37 : 317–332

Todd E A, Hunt P, Crowe P J, Royle G T 1984 What do patients eat in hospital. Human Nutrition : Applied Nutrition 38A, 294–297

Tones B K 1978 Effectiveness and efficiency in health education : a review of theory and practice. Scottish Health Education Unit, Edinburgh

Trowell H 1972 Ischaemic heart disease and dietary fibre. American Journal of Clinical Nutrition 25 : 926–932

Vir S, Love A H G 1979 Nutritional status of institutionalised and non institutionalised aged in Belfast. American Journal of Clinical Nutrition 32 : 1934–1947

Whitehead M S 1983 Nutrition of the hospital patient. Nursing Focus 4 (7) : 16–20

World Health Organization Expert Committee 1982 Prevention of coronary heart disease. Technical Report Series 678. World Health Organization, Geneva

Yudkin J 1957 Diet and coronary thrombosis : hypothesis and fact. Lancet 2 : 155 – 162

Yudkin J 1972 Pure, white and deadly. Davis Poynter, London.

15

Drug therapy

INTRODUCTION

The history of pharmacology is almost as long as that of man himself. The Greek word 'pharmakon', from which it is derived,was used to describe not only the curative drug but also generally to mean a poison, charm, spell or incantation.

Today the word 'drug' also has many meanings dependent on the context in which it is used. To the pharmacologist and the medical practitioner, a drug is a chemical which in minute doses can be therapeutic, i.e. it can reverse or inhibit a disease state or alleviate symptoms associated with a disease state. The production of such chemicals within this definition is subject to strict controls in many countries, although the standards agreed in one country are not necessarily those of another. Similarly, there are controls over their distribution, some drugs only being legally available by prescription from a registered medical practitioner, others being freely for sale without the supervision of either medical practitioner or pharmacist.

The relationship between the medical practitioner and the administration of drugs leads to an 'assumed' ratification of drugs, even when the drug in question can be obtained without a medical prescription.The terms 'drug' and 'therapeutic' are applied to a wide range of untested remedies available over the counter. Those who eschew 'chemical' medicines have developed 'natural' remedies, primarily from herbs. Many of these herbs have been grown, collected and used for medicinal purposes and some of these were the origins of modern drugs. For example, the foxglove was the source of digitalis, of which digoxin is a derivative. The use of drugs that are available only on medical prescription, by persons without that prescription, is 'illegal' clearly only in the countries where those laws apply: 'drug use', 'drug abuse' and 'drug addiction' are the words used. This highlights problems of classification, in that cultural and individual value systems affect the labelling not only of a substance as a 'drug', i.e. subject to legal controls (see above), but the acceptance of a drug as a legitimate remedy. This in turn affects not only the attitudes of the consumer to drug taking but the attitude of the medical practitioner involved in prescribing. At the extremes the patient may see a drug as something harmful, whereas the doctor sees it as essential.

The nurse's role

The nurse's role in relation to drugs is complex. On the whole she is not responsible for prescribing drugs (although she will be both prescriber and dispenser in some situations in developing countries, and may prescribe or alter the dose of a medically prescribed drug in specific situations even where legal controls are tight). However in hospital situations she is responsible for administering drugs to patients and, unless her role is seen as totally medically dependent, she must therefore have a responsibility for intelligent interpretation of medical instructions and the withholding of a drug where there is doubt over its prescription or where the condition of the patient has changed. She is also responsible with the hospital pharmacist for ensuring safe keeping, ordering and recording of drugs given. By contrast, in the community the patient is responsible for both storage and self administration. This situation can create problems of non-compliance after discharge from hospital, unless positive steps are taken to educate patients thoroughly prior to discharge about their required medication. This is explored in a later section of this chapter.

The complex role of the nurse in relation to the administration of drugs is a cause of conflict. Legally nurses in hospital have to depend on medical prescription for the most straightforward of remedies that can be bought over the counter, for example paracetamol for a headache, or mild aperients. In practice, for many such 'routine' remedies there will be a mutual agreement between senior ward nurses and medical staff as to their administration. Further difficulties can arise from patients' lack of knowledge of their disease condition and the inevitable questions that arise about drugs prescribed. Indeed, the nurse administering the drugs may disagree with the prescription in the absence of the patient's informed consent. The more mundane, but very practical, difficulty of illegible or unclear prescriptions has a much easier solution — while the nurse is responsible to the doctor and the institution for administering drugs, she is clearly responsible for ensuring the prescription is clear and should refuse to give anything that is not clearly prescribed.

History of drug development

Historically, pharmacology has relied heavily upon naturally occurring substances; some, like digitalis, are very potent while others are completely inactive. In the second half of the 19th century the new chemical industries started to produce new drugs and antiseptics. New ideas developed in pharmacology, the structure of compounds became related to their function and the ideas of receptors and selectivity appeared. In 1913 Paul Ehrlich, sometimes called the father of modern chemotherapy, made his much quoted statement in which he likens the drug to a 'magic bullet' which can seek out and destroy the parasite without harming the host.

From this first mention of a 'target' developed the whole modern theory of drug action — the receptor theory. The advent of the first sulphonamide drugs in the 1930s and the penicillins 10 years later opened a new era in the treatment of infection. Chemical synthesis has led to an explosion in the number of new drugs since then, which continues today. The United Kingdom is now one of the five largest manufacturers of pharmaceuticals. Although there has been a steady decline in drug innovation since the 1960s, the tendency is for companies to produce their own patent drug following each new discovery, so that every company has a very similar 'me too' drug in the new group (for example beta blockers and H_2 blockers). All these drugs have similar properties but are dissimilar enough to uphold the patent laws, so giving all companies a share in each new market. The main reason for this is to allow pharmaceutical industries to acquire a share in an otherwise monopolized market in order to ensure commercial viability. The cost of new drug development has rocketed in the last 10 years, therefore fewer companies are prepared to invest in drug development; when they do, they invest in fewer drugs within any possibly useful group. In addition to this, development tends to be concentrated upon drugs for illnesses which have a high frequency, such as infection, hypertension and rheumatism, where they will have a ready market, while many rare conditions remain untreatable by modern standards.

Drug use

Over the last 10 years there has been a steady increase in prescribing, which is most noticeable for genitourinary, cardiovascular, hormone and rheumatic diseases (Association of the British Pharmaceutical Industry, 1980). These trends can be related to the introduction of new drug groups such as beta blockers. The introduction of the benzodiazepine tranquillizers, although associated with a rapid increase in prescriptions, does not appear in the overall figures. This is because of the related reduction in prescriptions of barbiturates as sedatives (Williams, 1980).

The overall trend is that more people are taking more drugs and, with the development of gerontology and the associated medical speciality of geriatrics, there has also been an increase in the active treatment of elderly people. This has resulted in an apparent increase in adverse effects, the Adverse Drug Reaction register now having more than 40 000 adverse events experienced by people taking drugs. These reactions may not all be attributable to drugs, but those reporting them considered the association to be important enough to be recorded. Since the introduction, following the thalidomide tragedy, of the Medicines Act (1968) greater control has been placed on newly introduced drugs, and a systematic review of older drugs is taking place. The Committee of Safety for Medicines must be satisfied with the safety of any new drug and may ask for additional tests to be done before a clinical trial or product licence is issued. National differences in legislation, however, lead to differences in availability of drugs between different countries and to international dispute as to the relative safety and advocacy of particular drugs.

Since a greater variety of drug treatments is available and the results of their apparent achievements are well publicized, even though the achievements may be spurious and the apparent benefits may be later refuted, the patient's expectation of cure has been enhanced. Instead of expecting long-term medical and nursing attention to restore him to health he expects a few tablets to produce a miraculous cure. Although the physician has at his command this formidable array of treatments, there are, unfortunately, some ills which do not disappear on the administration of a pill; or, for that matter, on the administration of that pill which should bring about a cure. It is partly because of these problems associated with drug therapy that the discipline of clinical pharmacology has developed during recent years. The clinical pharmacologist is a doctor with special interest in the effects which drugs have on the human body in the clinical situation and with the effects which the human body can have on the drugs administered to it. It is only through this type of knowledge that the full benefit of drugs can be given to the patient.

In this chapter the principles of pharmacology upon which therapy is based will be outlined. Thus the chapter explores the mechanisms of drug action — receptors, absorption, distribution, metabolism and excretion; the way in which drug therapy is monitored; and factors influencing drug response, such as age and pathologies. The final two sections of the chapter are concerned with the increasing area of knowledge on adverse drug reactions and problems associated with drug therapy. Details of individual drug use and administration are not included because they are adequately covered in other literature. The reader is referred to specialized drug and therapeutics textbooks and to the frequently updated publication British National Formulary (BNF).

MECHANISMS OF DRUG ACTION

RECEPTORS

The theories of drug-receptor interactions are surrounded with considerable controversy. No receptor has been observed physically, nor is the exact relationship between the drug and receptor known. The relationship of the concentration of drug in the fluid surrounding the receptor and any given response has not been fully explained. Nevertheless, the present concept of receptors as the site of drug action goes some way to improve our understanding of how drugs act. The receptor theory originated in the work of Paul Ehrlich in the late 19th and early 20th century. He considered receptors to be the point of contact between cells and substances reaching them via the blood or tissue fluids. This idea was developed by Professor Langley in Cambridge who used the receptor concept to explain the functioning of the autonomic nervous system.

Interaction between a drug and a receptor occurs at molecular level; the interaction can produce either stimulation of a response or blockade of endogenous compounds. For example, histamine and adrenaline and their analogues act as agonists (stimulating the receptors) while some other compounds are antagonistic, blocking the receptors and preventing any effect. The drug in solution around the receptor must have an affinity for the receptor, so that it is attracted into association, in order to produce an effect. However, affinity alone need not produce an effect.

Type of response

Three types of response are possible when a drug

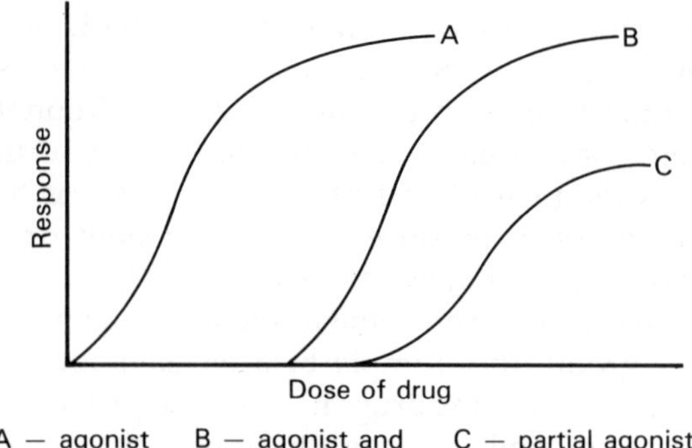

Fig. 15.1 Dose response curves.

and receptor combine in vitro, as shown in Figure 15.1. The response shown in curve A is the response to an agonist. Increasing doses of drug produce an increased response until a maximum effect results. Further increase of dose produces no increase in response, indicating that all possible receptors are activated. When an antagonist is administered no response can be seen. Because it occupies the receptor without producing any response, its affinity and ability to compete with agonists for receptors can be shown by adding doses of the known agonist. This combination shows a response which reaches the same maximum but which is shifted to the right (curve B), higher doses of agonist being needed to produce the same response. Curve C shows the response to doses of a partial agonist; this drug has affinity but reduced efficacy. Response develops slowly with increases in dose, the same maximum is not reached and blockade may follow.

The relationship between drug and receptor can be expressed as an equation:

Drug + receptor ⟵⟶ Drug receptor complex ⟶ Response

The size of the response is a function of the amount of drug in solution and the number of receptors. Maximum response would appear to be governed by the number of receptors. At this point, receptor theories diverge. On the one hand the occupancy of receptors is believed to govern response; on the other, the rate at which receptors are stimulated is considered to be of most importance. In either case, an optimal concentration of drug in the vicinity of the receptor is important. As a drug is absorbed from the site of administration, or circulates following direct administration into the circulation, it is distributed unevenly throughout the body. The most useful drugs are those which will concentrate in the target area thus avoiding unwanted effects in other tissues. Tests on animals before a drug is marketed show tissue distribution. In humans the main indicator is the concentration in the blood which can easily be sampled. Tissue levels can and have been measured where organs are removed during operation and the patient has previously required drug treatment (Kiss et al, 1976; Parsons et al, 1978).

The concentration of drug at the receptor depends on four main factors:

- absorption from the site of administration
- distribution within the body
- metabolism of the drug by the body enzyme systems
- excretion site and rate

Each of these factors is controlled to some extent by the chemical properties of the drug, the patient and his condition.

ABSORPTION

Route of administration

Before a drug can be absorbed it must be presented in a suitable form at the site of administration. It must therefore be soluble in body fluids and concentrated enough to allow administration in a small volume. The route of administration may be chosen for convenience; in this country we prefer the oral route. Some drugs, e.g. insulin and heparin, are unfortunately destroyed in the gastrointestinal tract and these must be given by injection. The rectal route is favoured in some countries for a wide range of drugs, but in the United Kingdom it is mainly confined to the administration of aminophylline in respiratory distress and phenylbutazone in arthritis. In common with the sublingual route which is used for glyceryl trinitrate and methyltestosterone, the rectal route has the advantage of avoiding the portal circulation,

Table 15.1 Main routes of administration for drugs

Local	Inhalation	Gastrointestinal	Parenteral
Dermal	Bronchial	Sublingual	Subcutaneous
Conjunctival	Alveolar	Oral	Intramuscular
Nasal		Rectal	Intravenous
Urethral			Intraspinal
Vaginal			

resulting in fast delivery to the site of action without prior exposure to the liver's metabolizing enzymes. Where fast effect is of vital importance the intravenous route is chosen. The main sites of administration are summarized in Table 15.1.

Methods of absorption

Except when given intravenously or applied locally, drugs must first be absorbed from the site of administration before they can enter the circulation and travel to their site of action. To achieve this the drug must pass through a series of cell membranes by one of four mechanisms (Schanker, 1961):

- passive diffusion
- active transport
- filtration
- pinocytosis.

Passive diffusion

Most drugs pass through membranes passively in solution. The speed and extent of movement depends on the concentration of the drug on either side of the membrane, the drug moving from high to lower concentration. As the body membranes are lipid structures, drugs which are lipid soluble will diffuse more readily. The polar nature of the membrane allows passage only to the non-ionized fraction of drug. Most drugs are weak acids or bases which in solution partly dissociate into ions. When the acidic drug for example aspirin, is least ionized in an acid medium (the stomach) diffusion will be rapid; on entry to the body fluids (pH 7.4) it becomes more ionized. The reverse is seen in the more alkaline environment of the small intestine, acidic drugs are more ionized and alkaline ones remain non-ionized. Theoretically this favours the alkaline drug but, in practice, because of the large surface area available for absorption and the length of time that the drug can remain in the gut, acidic drugs are more extensively absorbed in the intestine than in the stomach.

Active transport

Certain molecules, e.g. amino acids, are transported across membranes by energy consuming processes. Only the few drugs which closely resemble natural substances can be absorbed in this way. These include levodopa and methyldopa.

Filtration

Passage through pores within the membrane is only possible for drugs of a small molecular size. Absorption in this way is rapid, which accounts for the speed of ethanol action.

Pinocytosis

Small particles are engulfed by the cells, particularly of the gut wall. This route, although possible, cannot be relied upon as making a major contribution to drug absorption.

In general, absorption across a membrane depends on the concentrations on either side of the membrane, the surface area available for absorption and the time which the drug remains exposed to the membrane. The gut is ideally designed in all these respects to enable the maximum absorption of nutrients, and drugs are designed chemically with this fact in mind.

Factors which affect oral absorption

Bioavailability

The extent to which a drug is available for absorption depends on its physical preparation, the particle size, binding, compression and coating of the tablet or capsule. Laboratory tests ensure that disintegration takes place in the optimal time and in the body fluids with which the drug will come into contact. It is therefore important to remember that the tablet is made for a purpose. Where there is difficulty in swallowing, it is best to obtain a liquid formulation, unless the tablet is intended to be dissolved, e.g. soluble aspirin. In general, uncoated tablets may be broken or crushed but this will make them more unpleasant to take. Tablets with enteric coating and capsules should never be broken as the coverings are designed to prevent the drug coming into contact with the gut lining too soon.

It must always be remembered that changes in the formulation of a drug, as in preparations made by different companies or in different countries, can all affect bioavailability. The tablet administered does not consist of the drug alone; all sorts of additives are used to bind the components, make them dissolve and taste more pleasant. These additives vary and have been shown to affect bioavailability. This is important when small changes in concentration have a drastic effect on response. Such a change was demonstrated with phenytoin (Tyrer et al, 1970); when the excipient (tablet filler) was changed from lactose to calcium sulphate the steady state plasma concentration fell by 70%.

Food

Food and drink will dilute the drug and a meal will delay gastric emptying. Therefore, exposure of the drug to absorption sites leads to delay in the absorption of most drugs. Gastric emptying is not, however, an all or none effect, so that small amounts of drug will be absorbed within a short time of administration and dissolution (Prescott, 1974). Some drugs are better administered with food, notably levodopa which causes unpleasant nausea and vomiting if given on an empty stomach. The damaging effect of aspirin on the gastric mucosa is reduced if the drug is taken with food. In most cases the presence of food will not alter the overall absorption of drugs given in multiple doses, while locally-acting drugs such as antacids are given before or after food for reasons other than absorption. The main advantage of linking medication with meals is that it aids compliance — popping in a pill with a meal is

Table 15.2 Antibiotic absorption in malabsorption syndrome

Syndrome	Increased absorption	Decreased absorption	No change
A. Coeliac disease	cephalexin clindamycin erythromycin ethylsuccinate sodium fusidate	amoxycillin pivampicillin	ampicillin erthromycin stearate lincomycin
B. Crohn's disease	sulphamethoxazole	trimethoprim lincomycin	
C. Small bowel diverticulosis	cephalexin trimethoprim clindamycin		amoxycillin ampicillin sulphamethoxazole

easier to remember than taking it between times. Where the fast action of a single dose is important, between-meals administration is probably an advantage.

Malabsorption

Diseases which affect the gut may lead to malabsorption of nutrients due to the changes produced in the gut mucosa, motility and gut flora. Studies have shown that in conditions such as Crohn's disease, coeliac disease, small bowel diverticulosis and ulcerative colitis, the absorption of drugs differs from that in normal volunteers. The difference in absorption in coeliac disease is not always improved by a gluten-free diet. The alterations found are not always predictable, being increased with some drugs and conditions and decreased with others (Parsons et al, 1975a) (Table 15.2). Patients with malabsorption syndrome should be observed to ensure that the prescribed treatment is effective and does not cause toxicity.

DISTRIBUTION

Distribution through body

Once absorbed, a drug must rely upon the circulation to carry it to its site of action. Before reaching this site other membrane systems may have to be crossed, including the capillary endothelial cell walls and the target organ membranes. The transport across these membranes is governed by the same parameters which apply to absorption, i.e. lipid solubility,

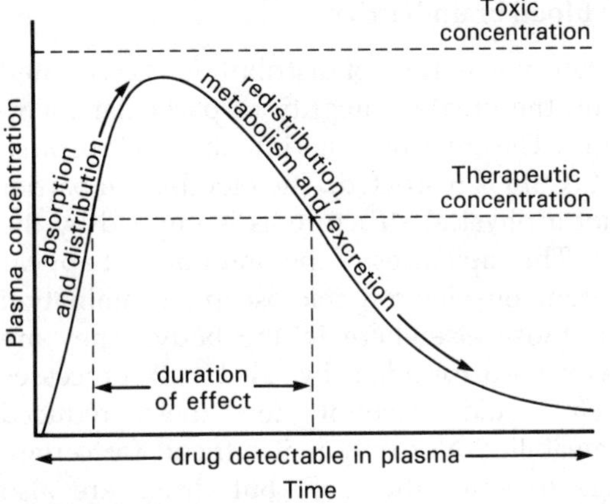

Fig. 15.2 Theoretical plasma concentration/time curve following a single oral dose of a drug.

ionization and concentration. In addition, a drug is usually transported in the blood in combination with plasma proteins. Such drugs are not biologically active or available to cross membranes, so that highly bound drugs do not become pharmacologically active until the binding protein is saturated. Following the initial rise in concentration due to absorption, redistribution contributes to a drop in the plasma concentration as the drug enters the tissue (Fig. 15.2). This redistribution is uneven because tissue uptake and binding ability varies. This can be useful therapeutically because drugs may concentrate in the tissue where they have their action. For example, mercurial diuretics accumulate in the renal cortex where they have their effect. On the other hand, the redistribution of drugs into adipose tissue removes these from the circulation and they are not available to act therapeutically. They are slowly released back into the circulation over a considerable period of time. For example barbiturates bind avidly to adipose tissue which accounts for the short duration of thiopentone action (Brodie et al, 1952). Originally it was thought that the short duration of anaesthesia achieved with thiopentone was due to rapid excretion, but in fact excretion of this drug from the fat deposit is very slow, taking several weeks. This may explain the prolonged general lassitude experienced by postoperative patients.

The blood brain barrier

Further unevenness of distribution is accounted for by the greater integrity of particular membranes. The entry of drugs into the cerebrospinal fluid (CSF) is restricted. The blood-brain barrier is not a physical structure as is implied by the term. The capillaries of the brain do not appear different on electron microscopic examination from those elsewhere in the body. They are however surrounded by glial cell processes which could account for their reduced permeability. Not only is it difficult for certain drugs to enter the CSF, but drugs are also actively removed into the plasma at the choroid plexus. Salicylates (aspirin) and the penicillins are amongst those excreted from CSF by a process similar to that which takes place in the renal tubules and which can be inhibited by probenecid. It is therefore important that drugs intended to act within the central nervous system should be administered directly, unless they can readily penetrate the blood-brain barrier (Creasey, 1979).

The placental barrier

Like the term 'blood-brain barrier', the term 'placental barrier' has developed because there appear to be some factors in the passage of drugs between the mother and fetus that are not seen in the passage of drugs across other body membranes. The same rules of passage apply as at other membranes, non-ionized, lipid soluble, low molecular weight structures will cross the placenta more readily than others. Protection is offered to the fetus by the placental ability to metabolize and inactivate endogenous substances. In the same way, drugs may also be metabolized; the products may not, however, be innocuous. In fact they could be toxic to the fetus. The most sound advice to a mother, therefore, is not to take any drugs during pregnancy, including patent medicines, unless they are strongly indicated and prescribed by a doctor who knows about the pregnancy (Creasey, 1979).

METABOLISM (BIOTRANSFORMATION)

The majority of drugs are chemically altered by the body. The usual effect of these changes is to make the drug inactive and more easily excreted by the liver or kidney thus preventing a build up of foreign compounds within the body. In some cases the metabolite may also be active, or an active metabolite may be produced from an inactive drug. It is this type of process which converts codeine to the more potent morphine, and imipramine to desipramine within the body. Drug metabolism can take place anywhere in the body, though most occurs in the liver (Remmer, 1970). This is not only because the liver has a vast capacity for enzyme activity but also because it is the first organ to which orally administered drugs are carried by the circulation. This so called 'first pass' metabolism removes large quantities of some drugs before they have reached their site of action.

Three main types of enzyme action take place:

- Non-specific intermediate enzyme action only affects drugs which are identical with, or similar to, substances naturally occurring within the body. The drug levodopa is acted upon to produce dopamine; histamine, adrenaline and noradrenaline are all dealt with in the same way as their endogenous counterparts.
- Another group of actions also takes place in the liver and is the product of the non-specific enzymes associated with the endoplasmic reticulum of the liver cells. These enzymes act as catalysts for a number of chemical reactions, mainly

oxidation, reduction or hydrolysis reactions. These reactions make the drug more water soluble. This is necessary to allow excretion to take place, and some drugs may be able to be excreted without further change. In addition, these reactions produce a chemically active site on the molecule which is necessary for conjugation to occur.
- The third type of action involved in drug metabolism is conjugation, also catalysed by enzymes found mainly in the liver. In conjugation the modified drug molecule combines with glucuronic acid (or acetic or sulphuric acid) to form a glucuronide (or acetate or sulphate). This increases still further the water solubility of the drug which can then be excreted readily in the urine or the bile.

It may seem strange that there is such a battery of enzymes waiting to metabolize drugs. They are, however, an integral part of the body's natural pathways for the breakdown of both intrinsic and extrinsic substances. Drugs can have an effect on this enzyme system, either damping down or increasing its activity. In normal conditions the system can cope, but when there is an overdose or where there has been liver damage the system is less capable of coping with demands and toxic reactions may occur. Thus a normal dose of barbiturate can induce hepatic coma in a patient with cirrhosis or infective hepatitis.

EXCRETION

Most drugs are excreted in the urine either as the parent drug or in the form of metabolites. They may also be excreted to some extent in the sweat (e.g. sulphonamides), expelled air (e.g. paraldehyde and anaesthetics), all parts of the gastrointestinal tract, breast milk and vaginal secretions. Some drugs are predominantly excreted in the bile (e.g. rifampicin). Knowledge of these facts can aid therapy; antibiotics excreted in the bile can be used to treat biliary tract infection. Where there is damage to the excreting organ (kidney disease, biliary obstruction or paralytic ileus), a build-up of drugs can take place. For excretion via the kidneys and gastrointestinal tract, including the biliary system, drugs must be water soluble to prevent reabsorption. Drugs excreted through the lungs are substances which rapidly vaporize and are therefore excreted unchanged.

Renal excretion

The factors which control absorption also define the ability of drugs to be reabsorbed in the renal tubule; lipid-soluble drugs of small molecular weight which readily enter the glomerular filtrate are as easily reabsorbed lower down the tubule. The more polar, water-soluble drug metabolites produced in the liver are of larger molecular weight and, though slower to enter the glomerular filtrate, remain there to be subsequently excreted. Excretion can be influenced to some extent by the urinary pH. The normally slightly acid urine favours the excretion of weakly basic drugs (amphetamine) which become ionized in the urine preventing their reabsorption; increasing acidity speeds the process of excretion. Giving sodium bicarbonate will render the urine more alkaline and prolongs the action of basic drugs by increasing their reabsorption into the body. The reverse applies with acidic drugs such as barbiturates giving rise to the concept of alkaline diuresis in cases of poisoning. The effect of these changes is not as great as had been expected, making therapeutic use of doubtful benefit.

Biliary excretion

While the majority of drugs are excreted in the urine via the kidney, the part played by the bile should not be overlooked. Drugs and their metabolites which concentrate in the bile may therefore be of value in treating biliary infections (e.g. rifampicin and ampicillin). Other drugs, e.g. stilboestrol and phenolphthalein, excreted as metabolites, can be reabsorbed into the circulation following reconversion to the parent drug by the gut bacteria. This enterohepatic circulation has an overall effect of prolonging the

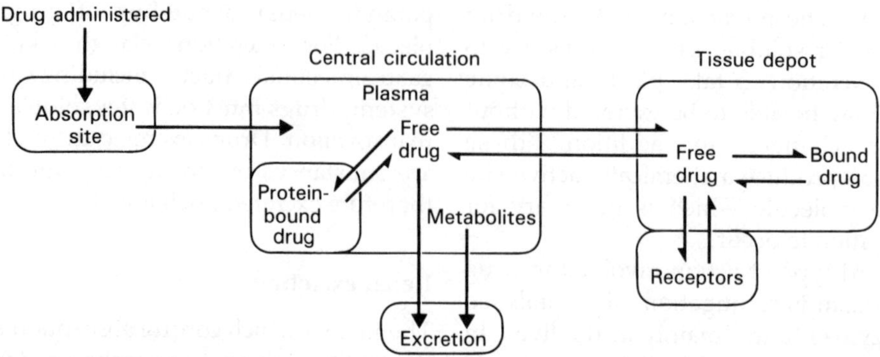

Fig. 15.3 The movement of a drug between body compartments

activity of the drug, but it is doubtful whether it can cause a post absorption peak in plasma concentrations.

PHARMACOKINETICS

Pharmacokinetics is about the application of mathematical principles to the movement (kinesis) of drugs within the body. Calculations of time, concentration, rate of movement and the volume in which the drug is distributed are included. This theoretical discipline is useful because it allows the calculation of rates of absorption, distribution, metabolism and excretion of drugs (see Fig. 15.2). In the development of new drugs it enables calculations to be made of dosage and dose interval. It is also of value in adjusting dosage regimes for individual patients with conditions such as renal or hepatic failure.

The interrelationships shown in Figure 15.3 can be calculated to give the rate constants for absorption, transfer between the main (blood) and other (tissue) compartments, metabolism and excretion. The number of compartments between which a drug is distributed can be computed from the shape of the curve derived by plotting plasma concentration against time. The volume in which the drug is distributed is the relationship between the total drug in the body and the plasma concentration. This volume of distribution can be in excess of total body water (41 litres) when the drug is concentrated in the tissues (i.e. less drug in the plasma). Accurate calculations of these kinetic parameters can only be made when drugs are given directly into the plasma compartment (intravenously) avoiding the variables of absorption.

Calculation of effective absorption by different routes can be made by comparing the area under the plasma concentration/time curve following the administration of the same dose, to the same individuals, by the two routes. Most drugs are not given in such large doses as to saturate the elimination process. Therefore, a constant fraction of the drug is excreted in any unit of time, regardless of concentration, so that the amount remaining can be calculated by subtracting the amount excreted from the amount administered. An alternative method of expressing elimination is by the half life ($t\frac{1}{2}$). This is the time required for the plasma concentration of the drug to fall by 50%. The half life is used by the clinical pharmacologist to calculate the interval between doses, while the actual dose of drug to be given is that which gives a concentration above the therapeutic and below the toxic level after multiple doses. Where elimination is a constant, depending on drug concentration, the steady state (plateau level) can be achieved after 4–5 doses when the dose interval is equal to 0.5 x the half life (Fig. 15.4). The time required to reach a therapeutic concentration will be measured in days, or for some drugs even weeks. To avoid this type of

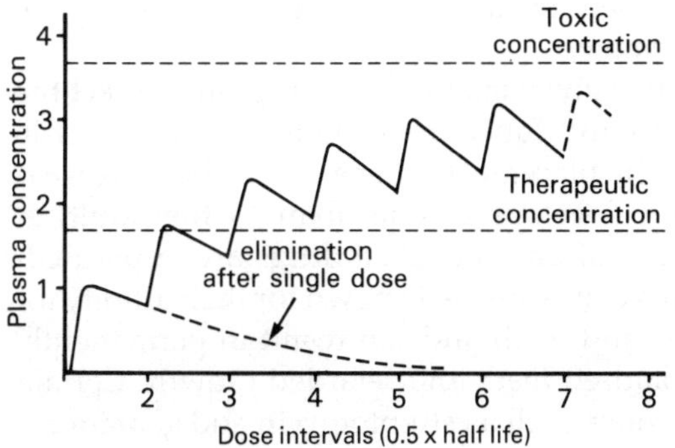

Fig. 15.4 The effect of repeated dosage at intervals of half the t½

delay in therapy a loading dose may be given, where it is safe to do so, to speed treatment.

Pharmacokinetic calculations are very helpful to those who plan drug therapy and study the effect of drugs in the human body. The theoretical models are the basis for demonstrating changes due to individual variation and the disease process.

MONITORING THERAPY

When a normal dose of drug is given to a patient, therapy is monitored by observing the pharmacological effect on the patient's condition. Antihypertensive treatment is monitored by taking the blood pressure at regular intervals, in the same way as the taking of a patient's temperature can indicate the success or not of antibacterial therapy. Dosage may also be determined by therapeutic effect, for example the anaesthetist injects thiopentone until the required depth of anaesthesia is achieved. With other drugs such observational methods are not possible, yet the need to know the effect may be of importance. When the therapeutic ratio is low (i.e.the range between a therapeutic dose and toxicity is small — see Fig. 15.2), regular monitoring of plasma drug concentration will be needed (phenytoin and lithium).

When a patient is acutely ill he may be receiving a number of drugs. At the same time his physiological functioning may be compromised and lead to alterations in the absorption, distribution, metabolism and excretion of drugs. In such circumstances it is valuable to monitor the concentration of drugs in the plasma. This helps to prevent the toxic effects of some drugs, such as gentamicin, which accumulate in a patient with renal impairment. Antibiotic assay, when the concentration of the drug is measured, is useful to confirm that the levels achieved are adequate for treatment. This is particularly important when there is doubt about the efficacy of intestinal absorption or when the drug is intended to cross the blood-brain barrier into the CSF.

The other use of drug monitoring is to determine the cause of failed treatment. It is possible to decide if failure is due to inadequate absorption, lack of compliance or lack of sensitivity to the drug. Drug assays do, however, require skill and time. They should not therefore be undertaken without consideration. If a patient's drug levels are to be tested it is essential that the drug should be given as directed (with or without food) and the dose, time of drug administration and time of blood sampling be recorded.

FACTORS WHICH INFLUENCE DRUG RESPONSE

No two human beings are the same. In spite of this fact drugs are usually administered in set standard doses. The likelihood that the set dose will have the exact therapeutic effect desired is as unlikely as finding a normal individual with a temperature of exactly 37°C. Individual variation in size, weight, absorptive, metabolic and excretory ability lies within a normal range. It is over this normal range that standard dosage generally applies.

Age

At the extremes of age special considerations apply.

Fetus and neonate

Drugs given to the pregnant woman may affect the fetus if they cross the placental barrier.

Substances present in the blood in sufficient concentration will reach the fetus to some extent, unless they are metabolized by the drug-metabolizing enzymes present in the placenta.

A considerable number of these substances will harm the embryo or fetus and they are discussed in detail by Ashton (1981). Since the disastrous damage caused by thalidomide, rigorous tests have been introduced in the United Kingdom to satisfy the Committee on Safety of Medicines before drugs can be marketed.

The specific effect is determined to a considerable extent by the stage of fetal development at which the drug is administered. During the first trimester of pregnancy the fetal organs are forming and undergoing rapid development. Teratogenic substances will cause malformation, which may be lethal, if given during this stage of pregnancy. The specific deformity which occurs is related to the particular organs developing at the time of administration of the drug, rather than to the individual drug given. After the first 3 months of pregnancy the fetal organs are completely formed and drugs can no longer be teratogenic, although function and growth can still be disrupted.

Some drugs are known to be teratogenic, for example anti-neoplastic drugs which are intended to destroy or damage the growing tumour cells will also damage the embryonic tissues. Some hormones have also been found to have a teratogenic effect and the use of the hormone pregnancy test has been withdrawn because of this. The use of hormones to prevent threatened abortion has been implicated in the birth of malformed babies but, in addition, daughters born of mothers given diethylstilboestrol in early pregnancy had a high incidence of vaginal carcinoma about 20 years later.

Many other drugs are suspected of being teratogenic. Drugs where the evidence is not conclusive include a wide range of substances including warfarin, anticonvulsants, anaesthetics, psychotropic drugs, alcohol, cigarette smoking and aspirin. It is not certain that any drug is safe in early pregnancy and medication should be kept to a minimum and only taken if prescribed by a doctor who is aware of the pregnancy.

Drugs given later in pregnancy may affect the growth and function of the fetus, as some will cross the placental barrier and may be more toxic to the developing fetus than to the adult. A number of anti-microbial drugs are implicated. Tetracyclines are well known for their affinity for bones and teeth and can result in permanently discoloured teeth and retarded growth. Certain antibiotics such as streptomycin and gentamicin may damage the eighth cranial nerve resulting in deafness. Chloramphenicol is another substance which readily passes into the baby but cannot be metabolized adequately and can result in circulatory collapse in the newborn (the grey baby syndrome). Sulphonamides displace bilirubin from the binding sites on the plasma proteins, and thus result in jaundice.

Some drugs, such as antithyroid drugs, will produce effects in the fetus which appear to be compensating for the drug action in an attempt to maintain homeostasis. The fetus within a mother being treated with antithyroid drugs will develop a goitre, but is usually euthyroid at birth. The effects of cigarette smoking and alcohol early in pregnancy have already been mentioned, but they are also harmful later in development leading to an increased risk of abortion and of restricted growth, particularly of the brain, when the mothers are alcoholic (Kessel, 1977).

Children

The treatment of children is specialized and beyond the scope of this book. However, it should be remembered that childhood is a period of continual change and the dose of drug given should be calculated according to size and maturity, rather than according to chronological age.

The elderly

Elderly patients are more prone to develop adverse reactions to the drugs administered. Hurwitz (1969) found an incidence of 15.4% of drug reactions among patients over 60 years compared with 6.3% in younger patients, and other studies (in Williamson, 1978) substantiate this finding.

Several factors contribute to this increase in drug reactions. There is a decrease in lean body mass in ageing and thus reduced dosage of many drugs is needed. Variation in absorption, distribution, metabolism and excretion also affect the concentration of free drug in the plasma.

The effect of ageing on drug absorption is not clear. It may be impaired if gut motility or blood flow is reduced. In distribution of the drug through the body, the reduced levels of plasma protein which may be found lead to decreased binding. Therefore, higher levels of the free drug within the plasma and an increased risk of toxicity occur (Hayes et al, 1975a and b).

The weight of the liver decreases with age after 50 years and it appears likely that the ability to metabolize drugs is also reduced. Therefore, higher levels of a drug will accumulate in the plasma. There is also a reduced ability to excrete drugs through the kidneys and Ewy et al (1969) found that this resulted in a prolonged half-life of digoxin in the plasma, 73 hours in men between 73 and 81 years compared to 51 hours in younger people.

The hazards of drug treatment in the elderly are discussed by Davison (1978). Many old people are on more than one drug, due to multiple pathology, and the likelihood of drug interactions occurring increases with the number of different drugs taken. The risks of this are now recognized and an effort is being made to keep the number of drugs prescribed to a minimum. This has the added advantage that the patient is more likely to remember to take the right drug at the right time.

Some old people become forgetful and muddled and will not be able to manage their own drug therapy after discharge from hospital. A relative or neighbour will need to be involved in the planning for discharge. Others may be able to manage if given adequate teaching and practice in self-administration before discharge. The preparation of a chart, making it clear which drugs are to be taken when, will help the patient to avoid mistakes. It is also easier to remember if the times that drugs are to be taken are related to meals. For some days before discharge the patient can be given the drugs for the whole day and his or her ability to take them correctly can be checked, so that the risk of errors after discharge are minimized.

Pathology

The disease state will in itself affect the body's homeostatic mechanisms. Water, electrolyte balance, acid-base status and body temperature all influence drug response. Nutritional depletion during prolonged illness can often reduce plasma proteins and bound drug concentration, thus leading to a rise in the concentration of free drug. Reduction in protein resources also leads to enzyme depletion,thus reducing metabolic capacity. Disorders of the gastrointestinal tract will alter absorption. This is not always seen as a reduction in concentration; increases in drug concentration are also possible. Considerable work has been done with patients with malabsorption syndrome, particularly in relation to antibiotic levels (see Table 15.2) (Parsons et al, 1975b; Parsons & Paddock, 1975). As these patients are prone to infections and these drugs rely on plasma concentration for their effect, knowledge of the difference in absorption of these drugs is important.

Liver disease

In liver disease, drug metabolism is decreased, therefore one would expect corticosteroids and barbiturates, which are extensively metabolized, to rise in concentration. However, barbiturates have the effect of increasing the production of liver drug-metabolizing enzymes (induction) and so speed their own metabolism (Beckenridge & Orme, 1971). This helps to reduce the expected effect of a damaged liver. Oral anticoagulant metabolism is reduced, but again the effect may be nullified by the damaged liver's reduced ability to produce clotting factors. In general, because the liver as an organ has such considerable reserves, the outcome of disease is unpredictable and cases must be assessed individually.

Renal damage

Renal damage has most effect on clearance and any drug which is extensively excreted by the kidney will have an increased half-life. The toxic effects of some of these drugs (aminoglycoside antibiotics e.g. streptomycin, neomycin, gentamicin, and digoxin) can be very damaging. It is now standard practice in patients with renal failure to calculate dosage of these drugs in relation to the patient's creatinine clearance (Dettli et al, 1971).

ADVERSE DRUG REACTIONS

IATROGENIC DISEASE

The intention of drug therapy is to cure or alleviate disease or symptoms; however in doing so adverse effects may be produced, some of which are in themselves diseases — iatrogenic (doctor-produced) diseases. A number of different types of adverse reactions to drugs can occur. These can be of varying severity — from minor, causing only interference, to severe, sometimes leading to death — and can affect any system of the body. In the United Kingdom the introduction of statutory requirements under the Medicines Act 1968 for the more rigorous testing of new drugs and the gradual review of older ones, together with the obligation now placed on doctors to report adverse reactions, has drawn attention to this problem.It is hoped that these measures will reduce the frequency with which they occur but it must be viewed against the trend to prescribe more drugs and multiple therapy. The types of adverse reactions can be classified under the following headings: side-effects, overdosage effects, and idiosyncratic and hypersensitivity reactions.

Side-effects

Side-effects are a normal or expected action of the drug,but one which is of no therapeutic use and may be unpleasant.The severity of side-effects may vary considerably between individuals, genetic factors contributing to the patient's reaction. Few drugs have a single specific action, so that their usefulness lies in the degree to which side-effects are acceptable. Some side-effects such as sleepiness (produced by antihistamines) and reduced reaction time (produced by benzodiazepines) are well known; patients taking these drugs should be told not to operate machinery or drive. Some drugs have severe side-effects but are still used when the results of not giving treatment will be worse than the adverse reactions; side-effects are considered acceptable in these circumstances.

Overdosage

An overdose leads to exaggeration of the therapeutic effects of the drug. However, individuals vary in the dose of drug required to produce overdosage symptoms, in the same way as they vary in response to therapy. Accidental or intended overdose may result in poisoning — this subject will be dealt with later.

Idiosyncrasy (genetic)

Genetic factors account for unusual drug reactions in otherwise normal individuals. A number of drugs are acetylated in the process of metabolism and some people have enzymes which perform this rapidly, while others carry out this reaction slowly. There is considerable variation in the proportion of fast to slow acetylators in different ethnic populations. When a drug is only slowly metabolized through this reaction, toxic effects are more likely to develop as the blood levels of the drug are high. Isoniazid, sulphonamides, procainamide and nitrazepam are examples of drugs dealt with in this way, and side-effects to them are found more commonly among 'slow-acetylators' (Karim & Price-Evans, 1976; Rawlins & Thompson, 1981). Sensitivity to suxamethonium (Scoline) is more dramatic — it is due to an abnormal plasma cholinesterase. Normally this enzyme will rapidly destroy circulating suxamethonium. The effect of this abnormality is to prolong the period of muscular paralysis for which the drug is given from a few minutes to several hours. Fortunately the frequency of this abnormality is low. Any history of abnormal reactions during anaesthesia should be recorded in the patient's notes and the patient should be informed in order to prevent the drug being used again.

In addition to this type of condition where drug response is altered by hereditary influences, there are also conditions which are genetically determined but are only revealed by drug treatments. About 10% of American Negroes will develop haemolytic anaemia when given primaquine, or a number of other drugs, due to a sex-linked lack of the enzyme glucose-6-phosphate dehydrogenase (Beutler, 1969). The development of acute porphyria in genetically susceptible individuals given barbiturates is also well known (Marver & Schmid, 1972).

Hypersensitivity reactions

Hypersensitivity or allergy is discussed in Chapter 5. The body can develop antibodies to drugs with which it comes in contact in the same way as to other antigens. There may have been previous exposure to the initiating drug; laboratory technicians, doctors, nurses and the relations of patients as well as the patient himself can all become allergic by careless drug handling. The reactions which develop may be of any of the types described in Chapter 5. Thus, reactions may range from the immediate anaphylactic reaction, necessitating emergency treatment, to the delayed hypersensitivity reaction developing 7 to 14 days after beginning treatment. Antibiotics in the penicillin and cephalosporin groups most commonly cause reactions but they may also be seen with streptomycin, barbiturates, chlorpromazine, sulphonamides, gold salts and many others. The occurrence of a reaction should be recorded in the patient's notes and the patient warned to avoid the drug in future.

SYSTEMS AFFECTED

Blood dyscrasias

Blood dyscrasias may be either of immunological origin or due to direct damage to the blood cells or their precursors.

Haemolytic anaemia

Drugs with oxidant properties, e.g. primaquine and nitrofurantoin, will induce haemolytic anaemia in most people when high doses are given. Those who are genetically more susceptible are affected at normal dosage. Immunological changes demonstrated by the development of a positive Coombs' test are seen during high dose penicillin treatment (White et al, 1968). Methyldopa is also associated with both a positive Coombs' test, in 20% of those receving it (Carstairs et al, 1966), and with the development of haemolytic anaemia in one out of every five of those with a positive Coombs' test. Fortunately these anaemias resolve after the withdrawal of treatment.

Aplastic anaemia

Some drugs are associated with the development of aplastic anaemia, usually after only a few doses, in those patients who are susceptible. The mechanism of this effect is not known and there seems to be nothing common to the causative drugs. These reactions are not commonly seen but occur most frequently with chloramphenicol, which is now used with caution, and following treatment with benzol derivatives (e.g. phenylbutazone), gold and sulphonamides.

Megaloblastic anaemia

Drugs which induce megaloblastic anaemia are structurally related (phenytoin, nitrofurantoin, primidone, phenobarbitone) and are thought to produce this anaemia by interfering with folic acid synthesis.

Agranulocytosis

Cytotoxic drugs induce agranulocytosis because of their antimitotic action. A more delayed reduction in white cell count develops in some people during treatment with aminopyrine, aspirin, sulphonamides, chloramphenicol, phenothiazines, antithyroid agents and gold salts (Orme, 1972). Patients receiving long-term treatment should be encouraged to contact the doctor if signs of infection such as sore throats develop.

Thrombocytopenia

In general, drugs which cause aplastic anaemia will also induce thrombocytopenia, as will quinidine and rifampicin which may induce thrombocytopenia without anaemia or leucopenia (Blajchman et al, 1970).

Clotting disorders

Blood clotting occurs through a series of reactions which may be disrupted at many points. This knowledge is used in anticoagulant therapy. Abnormal clotting can result from treatment with oestrogens for contraception and replacement therapy at menopause. The increases in clotting factors VII, VIII, IX and X together with an increase in platelets seen during pregnancy are mirrored during oral contraception. Genetic factors also appear to be important in the incidence of venous thrombosis during oral contraception, being more common in individuals of blood group O. The Committee on Safety of Medicines in the United Kingdom issued a warning in December 1969 about preparations containing high levels of oestrogen. Since then the high oestrogen 'pill' has disappeared from use in this country. The value and safety of low dose oestrogen tablets in hormone replacement therapy (HRT) during the menopause is not yet established.

Drug-induced diseases of the gastrointestinal tract

In view of the fact that most drugs are given by mouth, it is surprising how few cause gross damage to the gastrointestinal tract. Minor upsets, mainly diarrhoea with antibiotics or constipation with sedatives, are often seen and cause only passing discomfort. The more serious development of pseudomembranous colitis has been reported but has been shown in a retrospective study to be rare (Beavis et al, 1976), affecting only three out of 1158 orthopaedic patients treated with a variety of antibiotics. In long-term treatment, continuing diarrhoea can result in malabsorption of both food and drugs, for example the steatorrhoea which may occur with para-aminosalicylic acid could result in vitamin B_{12} deficiency during long term therapy.

Drugs which cause dyspepsia, notably the anti-inflammatory drugs, both steroid and non-steroid, are those which most frequently cause peptic ulceration. The therapeutic effect of these drugs can mask the painful symptoms of the condition so that the first demonstration of the ulcer is haemorrhage. Occult blood is frequently found in the faeces of patients taking aspirin and this drug is believed to cause gastric haemorrhage by destroying the protective mucus in the stomach. This can be prevented by the use of enteric coated tablets.

Liver disease

The metabolism of drugs occurs in the liver and its position at the receiving end of the portal system ensures that drugs are highly concentrated. The external sign of liver damage is jaundice, which can be due to obstruction (cholestasis) or interference with bilirubin metabolism, more usual in the very young where the system is not fully developed. Obstruction may develop over a period of months during oral testosterone therapy. The development of cholestasis is also associated with phenothiazines, notably chlorpromazine, with 1% of patients developing a jaundice which generally subsides within a few weeks of discontinuing treatment.

Although hepatitis is not a common complication of drug therapy, it carries a 20–25% risk of mortality. Diagnosis is difficult since it cannot readily be distinguished from viral hepatitis. Drugs which have been implicated in the development of this condition are mono-amine oxidase inhibitors and the anaesthetic halothane, which should not be used when frequent general anaesthetics are needed within a short period of time or when there is a previous history of sensitivity.

Drug-induced disorders of metabolism

Diabetes mellitus

Thiazide diuretics can induce a diabetic state

when treatment extends over a period of months. The extent to which this is due to the drugs is difficult to assess because many of these hypertensive patients already have an abnormal glucose tolerance. When treatment is discontinued the return to normal may take months or years.

Oral contraceptives also affect carbohydrate metabolism; 75% of normal women deteriorate in glucose tolerance (Wynn & Doar, 1969). The control of diabetics on insulin is also more difficult when they are taking oral contraceptives.

Salt and water retention

Many drugs can induce oedema, particularly the corticosteroids, phenylbutazone and carbenoxolone sodium (Baron et al, 1969). This appears during the first few days of treatment and can precipitate cardiac failure by increasing body fluid.

Osteoporosis develops during steroid treatment and prolonged heparinization; the increased excretion of calcium may result in aseptic bone necrosis.

Drug-induced renal diseases

Renal necrosis is precipitated by drugs which are excreted unchanged via the kidney, particularly the aminoglycoside antibiotics which cause necrosis of the proximal tubule. Prolonged intravenous dosage with tetracycline or the use of out-of-date tetracycline can produce the same damage. Mild analgesics, some of which are available 'over the counter', particularly phenacetin, aspirin and phenazone, are strongly implicated in the development of papillary necrosis (Burry et al, 1974). This poses two problems — first is finding alternatives for long-term treatment, and the second is the extent to which these drugs are available as constituents of 'over the counter' preparations. The symptoms develop only after a large quantity (1 kg of phenacetin) of the drug has been consumed, so that patients are not seen until they are in the final stages of renal failure. Because of this risk, phenacetin is no longer available.

Drug-induced diseases of the nervous system

The ototoxicity associated with the antibiotics streptomycin, neomycin, gentamicin and kanamycin (the aminoglycosides) has been well documented (Appel & Nev, 1977). The elderly and the very young are most at risk from these drugs, which are excreted unchanged through the kidney. Deafness due to damage to branches of the VIIIth cranial nerve may appear some time after the drug has been discontinued.

Peripheral neuropathy may be produced during isoniazid or nitrofurantoin therapy when plasma concentration is increased by genetically slow acetylation (isoniazid) or poor renal function (nitrofurantoin). Within the central nervous system extra-pyramidal reactions occur with phenothiazines (e.g. prochlorperazine, trifluoperazine, chlorpromazine) (Ayd, 1961). These appear as motor restlessness and dyskinesias similar to a Parkinsonian syndrome. An anti-Parkinsonian drug (e.g. levodopa) may be prescribed for the dyskinesia when treatment with phenothiazines must be continued. Phenytoin can also produce central effects such as nystagmus, ataxia and lethargy; this toxicity is more common in some patients who are slow to oxidize the drug. The difference between therapeutic and toxic plasma concentrations of phenytoin is very small, so that plasma concentration monitoring and appropriate dose adjustment are necessary to help prevent these symptoms from developing.

DRUG INTERACTIONS

It is now common practice in medicine to treat a patient with more than one drug at a time, particularly when one condition is coexistent with another. It is generally assumed that individual drugs will act separately and in many cases they do.However, in some combinations potentiation will occur, when two drugs together have a greater and rather different effect than the drugs given singly. For example, co-trimoxazole, a combination of sulphamethoxazole and trimethoprim, affects the metabolism of microorganisms at different stages, so reducing the dose of drug required. In other cases the effects of the drug may be prolonged as when insulin is combined with zinc. These types of reaction can be of considerable value in treatment.

On the other hand, drug interactions may be harmful when drugs antagonize each other's effect leading to a failure of therapy, or when the effect of interaction is not easily predicted and unexpected consequences occur. D'Arcy & Griffin, (1979, 1981) discuss in detail the adverse drug reactions known at the time their book was published, and hospital pharmacists can always be consulted about possible interactions.

Interactions may occur at any stage of treatment from the preparation of a medication to its excretion. Drugs should not be mixed in syringes or added to intravenous solutions until compatibility has been checked. Information on compatibility is contained on the data sheet of all injectable drugs. If this is missing, the information can be obtained from the pharmacy or the drug company's information service. Instilling drugs in infusions can also cause problems: tetracycline will inactivate penicillins if mixed in an infusion, and antibiotics, particularly penicillins, deteriorate rapidly if left to infuse over a prolonged period.For this reason intravenous penicillin, for example, is usually given as a bolus injection.

Interactions during absorption

Drugs which affect gut motility will alter the absorption of drugs administered at the same time. Propantheline bromide and tricyclic antidepressants reduce motility. This enhances the effect of drugs which are normally poorly absorbed (such as digoxin) by prolonging the time they remain in the gut. The reverse occurs with metoclopramide, which stimulates gastric emptying so reducing digoxin absorption. The pH of the gut is important, and antacids would be expected to reduce the absorption of acidic drugs. This effect is, in fact, not as great as would be expected because the length of time that the drug remains in the gut means that slow absorption can take place over a long time. The effect of antacids is, surprisingly, greatest on basic drugs which become less soluble in this medium and reduced in bioavailability. Charged compounds including some antacids, cholestyramine, iron and activated charcoal bind to some drugs preventing their absorption. Tetracycline can be inactivated in this way by iron, charcoal, or milk, and thyroxine absorption can be dangerously reduced if administered with cholestyramine.

Long-term treatment with para-aminosalicylic acid (PAS), neomycin or colchicine leads to the malabsorption of penicillin due to gut damage and an alteration in the gut flora (Pearson & Nestor, 1977).

Interactions during distribution

Most drugs travel in the circulation bound to plasma proteins; the extent and strength of binding depends on their chemical composition. Where two drugs, both of which bind to protein to a considerable extent, are administered simultaneously there is competition for binding sites. This will result in an increase in the free drug concentration of the least strongly- bound drug. For example, warfarin is displaced from plasma proteins by aspirin, resulting in an increase in anticoagulant activity. Aspirin will also displace tolbutamide causing hypoglycaemia. As aspirin is often self administered, patients should be warned that continuing use of this drug may upset their treatment and the doctor should be asked to suggest other analgesics for these patients.

At the receptor level, competition results when similar compounds are administered. This is used in the treatment of overdoses of narcotic analgesics when the non-narcotic drug, naloxone, competes for the receptor site and, by displacing the narcotic drug, reduces the toxic effects of the narcotic analgesics. The activity of coumarin, an anticoagulant, is affected by changes in the concentration of vitamin K, upon which it acts. The administration of antibiotics kills off the gut flora which produce this vitamin, reducing circulating levels and so enhancing the anticoagulant effect. Activity will also be augmented when drugs act within the same system; for example, antihypertensive activity is increased by central nervous system depressants, tranquillizers and anaesthetics.

Interactions during metabolism

Drug interactions can also take place in the process of metabolism by the liver drug-metabolizing enzymes. More than 200 substances will induce, or stimulate the formation of, these drug-metabolizing enzymes (Conney, 1967). By doing so the metabolism of the inducing drug is increased, but so is the metabolism of a number of other drugs whose activity is, therefore, reduced. Table 15.3 shows some examples of this. While this may cause no problems with some drugs, it can cause difficulty when the activity of such substances as anticoagulant, anticonvulsant or antidiabetic drugs is reduced.One example is that reported by Cucinell et al (1965). Phenobarbital increases the dosage of bishydroxycoumarin required for anticoagulant maintenance (Fig. 15.5). A patient stabilized on anticoagulants in hospital while receiving a barbiturate night sedative is at risk of haemorrhage after discharge when night sedation is no longer required. Fortunately, this is less likely now that barbiturates are rarely used for night sedation. Some hormones are metabolized by these same drug-metabolizing enzymes and induction will lead to more rapid metabolism and may lead to reduced effectiveness of the contraceptive pill. As bilirubin is metabolized in the same way, neonatal jaundice can be treated by provoking induction (Hunter & Chasseaud, 1976). Enzyme induction requires time to develop so that it is only seen as the result of a course of treatment, not of a single dose. It also takes time to disappear so that the resulting induction from a course of treatment can affect single doses given a week or so after treatment has been discontinued.

The action of drugs on enzymes is not limited to induction. They can also cause inhibition. Inhibiting activity does not generally require time to develop because the life of enzymes is short. Allopurinol inhibits the enzymes which metabolize warfarin and isoniazid, also those responsible for one stage in the metabolism of phenytoin. Inhibition leads to a reduction in metabolism and, therefore, to an increase in the active drug concentration and the possibility of overdosage (Table 15.4). The drugs most affected by enzyme changes are those which require the most extensive metabolism, often consisting of several reactions. The more drugs being taken, the greater is the risk of some interaction occurring between them. It is important that the nurse should be aware of the possibility of interactions and should report any unexpected reactions in the patient following the introduction of a new drug — Table 15.5 shows some of the more important interactions between commonly used drugs.

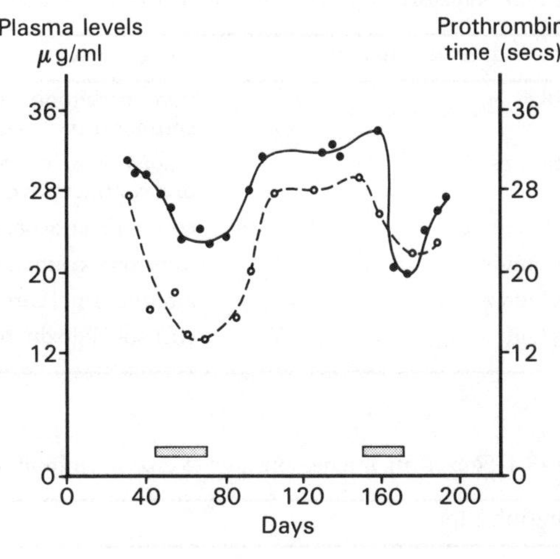

Fig. 15.5 The effect of phenobarbital on plasma levels of bishydroxycoumarin (from Cucinell et al, 1965).

Interactions during excretion

Drugs which are excreted mainly unchanged are most affected by interactions during excretion. Most metabolites are inactive so that a build-up within the body is not likely to cause any serious reaction. The main excretory interactions are due to competition for active transport systems and changes in urinary pH produced by drugs. In the

Table 15.3 Some drug interactions due to enzyme induction (adapted from D'Arcy & Griffin, 1979 & 1981)

Enzyme inducer (stimulator)	Drug activity reduced by enhanced metabolism
alcohol	pentobarbitone, phenytoin, tolbutamide, tricyclic antidepressants, coumarin anticoagulants
barbiturates	chlorpromazine, cortisol, coumarin anticoagulants, digoxin, oral contraceptives, phenytoin, testosterone, Vitamin D
chloral hydrate	coumarin anticoagulants
glutethimide	dipyrone, coumarin anticoagulants
phenylbutazone	amidopyrine, cortisol, digoxin
phenytoin	cortisol, digoxin, thyroxine, oral contraceptives

Table 15.4 Some drug interactions due to enzyme inhibition (adapted from D'Arcy & Griffin, 1979 & 1981)

Enzyme inhibitor	Drug activity increased by decreased metabolism
allopurinol	6-substituted purines (e.g. azathioprine, mercaptopurine)
aspirin, chloramphenicol, dicoumarol phenylbutazone, phenyramidol sulphaphenazole	tolbutamide
chloramphenicol, phenyramidol	dicoumarol
cortisol, testosterone	nortryptyline
dicoumarol, disulfiram, isoniazid PAS, warfarin	phenytoin
disulfiram, oxyphenbutazone	warfarin
MAOIs	barbiturates, phenindione, tyramine
methandienone	oxyphenbutazone, some anticoagulants
methyl phenidate	barbiturates, dicoumarol, phenytoin, primidone
phenothiazines	tricyclic antidepressants
prednisolone	cyclophosphamide

Table 15.5 Important interactions between commonly used drugs

Drug A	Drug B	Mechanism of interaction	Result
alcohol	barbiturates	enzyme inhibition	both enhanced
	disulfiram	enzyme inhibition	toxicity
	phenothiazines	potentiation at receptor	both enhanced
	trycyclic antidepressants	action in same system	alcohol enhanced
anticoagulants	barbiturates	enzyme induction	reduced anticoagulation
	cholestyramine	absorption in GI tract	reduced anticoagulation
	clofibrate	protein binding competition	increased anticoagulation
	glutethimide	enzyme induction	reduced anticoagulation
	non-steroid anti-inflammatory drugs (NSAI)	protein binding competition	increased anticoagulation
digitalis	beta-blockers	action in same system	increased beta-blockade
	ethacrynic acid	alteration in electrolyte balance	enhanced digitalization
	frusemide	alteration in electrolyte balance	enhanced digitalization
	thiazide diuretics	alteration in electrolyte balance	enhanced digitalization
oral hypoglycaemics	chloramphenical	enzyme inhibition	hypoglycaemia
	beta-blockers	influence glucose metabolism	hypoglycaemia
	steroids and oral contraceptives	altered glucose tolerance	hypoglycaemia
	phenylbutazone and NSAI	enzyme inhibition	hypoglycaemia

early days of penicillin, the blocking action of probenecid was used to preserve and prolong the drug's action in the body, but its inhibition of salicylate, indomethacin and PAS excretion can lead to toxicity. Bendrofluazide inhibits lithium carbonate excretion and this can be dangerous because lithium has a narrow therapeutic range (i.e. the dose which is needed to be effective is only slightly below that which is toxic). Hypoglycaemia can develop when levels of the anti-diabetic drug chlorpropamide are raised because its excretion is inhibited by dicoumarol. Alkalinization of the urine facilitates the excretion of acidic drugs (streptomycin, salicylates and phenobarbitone) while urine acidified by ascorbic acid will reduce the period of amphetamine activity (a basic substance) by increasing the rate of clearance from the body.

Other interactions

Some interactions do not fall readily into any category but are still of importance. Monoamine oxidase inhibitors (MAOIs) are used in the treatment of depression and act by blocking the catabolism of amines such as adrenaline, noradrenaline, serotonin and dopamine which act as neurotransmitters. However, the catabolism of these and other amines is blocked whatever the source of the amines, and if these are taken into the body they lead to increased stimulation of the adrenergic receptors resulting in a number of adverse reactions such as headache, cardiac dysrhythmias and hypertension, which may be severe. Patients should, therefore, be warned to avoid proprietary cold cures which contain such amines. Certain foods such as cheese, Marmite, red wine and broad beans can also precipitate a crisis due to their amine content. Since these reactions are well known, patients are supplied with a list of medicines and foods to avoid.

Changes in electrolyte balance can affect the action of drugs which rely upon their presence, digoxin toxicity being produced by hypokalaemia. Some drugs appear frequently in interaction reports; these are the ones which are used in long-term therapy (antibiotics, anticoagulants and antiepileptics) or those which may be bought without prescription (antipyretic analgesics and alcohol). It is therefore important that the patient should be educated about the drugs he is taking, what they are for, and side effects which may develop. This is an area in which the nurse may well develop her role in addition to those of the doctor and pharmacist. A small study by Burton (1980) demonstrated the ignorance of some patients regarding their medication, and Shulman & Shulman (1979) have shown how adverse reactions can be prevented by the pharmacist keeping individual records of his clients' prescriptions, previous reactions and over the counter purchases (George & Kingscombe, 1980).

PROBLEMS ASSOCIATED WITH DRUG TAKING

In our affluent society drugs are easily obtainable from the doctor, the hospital, the chemist or supermarket. Conditions can now be treated which would have been rapidly fatal before the advent of modern drugs such as antibiotics and insulin. This gives all patients a greater expectation of cure than they had previously. Many drugs once prescribed are continued as life-long therapy, and new drugs are added to the prescription as additional symptoms appear, leading to all the problems of polypharmacy. The stage is set for experimentation and new types of abuse to join the age-old problems of narcotic and alcohol addiction.

TOLERANCE AND DRUG DEPENDENCE

During long-term treatment the ability of the same dose of some drugs to produce the desired effect may diminish. This tolerance can develop because of the liver's increased capacity to metabolize the drug (enzyme induction). It is likely, however, that during long-term therapy tolerance is due to the body's adaption to the continued presence of the drug. When this takes place the patient becomes physically dependent upon the drug, absence of the drug leading to physical abnormality. This tolerance is important when treating patients requiring long-term analgesia. In the terminally ill, the use of narcotics is accepted on the basis that the increasing dose required to control pain is acceptable under these conditions. Pain due to arthritis, by contrast, must be managed without recourse to drugs of addiction. Habitual use of any addictive drug leads to this type of addiction, so that the heroin addict requires his 'fix' just as much as the nicotine or caffeine addict requires his cigarettes or coffee to feel normal. Less easily understood is the psychological type of dependence where the individual becomes convinced that it is only when he takes the drug that he can maintain his well being. Both physical and psychological dependence are components of addiction; both play an important part in alcohol, narcotic and barbiturate addiction. Where nicotine, amphetamine and anxiolytics (benzodiazepines) are concerned the physical element is less strong, while with LSD and marijuana it is absent. The drug addict is, in effect, caught up in a situation which prevents him from breaking out; he is completely dependent upon the drug in spite of the fact that it is damaging him physically, socially and financially.

The treatment of an addict depends on his co-operation and abrupt stopping of the drug can lead to very unpleasant withdrawal symptoms. These are real, physical and in some cases may be fatal. Psychological support is vital during the withdrawal period which usually involves gradual reduction of dose. In some cases drugs can assist with withdrawal or support the patient's resolve. The best known of these is disulfiram (Antabuse) used to reinforce alcohol withdrawal. This drug produces violent nausea if the patient takes any type of alcohol, and should only be used with the fully co-operative patient. Methadone can assist heroin and morphine withdrawal by substitution; the subsequent withdrawal from methadone produces far less violent symptoms.

SELF-POISONING

Overdose, like addiction and tolerance, may arise as the consequence of a therapeutic prescription, the drug used frequently being that given for treatment. The intention of the overdose may be suicide, manipulation or homicide, and of these suicide is the most common. The increasing incidence since the 1950s has been so rapid that the level reached has been described as a modern epidemic, although the incidence now appears to be stable.

Over the years changes have taken place in the drugs which feature in poisoning. This reflects the changes in pattern of drug prescription. Prior to the advent of diazepines, barbiturates were by far the most common of the drugs causing poisoning. They have now been superseded by other prescribed drugs including antidepressants, hypnotics and tranquillizers (Smith & Davidson, 1971). Poisoning with diazepines, although high in incidence, does not lead to the same fatality which accompanies that with barbiturates. A dose of 20 diazepine tablets results in a deep sleep from which the patient can be roused, rather than the severe illness which would follow a similar number of barbiturate tablets. Overdosage of paracetamol has now been shown to cause serious toxic effects which include acute liver failure, which carries a high mortality. The prevention of poisoning involves the unmasking and treatment of the underlying causes. Because potentially lethal drugs (salicylates and paracetamol) are available over the counter, there will always be a group of individuals whose vulnerability is not known until admission. Treatment depends on the drug or combination of drugs taken. Assistance with the diagnosis obtained during history-taking is available by blood analysis at one of the national Poisons Units. After the acute stage, rehabilitation and support are needed following suicidal or manipulative overdosage.

Accidental poisoning usually involves children, particularly those below school age. Prevention here rests on the education of adults in the importance of safe drug storage. The trend to experiment with drugs results in teenagers, unaware of the potency of a drug or their intolerance to it, suffering a 'bad trip' (LSD) which results in hospital admission. Solvent abuse causes similar problems but within a younger age group.

NON-COMPLIANCE IN DRUG TAKING IN RELATION TO MEDICAL PRESCRIPTION

The success of drug treatment depends on the drug reaching the target organ in the concentration which is optimal to obtain the desired results. In previous sections, the variables upon which this depends have been discussed. None of this is relevant unless the patient receives the correct dose of the correct drug by an appropriate route at the desired time. In hospital it is seen as the nurse's job to ensure this on the basis of the doctor's prescription. Once at home, however, it is up to the patient to maintain the prescribed drug-taking pattern. Studies have shown that as many as 41% of patients missed some doses of drugs in hospital (Bergman et al, 1979). The age and the number of drugs prescribed for the patients who missed doses were greater than for those who missed no doses. The main reason for missing a dose was that the patient refused the dose, but errors also occurred in administration, again in particular with elderly and long-term patients. Considerable work has been done to alleviate these problems in Dundee, using individualized and computerized systems with prescription checks by ward pharmacists (Johnston et al, 1976; Henney, 1977). All this assumes that the doctor's prescription is 'correct', i.e. that not only is the drug dose and route appropriate to the patient's needs, but that the time the drugs are to be taken in relation to factors affecting absorption, e.g. meals, is appropriate for optimal effect. Further, it is assumed that the interaction of drugs taken at the same time has also been taken into account. This cannot be assumed. A small informal study found that 30% of patients on an acute medical ward in a teaching hospital were prescribed drugs at times inappropriate in relation to meals or in inappropriate combinations (Champion, 1979).

The major problems of non-compliance, however, only appear when the patient returns home, 'non-compliers' falling into two groups; those who do not comply through non-comprehension and those who understand but still do not comply (Parkin et al, 1976). Individuals in the second group are difficult to identify and do not readily fall into any category — their non-compliance is a conscious disagreement with treatment. Clearly their non-compliance points to a need to discuss treatment more fully with patients prior to commencing therapy (or if emergency therapy was required, as soon as is feasible) in order that treatment is mutually agreed. In this way the patient becomes a full partner in the decision-making process, and is as committed to the therapeutic programme as the medical practitioner prescribing the drug. The non-understanders are more readily identified as those who are older and receiving more than one drug. Their failure to take the prescribed treatment is due to confusion: a new regime may have been established in hospital, drugs brought home are muddled with those already there, and other drugs which may have been obtained from the general practitioner, the local shop or even from friends or neighbours are added to the prescribed therapy.

The nurse can be of considerable use in alleviating this problem by ensuring that:

- the patient is not discharged home on unnecessary drugs
- the patient understands the regime, that is, can repeat instructions after a period of time
- the nurse looks at and knows what each drug is and when it should be taken
- the instructions on the bottle are legible to the patient
- the relatives understand the regime and can repeat it as above
- the patient is capable of taking his drugs without aid prior to discharge.

In a study of methods for training patients to take their drugs prior to discharge, it was found that a calendar on which the drug regime was written daily, and could be torn off when complete, together with instructions and understandable labelling of drugs, was the best method to reduce mistakes (Wandless & Davie, 1977). Alternatively, the calendar packs of drugs (such as those used for contraceptive pills) are now being used with success as an aide-mémoire for those on antidepressant and antihypertensive therapy. Compliance with therapeutic regimes is closely related to many areas of drug therapy, such as the effects of drugs in the elderly, interactions and side-effects. The nurse needs first to identify the patient who is unlikely to comply by finding the reasons why this may occur, then to act accordingly. In many instances, the procedures of drug administration in hospital mitigate against the patient either becoming familiar with the drugs he is taking or assuming responsibility for self-administration of drugs prior to discharge. Legal responsibilities, the variety of drugs available, poor drug-presenting practice and the traditional task orientation of the nurse have probably contributed to the development and continuance of the 'drug round' with its emphasis on 'checking'. The availability of individual patient/ dose dispensing methods, the increasing use of 'patient allocation' as a method of nursing work organization, and increasing discussion (if not action) of seeing patients as partners in, rather than recipients, of care, and nurses as concerned with promoting self-care, will hopefully lead to a more individualized and patient-managed system of drug administration in the future.

DRUGS AND THE ELDERLY

Old age is associated with several drug-taking problems. As mentioned above, compliance is a problem due to reduced mental agility and the additional problem of multiple prescriptions (or polypharmacy). National Health Service prescription expenditure for the elderly is 30% of the total, in spite of the fact that this group only comprises 15% of our population. Many of the prescriptions are repeated regularly and may amount to lifetime therapy and most patients also receive more than one drug (Garland, 1979). It is hardly surprising that many more of the elderly (Avery, 1976; Crooks & Christopher, 1979) suffer adverse side-effects, the figure being as high as 20%. There are sound physical reasons for this high incidence of reaction, just as there are sound medical reasons for treatment. With increasing age renal capacity declines, and drugs which are excreted via the kidney (digoxin, antibiotics) are likely to build up in the body. This is of particular importance with digoxin, whose effective dose is only slightly below that which is toxic. With age, body make-up changes so that fat replaces muscle. This alters the distribution of drugs so that high concentrations occur with water soluble drugs (aspirin), while the duration of action of fat soluble drugs (pentothal) is increased, leading to prolonged confusion after anaesthesia. In addition, the body's ability to detoxify drugs is diminished. Overall the effect is to increase concentration and prolong the time during which drugs remain in the body. In general, dosages for the elderly should be lower than for young adults. However, the problem arises as to when the dose should be reduced, since physiological age does not always mirror chronological age. The best way to find the correct dosage for an elderly patient is gradually to build up an individual dose. This requires skill and careful observation.

Old age is not a disease, but the physical and psychosocial processes involved in ageing frequently, but not inevitably, result in symptoms which may vary in effect from minor irritations to major problems, e.g. the pain of arthritis. The extent to which these problems may be relieved will often dictate whether the elderly person will be able to live a full life. However, as these symptoms are frequently multiple there is a tendency for doctors to add drugs to treatment as new symptoms develop. It is important for the nurse to encourage elderly patients to ask for a review of their drugs at intervals, and to check with the doctor that elderly patients need all the drugs they are taking, both on admission and discharge. This would go some way to reducing reactions due to interactions or confusion. A further problem area in which the nurse could become active is in relation to non-prescription drugs; as many as 21% of elderly patients regularly self medicate (Crooks & Christopher, 1979). A full drug history needs to be taken and an education programme initiated in relation to the drugs which the patient is prescribed. This is something which might well be encompassed within the nursing process.

CONCLUSION

The nurse's role in relation to drugs causes many anomalies. Nurses in hospital administer drugs which they do not prescribe, to patients who at home would perform this task for themselves. The nurse is legally responsible for the safe custody of these drugs and for ordering them, though not for preparing or packing them. As an intermediary between doctor, pharmacist and patient, the nurse is in a position to observe and report on the effects of drugs, as well as to spot errors. To do this effectively a nurse needs an understanding of how and where drugs act, their dosage and appearance; having gained this, he or she may then be led into ethical dilemmas, because, although the nurse has partial responsibility for the patient's welfare, he or she has no authority to change drug prescriptions.

Acknowledgement

We are grateful to The C.V. Mosby Company for permission to include in this chapter Figure 15.5 from Cucinell et al 1966 Clinical Pharmacology and Therapeutics, p. 423.

REFERENCES

Appel G B, Nev H C 1977 The nephrotoxicity of antimicrobial agents. New England Journal of Medicine 296:722–728
Ashton C H 1981 Disorders of the fetus and infant. In: Davies D M (ed) Textbook of adverse drug reactions. Oxford University Press, Oxford
Association of the British Pharmaceutical Industry 1980 The pharmaceutical industry and the nation's health. (Pamphlet) White Crescent Press, Luton
Avery G S (ed) 1976 Drug treatment. Churchill Livingstone, Edinburgh
Ayd F J Jr 1961 A survey of drug-induced extrapyramidal reaction. Journal of the American Medical Association 175:1054–1060
Baron J H, Nabarro J D N, Slater J D H, Tuffley R 1969 Metabolic studies, aldosterone secretion rate, and plasma resin after carbenoxolone sodium. British Medical Journal 2:793–795
Beavis J P, Parsons R L, Sanfield J 1976 Colitis and diarrhoea: a problem with antibiotic therapy. British Journal of Surgery 63:299–304
Beckenridge A, Orme M 1971 Clinical implications of enzyme induction. Annals of the New York Academy of Sciences 179:421–431
Bergman V, Norlin A, Wilolm B 1979 Inadequacies in hospital drug handling. Acta Medica Scandinavica 205:79–85
Beutler E 1969 Drug-induced haemolytic anaemia. Pharmacological Reviews 21:73
Blajchman M A, Lowry R C, Pettit J E, Stradling P 1970 Rifampicin-induced immune thrombocytopenia. British Medical Journal 3:24
Brodie B B, Bernstein E, Mark L C 1952 The role of body fat in limiting the duration of action of thiopental. Journal of Pharmacology and Experimental Therapeutics 105(4):421–426
Burry A F, Axelsen R A, Trolove P 1974 Analgesic nephropathy: Its present contribution to the renal mortality and morbidity profile. Medical Journal of Australia 1:31–34
Burton M 1980 The hospital patient and his knowledge of the drugs he is receiving. Project for BSc Nursing, Leeds Polytechnic
Carstairs I C, Beckenridge A, Dollery C T, Worlledge S M 1966 Incidence of a positive direct Coomb's Test in patients on methyldopa. Lancet 2:133–135
Champion R 1979 The administration of patient care. Unpublished MSc thesis, Welsh National School of Medicine, University of Wales
Conney A H 1967 Pharmacological implications of microsomal enzyme induction. Pharmacological Review 19:317–366
Creasey W A 1979 Drug disposition in humans. Oxford University Press, Oxford.
Crooks J, Christopher L J 1979 Use and misuse of home medicines In: Anderson J A D (ed) Self medication. MTP Press, Lancaster
Cucinell S A, Conney A H, Sansur M, Burns J J 1965 Drug interactions in man: lowering effect of phenobarbital on plasma levels of bishydroxycoumarin (dicumarol) and diphenylhydantoin (dilantin). Clinical Pharmacology and Therapeutics 6:420–429
D'Arcy P F, Griffin J P 1979, 1981 Iatrogenic diseases, Iatrogenic diseases update, 2nd edn. Oxford University Press, Oxford
Davison W 1978 The hazards of drug treatment in old age. In: Brocklehurst J C (ed) Textbook of geriatric medicine and gerontology. Churchill Livingstone, Edinburgh.
Dettli L, Spring P, Ryter S 1971 Multiple dose kinetics and drug dosage in patients with kidney disease. Acta Pharmacologica et Toxicologica 29 (Supplement 3):211–114
Ewy G A, Kapadia G G, Yao L, Marcus F I 1969 Digoxin metabolism in the elderly. Circulation 39:449–459
Garland M H 1979 Drugs and the elderly. Nursing Times, Extra, 75(9):3–6
George C F, Kingscombe P M 1980 Prevention of adverse reactions. Adverse Drug Reactions Bulletin 80:288–290
Hayes M J, Langman M J S, Short A H 1975a Changes in drug metabolism with increasing age: warfarin binding and plasma proteins. British Journal of Clinical Pharmacology 2:69–72
Hayes M J, Langman M J S, Short A H 1975b Changes in drug metabolism with increasing age II phenytoin clearance and protein bindings. British Journal of Clinical Pharmacology 2:73–79
Henney C R 1977 Drug administration 1. Nursing Mirror 142(14):73–79
Hunter J, Chasseaud L F 1976 Clinical aspects of microsomal enzyme induction. In: Bridges J W, Chasseaud L F (eds) Progress in drug metabolism. Wiley, London
Hurwitz N 1969 Predisposing factors in adverse reaction to drugs. British Medical Journal 1:536–539
Johnston S V, Henney C R, Bosworth R, Brown N, Crooks J

1976 The doctor, the pharmacist, the computer and the nurses. Medical Information 1(2):133–144
Karim A K M B, Price-Evans D A 1976 Polymorphic acetylation of nitrazepam. Journal of Medical Genetics 13:17–19
Kessel N 1977 The fetal alcohol syndrome from the public health standpoint. Health Trends 9:86
Kiss I J, Farago E, Pinter J 1976 Serum and lung tissue levels of cephradine in thoracic surgery. British Journal of Clinical Pharmacology 3:891
Marver H S, Schmid R 1972 The porphyrias. In: Stanbury J B, Wyngaarden J B, Fredrickson D S (eds) The metabolic basis of inherited disease. McGraw Hill, New York
Orme M 1972 Iatrogenic disease and drug interactions. Medicine, add on Series 4:302–316
Parkin D M, Henney C R, Quirk J, Crooks J 1976 Deviation from prescribed drug treatment after discharge from hospital. British Medical Journal 2:686–688
Parsons R L, Paddock G M 1975 Absorption of two antibacterial drugs, cephalexin and co-trimoxazole in malabsorption syndromes. Journal of Antimicrobial Chemotherapy 1 (Supplement):59–67
Parsons R L, Paddock G M, Kaye C M 1975a Drug absorption in malabsorption syndromes. Excerpta Medica, International Congress Series 383:193–202
Parsons R L, Hossack G, Paddock G 1975b The absorption of antibiotics in adult patients with coeliac disease. Journal of Antimicrobial Chemotherapy 1:39–50
Parsons R L, Beavis J P, David J A, Paddock G M, Trounce J R 1978 Plasma, bone, hip capsule and drain fluid concentrations of cephalexin during total hip replacement. British Journal of Clinical Pharmacology 5:331
Pearson R M, Nestor P 1977 Drug interactions. Nursing Mirror 145(19):Supplement i–iv
Prescott L F 1974 Gastric emptying and drug absorption. British Journal of Clinical Pharmacology 1:189–190
Rawlins M D, Thompson J W 1981 Pathogenesis of adverse drug reactions. In: Davies D M (ed) Textbook of adverse drug reactions. Oxford University Press, Oxford
Remmer H 1970 The role of the liver in drug metabolism. American Journal of Medicine 49:617–629
Schanker L S 1961 The passage of drugs across body membranes. Annual Review of Pharmacology 1:29–41
Shulman J I, Shulman S 1979 Operating a two card medication record system — a role for pharmacists in the 1980s? Pharmaceutical Journal 222:554–556
Smith J S, Davidson K 1971 Changes in the pattern of admissions for attempted suicide in Newcastle upon Tyne during the 1960s. British Medical Journal 4:412–415
Tyrer J M, Eadie M J, Sutherland J M, Hooper W D 1970 Outbreak of anticonvulsant intoxication in an Australian city. British Medical Journal 4:271–273
Wandless I, Davie J W 1977 Can drug compliance in the elderly be improved? British Medical Journal 1(6057):359–361
White J M, Brown D L, Hepner G W, Worlledge S M 1968 Penicillin-induced haemolytic anaemia. British Medical Journal 3:26–29
Williams P 1980 Recent trends in the prescribing of psychotropic drugs. Health Trends 12:6–7
Williamson J 1978 Principles of drug action and usage. In: Isaacs B (ed) Recent advances in geriatric medicine. Churchill Livingstone, Edinburgh
Wynn, V, Doar J W H 1969 Some effects of oral contraceptives on carbohydrate metabolism. Lancet 2:761–765

FURTHER READING

Baylis P F C 1980 Law on poisons, medicines and related substances. Studies in law and practice for health service management 9:50–76
Beard J R (ed) 1976 The menopause. MTP Press, Lancaster
Burgen A S V, Mitchell J F (revisors) 1972 Gaddum's pharmacology. Oxford University Press, Oxford
Crooks J, Stevenson I H (eds) 1979 Drugs and the elderly. Macmillan, London
Curry S H 1977 Drug disposition and pharmacokinetics. Blackwell Scientific, Oxford
David J A 1983 Drug round companion. Blackwell Scientific, Oxford
George C F 1980 Topics in clinical pharmacology. Kimpton, Medical, London
Goodman L S, Gilman A 1975 The pharmacological basis of therapeutics. Macmillan, New York and Baillière Tindall, London
Griffin J P, D'Arcy P F 1979 Adverse drug interactions. Wright, Bristol
Kessel N 1965 Self poisoning — Part I. British Medical Journal 2:1265–1270
O'Malley K, Crooks J, Duke E, Stevenson I H 1971 Effects of age and sex on human drug metabolism. British Medical Journal 3:607– 609
Smith S E, Rawlins M D 1973 Variability in human drug response. Butterworths, London
Stockley I 1981 Drug interactions. Blackwell Scientific, Oxford
Swonger A K 1978 Nursing pharmacology. Little, Brown, Boston
Turner P, Richens A 1982 Clinical pharmacology. Churchill Livingstone, Edinburgh

16

Radiotherapy

INTRODUCTION

The term radiotherapy is used when forms of ionizing radiation are employed in the treatment of disease.

Treatment may be delivered to the patient by exposure to the rays externally (teletherapy), or internally by placing radioactive material within a body cavity or within tissues (plesiotherapy). Radioactive materials may also be administered systemically, either intravenously or orally, so that they are distributed throughout the body by normal metabolic processes.

Radiotherapy is used almost exclusively to treat malignant disease; either as a first-line management, adjuvant treatment, or for palliative symptom control.

EFFECTIVENESS OF RADIOTHERAPY

The assessment of the (clinical) value of any form of treatment of cancer is invariably difficult, for three main reasons:

- the great variability of the natural history and behaviour of apparently similar malignant tumours in different patients
- the differences in the physical and mental responses of individuals to their disease and its treatment
- the length of time necessary to evaluate the results of treatment.

However, despite these difficulties there is a great deal of research material available indicating the value of radiotherapy as a primary treatment, and also as the major treatment in combined modalities. The examples discussed below illustrate the diversity of its uses in varying clinical situations.

First line management

Radical radiotherapy is intended to cure. It is given most commonly in the early stage of a disease where the tumour is localized with no evidence of metastatic spread.

Malignant disease of the cervix uteri, for example, is treated primarily by in vitro cavity irradiation supplemented by surgery or external irradiation to the pelvis (Hanks et al, 1983), or radiation therapy alone (Perez et al, 1983).

Basal and squamous cell carcinomas of the skin and other epithelial tissues can be treated by irradiation or surgery equally effectively. The choice of treatment is therefore more dependent upon convenience and the expected cosmetic result. For larger lesions, which would require extensive reconstructive surgery, radiotherapy is preferable.

Similarly, current thinking on breast cancer (summarized by Crile, 1975) suggests that radical and inevitably mutilating surgery is no more effective in treating clinical stage one breast cancer than less radical alternatives. Researchers in France (Pierquin et al, 1971) and in this country (Elliot, 1980) have developed and used, with some success, an afterloading technique with Iridium-192 wire implantation, and external beam therapy to treat the rest of the breast, including the iridium-irradiated volume. As this method of treatment effectively leaves the structural breast intact, it offers an enormous psychological advantage over disfiguring surgical techniques. It must be pointed out, however, that disfiguration of the breast can occur with radiotherapy treatment, and that, for example, the number of patients suffering from long-term effects of treatment such as lymphoedema are the same with radiotherapy to the axilla as they are with surgical excision.

Several authors have documented the dramatic improvements achieved in the cure rate of some of the rarer cancers following the advent of radical radiotherapy.

Radiation therapy for Hodgkins disease, for example, has improved considerably since the technique of mantle-irradiation (treating the major lymph node areas in the supra-diaphragmatic region) was introduced. This technique is illustrated in Figure 16.2 (the results have been reviewed by Liew et al, 1983).

The newer development of total body irradiation is now increasingly being used in the treatment of chronic lymphocytic leukaemia following bone-marrow transplantation (Lichter, 1980) and as a primary therapy for advanced lymphosarcoma (Johnson, 1975).

Patients who have refused surgery, or are considered unsuitable candidates, may be offered radical radiotherapy as an alternative. For example, it is uncommon for elderly patients (over 75 years of age) to be considered fit for a radical cystectomy, but they will usually tolerate external radiotherapy to the bladder satisfactorily.

Sometimes the long-term consequences of surgery outweigh its effectiveness as a first-line approach to treatment. Carcinoma of the larynx, for example, usually involves laryngectomy. Following surgery the patient has to go through the arduous process of learning oesophageal speech. A course of radiotherapy effects a cure in over 90% of cases in the early stages, and although the strength of the voice may be diminished in the process, there are no more serious side-effects or consequences (Crown, 1979).

Adjuvant treatment

In combination with surgery, for example, radiotherapy is valuable both pre- and postoperatively.

Some tumours are simply inaccessible due to their anatomical site, size, infiltrative nature, or fixation to adjacent tissues. Radiotherapy is often employed to reduce the tumour to a manageable size for excision. For example, in treating carcinoma of the rectum, Klugerman et al (1972) have reported some improvements in the survival of patients having irradiation before surgery.

Postoperatively, radiotherapy may be used both prophylactically, where no secondary spread of the disease is obvious, and therapeutically to irradiate remaining or recurrent cancer cells following an incomplete attempt at surgical removal of a tumour. There is still much controversy about the long term value of postoperative irradiation. Paterson and Russell (1962) were unable to demonstrate any improvement in survival when the mediastinum was irradiated following pneumonectomy. However, following mastectomy, the incidence of local recurrence on the chest wall is recognized to be lower if postoperative irradiation is given to the skin flaps and operation scar (Taply & Fletcher, 1970).

Radiotherapy is increasingly being used as an adjuvant treatment to chemotherapy. For example in Ewing's sarcoma and Hodgkin's disease (Timothy et al, 1979), initial chemotherapy aims to shrink the tumour mass so that high dose radiation is only given to the area of residual tumour. Subsequent chemotherapy then deals with residual disease or distant metastases.

Palliative radiotherapy

This is used to control distressing symptoms present in local disease before metastatic spread, and more commonly in advancing and terminal illness. A cure is not expected. The goal of treatment is to improve the quality of the rest of the patient's life. For example, some patients with carcinoma of the breast do not present for treatment until the tumour is inoperable, possibly fungating and there is a risk of haemorrhage. Palliative irradiation can promote healing in ulcerated lesions.

Some tumours cause distressing symptoms which can be controlled by palliative irradiation; for example, haematuria in carcinoma of the bladder, bleeding and mucous discharge in carcinoma of the rectum. Radiotherapy may also be used to relieve superior vena caval (SVC) obstruction in lung cancer, usually with good symptomatic relief.

In advancing disease, one of the commonest uses of palliative irradiation is the relief of pain for bone or skin metastases. In breast cancer, skeletal deposits are often extensive, and control of the pain is necessary whilst attempts to manage the generalized disease process continue.

Even when the disease is in its latter stages, palliative radiotherapy has a good psychological value for both the patient and his family who feel that 'something is being done'. Treatment courses are generally short, often only lasting until symptom relief has been obtained. The total radiation dosage may be lower to reduce the possibility of unpleasant side-effects. The general aim is to promote patient comfort, especially in cases where the natural course of the disease cannot be altered.

BIOLOGICAL AND PHYSICAL PRINCIPLES

PHYSICAL PROPERTIES

Naturally occurring radioactivity is found mostly in a few heavy elements, such as radium. Such elements are described as 'radioactive' because they possess unstable neutron-proton bonds which undergo spontaneous disintegration or decay in order to attain a more stable state. Energy released during this process is in the form of high speed electron and gamma rays capable of ionizing atoms in their path.

Naturally occurring radiation agents are expensive, and have been largely replaced in modern radiotherapy techniques by lower cost, artifically induced radioactive isotopes produced by nuclear bombardment in a cyclotron or nuclear reactor. One of the most useful of these radiation agents is radioactive cobalt (^{60}Co) which is used extensively in external irradiation. Others include radioactive iodine (^{131}I) used in systemic therapy, caesium (^{137}Cs) used in intracavity irradiation and iridium (^{192}Ir) used predominantly for implantation techniques.

BIOLOGICAL EFFECTS

In human tissue, ionizing radiation produces

physico-chemical changes in cells by interfering with the important function of cellular reproduction. The most significant cellular damage is produced when DNA (deoxyribonucleic acid) within the nucleus is damaged or destroyed. Such damage does not normally kill a cell outright, indeed, cellular function may continue for some time. Only when the time comes for cellular division to take place will the damage be revealed; mitosis will fail or be so severely abnormal as to culminate ultimately in cellular mitotic death.

Factors influencing cell damage

The degree of damage inflicted on a cell exposed to radiation depends on two major factors in addition to the radiation type and dosage:

- mitotic rate of the cell
- amount of oxygen in the tissues.

Mitotic rate

The ability of a cell to divide and thereby reproduce itself is a major characteristic of most (but not all) living cells. The period of time between each mitotic division is called the 'cell cycle time' and this varies with different types of cells. Cells comprising the skin, reproductive organs, bone-marrow and gut epithelium divide rapidly and grow quickly. The cells lining the intestine, for example, divide approximately once every 24 hours, whereas adult nerve cells do not divide at all.

Radiation destroys a greater proportion of cells where mitoses are frequent (in normal and malignant cells), therefore the rapidly dividing cells of the bone-marrow or reproductive organs are much more susceptible to irradiation than muscle or bone cells where the mitotic rate is slow.

Most courses of teletherapy are given as a fractionated course of treatment. By dividing the total calculated dosage of radiation to be given into smaller daily fractions, ongoing mitoses result in a fresh group of sensitive cells being present at each daily treatment, and consequently large numbers of malignant cells are likely to be destroyed.

Tissue oxygenation

The presence of oxygen at the time of irradiation also influences the susceptibility of a tissue to damage by irradiation. Vascular tissue (with its good oxygen supply) is more sensitive to radiation than tissue which is avascular. Actively growing tissue has a good blood supply, slow growing tissue is less well supplied. Although malignant tumours are usually rapidly dividing (active), they often possess a central hypoxic core which is resistant to radiation.

Several other factors reduce the amount of oxygen in the tissues:

- anaemia — a deficiency of haemoglobin in the blood affects the capacity of the blood to carry oxygen to the tissues
- scar tissue — resulting from surgery or previous irradiation, it has no capillary network
- sepsis or necrotic tissue in the irradiated zone.

Various ways of overcoming the oxygen defect are used.

Anaemia should be corrected prior to starting treatment. The lowest acceptable haemoglobin level in patients to be treated by radiation is 10 g per 100 ml. In severe anaemia, blood transfusion is the most rapid and effective method of raising the haemoglobin.

Hyperbaric oxygen therapy artificially increases the oxygen tension in the tissues by treating the patient in a pressurized oxygen-filled tank (hyperbaric tank). When oxygen is breathed under pressure the haemoglobin is 100% saturated. In addition, and more importantly, excess oxygen dissolves in the plasma from where it reaches the tissues by diffusion.

TREATMENT

RADIOCURABILITY

The radiocurability of a tumour depends upon a number of factors in addition to the rate of mitosis and presence of oxygen. These include:

- tumour size — a small, localized tumour is more likely to be eradicated than a larger, metastasizing one
- tumour site and accessibility
- the tolerance of surrounding tissues — a very radiosensitive environment, for example a testicular tumour, may limit the total dose of radiotherapy given.

Very large doses of prolonged radiation to living tissue eventually result in necrosis. Even at lower doses, sufficient damage could occur to impair the normal function of an organ.

PLANNING

The aim of radiotherapy in the treatment of cancer is to give either a lethal dose of radiation to malignant cells, or a dose which will render them harmless, with minimal effect on normal cells (Crown, 1979).

Two essential principles are employed in all treatment planning to minimize the side-effects of radiation to normal tissues:

- choice of treatment method and radiation energy, based upon a detailed diagnosis of the type of tumour and the extent of the malignancy
- the use of 'skin-sparing' techniques and shielding equipment during treatment sessions.

Choice of treatment method

Prior to deciding the most favourable treatment policy, patients must frequently undergo lengthy and sophisticated investigative procedures. Clinical, surgical and histological examinations, and grading of the malignancy can provide valuable information about the position of a tumour, its degree of differentiation and its liability to metastasise. Ultrasonic or isotope scans may also be requested.

Treatment plans are usually prepared using a 'simulator'. This specialized piece of equipment is designed to duplicate the movements and positions of the radiotherapy apparatus, without actually producing the treatment beam. Using X-ray opaque markers to provide a reference position, a representation of the internal anatomy is obtained which allows the radiotherapist to measure the dimensions of the area to be treated.

The distribution of radiation dose or possible 'treatment fields' is then calculated using Ellis's tables (published dosage data — Ellis, 1965).

Method of application

Where a very high cancerocidal dose is required, implants or intracavity sources are an advantage if the site of the tumour is appropriate, because only the local area is irradiated and the dose to the surrounding normal tissue is minimized. Tumours of the buccal cavity, for example, are often better suited to treatment by implantation because external beams would have to pass through the sensitive tissues of the cheek and mandible.

External beam therapy is generally used for the treatment of large tumours. In widespread disease the volume of malignancy could not be effectively irradiated by internal applicators or implants, and the numbers of needles necessary would be impractical.

In treating the head and neck region, where the slightest movement could jeopardize accuracy, perspex shells are made to fit the exact contour of the patient's head. These are worn throughout all planning and treatment procedures to ensure that the head is in exactly the same position each time. Small tattoos or indelible ink are used to identify the area to be treated (Cattell, 1979).

Type of radiation

Tumours can occur in any site in the body, and in a variety of shapes and sizes. Both the radiotherapy equipment and the treatment beam must be able to be manipulated accordingly. X-rays can be produced at different energies or voltages. The energy of a ray is partly responsible for the penetrating power of the beam.

Alpha rays are intensely ionizing positive particles, which are produced at low voltages and possess a low skin penetration value. They are sometimes used to treat non-malignant skin conditions such as psoriasis and eczema.

Beta rays are negative particles (electrons) whose penetration power varies according to the isotope emitting them. They are ideal for treating tumours of relatively few centimetres' thickness which overlie normal tissue. A different form of beta-ray therapy is systemic administration of a radioactive substance by either the oral or intravenous route.

Gamma rays are produced at greater voltages (4–20 megavolts, MV) by apparatus such as the linear accelerator; they have a correspondingly greater penetrating ability and are used in the very precise treatment of tumours which occur deeper in the body, for example carcinoma of the bronchus or oesophagus.

Research is currently investigating the effects of fast neutrons (particles found in the atomic nucleus in association with protons), and pi-mesons (heavy particles, with a negative charge and high energy value, which are produced artifically in large cyclotrons) upon normal and abnormal tissues. Neither are dependent upon the good oxygenation of cells for their effect, but the latter are very expensive, and available in only a few centres throughout the world (Deeley, 1980).

Skin-sparing techniques

The treatment machines are designed so that they can be moved in any direction around the patient. The radiation beam can be aimed from several different angles in order to minimize the dose to normal tissues while giving a maximum dose to the tumour. Careful planning can successfully avoid important structures such as the spinal cord or lungs. This technique is called 'multi-field irradiation' (Fig. 16.1).

The area to be irradiated may also be restricted by the use of 'cones' and specially prepared 'shields'. These consist of blocks of high density material, for example lead, which are placed in the path of the beam to absorb unwanted radiation. Figure 16.2 illustrates their use in the 'mantle-technique' used in the treatment of Hodgkin's disease.

The thickness and shape of the lead shields vary, depending upon the energy of the beam and the area needing protection. In the megavoltage range of beam energies, heavy blocks of lead 5–8cm thickness are required.

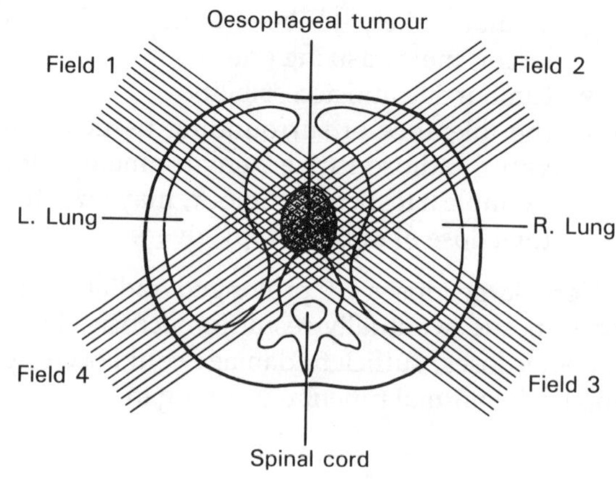

Fig. 16.1 Multi-field irradiation technique used to treat oesophageal carcinoma. The spinal cord is avoided, and although a portion of the lungs is unavoidably involved in the irradiation zone, the dose received is lower than the dose delivered to the tumour

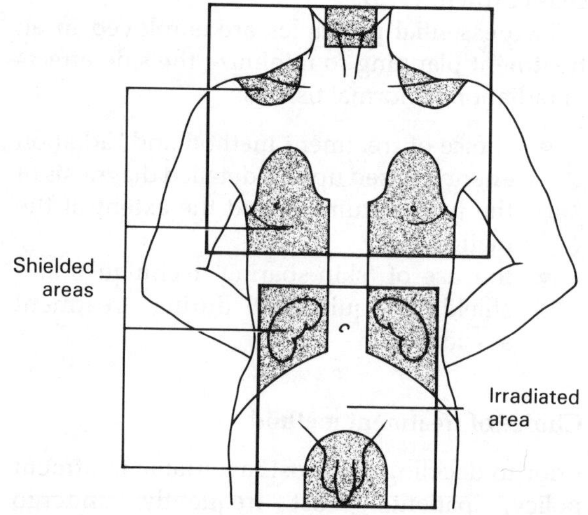

Fig. 16.2 Lymph node areas irradiated in the treatment of Hodgkin's disease, using the thoracic 'mantle' technique and an inverted 'Y' irradiation technique. Included in the treatment area are the cervical, supraclavicular, axillary, mediastinal, para-aortic and pelvic modes.

GENERAL EFFECTS OF RADIATION TREATMENT

It is inevitable that some normal tissue will be damaged in the course of treatment for cancer. The severity of the reaction will vary from individual to individual and be influenced by the type and volume of tissue being irradiated. The problem of massive skin reactions is not as great as it used to be before the development of megavoltage equipment, which delivers the maximum radiation dosage below the skin surface. However, about one-third of patients today are estimated to suffer from marked skin reactions during their treatment (Walker, 1982). Nearly all patients who receive radiotherapy to the skin intentionally, for example in post-mastectomy irradiation of the chest wall, will exhibit skin reactions to some degree. Similarly, nausea and abdominal discomfort are difficult to avoid if the gastrointestinal tract is included in the field of irradiation. When a large area of sensitive tissue is treated, for example the spinal column which contains bone-marrow, a severe systemic reaction can be anticipated, usually beginning 6–12 hours after radiation has been given. Common symptoms include tiredness, depression and lethargy, nausea, anorexia and bone-marrow suppression with a consequent drop in the blood count.

The effects of radiation upon normal tissue vary, not only according to the particular site of the body being irradiated, but also from individual to individual.

The aims of nursing care are twofold:

- to minimize unpleasant side-effects of treatment by teaching appropriate preventative actions
- to give support and encouragement throughout the treatment course.

SKIN

There are three basic stages of skin reaction to radiation:

- Erythema (reddening of skin) — caused by local vascular dilatation in response to the release of histamine-like substances from damaged germinal cells, hair follicles and sebaceous glands.
- Dry desquamation (scaling glands and basal columnar cells of irradiated skin) — caused by degenerative changes in epidermis. Results in sloughing of epidermis.
- Moist desquamation (denudation of skin with the subsequent leakage of and oozing of serum) — surface epithelium has been shed with the subsequent leakage of fibrinogen-rich fluid over the denuded area. When converted to fibrin, this forms a pseudo-membrane in which become enmeshed large numbers of leucocytes. This membrane constitutes the body's natural barrier against further physical, chemical and bacteriological injury, but is liable to rub off easily. Blister formation and local oedema may occur.

Management

It is important that patients are taught, and understand, the principles of good skin care. It may be impractical and uncomfortable to ask a patient to refrain from washing the area concerned, particularly if it includes the groin or axilla, and there is no evidence to suggest that water alone will predispose a skin reaction. However, the damage caused by friction during drying is well established and consequently it is sensible not to wet the irradiated area more often than comfort and cleanliness demand.

The following potential traumas are recognized by most authorities and should be avoided:

- vigorous rubbing with towels — washed treatment areas should be carefully patted dry with a soft towel
- wet shaving — an electric razor is preferred, as any cuts in the irradiated zone will be slow to heal and prone to infection
- pressure
- constrictive or abrasive clothing — loose cotton clothes, rather than those made of artificial fibres, are recommended
- the application of any type of soap,

perfumed talc or lotion, unless directed by a doctor — many lotions contain a zinc or lead base which increases the skin's sensitivity to irradiation
- exposure to direct sunlight, or the application of hot water bottles — ultraviolet light exacerbates any skin reaction.

The symptoms which patients have been found to complain of most frequently (Walter, 1978) are redness, peeling, itching, soreness, burning or tingling. There is a wide variety of preparations used commonly to treat these symptoms, but there is very little published research as to their effectiveness. However, Glees et al (1979) found that hydrocortisone cream 1% was soothing to many patients when used in all stages of treatment to control inflammation. A solution of calamine and tannic acid is used by staff at the Royal Marsden Hospital on itching erythematous skin (a mildly astringent agent, it cools and soothes the skin as the water component evaporates). Gentian violet is commonly used in skin reactions exhibiting moist desquamation although its actual effectiveness is unknown. It is bactericidal to some Gram-positive organisms such as staphylococcus, but stains skin purple and is removed only with vigorous washing.

GASTROINTESTINAL EFFECTS

Many patients begin a course of radiotherapy with the idea that nausea and vomiting always occur. In fact, this is not a universal experience; it depends upon many factors, including the site being irradiated, the dose of radiation, the number of fractions, the overall time in which it is given, and the general condition of the patient. Individuals with a malignant disease may experience nausea for a variety of reasons — for example, biochemical imbalances brought about by the disease itself. Hypercalcaemia (high calcium level in blood often associated with secondary skeletal deposits) and hyperuricaemia (high uric acid levels due to excess cellular breakdown) can both induce nausea. Adjuvant treatment by chemotherapeutic drugs and the patient's general anxious state may also be implicated.

Whilst it is important that patients appreciate that nausea does not occur to everyone, it is also reassuring to be told that it can be controlled and, to an extent, prevented by the skilful administration of anti-emetics, sedatives and anti-spasmodic drugs. Anti-emetics, for example metochlopramide, need to be given at least half an hour before meals and treatment sessions to be effective, and by intramuscular injection if necessary.

Nausea may considerably modify an individual's capacity to maintain an adequate level of nutrition and hydration. Small, attractively presented meals containing high protein and vitamin foods should be offered. Fluid intake should aim to exceed 2 to 3 litres in 24 hours (to assist in the elimination of toxic waste products, the result of tumour-breakdown, via the kidneys). If a patient does vomit, then accurate fluid loss must be charted and urea and electrolyte levels monitored. Mouth washes should always be offered, for example, glycerin and thymol, with ice or sips of preferred fluid as desired. The patient's hands and face should be sponged frequently, and a clean vomit bowl and tissues placed within reach to promote comfort and confidence in the nursing staff.

BONE-MARROW SUPPRESSION

Treatment involving the marrow-rich haemopoietic bones, such as the sternum and iliac crests, may cause a drop in the peripheral platelet and white cell counts in only a few days, and in red cell counts within a week. Treatment may need to be halted temporarily so that platelet or packed cell transfusions can be given — usually when platelets fall below 60 000 mm^3, white cell count below $2000/mm^3$ and the haemoglobin below 9–10 g/100 ml. Patients' full blood counts are normally obtained as a baseline, prior to commencing treatment, and then at weekly intervals as the course proceeds. Patients receiving radiotherapy to large skeletal areas may need their full blood count to be monitored more frequently and, in addition, the symptoms of bone-marrow suppression should be explained to them. An incident of bleeding gums, unaccountable bruising or weakness may otherwise be frightening, and interpreted as a sign of deterioration. These patients should be advised to plan rest periods and to avoid persons known to have infections of any kind. Electric rather than wet shaves should be recommended and the use of soft toothbrushes, which avoid trauma to the gums, should be advised. Staff must also be aware of the dangers of giving intramuscular injections to patients with bone-marrow suppression.

LETHARGY SYNDROME

Patients receiving radiotherapy often experience generalized malaise, lassitude and depression. This may occur in the absence of any physical signs of side-effects. One factor may be the presence of toxic products in the blood as a result of radiation, which circulate in the bloodstream before elimination via the kidneys. However, the patient's general condition and anxiety about their diagnosis and treatment must also be considered.

As a technique, radiotherapy is shrouded in mystery and misunderstanding. In comparison with other modes of treatment such as surgery, the principles of radiotherapy are not as readily understood, nor as well presented by the media. Among other concerns, patients have expressed fears of becoming radioactive or suffering from radiation burns, radiation sickness, and hair loss.

MANAGEMENT OF PATIENTS RECEIVING RADIATION TREATMENT

PREPARATION

It is essential that prior to treatment the myths and misconceptions of what the treatment will involve are replaced by clear, easily understood, factual information. This must include details of the equipment used, the length of treatment, any necessary skin-markings, sensations felt and anticipated side-effects. In addition, it is important that the patient has had the environment, or situation in which the treatment is going to take place, fully explained: for example, the need for isolation if implants or internal applicators are to be used, or the necessary isolation during teletherapy with the radiographer only in contact via an intercom system. Isolation for even a short period can be an upsetting experience for many patients, and the sympathetic understanding and reassurance of a nurse will be appreciated. One method of increasing patients' knowledge of radiotherapy was demonstrated in a learning experiment conducted by Mood & Israel (1972). Information was portrayed in a series of short film presentations relating to the procedures, side-effects and common emotional reactions of patients to radiotherapy. Learning was assessed by subsequent questionnaires and statistical analysis. Although this study provided no measure of how useful this information was to patients either in assisting with their treatment or reducing their stress, it was clear that patients were genuinely interested in viewing the presentations and were more knowledgeable when they did so.

PATIENTS WITH RADIATION SOURCES IN SITU

Protection of ward staff

Where radioactive sources in the form of implants or applicators are in position, or if a patient has had a recent therapeutic dose of an isotope such as ^{131}I, he or she carries a considerable radiation risk to others.

It is mandatory that all hospital staff involved in the care of such patients possess a thorough understanding of the risks and necessary safety precautions as laid down by the Department of Health and Social Security Code of Practice Regulations (1973). The official Code of Practice (HMSO, 1972) requires certain standards for the limitation of radiation dose, both to persons exposed to ionizing radiations during the course of their work and to members of the public. These standards follow the recommendations of the International Commission for Radiological Protection (ICRP, 1977). The ICRP recommendations recognize that some risk of inducing important biological effects, such as genetic or carcinogenic effects, extends to the lowest level of radiation dose, although at this level the risk to the individual is small.

Adequate isolation of patients receiving systemic or plesiotherapy is essential. Warning signs must be clearly displayed (see Fig. 16.3).

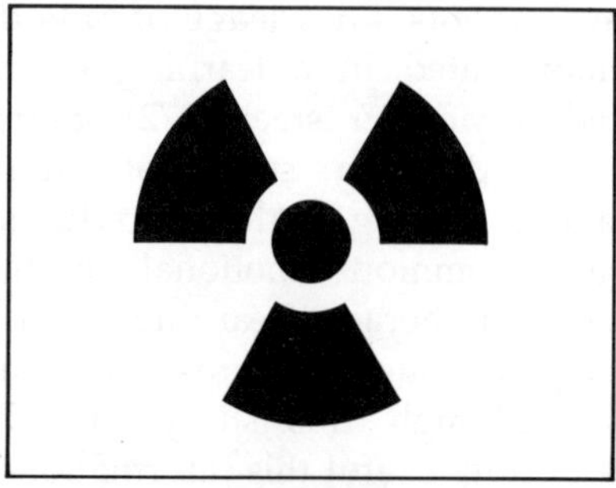

Fig.16.3 International radiation symbol.

All ward staff should be issued with a personal film badge which is then worn throughout all duty periods. The film detects radiation and is developed at regular intervals in order to monitor the amount of radiation to which the wearer has been exposed. The Code of Practice (HMSO, 1972) lays down the maximum permissible dose for workers in the United Kingdom.

Intelligent individual planning of patient care is essential to enable adequate nursing of the patient while not overexposing the staff to excessive radiation. All procedures must be carried out as quickly as possible and as far from the sources as is practicable. Radiations are subject to the inverse square law. That is, if a nurse stands 2 feet away from the source of radiation, she receives only one fourth as much exposure as when standing only 1 foot away. At 4 feet, she receives only one sixteenth of the exposure. Therefore, increasing the distance from the radiation source decreases the exposure.

Unsealed radioactive isotopes

Unsealed radioactive isotopes are used to treat cancer in two ways — either by injection as a non-absorbable solution, for example colloidal gold, into the pleural or peritoneal cavities, or alternatively systemic administration by either the oral or intravenous route.

Radioactive iodine-131 (^{131}I) is the most commonly used unsealed source for treatment purposes. It is given orally as a clear liquid in the treatment of well-differentiated thyroid cancer following total thyroidectomy (Harmer, 1979).

An initial ablation dose of ^{131}I destroys the majority of any remaining thyroid tissue. Further doses are repeated at regular intervals, as long as functioning thyroid deposits are present.

Treatment of this nature means that the patient becomes totally radioactive. Special precautions must be taken to prevent the transfer of radioactive material from saliva, sweat, urine and faeces to others. It is essential from the onset that patients fully understand the principles of the treatment that they are receiving, to enable them to comply with good radiation protection.

The main precautions for the patient concern safe personal hygiene. While the treatment is in progress, isolation within a single cubicle is desirable and the patient only allowed to leave for toilet purposes. A separate lavatory should be reserved whenever possible and clearly marked for that patient's use. Protective clothing should be worn, and the patient must be taught to flush the toilet twice after use to disperse the radioactivity. If the patient is confused or incontinent, catheterization will reduce the danger of contamination of the floor and bed. The medical physics department should be consulted about the emptying of the catheter bag, how often, and where the contents are to be stored. They should also advise what to do if spillage occurs of urine, faeces or vomit. An easily digested diet and mild anti-emetics are often routinely prescribed to reduce the risk of nausea and contamination by vomiting. Where they are able, patients should be instructed in the safe use of special bags for the disposal of uneaten food and soiled linen. Disposable cutlery and plates are useful as they can be safely discarded in these special bags. Alternatively, if personal cutlery is preferred, it must not be taken out of the patient's cubicle until it has been examined for residual radiation.

Successful management relies a great deal upon the teaching and supportive skills of the nurse. Each patient is entirely individual and levels not only of intelligence but also of tolerance and acceptance vary. To many patients, the concept of becoming totally radioactive, albeit temporarily, may be difficult to grasp and they may treat with suspicion assurances that the effects are negligible by the time of discharge. Family and friends must also be included in the teaching process. Their support and understanding is invaluable, but they must be instructed to avoid any physical contact with the patient or bed, and curtail their visits to within acceptable exposure times.

Plesiotherapy

Plesiotherapy is a form of treatment using small radioactive sources which can either be implanted into tissue itself, or be inserted into body organs or cavities using applicators. The source is then either removed after a period of time when the necessary dosage has been given or, if the half-life is a short one, then the implant may be left in situ permanently with no radiation hazard remaining after a few days. Tumours can be treated accurately, with minimum dosage to surrounding structures, and specifically, as the sources can be tailor-made to the organ or cavity to be treated. This is achieved by fitting the gamma ray source into specially designed perspex or plastic applicators.

The most common use of small, sealed source applicators is in the treatment of the cervix and uterine body. Although the applicators and methods used vary from centre to centre, the most frequently used radioactive source is ^{137}Cs. Most applicators are inserted in the operating theatre under general anaesthesia and held in position with a proflavine gauze pack and T-bandage. Treatment lasts approximately 48–72 hours.

Several precautions are taken to ensure that the tumour and surrounding organs receive a constant radiation dose. The patient is nursed almost flat in bed to prevent displacement of the sources, and an indwelling catheter is inserted to drain freely and prevent displacement of applicators during normal filling of the bladder and micturition. A high fluid intake is therefore encouraged. Special bowel management is required to prevent defaecation while the applicators are in position. A low residue diet is normally given for 48 hours before and during treatment, and suppositories or enemas used to ensure that the bowels are empty before the radioactive source is inserted.

The aims of nursing management are threefold:

- prevention and early detection of complications
- relief of pain and discomfort
- emotional support.

The patient's temperature and pulse should be monitored regularly. Pyrexia is usually indicative of a chest or urinary infection but occasionally is caused by an allergic reaction to the proflavine pack, or pelvic cellulitis. Very rarely peritonitis, due to perforation of the uterus, occurs.

Leg and breathing exercises should be taught as deep vein thrombosis is a common complication of bed-rest. Sources and applicators should be checked regularly. Any bowel movement or unavoidable movement by the patient should be reported to the medical physics department immediately. Applicators are sometimes re-X-rayed to ensure that they are in the correct position.

The treatment is essentially painless, but patients may suffer varying degrees of abdominal and back pain from the disease itself and the enforced restriction of movement. Analgesia of the appropriate strength should be administered when necessary, and turning from side to side encouraged several times a day with limb exercises to improve the patient's blood circulation.

The environment should be made as stimulating as possible by the provision of radio, television, books and drawing materials. Flowers, plants and pictures will all add colour to the room and help make the period of relative isolation more tolerable.

Radiation of any form which involves the vagina and reproductive organs represents a threat to a woman's sexuality, femininity and self-image. Intracavity irradiation causes considerable changes in the vagina. Inflammation is common and may take 6–12 weeks to subside. In some patients, adhesions and vaginal stenosis result which, if not treated, may be severe enough to impede both sexual intercourse and vaginal examination in the future. Many centres offer patients a vaginal dilator to be used daily for 6 weeks after treatment. Instruction in its use before discharge is essential.

Both the patient and, where possible, her partner must be forewarned that vaginal dryness and dyspareunia (difficult coitus) can be expected, as radiation damages the glands that produce vaginal lubricants. A water-based jelly may be useful and should be recommended where appropriate.

Sterility is an inevitable consequence of intracavity irradiation and a fact which may be particularly difficult for pre-menopausal women (and their partners) to accept. Assurances that other signs of premature ageing, e.g. greying hair and sagging skin, will not occur must be given, and every possible avenue of support mobilized.

CARE PLANNING

Introduction

Three broad categories must be considered when planning care for an individual about to begin a course of radiotherapy:

- the psychological impact of the disease upon the individual
- the physical limitations imposed by the disease process
- the physical and psychological implications of treatment.

The nursing process provides an ideal

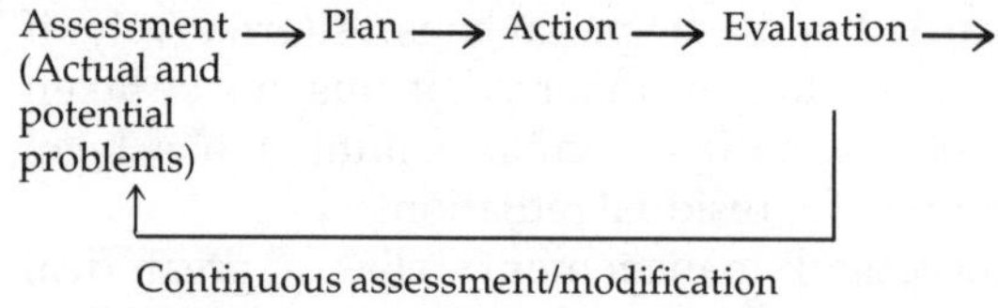

framework upon which to plan care.

The initial nursing assessment should not only aim to establish the general physical and mental condition of the patient (for example nutritional status, state of the skin, mouth and teeth) and identify any actual problems; in addition, the patient's fitness for radiotherapy should be considered with a view to anticipating the expected and possible side-effects of treatment (potential problems).

Insight into an individual's psychological needs may not be obtained at the first meeting. To most patients, the experience of admission to hospital and being separated from family and friends is traumatic and confusing (Franklin, 1974) especially when one considers the speedy referral system through which many patients requiring treatment for cancer are processed. The time interval between visiting a GP and admission to hospital is in some cases only a matter of hours, leaving very little time for the patient to become adjusted to the idea.

At the other extreme, some patients will be transferred for radiotherapy from another ward or hospital, only recently having undergone surgery. Maguire (1978) reported that referral for adjuvant treatment following mastectomy was a major contributing factor to the high incidence of depression and anxiety in his sample.

It may be several weeks, if it happens at all, before an individual feels confident enough to entrust their most intimate concerns and fears to a total stranger. What is important is that a relationship is initiated by at least one member of staff which will enable the patient to do so if he or she so wishes.

The aims of care planning are twofold.

- to begin to manage, prior to treatment, those actual problems identified in the initial assessment.
- to implement appropriate preventative measures where potential problems have been identified.

Patient teaching is an integral part of care. Most of the unpleasant side-effects of radiotherapy can be minimized by the patient when the principles of treatment are understood. Preventative actions performed by the patient restore, in part, an element of control over both his disease and his recovery. Wherever possible, relatives should be included in the teaching process. Involvement in their relative's care helps reduce the feeling of 'helplessness' and enables them to prepare for any continuous care the patient may require when discharged.

Many of the side-effects of radiotherapy are insidious and only develop or become troublesome in the latter stages of the treatment course. Continuous evaluation is essential and should continue after the completion of treatment. Patients should be encouraged to report new symptoms promptly so that early intervention can prevent more serious, often permanent, complications from developing.

Radiotherapy can modify an individual's capacity to perform activities of living. Anticipating this, the nurse can plan care accordingly.

Activities of living — effects and management

Breathing

Patients with disease arising from the larynx, pharynx and trachea may develop local oedema immediately following radiotherapy. Inflammation can obstruct an already narrowed airway making previous symptoms feel much worse, and in extreme cases may necessitate an emergency tracheotomy. Inflammation of the mucosa of the trachea and bronchial tree often causes tracheitis, chest discomfort and a dry, irritating cough sometimes proceeding to pneumonia if a portion of the lung is irradiated. Superimposed infection is a considerable risk. If left untreated, an acute reaction can lead to permanent pulmonary fibrosis and a reduction in functioning lung volume.

Any difficulty in breathing is frightening. Tension and fear only exaggerate the problem. It is important to assure the patient that the inflammation and concurrent breathing problems are only temporary, and provide the necessary support that is required until the symptoms subside.

Physical measures which may ease the problems include:

- positioning — to maximize ease of breathing
- the ready availability of oxygen
- medication — Mucaine gel and soluble aspirin mucilage suspension will help relieve soreness; tranquillizers and sedatives may be beneficial in some cases; ice-cubes produce a soothing local anaesthetizing effect when sucked
- planning — daily activities should be well spaced out; unneccesary exertion should be avoided; specific rest periods should be established.

Eating and drinking

The mouth and throat are lined with squamous epithelium which is highly sensitive to radiotherapy. Effects upon the buccal cavity include a dry mouth and hypogeusia (deterioration in taste perception) due to radiation damage to the microvillae of the taste buds (Donaldson, 1977; Rose, 1978). When the salivary glands and palate are included in the irradiation zone, stomatitis (inflammation of the mucus membrane of the mouth) and glossitis (inflammation of the surface of the tongue) are accentuated by the reduction of saliva and a change in its consistency. Inflammation of the mucosa of the oesophagus can cause dysphagia. Discomfort may lead to anorexia, poor nourishment and a low fluid intake, making the patient even more susceptible to infections such as pharyngitis, oesophagitis and thrush infections of the mouth.

Nursing goals are:

- to maintain the patient's energy and fluid intake at the required levels
- to reduce the risk of infection.

Copeland et al (1979) have demonstrated a statistically significant correlation between radiotherapy effectiveness and nutritional status. However, few individuals with sore and painful mouths and/or a diminished sense of taste look forward to meals. The dietician should be consulted so that a diet plan can be prepared with the patient, based upon their nutritional requirements but bearing in mind food likes and dislikes.

Frequent evaluation is necessary as treatment progresses, and dietary modifications made where necessary. In general, harsh crisp foods which are highly spiced or salted are replaced with high protein, bland alternatives which are cooled, pureed or liquidized as necessary.

A variety of commercial food supplements are available, for example, Fortimel (high protein), Fortical, Hycal, Complan and Build-up. Milk and egg beaten together provide a palatable savoury alternative if preferred.

Medication gels, such as Mucaine or aspirin-suspension mucilage, given prior to meals ease soreness and assist swallowing.

The patient needs constant encouragement to persevere, and assurance that symptoms will subside.

If the patient becomes unable to consume sufficient food by the normal processes it will be necessary to use alternative methods of feeding. Copeland et al (1979) recommend parenteral feeding (via a central venous catheter) when the nutritional side-effects of treatment become troublesome. They found that stomatitis was effectively reduced or eliminated during parenteral feeding. Naso-gastric tube feeding is another alternative but may not be well tolerated when the throat and tongue are very inflamed. Russell (1975) believes that enteral feeding (jejunostomy or gastrostomy feeding) has an important role to play in the management of elderly debilitated patients during radiotherapy.

The decision to employ alternative methods of feeding rests ultimately with the medical staff, but will involve nurses in its administration.

Measures to prevent infection are essential. The patient should be taught methods of maintaining good oral hygiene before treatment begins. Full oral irrigation may be given if gargling is difficult. Antiseptic mouthwashes, for example compound thymol glycerin, should be given liberally to remove viscous secretions. Some medical officers routinely prescribe an antibiotic syrup to reduce the risk of infection. Wherever possible smoking should be discouraged.

Dental care is of great importance, although a subject of some controversy. Radiotherapy causes the gums to shrink and exposes the vulnerable necks of teeth. This permanently increases the patient's susceptibility to dental caries. Extraction of a tooth from a part of the mandible which has received radiotherapy carries a high risk of bone necrosis. Consequently, some schools of thought advocate the routine extraction of all teeth in the path of the beam before starting treatment. Daley et al (1972), however, showed that pre-radiotherapy extraction is also a predisposing factor to osteoradionecrosis and the advisability of routine extraction is now questioned. Insistence on extraction adds further to the patient's distress and in some cases may even lead to refusal of treatment.

Eliminating

Bowels. Both the small and large bowel have a low tolerance to irradiation.

In a clinical trial by Trier & Browning (1966) oedema began to collect in the submucosa of the bowel wall within the first week of radiotherapy to the gastrointestinal tract. This was present in some cases for several weeks after treatment was completed.

Radiation enteritis leads to a reduction in the amount of food ingested, and the gut becomes less able to digest and absorb nutrients that do reach the small intestine. If left untreated, dehydration and avitaminosis develop.

Inclusion of the rectum in the irradiated zone may lead to tenesmus (painful, ineffectual straining to open the bowels) and mucus diarrhoea, possibly including some blood during the period of treatment. Persistent proctitis (inflammation of the rectum) with rectal bleeding are long-term complications of treatment.

Abnormal stools, particularly when they occur in association with abdominal 'colicky' pain, can be exhausting and debilitating. Minimizing the bowel reaction is essential for patient comfort and treatment success. A low residue diet should be given throughout treatment to rest the bowel as much as possible.

Fluids should be encouraged in excess of 3 litres daily in order to replace the fluids lost, and meticulous records of fluid balance must be maintained.

The frequency and nature of stools must be reported so that the nature of the problem and its severity can be correctly evaluated. Offensive or atypical stools should be sent for microbiological examination in case of infection. Anti-diarrhoeal agents, for example Lomotil (diphenoxylate) or codeine phosphate, delay the passage of gut contents so that there is time for more water to be absorbed. Both products are useful in the management of this problem. In addition, Mennie et al (1975) found calcium aspirin preparations valuable because of their anti-inflammatory effects.

Bladder. Irradiation which includes the bladder can cause radiation cystitis (inflammation) and may cause dysuria and frequency of micturition. If very severe, the patient may have to be catheterized. Fluid intake must exceed 3 litres in 24 hours. Support and supervision are required, as many patients may otherwise restrict their fluid input in the mistaken belief that this will minimize their symptoms.

Movement and self-protection

Unless specifically restricted by systemic or intracavity irradiation, radiotherapy does not normally prevent an individual from moving freely within his environment. However, debilitating side-effects of nausea or diarrhoea, for example, may indirectly reduce his inclination and capacity to do so.

Nurses must be acutely aware of how individual patients are responding to their treatment and the implications this has for their mobility and personal safety.

Resting and sleeping

Most patients admitted to hospital for any form of treatment experience difficulty sleeping (Hopkins, 1980). Those patients receiving radiotherapy are no exception.

Any of the unpleasant side-effects of treatment discussed earlier can prevent sleep. Frequency of elimination, difficulty in breathing and pain are all distressing and exhausting.

Anxiety and fear are often more pronounced at night when the busy daily routine is gradually winding down. Worries about the success of treatment and the significance of side-effects, as well as concern that there are no immediate signs of improvement, are common. Ward gossip and the exchange of symptoms in the dayroom are inevitable, but can be a source of great anxiety.

Nursing measures to promote sleep involve creating an environment which is conducive to rest. Establishing a comforting, relaxing, night-time routine is important. Many hospitals provide a hot milky drink in the late evening. The timely administration of appropriate medication may help in reducing the unpleasant side-effects of treatment. The time spent listening to patients, allowing them to express their anxieties, may be the single most important factor in promoting rest and sleep.

Seeking stimulation, reward and being motivated

> Human beings require an optimum level of sensory stimulation for behavioural efficiency. Too much is as detrimental as too little (Wright et al, 1970).

In 1969 Jackson identified several treatment situations in which patients were 'at risk' of developing clinical sensory deprivation:

- patients with perceptual disorders
- patients whose treatment restricted their movement
- patients isolated for the protection of others
- patients isolated for their protection from others
- patients confined for long-term rehabilitation.

Some methods of delivering radiotherapy will unavoidably place a percentage of patients 'at risk' of the effects of sensory deprivation. For example, perceptual disorders are common when treatment involves the head and neck region. The sensation of having one's head encased in a close-fitting 'jig' and secured to the treatment couch for any period of time is disturbing to most individuals. Lead shields covering and protecting the eyes prevent visual interaction with the environment and may cause a patient to feel vulnerable and helpless.

Strict bed-rest must be maintained for the duration of many forms of intra-cavity irradiation and all forms of systemic irradiation require isolation within a single cubicle.

Nurses must be aware of the problems associated with sensory deprivation, be able to identify those at risk, and implement preventative measures to reduce the problem.

Maintaining one's self concept

> Body-image is one of the subtly unique features of the individual personality . A person's conception of his own body, as a whole, and of different parts of the body, contributes greatly to his conception of his own personality and of his relations with other people (Bellak, 1952).

Radiotherapy may have both direct and indirect effects upon an individual's body-image.

Direct effects of radiotherapy on body-image. Radiotherapy can effect one's image of oneself through the visible effects of the treatment:

- hair-loss following irradiation to the brain can be most distressing to individuals of both sexes
- telangiectasis (dilatation of the capillaries in the skin) is a late effect of irradiation which affects most body surfaces. Radiation damage causes subcutaneous blood vessels to become fragile and brittle, and to run closer to the surface than normal. Although harmless they are often unsightly, and are seen commonly on the chest wall of women who have received post-operation irradiation following mastectomy
- erythema to visible skin areas, for example on the face, can be disturbing
- late fibrous changes often leave the skin feeling 'inelastic' and 'tough'.

In addition, some of the side-effects of radiotherapy will alter an individual's perception of his body-image; urinary frequency, for example, with occasional incontinence, may be totally unacceptable to a young person.

Indirect effects on body-image. In addition to these visible effects of treatment, the way in which one feels about oneself may be altered:

- any form of irradiation to the reproductive organs constitutes a threat to one's sexuality
- the concept of becoming 'radioactive', as during systemic therapy, may need considerable adjustment.

It is important that nurses recognize the importance of body-image to an individual and how it may be altered by specific treatments. Encouragement may be given by stressing the temporary nature of hair loss, for example, whilst the provision of a wig is of practical value. Where permanent changes are anticipated, for example telangiectasis, or where patients must be subjected to invasive, unpleasant procedures, the positive aspects of treatment should be stressed.

Relating to others

Radiotherapy may directly modify an individual's capacity to perform this function if any of the sensory organs or brain are in the irradiation zone (for example, the eyes or ears). The main implications for nursing care are to establish a means of effective communication with the patient, and prevent the distressing effects of perceptual deprivation.

CONCLUSION

Most patients who undergo a course of radiotherapy remain fairly well throughout treatment. The majority of unpleasant side-effects can be minimized considerably by the effective teaching and practice of simple preventative actions, and the prompt reporting of symptoms.

The psychological component of care is often

more complex. Discovering that one has cancer has been likened to a stressful life-event with major loss (Maguire, 1978). The anxiety begins from the time of diagnosis or when the first symptom is experienced, and exists regardless of whether the diagnosis is confirmed or evaded by the physician. In some cases acute psychological problems can occur, often related to diagnostic or treatment events (Levine et al, 1978), for example, following mastectomy (Dulcey, 1980; Morris, 1979).

Nurses caring for patients with knowledge of their disease may encounter a variety of emotional reactions including 'anger, depression, disbelief, self-pity and bitterness' (Lipowski, 1970; Brantner, 1974). Hostility (to the family, friends and hospital staff) and denial (of symptoms, diagnosis and prognosis) can occur. These latter responses are often difficult to cope with, and may require the skills and greater experience of trained counsellors.

It is essential to consider each patient as an individual, influenced by age, his or her personality, family and social obligations, site of disease and extent of spread and prognosis. Each response will be unique. In most cases, time spent talking with a patient is beneficial; sympathetic listening and reassurance may be all that is required.

Caring for a patient receiving any form of radiotherapy can be stressful and demanding, both physically and mentally, but the willingness of a nurse to become 'involved' with the patient, to begin to form relationships and to 'care', can make it one of the most rewarding and satisfying specialities in nursing.

REFERENCES

Bellak L 1952 The psychology of physical illness. Grune and Stratton, New York

Brantner J 1974 Life-threatening disease as a manageable crisis. Seminars in Oncology 1:153–157

Cattell A 1979 Technology in nursing. Radiotherapy 8: Dosimetry-Radiotherapy. Nursing Times 75(40) Supplement:29–32

Copeland E M, Daly J M, Ota D M, Dudrick S J 1979 Nutrition, cancer and intravenous hyper-alimentation. Cancer 43:2108–2116

Crile G Jr 1975 Results of Conservative Treatment of Breast Cancer at 10 and 15 years. Annals of Surgery 181:26–30

Crown V 1979 Principles of radiotherapy. In: Tiffany R (ed) Cancer Nursing–Radiotherapy. Faber and Faber, London

Daley T E, Drane J B, Maccomb WS 1972 American Journal of Surgery 124. Cited by Henk J M 1976 Neoplasms of the head and neck. In: Hope-Stone M F (ed) Radiotherapy in modern clinical practice. Crosby Lockwood Staples, London

Deeley T J 1980 Hypoxic cell sensitizers in clinical radiotherapy. In: Topical reviews on radiotherapy and oncology Vol 1. Wright, Bristol

Department of Health and Social Security 1973 The safe use of ionizing radiations. A handbook for nurses. DHSS, London

Donaldson S S 1977 Nutritional consequences of radiotherapy. Cancer Research 37:2407–2413

Dulcey M P 1980 Addressing Breast Cancer. Assault on Female Sexuality. Topics of Clinical Nursing 1(4):61–68

Elliot R 1980 Treatment without surgery for carcinoma of the Breast. A nursing care study. Nursing Times 76:958–960

Ellis R 1965 The relationship of biological effect to dose-time fractionation factors in radiotherapy. Cure — Topics — Radiation Results 4:357-397

Franklin B L 1974 Patient anxiety on admission to hospital. RCN, London

Glees J, Mameghan-Zadeh, Sparkes C G 1979 Effectiveness of topical steroids in the control of radiation dermatitis. Journal of Clinical Radiology 30:397–403

Hanks G, Herring D, Kramer S 1983 Patterns of care outcome studies. Results of the national practice in cancer of the cervix. Cancer 51: 959–967

Harmer C 1979 Technology in nursing. Radiotherapy 11: Radiotherapy: unsealed radioactive isotopes in treatment. Nursing Times 75(51) Supplement:41-44

Her Majesty's Stationery Office 1972 Code of Practice for the protection of persons against ionizing radiations arising from medical and dental use. HMSO, London

Hopkins S 1980 Silent Night? Nursing (1st series) 20 :870–873

International Commission on Radiological Protection 1977 Publication 26 Recommendations of the ICRP. Pergamon Press, London

Jackson C W 1969 Clinical sensory deprivation; a review of hospitalized eye surgery patients. In: Zubek J P (ed) Sensory deprivation: fifteen years of research. Appleton, Century Crofts, New York

Johnson RE 1975 Total body irradiation (TBI) as primary therapy for advanced lymphosarcoma. Cancer 35:242–246

Klugerman M M, Uroaneba N, Knowniton A, Vidon R, Hartman P V, Vera R 1972 in American Journal of Roentgenology 114:498–503. Cited by Newsholme G 1976 Tumours of the colon, rectum and anus. In: Hope-Stone H F (ed) Radiotherapy in modern clinical practice. Crosby Lockwood Staples, London

Levine P M, Silverfarb P M, Lipowski Z J 1978 Mental disorders in cancer patients. Cancer 42:1385–1391

Liew KH, Ding JC, Matthews JP et al 1983 Mantle irradiation for stage I and stage II Hodgkin's disease — results of a 10 year experience. Australia and New Zealand Journal of Medicine 13(2):135–140

Lichter AS 1980 Total body irradiation in bone marrow transplantation. International Journal of Radiation Oncology in Biology and Physics 6(3):301–309

Lipowski Z J 1970 Physical illness, the individual and the coping process. Psychiatry in Medicine 1:91–102

Maguire G P 1978 The psychological effects of cancers and

their treatment. In: Tiffany R (ed) Oncology for nurses, 2. Allen and Unwin, London

Mennie A J, Dalley V M, Dineen L C, Collier H 1975 Treatment of radiation induced gastrointestinal distress with acetylsalicylate. Lancet 2:942–943

Mood D W, Israel M J 1972 Three media presentations to patients receiving radiotherapy. Cancer Nursing 5(1):57–63

Morris T 1979 Psychological adjustment to mastectomy. Cancer Treatment Reviews 6:41–61

Paterson R, Russell M H 1962 in Clinical Radiology 13:141. Cited by Mantell B S 1976 Tumours of the chest and mediastinum. In: Hope-Stone H F (ed) Radiotherapy in modern clinical practice. Crosby Lockwood Staples, London

Perez C, Breaux S, Madoc-Jones H, Bedwinek N, Camel M, Purdy J, Walz B 1983 Radiation therapy alone in the treatment of carcinoma of uterine cervix. Cancer 51:1393–1402

Pierquin P, Chassagne D, Cox J D 1971 in Radiology 99:661–667. Cited by Jardine G W N 1976 Carcinoma of the breast in radiotherapy. In: Hope-Stone H F (ed) Radiotherapy in modern clinical practice. Crosby Lockwood Staples, London

Rose J C 1978 Nutritional problems in radiotherapy patients. American Journal of Nursing 78:1194–1197

Russell R J 1975 Elemental diets. Gut 16:68–79

Tapley W D, Fletcher C H 1970 Breast cancer, early and late medical diagnosis. Anderson Hospital Year Book Medical Publishers, Chicago. Cited by Jardine G W H 1976 Carcinoma of the breast. In: Hope-Stone H F (ed) Radiotherapy in modern clinical practice. Crosby Lockwood Staples, London

Timothy A R, Sutcliffe S B, Wrigley P F, Jones A E 1979 Hodgkin's Disease, combination chemotherapy for relapse following radical radiotherapy. International Journal of Radiation Oncology in Biology and Physics 5:165–169

Trier J S, Browning T H 1966 A morphological response of the mucosa of human small intestine to X-ray exposure. Journal of Clinical Investigations 45:194–204

Walker Y 1982 Skin care during radiotherapy. A review of topical preparations commonly used in the treatment of radiation dermatitis. Nursing Times 78:2068–2070

Walter J 1978 Cancer and radiotherapy. A short guide for nurses and medical students, 2nd edn. Churchill Livingstone, Edinburgh

Wright D S, Taylor A, Davies D R, Slackin W, Lee S G M, Reason J C (eds) 1970 Introducing psychology; an experimental approach. Penguin, London

17

Surgery and the implications for nursing

INTRODUCTION

Surgery is one of the most dramatic methods of medical intervention, and the implications for the patient, and therefore for nursing, are great.

Surgical intervention involves the manipulation of body tissues either manually or, more commonly, by using surgical instruments. Most operations require incision of the skin and underlying tissues to allow access to the particular part of the body that is diseased or deformed. Clearly this means that the patient is exposed to the danger of haemorrhage and therefore shock (see Ch. 10), to the risk of infection from microorganisms and to the experience of pain. Developments in surgical techniques have largely been made possible through developments in haemostasis, asepsis and anaesthesia which minimize these problems. These developments have made surgery very much safer than it used to be.

THE DECISION TO OPERATE

In reaching a decision about whether or not an operation will be performed, a number of issues are involved. The readiness with which a particular operation is performed will increase as the risks lessen in relation to the potential benefits, or as the risks of not performing the operation increase in comparison with the dangers of surgery.

The patient's decision whether or not to accept the advice to undergo surgery is reached as a result of a number of factors. Though a consideration of benefits compared to the likely side-effects and other risks of the operation seems a reasonable approach to take in reaching this decision, in many situations the patient will not have sufficient relevant information on which to base such a decision. Selection of a particular option will derive from the degree of trust in the surgeon, the emotional response to the thought of surgery (based at least partly on previous experiences), discussions with family and friends, who may or may not be well-informed, and cultural norms.

In some situations the decision is reached relatively easily as there is seen to be little choice. For example, acute appendicitis is 'known' to have dire consequences if surgery is not performed and the operation is not seen to be life-threatening or to have any adverse consequences. Other conditions are less clear-cut. The formation of an ileostomy may be seen as more difficult to tolerate than the effects of ulcerative colitis.

The system of health care and method of payment will also enter into this decision-making. If the patient is to pay, there may be some reluctance to undergo surgery unless there are clear benefits to be derived. On the other hand, profit to the surgeon may enter into the advice given to the patient.

Very considerable differences can be seen in the rate at which certain operations are carried out in different countries, even those of comparable levels of medical development. For example, hysterectomies are performed three times as often in the USA as in England and Wales (McPherson et al, 1981). Is it really the case that American women are so different from British women? Or does this reflect cultural and organizational factors related to health care? It seems unlikely that the risks to the patient are very different in the two countries.

Effectiveness of surgery

Surgical treatment is clearly the treatment of choice for some conditions, such as appendicitis (and the rates for this operation differ little between the USA and UK) or fractured neck of femur. However, where alternatives are possible there has been little evaluation of the effectiveness of surgical treatment as opposed to other methods of treatment, such as radiotherapy. Similarly, until recently there has been little, if any, careful comparison of different methods of surgical treatment of the same condition. For many years carcinoma of the breast has been treated by radical mastectomy. This operation involves removal of the breast with the underlying muscle of the chest and the axillary lymph nodes. It results in considerable deformity and loss of function as well as resulting in serious psychological difficulties in many women. Recent work appears to indicate that equivalent long-term survival rates can be achieved by much less drastic surgery, by simple mastectomy or partial mastectomy (tylectomy, lumpectomy) with retention of the nipple.

Consent

Some other methods of treatment, such as administration of drugs or radiotherapy, alter the cellular and organic functioning of the body and, in a sense, are assaults on the internal integrity of the individual which carry the risk of unwanted side-effects. However, surgery is a clear physical assault and, as such, could lay the surgeon open to legal proceedings. Therefore, the patient must give informed consent to the operation being carried out, and any further procedures which may be performed. The consent form signed by both patient and doctor is retained in the patient's notes. However, the term 'informed consent' is open to different interpretations. It would seem reasonable to assume that it means that the patient really understands what is to be done, what the risks are, what benefits can reasonably be expected from the operation, and what unwanted effects may result. It is at least questionable that all patients who sign consent forms have this degree of understanding.

CLASSIFICATION OF SURGERY

Operative treatment can be classified in several ways and some of these will be discussed, along with the implications for the patient.

DEGREE OF URGENCY

An operation may be described as elective, essential or emergency.

Elective surgery

Elective surgery is carried out to increase comfort and health, but is not essential for survival. Patients having elective surgery have had time to consider the idea of an operation and have had a real choice about whether or not to undergo the treatment. Time is available for adequate pre-operative preparation which, if the administrative procedures allow it, can be usefully carried out before admission to hospital. Anxiety levels are likely to be lower than immediately before surgery and learning is, therefore, enhanced (Fortin & Kirouac, 1976). Normally the operation will only be performed when the patient is in a satisfactory physical condition.

Essential surgery

This is carried out to remove or prevent a threat to life. The patients' choice is between accepting the treatment offered as it is necessary for continued health or survival, or refusing surgery with the implication that they may die in the fairly near future. For some there is no real choice as they want to continue to live if at all possible, but in some situations, perhaps because the proposed surgery is so mutilating, the patient may decide against undergoing surgery. Those who are to be admitted for operation will usually have some time to wait before it can be carried out. Some will be able to prepare themselves mentally, doing much of the 'work of worrying' in advance and coming into hospital in the moderate state of anxiety which results in the most satisfactory adjustment after operation (Janis, 1958). Others will be extremely anxious, while some may appear to have little anxiety on admission. In all cases it is valuable if they can be helped to achieve a realistic expectation of what is to happen. Time is normally available for adequate pre-operative care, and the operation may be able to be postponed until the patient is in a satisfactory physical state. Most operations in the UK fall into this category.

Emergency surgery

Emergency surgery has to be carried out with a minimum of delay to give the best possible chance of survival. The patient may have very little time to accept the necessity for surgery. There are a number of factors which may contribute to a high level of anxiety. The patient may well be worried about him or herself and the prognosis, but may be equally anxious about the family, work, or other responsibilities. It may be possible to relieve some anxiety and help the patient to undergo surgery in a better emotional, and therefore physical, condition, by contacting appropriate people for them.

Time for pre-operative preparation is clearly limited but psychological care can be given while carrying out physical measures. While the operation cannot be postponed for any length of time without increasing the risk for the patient, certain physiological disturbances, such as fluid and electrolyte imbalance, or severe anaemia, will usually be corrected by intravenous therapy before surgery.

TYPE OF LESION

Surgery can also be classified in the terms of the type of lesion being dealt with. These may be:

- an excess of tissue (tumours)
- a deficiency of tissue (defect)
- displacement of structures (deformity)
- non-living material (foreign bodies) (Myers et al 1980).

Tumours

A tumour may be due to a number of different pathological changes:

- neoplasia — which may be malignant or benign
- hyperplasia or dysplasia
- congenital hamartomas (a mass of tissue gone wrong (Myers et al, 1980) — malformations ranging from simple naevus to giant, complex malformations
- inflammatory masses
- cysts.

On first presenting for medical consultation, the patient with a tumour is likely to be anxious about whether or not he/she has cancer. Accurate diagnosis should be carried out without delay and the patient reassured when this is possible.

The type of condition diagnosed will have a number of implications for the patient. A malignant tumour is likely to need wide excision (possibly with resulting deformity) and may be followed by radiotherapy or chemotherapy with the resulting unpleasant side-effects. The patient will have to live with uncertainty about prognosis and may have to face further illness, operations, debility and death. It is not always possible to give an accurate diagnosis before operation and histological examination of the tissue.

On the other hand some other conditions may be treated surgically by excision or drainage or both but the surgery does not have to be so extensive. The patient may need prolonged treatment and have some residual change in function but can be reassured that the condition will not spread widely throughout the body. For some patients the operation and postoperative progress will be straight-forward and result in complete restoration to normal.

Tissue defects

Tissue defects are also of several types:

- tissue necrosis
- hernias (protrusion of an organ through an anatomical barrier which normally restrains it)
- congenital deficiencies.

Again the implications for the patient will vary. Tissue necrosis is due to reduction or complete loss of the blood supply to the tissue and can be caused by a number of different agents. Depending on the extent of the change, excision may result in simple scarring or marked deformity. Amputation of a limb affected by atherosclerosis will result in major problems of adaptation, both physical and psychological.

On the other hand, hernias and some congenital defects (such as hare-lip and cleft palate or atrial septal defect) when corrected by operation should enable the individual to return to, or achieve for the first time, a completely normal life style.

Some congenital defects cannot be corrected and surgery can only help to improve the functional abilities of the individual.

Deformities

These can be acquired or congenital. Trauma or certain diseases, such as rheumatoid arthritis or some orthopaedic disorders, result in acquired deformities, some of which can be treated surgically. Congenital deformities are often easier to treat than congenital deficiencies. Correction of deformities would be expected to have positive implications for the individual concerned.

Foreign bodies

Foreign bodies can be either extrinsic or intrinsic. Foreign material in contact with body tissues will often result in inflammation and infection and must therefore be removed.

Objects swallowed will often pass through the gastrointestinal tract without difficulty but the patient (and when the patient is a child, the parents) will have a period of anxiety while this takes place. Foreign bodies in other parts of the body, such as the bronchi, will need to be removed to relieve the airway obstruction that is the inevitable result.

Intrinsic foreign bodies are of three types:

- faecaliths

- calculi — most common are gallstones and renal calculi
- sequestra — separated piece of bone.

Any of these may result in chronic inflammation and infection, with resulting pain and malaise, and will need removal. However, some gallstones may cause no problems for many years.

AIMS OF SURGERY

Operative procedures can also be considered in terms of the aims of surgery:
- excision of diseased tissue
- repair or reconstruction of defect or deformity
- drainage of infective lesions or cysts
- modification of physiology
- investigation.

The first three of these are to deal with the type of lesion described above (Myers et al, 1980).

Modification of physiology

Surgery may be performed to modify the patient's physiology in an attempt to reduce the effects of some functional disorder. Some functional disturbances such as thyrotoxicosis or Cushing's syndrome are often associated with tumours and are treated by excision of the lesion (Ch.19). In other cases the cause of the disorder is less clear, but an alteration in physiology could be expected to modify the function in the direction of normality. For example, a vagotomy is carried out to reduce the acid secretion of the stomach thus promoting healing of peptic ulcers (discussed in Ch.23). Unfortunately this also inhibits gastric emptying so that a pyloroplasty is also performed when the stomach outlet is reconstructed allowing easier egress of gastric contents. Similarly, a sympathectomy is performed to reduce the vasoconstriction of blood vessels and to improve peripheral circulation. In a different way, the application of tubal clips via a laparoscope modifies normal reproductive physiology in the prevention of pregnancy.

Investigation

A number of investigative procedures (Ch.11) are also performed which expose the patient to some of the same risks as other operations. Many involve the insertion of a tube, an endoscope, through a body orifice or small opening made in the overlying tissues. This allows direct visual examination of the cavity and organs involved and permits the removal of small amounts of tissue (biopsy) for histological examination.

Some rigid endoscopes are still used and these carry some risk of damage to the patient's tissues. However, nowadays the flexible fibre-optic endoscopes are more commonly used. Frequently these procedures are carried out under local anaesthesia and sedation. A clear explanation of the events and sensations to be experienced reduces the stress experienced by the patient (Johnson, 1976) and makes it easier for him or her to relax and co-operate with the procedure.

A laparotomy, an abdominal operation, is performed when the diagnosis is not clear. In this situation the patient has to go through the unpleasant and potentially hazardous experience of an operation with the added uncertainty of not knowing the diagnosis. Clearly this is extremely stressful and the patient concerned will need considerable support (Chs 8 & 12).

Biopsy of cutaneous tissue may be undertaken without endoscopy. Similarly, aspiration of body fluids may be undertaken by inserting a trocar and cannula or a needle into the fluid-containing cavity without direct vision. While these are relatively 'minor' procedures they nevertheless still incur the risks of infection, haemorrhage and shock attendant on more extensive surgical intervention.

PRINCIPLES OF SURGICAL MANAGEMENT AND IMPLICATIONS FOR THE PATIENT AND NURSING

A satisfactory result from an operative procedure involves both the success of the operation and the prevention of complications and undue stress in the patient. There are four broad areas to consider:

- performance of the operation itself and the metabolic response
- the risk of haemorrhage and haemostasis, and circulatory disturbances
- the risk of infection and the need for maintaining asepsis
- anaesthesia and its complications.

The nursing implications are discussed throughout and form the basis for the pre-operative care plan (Table 17.1) and the postoperative care plan (Table 17.2) illustrated. These plans give an indication of the care necessary for any patient undergoing surgery, but do not include the management specific to a particular operation or deal with less common problems that patients may have on admission.

THE OPERATION

There are essentially four stages in achieving a satisfactory result from an operative procedure:

- excision of the pathological lesion
- rearrangement of local anatomy
- repair of tissue
- supportive treatment while healing takes place (Myers et al, 1980)

Excision

The lesion requiring surgery must be completely removed, with the excision extending into healthy tissue. Unless this is achieved satisfactorily, healing will not occur. In some situations this will only entail the removal of an encapsulated mass. However, if a malignant tumour is being dealt with, the excision of some surrounding tissue, and perhaps of the lymph nodes draining the area, is carried out in an attempt to remove the abnormal tissue completely. The patient may have considerable difficulty in accepting the resulting disfigurement. When appropriate, the provision of an appropriate prosthesis is important in helping the patient to present a normal appearance to the world. However, emotional support will be needed for some time as the patient begins to adjust to the change in body image (see Ch. 12).

Rearrangement of local anatomy

The second stage involves the rearrangement of body tissues to endeavour to achieve as near normal anatomical arrangement as possible following excision of tissue. When extensive amounts of tissue have been removed this may be difficult to achieve and require more than one operation. Tissues of the same type must be aligned and the continuity of hollow tubes restored in order to facilitate normal functioning. The blood supply to the damaged tissues must be satisfactory to allow wound healing to occur.

Sometimes normal structure cannot be achieved and the tissues are arranged to allow as near normal function as possible. For example, following a partial gastrectomy the remainder of the stomach is anastomosed to the duodenum to allow passage of food on through the alimentary tract. When this is not possible, as after an amputation or formation of a colostomy, a prosthesis which may be cosmetic or functional is used.

Repair of tissues

Various materials are used to keep tissues in alignment so that healing can occur. Screws and plates are used to immobilize bony joints, while sutures hold soft tissues together. Various types of suture material are available with a range of physical characteristics. Suture material to be used is selected with regard to the tension which will be exerted on it, the amount of tissue reaction which it may initiate and whether or not it is soluble. Sutures used externally can be removed but internal sutures need either to be removed by normal body mechanisms, as is catgut, or to be low in antigenicity thus causing little reaction by the tissues. Artificial materials used to replace diseased or damaged tissue, as in a hip replacement or repair of an aortic aneurysm, must also be of low antigenicity.

Supportive treatment

The aim of supportive treatment is to provide the conditions which facilitate wound healing following the surgical intervention. Wound healing and the nursing implications are discussed in Chapter 4, but one of the major areas to consider in promoting physical well-being is the nutritional care necessary to help the patient overcome the metabolic changes associated with surgery.

Metabolic response to surgery

The metabolic response to surgery has been discussed in detail by Moore & Ball (1952). In the immediate post-operative period the patient is in a catabolic state when the body reserves of carbohydrate, fat and protein are being used as an energy source. The protein releases essential and non-essential amino acids which are necessary for wound healing but which also act as a source of glucose essential for brain metabolism. The protein breakdown and its use as an energy source leads to an increase in the loss of nitrogen and the patient is in a state of negative nitrogen balance. Potassium is being lost from the body and sodium and water retained. While the protein breakdown leads to a loss in muscle mass and an expected fall in body weight, the retention of sodium and water may disguise this.

The duration and severity of these metabolic changes is related to the extent and severity of the injury. Moore & Ball (1952) described them as lasting approximately 4 days in a patient who has undergone gastrectomy. Following this the patient enters an anabolic phase during which structural protein is built up and the patient regains body weight. The metabolic changes described are very similar to those of stress (see Ch.8).

Recognizing that these changes occur, the nurse takes them into account when considering care of the patients. Canizaro (1981) states that a reasonably well-nourished, healthy person undergoing major surgery can tolerate the catabolic changes and partial starvation for one week after major, but uncomplicated, surgery. However, those patients already malnourished, or who are unlikely to be eating normally within that time, require additional nutritional support for satisfactory recovery to take place. The nurse should carry out a nutritional assessment to ensure that those patients requiring additional nutrient intake are identified. This is discussed in more detail in Chapter 14, along with methods used for increasing nutritional intake.

In the shorter term the period of pre-operative fasting must be controlled. The patient is necessarily fasted before going to theatre to ensure that the stomach is empty when he/she is anaesthetized in order to minimize the risk of vomiting and of inhalation pneumonia. Fluids pass through the stomach quite quickly and food rather more slowly, depending on the composition of the meal. Fat retards stomach emptying while carbohydrate passes through quickly. Hamilton-Smith (1972) found general agreement that the period of fasting should be at least 4 hours. Some of the sample of surgeons, anaesthetists and nurses would distinguish between fluids, which could be taken up to 4 hours before operation, and food which could only be eaten up to 6 hours beforehand. However, she found considerable variation in the periods of time for which the patients were reported to be fasted.

The short-term effects on the patient of prolonged fasting immediately before anaesthesia and surgery are not known.

During fasting the liver becomes depleted of glycogen as it is used to maintain the blood glucose level. Physiology texts vary widely in the reported time for which the glucose store is adequate but it appears that about 18 hours after food, the liver glycogen would be exhausted. By this time the body protein is being broken down to supply the brain, and fats are being used as an energy source for other tissues of the body. Excess fat breakdown will result in some degree of ketosis. As patients are necessarily fasted during and for a period after an operation, the pre-operative period of food deprivation should be kept to a minimum consistent with safety.

Postoperatively the patient should be given a high protein diet to minimize the degree and length of time of negative nitrogen balance.

Table 17.1 Pre-operative care plan

Actual (A) / Potential (P) Problems	Objectives/Expected Outcomes of Care	Plan of Care	Evaluation Criteria
(A) **Anxiety** due to:	Lack of behavioural and physiological signs of anxiety.		Able to relax and eat satisfactorily Pulse and BP stabilise
Uncertainty about diagnosis / prognosis	Able to discuss uncertainties and anxieties with member of staff or significant other	One nurse to work with patient and develop relationship to enable patient to discuss anxieties etc.	Able to interact freely with staff — particularly 'own' nurse.
Lack of knowledge about environment, ward routine, patient's role etc.	Able to function adequately within ward environment	Show round ward; explain routine, staff uniforms, staff's expectations of patient (e.g. not leave ward without checking); introduce to other patients	Able to find way round ward. Interacts appropriately with staff and patients
Lack of knowledge about procedures and experiences in pre- and post-operative period	Able to describe events that occur and sensations to be experienced during pre-operative procedures and postoperative circumstances, and own role in events	Teach about procedures, reasons for them, sensations to be experienced in pre- and postoperative periods: *Pre-operative* — fasting, skin preparation, bowel and any other special preparation, pre-medication, theatre clothing, journey to theatre, induction of anaesthetic *Postoperative* — recovery room, moved bed, intravenous infusion/transfusion, drains, catheters etc., details specific to operation, early mobilisation; pain, management of pain, patient's role	Able to describe events and sensations to be experienced, and own role in management of pain
Loss of control in running own life	Able to demonstrate activities to enhance recovery and to co-operate in own care	Teach deep-breathing and coughing, leg exercises, relaxation, and encourage practice pre-operatively, give choices whenever possible in care given and timing of events	Able to demonstrate breathing and leg exercises and relaxation
(P) **Haemorrhage/ Shock** peri- and postoperatively	Data available to enable rapid recognition of problem postoperatively	Record pulse and BP some hours after admission	Pulse and BP recorded
	Patient in good fluid balance and haemoglobin status	Encourage good fluid intake up to 4 hours before surgery	Urine volume high, specific gravity less than 10.15
		Check blood sample taken and sent to laboratory	Blood results obtained
	Patient in condition to enable anaesthetist to recognize condition	Ask patient to remove all make-up	No nail varnish or lipstick
(P) **Wound infection** postoperatively	Pre-operative procedures performed to reduce bacterial count on skin Low level of anxiety (see above)	Skin preparation — hair removed with depilatory cream only if essential: avoid shaving if possible Bath/shower with disinfectant (e.g. Hibiscrub), including hair, day before and day of operation Clean gown and sheets	Procedures performed Evaluation post-operatively — presence/absence of wound infection
(P) **Respiratory infection** postoperatively	Able to ventilate lungs fully and expectorate secretions Stopped smoking Low level of anxiety (see above)	Teach deep-breathing and coughing exercises (or co-operate with physiotherapist) (Fig. 17.1) Explain reasons for exercises and stopping smoking, and frequency (hourly when awake) of exercises	No smoking observed Able to demonstrate deep-breathing and exercises and state frequency to be performed

Table 17.1 Continued

Actual (A) / Potential (P) Problems	Objectives/Expected Outcomes of Care	Plan of Care	Evaluation Criteria
(P) **Deep vein thrombosis** postoperatively	Able to carry out activities to promote circulation (i.e. leg exercises)	Teach leg exercises (Fig. 17.1) and deep breathing, and importance of these and of early mobilization, and frequency to be performed	Able to demonstrate leg exercises and state frequency to be performed
(P) **Vomiting** and inhalation of vomit during anaesthesia	Stomach empty before anaesthetic	No solid food given 6 hours before anaesthetic	Food taken and withheld as planned No vomiting on induction of anaesthesia
(P) **Hypoglycaemia and ketosis**	Nutrient supply adequate to maintain normal metabolism	Easily digested food (low-fat) given up to 6 hours before anaesthetic	No acetone in urine postoperatively
(P) **Burns** from use of diathermy during operation	No foci available for passage of electrical current	Ask patient to remove all jewellery, hair grips or other metal objects Cover wedding rings with tape	All items dealt with
(P) **Hazards** of incorrect operation or treatment	Patient clearly identified and all necessary information available	Check arm band, notes and X-rays complete and available (check consent form completed)	All checks made
(P) **Harm** during operation due to presence of prostheses or aids	No prostheses or aids in position	Explain and ask patient to remove prostheses (e.g. false teeth, eyes) and aids (e.g. contact lenses, hearing aids)	All artificial aids removed

Table 17.2 Postoperative care plan

Actual (A)/ Potential (P) Problems	Objectives/Expected Outcomes of Care	Plan of Care	Evaluation Criteria
(P) **Airway obstruction**	Able to breathe adequately Tissues oxygenated	Ensure airway clear while unconscious by: placing patient in semi-prone position (if possible) Use of airway, hold jaw forward removal of secretions by suction or swabs (if necessary)	Breathing quiet and steady Colour normal
(P) **Haemorrhage/ Shock** (P) **Water intoxication** due to excess ADH following surgery	Fluid balance good and shock does not develop, or signs of and water intoxication	Management of intravenous infusion/ transfusion to ensure fluid intake, rota maintained Fluid intake and output recorded Observe for signs of dehydration and water intoxication	Fluid rota to time Urine output and specific gravity within normal limits Skin and mucous membranes moist, good turgor Breathing quiet, mental function normal
	Early indications of haemorrhage/shock recognized	Record pulse and BP and observe wound for haemorrhage at 15-minute intervals, increasing time intervals as condition stabilizes	Pulse and BP return to and remain at patient's normal No haemorrhage observed
	Adequate, prompt treatment of shock	If pulse rises and BP falls, raise foot of bed, inform medical staff, prepare additional IV fluids and plasma expanders or blood	BP and pulse return to normal
(A) **Pain** due to surgical trauma	Pain recognized — position, severity, etc.	Assess pain, patient's report about position, severity etc. Observe for rigidity, rise or fall in pulse or BP, pallor or other signs of pain	
	Pain relieved to enable rest and activities and exercises	Position patient and regulate environment (e.g. temperature, noise, light) for maximum comfort. Ensure IVI's, drains, catheters, dressings not pulling, rubbing, etc., bladder empty Reinforce patient's understanding of normality of experience Give analgesics, within limits of prescription, to minimize pain and prevent pain developing (i.e. give before mobilizing, physiotherapy, etc.) Make positive statements about effectiveness in minimizing pain If inadequate pain relief, request alteration of prescription	Patient reports comfort, is able to mobilize, deep-breathe, cough, etc.
(A) **Anxiety** due to: *Uncertainty about diagnosis/ prognosis*	No signs of anxiety seen *See under Anxiety,* Table 17.1		Appears relaxed in ward
Uncertainty about procedures and experiences	Understands events as they occur and is able to predict	Explain reasons for procedures, actions and sensations in advance and as they occur	Does not appear anxious when procedures performed
Loss of control in running own life	Able to contribute to activities which promotes recovery	Encourage deep-breathing, leg exercises, mobility, explain importance Give patient choice in care and timing of events when possible	Carries out activities conducive to recovery

Table 17.2 Continued

Actual (A)/ Potential (P) Problems	Objectives/Expected Outcomes of Care	Plan of Care	Evaluation Criteria
(A) **Restricted mobility** resulting in: (P) *Pressure sores* (P) *Restricted movement of joints*	Regains mobility No residual problems, e.g. pressure sores, restricted movement	Turn 2-hourly while incapable. Remind to move at frequent intervals to relieve pressure when in bed or chair	Pressure areas in good condition — no redness
		Help to carry out full range of movement exercises twice daily while mobility restricted	Full range of movements
		Help patient to increase mobility over some days according to ability: sit on side of bed, walk few steps to chair; walk round bed; walk to toilet, wheeled back; walk to and from toilet; increase mobility around ward till fully mobile and up all day	Satisfactory level of mobility in comparison with expectations for stage of recovery after particular operation
(P) **Deep vein thrombosis**	Good hydration state	Explain reasons and encourage fluid intake of 2000 ml/daily	Fluid intake of 2000 ml
(P) **Pulmonary embolus**	Good blood flow through legs	Encourage exercises (leg and breathing) hourly when awake Encourage mobility, (?) anti-embolic stockings applied, (?) IM heparin as prescribed	Carries out exercises without reminder
	Early signs of deep vein thrombosis identified	Observe for signs of DVT : slightly raised temperature, pain and/or swelling of calf, Homan's sign (calf pain when foot dorsiflexed and leg straight)	Presence or absence of signs of DVT
	Prevention of pulmonary embolus	If DVT develops, patient nursed on bed rest, anti-embolic stockings or legs bandaged Anti-coagulants administered as prescribed (patient observed for side-effects, e.g. bleeding gums, blood in urine)	
	Identification of pulmonary embolus, if occurs	Observe patient for : pain in chest, breathlessness, haemoptysis	Presence or absence of signs of pulmonary embolus
(P) **Chest infection**	Full ventilation of lungs and expectoration of secretions	Encourage deep-breathing and coughing hourly when awake, help patient splint wound	Breathing exercises carried out without reminder
	Signs of chest infection identified	Observe for : raised temperature, pulse and respiration; noisy respirations, breathlessness, discoloured sputum	TPR remain within normal limits
	If occurs, chest infection rapidly resolves with treatment	Sputum specimen obtained for micro-biological examination	
		4-hourly inhalations, co-operation with physiotherapist with regard to timing, position to aid breathing	After inhalation, sputum expectorated readily
		Administer prescribed antibiotics at correct time	Signs of infection clear
	Low levels of anxiety/ (see above)		
(P) **Delayed wound healing** due to:	Wound heals well — skin edges in apposition, no redness, swelling or oozing Suture line healed in 3—10 days (as appropriate)		Wound heals satisfactorily

Table 17.2 Continued

Actual (A)/ Potential (P) Problems	Objectives/Expected Outcomes of Care	Plan of Care	Evaluation Criteria
Infection	No signs of infection seen	Wound dressing used that maintains warm, moist environment at suture line, enables gaseous exchange, protects from infection Dressing left untouched unless necessary — sutures/clips removed aseptically when appropriate Wound drains managed aseptically, removed when no further drainage, 'strike-through' prevented	Infection does not occur
	Low levels of anxiety (see above)		
Poor nutritional or hydration status	Good nutritional and hydration state through good food and fluid intake	Encourage patient to drink 2000 ml fluid daily and to build up from light to high protein diet If inadequate food intake, give nutritional supplements	Food and fluid intake satisfactory Nutritional and fluid status good Minimal weight loss
(P) **Inability to pass urine** due to pain, awkward position etc.	Retention of urine recognized (if occurs)	Note urine output, inquire about sensation of full bladder palpate lower abdomen	Urine output adequate, no discomfort
	Able to pass urine satisfactorily	Ensure adequate fluid intake Provide bedpan/bottle when needed, assist into comfortable position, give privacy If difficulty — run taps, assist to commode or standing position If still unable, s.c. carbachol may be prescribed or patient catheterized	
(P) **Constipation**	Normal pattern of bowel function regained	Encourage fluid intake and high fibre diet (if possible) Encourage mobility, especially walk to toilet after breakfast. If bowels not open within few days (relate to patient's normal pattern), suppositories may be administered	Bowel function returns to normal pattern
(A) **Reduced ability to undertake activities of living**due to pain, immobility and feeling of insecurity	Pain minimal (see above) Mobility regained (see above) Regains independence within appropriate time	Give assistance with activities as necessary Encourage to undertake more for self each day, give support Explain what is permissible and what restrictions there may be	Regains ability to undertake activities of living within expected time following particular operation
(A) **Reduced/delayed self-care ability** after discharge due to lack of knowledge about expected progress and restrictions after discharge	Knows what to expect and to do after leaving hospital	Explain expected time-scale to full recovery, possible problems that may develop and how to deal with them Explain any restrictions on activity and length of time necessary, and how to gradually build up activity	Able to explain progress to expect during recovery and pattern of recommended activity

After surgery, particularly if the patient has been ill before operation, he/she may have little appetite and will need encouragement and tempting with attractive (but not too large) helpings of food that he/she likes. Nutritional supplements (see Ch. 14) can be a valuable aid in ensuring adequate nutritional intake.

HAEMOSTASIS, HAEMORRHAGE AND CIRCULATORY DISTURBANCES

In carrying out a surgical operation blood vessels, both large and small, are cut and blood is lost from the circulation. Loss of excess blood results in shock, discussed in detail in Chapter 10, but normal body mechanisms including blood clotting come into play to reduce blood loss. The initiation of these mechanisms increases the coagulability of the blood and the risk of development of complications associated with blood clotting.

Haemostasis

Normal haemostasis

The stages involved in haemostasis are described in detail in any physiology textbook. Normal haemostasis results from the balance between processes leading to coagulation and those which inhibit blood clotting.

The first stage after damage to a blood vessel is vasoconstriction due to the contraction of the smooth muscle caused by thromboxane (derived from prostaglandins) (Moncada & Vane, 1979). Thus, the volume of blood lost is reduced. Vasoconstriction is increased by cold. Thromboxane A also stimulates platelet aggregation at the end of the blood vessel and, at the same time, the laying down of a fibrin network begins. The fibrin and platelets form a blood clot which controls further haemorrhage as long as the pressure behind it is not so great that the blood clot is disrupted. The cascade system resulting in blood clotting is complex and not dealt with in this text. Inhibitory mechanisms normally prevent widespread blood clotting.

Techniques to promote haemostasis

The smallest blood vessels damaged in surgery will seal themselves without difficulty. Pressure exerted on them will hasten haemostasis and when tissues are approximated and sutured together that pressure alone will suffice to stop capillary bleeding in most cases.

Diathermy entails the use of an electric current passing through a finely pointed cutting tool or through a clamp which burns the blood vessels closed. When used as a cutting tool the capillaries are sealed as they are cut, while larger blood vessels are sealed by clamping them and then sending an electric current through the instrument. In preparing to use diathermy an electrolyte-soaked pad is attached to the patient's thigh. The electric lead from this is linked to the diathermy machine in the operating theatre; the voltage used is controlled from the machine.

Another lead from the diathermy machine goes to the instrument with insulated handles held by the surgeon, who can close the electrical circuit by means of a foot switch. When the circuit is closed the electrical current passes through the cutting tool or clamp to the blood vessel which is sealed, and then the current is dissipated through the patient's body fluids and through the diathermy pad, which spreads the current over a wide area and thus prevents skin damage. If diathermy is to be used, care must be taken to ensure that no part of the patient's skin is touching the metal theatre table. A wedding ring is covered adequately because, if the electrical circuit can be completed through a small area of skin, a burn will result. To protect the staff involved, metal instruments are released when diathermy is about to be used. While the use of diathermy as a cutting tool stops bleeding, it also reduces the blood supply to the damaged tissues. This inhibits wound healing and increases the risk of infection (Cruse & Ford, 1973).

Ligatures are used to tie off the cut ends of larger blood vessels.

Without these techniques much surgery would be impossible, as haemorrhage would endanger the patient's life.

Haemorrhage

The effect on the patient of haemorrhage depends on the volume of blood lost and the speed at which the loss occurs. When haemorrhage occurs into the tissues, the pressure exerted by the accumulation of blood within a confined area restricts the amount of blood loss. However, bleeding into a hollow organ such as the stomach or into a body cavity such as the peritoneal cavity is not limited in the same way and signs of haemorrhage may develop. Slow blood loss over a period of time results in anaemia, while the rapid loss of a fairly large volume can result in shock with resulting rise in pulse rate, fall in BP, pale, cold skin and anxiety. Bleeding may or may not be visible externally.

Blood accumulating in the tissues results in a haematoma which can cause pressure on other organs, with serious results. For example, respiratory obstruction can result from haemorrhage following thyroidectomy. If an accumulation of blood or serous fluid is allowed to remain, it may become infected and result in abscess formation. In addition, the cut tissue surfaces will be separated and wound healing inhibited. These are the reasons for the use of drainage tubes following surgery allowing fluid to drain into dressings or into some form of container.

Corrugated or Penrose drains have been frequently used to allow blood or serous fluid to escape by capillary action or by passing up the side of the drainage tube. In many situations now, surgeons use disposable polythene tubing with a number of holes in the side towards one end. This end is inserted into the operative field and low negative pressure suction applied at the other end with a Redivac or comparable disposable system in which the exudate collects in the suction bottle. The suction reduces the risk of fluid accumulating in the tissues.

Drains are usually brought out onto the surface of the skin through a separate 'stab' incision. This separation from the main wound reduces the risk of wound infection (Cruse & Ford, 1973).

Haemorrhage can be described as primary, reactionary, delayed or secondary.

Primary haemorrhage

This is the immediate blood loss that occurs during surgery and may continue if adequate steps are not taken to control it. Blood accumulating in the operative field is removed by the aspirating tube and accumulates in the suction bottle. It is important to observe the volume of blood in the bottle in addition to weighing used swabs in order to estimate blood loss accurately. Blood lost during operation is replaced by blood transfusion if it is extensive, e.g. in excess of 0.5 litres, or if the patient's condition indicates that this is advisable.

Reactionary haemorrhage

Reactionary haemorrhage occurs shortly after the operation is completed. It is usually said to be due to the bleeding occurring as the blood pressure rises after surgery and closed blood vessels re-open. However, it may also be due to a ligature slipping off a large blood vessel or to the arterial pressure forcing a blood clot out of the cut end of a blood vessel. In addition, instances of primary haemorrhage continuing at a fairly slow rate may not be identified until some time after the operation, when the body becomes unable to continue to compensate for the blood loss.

The nurse has the important responsibility of identifying signs of haemorrhage early in order to ensure rapid treatment. Pulse, blood pressure, possibly central venous pressure, and blood loss from the wound site are observed and recorded regularly following the completion of an operation.

Delayed haemorrhage

This is relatively uncommon following surgery. It occurs when haemorrhage is restricted within an organ and causes signs of haemorrhage when it eventually breaks out into a body cavity.

Secondary haemorrhage

This usually occurs some days after surgery and

is secondary to some underlying disease. It occurs as a result of erosion of a blood vessel and the commonest cause is infection, although neoplasia and chronic inflammatory disease are other causes. Management of such haemorrhage may require additional surgery to remove the diseased tissue and ligate bleeding vessels. Vigorous treatment of infection is essential.

Management of haemorrhage

The aim of management is to maintain an adequate peripheral circulation to continue to supply oxygen and nutrients to the tissues of the body. Management of shock resulting from severe haemorrhage is discussed in Chapter 10.

Simple fluid replacement will maintain the total extracellular fluid volume and in some circumstances may be adequate. However, if the blood loss has been of such a volume that the concentration of plasma proteins is markedly depleted, then the fluid will move out into the interstitial space. In such a situation a plasma expander, such as dextran, is needed. This contains large molecules which remain within the circulation and exert an osmotic pressure which attracts fluid back into the circulation from the tissue spaces and maintains the blood pressure.

Blood transfusion

If the haemorrhage is severe, then the oxygen-carrying capacity will be considerably diminished and blood transfusions will be necessary. Before operation the patient who may require transfusion will have his or her blood grouped and cross-matched. That is, his/her own blood group will be identified and this blood tested with the blood it is intended to transfuse.

The aim is to ensure complete matching of the transfused and the patient's own blood. However, the very large number of blood groups identified means that an absolute match is unlikely. In many situations this does not matter as in most blood group systems (the ABO system being the exception) an individual without a particular antigen does not carry the matching antibody and, thus, mismatching of blood with relation to that particular blood group system does not result in an antigen-antibody reaction. However, an individual receiving a foreign antigen in a transfusion will begin to form antibodies to that antigen. A patient who receives a considerable amount of blood may in time be transfused with blood containing an antigen which he or she has previously received and to which antibodies have already been produced. An antigen-antibody reaction will then occur, leading to haemolysis and the release of free haemoglobin into the bloodstream, which can result in renal damage. A patient receiving blood is observed frequently, usually hourly, for signs of reaction such as a sensation of heat along the vein into which the transfusion is running, chills and fever, headache, pain in the lumbar region, cramping abdominal pain, nausea and vomiting, tachycardia, hypotension and dyspnoea (Porth, 1982). Oliguria and acute renal failure can result.

Haemorrhagic complications. A patient who needs large volumes of blood (8–10 pints) is at increased risk of haemorrhage because stored blood rapidly loses platelets and other factors required for blood coagulation (except fibrinogen). This is prevented if possible by using fresh instead of stored blood (Myers et al, 1980).

Another condition which also results in excessive bleeding is Disseminated Intravascular Coagulation (DIC). In this condition, fibrinogen and other coagulation factors are depleted by widespread blood clotting throughout the microcirculation. This condition can be triggered by a number of conditions, including haemorrhagic shock, multiple injuries, obstetric complications and Gram-negative septicaemia. The underlying cause is treated, heparin given to prevent spread of the microthrombi, and all the necessary clotting factors are replaced (Myers et al, 1980).

Pre-operative measures

One of the aims of pre-operative care is that the patient should be in the best possible state to cope with the physiological effects of blood loss. Thus, if time permits, any anaemia will be treated before operation. Any fluid and electrolyte disturbances will be corrected beforehand and dehydration should be prevented by encouraging clear fluids up to 4 hours before the scheduled time of surgery.

Circulatory disturbances

Other than haemorrhage, the major complications of the circulatory system are concerned with blood clotting and the results. Conditions which may occur are:

- thrombophlebitis — venous thrombosis associated with considerable inflammation, possibly linked with infection
- phlebothrombosis — venous thrombosis associated with little inflammation
- thromboembolism — indicates the association of pulmonary embolus with venous thrombosis.

Following surgery, venous thrombosis occurs most commonly in the deep veins of the legs and pelvis, less commonly in the superficial veins. These may give rise to pulmonary emboli. Coon & Coller (1959) found that the sources of pulmonary emboli were:

- lower extremities about 80%
- pelvis 10%
- heart 5%
- unknown about 5%

More recently the use of long-term infusion and central venous lines with the associated risk of thrombosis has probably altered the proportions.

With more sensitive methods of diagnosis, the incidence of deep vein thrombosis has been found to be much higher than previously suspected. The use of ^{125}I fibrinogen (which is incorporated into the blood clot) and scanning techniques has shown that deep vein thrombosis (DVT) developed in 30–60% of surgical patients (Atkins & Hawkins, 1965; Kakker et al, 1969). However, symptoms were not present in half these patients.

Following DVT an embolus can break off and may end up in the pulmonary circulation where it may have fatal results. The reported incidence of pulmonary embolus following DVT varies, increasing with more sophisticated methods of diagnosis. Kistner et al (1972) reported 52% incidence, although three-quarters of the patients had no clinical symptoms. Morrell & Dunnill (1968) found that 62.8% of patients who died during the postoperative period had pulmonary emboli and 43% of these died as a result of the embolism.

A number of studies have examined the factors associated with increased incidence of thromboembolic disease and many of these are discussed in Miles (1975). Patients with certain conditions are at increased risk and require particular attention to prevention. These conditions are:

- previous thrombosis or embolus
- heart disease, particularly heart failure or atrial fibrillation
- malignant disease, particularly of the prostate and pancreas
- trauma to the leg
- obesity
- immobility
- blood types A, B, AB
- ileostomy for ulcerative colitis
- middle age and older
- operations on the great vessels and blood vessels of the legs
- possibly, taking oral contraceptives.

Development of deep vein thrombosis

The three major factors in the development of deep vein thrombosis were originally identified by Virchow (1856) as:

- stasis
- trauma
- hypercoagulability.

Patients undergoing surgery are exposed to all of these. Lying relaxed on the operating table for prolonged periods results in some degree of stasis of the circulation and this will be aggravated by any periods of hypotension. Postoperatively, immobility, which will be increased by pain, will similarly lead to some degree of venous stasis. The trauma of the operation leads to increased coagulability of the blood and thus the formation of a thrombus is readily initiated. Finally, pressure on the legs by instrument trays can cause trauma to the endothelial lining of the veins and thus precipitate thrombus formation.

Following development of a DVT, there are a number of possible eventualities:

- Spontaneous lysis occurs in almost a third of the patients in an average of 5.9 days (Flanc et al, 1969).
- The thrombosis may persist with a variable degree of venous obstruction.
- The thrombosis may embolize and a part of it will end up in the lungs – many pulmonary emboli are small and dealt with by fibrinolytic mechanisms of the body, but a large embolus can block a pulmonary artery and lead to death.

Identification of a deep vein thrombosis

In 30–50% of cases a DVT is silent, that is it causes no symptoms, and up to 75% of patients with pulmonary embolus may have no sign of DVT (Kakker et al, 1969; Kistner et al, 1972). However, signs and symptoms may be found if the patient is carefully observed and tested regularly. Miles (1975) suggests that unexplained tachycardia and anxiety frequently occurs with DVT and Homan's sign should be elicited. A positive Homan's sign is the occurrence of calf pain when the foot is dorsiflexed.

An extensive thrombosis is relatively readily identified as the patient complains of pain and tenderness of the limb. In addition, other signs can be observed, such as oedema and possibly bluish discolouration of the skin, distension of the superficial veins and probably a slight rise in temperature. However, the aim is to identify and treat this condition before a pulmonary embolus occurs, and daily observation and testing are necessary to attempt to identify the less severe forms of the condition. In those at particular risk the medical staff may use techniques such as scanning with radioactive fibrinogen, Doppler ultrasonography or venography to reach a diagnosis.

Prevention of deep vein thrombosis

The prevention of DVT can be considered in relation to the factors of Virchow's triad i.e. stasis, trauma and hypercoagulability.

Teaching the patient exercises to practise pre-operatively and carry out regularly post-operatively, and early mobilization, are part of the prophylactic management of these patients. In the operating theatre itself, measures can be taken to reduce stasis by raising the foot of the operating table or by using some form of rhythmic stimulation of the muscles. However, the evidence for the effectiveness of these measures is ambivalent. Flanc et al (1969) found that their intensive use made no significant difference to the incidence of DVT (except in the elderly) although the clots were dissolved more rapidly. Tsapogas et al (1971), on the other hand, found that these measures caused a considerable reduction in DVT development. Anti-embolic stockings are also advocated to reduce venous stasis and the risk of thromboembolic disease (Husni et al, 1970).

Trauma to the legs is reduced by care in positioning and handling the patient, and in avoiding pressure on the patient during the operation.

One important measure in preventing hyper-coagulability is ensuring adequate fluid intake. In addition, low doses of the anticoagulant heparin have been shown to reduce the incidence of DVT from up to 42% in control groups to between 4–10% in those treated (Smiddy, 1976). However, the patient is more likely to bleed and the operation may be more difficult than if heparin is not given.

Treatment

The treatment of DVT falls into four main groups:

- anticoagulant therapy
- antiplatelet therapy
- fibrinolytic substances
- rest.

Anticoagulant therapy, at first with heparin and later with warfarin, is used to prevent further spread of the thrombosis and reduce the risk of additional thrombus formation at other sites. Anticoagulant therapy is usually continued for about 6 months. Prothrombin time is regularly measured.

Antiplatelet drugs such as aspirin inhibit platelet coagulation and may be used in combination with anticoagulants for long-term therapy, or may be used alone when contraindications exist for the use of anticoagulants for a prolonged period.

Substances such as streptokinase or urokinase are sometimes used to break down the clot itself.

Initially, the patient with a DVT is nursed on bed rest with the legs elevated to improve the venous return and reduce oedema. Anti-embolic stockings or elastic bandages are applied.

Occasionally the clot may be removed by surgery.

Pulmonary embolus

The presentation of this condition is very variable, ranging from sudden circulatory failure and death to no symptoms at all. The classic symptoms of chest pain, dyspnoea and haemoptysis may only occur in a small proportion of these patients.

RISK OF INFECTION AND ASEPSIS

In performing most operations, the skin is cut and the internal tissues and organs exposed to the air and microorganisms within the environment. The skin is the patient's major defence against microorganisms entering the body and, therefore, the risk of infection in these patients is great. Since Lister started using carbolic acid as a disinfectant in 1876 much of the nurse's work in theatre has been concerned with minimizing this risk.

Infection and the body's response to microorganisms are discussed in Chapter 5. In this section the factors involved in the development of infection and the management of the patient and the surroundings to reduce this risk are discussed.

Factors in the development of infection

The development of infection in a wound occurs as a result of the interaction between the number and characteristics of the microorganisms involved and the resistance factors of the host (National Academy of Sciences, 1964).

Davidson et al (1971) have examined fifteen different factors to identify those of most importance in the development of wound infections. They found that the following were of major importance:

- the age of the patient
- the presence of bacteria in the wound at the end of an operation
- an open ward environment
- the duration of the operation.

Andriole (1966) also identified the length of stay in hospital pre-operatively as a factor which modified the risk of infection. The longer the patient was in hospital before surgery, the more likely it was that a wound infection would occur.

LeFrock & Klainer (1976) discuss the research showing that the sources of the bacteria resulting in postoperative wound infections are:

- the people in closest contact with the patient
- the things with which the patient is in contact
- the patient.

Management of care related to infection

The management of care in relation to infection needs to be concerned with two main aspects:

- enhancing the patient's immune response
- reducing the exposure of the patient and the patient's wound to bacteria.

Management of staff, environment, equipment, and the patient will be discussed. Wound management to enhance healing is discussed in Chapter 4.

Staff management

Staff dealing with the patient are a major pathway by which pathogenic bacteria reach the patient: they therefore need to be aware of methods by which they can minimize this risk. A high standard of hygiene, awareness of routes of infection, and the ability to carry out activities in such a way that pathogens are less likely to be transmitted, are all important. Careful hand-washing between caring for different patients is extremely important but research has indicated that this is not always performed adequately (Taylor, 1978). It has also been suggested that the wearing of rings, even wedding rings, considerably increases the number of bacteria carried on the hands (Hemstrup-Hansen, 1963; Jacobson et al, 1985).

In the operating theatre itself a number of additional precautions are taken. One of the sources of bacteria in the environment is from the staff shedding skin squames containing bacteria. All staff change into theatre clothing, the pattern and material of which is selected with the aim of minimizing this source of bacteria. Conventional cotton gowns have little effect on this. Closely woven theatre clothing which is closed at neck, wrists and ankles is fairly effective but sometimes uncomfortable. The more recently developed, disposable theatre clothing is effective (Whyte et al, 1976; Lidwell et al, 1978). Clean theatre wear is used every day.

The process of scrubbing up, gowning and gloving in sterile clothes by those involved in the operation, and the use of sterile drapes, is concerned with minimizing the risk of infection.

The hair is a major source of bacteria and must be completely covered by a surgical hat or hood to prevent dandruff or hair falling (Gruendemann & Meeker, 1983).

The use of surgical masks in theatre aims to trap the bacteria dispersed from the nose and mouth of the wearer. The mask should fit closely around the nose, side of face and under the chin so that air only passes out through the filter material of the mask. Used masks are highly contaminated and should only be handled by the strings and after removal should be disposed of immediately.

Management of the environment

In managing the environment, the aim is to minimize the number of air-borne micro-organisms. As microorganisms are found in dust and become airborne if the dust is disturbed, the first priority is cleanliness. Cleanliness of ward areas is very important in minimizing the risk of cross-infection but the highest possible standards of cleanliness are essential in the operating theatre. In the selection of furnishings and equipment, ease of cleaning is taken into account. In addition, operating theatres have positive pressure ventilation where the air is filtered as it enters the theatre at ceiling level to reduce the bacterial count. It leaves at floor level, thus carrying bacteria downwards away from the operating table.

There is evidence that the bacterial count in theatre increases with numbers and movement of staff. Therefore, the organization of work in the theatre suite should be such that numbers and activity of staff within the theatre itself are minimized shortly before and during the operation.

Management of equipment

The aim is to reduce the risk of microorganisms coming into contact with the patient's tissues. Again the first requisite is cleanliness as bacteria can be protected against sterilizing procedures by dried blood or tissue remnants on the instruments. All instruments and materials which will come into contact with the patient's tissues during operation must be sterile. The term 'sterility' implies the complete absence of dividing microorganisms and can be achieved in a number of ways.

The most common method of sterilizing reusable theatre equipment is autoclaving. The items to be sterilized are exposed to saturated steam under pressure for a specified length of time. The time required for sterilization to be complete varies with the pressure used and the temperature thus reached. Following sterilization the items are dried. Other methods of sterilization are used for items which cannot be exposed to the temperatures and pressures involved in autoclaving. Many disposable items are sterilized by radiation. Details of methods of sterilization can be obtained from any standard text on the subject, such as Gruendemann & Meeker (1983). Whatever method is used, it is essential that a form of indicator such as a heat sensitive strip is used to check that sterilization is adequate.

The instruments and materials sterilized in preparation for carrying out the operation must be managed in such a way that they do not become contaminated during the operation. Ensuring that procedures are carried out in order to achieve this is one of the main responsibilities of the scrub nurse during the operation and is discussed in detail by Gruendemann & Meeker (1983).

Management of the patient

Pre-operative management. Pre-operative management begins with keeping the patient out of hospital for as long as possible. It has been demonstrated that many wound infections in a surgical unit were caused by bacteria on the patient's skin before surgery (Loiseau et al, 1971), and the patient's upper respiratory tract and gut flora are a source of infection. Le Frock et al (1972, 1973) found that within 21 days of admission to hospital the normal throat flora had been replaced by Gram-negative bacteria in 23% of patients and in 47% of those treated with antibiotics. Similar changes were found in faecal flora with the addition of a thousandfold increase in *Staphylococcus aureus.* The bacteria found after a period of hospitalization were those which accounted for most of the infection in the postoperative period.

Reducing the number of bacteria on the skin reduces the risk of these entering the wound at operation, and skin preparation is carried out with the primary aim of reducing the bacterial count. In addition, for some operations it is necessary to remove hair from the site of operation and a wide area around the site to facilitate the work of the surgeons. Traditionally the hair has been removed by shaving the area concerned, frequently using a 'dry shave' method. There is electro-microscopic evidence that shaving of the skin results in minute abrasions and cuts (Hamilton et al, 1977), and the risk of wound infection is increased. Hamilton et al show one series of results comparing the infection rate in patients prepared by shaving, using a depilatory cream and without hair removal. It is recommended that, whenever possible, the body hair should not be removed. However, if it is necessary because the body hair is profuse and may hamper the surgeon, clipping the hair short and using a depilatory cream leads to infection rates comparable to those when the skin is not shaved. Unfortunately, these creams do cause skin irritation in some patients and a 'patch' test needs to be carried out before using them on a large area. In addition, at present there is not a preparation suitable for use in the genital area where they come in contact with the sensitive mucous membranes. If it is essential to remove the hair, then a wet shave, producing a thick lather and using a sharp, new razor blade, may be performed.

Following removal of the hair if necessary, a bath, or preferably a shower, should be taken. Use of a preparation like Hibiscrub has been shown to result in a marked reduction in bacterial count on the skin. The active ingredient leaves a residue on the skin and inhibits bacterial division for some time after use. When used according to the instructions there is a marked drop in bacterial count evident on arrival in theatre (Brandberg & Andersson, 1980).

Pre-operative preparation to minimize anxiety, and thus to reduce the biochemical and physiological changes of stress, has been found to reduce the incidence of postoperative infection (Boore, 1978).

Intraoperative care. The care within theatre builds on the pre-operative preparation which has already reduced the numbers of bacteria on the skin and endeavours to reduce the number still further. A wide area around the incision site is swabbed with a disinfectant, but this will still not sterilize the skin, and some surgeons use a semi-permeable membrane which adheres to the skin. A large sheet of this is applied to the disinfected area and the surgeon carries out the incision through this membrane. Bacteria on the skin are thus kept apart from the surgeon's hands and the risk of transmission into the wound is reduced.

Postoperative care. Postoperative care of the wound to prevent bacteria reaching the wound and to promote wound healing is discussed in

Chapter 4. Equally important is ensuring that the patient is adequately nourished and hydrated and that oxygenation of the tissues is enhanced by breathing exercises and promoting the circulation. These aspects of care, along with activites to minimize anxiety, will all help to enhance the patient's immune response.

Wound infection inhibits wound healing, increases the risk of secondary haemorrhage and of wound breakdown. Thus, it is important to identify any infection rapidly so that treatment can be started as soon as possible. Body temperature is often recorded 4-hourly for several days postoperatively but, with all the limitations of temperature recording discussed in Chapter 27, it is necessary to observe for other signs that may indicate the development of wound infection. The pulse and respiratory rates may be elevated as a result of the rise in body temperature. The wound is inflamed and tender and will become purulent. If a semi-permeable transparent membrane such as OpSite is used then the wound can be observed without exposure to bacteria in the environment.

ANAESTHESIA

Anaesthesia allows the surgery to be carried out without inflicting pain on the patient; local or general anaesthesia may be used. Local anaesthesia may block all sensation reaching the brain or may only prevent the passage of painful stimuli, when it is more accurately known as local analgesia.

In general anaesthesia there are three effects on the patient which occur to different extents with the different anaesthetic agents. These effects are:

- unconsciousness, which can range from deep coma to light sleep
- analgesia, which may be present before unconsciousness results or may only develop at deep levels of anaesthesia
- muscle relaxation, which occurs to a very variable degree with different anaesthetics — the use of muscle relaxant drugs allows achievement of the required degree of muscle relaxation without very deep levels of anaesthesia.

Stages of anaesthesia

There are four stages of anaesthesia, although they may be difficult to distinguish if the patient passes through them rapidly.

Stage 1 — the stage of analgesia

This is the stage when pain is relieved before unconsciousness develops and occurs readily with some anaesthetics such as trichlorethylene (Trilene) and nitrous oxide. Nitrous oxide 50% with oxygen 50% (as Entonox) is the commonest anaesthetic gas used to achieve this state outside the operating theatre. It is used extensively in midwifery when the mother controls her own intake of the gaseous mixture which is only obtained when the anaesthetic mask is held firmly in place during inhalation. Entonox is also used by ambulance men and in accident and emergency departments. It is easy and safe to use and there is considerable scope for extending its use into all areas where short, painful procedures are carried out.

Stage 2 — the stage of reflex excitement

During this stage the normal conscious control of many reactions is lost and exaggerated emotional responses may occur along with wild movements. While this stage is usually passed through very rapidly in the induction of anaesthesia this is not always so in the recovery from the anaesthetic, although the anaesthetist will aim to keep this stage as short as possible. During this stage the patient must be protected from harm and cannot be left alone safely.

Stage 3 — surgical anaesthesia

This is the stage during which surgery is performed. Regular respiration and fixed, central pupils indicate that this stage is being reached. As the patient descends into this stage of anaesthesia, reflex actions no longer occur so that the patient is no longer able to keep his/her own airway clear by coughing if regurgitation from the stomach occurs. The anaesthetist takes over this responsibility. Painful stimuli no longer cause any reaction and muscular relaxation is achieved. The anaesthetist is responsible for achieving the necessary level of anaesthesia within this stage to provide pain relief and muscular relaxation sufficient to allow the surgeon to operate.

The achievement of muscular relaxation requires a greater depth of anaesthesia than does adequate pain relief, so that the use of muscle relaxant drugs means that a relatively light level of anaesthesia will be satisfactory. Suxamethonium chloride (Scoline) is a rapid short-acting (2–3 minute) drug often used to allow the insertion of an endotracheal tube. Tubocurarine chloride (Tubarine) is a derivative of curare which starts acting more slowly but lasts for about 30 minutes. This is used to continue the relaxation and is 'topped up' as necessary to maintain appropriate relaxation. During this period the patient will have to be artificially ventilated. The antidote to tubocurarine is neostigmine methylsulphate, which is injected at the end of an operation. As only a light anaesthetic will have been necessary the patient wakes rapidly with functioning protective mechanisms.

Stage 4

This stage is never intentionally entered during a surgical operation. Analgesia and muscle relaxation increase but unwanted side-effects also occur. Depression of the respiratory centre and relaxation of respiratory muscles leads to overall depression of respiration. Cardiac output falls with inadequate perfusion of the tissues leading to renal and liver failure. Permanent liver damage can be caused by some anaesthetics particularly when used at dosages which result in this stage of anaesthesia. Respiratory and cardiac failure may cause death.

Administration of anaesthesia

General anaesthesia

Anaesthesia is usually initiated by intravenous injection of a short-acting drug such as thiopentone sodium (Pentothal), ketamine or methohexitone sodium (Brietal Sodium). A short-acting muscle relaxant then enables passage of an endotracheal tube through which an inhalation anaesthetic is normally administered for the rest of the operation. Intravenous diazepam (Valium) is also used to produce a light anaesthetic which is adequate for some procedures, such as endoscopies.

An anaesthetic machine facilitates the mixing of gases in accurate proportions at appropriate pressures for inhalation by the patient. It also controls the addition of anaesthetic vapours such as diethyl ether, halothane or trichloroethylene (Trilene) to the gas before inhalation. Cyclopropane and nitrous oxide are the commonest gaseous anaesthetics used.

Local anaesthesia

Nerve fibres are blocked to inhibit the transmission of pain and this blocking can be carried out at many stages of the nervous pathway (McFarland, 1980):

- topical analgesia is achieved when nerve endings are blocked by an anaesthetic solution penetrating the overlying membranes
- infiltration of local anaesthetic into a small area of the body blocks the nervous transmission from that part
- nerve block of a large nerve can anaesthetize a whole limb
- spinal anaesthesia is performed by injecting the local anaesthetic into the epidural space or into the subarachnoid space (into the cerebrospinal fluid); epidural anaesthesia is more difficult to carry out but safer for the patient — either of these methods block the nerves from the legs and abdomen as they enter the spinal cord.

The commonest local anaesthetic drug used for infiltration and nerve blocks is lignocaine hydrochloride (Xylocaine). It is often used in conjunction with adrenaline which delays absorption into the blood stream and thus reduces the amount of the drug required. The maximum safe dose is 200 mg, or 500 mg with adrenaline (Gilbertson, 1980).

When carrying out a spinal anaesthetic, the specific gravity of the anaesthetic drug in relation to the cerebrospinal fluid must be known. If it is heavier it will fall and the area of analgesia can be determined by positioning the patient so that the analgesia spreads downwards from the injection site.

An overdose of local (including spinal) anaesthetic can cause death preceded by vomiting, confusion, convulsions, hypertension, tachycardia and coma.

Preparation for anaesthesia

In preparation for anaesthesia a pre-operative medication is given about an hour beforehand. The drug given may be something like diazepam which helps to relieve anxiety or it may be a combination of an analgesic, such as morphine or pethidine, and an anti-cholinergic drug, such as atropine or hyoscine. The analgesic will also have the effect of relieving anxiety and making the patient drowsy. The anti-cholinergic drug will dry up secretions but is given primarily because it reduces the risk of bradycardia occurring due to vagal stimulation during passage of the endotracheal tube.

Complications or potential problems associated with anaesthesia

Administration of an anaesthetic leads to unconsciousness and potential problems associated with that condition, including loss of the ability to prevent injury or to maintain body temperature. In addition, the anaesthetic itself will affect the respiratory and circulatory systems.

Management associated with physical safety

During anaesthesia the patient is completely unable to look after him/herself and, therefore, one of the nurse's main responsibilities is to ensure the patient's safety throughout the whole event. Once anaesthetized the patient has no protective reflexes and must be protected from harm.

The patient must be moved carefully and positioned securely according to the surgeon's requirements. The limbs must be protected from harm. If the arm is allowed to drop over the edge of the trolley or is overextended, the brachial plexus can be damaged. Incorrect lifting into the lithotomy position can strain the lumbosacral muscles — the legs should be raised and abducted together and with care. A pre-operative visit by the theatre nurse offers the opportunity to collect specific information about the patient which necessitates modification of the standard care while under anaesthesia. For example, a thin, elderly patient requires specific care to reduce the risk of initiation of decubitus ulceration during the operation. Or a woman with arthritis will need careful moving and perhaps some modification of the normal position for some gynaecological surgery.

The temperature of the operating theatre must be maintained at a fairly high level as the patient will lose heat readily from exposed internal organs.

At the end of the operation the nurse supervises the lifting of the patient onto the trolley and transfer to the recovery room where the patient stays until consciousness has been regained and the condition is stable.

While unconsciousness continues, the nurse must continue to protect the patient from harm. The main danger is of obstruction to the airway.

If the patient is lying on his/her back, the respiratory tract can become obstructed by the tongue falling back and blocking the larynx, or by vomit entering the respiratory tract before the cough reflex returns. Both these risks are reduced by placing the patient in the semi-prone position at the end of surgery. However, this position is not always possible. An oro-pharyangeal airway helps to keep the airway clear, and normally remains in position until the patient is able to remove it; the tongue is prevented from falling back by lifting the angle of the jaw forward. If the patient vomits, the pharynx is cleared by suction.

Positioning the patient must be carried out with care to prevent undue pressure or abnormal positioning of the limbs. If unconsciousness is prolonged, and the following recovery of consciousness, the patient should be turned at regular intervals in order to relieve pressure and reduce the risk of pressure sore development.

During recovery from anaesthesia the patient's level of consciousness and response to speech and touch will be monitored. As the anaesthetic agents are metabolized and excreted he/she will become restless as the depth of anaesthetic lightens. The patient will need to be protected from injuring him/herself on the rails of the trolley and may have to be restrained during this period.

The patient can often be reassured simply by the knowledge of someone's presence. He/she will need to be told that the operation is over and that he/she has come through it.

After the patient has regained consciousness he/she will often fall asleep again or rest comfortably. However, some patients will be in pain or will be nauseated or vomiting. Analgesia will be given to relieve pain but these drugs also act as respiratory depressants. Therefore, sometimes only half the prescribed dose will be given at first and the patient observed carefully to estimate its effectiveness. An anti-emetic drug will probably be ordered to relieve nausea and vomiting. Andersen (1973) found that nausea was often associated with inadequate pain relief and recommended that adequate amounts of analgesia were given.

During and following recovery from anaesthesia, the patient's physiological status is closely monitored. Some of the observations are concerned with the risk of haemorrhage and have been previously discussed. However, the patient is at risk of disturbances of respiration and circulation because of the effect of the anaesthetic itself.

Circulatory disturbances due to the anaesthetic

Substances used as general anaesthetics tend to depress the activity of cardiac muscle, although the effect varies with different drugs. Diethyl ether and cyclopropane have only a slight effect on contraction of the heart but halothane and methoxyflurane have a considerable effect (Goldman & Wolf, 1980). The overall result depends on the effect of the drug on the sympathetic nervous system, which regulates vasoconstriction, as well as the effect on the heart itself. For example, diethyl ether has little overall effect on the blood pressure as the mild cardiac depression is counterbalanced by vasoconstriction due to stimulation of the sympathetic nervous system by ether. Halothane causes vasodilatation as well as cardiac depression and results in hypotension.

Some of the agents used for induction of anaesthesia also modify the blood pressure. Pentothal sodium causes vasodilatation while ketamine causes vasoconstriction and thus hypertension (Goldman & Wolf, 1980). Postoperatively the blood presssure is monitored until it returns to the patient's normal.

When his/her condition is stable, the patient is returned to the ward where observations are continued to ensure that his/her condition remains satisfactory.

Disturbances of respiration

Problems affecting the respiratory system are the commonest group of postoperative complications, particularly following thoracic and abdominal surgery (Webb, 1975).

In the immediate postoperative period respiration may be disrupted by obstruction of the respiratory tract or by depression of respiration due to the residual effects of the drugs used.

Respiratory depression may occur due to the residual effect of anaesthetic drugs on the respiratory centre or of muscle relaxant drugs on the respiratory muscles. In either case, artificial ventilation will be needed until the effects wear off, and this can be begun by using an Ambu bag.

The patient's respiratory rate, depth and sounds will be observed and the degree of oxygenation of the tissues assessed by observing skin colour, particularly looking for signs of cyanosis. Oxygen is often given postoperatively in fairly high concentrations, except in those with chronic lung disease (see Ch.24).

Oxygenation and perfusion of the tissues can often be improved markedly by asking the patient to take a few deep breaths and move his/her legs a little. If these exercises have been taught pre-operatively, the patient is often able to begin performing them very soon after recovery from the anasethesia.

Later complications are usually the results of retained secretions causing some degree of obstruction of the respiratory passages. Atalectasis (local collapse of a segment of the lung) and pneumonia are the commonest postoperative complications and it is possible to identify a number of factors which increase the risk of their development. These factors work in one or more of three ways:

- by changes in bronchial secretion
- by defective mechanisms for expulsion of secretions
- by reduction of calibre of the bronchioles.

A number of circumstances identifiable before operation have been found to be implicated. Smokers and bronchitic patients (the two are usually linked) (Piper, 1958) and older people (Clendon & Pygott, 1944) are at greater risk. Those with pre-existing respiratory disorders need vigorous physiotherapy and antibiotic therapy to get them into a suitable state for surgery. Postoperatively all these groups will need particular attention to minimize the development of respiratory complications.

A number of factors associated with the operation itself are also significant. Upper abdominal operations cause a reduction in respiratory measurements, with vital capacity falling by up to 60%. Operations which may be more severe but which do not involve the upper abdomen have only moderate and short-lasting effects (Anscombe, 1957). While adequate oxygenation may still be occurring, this reduction in respiratory movement and air flow through the respiratory passages may lead to the retention of secretions. Conditions which result in prolonged suppression of respiration or ability to cough vigorously increase the risk. The depth and duration of anaesthesia and the use of positions which inhibit respiration, for example, the Trendelenburg position in which the abdominal organs fall against the diaphragm, are both important factors.

Postoperatively, the prolonged use of narcotics, which inhibit the cough reflex, and the presence of pain, which may be exacerbated by the presence of drains, both enhance the development of respiratory problems.

Prevention. Pre-operatively, patients with any respiratory disturbance must receive vigorous treatment, but all patients who are to receive an anaesthetic are at risk of these complications. Patients or potential patients should be advised to give up smoking at least 2 weeks before (Webb, 1975) and should be taught deep-breathing exercises and coughing. While the physiotherapist is vitally important in cases with pre-existing respiratory disorders, she/he may or may not be involved with preparation of the 'fit' pre-operative patient. Therefore this must be part of the nurse's pre-operative plan of care for the patient. The nurse may either be doing the teaching her/himself or reinforcing that given by the physiotherapist. Lindeman & Van Aernam (1971) found that this form of preparation resulted in more effective lung function postoperatively.

Postoperatively, patients should be reminded to carry out these exercises regularly, at least every hour when awake, and should have adequate analgaesia to allow them do to so. Early mobilization will also be of benefit. While routine inhalations are sometimes administered postoperatively, even in those with no evidence of chest infection, their value has not been demonstrated.

THE PATIENT'S EXPERIENCE AND NURSE'S ROLE

A patient entering hospital to undergo surgery is going to pass through several different stages throughout this period in hospital. His/her situation and needs will alter considerably as he/she passes through the pre-operative, operative and postoperative stages. The nursing role will, similarly, alter considerably.

Although some generalizations can be made, each person is individual and the interaction between many factors contributes to a unique response to the situation. A number of factors are quite specific to the individual such as past experience, home and work background, intelligence and personality. However, some emotional responses can be related to the type of operation being performed.

EMOTIONAL RESPONSES

Embarrassment

Operations which involve the genitals or excretory organs have an innate 'embarrassment factor'. While some women who have experienced childbirth say that that experience has inured them to the necessary exposure during examination and preparation, others find the experience very difficult to cope with. Many men will not like young women, e.g. nurses, dealing with catheters. Patients will usually accept the necessity for the procedures being undertaken but can, perhaps, be helped by a sensitive, but matter-of-fact, approach.

Awkwardness

Some other operations may be relatively minor in absolute terms but, in the short-term, result in awkwardness in dealing with activities in daily living. Because they are in a condition of relative health, these patients may be reluctant to ask for the help they need. For example, an operation on a hand considerably reduces one's ability to wash, dress and eat. These patients should have help offered in advance.

Relief

A number of patients will feel a sense of relief at having pain relieved or dysfunction improved. Patients undergoing herniorrhaphy, cholecystectomy, ileostomy and many other operations may experience considerable satisfaction at the expected moderation of their symptoms. This emotion may well be combined with several other emotions.

Anxiety

Most patients will be anxious because of a strange environment, the prospect of undergoing an operation and the possibility of pain. However, some patients will have an additional cause of anxiety if there is the possibility that they have a malignant disease. Where this is a real possibility, the patient needs to be given the opportunity to talk through his/her feelings. However, some patients fear malignancy when this is certainly not the case and they also need help to recognize what is being said. After operation, patients who have had a malignancy removed may have to undergo unpleasant radiotherapy or chemotherapy and will need to come to terms with the possibility of recurrence. They will need help to cope with this situation and the approaches that can be used are discussed in Chapters 12 and 16.

Grief

When an operation results in disturbed body appearance or function, the patient may pass through several stages similar to those passed through in dying or grieving for a loved one. Kubler-Ross (1969) suggests that the dying person moves through five stages:

- denial and isolation
- anger
- bargaining
- depression
- acceptance.

Some patients may take a considerable period of time to reach the stage of acceptance and while in hospital should be given the support and help to begin the process.

Operations resulting in obvious mutilation, such as some facial surgery or amputation, affecting one's sexual identity, such as a mastectomy or hysterectomy, or altering one's manner of excretion, such as the formation of an ileostomy, are likely to result in more severe reactions (see Ch.25).

The patient's behaviour both during the pre-operative and postoperative period will be influenced by the emotional response which may be a mixture of several of those indicated.

PRE-OPERATIVE PERIOD

When patients are admitted into a surgical ward they are often relatively fit and independent in carrying out activities of daily living. They are used to being in control of their own lives. Each has made the decision to enter hospital and entrust his/her body, and even his/her life, to others. They usually find that they are expected to submit to complete loss of control over their own lives and to do what they are told, sometimes without explanation.

The patient is likely to have some degree of anxiety. Having made his/her decision to have the operation, he/she 'has to' trust the surgeon and medical team in order to reinforce his/her decision and reduce cognitive dissonance. In others, however, levels of anxiety may increase with waiting. This suggestion is supported by Hugh-Jones et al (1964) who found that emergency admissions were less anxious than those admitted from the waiting list. On the other hand, Wilson-Barnett & Carrigy (1978) found no difference in anxiety levels between the two groups. However, both these studies were carried out with medical, not surgical, patients. Wilson-Barnett & Carrigy in the same study found that, as one would expect, patients with a high N score, that is with a high level of emotionality on the Eysenck Personality Inventory, were more likely than others to report high levels of anxiety when admitted. Women under 40 years of age, those who had not been in hospital previously, those admitted for special tests and those with neoplastic, infective and undiagnosed illness were also particularly vulnerable to anxiety. This type of study helps the nurse to identify those patients particularly in need of focused psychological support.

Other researchers have examined the situations which give rise to anxiety. Franklin (1974) found that the causes in those surgical patients who were worried on admission were due to:

- did not know what to expect 32%
- worried about operation 31%
- worried about anaesthesia 18%
- worried about family 11%
- general dislike of hospitals 8%

Unfortunately, these results were obtained from a question about the main cause of worry. It is likely that several of these were anxieties for the same patients. Lazarus (1966) described six varieties of psychologically stressful stimuli:

- uncertainty about physical survival
- uncertainty about maintaining one's identity
- inability to control the immediate environment
- pain and privation
- loss of loved ones
- disruption of community life.

Other factors pertinent to surgical patients as causes of pschological stress have also been identified:

- disrupted physiological function (due to disease, loss of sleep, drugs etc) (Weitz, 1970)
- inability to interpret a situation
- inability to anticipate events (Lazarus & Averill, 1972)
- lack of control (Frankenhauser, 1975).

Thus, it is possible to recognize the types of situations which are likely to cause anxiety and to plan the appropriate pre-operative care.

Nursing care in order to minimize anxiety should aim to help the patient:

- to be familiar with the environment, including other patients and staff
- to understand the situation and events which occur
- to predict events which are going to happen and the sensations which he/she will experience
- to minimize disruption of circadian rhythm and other physiological functions
- to feel in control of him/herself and his/her situation
- to feel that he/she is a valued individual.

A great deal of research has been carried out which demonstrates the value of pre-operative preparation. Beneficial outcomes reported include a reduction in the amount of anaesthesia and analgesia required, lower corticosteroid excretion levels, fewer postoperative complications, less vomiting, stable pulse and blood pressure and a shorter stay in hospital (Aiken,

1972; Boore, 1978; Dumas & Leonard, 1963; Egbert et al, 1964; Hayward, 1975; Johnson, 1966; Linderman & Van Aernam, 1971; Schmitt & Wooldridge, 1973). The type of preparation which has been examined is of three types:

- information giving
- teaching specific activities
- developing and using purposefully an interpersonal relationship.

Information giving

Information giving about the situation, events and experiences enables the patient to understand, predict and feel in control of what is happening. The information to be given can be selected by reference to research findings. Hayward (1975) found that patients had experienced a number of anxiety-creating situations. These included:

- pre-operative preparation and pre-medication
- administration of anaesthesia
- waking up in an unexpected position in the ward
- intravenous infusions
- the experience of pain.

Johnson (1976) has undertaken a number of studies to find out what type of information is most helpful to patients. She carried out studies in the laboratory, with children having plaster casts removed, with patients before endoscopy and with pre-operative patients. Of the three comparison groups in each of these studies one was told exactly what was to be done to them. Another group received a description of the sensations they would experience and the third group received no relevant information. She found that a description of the experiences was most effective in relieving psychological stress, while describing the events also helped.

Johnson also found that the subjects in her studies gained as much (or nearly as much) relief from stress when given only most of the relevant information, instead of all of it. It was, however, important that the information received was accurate and the experience was compatible with the patient's expectations.

From such studies it is possible to identify that the information given to patients before operation should include:

- pre-operative procedures such as skin preparation, bowel preparation, fasting and the reasons for these
- immediate preparation, such as administration of pre-medication, induction of anaesthesia and what it feels like
- recovery from anaesthesia in the recovery room and return to a different position in the ward
- postoperative conditions such as the presence of intravenous infusions or drains, and why
- postoperative activities such as early mobilization and the importance of this
- pain — its normality, what it will feel like, how it will be managed and the patient's role in its management
- any additional information specific to the operation being performed.

The information must be given in such a way that it can be understood by the individual patient and repeated as necessary to ensure that the patient has clearly understood what he/she has heard.

Teaching activities

Teaching specific activities that patients can undertake gives them a positive role to play in their own recovery. It is suggested that, as well as the physiological effects, the feeling of control thus imparted will help to reduce anxiety.

The patient should be taught how to carry out the procedures, the reason for them, encouraged to practise them before the operation and given feedback on the correctness of his/her performance. The activites taught should include:

- deep breathing and coughing, which should be carried out hourly after the operation
- leg exercises to be carried out similarly
- relaxation of abdominal muscles and how to move in bed — the importance of changing position at least 2-hourly should be emphasised.

Repeat the following routine every 1 – 2 hours until you are up and about. Nurses will assist you if you have any difficulty or any questions.

Keep lungs functioning properly

Deep breathe and cough	1. Inhale as deeply as you can. 2. Hold for a second or two. 3. Exhale completely. 4. Repeat several times. Then: 5. Inhale deeply. 6. Produce a deep abdominal cough (not shallow throat cough) by short, sharp expiration. (Incision may be splinted with hands or bedclothes. Flexing knees relieves strain on abdominal muscles.)

Maintain good circulation.

Lie on each side as well as your back.

Change position	**To turn easily:** 1. Bend one knee, planting foot firmly on bed 2. Lift opposite arm overhead (in direction of turn). 3. Roll onto side, pushing bent leg (bedrails can be used to aid in turning). 4. If you need assistance, call one of the nurses. **To turn back again:** 1. Bend knee of upper leg. 2. Place palm of top arm solidly on the side of the bed. 3. Push yourself over onto your back.

Promote good circulation in your legs

Exercise feet and legs	Perform the following exercises fairly slowly, but with strong muscle contraction: 1. Push the toes of both feet toward the foot of the bed. Relax both feet. Pull toes toward the chin. Relax both feet. 2. Circle both ankles, first to the right, then to the left. Repeat three times. Relax. 3. Bend each knee alternately, sliding foot up along the bed. Relax.

Fig. 17.1 Patient instruction sheet to promote recovery after surgery

Interpersonal relationship

The development of a relationship between a specific nurse and the patient is important, as it reinforces the patient's feeling of individuality. It also gives the opportunity for him/her to ask questions, discuss anxieties and develop a feeling of trust in the nurse who will be caring for him/her after the operation.

The nurse developing this relationship needs to be knowledgeable enough to cope with questions and give the individual teaching required. She/he must also be able to cope with the emotional pressures, and there should be a support system available for the staff.

Organisation of care

While part of this preparation must be given individually there is evidence that group teaching is as effective and saves nursing time (Lindeman, 1972; Mezzanotte, 1970). The anxiety associated with hospital admission may inhibit learning. Fortin & Kirouac (1976) found that teaching sessions 15–20 days before admission were highly effective.

Pre-operative visits are now often made by the theatre nurse on the day before the operation. She/he has two aims:

- to minimize anxiety
- to identify factors which require attention during the operation.

The theatre nurse will try to ensure that the patient understands what will be experienced during his/her time in the operating theatre department, particularly in the anaesthetic and recovery rooms, and that this nurse will be looking after him/her during the operation. Lindeman & Stetzer (1973) found that a pre-operative visit by the theatre nurse reduced anxiety.

Pre-anaesthetic care in the theatre suite is of considerable importance. The patient needs reassurance and support during this period. He/she should be greeted by name on arrival in theatre, if possible by the nurse who has previously visited him/her on the ward, and should never be left to wait alone. Dumas & Leonard (1963) found that this period of waiting could be used effectively in promoting psychological well-being, and this reduced the incidence of postoperative vomiting. It is often helpful to hold the patient's hand during the induction of anaesthesia.

PAIN

One of the major aspects of the immediate postoperative experience of the patient undergoing surgery is pain, the management of which is discussed in Chapter 9.

The management of pain in these patients is undertaken with the aim of controlling the pain so that the patient is able to take part in the activities to promote recovery. Management begins before operation by ensuring that the patients are aware that pain is to be expected, but that it can be controlled, and that they have a part to play in this. Only the patients know what pain they feel, and they must know that they are expected to tell the nursing staff before it becomes severe. Less analgesia is required to prevent severe pain than to treat it. Many other techniques can be utilized as well, but analgesics should be used as required to control the pain. In the vast majority of surgical patients, their need for pain relieving drugs will diminish rapidly over the first few days and the risk of drug addiction developing is minimal.

Administration of analgesia before activities which may cause pain will allow the patient to participate fully in exercises and early mobilization. In addition, pain is more tolerable if one is rested, and the administration of analgesics to ensure a good night's sleep may reduce the amount needed the following day.

PROMOTION OF INDEPENDENCE

During the postoperative period the patient will initially need assistance with activities of daily living, but as he/she regains strength, he/she must be given encouragement to become independent again. To have the confidence to do this, the patient needs accurate information about what is expected of him/her at different stages in recovery. Involving him/her in deciding when and what he/she will do enhances this confidence.

Wilson-Barnett (1981) has highlighted the lack of adequate information given to patients before discharge following cardiac surgery. The teaching and information needed by patients before discharge will obviously vary according to the operation performed. The aim is to enable the patient to take care of him/herself out of hospital. For example, the patient who has had a stoma formed needs to be thoroughly competent at dealing with the stoma, needs to know how to get further supplies and how to dispose of used bags, as well as how to obtain help if required. All patients need advice on the amount of activity they should perform. While wound strength is still increasing they should not undertake heavy lifting.

THE NURSE'S ROLE IN RELATION TO SURGERY

The nursing care of the patient undergoing surgery has been discussed, but the nurse is also involved in the technical and procedural aspects of surgery.

Thus, the ward nurse checks that the identity band is in position, consent form signed correctly, operation site correctly identified and that the patient is transferred safely to the theatre with his/her notes and X-rays. The ward nurse then hands the patient over to the care of the theatre nurse, and ensures that that nurse is aware of the operation to be performed.

In the anaesthetic room, the nurse has two responsibilities — to the patient and to the anaesthetist. The nurse will have prepared all the equipment and drugs needed by the anaesthetist and will assist him/her in the induction of anaesthesia and the setting up of an intravenous infusion. At the same time, the nurse must ensure that the patient is kept informed about what is going on.

Most of the care the patient receives in the operating theatre department occurs between the time consciousness is lost as he/she is anaesthetized and the time he/she regains consciousness in the recovery room. However, this does not minimize the importance of the nurse's role in this department.

There are four aspects to the nurse's work in the theatre:

- care of the patient
- management of the environment

- care and preparation of equipment
- assisting anaesthetist and surgeon.

All of these are vital for the well-being of the patient as he/she passes through the reception area, anaesthetic room, operating theatre and recovery room, and in most situations the nurse will be concerned with several of these at the same time.

Operating Department Assistants will be available in some places to deal with some of the technical aspects of the work, but essentially responsibility is carried by the nursing staff. Much of the technical detail required by the nurse working in the theatre will not be discussed here. Warren (1983) gives a useful introduction to operating theatre nursing and *Alexander's Care of the Patient in Surgery* provides more detailed information (Gruendemann & Meeker, 1983).

The care of the patient whilst anaesthetized has been discussed previously. Much of the technical work in theatre is concerned with assisting the surgeon and anaesthetist, while at the same time having a wider awareness of the factors which will promote the patient's well-being. The nurse will aim to minimize the traffic through the theatre and thus the bacterial count in the air.

Another major area of responsibility is concerned with the equipment, drugs and lotions. The nurse deals with the preparation, management throughout the procedure and safe disposal of all equipment. If all is prepared, both in the anaesthetic room and the theatre, then everything runs smoothly, people do not get irritable, the period of anaesthesia may be shorter because the operation is completed expeditiously and the patient benefits. Clearly the nurse working in this area needs to be knowledgeable about the types of instruments, suture material, drains and dressings that are used, and is referred to Gruendemann & Meeker (1983).

The safety of the patient is paramount and the scrub nurse and circulating nurse together count and record instruments, swabs and packs in use during the operation. A final check is made to ensure that all are accounted for before the surgeon completes the suturing of the wound. The scrub nurse will also ensure that the sterility of all equipment and materials is maintained.

The patient is transferred to the recovery room and remains there until consciousness is regained and the physical condition is stable. The nurse has a number of responsibilities during this period and to carry them out fully she/he must ensure that she/he is quite clear about the procedure that has been carried out, any special care required and the condition of the patient on transfer to her/his care.

CONCLUSION

The achievement of a satisfactory outcome to surgery involves many different professionals and different types of skill. The nurse needs to be skilled at technical procedures but must be equally competent as a teacher to facilitate the best possible recovery.

REFERENCES

Aiken L H 1972 Systematic relaxation to reduce preoperative stress. Canadian Nurse 68:38–42

Andersen R 1973 Postoperative pain and nausea. Tidsskr Nor Laegeforen (English Abstract) 93:1368–1369

Andriole V T 1966 Treatment of opportunistic infections complicating surgery. Med Treat 3:1116–1128

Anscombe A R 1957 Pulmonary complications of abdominal surgery. Year Book Medical Publishers, Chicago

Atkins P, Hawkins L A 1965 Detection of venous thrombosis in the legs. Lancet 2:1217–1219

Boore J 1978 Prescription for recovery. RCN, London

Brandberg A, Andersson I 1980 Whole body disinfection by shower-bath with chlorhexidine soap. In: Newsom S W B, Caldwell A D S (eds) Problems in the care of hospital infection. Royal Society of Medicine, Academic Press, and Grune & Stratton, London

Canizaro P C 1981 Methods of nutritional support in the surgical patient. In: Yarborough M F, Curreri P W (eds) Surgical nutrition. Churchill Livingstone, Edinburgh

Clendon D R T, Pygott F 1944 Analysis of pulmonary complications occurring after 579 consecutive operations. British Journal of Anaesthetics 19:62–70

Coon W W, Coller F A 1959 Some epidemiological considerations of thromboembolism. Surgery, Gynaecology and Obstetrics 109:487–501

Cruse P J E, Ford R 1973 A five year prospective study of 23 649 surgical wounds. Archives of Surgery 107:206–210

Davidson A I G, Clark C, Smith G 1971 Postoperative wound infection: a computer analysis. British Journal of Surgery 58:333–337

Dumas R G, Leonard R C 1963 Effect of nursing on the incidence of postoperative vomiting. Nursing Research 12 (Winter):12–15

Egbert L D, Battit C E, Welch C E, Bartlett M K 1964 Reduction of postoperative pain by encouragement and instruction of patients. New England Journal of Medicine 270:825–827

Flanc C, Kakker V V, Clarke M D 1969 Postoperative deep vein thrombosis. Effect of intensive prophylaxis. Lancet 1:477–478

Fortin F, Kirouac S 1976 A randomised controlled trial of preoperative patient education. International Journal of Nursing Studies 13:11–24

Frankenhauser M 1975 Experimental approaches to the study of catecholamines and emotion. In: Levi L (ed) Emotions: their parameters and measurement. Raven Press, New York

Franklin B L 1974 Patient anxiety on admission to hospital. RCN, London

Gilbertson A A 1980 Anaesthesia. In: McFarland J (ed) Basic clinical surgery. Butterworths, London

Goldman L, Wolf M A 1980 The heart and circulation. In: Vandam L D (ed) To make the patient ready for anaesthetic: medical care of the surgical patient. Addison-Wesley, Menlo Park, California

Gruendemann B J, Meeker M H 1983 Alexander's care of the patient in surgery. C V Mosby, St Louis

Hamilton H W, Hamilton K R, Lone F I 1977 Preoperative hair removal. The Canadian Journal of Surgery 20:269–275

Hamilton-Smith S 1972 Nil by mouth. RCN, London

Hayward J 1975 Information — a prescription against pain. RCN, London

Hemstrup-Hansen R 1963 Do nursing personnel aid in the spreading of hospital infection by wearing rings on duty? Unpublished dissertation, Wayne State University College of Nursing, cited by: Beland I L, Passos J Y 1975 Clinical nursing: Pathophysiological and psychosocial approaches. Macmillan, New York

Hugh-Jones P, Tanser A R, Whitby C 1964 Patients' view of admission to a London teaching hospital. British Medical Journal 2:660–664

Husni E A, Ximenes J O, Goyette E M 1970 Elastic support of the lower limbs in hospital patients. A critical study. Journal of the American Medical Association 214:1456–1462

Jacobson G, Thiele J E, McCune J H, Farrell L D 1985 Handwashing, ring-wearing and number of microorganisms. Nursing Research 34:186–188

Janis I L 1958 Psychological stress; psychoanalytic and behavioral studies of surgical patients. Wiley, New York

Johnson J E 1966 Influence of purposeful nurse-patient interaction on the patient's postoperative course. In: Exploring progress in medical-surgical nursing practice, No 2, 16–22. Presented at the 1965 regional Clinical Conference sponsored by the American Nurses' Association in Washington and Chicago. American Nurses' Association, New York

Johnson J E 1976 Stress reduction through sensation information. In: Sarason I G, Spielberger C D (eds) Stress and anxiety 2. Halstad Press, New York

Kakker V V, Howe C T, Flanc C, Clarke M B 1969 Natural history of postoperative deep vein thrombosis. Lancet 2:230–232

Kistner R L, Ball J J, Nordyke R A, Freeman G C 1972 Incidence of pulmonary embolism in thrombophlebitis of the lower extremities. American Journal of Surgery 124:169–176

Kubler-Ross E 1969 On death and dying. Macmillan, New York

Lazarus R S 1966 Psychological stress and the coping process. McGraw-Hill, New York

Lazarus R S, Averill J R 1972 Emotion and cognition with special reference to anxiety. In: Spielberger C D (ed) Anxiety: current trends in theory and research. Academic Press, New York

LeFrock J L, Ellis C A, Weinstein L 1972 The impact of hospitalization on the aerobic fecal microflora. Presented at the 53rd Annual Meeting of the American College of Physicians in Atlantic City, NJ, April. Cited by LeFrock J L, Klainer A S (1976) Nosocomial infections: current concepts, a scope publication. Upjohn, Kalamazoo, Michigan

LeFrock J L, Ellis C A, Weinstein L 1973 The relation between fecal and pharyngeal microflora in hospitalized patients. 13th Interscience Conference on Antimicrobial Agents and Chemotherapy, Washington, DC, September. Cited by LeFrock J L., Klainer A S (1976) Nosocomial infections: current concepts, a scope publication. Upjohn, Kalamazoo, Michigan

LeFrock J L, Klainer A S 1976 Nosocomial infections: current concepts, a scope publication. Upjohn, Kalamazoo, Michigan

Lidwell O M, Mackintosh C A, Towers A C 1978 The evaluaton of fabrics in relation to their use as protective garments in nursing and surgery. Journal of Hygiene (Cambridge) 81:453–469

Lindeman C A 1972 Nursing intervention with the presurgical patient effectiveness and efficiency of group and individual preoperative teaching — phase 2. Nursing Research 21:196–209

Lindeman C A, Stetzer S L 1973 Effect of preoperative visits by operating room nurses. Nursing Research 22:4–16

Lindeman C A, Van Aernam B 1971 Nursing intervention with the presurgical patient — the effects of structured and unstructured preoperative teaching. Nursing Research 20:319–332

Loiseau M M L, Hemmer C, Boisivon A, Gerbal R 1971 Source of surgical wound infection. Contribution à l'étude de l'origine d l'infection en milieu chirurgical. Pathologica Biologica 19:847–855

McFarland J 1980 Basic clinical surgery. Butterworths, London

McPherson K, Strong P M, Epstein A, Jones L 1981 Regional variations in the use of common surgical procedures: within and between England and Wales, Canada and the United States of America. Social Science and Medicine 15:233–288

Mezzanotte E J 1970 Group instruction in preparation for surgery. American Journal of Nursing 70:89–91

Miles R M 1975 Complications of surgery that involve the venous system. In: Artz C P, Hardy J D (eds) Management of surgical complications. W B Saunders, Philadelphia

Moncada S, Vane J R 1979 Arachidonic acid metabolites and the interaction between platelets and blood vessel walls. New England Journal of Medicine 300:1142–1147

Moore F D, Ball M R 1952 The metabolic response to surgery. Charles C. Thomas, Springfield, Illinois

Morrell M T, Dunnill M S 1968 The post-mortem incidence of pulmonary embolism in a hospital population. British Journal of Surgery 55:347–352

Myers K A, Marshall R D, Freidin J 1980 Principles of

pathology in surgery. Blackwell Scientific, Oxford
National Academy of Sciences 1964 Postoperative wound infections. Report of an ad hoc committee of the Committee on Trauma division of Medical Sciences, National Academy of Sciences, National Research Council. Annals of Surgery 160(2):supplement,
Piper D W 1958 Respiratory complications in the postoperative period. Scottish Medical Journal 3:193–198
Porth C 1982 Pathophysiology: concepts of altered health status. Lippincott, Philadelphia
Schmitt F E, Wooldridge J 1973 Psychological preparation of surgical patients. Nursing Research 22:108–116
Smiddy F G 1976 The medical management of the surgical patient. Edward Arnold, London
Taylor L J 1978 An evaluaton of hand-washing techniques 1 and 2. Nursing Times 74:54–55,108–110
Tsapogas M J, Goussous H, Peabody R A 1971 Postoperative venous thrombosis and effectiveness of prophylactic measures. Archives of Surgery 103:561–567
Virchow R 1856 Weitere Untersuchungen über die Verstopfung der Lungenarterie und ihre Folgen. In: Gesammelte Abhandlungen zur Wissenschaftlichen Medizin 227, from Traube's Beitr z experiment Pathologie und Physiologie 2:21
Warren M C 1983 Operating theatre nursing. Lippincott Nursing Series, Harper and Row, London
Webb W R 1975 Postoperative pulmonary complications. In: Artz C P, Hardy J D (eds) Management of surgical complications. W B Saunders, Philadelphia
Weitz J 1970 Psychological research needs in the problems of human stress. In: McGrath J E (ed) Social and psychological factors in stress. Holt, Rinehart and Winston, New York
Whyte W, Vesley D, Hodgson R 1976 Bacterial dispersion in relation to operating theatre clothing. Journal of Hygiene (Cambridge) 76:367–378
Wilson-Barnett J 1981 Assessment of recovery: with special reference to a study with postoperative cardiac patients. Journal of Advanced Nursing 6:435–445
Wilson-Barnett J, Carrigy A 1978 Factors affecting patients' response to hospitalisation. Journal of Advanced Nursing 3:221– 228

SECTION THREE

Disturbances of systems' functions

This section focuses on the nursing of patients with disturbances of physiological functioning. It begins with two chapters dealing with disturbances of control mechanisms, the nervous and hormonal systems. Protective mechanisms are then considered in the following three chapters. These in turn examine disorders of the skin, which acts as a barrier between any being's internal and external environment; the immune system, which protects the body against infection and deranged cells within the internal environment; and the musculoskeletal system, which enables the body to move away from potential danger in the external environment.

The next four chapters examine disorders of the systems concerned with the intake and supply of oxygen and nutrients to the body tissues, and the excretion of waste from the body. This section, therefore, includes disturbances of transport, of nutrient supply, of oxygen supply and carbon dioxide excretion, and of the excretion of other waste products.

The final chapters in this section of the book examine disturbances of homeostasis related to fluid and electrolyte balance and temperature regulation.

Throughout, the aim has been to draw out the principles underlying the disorder and its management and to examine the nursing implications.

18

Disturbances of neurological control mechanisms

INTRODUCTION

The nervous system is one of the two major controlling systems of the body, the other being the endocrine system (Ch. 19). Through neurological mechanisms a rapid response to external or internal stimuli takes place; glandular and muscular activity are initiated. The action of the nervous system thereby underlies all behaviour. Memory, learning, emotion, motivation, intelligence and personality are all functions for which the nervous system is responsible. Add to this the control of life-maintaining mechanisms such as the cardiac output, blood pressure, respiration and temperature, and it can be seen that pathological conditions of the nervous system may have quite devastating and life-threatening consequences. There will almost certainly be severe psycho-social effects as well. However, it is difficult to identify the extent to which this is the individual's response to the knowledge that such a vital part of the body is affected, vital to both physical functioning and to one's self identity, or whether it is due directly to the disruption of neural cells and nervous pathways. However, just imagine for a moment how you would feel if you wished to pick up a cup of tea and your hand and arm failed to move, or your arm moved wildly and uncontrollably so that your hand missed the cup altogether. We carry out innumerable highly-skilled movements every day without consciously thinking about them. It becomes difficult to imagine how it must feel to have such movements disrupted, but the consequences of loss or abnormality of everyday movements are not only functional but also have great social impact.

It is perhaps easier to empathize with patients suffering from headache, since this is one of the commonest symptoms suffered by the population as a whole (Walton, 1977). It is important to note that whilst pathology of the central nervous system is frequently associated with headache, only a very small proportion of people suffering from headaches have any underlying central nervous system lesion. Most people also experience temporary sensory loss when they have accidentally exerted pressure upon a peripheral nerve, for example, by carelessly leaning with the back of a chair pressing upon the upper arm.

Perhaps, however, one of the most potentially shaming effects of pathology of the nervous system is the possibility of becoming incontinent and completely dependent upon others to carry out the simplest actions on one's behalf. The burden on the relatives of a completely dependent person may be rendered horrific by personality changes due to nervous system pathology. This drastically alters the quality of all interpersonal interactions and thus the essential nature of the relationship. The loved one may become, not merely a stranger, but a hostile, unlikeable stranger.

Not all diseases of the nervous system have dramatic effects, but nurses working in this type of nursing need the ability to cope with emergency life-threatening events, highly dependent patients, and the chronically disabled, whilst not neglecting those patients who are admitted for what is to the nurse (but not to the patient) a comparatively minor and unproblematic investigation or operation.

STRUCTURE AND FUNCTION

In considering lesions of the nervous system it is useful to start by considering some important aspects of the structure and function of the nervous system, in particular its many unique features.

CELLS OF THE NERVOUS SYSTEM

Neurones are the functional units of the nervous system (Hilgard et al, 1979) (Fig. 18.1). Compared with cells elsewhere in the body, neurones are large, some being the largest cells to be found in the body. They display an immense variety of shapes, although most have a central body (or soma) containing the nucleus and one or more elongated processes. These processes are usually described as being dendrites or axons. Dendrites may be numerous and branching and are said to receive and pass on the stimulus input into the cell. Cell bodies also receive stimulus inputs from other cells. Each neurone usually has only one axon which in vitro has the function of transmitting the nerve impulse on to the next cell, i.e. the axon is the output unit of the cell. Whilst the total dendritic surface area of the neurone may be great due to the sheer number and extensive branching of the dendrites, one of the characteristics of many axons is their enormous length. Some are several metres in length (Jewett & Rayner, 1984). Since both dendrites and axons have a very small diameter it follows that the cell membrane occupies a large proportion of the structure of these processes. The membrane is functionally as well as structurally of immense importance, since it is the highly selective permeability of this membrane which is the basis of the transmission of the nerve impulse (Lamb et al, 1980).

Although the diameter of the axon (or neural fibre) is very small compared with its length, there are variations in diameter. The larger the diameter is, the more rapidly the nerve impulse is transmitted (Jewett & Rayner, 1984). A large number of axons become myelinated on leaving the grey matter of the brain, brain stem, or spinal cord and this also increases the speed of nerve impulse transmission.

Study of the neural synapse has proved to be of crucial importance not only to our understanding of the function of the nervous system but also in the development of drugs and our

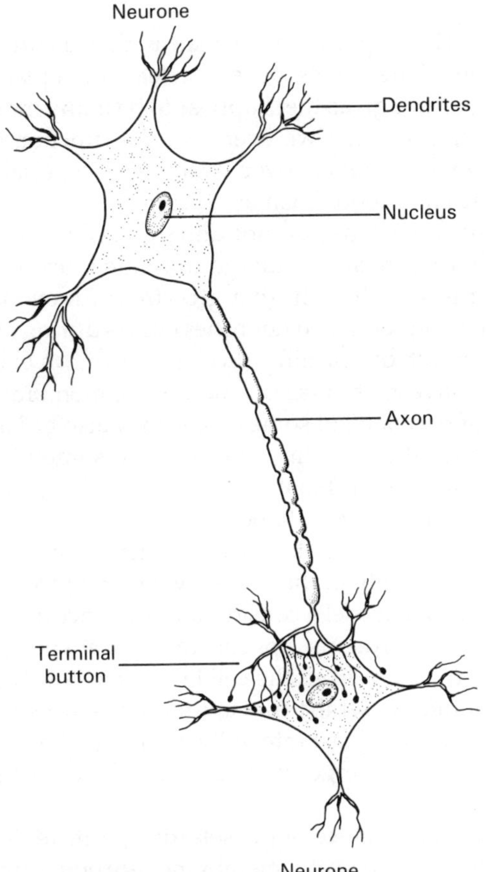

Fig. 18.1 Structure of a neurone and how it may synapse with another neurone.

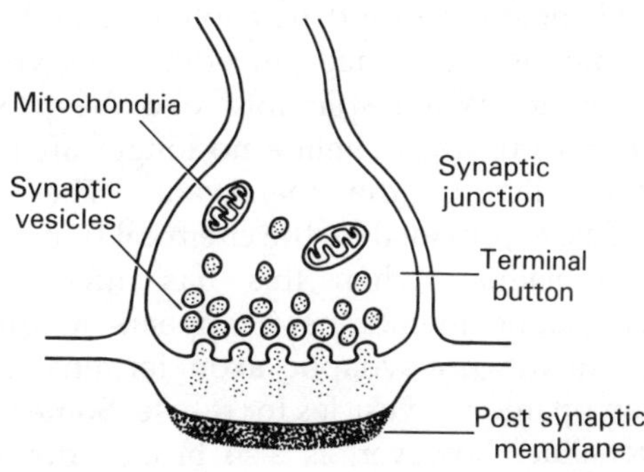

Fig. 18.2 Synaptic membrane

understanding of their pharmacology. The synapse is the junction between two neurones in series with one another, in mammals close juxtapositions of two separate discontinuous structures (Fig. 18.2). Whilst there are synapses where the transmission of the impulse across the gap is electrical, in a significant number the functional connection between the two cells is a chemical transmitter, which is only released in any quantity by the pre-synaptic cell in response to a nerve impulse which has travelled along the axon (Lamb et al, 1980). This chemical transmitter diffuses across the synapse to attach itself to the specially adapted membrane of the postsynaptic cell, altering the architecture of the membrane and thus its permeability. In turn the alteration in permeability changes the electrical potential across the membrane, either in the direction of greater polarity (hyperpolarization) or reduced polarity (depolarization). If a sufficient quantity of excitatory transmitter reaches the postsynaptic membrane it may reach a critical level of depolarization which triggers a nerve impulse spreading rapidly from that point over the whole membrane of the cell (Eccles, 1957). Conversely an inhibitory transmitter may induce a level of hyperpolarization which prevents the depolarization of the membrane by excitatory transmitters released by other pre-synaptic cells. As far as we know, a pre-synaptic neurone always manufactures, stores in vesicles and releases just one type of transmitter, either excitatory or inhibitory. Up to 1000 pre-synaptic nerve cell endings (from axons) may impinge upon a single postsynaptic cell (Thompson, 1967). There are estimated to be approximately 12 billion neurones in the human brain. It is thought that it is due to this vast interconnectedness of neurones that the exquisite variety of neural function occurs, as well as its ability to change (or learn) with time (plasticity) (Hilgard et al, 1979; Konorski, 1948).

Having attached itself to the postsynaptic membrane and altered its permeability and thus the electrical potential, the transmitter substance must be removed or neutralized in some way, otherwise the cell would continue in a state of excitation or inhibition for ever (or until its metabolic processes were exhausted). There seem to be at least two mechanisms for the removal of chemical transmitters. The case of acetylcholine provides an example of one of these methods. Acetylcholine is split into an acetyl group and a choline group by the enzyme acetyl cholinesterase (true cholinesterase). This enzyme is contained in the postsynaptic membrane. When split into two the product molecules of acetylcholine no longer affect the permeability of the membrane. The other example is provided by the chemical transmitter noradrenaline. When this has affected the postsynaptic membrane it appears to diffuse back to the pre-synaptic axon terminal to be taken up into the vesicles for re-use. Some of the adrenaline, however, is also broken down by enzymes, examples of two of these being monoamine oxidase (MAO) and catecholo-methyltransferase (Ganong, 1983). These both have a relatively slow action and so it is unlikely that they bring about a termination of the action of noradrenaline at the postsynaptic site. Adrenal-ine can also act as a chemical transmitter on synaptic membranes, although it is noradrenaline which is released at the adrenergic neuronal endings. It will be realized that both adrenaline and noradrenaline are released from the adrenal medulla into the bloodstream and it is by this means that adrenaline (and additional noradrenaline) can reach peripheral synapses.

This leads to a consideration of the action of the many drugs which have been found to be similar in structure to chemical transmitters. They may have their effect by attaching themselves to the postsynaptic membrane and altering its permeability. Some may prevent the chemical transmitter from acting by occupying or competing for the receptor sites. Other drugs act by preventing the release of the transmitter or prolonging its action by inhibiting the enzymes involved in transmitter degradation. Increasing identification of the neurotransmitters and their action has led to a search for pharmacologically similar substances to be used as drugs (Ganong,1983).

Metabolism of neurones

Research suggests that one of the important differences between neurones and other cells in the human body is that we have our full complement of neurones at birth and these are not replaced by cellular division (Lamb et al, 1980). The implication for man is that death of functional neurones does not lead to replacement, although as there appear to be many more cells present than we ever use, the function of cells may be taken over by others, especially during childhood (Lashley, 1929).

Whilst neurones do not undergo cell division their structure does undergo continued turnover and it is also thought that growth of functional connections between neurones occurs during life as a result of learning (Eccles, 1961). Myelin, which invests, but is not a part of the membrane wall of part or all of some axons, may also be laid down for the first time after birth in some fibre tracts (McIlwain, 1966).

The size and shape of neurones have implications for metabolism. Protein synthesis takes place only in the cell body, yet the product may need to travel a considerable distance down the axon. Proteins appear to be transported down the axon from the cell body at a slow rate (1–2 mm/day) whilst transmitter substances are transported at a fast rate of 100 mm/day (Walton, 1983), with a range of 50–2000 mm/day (Ochs, 1972).

The maintenance of the selective permeability of the whole cell membrane through the mechanism of the sodium pump uses a great deal of energy obtained from ATP. In turn, the ATP is manufactured in mitochondria which are found in the axon as well as the soma. Neurones are unusual in the fact that they appear able to use only glucose aerobically to produce this ATP, whilst only minute stores of glycogen can be found in neurones. Thus they are critically and sensitively dependent upon blood levels of glucose and oxygen. The metabolic requirements of brain tissue are remarkably constant (Thompson, 1967). Although the brain is about 2.5% of body weight, during resting metabolism 25% of the total oxygen consumption of the body occurs within the brain. Amino acids and lipids are utilized by neurones in the maintenance of membrane structure, cytoplasm, enzymes and the production of transmitters. Rare inborn errors of lipid and amino acid metabolism may have crucial implications for development and result in a grossly abnormal nervous system (McIlwain, 1966).

Glial cells

In discussing the metabolic requirements of the brain and spinal cord it is important to realize that many other cells apart from neurones go to make up central nervous system tissue. In the brain these other cells outnumber neurones by 9 to 1, although since they are smaller than neurones they comprise only 50% of the brain weight. These other cells are collectively called glial cells. They closely surround and invest nerve cells and fibres. They differ greatly from one another in shape. The three main kinds are astrocytes, oligodendrocytes and ependyma. Some astrocytes appear to rest part of their structure in the walls of capillaries and are thought to be concerned in acting as an exchange medium between the blood and neurones. On electron microscopy they appear to occupy what would otherwise be the extracellular space of neurones. Ependyma line the ventricles, while oligodendrocytes are concerned in the formation of myelin within the CNS (Lamb et al, 1980).

Glial cells do undergo cell division, and for this reason brain tumours arise from these cells or from the connective tissue coverings of the brain and spinal cord, and not from neurones. Glial cells serve the supportive functions of connective tissues in other areas of the body. A further type of cell is the equivalent of phagocytic cells in other tissues. This is the microglial cell, and it probably serves the function of protecting the neurones from microorganisms and particulate matter. The Schwann cell forms myelin in the peripheral nervous system while the oligodendrocyte performs this function in the central nervous system (Jewett & Rayner, 1984).

Although the function of glial cells is not fully understood it is important to remember that as far as our current state of knowledge goes they are crucially different from neurones in that they do not transmit a nerve impulse (Jewett & Rayner, 1984). It is the nerve impulse transmitted along neurones and across synapses which underlies all behaviour.

PROTECTIVE STRUCTURES

Since functional neurones are so important to the continued existence of the individual and the species, it is not surprising that special structures have evolved which protect them. Many other unique features of the nervous system arise from these protective structures.

Blood-brain barrier

The blood-brain barrier is the term used for a conceptualized structure which was first demonstrated functionally and has now been identified as the specialized tissue surrounding cerebral vessels.

Surrounding the cerebral blood vessels is a thin covering formed by the processes of astrocytes. Plasma in the capillaries is separated from nervous tissue by the endothelium, with its basement membrane and the perivascular processes of astrocytes. This is the blood-brain barrier (Walton, 1983).

Whilst all other cells in the body come to reflect the chemical content of blood plasma, brain cells do so only very selectively. This barrier sequesters the brain and prevents the diffusion of some substances from the blood plasma to the brain (Thompson, 1967). This helps to protect brain cells and ensures a stable chemical environment. The barrier has been studied to identify those substances which cross easily and those which do not. Water, carbon dioxide, oxygen and some lipid soluble anaesthetics cross freely. Electrolytes such as sodium and potassium take a long time to cross and some drugs also take a long time, whilst others fail to cross at all. It is necessary to know which drugs cross into the brain readily and which do not, to determine the route of drug administration in the treatment of brain conditions. Drugs which do not cross the blood-brain barrier readily have to be administered directly into the cerebrospinal fluid (CSF) if they are to be effective. The blood-brain barrier breaks down functionally at the site of tumours in the brain. This allows their identification through the use of radioactive isotopes and also is an aid in treatment.

Protective coverings and cerebrospinal fluid

Alongside the evolution of the brain and spinal cord, a complex series of connective tissue coverings have evolved to protect the delicate nervous tissue. The skull and dura mater are of particular interest. In effect, in the adult the brain is enclosed within a hard box with only one outlet through which pass the medulla oblongata/spinal cord, all blood vessels and CSF channels.

Separating the cerebrum from the cerebellum and the brain stem is the tough, hard sheet of dura mater called the tentorium cerebri which functions for all intents and purposes as the floor of the skull, having one central foramen in which lie the midbrain, blood vessels and CSF channels.

In erect man these two outlets normally lie at the base of their respective compartments, although in animals they lie posteriorally.

Raised intracranial pressure

The rigid nature of the skull and dura mater means that any pathological conditions which increase the volume of the tissue contained within them does not cause swelling, as it might if it occurred in the abdomen for example, but causes pressure effects instead. Such pathological conditions are collectively termed space occupying lesions and are potentially serious. Three main constituents contribute to increased volume (Plum & Posner, 1980):

- brain tissue
- CSF
- blood.

If any one of these increases in volume it causes pressure on blood vessels in particular, unless there is a compensating decrease in one of the other constituents.

A degree of compensation can occur very temporarily through constriction of blood vessels. Other small compensating mechanisms are increased shunting of cerebrospinal fluid to the spinal dural sac, reduced production of CSF, and increased reabsorption of CSF. Increased intracranial pressure is important because it may lead to reduced blood perfusion of cerebral tissue and consequent reduction in O_2 and glucose supplied to neurones. This occurs when the intracranial pressure is from 15–40 mmHg. At 40 mmHg perfusion ceases (Jennet, 1981). Due to the compensatory process there may be little or no clinical change in the patient as intracranial mass increases, and only when compensation becomes increasingly ineffective do the signs of pressure develop, such as headache and drowsiness (Walton, 1983). Consequent changes in the patient's condition may not be detected by neurological assessment until massive shifts in the position of the intracranial contents have taken place. Thus it is vital to monitor the intracranial pressure directly in patients who are at risk, in order to detect changes in condition at an early stage.

A severe increase in intracranial pressure leads to shifting of the brain structures. The presence of a space-occupying lesion in the left cerebrum can cause a movement to the right of the midline structures. Pressure may be exerted on the right cerebrum as it is forced against the skull and dura mater, causing symptoms of an apparently right-sided lesion (contrecoup). Traction on cerebral blood vessels can cause tearing, small haemorrhages, infarction and oedema (cf the development of pressure sores – Ch.20) which in turn increase the pressure inside the cerebral compartment.

If pressure continues to rise, compensation fails and the brain will herniate downwards through the foramina in the rigid structures around the brain. A lesion in the cerebral hemisphere may cause herniation of the temporal lobe on the same side through the tentorial hiatus, creating intense pressure on the midbrain (Fig. 18.3). In particular the nucleus of the third cranial nerve (oculomotor) will be affected. If the lesion is in the posterior fossa (i.e. below the tentorium but within the cranium) then the cerebellar tonsil is the structure which commonly herniates into the foramen magnum, causing pressure on the medulla oblongata (Fig. 18.4). This affects in particular the centres within the medulla which control vegetative functions.

These two types of clinical (and human) disaster are commonly called 'coning'. The

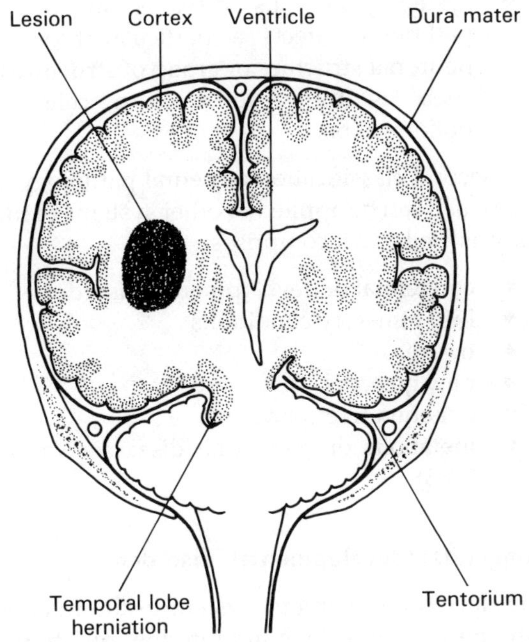

Fig. 18.3 Effect of lesion in the cerebral hemisphere causing shift of midline structure and temporal lobe herniation.

importance of preventing them cannot be overemphasized. Prevention in this case is the task of the medical staff through the use of drugs or surgical techniques to reduce intracranial pressure. Above all, lumbar puncture must be avoided for anyone who is suspected of suffering from increased intracranial pressure. The cardinal sign of such pressure is papilloedema. Lumbar puncture reduces pressure below the foramen magnum and in the presence of increased intracranial pressure has a high risk of literally pulling the brain down through the foramina.

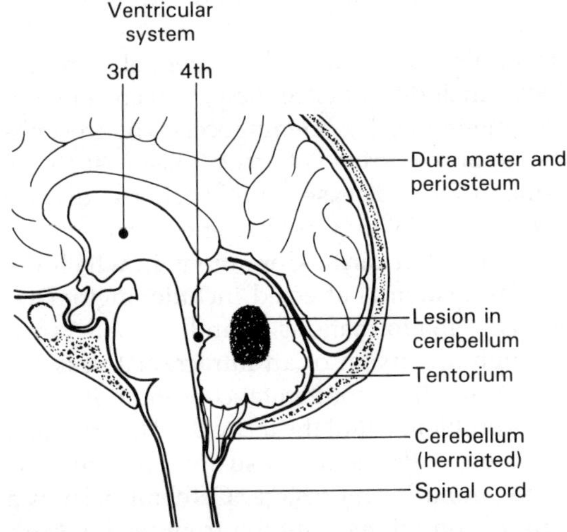

Fig. 18.4 Effect of a space-occupying lesion within the cerebellum causing cerebellar herniation.

The nursing role is to assess the patient's condition continuously, to report any increased CSF pressure if this is being monitored and to report any deterioration in the patient's neurological condition or conscious level. Blood pressure level, pulse and respiratory rate must also be monitored frequently. (For a full discussion of neurological assessment see pages 434–445). If there is any cause for concern, preparation must be made to help the doctor in measures to reduce the pressure in an emergency.

Medical intervention involves the use of hypertonic solutions of urea, mannitol or glycerol given intravenously, whilst surgical intervention requires the removal of CSF directly from the lateral ventricles. This latter procedure cannot be carried out, of course, unless burrholes have already been made in the skull. Muscle relaxants, hypothermia and coma induced by barbiturates have also been used to reduce intracranial pressure (Miller, 1979).

Longer term prevention and treatment is through the injection of the corticosteroid dexamethasone, which has a strong anti-inflammatory effect but very little mineralocorticoid activity so that fluid retention is minimal. This takes at least 12 hours before it is effective (Walton, 1977, 1983).

Hypercapnia. When intracranial pressure is increased it may take only a small additional increase of pressure to cause irreversible changes. Higher than normal plasma PCO_2 levels cause dilatation of cerebral blood vessels (Grubb et al, 1974) and this may be all that is necessary to cause deterioration of the patient's condition. Careful monitoring of PCO_2 levels is important in unconscious patients with increased intracranial pressure (Walton, 1983). Occasionally a tracheostomy is performed to reduce respiratory dead space and thus to improve the alveolar PCO_2 and consequently plasma PCO_2 levels. A tracheostomy also allows the use of an artifical ventilator and more efficient suction of secretions (Clarke, 1983).

FUNCTIONAL AND ANATOMICAL SPECIALIZATION

Cell bodies of neurones subserving a particular function tend to be aggregated together in the central nervous system. For example, the neurones concerned with the initiation of voluntary movement lie together in the cortex along the precentral convolution of the cerebrum (Solomon & Davis, 1983). Cells concerned with the interpretation of visual stimuli lie in the cortex of the occipital lobe. Similarly, fibres of neurones subserving a given function travel together in 'tracts' through the brain stem and spinal cord. It is well known that the majority also cross the midline with the consequence that the left side of the cerebrum controls function of the right side of the body and vice versa.

This functional and anatomical specialization has the consequence that a relatively small lesion in an area subserving a crucial function may have an effect which is more devastating than a larger lesion in a less crucial area. A knowledge of the anatomy and physiology of the CNS allows clinicians to localize the lesion accurately by careful examination of signs and symptoms. This aids diagnosis and prognosis. A knowledge of the history of the onset of the illness helps to indicate the nature of the lesion or disease (Walton, 1983).

PATHOLOGICAL CONDITIONS AFFECTING THE NERVOUS SYSTEM

Pathology of the nervous system can be classified in two ways. The first classification divides disorders of structure and function into:

- focal lesions which cause localized disturbance (at least initially)
- diffuse or generalized pathology
- systemic nervous diseases in which pathology affects a particular type of neuronal structure or group of structures, such as the anterior horn cells in poliomyelitis.

A second classification of neural pathology is one which can be applied to other systems of the body as well and it comprises:

- congenital or developmental disorders
- inflammatory conditions
- trauma
- new growths
- degenerative conditions
- metabolic or endocrine disease (Walton 1983).

Congenital (developmental) disorders

The developing nervous system in the fetus is extremely vulnerable to intrauterine conditions, including drugs and microorganisms with the ability to pass through the placental barrier into the fetal bloodstream. Severe abnormalities result in death, but less severe ones allow survival of the fetus with variable degrees of defect at birth. Some chromosomal abnormalities also result in neural defects. Anomalies of cerebral blood vessels may cause problems, often later in life. Finally, trauma to delicate nervous tissue during birth can result in functional disorder.

Examples of structural congenital abnormalities include anencephaly, microcephaly, myelomeningocele, meningocele, hydrocephalus. Inborn errors of metabolism such as Niemann-Pick disease or Gaucher's disease (McIlwain, 1966) may not become apparent until some time after birth. Conditions in which the vascular system is affected include angiomata, venous malformations and aneurysms. Although aneurysm of an intracranial vessel is very frequently a congenital condition, it rarely causes problems until the individual has reached adulthood. Problems usually present as subarachnoid haemorrhage. Cerebral palsy is a group of conditions resulting from fetal or birth injury in which there is non-progressive motor dysfunction. Incidence in this country is approximately 2/1000 live births (Walton, 1983). Epilepsy can be primary (idiopathic) with no evidence of underlying disease. Primary epilepsy is thought to be a functional disorder with a genetic component. It is characterized by the discharge of a periodic, sudden excessive burst of electrical activity of the brain which completely and violently disrupts the normal EEG picture. The individual displays typical grand mal attacks. A much milder form of the condition produces petit mal attacks, in which the individual momentarily appears unaware of his surroundings. Epilepsy can also be a symptom of brain pathology. Onset of attacks in later life should always be investigated, especially if the attacks show features of localization.

Inflammatory conditions

Inflammatory conditions of the nervous system may be generalized, e.g. meningitis or encephalitis, or localized into an abscess. Tabes dorsalis of syphilis specifically affects the area around the entry of the posterior spinal roots and the ascending posterior columns of the spinal cord, whilst allergic encephalomyelitis affects white matter in particular (Walton, 1983).

Bacterial meningitis is less common than it once was, although it is still serious if it does occur. Viral meningitis or other viral infections may be difficult to treat. The incidence of acute anterior poliomyelitis has dropped dramatically in the Western world since the introduction of vaccine in the 1950s (Houston et al, 1985). Herpes zoster or shingles is a virus infection of the spinal cord ganglia and grey matter.

Trauma

Trauma of the nervous system is quite frequent in spite of the protection afforded by bone, CSF and meninges. Damage may be direct as in a blow to the head. A fall on the head may cause both an acceleration and a deceleration injury, as well as bone fracture and injury at the site of impact (Walton, 1983). Indirect injury occurs due to movement of one area of the brain on impact whilst other areas are fixed (e.g. the brain stem). This may cause disruption of tissue at a distance from the site of impact.

Blood vessels may be among the tissues damaged in head injury. If these bleed inside the skull, secondary pressure effects may occur, increasing the extent of the trauma and threatening life. Laceration of the meningeal artery can cause an extradural haematoma which accumulates rapidly and is fatal unless it is evacuated immediately. Subdural haematoma usually develops more gradually, often allowing some accommodation of the skull contents (Houston et al, 1985). Diagnosis is important and surgical treatment is necessary. Small, widespread haemorrhages due to tearing of vessels during brain movement may cause areas of infarction having a widespread and devastating effect. Impact damage to brain cells with oedema is irreparable.

Infection may occur as another secondary effect of head injury if a fracture of the skull combined with external soft tissue injury allows the entry of microorganisms. For this reason patients with open skull fractures should be reverse barrier nursed. Sometimes, if the fracture is in the base of the skull, the fact that there is a tract for infection to enter is not immediately obvious. Any leakage of liquid from the nose, eyes or ears could be CSF and immediate precautions should be taken to prevent infection by the use of reverse barrier nursing.

Spinal cord injuries may also result from penetrating or crushing injury, spinal column dislocation, compressing tumours or prolapsed intervertebral discs. Apart from direct tearing and pressure on cells and fibres the main damage is caused by haemorrhage, oedema and disruption of the blood supply to the cord.

Injury to peripheral nerves may occur as part of a traumatic lesion of the body in general.

Neoplasms

Tumours of the nervous system may be benign or malignant. Benign tumours include meningioma and neuroma arising from the meninges and the neurilemma respectively. These cause symptoms through the exertion of pressure and, in particular, may cause increased intracranial pressure. Pituitary adenoma which is benign may cause neurological symptoms, especially visual defects as it is likely to compress the optic chiasma. If untreated it can lead to irreversible blindness.

Malignant tumours of the nervous system arise from glial cells. In adult life the common malignant tumours are the astrocytoma and the oligodendroglioma, whilst in childhood ependymomas and medulloblastomas are more common.

It is worth noting that from 10–20% of all intracranial tumours are metastatic from outside the nervous system (Walton, 1983). Carcinoma is more common than sarcoma and the commonest primary sites giving rise to intracranial metastases are the bronchus or breast.

Symptoms of tumours may be due to pressure, but the malignant and metastatic tumours also cause direct destruction of brain tissue, oedema and disruption of the blood supply (as does a brain abscess).

Degenerative conditions

Degenerative conditions of the nervous system include multiple sclerosis, Parkinson's disease, Huntington's chorea, myasthenia gravis, syringomyelia and dementia.

In multiple sclerosis there is progressive demyelination of nerve fibres within the central nervous system in general and the spinal cord in particular. If the brain stem is also affected the disease is more acute and more rapidly fatal.

Parkinson's disease may be due to one of several causes. It used to be fairly common as a consequence of epidemic encephalitis. It can also occur as a side-effect of long-term treatment with drugs such as reserpine, phenothiazide and haloperidol, but in this case the symptoms usually disappear when the drug is discontinued. Parkinsonian symptoms may occur as part of more general cerebral atherosclerosis. Most commonly there is no obvious cause of the disease. Anatomically the disease affects the basal ganglia and the substantia nigra, whilst biochemically there appears to be a dopamine deficiency in these structures. Motor function is affected with tremor. There is a characteristic posture and gait and rigidity of the musculature.

Huntington's chorea is hereditary. It affects the basal ganglia and cerebral cortex. Typically symptoms do not appear until adult life, usually after the age of 30 years (Walton 1983). Symptoms are of three kinds: emotional disturbance, mental deterioration, and choreiform movement. There is no effective treatment for the disease but symptomatic relief of the abnormal movement can be gained by the use of haloperidol. Death usually occurs about 15 years after the onset of symptoms.

Syringomyelia is thought to be a developmental anomaly but symptoms often do not appear until the age of 30–40 years (Walton, 1983). Symptoms are caused by the development of cavities filled with yellow liquid within the substance of the spinal cord. These occur frequently within the cervical cord. Symptoms include loss of muscle power, sensory loss and disturbed bladder control. Syringobulbia is a similar condition where the cavities appear within the medulla oblongata. The tongue and face may be affected. No effective treatment is available but surgical drainage of spinal cord cavities may produce symptomatic relief. When once the diagnosis has been made the patient must be given a great deal of psycho-social support. Teaching is aimed at helping him/her to compensate for the loss of sensation, including pain, otherwise severe injury could occur.

Myasthenia gravis is characterized by fluctuating weakness in voluntary muscle, especially those muscles supplied by cranial nerves. The main defect is at the neuromuscular junction where there is a decrease in the number of acetylcholine receptor sites on the postsynaptic muscle membranes. It is thought that this is due to an autoimmune response triggered through the thymus gland. Treatment may be medical or surgical. Medical treatment involves the use of anticholinesterase drugs which prolong the action of acetylcholine at the neuromuscular junction by blocking cholinesterase. Corticosteroids may also be used to suppress the symptoms. Surgical treatment involves the removal of the thymus glands and empirically this brings about a marked improvement in the symptoms in a high percentage of patients.

Dementia is a condition in which there is a progressive deterioration of intellect, memory and power of abstract thought (Walton, 1983). It can arise from many causes including arteriosclerosis of cerebral vessels, chronic alcoholism and neurosyphilis. In some cases there is no obvious cause. Normal ageing brings about a progressive deterioration of certain cortical and spinal neurones and this is associated with neurofibrillary tangles and argyrophilic plaques at the sites affected. Such lesions seen in profusion are diagnostic of senile dementia and if they occur at a relatively early age the condition is called presenile dementia. Persons with dementia present a particularly difficult problem for relatives, friends and for nurses, since their behaviour disintegrates. They may suffer delusions and hallucinations, disorientation, agitation, hostility, incontinence, and become socially disruptive. The condition is progressive. When once a treatable cause has been eliminated, nursing management of symptoms and good care is all that remains to help these patients.

Metabolic and endocrine disorders

Certain metabolic and endocrine disorders can result in disturbances of the nervous system.

Coma results when the body temperature falls below about 30°C and hypothermia of this degree of severity can develop, in the absence of cold, when the metabolic rate is depressed by myxoedema or hypopituitarism.

Wilson's disease is a genetic disorder of copper metabolism which, in the cerebral type of the disorder, causes choreiform movements, sometimes Parkinsonism and usually dementia.

Certain nutritional deficiencies will affect specific cells, including nerve cells, according to individual characteristics of their metabolism, and result in damage to the cell bodies and dying back of the neurones. Subacute combined degeneration of the cord is due to the vitamin B_{12} deficiency of pernicious anaemia and consists of degeneration of the posterior and lateral columns of the spinal cord. Initially the patient suffers sensory disturbances and later motor disturbances of the limbs. Thiamin deficiency results in Wernicke's encephalopathy in which there are disorders of cortical function with confusion which may progress to stupor or coma (Macleod, 1981).

Vascular lesions of cerebral vessels

Whilst vascular lesions are not primarily lesions of nervous tissue, if they occur within the skull or spinal canal they can cause severe neurological disturbance. Subarachnoid haemorrhage from an aneurysm or angioma has already been mentioned. This classically causes meningeal symptoms if the bleeding is directed into the subarachnoid space. Bleeding can also be directed into the brain substance to form a haematoma, causing local pressure symptoms. One of the most common vascular lesions is 'stroke' or cerebrovascular accident. Indeed this is the third most common cause of death in the UK (Myco, 1983).

'Stroke' includes the following types of lesion:

- occlusion of a cerebral blood vessel by a thrombosis or an embolus causing infarction
- intracerebral haemorrhage from a ruptured intracranial vessel
- transient interruption of the cerebral blood flow causing ischaemia and possibly infarction.

The most common underlying pathology in these conditions is athero- or arteriosclerosis and hypertension.

In theory, since any cerebral blood vessel could be involved, many different patterns of symptoms could occur, but in practice the classical symptoms of an intracerebral haemorrhage or occlusion due to embolus are:

- sudden onset
- coma
- hemiplegia

unless death occurs instantly.

The classical picture in an occlusive lesion due to thrombosis is:

- onset over several hours
- hemiplegia
- loss of consciousness relatively uncommon.

If the right side of the body is affected there is usually an accompanying speech defect.

Patients with 'stroke' are usually elderly. Recovery is possible but the process is very lengthy and a good deal of morbidity is associated with the condition.

NURSING CARE

Nursing care of the patient with a neuromedical or neurosurgical condition is very challenging. The quality of that care is frequently the critical factor in determining whether the patient will live or die; and for those who live, the quality of that life. Nonetheless, the basic skills required are those used in other forms of nursing, i.e. the skills of the nursing process; obtaining a nursing history, nursing assessment, nursing problem identification, care planning, giving the planned care, and evaluation of the outcome.

Aspects of the nursing process which are particularly important are:

- assessment and monitoring of the patient's condition (this may be carried out at very frequent intervals)
- planning and giving care to prevent potential problems of immobility
- attention to activities of daily living which the patient is unable to cope with him/herself.

Neurosurgical nursing may well require the nurse to take on the values and attitudes appropriate to the care of the young patient with long-term chronic illness alongside the highly technical care more usually associated with intensive care units.

The successful neurosurgical nurse requires the knowledge and ability to manage highly technical apparatus whilst maintaining the human dignity of the patient and remaining sensitive to psychological and social aspects of care.

ASSESSMENT AND MONITORING

Deterioration in a patient's condition may be rapid. As a general rule the more rapid such deterioration, the greater is the threat to the patient's life. Detailed assessment of the patient's condition on admission is important to obtain criteria on which to judge the often very small changes which can forewarn of a significant deterioration in condition. Subsequent frequency of assessment depends on the degree of risk to the patient. Judgement of risk needs to take account of the patient's history, especially recent history, and the known or suspected diagnosis.

GENERAL ASSESSMENT

General assessment of the patient's condition should not be neglected, e.g. skin integrity, mouth condition, weight, appetite, urinalysis. Here we concentrate upon assessment specific to the neuromedical/surgical patient; namely neurological assessment.

NEUROLOGICAL ASSESSMENT

Details will be given of the dimensions of assessment, and the possible implications of abnormal findings. The order in which each item of assessment is carried out may be left to the preference of the nurse or to ward policy. For example, one could proceed according to some priority structure or by assessing from the head, working down the body to the legs and feet last of all. Sometimes the patient's condition forces priorities upon the nurse and may be so critical that only a very brief initial assessment is possible. However, whatever the state of the patient, unless his/her life is threatened or he/she is deeply unconscious, it is useful to start by assessing the patient's conscious level and mental state since this can be combined with the process of greeting the patient, introducing oneself, explaining the procedure to the patient and enquiring about his/her feelings.

In recording the outcome of assessment, it is better to write an accurate description of the patient's behaviour and responses independently of the inferences which are made from the observed behaviour. Inferences are subjective and may be misleading.

Symptoms of neurological disturbance may be positive or negative. Positive symptoms are those increased or abnormal sensations or actions which arise from irritation of the nervous system or from the release of neuronal activity from the normal inhibitory control. Examples are epileptiform attacks and abnormal movements such as athetosis. Negative symptoms are those which arise from the depression or abolition of function, which may be temporary or permanent. Paralysis or sensory loss are examples of negative symptoms. Hughlings' Jackson's law of dissolution states that functions or skills most recently acquired during evolution or during the individual's lifespan are the first to be lost in cortical disorders (Walton, 1983). Primitive or long-learned and practised behaviour persists longer. This also applies in temporarily depressed cortical function induced by drugs. One example is that a second language may be lost whilst the first is retained. This is important when nursing patients who are not native English speakers. Another example is the loss of man's precision grip but the retention of the more primitive power grip (Walton, 1983).

Assessment of awareness and mental state

Normal adults are fully aware of their own identity, their past history and their location in time and place. Their interpretation of the environment agrees with that of other normal individuals. An adult has a sense of self determination, is able to interpret his/her own mood and emotions and has a self-concept which is stable over time. The mood and emotional state of an individual is relatively stable and his/her emotional response can be predicted from a knowledge of the event and of the characteristics of the person concerned. Direction and integration of the individual's activities and being is derived from the possession of one or more aims and goals for the future.

A normal person is either alert or arouses easily when his/her name is spoken. In conversation his/her posture, facial expression, eye contact and verbal response is appropriate to the setting, the topic of conversation and the immediately preceding circumstances.

Socially unacceptable behaviour and speech e.g. physical aggression, swearing, sexual approaches and exposure of the body other than when requested, are normally suppressed and inhibited within a setting such as a hospital. Verbal responses are appropriate both to the relationship between the respondent and the other individual(s) involved and to the words which are actually said. During a prolonged verbal exchange, as in giving a nursing history, a patient is normally able to display short-term and long-term memory, the ability to conceptualize and the ability to pay attention over a period of time. Responses are structured into words which are meaningful and sentences conform to the grammatical rules of a known language.

Any or all of these abilities may be affected in a patient with a neurological disturbance, and they can be assessed during the first stage of taking a nursing history.

Some of the abnormalities of function which can be observed when present will now be defined and described briefly. It is not possible to relate all signs and symptoms of disorder in the higher functions to localized lesions of the brain, since our knowledge is still inadequate. Such functions appear to depend upon complex interactions of many parts and are not only a function of intact cortical areas but also the tracts and association areas which create the interconnectedness of the brain.

Disorders of personality, mood and emotion

Psychosis and neurosis are less clearly distinct from one another than was once thought (Walton, 1983). Psychosis is a serious derangement of thought processes and can occur as a result of organic disease diffusely affecting the brain. In particular it can occur as a temporary state induced by psychoactive drugs such as LSD or by the withdrawal of drugs such as the amphetamines.

Dementia is the disintegration of previously normal intellect (Walton, 1983) resulting from organic brain disease such as cerebral atrophy. Hallucinations are mental impressions of sensory events occurring without an external stimulus, but appearing to be located and to possess a cause external to the individual experiencing them. They may be experienced in relation to any of the special senses but are most usually visual or auditory. They appear to be associated with disorders of function of the reticulohypothalamic pathways. Occurrence is associated with hypnagogic states, sleep disorders, perceptual deprivation over a period of time, organic disease of the sense organs and toxic states affecting the CNS such as generalized acute infections and the taking of drugs such as LSD and mescaline. They may also occur as part of the withdrawal symptoms of amphetamines and barbiturates.

A delusion is a false idea or thought which has no substance in fact. Ideas of reference are delusions that one's actions are being controlled by some external force or conspiracy (through the medium of water pipes, the radio or TV, for instance).

Temporal lobe lesions may give disorders of perception, feelings of unreality and depersonalization, déjà-vu, or of observing oneself from outside as an object.

Delirium is a state of severely clouded consciousness in which patients are disorientated in time and space and the attention span is limited. Thought processes are so disordered that the sufferer cannot appreciate present circumstances and relate them to past experience. Delusions and hallucinations are common in delirium. There is a fluctuation in the mental and physical state in which periods of restlessness and shouting may alternate with drowsiness and muttering. Delirium occurs in acute generalized infections and metabolic disorders, drug psychosis, alcoholism and ence-phalitis. A less severe condition with fluctuating incoherence and disorientation is called a confusional state and can occur in head injury.

Emotional instability or lability also occurs in diffuse lesions, e.g. head injury, massive cerebral infarction and diffuse cerebral arteriosclerosis. It appears to result from an impairment of the control which the cortex normally exercises over the limbic system.

Apathy or emotional flatness can occur in Parkinson's disease due to encephalitic lethargy (Walton, 1983). It may be due to general mental deterioration as in senile or presenile dementia. Euphoria is a mood characterized by feelings of happiness and a sense of mental well-being. It occurs sometimes in multiple sclerosis, frontal lobe and temporal lobe lesions, especially those due to tumours.

Anxiety can be seen in organic brain disease, toxic drug states and head injury. It can accompany hallucinations.

Impulsive disorders of conduct are more frequently seen in children or adolescents, due to general brain damage or temporal lobe disorders.

A frontal lobe syndrome was first described after the 1848 accident to Phineas Gage. It comprises aimlessness, improvidence, loss of tact, loss of sensitivity and self control, impulsiveness, and a failure to appreciate the consequences of one's behaviour for oneself or others.

Nonetheless one frontal lobe can be amputated with little or no effect upon the personality. Frontal leucotomy which separates pathways between the dorso-medial nuclei to the frontal cortex and the antero medial nuclei to the cingulate gyri can relieve anxiety and obsessional behaviour.

Loss of memory or amnesia appears to be associated with bilateral temporal lobe disease. It may occur after head injury and in dementia. Korsakoff's syndrome comprises loss of neurones, demyelination with gliosis and haemorrhagic lesions in the thalamus, mamillary bodies and midbrain. It is thought to be due to vitamin B_1 deficiency and is most common in alcoholism. There is a loss of the ability to register new events and remember them. The individual appears lucid and alert but forgets within minutes. This results in disorientation in time and place. Elaborate fantasies are concocted to fill the memory gap (confabulation). The memory of remote events is intact. Hysterical amnesia also occurs, i.e. there is no organic lesion to account for it.

Speech and conceptual thought

Speech is a very complex function. During the development of language, nouns are acquired first, but verbs and adverbs etc. qualify the meaning of nouns which represent objects in the environment. Non-noun parts of speech refer to the manipulation of objects in time and space and are essential to the development of conceptual thought. Later the capacity to internalize speech develops and this becomes thought (Vygotsky, 1962). Rules of grammar are also acquired by the child before becoming a full conversant in his/her native language. Movements of the speech organs and the ability to write and read are also involved in language.

Speech requires the formulation of thoughts, their conversion into words, the use of grammatical rules and the use of the muscles of speech. The brain representation of speech is not localized to any one point as numerous cortical areas, association areas and pathways are involved. However, in right-handed people the overall control of speech is located in the left hemisphere of the brain, as it is in 60% of left-handed individuals (Walton, 1983). Broca's area, which is found at the posterior end of the inferior frontal convolution, is especially con-cerned with the spoken word (it lies near the motor area for the muscles of speech). Wernicke's area lies in the posterior third of the superior temporal convolution and is important for the understanding and interpretation of word symbols. The area connecting the two is the external capsule and accuate fasciculus which then passes round the posterior part of the sylvian fissure and then runs forward in the white matter of the inferior parietal lobe. It makes connections deep in the angular gyrus with visual association fibres.

Phonation is the production of sound through the controlled passage of expired air over the vibrating vocal cords. Articulation is the modification of that sound by movements of the lips and tongue.

Aphasia means the complete absence of speech. It is loosely used in place of the more accurate term dysphasia to refer to disorder of the use of words and symbols. Walton (1977) has classified aphasia (see Table 18.1).

Table 18.1 Classification of aphasia (Walton 1983)

1. Broca's aphasia (expressive or motor aphasia, anterior aphasia)
2. Wernicke's aphasia (sensory or receptive aphasia: pure word-deafness
3. General or total aphasia
4. Conduction aphasia (central aphasia of Goldstein, syntactical aphasia)
5. The Posterior (Association) aphasias
   a. The syndrome of the isolated speech area
   b. Nominal, anomic or amnesiac aphasia
6. Related disorders of language: agraphia, alexia, acalculia, amusia

Anarthria and dysarthria mean slurred, indistinct production of speech sounds in the presence of the correct use and understanding of words. Muscles of articulation can be affected by:

- upper motor neurone lesion (e.g. in stroke)
- disorders of co-ordination (e.g. a cerebellar lesion)
- disorders of the extrapyramidal system (e.g. in Parkinson's disease)
- by lower motor neurone lesions.

A cerebellar lesion gives incoordinate, jerky, explosive speech, with undue separation of syllables — called 'scanning' speech.

Mutism is the total inability to speak. This is usually functional, but can occur very rarely in an upper brain stem lesion.

Aphonia is usually hysterical but can arise from paralysis of the vocal cords due to a lesion in the throat.

Assessment of conscious level

Whilst the cerebral cortex is essential to the awareness of self and surroundings, alertness and receptivity to stimuli is a function of the ascending reticular activating system (ARAS) (Fig. 18.5). This relays to the cerebral cortex in two ways:

- by specific sensory projections (via the

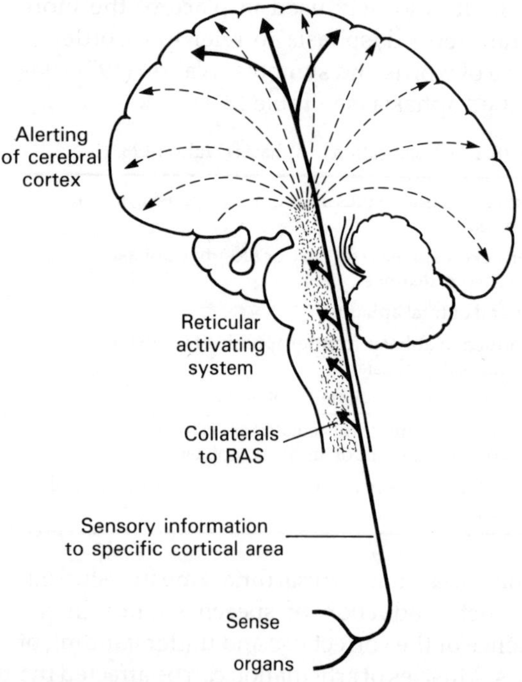

Fig. 18.5 Ascending reticular activating system and its alerting action.

thalamus) to the cortex related directly to the sensory stimulus concerned, e.g. auditory cortex for a sound stimulus
- by non-specific projection fibres to the cortex via the hypothalamus and thalamus: this has a general alerting and arousal function upon the cortex.

Sleep is the normal opposite of arousal but lesions or drugs which interrupt or depress function of the non-specific projection system cause loss of consciousness.

Plum & Posner (1980) have outlined several principles relating to consciousness vs unconsciousness.

- Lesions destroying the reticular formation below the level of the lowest third of the pons do not produce coma.
- Above this level the lesion must be bilateral to interrupt conciousness.
- Sleep is an active physiological process not a mere failure of arousal and is clearly different from loss of consciousness.
- Sleeping/waking can occur in man even after total bilateral destruction of the cerebral hemisphere.

Assessment of conscious level comprises several elements:

- general arousability
- movement
- eye and pupillary responses
- protective reflexes
- respiratory pattern
- pulse and BP level.

These can be related to the pathophysiology of 'coning' which affects the ARAS through shearing strain and displacement effects upon the brain stem.

General arousability. Whilst various degrees of loss of consciousness are given specific labels such as stupor, semi-coma and coma, each term covers a range of lost ability. It is more precise and therefore more effective to describe accurately the best responses which can be elicited from the patient on each dimension at the time of assessment. The Glasgow coma scale (Jennett, 1981) (see Ch.10) is a useful way of monitoring changes and incorporates these principles.

The assessment of conscious level starts by the determination of the strength of stimulation required to produce arousal. Obviously the individual may be alert on the nurse's approach, but if not it is normal to rouse as approached. Even in deep sleep we arouse if our name is called (Oswald, 1974). Touch stimuli should be used before attempting a painful stimulus to rouse the unresponsive patient. Verbal response to stimulation should be recorded.

Eye responses are part of the general arousal to stimulation unless the individual has some lesion specifically affecting the eye or the The amount and type of stimulation required to produce eye opening on at least one side should be recorded. Spontaneous eye opening should be distinguished from eye opening to command. Blinking suggests that the pontine region is intact. An individual can be unconscious with the eyelids in the open position.

Movement. Motor responses of the limbs can also be elicited by the methods already mentioned. The record of the observations made should state whether movement is spontaneous, in response to command, to touch, or in response to a painful stimulus. Any difference in strength or type of response between the four limbs should be noted.

Motor reflexes should be noted. The grasp reflex is a natural reflex and is a function of the frontal lobe. Localization response to pain should be recorded. This is a purposeful movement toward the spot at which the stimulus was applied. Flexion withdrawal of each limb in response to a locally applied painful stimulus may be observed.

Signs of decorticate or decerebrate rigidity are prognostically grave. These signs may be elicited in response to pain applied centrally, a painful stimulus applied to each limb in turn, or through the elicitation of tonic neck reflexes. They may also occur spontaneously either intermittently or as a continuous postural position, which is extremely serious.

Decorticate rigidity consists of flexion and adduction of the arm, wrist and fingers, with leg extension and plantar flexion of the foot. (Note: This is frequently the position seen on the affected side in hemiplegia due to 'stroke'.) The presence of tonic neck reflexes on turning the head and neck to one side is displayed by extension of the limbs on the side toward which the head is turned and flexion of the limbs on the contralateral side.

The decerebrate posture/response consists of extension and internal rotation of all four limbs with plantar flexion of the feet.

Failure to respond at all to painful stimuli reveals severe depression of brain stem function.

Eye and pupillary responses. Pupil size and reflex responses to light and accommodation depend upon the optic nerve, the oculomotor nerve and sympathetic fibres from the superior cervical ganglion. In response to light, sensory fibres of the optic nerve not only conduct impulses to the occipital lobe of the brain but also relay to the corpora quadrigemina, from whence there is transmission to the nuclei of the third, fourth and sixth cranial nerves. Pupil size depends upon the balance of parasympathetic stimulation (constriction and accommodation for near vision) and sympathetic stimulation (dilatation and accommodation for far vision). Both light and accommodation to near vision cause pupillary constriction.

Posterior and ventrolateral hypothalamic damage causes ipsilateral pupil constriction, ptosis, and lack of sweating of the face (Horner's syndrome). This may be a very early sign of tentorial coning. Later with herniation of the temporal uncus comes a fixed dilated pupil due to pressure upon the nucleus of the oculomotor nerve. Damage to the midbrain produces loss of reflex response to light, whilst the response to accommodation may be preserved. There is normally a consensual response to light, i.e. the other pupil constricts in response to light shone into one pupil. This response can help to distinguish whether an unresponsive pupil is due to damage of the optic nerve pathway or whether it is due to damage of the motor pathways to the pupil.

Drugs and generalized conditions of the brain affect both pupils equally. It follows that a change in the size and reaction of one pupil is likely to be a highly significant clinical sign. Ocular movements are controlled by the third, fourth and sixth cranial nerves (oculomotor, trochlea, abducens) and brain stem pathways. Movements of the eyes can be reflex when such reflexes are released from the voluntary control of the cortex. Destructive lesions of one hemisphere are characterized by lateral deviation of the eyes to the same side as the lesion. This can be seen in stroke where the lesion is affecting less than a complete hemisphere. A positive sign of an irritant lesion in a hemisphere is deviation of the eyes to the side opposite from the lesion. Eye deviation toward the paralysed side of the body suggests a pontine lesion.

The oculocephalic reflex can be elicited by holding the eyelids open and briskly rotating the head of the patient from side to side, pausing briefly on each side. The normal response is conjugate deviation of the eyes to the opposite side. Brisk flexion or extension of the neck results in the deviation of the eyes upwards and downwards respectively.

Protective reflexes. Swallowing, coughing, sneezing, gagging and vomiting are reflex responses integrated in the medulla oblongata (Ganong, 1983). The deeper the level of coma, the less likely it is that these reflexes will be present. Even a drowsy or stuporous patient will fail to swallow liquid given to him. It is important to exclude any possibility of a patient being given fluid or food when his conscious level places him at risk from choking. It is even more vital to avoid the risk of fluids or natural secretions from blocking the airway of a patient who has lost his coughing reflex. Alternative methods of ensuring nutrition, as well as suction of airways, is needed for such patients.

The corneal reflex, mediated by the fifth cranial nerve, the oculomotor nerve and the facial nerve is lost in the unconscious patient. Care is needed to avoid damage to the delicate corneal tissue in the absence of this reflex.

Respiratory pattern. Both the depth of respirations and their pattern are altered in severe lesions of the cerebrum and brain stem. A lesion in the basal ganglia or deep in the cerebral hemispheres (bilaterally) may cause Cheyne-Stokes respirations. Cheyne-Stokes respirations are cyclic. Periods of apnoea change in a smooth crescendo to periods of hyperpnoea, dying down again to apnoea. The hyperpnoeic phase is usually of longer duration than the period of apnoea.

Hyperventilation is thought to be a reflex response in increased intracranial pressure since it reduces the calibre of intracerebral blood vessels, thus reducing blood flow and preventing even greater intracranial pressure. It is associated in particular with lesions of the midbrain and pons.

Lesions occurring in the lower part of the pons with extensive lower brain stem damage are associated with apneustic respiration. Cramp-like inspirations occur with only rare expiratory movements.

Medullary lesions occurring in the upper area lead to cluster breathing where irregular respiratory bursts alternate with periods of apnoea. Low medullary damage leads to an ataxic respiratory pattern in which respirations are deep or shallow in a random way with periods of apnoea.

Changes in the pattern of respirations are very grave prognostic signs, since they indicate damage of the areas which are essential to the maintenance of the vital functions (of which respiration is itself an example).

Pulse and blood pressure. Hypertension can occur as the primary lesion in a patient who has had an intracerebral or subarachnoid haemorrhage. It may also occur as a consequence of increased intracranial pressure. Bradycardia is also recorded, this occurring as a homeostatic reflex, compensating to some extent for the increased blood pressure.

When increased intracranial pressure is present hypertension, bradycardia and increased pulse pressure (Cushing's reflex) are grave prognostic signs, indicating compression of the medulla. Unless this can be relieved, rapid pulse and low blood pressure follow, prior to death. The absence of Cushing's reflex, however, does not necessarily mean the absence of threat to the patient from increased intra-cranial pressure as it may only be present in a small percentage of the patients at risk (Ricci, 1982).

Motor and sensory function

Assessment of the function of the cranial nerves

The cranial nerves are the sensory and motor nerves supplying the head and face; neck and shoulders; and (via the vagus nerve) the viscera of the thorax and abdominal cavity. Their importance is obvious but since they arise from or relay to the brain stem, dysfunction of cranial nerves may well indicate a lesion in the brain stem which is always extremely serious. In the following paragraphs, the function of each cranial nerve will be described briefly, with an indication of the effect of disturbed function.

The olfactory nerve is the sensory nerve which responds to dissolved molecules reaching the nasal mucosa. Impulses from the fibres of the olfactory nerve are interpreted as smell. This sense is tested by asking the patient to name volatile substances which are presented to each nostril separately by uncorking tubes containing the relevant solution, e.g. peppermint. Loss of the sense of smell is called anosmia and may indicate a frontal lobe lesion. It is important to remember that smell is a very important component in the tastiness of food and an anosmic person may lose interest in eating. Depression of the sensation of smell can occur in local lesions of the nose, e.g. common cold. Olfactory hallucinations indicate a temporal lobe lesion and appear to be particularly unpleasant, causing the patient great anxiety.

The optic nerve has already been mentioned. It carries the impulses coding for light to the occipital lobe. Visual acuity and the shape and size of the visual field are functions of the optic nerve, as is the blink reflex. It is concerned in pupillary reflexes, as already mentioned.

Defects of visual acuity are tested by distance/near visual charts. Mapping of the visual field carried out by the doctor requires the use of perimetry apparatus and time, but gross defects can be identified by moving a finger or a pencil from different directions in toward each eye in turn (with the other closed) and asking the patient to say when he can see it (Fig. 18.6).

Hemianopia is the name given to the defect when a half of each visual field is lost. One form is bilateral temporal hemianopia, where the external half of each field is lost, causing defec-tive peripheral vision. This creates great problems for the patient in moving about. It occurs when there is a midline lesion in the region of the optic chiasma, e.g. pituitary adenoma.

Involvement of the optic tract on one side beyond the optic chiasma gives a homonymous hemianopia in which the same half of each visual field is lost on the side of the lesion, e.g., a left-sided lesion means that the left side of the visual field is lost from the right eye and the left eye. Vascular lesions not uncommonly cause this problem.

The point at which the optic nerve leaves the retina (the optic disc, functionally the blind spot) can be seen through an ophthalmoscope. This gives an opportunity for the doctor to identify papilloedema which is the cardinal sign of increased intracranial pressure. Papilloedema develops to a very severe level before it affects eyesight.

The oculomotor, trochlear and abducens nerves (third, fourth and sixth cranial nerves) will be discussed together, as jointly they supply

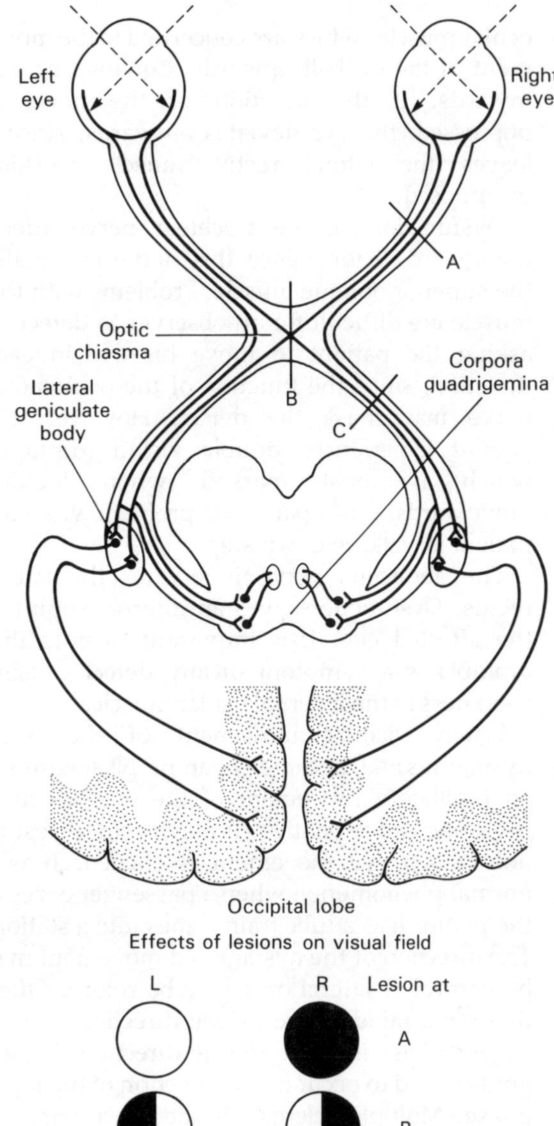

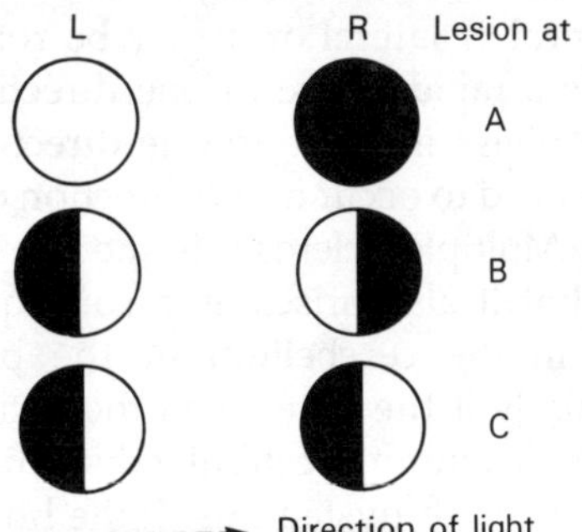

Fig. 18.6 Defects of the visual field occurring due to lesions at points along the optic tracts.

the external ocular muscles and are therefore concerned with eye movements. Most of the functions of the oculomotor nerve have been discussed in the previous section. In addition it innervates the medial rectus, superior and inferior recti and the inferior oblique external ocular muscles which are concerned in the movement of the eyeball upwards, downwards and inwards. If the function of the nerve is depressed, the eye deviates outwards, since it leaves the lateral rectus muscle working unopposed.

Dysfunction of the trochlear nerve affects downward vision, since this nerve innervates the superior oblique muscle. Problems with this muscle are difficult for an observer to detect on asking the patient to move his eye in each direction, since the function of the oculomotor nerve may mask the defect. However, the patient experiences double vision (diplopia) which is most marked when looking downwards. It is a particular problem when the patient is walking down steps.

The abducens nerve innervates the lateral rectus. Dysfunction gives an internal squint of the affected eye. It is important to note that diplopia is a symptom of any defect causing weakness of the external ocular muscles.

When eliciting movement of the eyes, nystagmus may become apparent. Nystagmus is an oscillatory movement of the eye which is rhythmic and repetitive. It may occur at rest or only when eye movement is elicited. It is a normal phenomenon when a passenger gazes at the platform as a tube train comes into a station. The direction of the nystagmoid movement may be vertical or lateral or it may be rotary. Often there is a rapid phase in one direction, with a slower phase in the opposite direction. Nystagmus is said to occur in the direction of the rapid phase. Multiple sclerosis is the most common cause but it also arises as a consequence of a lesion in the cerebellum or the brain stem, particularly if the latter is in the vicinity of the foramen magnum. Vestibular disturbance is also associated with nystagmus. If the horizontal canals are affected lateral nystagmus results, whilst rotary nystagmus occurs if the vertical canals are involved. Unilateral cerebellar lesions give lateral nystagmus toward the side of the lesion.

The trigeminal nerve is a motor and sensory nerve of the face. It carries touch, pain, temperature and proprioceptive information from the face, cornea, nasal and oral mucosa, sinuses, teeth, tongue, external auditory canal and the meninges. Its motor fibres supply the masseter and temporal muscles controlling the opening and closing of the jaw. Depression of the function of this nerve can put the eye at risk from corneal ulceration with the loss of the corneal reflex. This is the nerve which is affected in tic doloureux (trigeminal neuralgia), a condition of intermittent, brief, extreme pain which occurs in bouts lasting several weeks or months. It is more common in the elderly.

The facial nerve is also both motor and sensory. It innervates the muscles of facial expression, the motor component of the blink reflex, the lower eyelid and the salivary and lachrymal glands. The sense of taste from the anterior two-thirds of the tongue is carried by this nerve. Depressed function of the facial nerve causes facial asymmetry and sagging of the lower eyelid with inability to close the eye properly. An upper motor neurone lesion spares the forehead as this is doubly represented at cortical level. The side opposite to that of the lesion is affected. A lower motor neurone lesion affects the whole side of the face on the same side as the lesion. The patient is unable to whistle and has difficulty in showing his teeth. There is a tendency to drool and difficulty in feeding. Taste is tested by solutions of sugar, salt, quinine and lemon.

The auditory or acoustic nerve is sensory and codes information about sound and position in space from the vestibular organs. Hearing is tested by comparing conduction of air vibration via the ear drum with that of bone conduction of vibration. Cochlear nerve involvement produces a depression in both air and bone conduction. If bone conduction is better than sound this suggests an obstructive lesion of the external auditory canal or middle ear disease. In Weber's test the vibrating tuning fork is placed on the forehead in the midline. The sound is referred to the opposite side in cochlear nerve deafness. Disturbance of the semi-circular canals gives vertigo and nystagmus. These responses are elicited as a normal but brief reaction if the ear is irrigated with cold water (calorific test). This test is highly specialized but allows the diagnosis of depressed or abnormal vestibular function.

The glossopharyngeal is a sensory nerve carrying taste from the posterior one-third of the tongue. It is also responsible for the sensory side of the gag and carotid sinus reflexes.

The vagus nerve is large and important. It is both motor and sensory, also carrying parasympathetic fibres. It supplies the muscles of the larynx, pharynx and soft palate. Its parasympathetic fibres are distributed to the organs of the thorax and abdomen. Whilst sensory fibres of the vagus nerve carry information from the heart and respiratory system in particular, above all it is the vagus which is responsible for the slowing of the cardiac rate. Vagal impairment affects phonation and articulation and produces dysphagia. Movement of the soft palate can be tested by observing whilst the patient says 'Ah'. In paralysis of the soft palate the uvula is pulled toward the unaffected side.

The spinal accessory nerve innervates the sternocleidomastoid muscles and the trapezii responsible for flexion and turning of the head and elevation of the shoulders. A lower motor neurone lesion gives a flaccid weakness on the side of the lesion.

The hypoglossal nerve is the motor nerve of the tongue. Its function can be tested by getting the patient to stick out his tongue and to move it from side to side. A lower motor neurone lesion causes a deviation of the tongue from the midline toward the affected side. An upper motor neurone lesion may cause tremor and weakness of the tongue with slow, spastic and incoordinate movement.

Motor function generally

The motor cortex, basal ganglia and cerebellum are heavily involved in the initiation and control of movement. Pyramidal and extrapyramidal tracts converge upon the cell bodies of the lower motor neurone (anterior horn cell) in the spinal cord. Fibres of the lower motor neurones transmit to the motor end plates of muscles. Assessment of motor function involves noting muscle bulk, strength and willed active movements. It is important to record muscle tone (resistance to passive movement), co-ordination of movement, posture and gait. The presence of any abnormal movements should be noted.

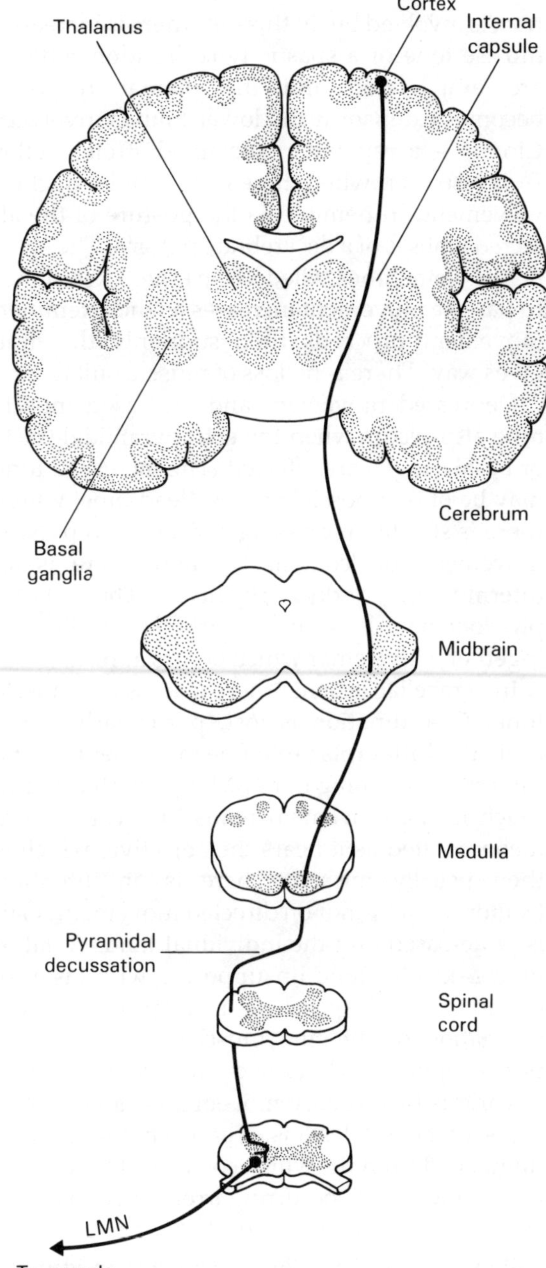

Fig. 18.7 The pyramidal tract (LMN = lower motor neurones)

Loss of muscle bulk implies muscle disease or a lower motor neurone lesion. There will be an associated weakness. Muscle tone is reduced (flaccid weakness) in lower motor neurone lesions and tendon reflexes are diminished or absent.

Weakness also occurs when the pyramidal

tract is involved but in this case there is increased muscle tone of a spastic type. Tendon reflexes are exaggerated and the plantar response becomes extensor if the lower limb is involved. Clonus — a repetitive, sustained stretch reflex — is also seen when there is pyramidal tract involvement. In hemiplegia the posture of the affected limbs is of a decerebrate pattern. The spasticity is sometimes called 'clasp knife'. Resistance to passive movement increases as the attempted movement proceeds then suddenly the limb gives way. There is no loss of muscle bulk.

Depressed movement and increased muscle tone also occurs when the extrapyramidal tracts or basal ganglia are affected. The increased tone may be of two possible types: 'lead pipe' where there is steadily increasing resistance to passive movement, or 'cogwheel' where there is an intermittent, jerky rigidity. This latter phenomenon is seen in Parkinson's disease, together with tremor which occurs at rest.

In cerebellar lesions, there is a loss of muscle tone. Co-ordination is lost, particularly if the individual attempts rapid fine movements of the fingers. On homing in to pick up an object or to touch it, the movement tends to become more incoordinated as it nears the objective, which is then usually missed. There is an intention tremor, i.e. a tremor on directed movement. Gait is wide-based and the individual tends to fall if he is asked to stand unsupported with his eyes closed. Slurred speech is a symptom of incoordination of the fine muscles. Typically the person appears to have had 'one over the eight'.

Various involuntary movements can occur as signs of neural lesions. These should be distinguished from tic, which consists of twitching, jerky movements occurring irregularly, particularly among muscles around the eyes, face or shoulders. Tics are related to anxiety or fatigue. Tremor, which has been mentioned above, is a rapid, rhythmically repetitive movement of muscles, consistent in pattern, amplitude and frequency (Walton, 1983). It consists of intermittent contraction of a muscle group alternating with contraction of the antagonist group.

The involuntary movements of chorea look semi-purposive and show a high degree of organization, e.g. facial grimace, raising of the eyebrows, rolling of the eyes, curling of the lips, protrusion and withdrawal of the tongue. In the limbs the movements are peripheral with intermittent wriggling and squirming of the fingers and toes. In contrast, limb movements in athetosis are proximal. The writhing is slower and of greater amplitude than in chorea. Athetosis results from degenerative changes in the corpus striatum. Torsion spasm also appears to be associated with lesions of the corpus striatum. This comprises increased muscle tone with frequent, irregular, spasmodic contraction of muscles of the neck, back, abdomen and limbs, giving bizarre alterations in posture. Spasmodic torticollis comprising spasmodic turning of the head and neck to one side is thought by some authorities to be a fractional variety of torsion spasm (Walton, 1983).

Sensory function generally

Assessment of sensory function depends upon the patient being alert, articulate and co-operative. Detailed sensory testing is performed by the doctor in this country, but it is crucial for the nurse to know the type and distribution of any sensory loss in order to help to prevent damage to the patient's skin or joints. Sensory loss occurring at the level of individual nerves will be distributed according to 'dermatomes'. Lesions in spinal cord tracts affect particular functions below the site of the lesion, since touch, tactile discrimination, joint position sense and pressure are served by the anterior spinothalamic tract whilst pain and temperature are carried in the lateral spino-thalamic tracts. Sensory pathways synapse in the thalamus before transmission upwards to the parietal cortex. Cortical lesions therefore impair the perception of sensation on the opposite side of the body. This type of lesion will affect the ability to recognize form, texture, size and weight of objects (agnosis) and changes in position of the individual's body on the affected side. Distortion of the body image may occur and there may be confusion between right and left sides. Sometimes patients deny that the affected side of the body belongs to them, as occurs with some stroke patients. The ability to relate sensory data to past experience is lost. Localization and discrimination between two stimuli is affected. 'Crude' sensations of pain, temperature and touch are retained.

Abnormal sensations may occur. Trigeminal neuralgia has already been mentioned. Causalgia is a particularly unpleasant burning type of continuous pain which may follow a peripheral nerve injury or arise in lesions of the spinal root of a sensory nerve. Postherpetic neuralgia is also extremely unpleasant and consists of a burning pain within the skin distribution of the nerve(s) which were affected by the herpes virus.

Thalamic pain is thought to be due to an infarctive lesion of the thalamus (Walton, 1983). Intense, burning, continuous pain occurs on the contralateral side of the body, particularly around the corner of the mouth, the cheek, the hand or the foot. The patient may describe it as tearing or grinding.

Crude testing of sensation may be carried out with the patient's eyes closed. He is asked to say when he is touched, whether he is touched in one or two places at once, in which direction his toe is moved, etc. More accurate information may be obtained from the patient's notes when the doctor has carried out a thorough neurological examination.

Bowel and bladder function

Incontinence or retention of urine or faeces gives important information about the patient's neurological state. Such information is also important for the planning of nursing care. Incontinence with overflow in an unconscious patient may mask retention and so percussion in the suprapubic area or rectal examination may be necessary to eliminate this possibility.

DIAGNOSTIC INVESTIGATIONS

Straight X-rays

These are probably the most frequently performed investigations of the skull and spine. They show up any bony deformity or fracture. Provided the pineal gland has calcified, straight skull X-rays may reveal a space-occupying lesion if it has caused a shift of midline structures. Any obvious foreign body such as a bullet also shows up on straight X-ray.

Straight X-rays are 'routine' from the perspective of the nurse. Patients do require explanations, however. Whilst most people have undergone an X-ray of some kind during their lifetime, the positions they may have to assume, the fact that staff disappear from the X-ray room as the film is taken, and the journey to X-ray (possibly on a trolley) all require explanation.

Computerized axial tomography scan (CAT scan)

This is also performed frequently and replaces the invasive techniques of previous decades in giving accurate information about the position, size, and possibly the type of brain lesion. Occasionally contrast media is injected into the arm during the procedure (Ramsey, 1977). A patient will require information about the procedure since he/she will have to remain in a still position for some time. Occasionally the head is held in position in a 'cap' (Rudy, 1984). The procedure may last as long as 45 minutes or one hour, during which time the patient may be alone with only the whirring of the machine. Such conditions are conducive to the development of anxiety or sensory deprivation. If contrast media is to be used, the patient must be asked about any known allergies. He/she is likely to experience a warm flush and a metallic taste in the mouth as the material is injected, and should be warned about this.

Observations should be made for any reactions to the contrast media such as restlessness, tachycardia, increased respirations, flushing of the face, urticaria, nausea and vomiting.

A brain scan

A brain scan involves an injection of a radioactive isotope followed by the scan itself, using a machine. From the patient's point of view, apart from the intravenous injection the technique is non-invasive. However, he/she will need to stay still whilst the scan is done.

Electroencephalography (EEG)

This is a method whereby the minute voltage changes involved in normal (or abnormal) brain activity are picked up and amplified. A pen and ink recorder displays them on paper so that this can be 'read' to detect any abnormalities which are characteristic of epilepsy or pathological lesions (Walton, 1983). The EEG is also used to confirm or detect brain death.

Explanation to the patient should include the information that there is no invasion of tissue, but that electrodes are placed in contact with the scalp and contact is made by electrode paste or jelly. Any patient who has previously had an ECG will understand this point. During the recording of the EEG the patient will be asked to sit or lie comfortably and may be asked to open and close his/her eyes. Sometimes stimuli are presented. After the investigation is complete the patient may wish to wash his/her hair, otherwise the paste must be removed, possibly using nail varnish remover.

Cerebral angiography

Cerebral angiography is used in the identification of cerebrovascular lesions (Walton, 1983). Contrast medium is injected into the carotid or brachial artery. Alternatively a catheter may be inserted into the femoral artery and passed up to the aortic arch.

The invasive procedure is carried out in the X-ray department itself and the patient may experience a burning sensation lasting for some seconds when the medium is introduced. Any known tendency to allergy should have been identified well before the procedure was planned. A consent form should be signed before the procedure is carried out since the procedure is not only invasive but the contrast medium may exacerbate the patient's symptoms. The whole procedure may exhaust an ill patient, who will need careful observation, information and reassurance throughout the investigation.

On return to the ward, frequent observation of vital signs and neurological status is necessary. Ice should be applied to the puncture site to prevent a haematoma occurring. In the rare instance where the carotid artery itself has been the site of the puncture then observation of the neck for swelling and for any sign of respiratory distress should be included in the general care of the patient. If the femoral artery was used the leg should be kept straight for six to eight hours afterwards. The patient should remain in bed for twenty-four hours following the investigation.

Lumbar puncture

Lumbar puncture is carried out in order to obtain a specimen of cerebrospinal fluid for examination or to check for blockage of subarachnoid channels. It is a distressing procedure to a patient. Potentially infection could be introduced, and if the patient should have increased intracranial pressure which has not been recognized it is extremely dangerous. For these reasons the procedure will be avoided unless absolutely necessary. It should be carefully explained to the patient. Explanation should include the fact that a nurse will be with him/her throughout and will keep him/her informed about what is going on (Clarke, 1977).

The patient should be lying in the lateral, curled up position, and this should be explained. He/she should be told that he/she will feel the application of skin cleansing lotions and the injection of local anaesthetic. Thereafter he/she should feel nothing, except a very brief pain sensation as the needle punctures the dura mater.

The nurse should be prepared to help the doctor in the collection of CSF. If a Queckenstedt test is required, the nurse will also assist by compressing the jugular vein on both sides serially for about ten seconds, before pressing both together.

A small dressing should be placed over the lumbar puncture wound after the needle has been withdrawn. The patient should be advised to rest in the head flat position and to take plenty of fluids. If headache occurs analgaesics may be given.

Myelogram

Myelogram involves the use of a lumbar puncture. This technique requires the insertion of an oil or water based contrast medium to show up the spinal subarachnoid space on X-ray films, thus revealing the presence of lesions of the spinal cord. The procedure causes more problems for the patient if an oil-based medium is used since CSF has to be removed to allow the medium to replace it. (The medium must then be removed as far as is possible after the X-rays have been taken.)

The patient's head should be kept raised afterwards to prevent any remaining dye from moving to the cerebral meninges which could cause a non- infective meningitis, and this is also true if a water-based medium has been used. The water-based type is excreted, however, within 24 hours or so and thus there is no need for it to be removed by lumbar puncture. The most frequent post-investigation problem is headache. Careful explanation is required, including the reason for maintaining the head up position afterwards.

Ultrasound investigation

Ultrasound investigation may be used for investigation of patients with suspected brain lesions. Explanation is required, but the procedure itself causes little or no disturbance to the patient.

Air encephalography

Air encephalography has been almost completely replaced by CAT scanning. Occasionally it is still used to identify lesions affecting the circulation of CSF itself (Rudy, 1984).

There are two methods of instilling air into the ventricular system. One is through a lumbar puncture. The procedure itself is similar to that described for myelogram. However, the patient should be nursed in a flat or head down position after the investigation has been completed to allow the air to move to the spinal area. Headache, nausea, and vomiting are common after this investigation and the patient should be encouraged to take plenty of fluids as soon as he/she is able. This helps to reduce headache. The other method of instilling air is directly into the ventricles. In this case burrholes are needed in the skull to allow the passage of a soft, blunt-ended needle through the brain tissue to the ventricles. The procedure is carried out under general anaesthesia in the operating theatre. A consent form must be signed and the usual preparation for anaesthetic carried out. The patient must be prepared very carefully for the body image impact of a partial head shave. Postoperatively reassurance is needed, as is careful observation of vital signs and neurological status.

In practice the surgeon is likely to be prepared to proceed immediately with a craniotomy when once the X-rays have been seen, and whilst the patient is still under anaesthetic. Obviously this requires very careful explanation, not only to the patient but also to the next of kin.

CARE OF PATIENTS WITH NEURO-MEDICAL OR NEUROSURGICAL DISTURBANCES

In this section, rather than consider the care of the unconscious patient, the hemiplegic patient, the patient with head injury, multiple sclerosis, etc., the focus will be upon problems affecting physiological systems or behaviour which have implications for nursing. Each of these problems could be displayed by patients with a variety of different diseases.

INCREASED INTRACRANIAL PRESSURE

This is perhaps the most important single aspect of neurosurgical nursing to be understood, since it can affect many other aspects of care and is life-threatening if severe. It can occur due to any space-occupying lesion within the skull, including cerebral oedema. Cerebral oedema may occur after operation or other trauma and following any condition which compromises the cerebral circulation.

The nursing assessment for increased intracranial pressure is based upon assessment of the patient's conscious level and general neurological signs, including pulse, respiratory rate and BP. Medical notes should be scrutinized to check if the patient has papilloedema.

However, it should be noted that the occurrence of the classical neurological signs of increased intracranial pressure occur too late to detect its presence at an early enough point to be useful (Mitchell, 1982) and the only reliable method is constant monitoring of the intracranial pressure. A closed-circuit, fluid filled, pressure resistant tubing with a transducer linked to a digital monitor and/or paper recorder is used. It is calibrated in mmHg or mmH_2O. The actual intracranial pressure is detected by means of a catheter placed into one of the lateral ventricles, or the subdural, epidural or subarachnoid space. An opening in the skull will be needed to allow this (burrhole). The pressure monitor should be placed at the level of the cerebral blood vessels.

Neurosurgical patients may be at risk from increased intracranial pressure because their brain cells are already damaged or ischaemic. Compensatory mechanisms may be at their limit allowing no further accommodation (Walton, 1983).

Intraventricular cannulation may be difficult since the lateral ventricles may be very small if the brain tissue is oedematous. Subdural, epidural or subarachnoid devices may get blocked because of oedema, giving false readings.

Pressure waves

The record of intracranial pressure obtained may show three different types of waves:

- A waves are plateau waves which occur in response to sudden increases in intracranial pressure. They occur paroxysmally and are associated with headache or other signs of pressure. The pressure increases by 50–100 mmHg for 5–20 minutes. These waves are of great clinical significance and they may be accompanied by hyperventilation.
- B waves are short duration intracranial pressure waves. They are rhythmical and occur at ½–2 per minute. They do indicate changes of pressure-volume relationships but are of less clinical significance than A waves. They may occur in sleep and are thought to be due to periodic breathing.
- C waves occur at a rate of 4–8 per minute and correlate with normal fluctuations of the systemic arterial pressure (Meyer, 1979).

Compliance/elastance

If one considers the skull to be a closed box, changes of volume within the skull have

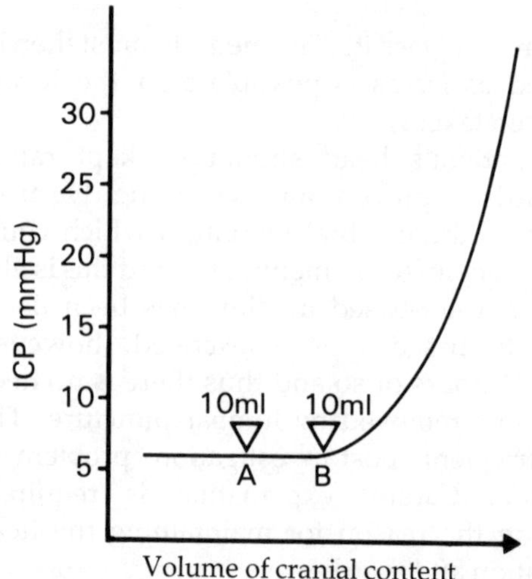

Fig. 18.8 Principle of elastance shown by response in terms of pressure to the addition of 10 ml of fluid. Addition of 10 ml of fluid at A causes no or minimal increase in ICP; at B, however, there is a significant increase (after Snyder, 1983)

pressure consequences and vice versa. It is these relationships which are used to estimate the compensatory mechanisms which are still possible and therefore the degree of risk to the patient from any further increase in pressure. Two concepts are important: compliance and elastance. Compliance is defined as the change in volume which occurs in response to a change in pressure, whilst elastance is the change in pressure which occurs as a consequence of a change in volume.

$$\text{Therefore: Compliance} = \frac{\text{change in volume}}{\text{change in pressure}}$$

$$\text{Elastance} = \frac{\text{change in pressure}}{\text{change in volume}}$$

High elastance is dangerous since it means that compensating mechanisms are exhausted.

Volume-pressure relationships can be measured. The volume pressure response (VPR) test (Miller & Garibi, 1972) is measured by identifying the immediate intracranial pressure response to a known volume of saline injected over one second. A VPR of two or more is significant. As an example: if 2 ml of saline were injected in 1 second and the response was a rise of 4 mmHg pressure (4 torr), then the VPR would be 4/2 = 2.

An alternative method of measuring the danger to the patient is by the use of the pressure volume index of Marmarou (PVI) (Marmarou et al, 1978). This is defined as the volume which must be added to produce a tenfold increase in intracranial pressure. The reader will be relieved to know that one does not actually attempt to produce a tenfold increase but a formula is used to extrapolate. This is

$$PVI = \frac{V}{\log P_p / P_o}$$

where P_p is peak pressure
and P_o is baseline pressure.

Supposing the baseline pressure was 10 torr (10 mmHg) and 0.5 ml saline was injected. The response was peak pressure of 20 torr. Then PVI would be:

$$\frac{0.5}{\log 20/10} = \frac{0.5}{\log^2} = \frac{0.5}{0.30} = 1.67$$

This means that only 1.67 ml of fluid are needed by this patient to raise intracranial pressure by a factor of 10. Therefore elastance is high. The normal PVI for an adult is 25 ml.

The major problem of increased intracranial pressure with high elastance is the danger to cerebral perfusion pressure. Without adequate blood perfusion of cerebral cells, neuronal death occurs.

The cerebral perfusion pressure is the mean BP minus the mean intracranial pressure.

Mean intracranial pressure (calculated in same way as mean BP) =

$$\frac{\text{systolic ICP} - \text{diastolic ICP}}{3} + \text{diastolic ICP}$$

Treatment

The goals of treatment are:

- early detection of increased intracranial pressure, but especially of reduced compliance, increased elastance
- to remove cause of increased intracranial pressure
- reduction by temporary measures of the intracranial pressure to levels which allow adequate blood perfusion
- prevention of transient sudden increase of intracranial pressure in patients caused by nursing care or other environmental stimuli.

Increased intracranial pressure is called intracranial hypertension. Treatment is indicated in patients whose baseline pressure reading rises to 20–25 torr, patients who have pressure waves (A waves) occurring more than one an hour and higher than 20–25 torr, or when a single wave is present exceeding 30 torr (Mitchell, 1982).

General aspects

The following aspects of management deal with general maintenance of certain homeostatic parameters:

- hypoxaemia and hypercapnia must be prevented or corrected
- the systemic BP must be maintained
- systemic hypertension must be treated
- fluid replacement using non-osmotic IV fluids must be avoided
- serum electrolytes and osmolality must be monitored.

Specific treatment

1. If possible the cause of the increased intracranial pressure is corrected surgically. This may involve the removal of a space-occupying lesion or the correction of an abnormality blocking the free flow of CSF, for example. Such operations are major and require preparation. Other methods of reducing intracranial pressure are used until surgical correction can be carried out. In cases where surgical intervention is not possible, more conservative methods are used to aid the physiological compensatory methods until the problem resolves itself (or otherwise).
2. Hyperosmotic substances such as mannitol 20% (Miller & Leech, 1975), urea or glycerol are used provided that the patient has an intact blood-brain barrier, otherwise the substance will cross into the brain, increasing brain oedema. Mannitol is most

frequently used as it carries the least risk of rebound swelling. Usually it is administered intravenously over 30–60 minutes as 500ml of 20% solution. Alternatively it can be administered as 50–100g IV (dose 0.5–1.5g/kg of body weight). Mannitol tends to crystallize and should be administered using a blood filter. It can be immersed in warm water prior to use to dissolve crystals or the unit can be placed in a warming jacket during administration. It is effective within 5–15 minutes of administration for several hours. When mannitol or any other hyperosmotic substance is used serum osmolality must not be allowed to rise to 315mosmol/l or more, otherwise renal failure will occur with the risk of seizures which would further compromise cerebral function through the increased demand created by high levels of cell metabolism.

3. Frusemide or other diuretics may be ordered.
4. Dexamethasone 5 mg 4-hourly is used to prevent increased intracranial pressure. It takes 12 hours before it is effective (Walton, 1983).
5. Coma may be induced by the administration of large doses of barbiturates (Ricci, 1979). This acts by reducing the metabolic requirements of brain cells and cerebral blood flow. It also reduces the patient's response to environmental stimuli. Patients treated in this way will require the intensive nursing appropriate to unconscious patients.
6. Hypothermia may also be induced to lower the metabolic requirements of brain cells, especially in children. Pancuronium and morphine sulphate may be used as adjuncts to hypothermia or barbiturate coma to decrease the responsiveness of skeletal muscle and central nervous tissues to procedures such as suctioning or turning.
7. If there is a catheter within the lateral ventricle (to measure intracranial pressure) then cerebrospinal fluid may be drained off from the head intermittently. Alternatively it may be drained continuously against positive pressure.

Nursing care

It is usual to nurse a patient with increased intracranial pressure with the head of the bed raised at an angle of 15–30°. Flattening of the head of the bed has been shown to increase ICP. It should be noted that transient increased ICP is not dangerous in itself. We all experience such transient increase during coughing, sneezing, straining during defaecation, etc. Compensatory mechanisms quickly reduce the pressure under normal circumstances. The neurological patient, however, may be at risk from such increases because the brain cells may already be damaged or ischaemic, cerebral blood flow may be altered and compensatory mechanisms may be impaired. Apart from the activities mentioned above, many nursing activities have been shown to increase intracranial pressure in vulnerable patients. These include turning, flexion, extension and rotation of the head (Lipe & Mitchell, 1980); tracheal suction; positive end expiratory pressure respiration; the use of the prone position; and combining several activities in succession. It is worth noting this last point, particularly since it is common to attempt to carry out many nursing activities for the same patient at one time 'to avoid disturbing him'! It has also been found that speaking over the patient's bed without including him/her in the conversation increases intracranial pressure, as does emotionally disturbing conversation (Mitchell & Mauss, 1978).

Patient activities which affect the pressure include chewing, coughing, REM sleep, periodic breathing and restlessness.

It follows that nursing care should be given in a way which minimizes rises in intracranial pressure (Johnson, 1983). Extreme sudden stimuli must be avoided (Johnson, 1983). Movement of the patient's head must be carried out very carefully. If pressure is higher than expected after the patient's position has been changed, then a further adjustment of position should be tried. All nursing care should be explained carefully before it is given. Constipation must be avoided. Suction should be carried out in several short periods of 15–20 secs rather than long periods (Mitchell et al, 1980).

It is worth noting that signs of decreasing compliance and high elastance can be detected by observing the pressure response to nursing care on the monitor. If the response lags, giving a rounded upward sweep rather than a straight vertical line, it indicates low compliance (Portnoy & Clopp, 1980).

NURSING PROBLEMS

Environment for care

Henderson (1960) has stated that one aspect of the role of the nurse is to be the consciousness of the unconscious. This can be translated into action specifically in relation to the unconscious patient's inability to respond to the environment. Nursing care involves being conscious of the ways in which the environment could potentially harm the patient, and preventing harm by constant vigilance. This aspect of awareness is also important in relation to patients who are paralysed, suffering from sensory loss, confused patients, and patients with mobility problems.

Care needed in respect of extreme environmental stimuli acting upon patients with increased intracranial pressure has already been mentioned. Similar considerations pertain to patients who have irritation of the meninges.

Patients with disturbances of temperature control, open skull fractures and loss of protective reflexes (with or without loss of consciousness) are also particularly susceptible to environmental stimuli which would not in any way threaten an intact individual. Assessment of the environment should be carried out regularly when such vulnerable patients have been admitted to hospital. This includes noting the temperature of objects and liquids in the vicinity of the patient, care with sharp or rough objects, electrical apparatus, and so on. Whenever a patient who cannot speak is having medicinal gases administered, especial care must be taken to ensure that the type of gas and the rate of administration are appropriate.

In modern hospitals the thermal gain from glazed windows may be excessive, causing the environmental temperature to soar on sunny days. Patients who have disturbances of temperature regulation must be protected from this.

Care should be taken with open windows and fans for patients who have lost their corneal reflex.

Any patient with a head or spinal wound is at risk from infection which could track into the central nervous system. Therefore strict aseptic techniques and reverse barrier nursing are needed for vulnerable patients.

When patients with mobility problems are relearning skills of sitting, walking or standing, care is needed to ensure the correct choice of furniture, floor material and mobility aids. Signs which label toilets, bathrooms, and day rooms etc., must be large and clear.

Assessment of environmental stimulation should be made in relation to the optimum level of environmental stimulation for that individual patient. A patient with meningism or intracranial hypertension will require a low level of environmental stimulation whilst an elderly patient following a stroke may require a higher level (Myco, 1983).

Finally, the total environment in which the patient is being nursed should be considered in relation to his/her needs. For example, a critically ill patient requires a safe environment above all, and this is what should be provided. On the other hand, to a patient who has a long-term chronic illness such as multiple sclerosis but who has to be in hospital for social reasons, the ward is home and should be as stimulating and comfortable as possible. It is legitimate for safety in relation to choice of furniture, floor covering, etc., to give way to the prime consideration that the patient's life should be normalized, including taking decisions for him/herself.

Respiratory problems

Problems of respiration will be considered first since they are fairly common among neuromedical/neurosurgical patients and may be life threatening if they are not recognized and dealt with (Sanford, 1982).

Possible respiratory problems include respiratory arrest, acute obstruction of the airways,

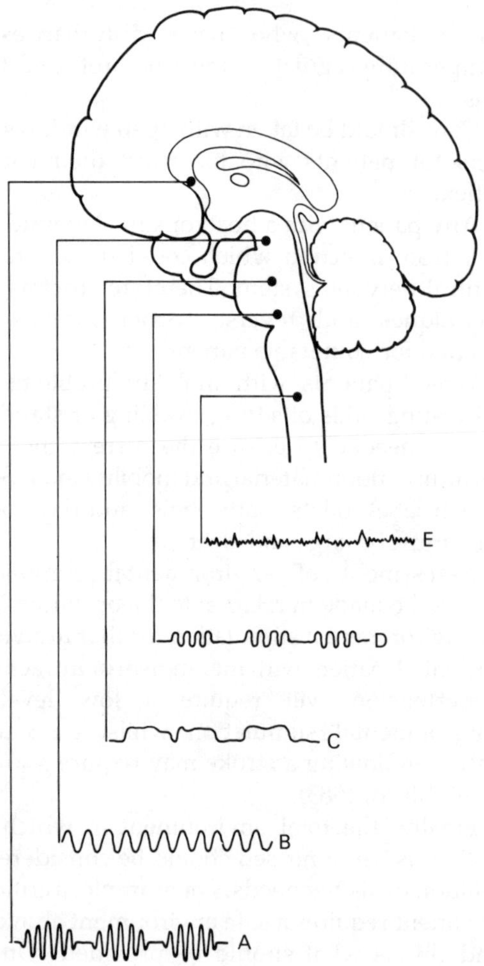

Fig. 18.9 Patterns of abnormal breathing associated with different brain lesion sites (A) Cheyne-Stokes respiration associated with lesions deep inside cerebral hemisphere (B) Central neurogenic hyperpnoea associated with lesions in lower mid-brain to middle pons area (C) Apneusis associated with lesions in lower and middle pons area and extensive brain damage (D) Cluster breathing associated with lesions in upper medulla (E) Ataxia. Irregular and random breaths and pulse associated with lesions in lower medulla (adapted from Johnson L V 1983)

respiratory infection, atelectasis, ventilation/perfusion mismatch, pulmonary oedema, paralysis or weakness of the muscles of respiration. Hypoxaemia, hypercapnia and hypocapnia may occur as a result of respiratory problems and will further jeopardize any brain cells which are already at risk from the primary condition.

Nursing recognition of potential or actual problems may be through the nursing history or by direct observation and assessment of respiratory function. Any patient who has developed a neurological problem and who has a history of chronic bronchitis or emphysema will be at risk of developing a chest infection. It should also be remembered that bronchial carcinoma is a site from which secondaries frequently metastasize to the brain. Unconscious and semiconscious patients in particular are vulnerable to the development of partial or total obstruction of the respiratory airway.

Obstruction/arrest

Noisy respirations must always be recognized immediately and investigated since they indicate respiratory obstruction in some degree. Careful counting and recording of the patient's respiratory rate is important. The pattern of respirations should also be noted. Is the pattern regular? Are the respirations of uniform depth? Are the muscular movements equal on each side? Is the diaphragm being used properly in respirations? Are accessory muscles of respiration being used? The patient's colour should be noted and any cynanosis recorded, but hypoxaemia or hypercapnia can exist without obvious changes and so medical staff will monitor blood gas levels in vulnerable patients. Monitoring of the patient's temperature will show any pyrexia which may indicate chest infection.

Respiratory arrest may occur if the respiratory centre in the brain stem is affected by lack of oxygen and/or glucose, or if its blood supply is affected. This may occur due to pressure effects from lesions elsewhere within the cranium (Mitchell & Mauss, 1976). Artificial respiration will be required as an emergency measure until medical staff can institute medical management of the patient's condition.

Respiratory obstruction may occur through blockage by a foreign body if the patient should lose consciousness suddenly. In an unconscious patient the tongue can fall back, so if there is any risk of this occurring the patient should be nursed in the semi-prone position or must have an airway inserted. Regurgitation of the stomach contents, respiratory secretions, even excessive salivation may cause problems in a patient who has lost swallowing and cough reflex. Laryngeal spasm may also occlude the airway, as may bleeding following a carotid angiogram, if that has been performed by injection directly into the carotid artery in the neck. Immediately any degree of obstruction has been recognized and the cause ascertained, the obstruction should be removed if possible by positioning the patient, employing suction, etc. If the problem cannot be reversed by these means then, provided the obstruction is partial, oxygen should be given until the medical officer can carry out an endotracheal intubation or a tracheostomy.

Infection

Respiratory infection may occur, not only because the patient is at special risk due to pre-existing chest problems, but because of poor ventilation of the lungs during bed rest, depression of conscious level, or weakness of respiratory muscles. Mouth infections or regurgitation of stomach secretions can also lead to a risk of chest infection, as can depression of the ciliary activity of the respiratory endothelium or depression of the cough reflex. Prevention involves the physiotherapist who should teach the patient deep breathing (if conscious). Postural drainage and physical movement of secretions by shaking or percussion of the chest wall may also be carried out. Postural drainage in the head down position may not be possible since it increases intracranial pressure. Antibiotics will be prescribed for patients with chest infection. Good suction technique to prevent trauma to the respiratory endothelium, and to prevent the carriage of infection from the mouth or nose downward, is essential. If the patient has a tracheostomy or an endotracheal tube, humidification of respiratory gases may be required to aid the removal of particulate matter along the airways.

Hypoxaemia, hypocapnia, hypercapnia

Hypoxaemia, hypocapnia or hypercapnia may arise as a consequence of any of the conditions mentioned already. If so, a tracheostomy may be performed to reduce respiratory dead space. The administration of prescribed amounts of O_2 and physiotherapy may be ordered to correct hypoxaemia and hyperapnia. A positive pressure respirator may be used to ensure adequate lung ventilation. The type of choice is often a positive end expiratory pressure respirator (Sanford, 1982). Hypoxaemia can be the additional factor leading to brain cell death and it must be corrected as a matter of urgency. Hypercapnia leads to dilatation of cerebral blood vessels which in turn can increase intracranial pressure to a critical level in a patient who is at the limit of compensatory mechanisms (Walton, 1983).

Ventilation/perfusion mismatch

Ventilation/perfusion mismatch is thought to occur as a direct consequence of increased intracranial pressure. It is suggested that it is initiated by intense sympathetic discharge (Cohen et al, 1977). This decreases pulmonary compliance by altering the surfactant in the alveoli.

It is possible that a further factor operates, as adrenergic stimulation causes intense peripheral vasoconstriction. The consequent increased peripheral resistance forces blood into the relatively low pressure pulmonary circulation, giving increased pulmonary capillary pressure. The vasoconstrictive agent, however, affects pulmonary venules, leading to capillary pooling. This damages pulmonary vessels. Fluid leaks into the alveoli causing pulmonary oedema (Moss, 1976).

If this mechanism is thought to be a potential problem, adrenergic blocking agents may be ordered as well as phenytoin. Obviously the prevention or treatment of increased intracranial pressure will be the most effective method of preventing this problem.

Paralysis or weakness of respiratory muscles

Paralysis or weakness of respiratory muscles may occur in the presence of cervical or thoracic spinal cord damage, and in poliomyelitis and myasthenia gravis. In spinal cord lesions the respiratory muscle weakness leads to reduced lung volumes and capacity, poor O_2 exchange and CO_2 retention. Lack of muscle power reduces the patient's ability to cough and to blow his/her nose. There is a decline in lung compliance and elastic recoil. Coughing and deep breathing exercises are taught by the physiotherapist. The patient may have to be assisted to cough hourly, so the nurse must learn the technique from the physiotherapist. It consists of sitting the patient well forward and putting one's arms round the patient at the level of the lower ribs/diaphragm, from behind, and clasping them over the patient's diaphragm. The nurse presses the diaphragm as the patient breathes out and attempts to cough (Lavigne, 1979). It may be necessary for assisted respirations to be started using a volume respirator. Breathing can be assisted by the use of a rocking bed. A motor automatically and alternately raises the head and then the foot of the bed at the rate and to the angle prescribed for the patient. In the head up position, the abdominal organs fall from the diaphragm allowing diaphragmatic expansion of the chest volume. When the foot is raised the abdominal organs move upwards forcing the diaphragm upwards. This expels air from the lungs. The patient must be taught to breathe in as the head is raised and out as the foot of the bed is raised. Problems which may be created by the use of this bed include dizziness, insomnia, and loss of appetite.

In myasthenia gravis the patient may suffer sudden crises in which respirations are in jeopardy with dyspnoea, nasal flaring and respiratory distress. If this occurs a nurse must stay with the patient to assure him/her of help. The emergency equipment with Ambu bag, respirator and emergency tracheostomy set will be required, together with syringes and needles for the administration of drugs. The crisis can be due to the disease itself, in which case neostigmine will be administered. It may also, however, be due to sudden spontaneous improvement in the patient's condition. In this case the cholinergic drugs he/she has been given for treatment swamp the system and atropine will be administered (Mastrian, 1984).

Nursing care

Whenever the patient's respirations are in jeopardy he/she will require assurance that something is being done to help. This is an element of care which is as important as the physical measures taken to remedy the problem.

Nurses who work with acutely ill neuromedical or neurosurgical patients need to understand the importance of the correct blood levels of respiratory gases for the patient's survival. The dynamics of the respiratory system should also be well understood. Respirators are frequently in use with neurological patients and nursing staff must be skilled in the management of both the patient and the apparatus. It is literally a matter of life or death for the patient.

After the acute phase of the respiratory problem is over, the patient will need to learn gradually to manage without the artificial support of a ventilator. Again patience and reassurance through the constant presence of a nurse will be needed as the patient learns first to cope in the daytime with longer and longer periods off the ventilator. Later he/she will learn to sleep without it. A similar rehabilitation regime will be required after tracheostomy. This may be plugged off for increasing periods of time until the patient can manage sufficiently well for it to be removed. Occasionally keloid scarring may cause problems at the site of a tracheostomy, so it is important that early wound care is meticulously carried out.

Cardiovascular problems

From what has been said above about the importance to the viability of normal tissue of the cerebral perfusion pressure, it follows that any general cardiovascular problem may add to neurological problems, even though there are physiologically different arrangements for the control of cerebral blood vessels and blood vessels elsewhere. Consequently staff must be aware of general cardiovascular problems (such as shock due to haemorrhage, or pre-existing mild heart failure, for example). General measures to control such problems must be instituted.

There is some evidence that cerebral lesions affect the cardiovascular system, and this is particularly so in any condition which affects the cardiac or pressure controlling centres. The result may be hypertension, hypotension, or cardiac arrhythmias (McCarthy, 1982). Some cardiovascular conditions, for example atherosclerosis, include a high risk of concomitant cerebrovascular lesions such as subarachnoid haemorrhage, stroke, or embolus (Myco, 1983).

Disturbance of motor function

Disturbance of motor function is very common amongst patients following stroke, spinal cord injury, accompanying cerebral space occupying lesions, multiple sclerosis, and myasthenia gravis, as well as less common conditions.

The aims of care are:

- to prevent joint stiffness which could lead to joint rigidity through ectopic calcification
- to prevent muscular contracture which could lead to shortening of connective tissue and permanent contracture deformity
- to prevent abnormal reflex activity
- to facilitate normal motor response
- to facilitate mobility
- to facilitate functional independence
- to maintain or help restoration of normal body image.

The most common problems of motor function seen in neuromedical or surgical nursing are disturbances of control rather than true muscular weakness (Dardier, 1980). Disturbance of control invariably results in exaggeration of postural and tonic reflexes. Consequently patients have problems of posture and balance, difficulty in co-ordinating movement, difficulty in carrying out fine movement and an inability to carry out isolated movements.

True muscular weakness comprising flaccidity, loss of tone, and loss of muscle bulk is seen rarely. It occurs when there is a lower motor neurone lesion (e.g. peripheral nerve damage, severe prolapsed intervertebral disc, poliomyelitis (Rudy, 1984)). Some loss of tone is also involved when there is a cerebellar lesion; however, there are also postural problems and problems of fine movements in this case.

Physiotherapists and occupational therapists are the specialists who teach the patient to maintain and improve muscular function. Nursing staff should understand the work of such therapists and co-operate. Nursing staff are with the patient in hospital continuously whilst members of the remedial professions usually work only from 9 to 5, Monday to Friday. Unless nursing staff understand the principles of care and can help to motivate the patient to carry out exercises in between the physiotherapist's visits, a great deal of harm may result for the patient. This can happen through allowing the patient to get into bad habits by positioning the patient badly or by doing for the patient things he/she should be doing for him/herself.

The most important thing a nurse can do for a patient with regard to movement is to learn from the physiotherapist how to position the patient, how to help the patient to move and what exercises and activities the patient should carry out so that the nurse can remind the patient to practise them. Motivating the patient by praise when he/she achieves the goals which have been set is important. Correcting the patient if he/she carries out exercises incorrectly is also important, so he/she is not allowed to get into bad habits. Psychologically, praise for achievement is more effective than scolding.

Some principles of positioning and moving patients can be stated (Dardier, 1980). These are based on what we know about reflexes which are released when cerebral centres controlling movement are affected. These are relevant to patients with brain lesions affecting movement on one side of the body (hemiplegia) rather than to paraplegic patients. Use is made of such knowledge to prevent contracture and deformity.

When a patient is unconscious or paralysed and so has no ability to move, it is important to take each affected joint through a full range of passive movements. In carrying out passive movements and positioning the patient, no joint must be stretched beyond its normal range.

The patient's resting position must be such that it does *not* reinforce the dominant spasticity (Bobath, 1971).

Positioning and moving the patient

Positioning the patient into the supine

position (Dardier, 1980). The head should be supported with the neck slightly flexed using one pillow only to prevent the initiation of the tonic labyrinthine reflex (Bobath, 1977). A pillow should be placed under the affected arm to draw the scapula forward around the chest wall. The lower limbs should be placed with a small pillow under the knees to prevent hyperextension and a pillow or roll of blanket by the side of the leg to prevent external rotation. A bed cradle should be used to keep the weight of bedclothes from the legs. No support should be given to the sole of the foot or it may stimulate reflex extension of the hip and knee with plantar flexion of the ankle. This would create great difficulty for walking later.

If the patient's head must be turned to one side then it should be turned toward the affected side. This then makes use of asymmetrical tonic neck reflexes, and increases the extensor tone of the affected upper limb thus counteracting the tendency to hyperactivity of the flexors in the upper limb.

If sensory loss or hemianopia is a problem then staff and relatives should be asked to approach the patient from the affected side. This should be explained to the patient. It is to help him/her to relearn awareness on the affected side.

Use of the lateral position (Dardier, 1980).

Lying on the unaffected side. Obviously if the patient has a problem of mobility he/she cannot lie supine the whole time or he/she will develop pressure sores or chest infection, etc. Therefore he/she will have to be moved from side to side.

The position in which the patient should be placed when lying on the unaffected side will be described.

If his/her head is to be raised this should be done by raising the head of the bed rather than using a lot of pillows. Only one pillow should be used under the patient's head, which should be supported in normal alignment in relation to the trunk and shoulders. A pillow may be placed at his/her back longitudinally pressed against the rib cage to help the maintenance of position.

The uppermost arm (affected arm) should be placed on a pillow at right angles to the chest. His elbow and wrist should be semi-extended and the wrist and hand supinated. The unaffected (underneath) arm should be comfortable. The affected lower limb should be supported on a pillow to maintain a natural position of abduction at the hip, slight flexion of knee, dorsiflexion at ankle and slight eversion of the foot.

The good leg should be straight or partially flexed and placed slightly behind the uppermost leg to prevent the pelvis from rolling back.

Lying on the affected side. In this position there is constant sensory stimulation to the affected side and this is beneficial.

The position is similar to that described above except that the affected area should be drawn forward and lie partially extended, fully supported on a pillow.

Changing position. To change the patient's position, the patient should be rolled and encouraged to help as soon as possible. His/her head should be supported only if the neck is completely flaccid and support is necessary. Initiation of rolling should be by moving the patient's shoulder girdle and pelvis in the desired direction.

First the patient should be moved to the side of the bed. The arm which is to be uppermost should be supported from wrist to elbow with a helper's arm. The nurse's other hand should be placed behind the scapula, and the shoulder girdle gently moved toward the nurse. If righting reflexes are present then the pelvis and leg will follow the shoulder. If not, the leg which will be uppermost should be bent and supported over by another nurse.

Limbs must *never* be pulled.

If the pelvis is used to initiate rolling then the leg which will be uppermost is supported in a flexed position from the ankle to the knee on the nurse's lower arm. The other hand is placed below the pelvis and the patient is rolled gently.

Range of movement exercises. These are difficult to describe meaningfully. Since it is important that they are carried out correctly the reader should learn how to perform this skill from a physiotherapist, first by watching, then by working under the supervision of the physiotherapist. The aim of such exercises for the upper limb and shoulder girdle is to promote mobility, whilst the aim for the lower limb is to maintain and encourage stability. The reader is referred to Dardier (1980), to Myco (1983) and to Chapter 13 for more information.

Sitting on a chair. The choice of chair to be used by the patient is important. It should give good support to the back and allow the feet to reach the floor with knees, hips and ankles at right angles.

When sitting, the body weight of the patient should be evenly distributed on both buttocks. The head and trunk should be aligned with each other with the midline. The affected arm should be forward at the shoulder and supported by pillows on a side table.

Standing. When the patient stands he/she should be reminded to hold his/her head in the midline, looking straight ahead with the chin well up. The affected leg must be properly placed with the whole foot in contact with the floor.

Transferring from the bed to a chair (Dardier, 1980). First the patient should be helped to roll on to the affected side. He/she should then be helped to sit using the affected side for weight bearing. His/her legs are then swung over the side of the bed. He/she then stands before sitting in the chair.

Important points to remember are to be gentle, to support the patient's limbs and never to pull.

The paraplegic patient with spinal cord injury

Detail has been given of the patient with hemiplegia. Hemiplegia frequently results from 'stroke' and this is one of the most frequent problems for which patients are admitted to hospital.

However, nurses may also encounter patients with paraplegia or tetraplegia. The most severe form of this is encountered in patients with severe spinal cord injury. Fortunately the condition is comparatively rare and patients are likely to be transferred to special spinal units after the immediate danger to the patient's life has subsided.

During the acute phase nursing principles are those mentioned earlier: to prevent deformity of limbs by careful positioning. The physiotherapist should advise on this and also initiate passive movement. Prevention of pressure sores is also of great concern at this time. Later care in developing mobility calls for intensive work by the physiotherapist and occupational therapist. A focus of concern will be the development of the ability to sit and balance. In the case of the paraplegic patient the power of the arms and shoulder girdle is developed.

Disturbance of sensory function (touch, temperature and kinaesthesia)

The extent of any loss of sensory function should be carefully assessed and recorded. There is no method of actively helping recovery. All one can do is to prevent further problems from arising whilst sensory loss is present and help the patient to adjust and cope with residual loss when progress becomes so slow as to be imperceptible.

Principles of care

Principles of care are:

- To avoid injury to the skin by taking care with hot, cold, sharp, or rough objects within the vicinity of the patient.
- Positioning of the patient is particularly important to ensure that no stretching or contracture of muscles and joints occurs.
- Prevention of pressure sores is also crucial as vasomotor reflexes may be affected, increasing the patient's vulnerability to pressure. Great care is needed when touching and moving the patient to prevent accidental injury to tissues.
- Whenever the affected part is being touched or moved it is vital to warn the patient and to ask him/her to concentrate to see if he/she can begin to develop awareness (Dardier, 1980).
- As far as possible, the patient should be encouraged to use the affected part of the body. Staff and visitors should be encouraged to approach the patient from the affected side, since there is a danger that the part may be neglected or denied

unless the patient is made aware of it (Myco, 1983).

This latter point is particularly important for patients who have a distortion of their body image which is associated with the brain lesion and does not arise solely from the lost sensation.

Especial care should be taken when the patient is sitting in a chair, to place limbs correctly and maintain the approach from the affected side. Overall levels of sensory input must be monitored to ensure that optimum levels of stimulation are provided.

Above all the patient will require encouragement and praise to motivate him/her to cope with what is a very distressing condition. When it becomes obvious that little or no further improvement will take place, a great deal of patient teaching will be needed to ensure that the patient can cope with his/her own skin care and positioning.

Confusion; memory loss; aggression or agitation

Again, the major aim of care is to prevent complications from occurring until some recovery occurs, but also to structure the environment in a way which is helpful to the patient.

It is important to identify all sources of stimulation and to adjust total levels of stimulation to an optimum level for the patient, with clear contrast between day and night. Stimuli should be structured. Activities throughout the 24 hour cycle should occur at regular times and the patient should be kept informed of the time as each activity occurs and reminded about the next activity. A memory board can be used to aid this process if the patient's visual acuity is satisfactory. A clock and a calendar should also be provided. It is important to ensure that the patient is in a room with outside windows, so that daylight enters to help orientation to the difference between day and night.

A limited number of regular staff should be allocated to care for the patient so that helpful relationships can be built up. As far as possible, staff with calm personalities should be used, each developing a consistent approach. It is worth providing music of a kind liked by the patient, but choosing the quieter, more soothing pieces within the general repertoire (Brigman et al, 1983).

In interaction, short sentences with simple words, clearly enunciated, should be employed. Each member of staff should say who they are on approach and the patient should be addressed by his or her correct name and title. Confusions should be corrected as they occur. The patient should be reminded of the date and the day and the weather can be reported to him/her (Brigman et al, 1983).

If aggression or agitation is a problem then careful observation is needed to identify circumstances which trigger such behaviour. This should be recorded so that such circumstances can be avoided or modified.

Brigman et al (1983) have described a method of nursing a patient who was very aggressive, restless and self-destructive. This involved nursing the patient on a mattress placed on the floor, surrounded by mattresses standing up around the floor mattress in a locked unit. Mittens were placed on the patient's hands to prevent him from tampering with tubing. These had to be removed from time to time to allow finger exercises.

In dealing with such a patient Brigman et al (1983) argue that a calm, confident approach is needed by staff and there should always be at least two or three staff in attendance. Each person present should speak to the patient so that he/she realizes there is more than one person there. Eye contact should be used, and if the patient appears threatening, state 'I am not going to allow you to hurt me'. Attention must always be directed at the patient and clear explanations of what is to be done must be given. It is important not to laugh or joke in case this is interpreted as laughing or joking at the patient.

The relatives of a patient who has memory loss or a personality change will need a great deal of understanding and support. They should be taught about what to do and to say so that their approach is consistent with that of staff. If their visits can be made at a time which is consistent with the daily routine and included on the memory board, this is helpful.

It is extremely upsetting if the patient no longer recognizes a relative, forgets incidents in the past, suddenly appears aggressive, or perhaps loses rigid standards of behaviour which were a consistent part of his/her personality. A great deal of explanation, counselling and support will be needed if the relatives are to be able to cope with the situation.

Speech problems

The speech therapist will be the most important professional in the treatment of the patient with a problem with speech. Often, however, the time of this expert is at a premium. For consistency, nursing staff should learn from the speech therapist the approach which is needed with the particular patient so that it can be continued between therapy sessions.

In caring for a patient with dysphasia or aphasia the following points should be noted. Time and patience are required, whilst showing respect toward the patient as an individual. Attention should be paid to the choice of sound environment for any interaction between nurse and patient, so that it occurs during quiet and without background distractions or masking noises.

Non-verbal gestures can be used to reinforce what is being said, provided that their meaning is clear and consistent. In talking with the patient simple sentences and simple words should be used. It is better to use words in common usage rather than rare ones. In using nouns, objects to which they refer can be pointed out. When asking the patient a question it should be phrased in such a way that it is impossible to answer with a 'yes' or 'no' unless the patient's progress is so poor that this approach causes great distress and frustration to him. In that case it is important to help him to communicate in any way possible. Anticipation of the patient's needs should be increasingly withdrawn as progress is made. If anticipation is used too accurately and frequently it may preclude the need for speech and thus retard the relearning process.

It goes without saying that all patients must be treated as adults and the temptation to shout must be avoided. Clear articulation is important however. If what the patient has said cannot be understood, this should be made clear with no pretence (Myco, 1983). Prompting the patient to practise skills which are being developed by the speech therapist is useful. Giving praise for small achievements and progress is helpful in motivating the patient to persist in his/her efforts. The patient's relatives should be included in the process of helping with speech, and they may need both support and positive teaching, since eventually they may have to take over the role of caring for the patient (Myco, 1983).

Problems of nutrition and fluid intake

Special consideration of the nutritional and fluid status of patients with a neuromedical or neurosurgical condition is frequently necessary. Confused, drowsy patients may eat or drink amounts which are quite inadequate for their needs. Any patient who has an impaired swallowing reflex must be fed by nasogastric tube or parenterally. This, of course, includes unconscious patients. Since nutritional and fluid status may be problematic, it follows that careful initial assessment and continued monitoring of the patient's condition with reference to these dimensions is required.

Nutrition

Methods of assessing an individual's nutritional status include weighing, measuring skinfold thickness and upper arm circumference and carrying out an estimation of urinary N_2 excretion levels. The former two methods are within the competence of the nurse.

For patients who are able to take food and fluid by mouth, the presentation of food is important. By giving help with feeding as necessary and carefully observing the amount and nutritional value of food actually eaten it is possible to prevent protein-calorie deficiency with the possible consequent delay in the patient's recovery (Coates, 1982).

For patients who are being tube-fed, the nutritional content of the food should be calculated carefully in co-operation with the dietician. Any feed which is not given or not absorbed for any reason must be reported so that the nutrients can be administered in some other way (Jones, 1975). If a patient is unconscious for any length of time it is likely that the initial intravenous infusion will be replaced by nasogastric feeding, although parenteral nutrition is a possibility. When administering a nasogastric feed the following points should be noted:

- Using gentle aspiration, a check should be made before the administration of the feed to ensure that the previous feed has been absorbed. If it has not, then the presence of bowel sounds must be ascertained. Provided they are present, the reason for the non-absorption of the previous feed must be sought, e.g., length of time which has elapsed, position of the patient since last feed, type of feed given. If bowel sounds are absent medical staff will be informed as this indicates paralytic ileus.
- A careful check should be made to ensure that the end of the nasogastric tube rests within the stomach before the feed is given (Clarke, 1983).
- Administration of tube feeds should be carefully co-ordinated with any turning or other position changing programme, so that the patient's position is changed before the feed and not immediately afterwards. If possible the patient should be nursed in the head up position for one hour after the feed has been given.
- If diarrhoea should occur, it is useful to consult the dietician so that the type of feed can be changed.

Feeding a patient by mouth. When feeding a patient by mouth who has a facial weakness, or who is relearning to eat after having had tube feeds, it is important to ensure that the person helping the patient allocates plenty of time and ensures that it is a pleasant and rewarding experience for the patient. Pains should be taken to provide food which the patient likes and it should be attractively presented. If the meal is a hot one, small portions only should be presented whilst the remainder is kept hot until needed. The patient should be made physically comfortable before the meal and should be sitting up well at a table or in bed. A mouthwash given before the meal helps to refresh the mouth, and dentures should be in position. Some authorities (Cockcroft & Ray, 1985) advocate that sucking ice immediately before a meal helps to stimulate palatal movement.

As food is placed in the patient's mouth the swallowing reflex can be stimulated by gentle, slight pressure on the tongue with the spoon or fork. If the food is to be chewed then chewing may be stimulated by placing the food on the back teeth (Cockcroft & Ray, 1985).

If the patient has a facial weakness, the food should be placed into the good side of the mouth. One should get the patient to explore his/her mouth with his/her tongue (if possible) to ensure that food does not get trapped in the cheek on the weak side (Myco, 1983). Cockcroft & Ray (1985) suggest that the nurse or therapist should stand slightly behind the patient who has difficulty with jaw movement and use a jaw grip with one hand to help in the opening and closing of the patient's mouth during feeding. A record should be kept of the patient's food intake.

Patients should be encouraged to feed themselves as soon as possible with the use of aids supplied by the occupational therapy department. Food which can be eaten with the fingers is useful. Paper tissues and a receptacle for used ones should be supplied.

Paralytic ileus. This was mentioned above with relation to tube feeding but it is a comparatively frequent complication in the acute stage following spinal cord injury (Rudy, 1984). Signs include distended abdomen and loss of bowel sounds. Monitoring should be carried out every eight hours to ensure that intestinal sounds are present, since the patient will not necessarily be aware of symptoms due to sensory loss. Unless the development of the condition is identified early the patient may vomit, develop electrolyte imbalance and possibly respiratory complications. Management includes the use of a nasogastric tube to aspirate the contents of the stomach and an intravenous infusion to maintain hydration. A rectal tube may be used to remove flatus. Only when bowel sounds have returned should oral feeding be reinstated.

The possibility that a patient with acute neurological disorder may develop a peptic ulcer due to stress should be kept in mind (Rudy, 1984).

Fluid balance

A careful record of fluid intake and output should be kept for any patient who has difficulty in reaching liquids or feeding him/herself, or swallowing. Such a record is also needed for patients who are given dehydrating drugs or solutions to reduce or prevent increased intracranial pressure.

Assessment of a patient's fluid balance includes urine testing, especially for the specific gravity, and the identification of any signs of dehydration such as sunken eyes or alterations in skin plasticity. Medical staff will monitor serum electrolyte levels if signs of imbalance occur and will initiate the administration of intravenous fluid containing the appropriate electrolytes.

DISTURBANCES OF BOWEL FUNCTION

There are three important types of problem which may occur in patients with a neurological condition. First, straining at stool may increase blood pressure and intracranial pressure within a patient whose physiology is already compromised. Secondly, patients who are not fully conscious may develop diarrhoea or constipation. Thirdly, patients with spinal cord injury have special problems which will be discussed later.

For the first group of patients identified above, the use of stool softeners and suppositories prevents straining (Gray, 1983). Enemas should only be given on a written doctor's order since they can be dangerous in the presence of increased intracranial pressure (Rudy, 1984).

For patients with depressed levels of consciousness one of the most important nursing measures is very careful observation and recording of not only the fact of bowel movement, but the amount and consistency. A potential problem which may occur is apparent faecal incontinence which is superimposed upon constipation severe enough to have led to impacted faeces. The problem may be prevented by using stool softeners followed by the insertion of suppositories every third day.

Occasionally, as mentioned already, a patient who is being tube fed develops diarrhoea. This must be distinguished from faecal impaction with overflow. Genuine diarrhoea requires investigation to ensure that it is not due to infection. Provided that gastroenteritis can be eliminated then a change of the feed being given may solve the problem.

The usual problems of being in hospital may affect the neurological patient as any other. These include the administration of drugs which are constipating, lack of exercise, the use of positions in which defaecation is difficult, a diet which is low in fibre, general depression and embarrassment.

After a period of depressed consciousness a lengthy period of retraining may be required before the patient can cope with defaecation for him/herself.

In the management of a patient who is regaining control of the bowel after loss of conciousness or hemiplegia, it is vital to let the patient know where the toilet is and to place his/her bed or chair in such a position that he/she can reach it easily (Myco, 1983). In so placing the patient, the length of time it takes the patient to get to the toilet should be taken into consideration and he/she should be advised to allow plenty of time. He/she should also be encouraged to attempt to defaecate at the same time each day so that a routine is set up. Help must be available promptly when needed. All equipment needed to ensure cleanliness must be provided and the patient's self respect and modesty must be preserved. Nonetheless it is helpful to take discreet interest in this progress and praise achievement. Provided there are no medical contraindications the intake of plenty of fluids and dietary fibre is helpful.

Bowel dysfunction associated with spinal cord damage (Schaupner, 1982)

If the damage involves spinal cord segments or nerve pathways controlling reflex activity of the lower bowel, rectum or anal sphincter, there is difficulty in expelling hard faeces and in retaining soft faeces. Lesions at T12 downwards cause some impairment. Complete impairment occurs if the S2, 3 or 4 segments are affected. If the damage is at a higher level than this, reflex activity of the bowel is retained but it is completely disconnected from any voluntary control.

When once the site and severity of neurological damage have been assessed and the prognosis for recovery ascertained, then the task is to teach the patient to manage bowel function him/herself or to give sufficient information and awareness so that he/she can teach someone of his/her choice to cope for him/her.

Motor function of the upper limbs, the patient's ability to get on and off the toilet and his/her balance when sitting, determines whether he/she will be able to cope unassisted. Balance is helped if a bar is placed in front of the toilet seat. The patient can use it to steady him/herself. This usually requires a structural alteration to the toilet.

Aims of bowel management. The aims of bowel management, both the nursing management during the acute phase and for the patient when he takes over, are:

- that faeces should be soft and well formed
- that frequency of bowel movement should conform as much as possible to the patient's pre-injury routine but in any case should be at least once every three days
- no bowel movement should occur at unplanned times
- bowel movement should occur within one hour of a stimulus to bowel movement
- management of diet and fluids should be used to produce the correct consistency of stool
- symptoms of impaction and its treatment should be clearly understood.

Principles of management. Principles of management include the following:

1. Meals or snacks stimulate the gastrocolic reflex, moving colonic content on into the rectum and therefore bowel movement should be planned to occur within ½–1 hour after eating.
2. A stimulus to bowel movement should be provided at the same time each day. During the rehabilitation phase this may be required for four to eight weeks until training is complete.
3. The trigger or stimulus to bowel function should be chosen individually by finding out which works best with the individual. Possible stimuli include the insertion of a well-lubricated gloved finger into the rectum, touching the wall of the rectum; or the use of suppositories. Since the patient ultimately must learn to do this him/herself, provided he/she has upper limb movement, a mirror should be provided and the patient should be allowed to practise. Bowel movement should take place within one hour of the insertion of suppositories.
4. The position for defaecation is important and use is made of gravity if the patient can sit on a toilet or commode. If this is quite impossible then the side lying position in bed is used (Note: Metal bedpans must be avoided for their deleterious effect upon devitalized skin and the difficulty the patient has in balancing.)
5. If the patient cannot take fibre in the diet then bulk forming medications may be needed.
6. The symptoms of faecal impaction are the absence of bowel movement for five days (provided food is being taken) with seeping of liquid stool. In patients with lesions above the level of spinal segment T6, there may be headaches and profuse sweating. Impaction is managed by manual removal. Gentle palpation of the abdomen should be used to check that all faeces have been removed and if not then two Senokot tablets may be given followed by the insertion of suppositories 8 to 10 hours later. If the problem remains

intractable, medical staff may order an enema or rectal washout. Administration of this should be stopped if the patient complains of headache.
7. The patient should be taught how to recognize impaction for himself and what to do about it.
8. Patients need to learn how to clean themselves after bowel movement. Again the use of a mirror is required.

It should be noted that whilst the aims and principles of management have been detailed here, this is a highly skilled area of care in which much sensitivity is required, together with a high level of assessment and teaching skills.

Problems of urination

The patient with impairment of conscious level

The patient with impairment of conscious level presents a rather different problem as regards management of bladder function compared with a patient who has a spinal cord lesion.

Aims and principles of care. Aims and principles of care for such a patient who is invariably incontinent of urine are:

1. To assess frequently enough to identify if retention of urine is present (with or without overflow).
2. To maintain a fluid balance chart on which is recorded the frequency of incontinence with an estimate of amount voided. In male patients it is possible to measure the amount.
3. To prevent skin breakdown due to contact with urine. For men this can usually be achieved by the use of a urinal placed in position, or the use of a penile sheath or condom and tubing running into a drainage bag. For women frequent monitoring of the bed linen is necessary. It should be changed as soon as the patient voids. Catheterization may be necessary, but this introduces a further potential problem, that of infection.
4. To avoid urinary infection, closed circuit drainage is used if the patient is catheterized. Walsh (1968) and Guttmann (1973) recommend that intermittent catheterization is less likely to lead to infection than an indwelling catheter. The importance of aseptic precautions and skilled atraumatic technique in the carrying out of catheterization cannot be overemphasized.
5. Retention of urine, whether absolute or due to incomplete emptying of the bladder must be treated by catheterization.
6. Bladder tone should be maintained if the patient has a self-retaining catheter, by clamping off the closed circuit system, allowing the bladder to fill, then unclamping the system every 1–2 hours and allowing the bladder to empty. Whilst few people void every 1–2 hours, if the patient's bladder is allowed to fill to too great a level then incontinence may occur around the catheter.

Provided that normal bladder tone has been maintained and infection has been avoided during the severe phase of the patient's condition, the bladder will be normal when consciousness is regained and retraining for normal conscious control of voiding should not take long.

Management of this phase includes careful, co-ordinated timing of fluid intake, and the provision of an opportunity to pass urine. The normal position for voiding should be used if possible: standing for men, sitting for women. All requests to be taken to the toilet, or to use a commode, should be attended to immediately. The patient should be placed within reasonable distance of the toilet. Praise should be used to reinforce progress in control.

Management in spinal cord lesions

The effect of spinal cord lesions depends upon their level and their severity (Schaupner, 1982), but, whilst the type of bladder dysfunction is closely associated with the type of lesion, it is the residual bladder function itself which determines the method of management. Investigations to identify bladder functional levels include cystogram, cystometrogram and electromyography. Outcomes of these investigations determine the management, but where there is a choice of method it should be reached by taking account of the patient's wishes, his or her lifestyle, body image and so on.

Incomplete spinal lesions or multiple sclerosis lead to uninhibited contractions of the bladder which produce incontinence. In this case management includes retraining the patient as outlined above, together with the possible use of anticholinergic drugs.

Lesions which completely block the transmission of impulses between the spinal cord reflex centre for bladder function and the cerebrum result in reflex spontaneous voiding when the urine in the bladder reaches a certain level. Management is possible using condom drainage for men. For women there must be regular toileting combined with stimulation techniques. Stimuli include stroking the perineal area, tapping the abdomen or stroking the thighs. Careful control of fluid intake is important. The danger for a patient with this type of bladder is that emptying may be incomplete and the retained urine may build up within the bladder. A patient must learn how to estimate the amount of urine to expect. For example, if the total fluid intake in 24 hours is 2500 ml then 3-hourly voiding of 300 ml during the day should follow (this allows for perspiration, etc.).

If retention occurs then catheterization is necessary, intermittent self-catheterization being the method of choice. Cholinergic drugs may be prescribed to aid bladder emptying.

When the lesion directly affects the sacral segments or nerves involved in bladder reflexes then the problem is usually that of an inability to void at all with severe retention of urine. The management of choice for both sexes is intermittent catheterization. Patients are taught how to carry it out for themselves. If they are unable to do this themselves for any reason, such as quadriplegia, then a relative, friend or other contact of the patient's choice is taught to carry out the technique. Fluid intake is calculated carefully to prevent more than 300 ml of urine building up in the bladder before the catheterization, otherwise oedema of the bladder wall may occur (Schaupner, 1982).

There are patients for whom intermittent catheterization is neither practicable nor desirable. Here urinary diversion operations may be preferred or the use of a self retaining catheter may be advocated. In the latter case a fluid intake of 3000 ml or more in 24 hours is needed to help in the prevention of infection.

Potential damage to patients' eyes

A patient with a lesion of the trigeminal nerve will have lost the corneal reflex, as will a high proportion of unconscious patients. In such circumstances great care must be taken to prevent the contact of foreign bodies with the cornea. Even the drying effect of a fan or breeze from an open window can lead to problems if the eye is not protected by the eyelid or some other method. Awareness of the potential for damage to the cornea is essential when placing an unconscious patient into the semi-prone position. It is best to avoid placing a pillow under the head. Eyedrops may be instilled on the doctor's prescription. Conscious patients with a trigeminal nerve lesion may be advised to wear an eyeshield. They must be warned to maintain it in a correct position at all times or the edge of the shield may itself damage the cornea.

During craniotomy, tissue fluids released by trauma invariably track to the periorbital area leading to a swollen and bruised eye on the side of the operation. Surgeons may place a compression dressing over the eye before the patient leaves theatre to help to prevent this. This makes the assessment of the pupillary response difficult; however, this is equally difficult if the eyelids swell. Patients must be warned about this occurring as it may upset them if they regain consciousness to find that their eye is painful or that they are unable to see out of it.

Patients who have sustained head injury may also develop severe swelling and bruising of the eyelids.

THE CARE OF PATIENTS WITH INJURY

Patients who are admitted with head injury or spinal injury may have sustained other bony or soft tissue damage as well. Identification of other injuries is often made difficult because the patient is unconscious or has lost the sensation from a part of the body. Acute awareness of the possibility of other injury is vital when the patient is being moved, to ensure the utmost care. Both the doctor examining the patient and the nurse assessing the patient on admission must identify any signs of shock, bruising or abnormal function which are present.

Patients who have suffered a fracture of the base of the skull may develop leakage of cerebrospinal fluid from the ear, eyes, nose or mouth. Any clear liquid which seeps from any one of these sites should be treated as if it were CSF until proved otherwise. This means that the patient should be reverse barrier nursed, and that no nasogastric tubes should be inserted to prevent the possibility of infection tracking into the CNS. Antibiotic cover will doubtless be prescribed.

Any scalp injury must be noted and the area shaved and cleaned. Foreign bodies within the wound are usually removed in theatre. Suturing is also carried out in the operating theatre.

PAIN

Types of pain

Headache is not only one of the most common types of pain encountered within neurological nursing, it is also one of the most common types of pain amongst the whole population (Walton, 1983). The central nervous system itself is relatively insensitive to pain, and pain from within the cranium arises mainly from blood vessels and the dura mater. Headache also occurs as a result of tension within extracranial structures such as the air sinuses, muscles and extracranial blood vessels.

Headaches can be classified according to the structures involved (Vogt et al, 1985).

Vascular headache

Migraine. Migraine is a very common example of this, but allergic 'cluster' headaches may display very similar symptoms. Migraine is still incompletely understood (Walton, 1983) and is the subject of continuing research. It appears to result from an inherited predisposition, together with the occurrence of trigger factors of which there are a great number. Trigger factors include stress, the sudden reduction of stress, abrupt changes in barometric pressure, abrupt falls in oestrogen levels associated with the menstrual cycle, fever, low blood sugar levels, regularly flickering or flashing light. Many food substances have been cited as triggers, e.g. amines in cheese, chocolate, citrus fruits, alcohol, especially red wine, smoked fish and food additives such as nitrates, nitrites and monosodium glutamate. The condition is best managed by the victims who learn what precipitates the attacks in their own case and avoid these triggers as far as possible. Attacks are treated by ergotamine compounds, caffeine and analgesics. Some migraine sufferers gain relief from the use of propanolol.

Hypertension headaches. Such headaches indicate severe hypertension which requires immediate action to reduce the blood pressure. Hypertension is usually symptom-free, at least in the early stages.

Temporal arteritis. Pain in this condition occurs in elderly people and is due to swollen, tender temporal arteries. It is experienced as a throbbing unilateral pain, producing visual loss and occasionally fever. It is treated by corticosteroids to reduce inflammation of the blood vessel.

Tension headaches

These are often called psychogenic headaches, since they are frequently associated with psychological factors. Nonetheless the underlying mechanism is physical, since they are caused by prolonged contraction or tension of neck, head and/or facial muscles. The pain which arises tends to be bilateral in distribution, and unlike vascular headaches is not throbbing in character. Such headaches may be associated with anxiety and depression. Management includes the relief of headache with analgesics such as paracetamol and aspirin. Measures are needed which help the sufferer to relax. Tranquillizing drugs may be used but methods which give the individual an active coping method should be taught if possible. Examples of active coping methods include autogenic training, relaxation therapy, biofeedback and massage (see Ch. 12). Another immediate cause of stress headaches occurs in people who grind their teeth.

Traction and inflammation

These are the types of headache which are encountered amongst patients with neuropathology. Increased intracranial pressure causes traction on blood vessels and the dura mater within the skull. Meningitis also causes severe headache. Extracranially, inflammation of the sinuses causes this type of headache. It follows that such headache is clinically significant. The cause must be treated. However until that is possible the headache will be managed by the administration of analgesic drugs.

Management of acute pain

Apart from headache, patients with neuropathology may suffer pain from muscle contractions or spasms, spinal lesions or after spinal surgery. Patients with pain in their wrist, hand and fingers due to a carpal tunnel syndrome may be admitted to a neurosurgical ward for operative relief through freeing the nerve within the carpal tunnel. Such patients require analgesia in the pre- and immediate postoperative period.

The nursing assessment of pain is important. The most important thing to bear in mind is that there is no such thing as an objective measure of pain. Pain is whatever the patient says it is and it occurs whenever the patient says it does (McCaffery, 1979). Various methods may be used in making public the essentially private and subjective experiences of pain. These include the use of questionnaires (e.g. the McGill-Melzack pain questionnaire — (Melzack, 1975), the pain thermometer (Hayward, 1975), or other analogue rating scales (Rudy, 1984).

As far as nursing management is concerned it is always better to administer analgesia in a sufficient dose to render the patient pain free before the pain has reached such an aversive level that a 'normal' dose of analgesia is relatively ineffective.

Nursing adjuncts to pain relief are helpful, e.g. ensuring a quiet environment, distraction techniques, use of imagery, use of warmth or cold packs, relaxation, positioning, allowing the patient to talk.

For patients with an intracranial lesion, or postoperatively following a craniotomy, the doctor may be afraid of masking symptoms of respiratory failure (indeed, of precipitating respiratory failure with a vulnerable patient) by the use of an analgesic such as morphine which depresses respirations. Pethidine or codeine phosphate are alternatives which are less likely to endanger respiratory function. Alternatively a drug which antagonizes the respiratory effects of morphine (e.g. nalorphine) may be administered with morphine.

Relief of pain caused by muscular spasms calls for the use of antispasmodics.

Chronic pain

This is a more problematic medical problem than acute pain. It is mentioned here since patients with chronic pain may be admitted to neurosurgical wards for surgical procedures to relieve intractable chronic pain. Very careful assessment is needed before the operation is carried out. Whilst this is the clear responsibility of the medical team, it is nonetheless true that a nurse may be able to make more continuous observations than the doctor, as well as seeing the patient in a wider variety of situations.

Surgical management

Surgical procedures which may be carried out include the following:

Nerve block. This involves the injection of local anaesthetic close to the relevant nerve trunk. The effect of such an injection wears off, but it may be used to evaluate the pain relief gained before a more permanent injection of alcohol or phenol is carried out at the same site. Alcohol is used in particular for the pain of trigeminal neuralgia (Onofrio, 1977) and the painful muscular spasms which may occur in multiple sclerosis.

After such an injection into the trigeminal nerve, great care is needed since a part of the affected side of the face will be numb and the corneal reflex may be abolished.

Neurectomy. Neurectomy is the destruction of a sensory nerve by cutting or cryosurgery. The recent development of microsurgical techniques allows this as a possible treatment for trigeminal neuralgia (Vogt et al, 1985). The pain and temperature fibres of the nerve are transected but touch and the corneal reflex are left intact. In the case of the cranial nerves (including the trigeminal) a craniotomy is required to allow access to the nerve.

Rhizotomy or sensory nerve root destruction. Here the sensory nerve fibres are surgically interrupted between the dorsal root ganglia and the spinal cord. Usually several nerve roots are involved. If the operation is to be accurate, to prevent extensive sensory loss, a laminectomy must be performed with all the potential problems posed in undergoing major surgery.

Cordotomy. This is the interruption of nerve tracts subserving pain sensation within the spinal cord. Again laminectomy is involved. Postoperatively, temperature sense will be lost in the affected area since this sensation is carried in the same tract as pain. Often the pain recurs within several months, changed in nature and particularly distressing. For this reason percutaneous cordotomy is preferred (Rudy, 1984). An electrode is placed into the spinal cord by a closed technique and under radiological control. Radio frequency coagulation is used to destroy the anterior spinothalamic tract in gradual increments guided by the patient's response.

Sympathectomy. Here afferent pathways are interrupted in the sympathetic division of the autonomic nervous system. Blood vessels are affected, increasing peripheral blood supply and preventing vasospasm. This operation may be used for Raynaud's disease as well as to relieve pain of vascular origin.

Cerebral surgery. Cerebral surgery such as lobotomy, thalamotomy and cingulotomy may be used in the treatment of pain from head or neck cancer.

The reader will recognize that these drastic surgical measures are reserved for patients where all else has failed. It says much for the disruption to life caused by pain that patients are willing to undergo such procedures to gain relief.

CARE OF THE PATIENT WITH EPILEPTIFORM SEIZURES

Epileptic seizures may be primary and idiopathic, or secondary and symptomatic of a central nervous system lesion.

There is an international classification of seizures (Rudy, 1984) and this can be seen in Table 18.2.

Table 18.2 International classification of seizures

I. Partial or focal seizures
- A. Elementary
  1. Motor symptoms
  2. Sensory symptoms
  3. Autonomic symptoms
  4. Mixed symptoms
- B. Complex (temporal lobe or psychomotor)
  1. Impaired consciousness only
  2. Cognitive symptoms
  3. Affective symptoms
  4. Psychosensory symptoms
  5. Psychomotor symptoms
- C. Partial seizure that becomes generalised secondarily

II. Generalized seizures (without focal onset)
- A. Tonic-clonic (grand-mal)
- B. Status epilepticus
- C. Absence attacks (petit-mal)
- D. Tonic
- E. Clonic
- F. Myoclonic
- G. Atonic
- H. Akinetic

III. Unclassified

Patients may be admitted to hospital with seizure disorder for one of the following reasons:

- for assessment and the establishment of medical control of attacks in primary epilepsy
- for diagnosis after a first attack
- for establishment of the cause and treatment in secondary epileptic attacks
- as an emergency to control status epilepticus.

Nursing management

During an attack the objective of care is to prevent the patient from injuring him/herself. Any object within the patient's vicinity which could cause harm during the clonic phase in particular should be moved well beyond the range of violent movement. If the patient is in bed, padded bedsides should be put up. Any constrictive clothing should be loosened and a soft pillow or folded towel, etc., placed under his/her head.

During the tonic and clonic phases, it is rarely possible to attempt to place anything into the patient's mouth to prevent tongue biting, since the onset is usually such that the jaw becomes tightly clenched before any measures can be taken. Any attempt to force anything into the patient's mouth will lead to injury. It becomes possible to insert an airway after the clonic phase has finished, if it is necessary.

The patient's respiratory status and oxygenation levels should be observed carefully. During the tonic phase, hyperextension of the jaw to prevent airway obstruction by the tongue could be tried. The head should be turned to one side if vomiting occurs. O_2 should be given if the patient becomes cyanosed and it is possible to give it.

Observation

Careful observation of the attack may aid diagnosis. The following points should be recorded:

- the activity in which the patient was engaged immediately before the attack
- whether there was any warning
- the posture during the tonic phase; any respiratory difficulty; how long this phase lasts
- during the onset of the clonic phase, whether this started from a focal point and spread or if it was generalized to begin with
- the violence of the movements; the limbs involved, the individual muscles involved and the length of this phase should be noted
- assessment of conscious level during any period of unconsciousness
- it is particularly important to note and record any incontinence, frothing at the mouth, and tongue biting
- the patient's behaviour on recovery should be noted and his/her mental state and mood.

Throughout the attack it is important to maintain the patient's privacy (if possible) and dignity. Other patients should be reassured and kept away. On recovery the patient should be reorientated. If the attack should be prolonged, medical help should be sought so that drugs may be prescribed to control the attack.

Rehabilitation

For any newly diagnosed patient with primary epilepsy, the knowledge of having this condition may prove very distressing, since it is still a stigmatizing condition in our culture. Even without that aspect there may be issues to be faced about choice of occupation and leisure activities, since there are some jobs which are not available to anyone who is liable to epileptiform attacks. Legally the individual is not allowed to drive until he/she has been free of daytime attacks for 3 years (Hopkins, 1981).

A great deal of teaching and support will be needed from the nursing staff so that the patient (or in the case of a young child, the family) learns to manage his/her own medication and life style within safe limits (Hopkins, 1981).

NEUROSURGERY

Procedures performed

After the fontanelles have closed in infancy, the central nervous system is completely protected by bone. It follows that bone must be removed to allow access for surgery.

Operative procedures which allow access to the CNS are:

Burrholes

Bone is drilled from small circular areas of the skull, allowing the passage of electrodes, cannulas, catheters, etc. Most commonly they are made over the posterior parietal region of the cerebrum and may be unilateral or bilateral.

Craniotomy

This is carried out by removing or turning back a flap of bone, usually in the frontal region. The bone is then replaced after the surgical procedure has been carried out.

Craniectomy

This involves the removal of an area of bone varying in size according to the surgical manipulation which is to be carried out. This operation is used for lesions within the posterior fossa (i.e. below the tentorium cerebri) and it therefore occurs toward the back and base of the skull. Structures lying within the posterior fossa include those controlling vital vegetative functions, and these structures must be identified and avoided in any procedure.

Laminectomy

Laminectomy involves the removal of one or more vertebral laminae to allow access to the spinal cord, the spinal dura mater, or an intervertebral disc.

Other operations

Other operations which may be carried out include spinal fusion to stabilize the spine, and operation for carpal tunnel syndrome. The latter operation involves exploration and surgical repair of the carpal canal in the wrist to relieve pressure on the median nerve arising from the transverse carpal ligament.

PRE- AND POSTOPERATIVE CARE

Careful assessment of both the patient and the family or friends includes exploration of how the prospect of operation is viewed. Whilst pre-anaesthetic care is normally similar to that in other surgical wards, the informational and psychological preparation is different and extremely important for recovery (Hayward, 1975; Boore, 1978).

Cranial surgery

In the case of surgery to the head, shaving of at least a portion of the scalp will be necessary. This will involve a change of body image for the patient and a change in the way the patient appears to relatives and friends. Surgeons differ in whether or not they are willing to allow some hair to remain when they carry out a craniotomy or craniectomy. Although a complete head shave may be more upsetting for the patient and family, it is often easier to fit a wig afterwards than if only a partial shave has been carried out. In either case, the psychological preparation for the head shave must be handled sensitively.

Postoperatively, the development of a swollen and severely bruised eye on the side of the operation is virtually inevitable after a frontal craniotomy. The extent of this may be reduced by the use of a compression dressing. In any case the vision of one eye will be obscured for some time, and this must all be carefully explained before operation. Patients and relatives will also require warning about the head dressing, intravenous infusion or nasogastric tubes etc.

One of the most significant aspects of postoperative care following head surgery is the frequent (possibly 15-minutely) neurological assessment and recording of TPR and BP. The patient should be prepared for this and the best method of preparation is to allow the patient to experience the assessment pre-operatively if it has not already been carried out.

Headache is likely postoperatively and warning should be given about this, together with assurances about the availability of analgesia. Other drugs such as anticonvulsants or antibiotics may be started postoperatively and these require explanation.

Quite quickly after the end of the operation the patient may be nursed in the head up position, and patients should be warned about this too. Together with the frequent assessments, this will disturb the patient's rest quite considerably.

Under normal circumstances the scalp heals rapidly and sutures are normally removed within 48 hours of operation. This is something very positive that the patient can be told. As with any other surgical patient, it is customary to allow those who have had brain surgery and are well enough to sit out of bed on the first postoperative day. This, of course, helps to prevent the formation of deep vein thrombosis and this should be explained, as it has been shown that some patients believe it is for the convenience of the nurse (Hayward, 1975).

Pre-operatively leg and deep breathing exercises should be taught and the patient reminded to practise them postoperatively (Boore, 1978).

Spinal surgery

The usual explanations about preparation for anaesthetic will be needed and so will teaching of leg and deep breathing exercises.

Special explanations which are needed include a description, or better still an experience, of the position which will be used for nursing the patient postoperatively. This will be flat on the back with good central spinal alignment and limbs carefully positioned. Depending upon the exact operation performed and the particular surgeon, the patient may have to maintain this position for about 2 days postoperatively. In this case, relief of pressure to prevent sores will require 'log-rolling' with the assistance of many nurses (Agee & Herman, 1984). Pre-operatively, the patient should be allowed to experience this. Occasionally a patient will be nursed on a plaster bed postoperatively. He/she must be allowed to acclimatize to this for increasing periods of time pre-operatively, since a considerable amount of adaptation is required.

As with the person undergoing surgery of the brain, any assessment procedure which will be adopted postoperatively should be experienced by the patient pre-operatively. Occasionally an indwelling catheter will be inserted into the bladder in theatre and if this is a possibility it must be explained, as must the possibility of an IV line. Pre-operatively, measures will be taken to ensure bowel evacuation and postoperatively careful assessment is needed to identify any problems of bowel function (and indeed bladder function in an uncatheterized patient). This requires explanation.

SOME PSYCHOLOGICAL ASPECTS OF CARE

There is a high probability that patients with neurological problems will at some time lose consciousness, suffer one or more neurological deficits or become changed in appearance through sensory or motor changes. It is, therefore, exceptionally important that nurses continually maintain their awareness of the patient as a human being embedded within a network of family and friendship relationships. Throughout the period of dependence the patient's dignity should be preserved, and he/she should never be treated in any way which would shame or embarrass if he/she were fully aware. As far as is possible the patient's identity as a unique individual, recognizable to his/her family and friends, should be maintained. The patient's usual hairstyle, hygiene and standards of grooming contribute to this, and should be included in the care plan as far as this is compatible with safety and treatment objectives. He/she should be greeted and spoken to by name. Great sensitivity is needed to cope with incontinence, vomiting or behaviour which is unlike the normal personality of the individual.

For unconscious patients it remains important to maintain adequate levels of sensory input and to speak to such patients, explaining nursing actions and so on, as one would with a conscious patient. Relatives can contribute by being encouraged to talk to unconscious patients, since evidence suggests that sound stimuli may be registered during coma (Myco, 1983).

The nurse's attitude towards a patient with a chronic neurological condition is important. It should be remembered that the patient acquires a good deal of knowledge not only about the disease process but about its management in his/her own case. This knowledge is likely to be far greater than that of the nurse on many occasions. A goal of care must always be to maintain or improve a patient's independence.

Giving information has been mentioned in relation to pre-operative care but it is important throughout a patient's contacts with doctors and nurses. A patient requires information about the ward environment, routines and staff when he/she is admitted to hospital. Thereafter he/she must be prepared for every event in which he/she will be involved. In relation to procedures and treatments, the patient needs information on:

- the reason, purpose or objective of the procedure
- what it will feel like
- what he/she must do to help (Altschul & Sinclair, 1981)
- any aspects on which he/she should report
- when it will happen
- how long it will take.

If the procedure is a complex one, the patient should be given the opportunity to practise any subskills required of him/her. Assessment of a patient's information needs forms the first important step in giving information.

In addition to information and teaching, the patient will require counselling and almost certainly the relative or friend will need counselling too. Counselling skill includes a high level of social skill, the ability to listen actively, to ask open-ended questions and to reflect. Plenty of time must be put aside to carry out counselling. Both patient and relatives need a good deal of support to come to terms with some of the issues raised by diagnosis and treatment. Denial is one mechanism used quite often by patients to cope with the reality of devastating illness (Lazarus, 1979). This appears to be helpful, but the nurse must be ready to give the necessary support when denial is given up and the patient begins to come to terms with reality (Clarke, 1984).

People suffering from some neurological conditions require a very lengthy period to regain what were once automatically performed skills involved in the activities of daily living. They may become very depressed and likely to give up. It is important to set goals with them which require only a small step of improvement and which are fairly easily achieved by the patient. An achievement, however small, should be commended. He/she can be reminded about what has been achieved so far, rather than how far there is yet to go. A patient who feels that he/she is not making much progress should be encouraged to talk about his/her feelings. Whenever possible the patient should be given control of decision making on issues relating to his/her own activities of daily living and treatment. Relatives should be encouraged to include the patient in family plans for the future and also to make an explicit effort to give the patient a role in decision making.

Neurological and neurosurgical nursing is one of the most challenging of nursing specialities. It requires a high level of clinical nursing skill, together with sensitive awareness of the impact that disorders of the nervous system can have upon both patient and the family. It is an extremely rewarding type of nursing however, since frequently it is the quality of the nursing care which determines whether the patient will live or die, and if he/she lives, the quality of the life he/she will lead thereafter.

Acknowledgement

We are grateful to Blackwell Scientific Publications Limited for permission to reproduce Figure 18.9 from Snyder M 1983 Relation of nursing activities to increases in intracranial pressure. Journal of Advanced Nursing 8:274.

REFERENCES

Agee B L, Herman C 1984 Cervical log rolling on a standard hospital bed. American Journal of Nursing 84:314–318
Altschul A, Sinclair H C 1981 Psychology for nurses. Baillière Tindall, London
Bobath B 1971 Abnormal postural reflex activity caused by brain lesions, 2nd edn. Heinemann, London
Bobath B 1977 Treatment of adult hemiplegia. Physiotherapy 63:310–313
Boore J 1978 Prescription for recovery. RCN, London
Brigman C, Dickey C, Jimmzieger L 1983 The agitated aggressive patient. American Journal of Nursing 83 (10):1408–1413
Clarke M 1977 Practical nursing, 12th edn. Baillière Tindall, London
Clarke M 1983 Practical nursing, 13th edn. Baillière Tindall, London
Clarke M 1984 Stress and coping. Constructs for Nursing. Journal of Advanced Nursing 9 (1):3–14
Coates V 1982 An investigation of the nutritional care given by nurses to acute medical patients and of the influence that ward organisational patterns may have upon that care. Unpublished M.Phil thesis, University of Hull
Cockcroft G, Ray M 1985 Feeding problems in stroke patients. Nursing Mirror 160(9):26–29
Cohen H B, Gambill A F, Eggis G W N 1977 Acute pulmonary oedema following head injury: two case reports. Anaethesia and Analgesia 56:136–139
Dardier E 1980 The early stroke patient. Baillière Tindall, London
Eccles, Sir J C 1957 The physiology of nerve cells. Johns Hopkins Press, Baltimore
Eccles, Sir J C 1961 The nature of central inhibition. Proceedings of the Royal Society Series B, 153:445–476
Ganong W F 1983 Review of medical physiology, 12th edn. Lange Medical Publications, Los Altos, California
Gray R 1983 Caring for patients with cerebral aneurysms. AORN Journal 37 (4):631–642
Grubb R L, Raichle M G, Eichling J O et al 1974 The effects of changes in $PaCO_2$ on cerebral blood volume, blood flow and vascular mean transit time. Stroke 5:630–639
Guttmann Sir L 1973 Spinal cord injuries: comprehensive management and research. Blackwell, London
Hayward J 1975 Information, a prescription against pain. RCN, London
Henderson V 1960 Basic principles of nursing care. International Council of Nurses, Geneva
Hilgard E R, Atkinson R C, Atkinson R L 1979 Introduction to psychology, 7th edn. Harcourt Brace Jovanovich, New York
Hopkins A 1981 Epilepsy. OUP, Oxford
Houston J C, Joiner C L, Trounce, J R 1985 Short textbook of medicine, 8th edn. Hodder & Stoughton, London
Jennet B 1981 Management of head injuries. Davis, Philadelphia
Jewett D L, Rayner M D 1984 Basic concepts of neuronal function. Little, Brown & Co., Boston
Johnson L V 1983 If your patient has increased ICP your goal should be: no surprise. Nursing 83 June: 58–63
Jones D 1975 Food for thought RCN, London
Konorksi J 1948 Conditioned reflexes and neuron organisation. Cambridge University Press, London
Lamb J F, Ingram C G, Johnston I A, Pitman R M 1980 Essentials of physiology. Blackwell Scientific Publications, Oxford
Lashley K S 1929 Brain mechanisms and intelligence. University of Chicago Press, Chicago
Lavigne J M 1979 Respiratory care of patients with neuromuscular disease. Nursing Clinics of North America 14:133–143
Lazarus R S 1979 Positive denial: the case for not facing reality. Psychology Today, November: 44, 47, 48, 51, 52, 57, 60
Lipe H P, Mitchell P H 1980 Positioning the patient with intracranial hypertension: how turning and head rotation affect the internal jugular vein. Heart and Lung 9:1031–1077
Macleod J (ed) 1981 Davidson's principles and practice of medicine. Churchill Livingstone, Edinburgh
Marmarou A, Shulman K, Rosende R 1978 A non-linear analysis of ventricular fluid pressure. Journal of Neurosurgery 48(3):332–334
Mastrian K G 1984 The patient with an autoimmune disease affecting the nervous system. In: Rudy E B (ed) Advanced neurological and neurosurgical nursing. CV Mosby, St Louis
McCaffery M 1979 Nursing management of the patient with pain, 2nd edn. Lippincott, Philadelphia
McCarthy E 1982 Cardiovascular complications of intracranial disorders. In: Nikas D L (ed) The critically ill neurosurgical patient. Churchill Livingstone, Edinburgh
McIlwain H 1966 Biochemistry and the central nervous system. Churchill Livingstone, London
Melzack R 1975 The McGill pain questionnaire. Major properties and scoring methods. Pain 1:277–299
Meyer N 1979 Nursing the critically ill adult. Addison–Wesley, Menlo Park, California
Miller J D 1979 The management of cerebral oedema. British Journal of Hospital Medicine 21 (2):152–166
Miller J D, Garibi J 1972 Intracranial volume/pressure relationship during continuous monitoring of ventricular fluid pressure. In: Brock M, Dietz H (eds) Intracranial pressure. Springer-Verlag, Berlin
Miller J D, Leech P 1975 Effects of mannitol and steroid therapy on intracranial volume/pressure relationships in patients. Journal of Neurosurgery 42:274–281
Mitchell P H 1982 Intracranial pressure: dynamics, assessment and control. In: Nikas D L (ed) The critically ill neurosurgical patient. Churchill Livingstone, Edinburgh
Mitchell P H, Mauss N K 1976 Intracranial pressure: fact and fancy. Nursing 76:53–57
Mitchell P H, Mauss N K, Ozuna J, Lipe M 1980 Relationship of nurse/patient activity and ICP variation. In:Shulman K, Marmarou A, Miller J D, Becker DP, Hochwald G M, Brock M (eds) International pressure IV. Springer- Verlag, Berlin
Mitchell P H, Mauss N K 1978 Relationship of patient–nurse activity to intracranial pressure variations: a pilot study. Nursing Research 27:4–10
Moss G C 1976 Respiratory distress syndrome as a manifestation of primary CNS disturbance. In: McLaurin R L (ed) Head injuries: Second Chicago symposium on neural trauma. Grune & Stratton, New York
Myco F 1983 Nursing care of the hemiplegic stroke patient. Harper & Row, London
Ochs S 1972 Fast transport of materials in mammalian nerve fibres. Science 176:252–760
Onofrio B M 1977 Pain control by injection techniques; enzymes, phenol and steroids. In: Lee J F (ed) Pain

management. Williams and Wilkins, Baltimore
Oswald I 1974 Sleep, 3rd edn. Penguin Books, Harmondsworth
Plum F, Posner J 1980 Diagnosis of stupor and coma, 3rd edn. Davis, Philadelphia
Portnoy H D, Clopp M 1980 Spectral analysis of intracranial pressure. In: Shulman K, Marmarou A, Miller J D, Becker D P, Hochwald G M, Brock M (eds) Intracranial pressure IV. Springer-Verlag, Berlin
Ramsey R G 1977 Computed tomography of the brain, vol. 9. Advanced exercises in diagnostic radiology. WB Saunders, Philadelphia
Ricci M M 1979 Intracranial hypertension: barbiturate therapy and the role of the nurse. Journal of Neurological Nursing 11:247–252
Ricci M M 1982 Neurological examination and assessment of altered states of consciousness. In: Nikas D L (ed) The critically ill neurosurgical patient. Churchill Livingstone, Edinburgh
Rudy E B 1984 Advanced neurological and neurosurgical nursing. C V Mosby, St Louis
Sanford S J 1982 Respiratory complications of intracranial disorders. In: Nikas D L (ed) The critically ill neurosurgical patient. Churchill Livingstone, Edinburgh
Schaupner C J 1982 Teaching neurologically impaired individuals bowel and bladder management. In: Van Meter M J Neurologic care: a guide for patient education. Appleton-Century-Crofts, New York
Solomon E P, Davis P W 1983 Human anatomy and physiology. Holt-Saunders, New York
Snyder M 1983 Relation of nursing activities to increases in intracranial pressure. Journal of Advanced Nursing 8:273–279
Thompson R C 1967 Foundations of physiological psychology. Harper & Row, New York
Vogt G, Miller M, Esluer M 1985 Mosby's manual of neurological care. CV Mosby, St Louis
Vygotsky L S 1962 Thought and language. MIT Press, Cambridge, Massachusetts
Walsh J J 1968 Intermittent catheterisation in paraplegia. Paraplegia 6:168–171
Walton J N 1977 Brain's diseases of the nervous system, 8th edn. OUP, Oxford
Walton J 1983 Introduction to clinical neuroscience. Baillière Tindall, London

19

Disturbances of hormonal control mechanisms

OVERVIEW OF HORMONAL REGULATION OF HOMEOSTASIS

Hormonal regulation of homeostasis is carried out largely through the distinct structures known as endocrine glands. However, it is important to realize that a number of organs of the body have an endocrine activity in addition to their other functions. For example, the pancreas contains discrete structures, the islets of Langerhans, which secrete hormones involved in the control of glucose metabolism. The kidney is less commonly recognized as an endocrine gland but plays a major role in the regulation of serum calcium levels by the activation of vitamin D (a hormone secreted by the skin) and the secretion of the hormone erythropoietin which regulates the formation of erythrocytes. The endocrine function of the gut is specifically involved in the control of digestion and absorption of nutrients. The thymus gland is a discrete endocrine gland with a role in the immune defences of the body. The objective of this chapter is to examine the disorders of the major endocrine glands involved in homeostasis.

There is a close interrelationship between the endocrine and neural systems, with some endocrine cells derived from embryonic neural crest cells, being both conductive and secretory. Other endocrine cells are derived from neural tissues which have lost the ability to conduct an impulse. Because of this relationship, many features of endocrine malfunction are reflected in neurological symptoms, and these symptoms are often a primary facet in the nursing care of patients with endocrine malfunction.

Hormonal structure

Although the reader of this chapter is expected to have knowledge of normal anatomical structure and physiological function, it would appear useful to emphasize a number of key issues. Hormones are of two basic types, peptides and steroids.

Peptide hormones. These are composed of sequences of amino acids, which may be as few as eight amino acids (e.g. angiotensin II). Most peptide hormones are derived from larger inactive peptides (pre- or prohormones) and activation occurs following proteolytic cleavage by specific enzymes. Many peptide hormones have common sequences of amino acids which may result in apparent cross-reactivity. For example, luteinizing hormone (pituitary) and chorionic gonadotrophin (placenta) have similarities in peptide structure to thyroid stimulating hormone, and the resulting cross-reactivity can cause enlargement of the thyroid gland during pregnancy.

Steroid hormones. These are organic molecules, with cholesterol being the parent compound from which all other steroids are synthesized. Although steroid hormones are complex molecules, small changes in structure markedly influence the shape and thus the biological activity of the molecule. This is of particular importance in the design of synthetic steroid hormones to be used in additive therapy following hormonal ablation.

Hormones as metabolic regulators

Hormones have a series of distinctive properties which characterize their regulatory functions:

- They have no direct effect upon the organ secreting them.
- They are produced in small amounts by endocrine glands (1×10^{-9} to 1×10^{-3}g per day), and in the healthy person, this rate of secretion is determined by the need for that hormone.
- Hormones may exert their effect on specific cells within an organ, or on cells throughout the body.
- The metabolic reaction to the hormonal stimulus is age-dependent: for example, in adults growth hormone regulates the release of the fatty acids from adipose tissue, whereas in young children it stimulates body growth.
- The reactions that hormones initiate continue long after the maximal concentration of hormone in the plasma has occurred.

These distinctive features of hormones are reflected in their sensitive regulation of metabolism. This is best explained in terms of self-adaptive feedback systems, an example of which is shown in Figure 19.1. This illustration shows how hormone release and activation are regulated through negative feedback, the parameters being modified in a controlled, self-regulated fashion. It is only when this self-adaptive feedback system is disrupted that normal homeostatic regulation is perturbed.

Hormones also provide mammals with an integrative capacity that may parallel or supplement the role of the central nervous system. In response to stress the nervous system can activate the hypothalamus which, in turn, by neural impulses stimulates the adrenal medulla to secrete adrenaline (epinephrine) and noradrenaline (norepinephrine). These hormones stimulate the liver to release glucose into the blood to maintain brain metabolism. A further metabolic control is exerted by some hormone systems in that they are unable to exert their metabolic directives in the absence of a second hormone. For example, adrenaline is unable to release hepatic glucose into the circulation in the absence of thyroid hormones.

In view of the widespread nature of the functions of the endocrine system, disturbances of this system are clearly going to have widespread effects on the individual. This is particularly so during periods of growth and development, with hormone imbalance during

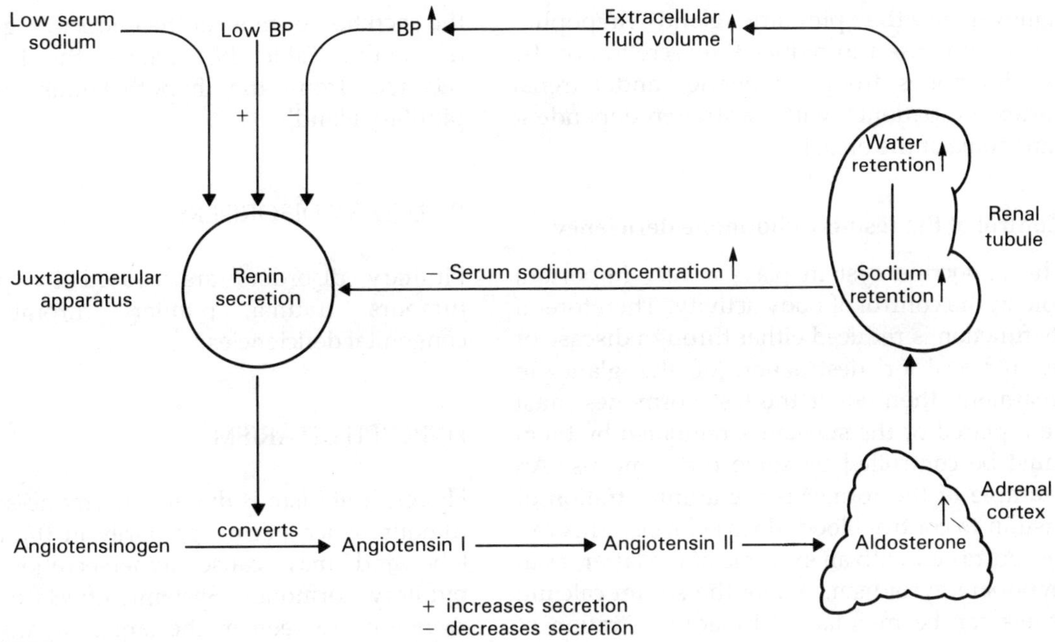

Fig. 19.1 The renin-angiotensin-aldosterone axis in control of extracellular fluid volume.

these periods resulting in considerable abnormality.

PRINCIPLES OF TREATMENT OF ENDOCRINE DISORDERS

Due to the nature of the endocrine system, certain underlying principles of management can be identified.

Utilization of substances essential for normal gland function

Where a gland preferentially extracts a substance from the blood, this fact can be used both in diagnosis and treatment. The major example of this is the thyroid gland which removes iodine from the blood against a concentration gradient. Radioactive iodine is concentrated in the gland so a small dose can be used in diagnosis of thyroid malfunction, although this has been largely supplanted by more precise tests of thyroid function. For radiation treatment of the gland a larger dose of radioactive iodine is given, becomes concentrated in the gland, and destroys thyroid tissue.

Replacement of hormone deficiency

When there is a hormone deficiency because of gland malfunction the output of that gland can be replaced. Steroid hormones, which are not modified by the enzymes of the gastrointestinal tract, can be given orally; the peptide hormones, which would be digested by the enzymes, have to be injected. Unfortunately the normal regulatory mechanisms cannot function in this situation, therefore careful monitoring of the blood levels and the effects of the dose being administered is necessary.

Utilization of trophic hormones

The output of a number of the endocrine glands is regulated by the trophic hormones from the anterior pituitary gland. When an increased blood level of the hormone secreted by the target gland is required, the same effect can be achieved either by administering that hormone, e.g. cortisol, or by administering the trophic hormone, ACTH (adrenocorticotrophic hormone), which will stimulate secretion of glucocorticoid hormones (mainly cortisol). This same principle can be used in reverse when the removal of the pituitary gland (hypophysectomy) is used to reduce the secretion of the sex hormones from the ovaries and adrenal cortex in patients with oestrogen-dependent carcinoma of the breast.

Control of the results of hormone deficiency

The endocrine system plays a very important role in the control of body activity. Therefore, if its function is reduced either through disease or by removal or destruction of the gland in treatment, then either the lost hormones must be replaced or the substance regulated by them must be controlled by some other means. An example of the former is the administration of insulin to control blood glucose levels. This can be contrasted with an example of the latter, as in hypoparathyroidism, where the serum calcium levels can be maintained by administration of calcium itself.

DISTURBANCES OF PITUITARY AND HYPOTHALAMIC FUNCTION

PITUITARY PHYSIOLOGY AND FUNCTION

The pituitary gland is located on the floor of the skull and is connected to the hypothalamic area of the brain by a stalk. Developmentally it has two origins; the posterior pituitary gland (neurohypophysis) forms from a downgrowth of the brain, while the anterior gland (adenohypophysis) is formed from an upgrowth of the buccal cavity. As expected from the developmental origins the posterior pituitary has nerve fibres passing down it from cell bodies in the hypothalamus. Hormones are synthesized in the cell bodies, pass down the axons and are released from the nerve fibres in the posterior pituitary when the nerves are stimulated. The anterior pituitary gland has no such direct link with the brain, but the hypothalamo-hypophyseal portal system carries hormones secreted from the hypothalamus into the blood to the anterior pituitary gland. These hormones regulate the secretion of the hormones of the anterior pituitary, which in turn regulate the secretion of most of the endocrine glands of the body. Table 19.1 shows the hormones secreted from the hypothalamus and the pituitary gland.

PITUITARY DISORDERS

Pituitary disorders are caused by pituitary tumours, trauma, pituitary thrombosis or congenital deficiencies.

HYPERPITUITARISM

Hyperpituitarism is due to a hormone-secreting tumour which occurs primarily in the anterior lobe and may cause hypersecretion of all pituitary hormones. Systemic effects of hypersecretion are seen in the larger organs, while local effects include blindness and headaches due to pressure effects of tumour growth.

Systemic effects

Systemic effects arise in three different ways:

1. Increased secretion of a specific pituitary hormone can have a direct effect on the tissues. For example, the particularly dramatic results of excess production of growth hormone are seen as gigantism in children and acromegaly in adults (Glick, 1979). In children, the long bones extend before the epiphyses close, while in adults the bones thicken and soft tissue hypertrophies, leading to different presentations of the same condition.
2. Increased secretion of the trophic hormones will lead to a rise in the production of the hormones of the target endocrine glands. This may be the cause of hyperthyroidism, Cushing's syndrome (increased corticosteroid secretion) and androgen hypersecretion.
3. Specifically, growth hormone is antagonistic to insulin; therefore, increased secretion of this hormone can lead to the development of diabetes mellitus.

Table 19.1 Hypothalamic and pituitary hormones

Hypothalamus	carried in blood stream and regulates secretion of	Anterior pituitary
Corticotrophin-releasing hormone	→	Adrenocorticotrophic hormone
Thyrotrophin-releasing hormone	→	Thyroid stimulating hormone
Growth hormone-releasing hormone; Growth hormone-release-inhibiting hormone	→	Growth hormone
Prolactin-releasing hormone; Prolactin-release-inhibiting hormone	→	Prolactin
Luteinizing hormone — releasing hormone; Follicle stimulating hormone (? 2 separate or one Gonadotrophin-releasing hormone)	→	Luteinizing hormone or Interstitial cell stimulating hormone; Follicle stimulating hormone
Melanocyte stimulating hormone-releasing hormone; Melanocyte stimulating hormone-release-inhibiting hormone)	→	Melanocyte stimulating hormone
Hypothalamus	**carried down nerve fibres and released from**	**Posterior pituitary**
Antidiuretic hormone (Vasopressin)	→	
Oxytoxin	→	

Treatment

Treatment involves ablation of the pituitary gland either by surgery or radiotherapy (Brady et al, 1979).

HYPOPITUITARISM

Hypopituitarism is a deficiency in the secretion of one or all of the pituitary hormones (Schneeberg, 1979). The latter condition is referred to as panhypopituitarism. Hypopituitarism may be caused by surgical trauma including hypophysectomy for the treatment of other disease, genetic conditions, non-secreting pituitary tumours, postpartum pituitary necrosis or malnutrition. Dwarfism is the congenital form of hypopituitarism which, if diagnosed early, can be treated by administration of growth hormone.

Systemic effects

Systemic effects of hypopituitarism include adrenocortical insufficiency, hypothyroidism and sexual and reproductive inadequacies.

Treatment

Treatment is by the administration of the deficient target organ hormones. These can be given by mouth, whereas pituitary hormones are destroyed in the gastrointestinal tract.

Nursing care of patients undergoing pituitary ablation

Hypophysectomy is performed to reduce hormonal stimuli throughout the body for diseases such as Cushing's syndrome, cancer of the breast and ovaries and (very rarely) to treat diabetic retinopathy as well as to treat tumours of the pituitary gland. Ablative methods include partial or total surgical removal of the gland, irradiation, cryosurgery, radiofrequency coagulation and transsphenoidal microsurgical hypophysectomy (Stowe, 1973).

Pre-operative care

In addition to the usual pre-operative care of patients, the emphasis medically will be on identifying the precise location, size and effect of the lesion. Because the pituitary gland is both structurally and functionally closely related to the brain, many patients exhibit neurological motor and sensory defects. A full baseline assessment is particularly important in this situation in order to make postoperative comparisons. In addition, nursing attention will need to take account of these defects, e.g. disorders of orientation, sight, movement and sensation. Of central importance is the realization that there is a risk of brain damage arising from surgery, and that the patient may well be fully aware of this.

Postoperative care

Postoperative care centres around factors related to the location of the wound, the possibility of cerebral oedema, possible damage to the brain by surgical trauma, and hormone deficiencies.

Wound location. The usual surgical approach for this operation is through the nose or the sphenoid bone of the face. This can give rise to oedema of the nasopharynx with some oozing of tissue fluid or blood. Careful observation for respiratory problems is required, and tracheopharyngeal suction may be necessary to remove secretions. Oedema of the periorbital tissues is common; ice packs may be used to minimize the swelling and petroleum jelly used to lubricate the eyelids. Occasionally cerebrospinal fluid (CSF) may leak down the nose and can be distinguished from mucus by the use of Clinistix, as CSF contains glucose. In this situation there is a risk of infection tracking back up to the brain. The patient is warned to avoid noseblowing and coughing, as these increase intercranial pressure and more CSF will escape. Care must be taken to minimize the risk of introducing infection by using sterile equipment and an aseptic approach to all activities.

Cerebral oedema. Cerebral oedema may develop after hypophysectomy. As soon as consciousness is regained the patient's head is raised to promote venous return and minimize this oedema. The patient may also be kept slightly dehydrated to control such oedema, and this is monitored by regular measurement of urinary specific gravity and serum electrolyte levels. Intravenous mannitol may be used to achieve the desired state of dehydration and fluid intake is controlled accordingly. Neurological observations are carried out at frequent intervals to monitor brain function (see Ch. 18).

Brain damage. Surgical trauma to the brain may lead to dysfunction of both the temperature regulating centre in the hypothalamus and specific motor and sensory nervous pathways. This may be only temporary due to localized swelling of tissues. Frequent monitoring of body temperature and motor and sensory function is necessary.

Hormone deficiencies. Systemic pituitary hormonal deficiencies may also develop, and symptoms of hypothyroidism, adrenal insufficiency and diabetes insipidus should be monitored. Hormone replacement therapy will be required with thyroid and adrenocortical hormones or the relevant trophic hormones. Antidiuretic hormone may be needed for some time, but often the hypothalamus will take over the secretion of this hormone.

Diabetes insipidus

This condition is the result of a disorder of the posterior lobe of the pituitary gland and is due to a deficiency of antidiuretic hormone. This hormone stimulates renal water reabsorption and regulates the osmotic pressure of the extracellular fluid. Deficiencies of this hormone may be due to familial hormone deficiencies, pituitary tumours or trauma. A similar clinical picture may be due to an inherited inability of the kidneys to concentrate urine. Patients may excrete up to 40 litres of fluid each day. Replacement of such volumes of fluid by drinking is a major problem and patients are therefore in continuous danger of dehydration and hypovolaemic shock.

Management

Management is directed to replacement of antidiuretic hormone (vasopressin). In short term conditions when at least some recovery is expected, e.g. after head injury or pituitary

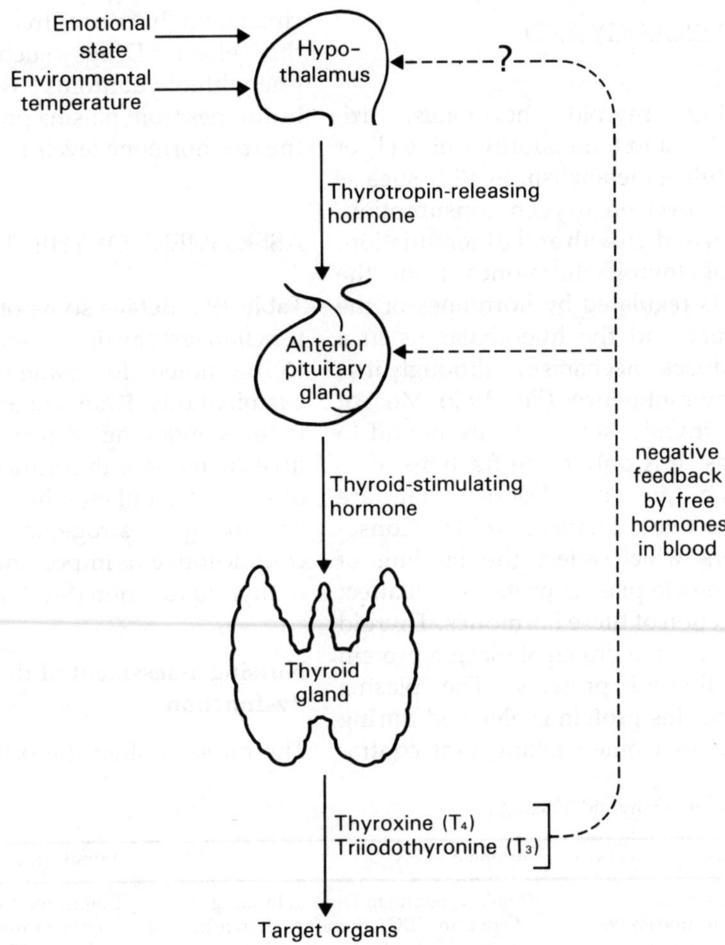

Fig. 19.2 Metabolic regulation of thyroid hormone synthesis and release.

surgery, aqueous vasopressin subcutaneously is used. Vasopressin tannate (pitressin tannate) in oil is no longer available in the UK, but if still used the vial needs to be warmed and thoroughly mixed before injection. Patients will need to be instructed on the preparation, injection procedure, rotation of sites and symptoms of overdose in the same way as insulin-dependent diabetic patients. Vasopressin can also be absorbed topically via nasal sprays. The synthetic form (DDAVP i.e. 1-deamino- 8D-arginine-vasopressin) is longer acting and is now the most commonly used drug for treatment. It only needs to be administered once or twice a day. Chronic rhinopharyngitis is a possible complication. As vasopressin administration may well be required for life the nurse should develop a teaching programme with each patient.

Patients with diabetes insipidus due to renal dysfunction sometimes benefit from use of the benzothiadizine diuretics. These probably reduce urine volume by causing mild sodium depletion, thus increasing reabsorbtion of sodium with water in the renal tubule. Potassium supplements will be required to replace the potassium lost as a result of the action of the diuretic.

DISORDERS OF THE THYROID GLAND

THYROID PHYSIOLOGY AND FUNCTION

The circulating thyroid hormones, triiodothyronine (T_3) and tetraiodothyronine (T_4 or thyroxine), regulate metabolism in all tissues as shown by the effect on oxygen consumption, heat production and growth and differentiation. The release of thyroid hormones from the thyroid gland is regulated by hormones of the anterior pituitary and the hypothalamus in a controlled feedback mechanism, although it is modified by other influences (Fig. 19.2). Most of the circulating thyroid hormones are bound to plasma proteins. It is only those fractions of T_3 and T_4 which are not bound that are metabolically active (Gharibe, 1974). Consequently, factors which affect the binding of thyroid hormones to plasma proteins will affect the metabolic action of these hormones. Thyroid binding globulin is the principal plasma protein which binds thyroid proteins. The plasma concentration of this protein is elevated during pregnancy and in women taking oral contraceptives leading to a rise in total T_4 in the circulation, but not of free T_4. Androgens reverse this effect. Drugs such as salicylates and phenylthiohydantoins will displace thyroid hormones from plasma proteins, thus increasing the free hormone levels in the blood.

ASSESSMENT OF THE THYROID FUNCTION

Table 19.2 details some of the different thyroid function tests available, and nursing precautions to be noted for patients undergoing these examinations. Knowledge of a history of taking iodine-containing drugs, recent radiographic investigations with contrast media, a high intake of seafoods, and whether the patient is pregnant or taking oestrogenic medication or oral contraceptives is important in correct assessment of thyroid function (Sterling, 1975).

Nursing assessment of the patient with thyroid dysfunction

The nurse is often the primary point of contact

Table 19.2 Assessment of thyroid function

Diagnostic procedure	Rationale	Nursing measures
T_4, T_3: Measured in serum by radioimmunoassays TSH, TRH: Measures total amount of hormone in blood by using radioactively-marked antibodies to specific hormone	99.96% T_4 bound to Thyroid Binding Globulin (TBG), therefore change in total T_4 may be due to change in TBG. Levels of free-binding sites on the TBG can be measured by T_3-resin uptake test thus allowing calculation of free T_4. Free T_4 ↑ –hyperthyroidism, Free T_4 ↓ hypothyroidism T_3 ↑ –T_3-toxicosis, T_3 ↓ –hypothyroidism Measurement of TSH and TRH allows diagnosis of specific alteration causing thyroid hormone level disturbances	Determine whether patient is pregnant or on oral contraceptives as either will change TBG levels and total T_4 levels Check whether thyroid drugs taken in last 2 weeks — inform medical staff Explain procedure to patient Ensure patient given results and explanation of them
T_3 — Resin Uptake test measures free binding sites on TBG by adding T_3 (radioactively labelled) and resin which binds T_3 to serum	The more protein binding sites available on TBG, the less T_3 will bind to the resin. Allows calculation of free T_4 levels in serum — the free thyroxine index (FTI)	As above
Thyroid scanning — radioactive iodine or technetium becomes concentrated in thyroid: Areas of uptake shown by scanner	Areas of increased or decreased uptake demonstrated Functioning nodules (i.e. which pick up radioactive substance) may be benign adenoma or localized goitre. Non-functioning nodule may be cyst, carcinoma, non-functioning adenoma, etc	As above Patient may need to be fasted before test, allowed to eat 45 minutes after.

Table 19.3 Features of thyroid dysfunction

	Features of overactivity	Features of underactivity
Metabolism	Intolerance to heat Raised temperature Weight loss with increased food intake	Intolerance to cold Reduced temperature Weight gain with decreased food intake
Cardiovascular and respiratory systems	Tachycardia, palpitations Increased respiratory rate, breathlessness Warm extremities	Bradycardia Decreased respiratory rate Cold peripheries
Gastrointestinal tract	Diarrhoea	Constipation
Neuromuscular system	Hyperactivity Muscular tremor Anxiety, irritability Insomnia Muscle wasting	Slow clumsy movements Impaired memory Increased sleep, tiredness, general 'flabbiness'
Other features		
Skin tone and texture	Pretibial myxoedema Moist skin	Dry, coarse, flaky skin Yellow cutaneous deposits Hair loss
Face, neck and voice	Exophthalmos (Infiltrative ophthalmopathy) Rapid speech Enlarged thyroid	Oedema of eyelids, thick lips and tongue Thick slurred speech, deep husky voice Thyroid could be enlarged
Menstruation	Disordered	Disordered

with the patient with thyroid dysfunction and thus plays a major role in noting and interrelating apparently unrelated symptoms in these patients. Community nurses dealing with pregnant or nursing mothers or the elderly should be particularly aware of the symptoms of, and need for, detection of thyroid dysfunction. School and community nurses should also consider thyroid dysfunction when assessing the health, cognitive and manipulative ability of children. Table 19.3 shows some of the features of thyroid dysfunction.

HYPOTHYROIDISM

Classification of the disease

Hypothyroidism has been classified in two schemes (De Groot & Larsen, 1984). The first classification is based upon the site of the thyroid malfunction. In this classification, primary hypothyroidism refers to defects within the thyroid gland, and secondary hypothyroidism is due to damage to the anterior pituitary gland following pregnancy, severe influenza or malignant growth. Tertiary hypothyroidism originates in the hypothalamus and may be due to hereditary defects or malignant invasion.

The second classification of hypothyroidism is based upon the age of the patient when clinical symptoms become apparent. Congenital cretinism is due to complete or incomplete embryonic hyposecretion of the fetal thyroid. The treatment of pregnant women with antithyroid agents may give rise to fetal goitre or other damage to the fetal thyroid gland. In childhood, the most common disorder is Hashimoto's thyroiditis (chronic lymphocytic thyroiditis); this is also the most common hypothyroid disease of middle-aged females. It is believed to be an autoimmune disease, and genetic predisposition may also play a role in the aetiology of the disease. Adult forms of hypothyroidism (myxoedema) may result from thyroid atrophy, treatment of hyperthyroidism with radioactive iodides or partial thyroidectomy, lithium carbonate administered in psychiatry, or hypothalamic or pituitary malfunction.

Effects of hypothyroidism

Thyroid hormones influence every body system and the symptoms of hypothyroidism are thus widespread. However, the expression and severity of the manifestation of these symptoms will vary from patient to patient.

Changes in extracellular fluid and skin

Deficiencies in thyroid hormones are clearly manifested in peripheral tissues. In particular, total body fluid and extracellular water are increased. This increase in body fluid content is reflected in oedema of the eyelids and extremities, which may also extend to the heart, vocal cords and tongue. Fluid retention distends the tongue, causing speech to become thick and slurred and swelling of the vocal cords results in a hoarse voice. Decreased water intake with a subsequent fall in urinary output are common features. Skin tone and texture also change due to plugging of hair follicles with mucoprotein and cutaneous deposits of yellow carotene may be present. Fat tends to be deposited subcutaneously and hyperkeratosis of the epidermis may also occur. Dry, rough skin and brittle nails, swollen hands and eyelids are therefore characteristic of the person with hypothyroidism. The thyroid gland may be palpably enlarged.

Neurological disturbances

Because of the close interrelationships between thyroid hormones and the nervous system, many symptoms of hypothyroidism present as neurological disturbances. Mental dullness, impaired memory and sleepiness are common symptoms which are associated with an elevation of the protein content of cerebrospinal fluid. Slow and clumsy motion may result from oedematous separation of muscle fibres and this is reflected in a delayed relaxation time of the Achilles tendon. Similarly, oedematous compression of the median nerve can result in sensory changes leading to numbness and tingling in the extremities.

Cardiovascular changes

As a consequence of an overall decrease in metabolic activity, and thus a lesser demand for oxygen, cardiac output is reduced with subsequent bradycardia and peripheral resistance to blood flow is increased. The rate of synthesis of erythrocytes is reduced, resulting in a normocytic, normochromic anaemia. Concurrent deficiencies in the metabolism of iron, folate or vitamin B_{12} can exacerbate this anaemia. Excessive bruising due to capillary fragility may occur. Enlargement of the thyroid gland, particularly in Hashimoto's thyroiditis, can result in respiratory distress and dysphagia.

Metabolic changes

Hypothyroidism causes an overall depression of the metabolic rate, which ultimately lowers body temperature and results in intolerance to cold. A common feature is decreased peristalsis with consequent constipation. Food and vitamin malabsorption may also occur. Liver function is impaired with elevated levels of serum cholesterol, beta-lipoproteins and some enzymes, while the synthesis of vitamin A from carotene is diminished. Decreased hepatic detoxification results in increased sensitivity to normal doses of drugs such as barbiturates, phenothiazines and digoxin.

Changes in the reproductive systems

In females, irregular and abnormal menstrual bleeding occurs because of decreased progesterone regulation of endometrial cell growth.

Clinical laboratory assessment

Estimation of the thyroxine index (see Table 19.2) allows diagnosis of hypothyroidism. In primary hypothyroidism, when the thyroid gland itself is not functioning normally, the thyroid hormone level will be low whilst the TSH levels in the serum are high due to the lack of negative feedback to the pituitary gland and hypothalamus. In secondary or tertiary hypothyroidism, the TSH levels, as well as the thyroid hormone levels, will be low.

Nursing care of the hypothyroid patient

General issues

Myxoedema is common, particularly in the elderly. Due to its insidious onset, hypothyroid patients who require hospitalization usually present with advanced disease with many diverse symptoms. Such patients may present in a stuporous state. Low temperatures during winter may precipitate myxoedematous coma. These patients present with hypothermia, concomitant hypoventilation, hypoglycaemia and hyponatraemia which may precipitate shock and death.

Patients admitted with myxoedema may have a diminished ability for self-care due to impaired cerebral function. The nurse should therefore restrict his or her demands and be attuned to the capacity of these patients to respond to simple requests. In particular, they will require assurance, comfort and encouragement in performing for themselves the tasks of daily living, as thyroid-replacement therapy progresses. Patient stress should be minimized to lessen the risk of dyspnoea and excess cardiovascular load. Many hypothyroid patients undergoing therapy are sensitive to cold and complain of numbness particularly in the fingers. Woollen gloves and socks may help alleviate these symptoms, and a warm environment is important. As hepatic metabolism is depressed these patients often exhibit hypersensitivity to prescribed dosages of antidepressants.

Nursing care of the advanced myxoedematous patient

These patients are often admitted to hospital in a comatose condition. The survival rate is 50% (Hoffenberg, 1983). They may present with ischaemic heart disease and atherosclerosis. If not comatose, they may exhibit a schizoid paranoid condition referred to as myxoedema madness. Hypoventilation, hypothermia, signs of cerebral hypoxia and increased susceptibility to hypnotic and sedative drugs are common features. Initial management is concerned with the maintenance of vital functions and administration of thyroid hormones to achieve a euthyroid state. Assisted ventilation with controlled oxygen is maintained to reverse hypoventilation and respiratory acidosis. Hypothermia should be treated by slow rewarming, as discussed in Chapter 27. Thyroid hormone replacement therapy is commenced with 400–500 micrograms of thyroxine intravenously or via a nasogastric tube. Thyroxine (T_4) is rapidly converted to T_3, the active hormone, in the tissues so that it is unimportant which is given (Hoffenberg, 1983). Glucose is administered through a central venous line in concentrated amounts to prevent fluid overload. Recognition of sensitivity to hypnotics and tranquillizers, treatment of infection and compassionate care of depressed or disturbed patients will minimize cardiovascular damage. Lubricants should be applied to the dry, scaly skin. After the crisis of admission, constipation is a frequent problem and a high fluid intake, dietary roughage and stool softeners may be necessary. Low calorie meals are often recommended to reduce excess body weight.

Continuing nursing care

Thyroid replacement therapy is always commenced slowly and conservatively. This is done to minimize excess demand on the cardiovascular system in response to an overall increased metabolic rate. Excessive medication can result in arrythmias and congestive heart failure. Careful detailing of body temperature, skin colour and tone, locomotor co-ordination, blood pressure, pulse rate, fluid intake and urinary output are necessary in monitoring therapy (Wake & Brensinger, 1980). Diuresis rapidly follows the commencement of thyroid therapy and is accompanied by weight loss. Symptoms of extracellular fluid imbalance, particularly oedema, disappear. Tissues which have been oedematous are susceptible to decubitus ulcer formation and should be regularly inspected for redness or tissue breakdown. Regular turning of the patient and use of other pressure relieving aids can help prevent ulcer formation. Patients should be kept warm and a low calorie, high fibre diet with high fluid intake should be encouraged to prevent constipation and faecal impaction. Guidance should also be given to the patient to encourage a normal return to, and self-confidence in, performing personal care and hygiene as well as coping with normal life. This may be a major problem in elderly patients with advanced hypothyroid dysfunction.

Once successful replacement therapy has been initiated the nurse, particularly the community nurse, plays a major role in maintaining the success of the therapeutic protocol primarily through teaching. This involves ensuring that the family and friends of the patient understand the rationale for continuous therapy and the need for following the programme rigorously. Both the patient and family or friends should be aware of side effects and signs of therapeutic overdose. Symptoms such as headache, palpitations, excessive sweating and heat intolerance should be described as warning signs which should immediately be reported to a physician. A teaching plan should be prepared with each patient with particular emphasis on the need for regular evaluation by a physician of the efficacy of treatment.

HYPERTHYROIDISM

Classification of the disease

With the exception of diabetes mellitus, the incidence of hyperthyroidism is more prevalent than all the other endocrine diseases combined. It is a disease predominant in females occurring in the third and fourth decades in life. There are six categories of hyperthyroidism. Graves' disease is the most common form and is an autoimmune disorder. An antibody of the IgG class termed long-acting thyroid stimulator (LATS) is often present in the serum of patients with this disease. It has been suggested that severe emotional disturbances trigger this form of hyperthyroidism but the evidence is unconvincing (Hoffenberg, 1983). Toxic multinodular goitre is believed to be a variant of Graves' disease and is common in elderly patients. Toxic thyroid nodule or toxic adenoma is a single hyperfunctioning nodule which suppresses the rest of the thyroid gland. This disease primarily occurs in younger adults and surgical removal of the toxic nodule usually results in return to normal thyroid function. In T_3-toxicosis elevated levels of unbound T_3 are found. It is not clear whether this is different from the more usual thyrotoxicosis or is just the early stage of the condition. Exogenous thyroxine administration can result in hyperthyroidism due to overdose of thyroid replacement therapy.

Effects of hyperthyroidism

The features of hyperthyroidism are widespread (see Table 19.3).

Changes in extracellular fluid and skin

Disturbances of regulation of extracellular fluid result in two of the features of Graves' disease. Infiltrative ophthalmopathy (exophthalmos) is due to inflammatory oedema of the orbit, lid and periorbital tissues resulting in protrusion of the eyeball and paralysis of the extraocular muscles (Kriss, 1975). Localized pretibial myxoedema is due to deposition of mucopolysaccharide, particularly in the skin of the lower legs. These deposits cause localized oedema with accompanying thickening of the skin.

Neurological disturbances

The excess production of thyroid hormone stimulates the central nervous system resulting in hyperactivity, anxiety, irritability, insomnia and other emotional problems. Muscular activity is increased as evidenced by a faster Achilles tendon reflex and muscle tremors are common. This is well demonstrated by observing the patient attempting to balance a sheet of paper over the tips of the fingers of the outstretched hand. Non-infiltrative ophthalmopathy is due to spasmodic eyelid movement which gives the patient a 'popeyed' appearance. This is a disturbance of eyelid musculature and not oedema.

Cardiovascular changes

In an attempt to lower the excess body heat, cutaneous vasodilatation occurs which is manifest by sweating, hot and moist skin and intolerance to heat. An increase in cardiac output occurs which may result in tachycardia, palpitations and congestive heart failure.

Metabolic changes

As a result of excess thyroid hormone production, normal intestinal function is disrupted, with hyperperistalsis and diarrhoea (Neumark, 1976). Resultant malabsorption of vitamin B_{12} and/or iron can lead to anaemia. The elevated metabolic rate results in increased protein, glucose and fat catabolism. Muscle wasting and weakness, thinning of hair and nails, increased appetite, lowered serum cholesterol and rapid glucose absorption all reflect an accelerated metabolic rate.

Disturbances of the reproductive systems

Disturbances in other endocrine systems occur which may impart impotency in the male, while in the female the menstrual cycle may become irregular or cease.

Clinical laboratory assessment

Initially a free thyroxine index is determined. If elevated, this is suggestive of hyperthyroidism. Elevated T_3 levels indicate T_3-toxicosis. In marginal cases, a TRH challenge test may be performed. If, following administration of TRH, circulating levels of T_3 and TSH do not increase, autonomous production of T_3 by the thyroid gland is indicated. Iodine uptake and thyroid scans may then be employed to identify specific malfunctioning thyroid nodules.

Nursing care of the hyperthyroid patient

General issues

Many hyperthyroid patients do not require hospitalization, but a stable, restful home environment is of value during therapeutic management. This is of particular importance for patients suffering from hyperactivity and insomnia. Heat intolerance is a common symptom which can be alleviated by appropriate clothing and cooling systems. If the patient is suffering from diarrhoea or weight loss, a dietician should be requested to advise upon suitable diet. In the hospital situation a similar approach to care is necessary.

Nursing care during antithyroid therapy

This therapy is employed to induce a euthyroid state. Drugs commonly used are propylthiouracil and methimazole, both of which block the synthesis of thyroid hormones. As the release of thyroid hormones synthesized before treatment is not blocked, thyroid hormone stores may not be reduced until about a month after commencement of drug therapy. After an initial high dosage of antithyroid medication, the dose is reduced and adjusted until the lowest possible dosage which will maintain the euthyroid state is achieved. As this process of adjustment may take in excess of 12 months, patients and their families should be advised on the need to take the medication as prescribed and to visit the physician routinely for assessment of the therapeutic protocol. Toxic reactions to these medications may occur, usually presenting as skin rashes, pain, swelling or fever. The patient should be told about the significance of such symptoms and advised to seek immediate medical assistance. Drugs such as reserpine and guanethidine, which deplete catecholamines, and beta-adrenergic blockers, such as propranolol, may be prescribed to alleviate the sensory and locomotor dysfunctions of the hyperthyroid patient. Such medications alleviate the symptoms but do not modify the thyroid malfunction.

Nursing care during radioiodine therapy

By use of a strong gamma-emitting source of iodine (^{131}I), active and particularly hyperactive thyroid follicles are destroyed when these isotopes are concentrated in the thyroid gland.

Patients administered this medication as outpatients should not consume food for at least three hours after swallowing the radioactive iodine to ensure adequate absorption, and they should also be advised to increase their fluid intake to at least 2 litres a day and to pass urine as often as possible during the first day of treatment in order that the free circulating ^{131}I should be excreted as rapidly as possible. Nursing mothers should cease breast feeding for 7 days and be taught how to express milk, which must then be discarded. Parents should remain isolated for 24 hours to minimize radiation damage to, or contamination of, children. All patients should be warned of the possibility of the development of a painful thyroid gland during the early stages of medication, and of the later development of hypothyroidism (see Ch. 16 for further discussion of radiation hazards and related nursing).

Nursing the patient in thyroid crisis

Some patients with advanced hyperthyroid disease may be admitted to hospital in thyroid crisis. This condition is stimulated by emotional stress, cardiovascular disease or infection, and as a result all symptoms of hyperthyroidism are exaggerated. In particular emotional instability, restlessness, fever, tachycardia, atrial fibrillation and heart failure may be present on admission. Nursing care is directed toward rapid lowering of the metabolic rate to alleviate the exaggerated symptoms, while thyroid hormone release is inhibited in a feedback mechanism by administering saturated potassium iodide solutions. Beta-blocking agents are administered to depress myocardial excitability. Adrenal corticosteroids may also be administered to replace glucocorticoids metabolized in response to the thyroid crisis. Failure to administer corticosteroids could precipitate an Addisonian condition. In spite of the emergency of the situation, it is vital to reduce all external stimulation that might exacerbate the crisis. A quiet environment and a calm, supportive approach is therefore important. Room temperature should be cool and frequent sponging may be required to reduce body temperature. Prompt attention to patient requests minimizes frustration and tension. Throughout periods of thyroid crisis, heart failure is a major potential problem and myocardial function should be closely monitored.

Nursing care of the patient undergoing thyroid surgery

Hyperthyroid patients are only admitted for surgical intervention if:

- the patient has not responded to drug therapy or radioiodine administration
- the patient has a goitre which is compressing structures around the gland
- carcinoma of the thyroid is suspected.

Subtotal or total thyroidectomy can be employed in all three circumstances.

Preoperative care. Preoperative nursing care has two aims:

- the achievement of a stable euthyroid condition
- teaching the patient about the reason for the pre- and postoperative procedures, and the need to minimize strain to the thyroid gland and adjacent structures.

Antithyroid drugs are administered to induce a euthyroid state, and beta-blockers may be used for short-lasting control of symptoms. A saturated solution of potassium iodide is prescribed to inhibit both the release of thyroid hormones and to harden the texture by reducing vasculature in the gland. During this period the nurse should endeavour to keep the patient calm and relaxed. The patient should be reassured that the surgical scar will not be a major disfigurement and should be shown how to sip fluids and cough with minimum tension on the thyroid gland and trachea. The patient's dietary intake should be increased to at least 16.8 MJ (4000 Calories) daily to compensate for excessive metabolic activity, and stimulants such as tea and coffee should be avoided.

Postoperative care. Postoperative care is concerned with the promotion of wound healing, the early detection and management of postoperative complications, and rehabilitation.

In the immediate postoperative period, the patient should be moved carefully and placed in a semi-upright position with the head supported by pillows as soon as consciousness is regained and the blood pressure is stable. As haemorrhage and respiratory obstruction may occur, the patient should be routinely examined for symptoms of distress. Pulse, blood pressure and observation of dressing for evidence of bleeding should be undertaken half-hourly during the first 24 hours. Signs of irregular breathing and choking should be carefully monitored and clip removers must be available at the bedside for use in emergency. A tracheotomy set should also be available on the ward. The tone and strength of the patient's voice should be regularly noted, as prolonged hoarseness or weakness of the voice may indicate damage to the laryngeal nerves.

Serum calcium levels should be routinely determined, particularly if parathyroid glands have been removed or damaged. Twitching of facial muscles, tingling of toes and fingers, Chvostek's sign (twitching of the face on tapping the facial nerve) or Trousseau's sign (carpopedal spasm provoked by constriction of a limb) are all indicative of tetany, and calcium gluconate should be available.

Patients should be encouraged to take fluids by mouth, and if nausea or vomiting ensues oral intake is reduced and the prescribed antiemetic administered. Narcotics can be administered to patients with pain in the throat. Mist inhalation eases breathing and liquifies mucous secretions. Temperature should be regularly checked as pyrexia often precedes thyroid crisis. Radioactive iodine treatment may be prescribed following a total thyroidectomy for malignant disease, to ensure that all thyroid tissue is removed or destroyed. The nurse should observe the patient for manifestations of hypothyroidism.

Subsequent postoperative care should be directed towards supporting the patient and evaluating the efficacy of the therapeutic regime. Before discharge from hospital a teaching plan should be drawn up explaining the symptoms of hypo- and hyperthyroidism that may develop, and emphasizing that should such symptoms develop the patient should immediately notify a doctor. The patient should be advised about cosmetic creams and preparations which may be used to mask the scar but which are unlikely to promote an inflammatory response. Arrangements will also be confirmed for regular evaluation of treatment.

OTHER THYROID DISORDERS

Goitre

This term refers to any thyroid enlargement whatever the cause, and may be associated with over- or undersecretion of thyroid hormones. A cause of diminishing significance is deficiency of iodine in the diet when the gland hypertrophies in an attempt to compensate. Before the introduction of iodised salt into the Western diet the incidence of goitre was high in areas where there was little iodine in the environment. It is still endemic in some regions of the world. Today a goitre is usually indicative of thyroid malfunction rather than being dietary in origin.

Apart from being unsightly and creating associated hormonal disturbances, a goitre can cause considerable local problems by exerting pressure on the trachea and, if large enough, on the oesophagus. Surgical removal will be indicated in such situations.

Thyroid tumours

Thyroid tumours are a common cause of thyroid enlargement. Benign follicular adenomas occur in patients of all ages and may cause discomfort by pressing against the trachea. Malignant thyroid tumours can be either hormone secreting or non-hormone secreting. Surgical thyroidectomy is the primary mode of treatment followed by radioiodine treatment to destroy residual thyroid tissue. Nursing care for these patients has already been discussed.

Thyroiditis

Thyroiditis is a general term used to describe an inflammation of the thyroid gland which may be due to infection or autoimmune disturbance. Subacute thyroiditis is a limited inflammation of the thyroid gland induced by viral agents. Severe pain in the thyroid region is accompanied by fever, coughing and symptoms of hypothyroidism may develop. Analgesics and anti-inflammatory agents such as corticosteroids are administered, after which thyroid function normalizes.

Acute suppurative thyroiditis is due to bacterial infection of the thyroid gland and is associated with acute thyroid pain, fever and malaise. Antibiotics are used to treat this condition. Hashimoto's disease (lymphocytic thyroiditis) is an autoimmune disorder common in middle-aged females and often results in hypothyroidism. It is usually treated with short term steroids and thyroid hormones.

DISTURBANCES OF THE PARATHYROID GLANDS

PARATHYROID FUNCTION AND CALCIUM METABOLISM

The parathyroid glands develop as two pairs of small, yellowish bodies embedded in the posterior section of the thyroid gland. They secrete parathormone which, along with calcitonin and vitamin D, regulates the levels of calcium and phosphate ions in the serum (Fig 19.3).

Parathormone

Parathormone increases the level of calcium ions and reduces phosphate ions in serum. It achieves this by increasing the release of calcium and phosphate from bone into the extracellular fluid and increasing calcium reabsorption from the renal tubules, but at the same time increasing the excretion of phosphate. It also increases activation of vitamin D by the kidneys.

Vitamin D

Vitamin D also increases the amount of calcium ions in the extracellular fluid. This substance is either produced in the skin through the action of ultraviolet light or is ingested. It is metabolized in the liver before activation in the kidney. The activated vitamin increases calcium absorption from the gut, reabsorption from the renal tubules and release from bone. Reabsorption of phosphate in the kidneys is also increased, but this is masked by the effect of parathormone.

Calcitonin

The third hormone involved is calcitonin, produced in the thyroid gland. This has an action which opposes that of the other two hormones, causing a fall in calcium ion and a rise in phosphate ion concentration in the serum. However, in adults it is of less importance than the other substances.

HYPERPARATHYROIDISM

Causes

There are a number of causes of hyperparathyroidism. Primary hyperparathyroidism is usually due to adenoma, but can be the result of general hyperplasia or carcinoma. Hyperparathyroidism can also occur secondary to conditions which cause hypocalcaemia. Hypocalcaemia is due to conditions such as chronic renal failure, when calcium is lost in urine, reduced intake of calcium or lack of vitamin D. Whatever the cause, hyperparathyroidism eventually results in hypercalcaemia with consequent decreased serum phosphate resulting in neuromuscular irritability (Hoffman & Newby, 1980).

Effects and treatment

Clinical symptoms of bone decalcification are manifested as backache, skeletal pain, bone curvature and pathological fractures. Calcium-containing renal stones may also develop due to high calcium output in the urine. This may cause polyuria with the risk of dehydration, although the resulting polydipsia is likely to prevent this. Neuromuscular co-ordination is often impaired with fatigue, nausea, depression, mental dullness and cardiac dysrhythmias. Peptic ulceration may also occur. Clinical diagnosis relies on laboratory evaluation of plasma calcium

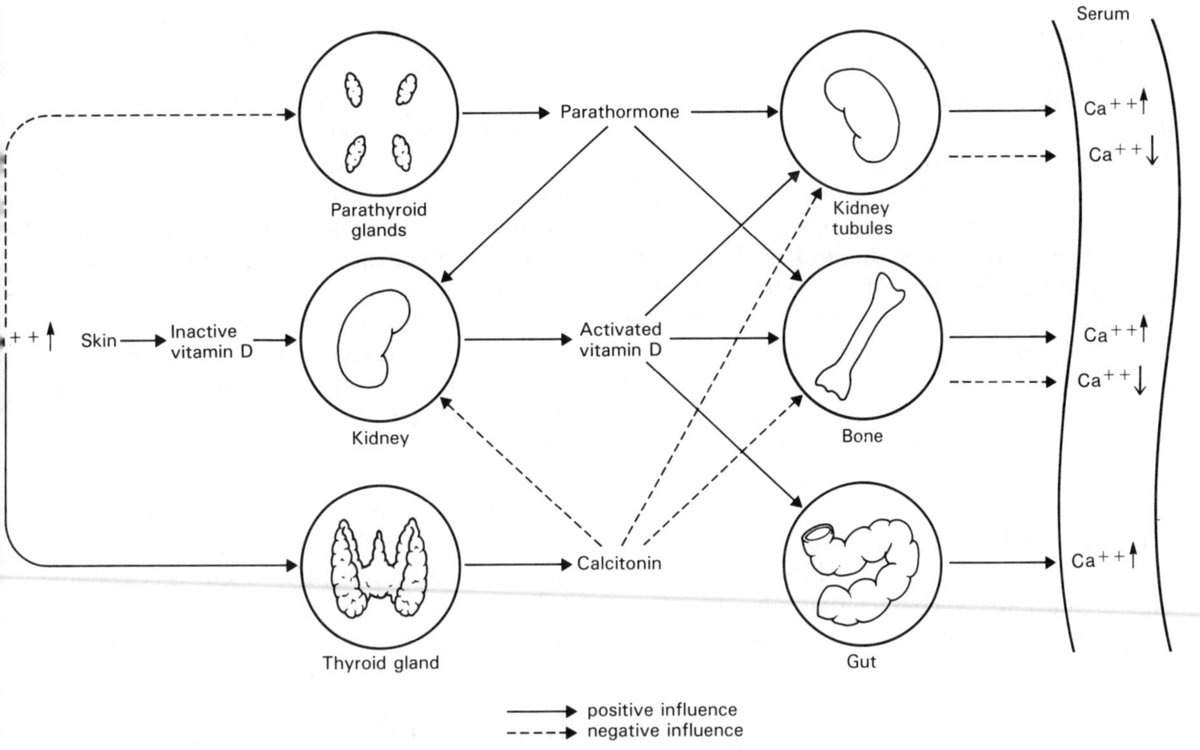

Fig. 19.3 Regulation of serum calcium levels.

and parathyroid hormone levels, as well as X-ray examination of phalanges and skull which show typical bony changes. Adenoma may be diagnosed by arteriography. Treatment involves surgical ablation of the adenoma or excess glandular tissue.

Nursing management

Pre-operative care

Pre-operative nursing care is directed towards lowering calcium concentrations. To minimize the risk of calculi formation, 2–3 litres of fluid per day should be taken. In order to increase the solubility of calcium the urinary pH should be lowered by giving acidic fruit juices. Low calcium and low phosphate diets, i.e. low in milk and milk products, should be provided and the patient encouraged to mobilize to reduce the constipation which may result from the neuromuscular depression. If the patient suffers from peptic ulcers, other types of protein, which reduce acid concentration by their action as buffers, will have to be substituted for milk and milk products. Antacids containing calcium will also have to be avoided.

If a simple increase in fluid output does not lower serum calcium levels sufficiently then loop diuretics such as frusemide, which decrease renal calcium reabsorption by the renal tubules, can be administered. Thiazide diuretics which decrease renal secretion of calcium should not be used. It is particularly important to protect patients from accidents, as pathological fractures easily occur.

Postoperative care

Postoperative care is similar to that prescribed for patients following thyroidectomy. Fluid input and output should be continuously monitored and care should be taken not to overhydrate the patient. Signs and symptoms of tetany should be carefully evaluated. When calcium levels decrease, calcium lactate or gluconate can be administered orally if necessary. If the gastrointestinal tract cannot absorb sufficient calcium, calcium gluconate can be administered intramuscularly or intravenously. Vitamin D can be given to increase absorption of calcium. Hyperparathyroid crisis, due to handling of the gland during surgery, where extreme hypercalcaemia develops postoperatively, is rare and is characterized by extreme neuromuscular disorder.

The patient should be reassured that the continuing skeletal pain will regress as bony recalcification occurs, and should be encouraged to ambulate to accelerate this process.

Patients with bone disease may develop 'hungry bones' syndrome following surgery. This syndrome is characterized by hypocalcaemia and severe tetany due to rapid utilization of calcium by the bones. These patients are maintained on high calcium diets with oral calcium preparations given for long periods whilst skeletal tissues are rebuilding. Tetany is treated with injections of calcium gluconate. Although the symptoms of bone pain may be alleviated following surgery, renal damage is irreversible and progressive.

HYPOPARATHYROIDISM

Causes and effects

Hypoparathyroidism is due to either surgical damage to the parathyroid glands during surgery or to autoimmune reactions, similar to Hashimoto's thyroiditis. The decreased bone reabsorption due to lack of parathyroid hormone results in hypocalcaemia and hyperphosphataemia causing increased neuromuscular activity. Acute symptoms include tetany with Chvostek's sign, Trousseau's sign and laryngeal spasm. Anxiety and apprehension are evident and chronic idiopathic symptoms include dry skin, brittle nails and renal colic. Clinical diagnosis involves laboratory examinations similar to those employed in hyperparathyroid patients.

Management

Management of the hypoparathyroid patient is directed towards elevating serum calcium concentrations. For rapid relief of the symptoms of tetany calcium chloride (10% w/v) can be infused slowly. In this form calcium is a marked irritant, causing thrombosis, whereas calcium gluconate administered intravenously does not suffer this disadvantage. In acute cases patients should rebreathe into a paper bag to induce respiratory acidosis which elevates blood calcium. Anticonvulsant drugs may be prescribed to control tetany and a tracheotomy may be required.

Patients with chronic hypoparathyroidism will require teaching about techniques to maintain blood calcium concentrations in excess of 2.5 mmol/l (Table 19.4). Complete recovery from the effects of hypoparathyroidism is dependent upon the time of diagnosis, and life-long management may be required for some patients.

DISTURBANCES OF PANCREATIC ENDOCRINE FUNCTION

PANCREATIC ENDOCRINE ACTIVITY

The islets of Langerhans in the pancreas secrete three hormones which are involved in the regulation of blood glucose levels, with insulin and glucagon playing major roles.

Insulin is a polypeptide hormone synthesized as proinsulin in the beta cells and converted to insulin before secretion. Glucagon is also initially formed as a precursor molecule and converted to the active hormone in the alpha cells. The third substance, somatostatin, is synthesized in many parts of the body, including the delta cells of the islets of Langerhans. It is thought to act as a general intra-islet regulator, as it inhibits the secretion of both the other hormones (Grodsky, 1981).

The metabolic effects of insulin and glucagon are antagonistic, both having an important role in the control of blood glucose. Insulin is released in response to a rise in blood glucose levels, the amount released being dependent on both the concentration of glucose in the blood and the

Table 19.4 Aspects of management of hypoparathyroid patients

Therapeutic management	Teaching aspects
1. Obtain laboratory determination of serum calcium concentration three times each year	Explain the need for vitamin D and oral calcium dosage if needed
2. Optimize dosage of vitamin D and oral calcium salt before patient is discharged	Ensure that the patient is conversant with the symptoms of hypo- and hypercalcaemia
3. Request dietician to prescribe appropriate diet, high in calcium and low in phosphorus	Teach the patient about the need to adhere strictly to diet plan
4. If necessary prescribe aluminium gels before meals to lower phosphate absorption	Ensure that the patient is evaluated regularly by a clinician

rate of change in that concentration. By stimulating utilization of glucose, storage as glycogen and conversion to fats, it causes a fall in blood glucose to normal levels. Conversely, glucagon and some other hormones (e.g. adrenaline, growth hormone, corticosteroids) act to increase the blood glucose levels by stimulating the breakdown of glycogen and the formation of new glucose (gluconeogenesis) from protein. However, insulin secretion responds rapidly to a change in blood glucose levels, while glucagon secretion remains fairly constant in subjects who are eating a normal mixed diet, and the other hormones are secreted mainly in response to stimuli unconnected to blood glucose levels (except in unusual states of hypoglycaemia). Therefore, it appears that insulin, rather than the other hormones, plays the major role in the regulation of glucose metabolism (Cryer, 1984).

DIABETES MELLITUS

Diagnosis

Diabetes mellitus is a disorder characterized by a degree of hyperglycaemia. In the healthy adult the fasting blood glucose level is normally between 4.0 and 6.0 mmol/l, and a random blood sample should contain less than 10.0 mmol/l (Giles & Ross, 1983). The criteria endorsed by the WHO (1980) for diagnosis of diabetes mellitus are as follows (Welborn, 1984):

- In a patient with acute symptoms
  — a fasting venous blood glucose of 7.8 mmol/l or above
  — a post-absorptive (2 hours after eating) blood glucose of 11.1 mmol/l or above
- In a person without symptoms of diabetes
  — two abnormal values as above
- An abnormal oral glucose tolerance test. This test can precipitate the development of hyperosmolar coma and is unnecessary if the previous conditions are met. It should only be used in diagnosis where ambiguous blood glucose values are obtained, when gestational diabetes is suspected or to exclude diabetes mellitus.

The subject of a glucose tolerance test will have received a normal diet before fasting overnight. Blood glucose levels are measured at the time when 75g of glucose are taken orally and at 30 minute intervals for 2 hours afterwards. Diabetes mellitus is diagnosed when the 2-hour sample and one other sample have a glucose concentration of 11.1 mmol/l or above. Impaired glucose tolerance is identified by one 2-hour level of between 7.8 and 11.1 mmol/l, and one sample with a glucose concentration of 11.1 mmol/l or more. These people have an increased risk of developing diabetes mellitus.

Diabetes mellitus is a syndrome in which the patient has a relative or absolute lack of insulin, but in different cases there are varying aetiological factors and the presentation differs. Some patients initially present with what are usually thought to be complications of diabetes such as atherosclerosis, eye, renal or nervous conditions. Table 19.5 shows the classification and aetiology of this disorder. The two major groups of patients are those who require insulin (type 1) and those who usually do not need insulin (type 2) to control their blood glucose level.

Clinical features

Due to the inadequate amounts of insulin present, changes take place in glucose metabolism that affect total body physiology (Fig. 19.4). In the liver the glycolytic enzymes required for the breakdown of glucose for energy are inhibited. At the same time the gluconeogenic enzymes are activated and the amino acids released by protein breakdown are used to form glucose. The overall result is that additional glucose is liberated into the bloodstream. However, without insulin, glucose is unable to cross the cell membranes into muscle and fat cells. The blood glucose level continues to rise causing hyperosmolarity of serum.

The blood glucose level eventually exceeds the renal threshold (usually about 10 mmol/l) and is excreted in the urine. Glucose is an osmotically active particle so that additional fluid is excreted, giving rise to polyuria. The resulting dehydration and thirst gives rise to polydipsia. Dehydration results in some of the signs found in uncontrolled diabetes, such as hot, dry skin and rapid pulse rate. If severe, the hyperosmolar state and dehydration can lead to coma — hyperosmolar, non-ketotic coma. This is sometimes the presenting condition in patients with type 2 diabetes. After initial treatment these people often do not need insulin to maintain their blood levels of glucose within normal limits.

At the same time that the levels of blood glucose rise, a total lack of insulin allows an increase in the release of fatty acids from adipose tissue to act as an energy source. In the liver some of the fatty acids are used to form ketones, which are utilized for energy by many tissues of the body. However, there is a limit to the amount of ketones which can be used by the body tissues and, in uncontrolled diabetes, these may be produced in excess. Ketones will then be excreted in the urine and will be smelt on the breath as they are excreted through the lungs. In addition, ketones are acidic substances and the resulting lowered pH will affect enzyme activity and, therefore, many metabolic functions. Brain function will become deranged and coma may result — a hyperglycaemic, ketotic coma.

The increase in protein and fat breakdown will lead to weight loss even though the patient is eating well.

The other features of this disorder are usually considered as complications, but may be the presenting conditions, particularly in those with type 2 diabetes.

Complications/other presentations

Diabetic patients are prone to a number of complications which are more common in those whose blood glucose levels are poorly controlled. It is these complications which result in the excess mortality found in diabetics. A study of 370 diabetics showed that 60% had died after 40 years of the disease. The mortality rate was between two and six times that in an age and sex-matched non-diabetic population (Deckart et al, 1978). Good blood glucose level control was linked with increased survival time.

There is still controversy about whether hyperglycaemia is the cause of these complications. On the whole, the evidence suggests that the development of retinopathy, neuropathy and glomerulosclerosis is related to the degree of hyperglycaemia. The evidence is less strong, but still suggestive, of a relationship between cataract and vascular disease and high blood glucose levels. However, genetic and environmental factors are also involved in the aetiology of the long-term complications of diabetes (West, 1982)

The complications which develop involve a number of different systems and tissues of the

Table 19.5 Classification and aetiology of diabetes mellitus (adapted from Alberti & Hockaday, 1983)

Classification	Other names	Characteristics	Aetiology
Type 1	Insulin dependent diabetes Juvenile onset diabetes Ketosis prone diabetes	No endogenous insulin secretion after early phase Usually young when diagnosed Weight loss May develop ketoacidosis	Genetic predisposition Possible autoimmune disorder — antibodies to islet cells found May be provoked by infection
Type 2 (non-obese)	Non-insulin dependent diabetes Maturity onset diabetes Maturity onset diabetes of young	Some insulin secretion continues Tendency to insulin resistance may become ketoacidotic with severe illness — not on withdrawal of insulin	Stronger genetic component than Type 1 ? Precipitated by environmental factors
Type 2 (obese)	as Type 2 (non-obese)	Some insulin secretion (may be high) Insulin resistance	As for Type 2 (non-obese) Obesity — glucose tolerance may be normal after weight loss
Impaired glucose tolerance	Asymptomatic diabetes Chemical diabetes Borderline diabetes Latent diabetes Subclinical diabetes	Increased risk of vascular disease Likely to be obese	Mild glucose intolerance from any cause
Gestational diabetes		Impaired glucose tolerance or more severe forms of glucose intolerance	Pregnancy (normal Glucose Tolerance test beforehand)
Secondary causes			
Pancreatic disease		Often underweight, history of malnutrition Mainly in tropical countries and non-Caucasians ? Severe insulin resistance	Chronic pancreatitis Pancreatic calcification — ? alcohol involved Malnutrition, Cassava consumption
Hormonal		Obvious signs of hormonal excess Diabetes mild	Corticosteroid excess Glucagonoma Agromegaly Thyrotoxicosis Phaeochromocytoma ? Hypothalamic lesions
Drug induced			Diuretics, analgesics, psychoactive drugs, catecholamines
Insulin-receptor abnormalities			
Genetic syndromes			e.g. Glycogen storage disease Huntington's chorea

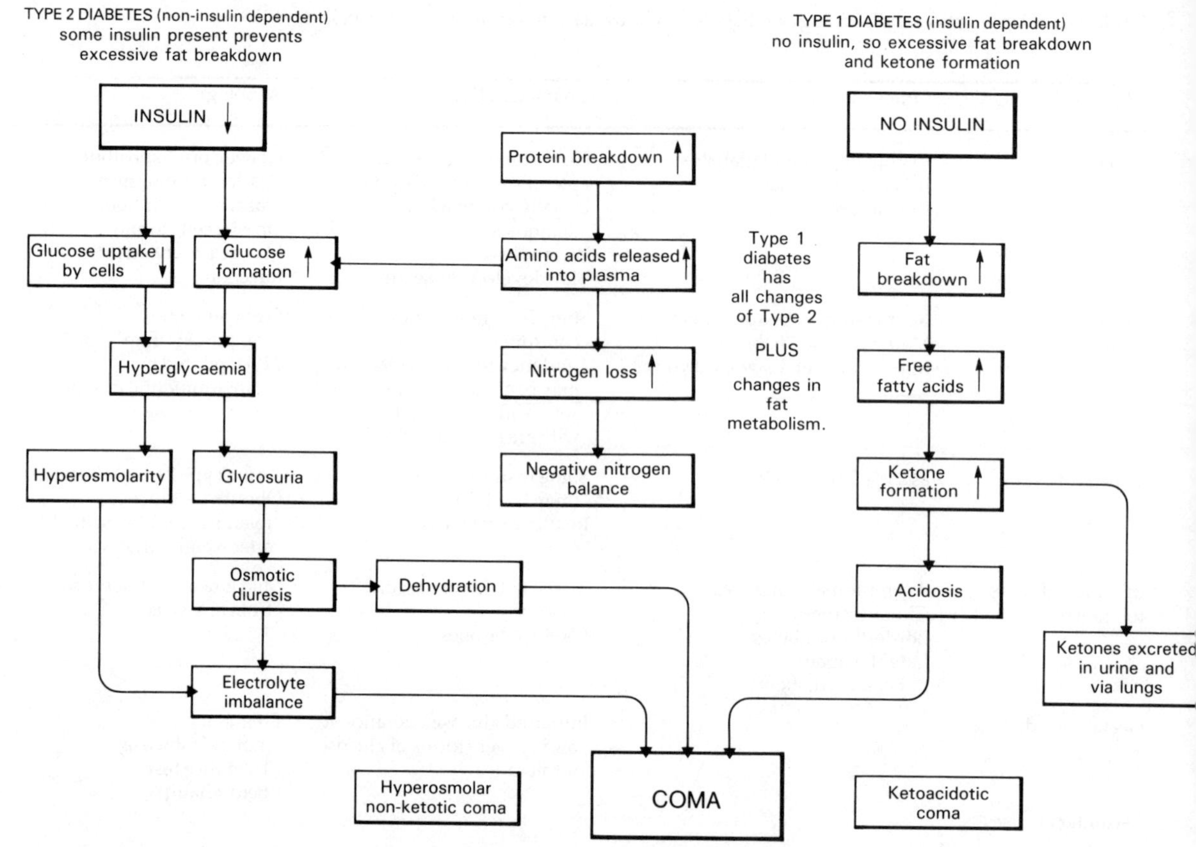

Fig. 19.4 Physiological effects of diabetes mellitus

body and the major ones will be considered in turn.

Immune system. There seems to be good evidence that the body's defence mechanisms are impaired in poorly controlled diabetes, probably due to defective energy metabolism in the polymorphonuclear leucocytes (Alberti & Hockaday, 1983). In the well controlled patient the response to infection is satisfactory.

A number of infections are more common in diabetics, particularly urinary tract infections and tuberculosis. Fungal infections are common, particularly *Candida albicans* of the vulva and/or vagina. Many female patients first present with this condition (Alexander, 1982). Infected skin lesions, particularly of the feet, occur frequently in those with poor diabetic control. Foot lesions are likely to be exacerbated by impaired circulation and may progress to osteomyelitis, requiring surgical treatment. To minimize this risk patients should recognize the importance of good control of blood glucose levels and should be taught about the importance of foot care as shown in Table 19.6 (Chandler, 1976).

Infection, particularly bacterial, results in the stress response (discussed in Chapter 8), causing hyperglycaemia. Type 1 diabetics will need increased insulin and type 2 diabetics often require insulin to control their blood glucose levels during this period. Maintenance of blood glucose within normal limits is essential if treatment for the infection is to be effective. During the illness, careful monitoring of blood glucose levels is necessary in order to determine the amount of insulin needed at any particular time.

Cardiovascular system. Diabetics are considerably more likely to develop disease of the arteries than the general population. The

Table 19.6 Plan of skin and foot care for diabetic patients

Purpose of care	Physical aspects of care	Educational aspects of care
Hygiene of the skin and feet	1. Massage dry feet with lanolin	1. Explain the circulatory and sensation changes that may occur with diabetes
	2. Use powder in web spaces	2. Wash feet daily with mild soap and lukewarm water: pat dry, do not rub, skin dry
	3. Insert lamb's wool between toes	3. Instruct patient to massage feet upwards from the tips of toes
	4. Soft feet should be rubbed weekly with alcohol	4. Wear well-fitting low-heeled shoes with wide toes
	5. Examine for tinea pedis between toes and onchomycosis in the nails	5. Wear clean nonrestrictive stockings and shoes
		6. Trim toenails straight across with emery board to prevent paronychia
Treatment of corns and calluses	1. Check that shoes fit correctly	1. Instruct patient on curling and stretching foot exercises
	2. Never cut corns and calluses	2. Instruct patient to see a chiropodist if corns and calluses need attention
Treatment of skin abrasions	1. Commence immediate first-aid treatment	1. Instruct patient that abrasions become ulcerous and gangrenous unless rapidly treated
	2. Examine for any redness, blistering or swelling	2. Instruct the patient about the symptoms of athlete's foot and the need to seek assistance
	3. Avoid irritating antiseptics	
	4. Keep abrasions covered with sterile gauze	
Treatment of imperfect circulation	1. Compare skin colour and temperature of each foot	1. Instruct patient to keep warm with clothing: hot water bottles and heating pads should not be used because of potential skin damage
	2. Examine digital and midtarsal areas for cyanotic colour	2. Instruct patient not to wear garters or to cross legs, which reduce blood flow
	3. Palpate the dorsalis pedis and posterior tibial arterial pulses Weak pulses indicate atherosclerosis	3. Prescribe exercises to increase circulation
		4. Smoking should be discouraged because of the vasoconstrictive properties of nicotine

initial lesion is an abnormality of the basement membrane of the capillary (diabetic microangiopathy). It has been suggested that this may be the primary disturbance in diabetes (Williamson et al, 1971) and many of the other complications of diabetes mellitus are associated with this.

Atherosclerosis is common and develops at a younger age in the diabetic than in the non-diabetic. It affects the major arteries throughout the body and tends to be more widespread and peripheral in diabetic patients. The presentation of the disease is similar to that in other patients although diabetics are more likely to have a painless myocardial infarction, possibly due to autonomic neuropathy (see below). As the disorder tends to spread peripherally to a greater extent than in non-diabetics it is more difficult to treat by arterial surgery. A large proportion of those undergoing leg amputation for atherosclerotic disease are diabetics. Due to this risk the importance of foot care and of not smoking must be emphasized to newly-diagnosed diabetic patients (Jarrett et al, 1982).

Renal system. The kidneys may be affected by the microangiopathy already mentioned, as well as being more prone to damage as a result of infection. Nodular glomerulosclerosis (Kimmelstiel-Wilson's disease) can lead to proteinurea, oedema, hypertension and uraemia. The development of the disorder is usually slow, taking many years, and few signs and symptoms may occur until signs of uraemia and oedema develop. Management of these patients will involve the same approaches as for others with renal failure, but may be more difficult because of arterial changes and increased risk of infection. Dietary control is more complex because it is necessary to take into account the diabetes mellitus (Ireland et al, 1982).

Nervous system. Somatic sensory and motor nervous supply and the autonomic nervous system may be affected in diabetes (Thomas et al, 1982). Somatic sensory neuropathy gives rise to decreased vibration and position sense and disturbances of sensation such as numbness, tingling, warmth or cold, etc. This may become very painful and the patient, in addition to analgesia, will need to experiment to find the situation of most comfort to allow him or her to sleep. People vary considerably and some find that having the foot of the bed raised, or the head of the bed elevated, the feet exposed or wearing bedsocks adds to their comfort. This dysesthesia becomes less troublesome as the neuropathy progresses and the feet become numb. However, once this has occurred the feet are at risk of becoming damaged without the patient being aware of the trauma. This can lead to deformities and ulcers of the feet, which heal with difficulty. The patient needs to understand this risk and be prepared to visually examine both feet every day.

Motor neuropathy occurs most commonly in those with type 2 diabetes and causes sudden weakness, usually of the hip and knee. A considerable degree of recovery is usual within 12–24 months.

Autonomic neuropathy initially causes few symptoms but later may cause severe, even life-threatening, problems. Postural hypotension, diarrhoea, urine retention and impotence are all problems that can occur. It is also possible that cardiac autonomic disturbances may lead to cardiac arrest, particularly after anaesthesia. The management of these problems is not always easy, although there are some simple actions which sometimes help.

Postural hypotension may be minimized by teaching the patient to move to an upright position slowly. Encouraging a high fluid intake and administering a low dose of a synthetic mineralocorticoid may be helpful, as they prevent a drop in extracellular fluid volume thus minimising postural hypotension. Codeine and increased bulk in the diet can be used in an attempt to control bowel function after other causes of diarrhoea have been excluded and treated.

Urinary retention is treated by drugs, anticholinesterases or cholinergic agents, but sometimes surgery may be needed. Impotence may have profound social and psychological implications for the patient. Patients with autonomic neuropathy have a poor prognosis (Scarpello & Ward, 1984).

Eyes. Disorders of the eyes in diabetic patients are the major cause of blindness in the UK in those between 30 and 64 years of age (Kohner et al, 1982). The commonest disturbances are diabetic retinopathy and cataract.

Diabetic retinopathy results from a number of contributory factors which lead to disturbances in the blood vessels of the retina. Some blood vessels become blocked, new blood vessels are formed, retinal exudates are seen and sometimes haemorrhage. There are three types of diabetic retinopathy:

- Simple (background) retinopathy. The veins are increased in size and are tortuous. Small haemorrhages and small areas of exudate are seen. These characteristics may remain unchanged for many years. The vision is unaffected.
- Proliferative retinopathy. In this condition areas of neovascularization are seen, sometimes throughout the retina, and haemorrhage is not uncommon. Retinal detachment sometimes occurs. Smoking and hypertension exacerbate this condition.
- Exudative retinopathy. The retina does not always appear very unusual in this

condition, although vision may be deteriorating. Exudates and oedema occur, sometimes over the macula with serious effect on vision. Exudates occurring elsewhere on the retina have less serious results.

People with diabetes must have their visual acuity checked at regular intervals, annually after 10 years from diagnosis and in those over 40 years of age. Control of blood glucose levels is the major factor in prevention and minimizing progression of the condition. Smoking should be discouraged and hypertension and hyperlipidaemia (which may increase exudates) should be controlled. Retinal damage is limited by photocoagulation.

Cataract is also common among these patients and, at present, is treated by surgery.

Monitoring of blood glucose level

There is now a considerable amount of evidence to indicate that the development of the above complications is reduced in those patients whose blood glucose levels have been well controlled (Scobie & Sönksen, 1984). In addition, some of the abnormalities discussed are at least partially reversible if normal blood glucose levels can be achieved.

Methods of monitoring blood glucose levels are essential if normal values are to be maintained. Until recently the adequacy, or otherwise, of control was monitored by patients carrying out urine testing for sugar and ketones several times a day. Some patients, particularly the elderly, continue to monitor their progress in this way. However, under normal conditions glucose should not appear in the urine at all, so that it is not possible to gain any indication of blood glucose levels until they are high enough to exceed the renal threshold. In addition, considerable variation in renal threshold for glucose has been reported (Tattersall et al, 1980). Urine testing is therefore no longer considered adequate.

Many diabetic patients now monitor their control of blood glucose levels by using reagent strips to which capillary blood is applied. The colour which develops on the strip is then compared with a standard, either visually or with a reflectance meter. Patients need to learn how and when to carry out this procedure, and also what the results mean and how to use them. The most important factor is that the patient should accept the importance of meticulous control of blood glucose levels, and realize that the use of this technique gives the feedback needed to achieve this control.

It is now possible to estimate the adequacy of diabetic control over the previous 8–10 weeks by measuring the concentration of glycosylated haemoglobin in the blood. The formation of this occurs irreversibly at a rate dependent on the average blood glucose concentration. High levels of glycosylated haemoglobin indicate poor control of blood glucose levels, while particularly low levels are indicative of hypoglycaemia, possibly nocturnal. False results will be obtained if the survival of red blood cells is altered (Scobie & Sönksen, 1984).

Principles of management

The principles of management of diabetes mellitus are to maintain the blood glucose level within normal limits and to enable the person with this condition to live as normal a life as possible.

The blood glucose level is regulated by balancing the food intake, exercise and insulin. The insulin may need to be given by injection, secretion may be stimulated by the use of drugs, or endogenous secretion may be adequate if diet and exercise are regulated. Recently there has been a major change in the approach to both diet and the use of insulin in the management of the disorder. The aim is that the patient will achieve a thorough understanding and acceptance of the condition and the factors which alter blood glucose levels, and will be able to adjust these appropriately. Patients will be in control of their own lives. The nurse's role, with that of the physician and dietician, is to help patients to achieve this goal.

Diet

Manipulation of the diet is an important aspect of diabetic control in subjects with both type 1 and type 2 diabetes. The individual with type 1 diabetes has to carefully balance food intake and injected insulin, and must time meals to prevent the development of hypoglycaemia. The dietary programme needs to be planned with the patient. He or she is more likely to comply with the planned diet if it is similar to the pre-illness diet and fits into his or her normal lifestyle. The amount to be ingested should be based on the requirements of someone of the same age, sex and activity.

The patient with type 2 diabetes is still producing some insulin and is more able to respond to fluctuations in nutritional intake. As long as the overall intake is controlled, adherence to a rigid schedule is not necessary. However, the endogenous insulin secreted will be utilized most effectively if food intake is divided into several meals spread throughout the day. The obese patient with type 2 diabetes will be encouraged to lose weight, as this often results in a lowering of blood glucose levels. This is partly due to regaining normal sensitivity to insulin (Olefsky, 1976).

Until recently the amount of carbohydrate in the diet has been strictly controlled and much of the energy requirement was taken in the form of fat. However, it is now thought that the amount of fat taken may be implicated in the development of atherosclerosis in these patients, and the recommended diet for diabetics is changing. There is evidence that a diet high in carbohydrate can improve diabetic control as long as the carbohydrate required is taken in a high-fibre form, with only small amounts of simple sugars (Kiehm et al, 1976; West, 1980). The value of a high-fibre, high carbohydrate diet in lowering blood glucose levels in diabetics and in reducing the amount of insulin required is clear (Horwitz, 1984).

It is now recommended that fat should provide only 20–38% of the energy in the diet, with less than 10% from saturated fats and up to 10% from polyunsaturated fats.

Exercise

Many people enjoy sport and exercise and do not wish to be restricted by their medical condition. In addition to this, there is some evidence that exercise is of value to diabetics.

Diabetics not requiring insulin have been found to improve medically, in terms of blood glucose control, as a result of exercise. It appears possible that there may be an increase in sensitivity to insulin (Kemmer & Berger, 1984).

In type 1 diabetics, the management of exercise is more complex. During exercise the uptake of glucose by muscle cells is increased and injected insulin may be absorbed more rapidly from the tissues, leading to hyperinsulinaemia. Both these factors will contribute to the development of hypoglycaemia. Theoretically, exercise should be planned into each day's programme and balanced with dietary intake and insulin. However, this is often not possible and it is important that diabetics learn to balance the three factors under varying conditions. To prevent the development of hypoglycaemia following exercise the patient needs to increase nutritional intake or reduce insulin dosage.

Kemmer et al (1982) has found that a reduction in insulin dosage of more than 60% before breakfast prevented the development of hypoglycaemia for 3 hours of exercise after breakfast. On the other hand, increasing carbohydrate intake only prevented it for 30 minutes. Initially the patient will have to monitor the blood glucose level frequently and will need encouragement and support, but will become more experienced and able to adjust personal requirements.

Insulin

Insulin is the third major factor involved in the regulation of blood glucose levels as it is essential for the normal metabolism of glucose.

Type 2 diabetics still produce some insulin, and a number of these subjects will be able to control their blood glucose level simply by regulation of diet and exercise. The endogenous insulin secretion can then be used more

Table 19.7 Properties of oral antidiabetic agents

Agent	Duration of action (hr)	Daily dosage/mg	Adverse reactions	Contraindications
Sulphonylureas — stimulate insulin release				
Tolbutamide	6–12	500–3000	Hypoglycaemia Digestive disorders Liver toxicity Skin rashes	Hepatic and renal disease
Acetohexamide	6–24	250–1500		
Tolazamide	6–18	100–750		
Chlorpropamide	24–72	100–500		
Glibenclamide	intermediate between Tolbutamide and Chlorpropamide	2.5–15		
Biguanides — potential insulin action by inhibiting glucose absorption from gut				
Metformin	8–12	1000–2000	Lactic acidosis Digestive disorders	Hepatic and renal disease Heart failure

efficiently. Particularly if the patient is obese, dietary measures leading to weight loss may be all that is required.

Oral antidiabetic agents are used to regulate blood glucose concentrations when dietary regulation is inadequate (Fletcher, 1976). These agents are of two types (Table 19.7), which are the sulphonylureas and biguanides. Controversy has arisen following a study of these agents by the University Group Diabetes Program in the USA. This study concluded that patient longevity was not increased, and that the incidence of cardiovascular disease was significantly elevated in patients administered these drugs (Klimt et al, 1970). Although these doubts do exist, many patients can be controlled by these drugs without recourse to insulin administration (Podolsky et al, 1980).

Insulin dependence in type 2 diabetics occurs when diet and/or oral antidiabetic agents are no longer effective in maintaining blood glucose concentrations. This is usually caused by a gradual destruction of the islets of Langerhans. The onset of symptoms is not as severe as in type 1 diabetes and can be largely controlled by a low dosage of insulin with adequate dietary control. Many patients who develop this form of diabetes are elderly, and precautions must be taken with these patients to prevent hypoglycaemia (Small, 1976). When insulin requirements are not high (less than 40 units per day) one injection a day of a long-acting insulin may be acceptable (Scobie & Sönksen, 1984).

Type 1 diabetics produce no insulin, or virtually none, and will need it administered for the rest of their lives. Because insulin is degraded by the proteolytic enzymes of the gastro-intestinal tract, it must be given by injection. The aim of diabetic management is to maintain the blood glucose levels within normal limits, i.e. between 2.5 and 7 mmol/l. This has only become possible with the development of home blood glucose monitoring and requires a high degree of motivation in the patient.

Many types of insulin are available, and some are shown in Table 19.8. Short, intermediate and long-acting insulins may be used in combination to achieve the control desired. In order to attain this precise control of blood glucose levels a number of insulin injections will be required during the day. Two or even three injections a day before meals may be needed. Twice daily injections of intermediate acting and short-acting insulin can be used, but may lead to nocturnal hypoglycaemia. Giving the short-acting insulin before the evening meal and the intermediate one on going to bed deals with this problem (Scobie and Sönksen, 1984). An alternative regime of injecting a long-acting insulin before breakfast and two or three doses of short-acting insulin before meals has given good results (Ward et al, 1981). Mixtures of some of these

Table 19.8 Properties of insulin preparations

Action	Preparation	Time of onset (hrs)	Peak (hrs)	Duration	Anticipate hypoglycaemic response*
Short-acting	Soluble or regular Neutral	1	2–4	6–8	before lunch
Intermediate-acting	Isophane insulin	1–2	5–8	18	late afternoon
	Insulin zinc suspension (amorphous — semi-lente)	1	4–6	14	late afternoon
	Insulin zinc suspension (Lente)	2	8–12	24	late afternoon
Long-acting	Insulin zinc suspension (crystalline — Ultralente)	3	8–12	60–80	night and early morning
	Protamine zinc insulin	3	8–12	30–40	night and early morning
	Combinations of some of these insulins are also available				

*based on insulin administered before breakfast

insulins are available and are useful for some patients, but the same degree of control is unlikely to be achieved.

In the last few years, methods of administering insulin have been developed which aim to achieve control of blood glucose levels which is more similar to that in non-diabetics. Pumps can be used to administer a basal level of insulin with a bolus of the hormone at each meal. This bolus can be adjusted according to the needs of the individual and can be preprogrammed or initiated manually (Guthrie & Guthrie, 1983). The pump is usually external to the body and administers insulin subcutaneously or intravenously. Some, mainly experimental, pumps are implanted in the body, operated by radio, and infuse insulin into the peritoneal cavity. The administration of insulin intra-peritoneally mirrors the normal distribution of insulin more acurately than when given by other routes. The insulin passes directly to the liver, as it does when normally secreted by the pancreas, and a large fraction of it is removed at this point. The liver is then exposed to higher levels of insulin than the peripheral tissues and metabolic control parallels normal homeostasis (Alberti & Hockaday, 1983).

Research is continuing in two main areas. First, the development of an artificial pancreas would be of considerable value but, as yet, small enough equipment has not been achieved. It must consist of a device for sensing the blood glucose level, a control unit, and a pump which will administer the necessary amount of insulin. Secondly, work continues on the transplantation of either the pancreas or only islet cell tissue. Successful transplantation would provide a cure for diabetes mellitus.

Another distinction to be made between insulins is between the conventional and the highly-purified preparations. The highly-purified types appear to be less likely to provoke antibody formation. The formation of antibodies to insulin will lead to a delayed release of insulin into the blood, as it is only gradually released from combination with antibodies. If high levels of antibodies develop, large amounts of insulin will be needed, and as the insulin is released hypoglycaemia may occur. Some of the complications of insulin treatment develop less commonly in patients receiving the highly-purified type.

Complications of insulin therapy. Complications of insulin therapy should be thoroughly explained to each patient and to the patient's immediate family. Initially, patients may experience blurred vision because alterations in blood glucose concentrations cause ocular osmotic changes. Patients should be advised that this may happen and that these symptoms will subside after about 8 weeks. Initial allergic reactions may occur at injection sites, but these usually subside. Insulin allergy may, however, persist in patients allergic to either cleansing alcohol or to the protein components of insulin preparations. Such patients may require alternative insulin preparations. Syringes may be boiled (or disposable ones used) and alcohol wipes are by no means essential for cleansing. Disposable syringes may be used for up to a month, as long as they are kept in the refrigerator between use.

Tissue hypertrophy or atrophy may occur at injection sites. These lipodystrophies manifest as dimpling, skin thickening and depressed craters at the site of injection and usually result from injection of cold insulin, failure to rotate injection sites, or injection of insulin into fat or muscle tissue. The patient should be taught to recognize these features and how to avoid them. Apart from cosmetic disfigurement, these lipodystrophies decrease the absorption of insulin and diminish sensation in the areas affected. These complications are less common if a highly-purified insulin is used.

Insulin care. Insulin preparations should be stored at temperatures less than 25°C but must be warmed to room temperature before use. The injection of cold preparations can cause tissue reactions (Hayter, 1976). Insulin preparations have now been standardized to 100 units per ml (U-100) and insulin syringes are calibrated in units of insulin. A 12 or 16 mm (25 or 27 gauge) needle is recommended for injection. The insulin preparation should be thoroughly mixed before drawing up the injection by rotating the bottle between the palms of the hands. Shaking of preparations may denature the hormone. Insulin is normally administered subcutaneously, and sites suitable for injection with a suggested rotation scheme are shown in Figure 19.5. Insulin may also be injected intramuscularly and, in emergency situations, intravenously. Rapid-acting insulins are injected about 30 minutes before a meal and should always be related to ingestion of food, not specific time periods. Long-acting insulins are normally injected before breakfast, whereas the intermediate insulins may be used more flexibly to achieve control of blood glucose levels.

Balance

It is recommended that patients develop a routine which balances diet, exercise and insulin which can be maintained on normal days and achieves good control of blood glucose levels. At weekends, holidays and during menstruation when activities may alter, diet and insulin should be adjusted. To achieve this flexibility a considerable degree of understanding of the condition is required. The major role of the nurse therefore is an educative one (Hartman, 1979).

Education of the diabetic patient

To be informed that one has diabetes will be extremely traumatic for most people and depression, apathy, decreased self-esteem and feelings of helplessness and hopelessness have all been reported (quoted in Scobie & Sönksen, 1984). However, if the patient is to be able to regain self-reliance in managing his/her life he/she must accept the condition and the changes in life style that go with it, and acquire a considerable amount of knowledge and new skills.

Considerable lack of success in patient education has been demonstrated (Miller et al, 1978), but Dupuis (1980) found that a well-planned, rigorous education programme resulted in diminished anxiety, better acceptance of their illness, greater self-reliance and better diabetic control in a group of insulin-dependent diabetics. These findings demonstrate the importance of a well-planned programme both of teaching and of counselling, to help the patient come to terms with the changes in his/her life. It may be equally important to involve other members of the family in these sessions, as the diagnosis of diabetes may have considerable repercussions on the family as a whole; they also need to adjust. Some guidelines for an educative programme for these patients and their families are given in the Appendix to this chapter. One of the areas in which they have to become knowledgeable is the prevention, recognition and management of crises.

Crises

There are two major crises which can develop as

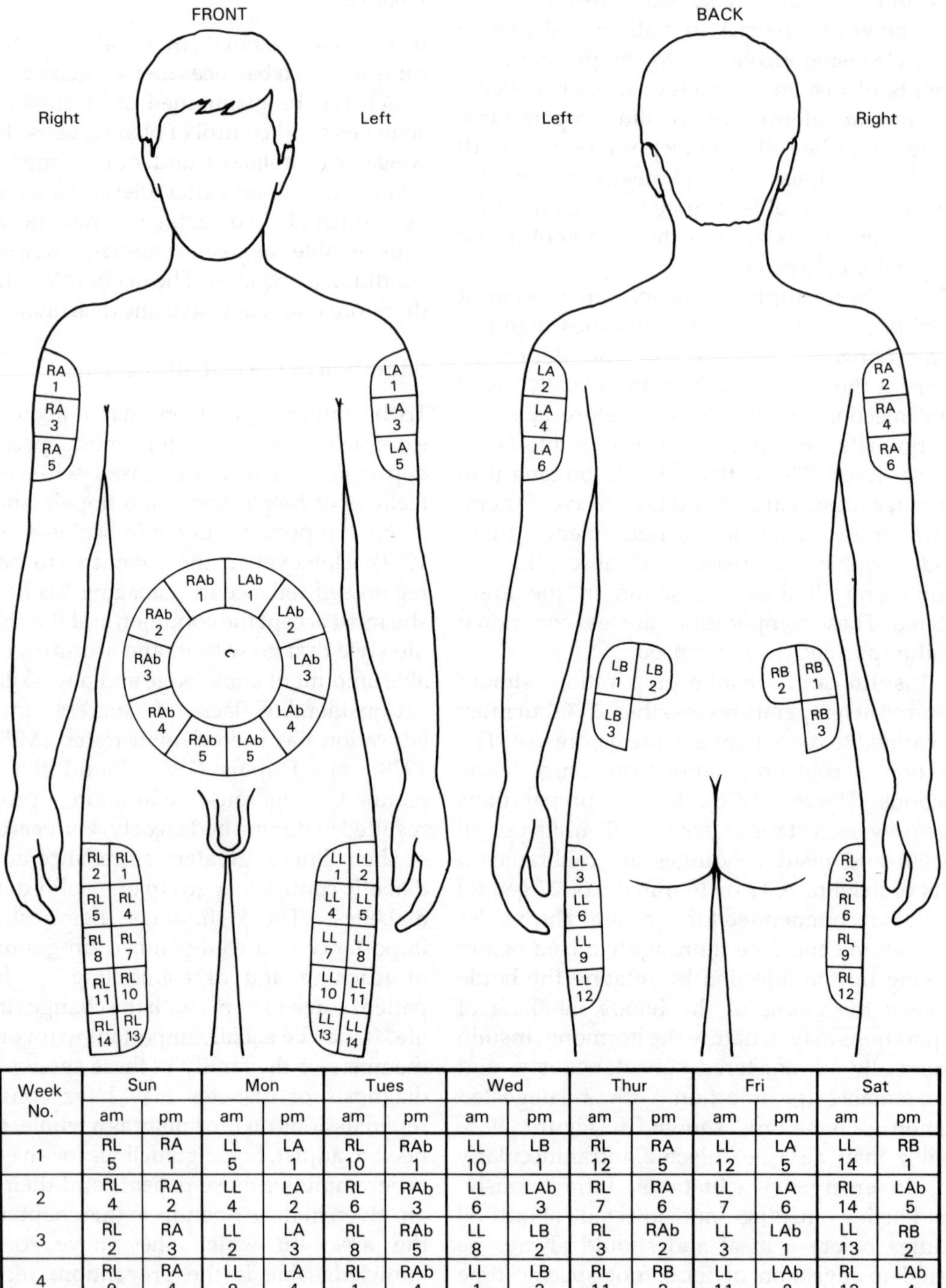

Week No.	Sun		Mon		Tues		Wed		Thur		Fri		Sat	
	am	pm	am	pm	am	pm	am	pm	am	pm	am	pm	am	pm
1	RL 5	RA 1	LL 5	LA 1	RL 10	RAb 1	LL 10	LB 1	RL 12	RA 5	LL 12	LA 5	LL 14	RB 1
2	RL 4	RA 2	LL 4	LA 2	RL 6	RAb 3	LL 6	LAb 3	RL 7	RA 6	LL 7	LA 6	RL 14	LAb 5
3	RL 2	RA 3	LL 2	LA 3	RL 8	RAb 5	LL 8	LB 2	RL 3	RAb 2	LL 3	LAb 1	LL 13	RB 2
4	RL 9	RA 4	LL 9	LA 4	RL 1	RAb 4	LL 1	LB 3	RL 11	RB 3	LL 11	LAb 2	RL 13	LAb 4

Fig. 19.5 Sites for insulin injection.

a result of unsatisfactory control of blood glucose levels; hyperglycaemiac (or diabetic) coma and hypoglycaemic (or insulin) coma. On the whole these conditions can be prevented if the patient and his or her family are aware of predisposing factors and are able to recognize the onset of the condition and take appropriate action (Moorman, 1983).

Hyperglycaemic coma

Hyperglycaemic coma is often precipitated by stress, commonly an infection. This can occur in diabetics of both type 1 and type 2, but the presentation is rather different.

The type 2 diabetic still produces some insulin and does not develop the major disturbances of fat metabolism leading to ketone formation and ketoacidosis. As described previously, these patients will develop a hyperosmolar, non-ketotic coma. They will show signs of dehydration, having passed large volumes of urine, and will have electrolyte imbalances.

The type 1 diabetic is more likely to develop ketoacidosis and coma will be due to acidosis as well as the effects of hyperosmolarity and dehydration. Ketones will be smelt on the breath and respirations will be deep and rapid (Kussmaul respirations) in an attempt to control acidosis (see Ch.26).

The management of these patients is concerned with correcting fluid and electrolyte imbalances, lowering blood glucose levels to normal and preventing complications of unconsciousness. After recovery from coma the aim is to restore the patient's confidence and help achieve metabolic control.

Intravenous fluids will be given. Normal saline will correct dehydration and in the ketoacidotic patient this may be all that is required to enable the kidneys to correct the acidosis. Sometimes sodium bicarbonate may be given in small amounts. Intravenous short-acting insulin will be given in order to return the blood glucose levels to normal. Inherent in the rapid and effective action of insulin is the danger that the patient will become hypoglycaemic. After the initial rapid drop is achieved, 5% dextrose is given and the insulin dose reduced in order that blood glucose levels may return to normal more slowly. During hyperglycaemia and electrolyte disturbances, potassium will have been lost from the cells of the body and excreted in the urine. When the blood glucose levels fall as glucose is deposited as glycogen, potassium also re-enters the cells. This can result in hypokalaemia, so that signs of low serum potassium levels should be noted, e.g. muscle weakness. Serum electrolytes must be monitored frequently and intravenous potassium administered as indicated.

During the period of unconsciousness the circulation will be poor, due to the reduced volume of the extracellular fluid. Thus perfusion of the tissues will be poor. In addition, body temperature will be elevated due to dehydration and the metabolic rate thus increased. Both these factors increase the vulnerability of the tissues and frequent turning is essential. The propensity to develop infections, particularly when the blood glucose levels are high, requires that emphasis is placed on reducing this risk. The intravenous site must be dressed aseptically, the giving set changed at least 48-hourly and care taken with handwashing. Those with any infection should not care for these patients.

Hypoglycaemic coma

Hypoglycaemic coma develops when too much insulin, too little or delayed food intake or too much exercise is taken. The condition develops rapidly with initial symptoms such as hunger, pallor, tachycardia, yawning and nausea due to adrenergic effects resulting from deficient glucose metabolism by the brain. The effect on the central nervous system is demonstrated by mental confusion and abnormal behaviour, often aggressive. If the hypoglycaemia is not corrected rapidly the patient will become comatose. If coma is prolonged permanent brain damage will result or death may ensue. The symptoms develop more slowly with overdose of intermediate and long-acting insulins, and personality changes, emotional instability and nightmares may precede the more obvious symptoms of hypoglycaemia. The aim of management is that the patient should recognize the onset of hypoglycaemia and prevent its development. Patterns of hypoglycaemic reactions vary between patients, and a newly-diagnosed diabetic must be allowed to experience the early stages of hypoglycaemia under supervision. Reversal of the symptoms of hypoglycaemia can be achieved by the immediate administration of simple sugars in the form of glucose, sweets or honey. These foods are readily absorbed and for this reason are particularly suitable for achieving rapid reversal of hypoglycaemia. Insulin-dependent diabetics should always carry one of these rapidly-acting forms of carbohydrate. Treatment of established hypoglycaemic coma is aimed at raising the blood glucose level either by administering intravenous glucose or intravenous glucagon.

The Somogyi effect is a major complication which may follow a hypoglycaemic episode (Keyes, 1977). Adrenaline, glucocorticoids and growth hormone are released causing gluconeogenesis and an increased blood glucose level. The administration of further insulin under these circumstances will induce a major hypoglycaemic reaction and the correct treatment is to lower, not increase, the insulin dosage.

Periods of metabolic change

Diabetes in adolescence

The symptoms of diabetes in these young patients are usually severe, and polydipsia and polyuria are usually dramatic at the onset of the disease. Considerable weight loss occurs. Diabetic ketoacidosis may develop which can induce vomiting and exacerbate the weight loss (Felig, 1974). This disorder requires a considerable degree of planning and self-control to balance diet, insulin and exercise. The life style of many people of this age is not conducive to achieving this. They may deny the changes required and thus have episodes of hyperglycaemia and hypoglycaemia. Some patients experience difficulties in social interaction because of the changes in diet required and the fear of hypoglycaemic episodes (Thomas, 1976). They will need a lot of support, counselling and teaching to help them to accept the co-ordination and the changes required in their life style, and to acquire the knowledge necessary to keep these changes to a minimum (Hoette, 1983).

Diabetes during pregnancy

Diabetes and pregnancy interact to affect both maternal and fetal health, although improvements in the management of diabetes with advances in obstetric and paediatric care have considerably reduced perinatal mortality (Wright, 1984).

Before the discovery of insulin, most diabetic women could not conceive and the mortality rate was high for pregnant diabetic women. Today the incidence of infertility among controlled diabetic women is no greater than is seen in non-diabetic women (Felig & Tyson, 1975). However, women known to be diabetics at the time of conception are two to three times more likely to have babies with major congenital abnormalities and therefore contribute considerably to the perinatal mortality rate. Organ development occurs within the first 7 weeks of pregnancy and few diabetic mothers receive particularly careful observation and management during this period. Using glycosylated haemoglobin as an indication of diabetic control in early pregnancy, Miller et al (1981) found that those with poor control (glycosylated haemoglobin over 8.5%) had 22.4% major abnormalities, while good control (less than 8.5% glycosylated haemoglobin) resulted in only 3.4% major congenital abnormalities. This compares with the rate in the general population. As organogenesis occurs during such a short period at the beginning of pregnancy, it is suggested that a clinic for diabetic women to allow discussion of management, problems, etc., before conception occurs may be valuable (Steel et al, 1980).

During a normal pregnancy, glucose metabolism is altered with lower fasting blood glucose levels (3.6 compared to 4.1 mmol/l mean values) and greater variation in blood glucose levels in relation to nutritional intake (Wright, 1984). In diabetic women the changes due to pregnancy will increase the difficulties of diabetic control. Fetal utilization of glucose can cause maternal hypoglycaemia and to counter this, the hormones synthesized during pregnancy tend to induce hyperglycaemia. The oestrogens act as insulin antagonists, and progesterone decreases the peripheral action of insulin. Cortisol stimulates gluconeogenesis and human placental lactogen mobilizes fatty acids. The high concentration of these hormones circulating during pregnancy creates a diabetogenic effect which can further exacerbate the management of the diabetic patient. During the first trimester, the fetal need for maternal glucose may decrease the diabetic stress in the mother, but in the second and third trimesters the diabetogenic effects of hormone synthesis during pregnancy exert a major influence (Cranley & Frazier, 1973). The most serious complication is maternal acidosis because it can retard the neurological development of the fetus and can lead to fetal death.

Management during pregnancy. The aim of management is to maintain the blood glucose levels within normal limits (here, the limits normal in pregnancy). The approach used is similar to that with non-pregnant diabetics, but the changing physiological state will require monitoring and adjustment of diet, exercise and insulin throughout pregnancy. Satisfactory results in terms of blood glucose can be achieved by giving subcutaneous insulin two, three or four times daily or by continuous infusion. A twice-daily injection of a mixture of short and intermediate acting insulin is usually adequate. Administering the intermediate-acting insulin last thing at night seems to reduce the risk of nocturnal hypoglycaemia (Wright, 1984). It has been shown that diabetic control with self-monitoring of blood glucose levels can be as satisfactory at home as in hospital (Peacock et al, 1979; Stubbs et al, 1980).

Diabetic women are more susceptible to the development of pre-eclampsia and regular monitoring of blood pressure, urine (for albumin) and weight are essential. Adequate rest with reasonable activity should be advised. Accurate assessment of the progress of pregnancy is essential in planning the date of delivery. Babies of diabetic mothers are sometimes particularly large, while in other cases the placenta may be inadequate leading to a 'small-for-dates' baby. In either case postmaturity should be avoided. They are also more prone than usual to develop respiratory distress syndrome so prematurity should also be avoided if possible. Delivery at 38 weeks gestation is frequently the planned goal.

Labour. Care of the diabetic woman during labour requires special attention (Wimberly, 1979). The demands of labour increase glucose utilization by the muscles and insulin levels may exceed the metabolic needs of the body and lead to hypoglycaemia. To prevent this, insulin dosage is reduced prior to commencement of labour. Blood is regularly monitored for glucose and ketone levels during labour. The mother's vital signs should be noted every hour, particularly examining for symptoms of shock, hyperglycaemia or hypoglycaemia. Fetal heart rate should be recorded every 15 minutes. Intravenous fluids are usually administered and, if needed, insulin can be infused in this fashion. The bladder should also be regularly checked for distension. Particular care of the mother is required after delivery of the baby and placenta, as stress complications may trigger a hypoglycaemic response. Should this occur an increase in the intravenous administration of glucose will be required. Wherever possible during labour, the nurse should keep the mother informed of the fetal status, treatments, and reassure her to minimize stress.

Postnatal care. Postnatal care of the diabetic woman is initially directed at maintenance of blood glucose concentrations and prevention of postpartum complications, as residual circulating human placental lactogen proteolytically degrades insulin (Rancilio, 1979). During the immediate postnatal period insulin may need to be administered and regular blood samples (2-hourly) are taken and examined for glucose and ketone levels. However, within about 72 hours of delivery the anti-insulin activity of the maternal hormones has disappeared, and the postpartum catabolic activity will decrease the need for insulin and may induce an insulin reaction. If possible, the patient should be controlled by diet, but if this proves unsatisfactory a new insulin regime may need to be established. Because of the violent fluctuations of insulin during the first 4 days postpartum, careful monitoring of the vital signs is essential. Hypertension, toxaemia, haemorrhage and infections are common postpartum complications in diabetic women and require rapid treatment. The dietary intake of the mother should be increased because of the increased postpartum energy requirements.

Babies of diabetic mothers are particularly at risk and are usually cared for initially in the special care baby unit until their condition is stabilized. Both parents will need particular support at this time.

Postnatal teaching and advice are extremely important. Discussions on birth control should take into account the diabetogenic effect of some oral contraceptives. Nutritional intake will require discussion as needs may be altered, particularly if the woman is breast-feeding her baby. Both parents must be informed that their child may develop diabetes mellitus (Goldstein & Podolsky, 1980) and should be aware of the symptoms of juvenile onset diabetes and seek medical consultation if these symptoms develop. Children with a strong family history of diabetes should be examined each year.

Diabetes in the elderly

Elderly people with diabetes are likely to have a number of problems which are less common in younger patients. These may be specifically related to the diabetes, or simply due to ageing, although many of the changes which occur with ageing are exacerbated by diabetes.

These patients often present with some of the complications of diabetes. They are likely to have atherosclerosis and any damage to their feet tends to heal badly. Sensory neuropathy may mean that they do not feel the damage that occurs. They need to know how to examine and care for their feet and any problems such as bunions or corns must be dealt with by a chiropodist.

Disturbances of vision are also common and should be monitored by annual eye examinations (Miller & White, 1980). Diabetes is one of the commonest causes of blindness in this country and results in difficulty in management of the diabetic's condition. Fixed volume syringes may still allow such patients to administer their own insulin.

Decreased energy requirements and reduced appetite in the elderly will mean that their diet may need altering so that they have smaller, more frequent meals. In addition, other disorders may mean that their diet will need to be modified in other ways, such as by alteration of sodium or protein content.

These patients may have difficulty in monitoring their blood glucose levels accurately and be unprepared to change from urine to blood testing, even if their vision is adequate for the task. Patients in this age group may need to change from taking oral antidiabetic drugs to insulin, or need to change their insulin from single to multiple dose administration. The acquisition of new skills and the adjustments required are particularly difficult at this stage of life. Careful assessment of their ability to manage their own condition is essential. It may be that members of the family or a neighbour will need to take over the responsibility for supervision and will need teaching and the support of the community nursing service (Marchesseault, 1983).

The diabetic patient undergoing surgery

A diabetic patient undergoing surgery requires particular care for two reasons. First, the metabolic disturbances associated with anaesthesia and surgery alter diabetic control. Secondly, many of the complications of diabetes, or conditions associated with diabetes, increase the risk of surgical complications. Type 2 and older diabetics are more likely than the general population to have cardiovascular disease or neurological impairment, and obesity is also more common. All these factors increase morbidity.

As part of the stress response and the catabolic response to surgery there is increased secretion of ACTH, glucocorticoids, catecholamines and growth hormone. These hormones are antagonistic to insulin and thus blood glucose levels rise in proportion to the severity of surgery. Gluconeogenesis contributes to

Table 19.9 The management of Type 1 (insulin dependent) diabetics during surgery (from Alberti and Hockaday, 1983)

A. Pre-operative

1. Admit to hospital 2–3 days before operation
2. Stop long-acting insulins and stabilise on either twice daily short- and intermediate-acting insulins or thrice daily short-acting insulin with intermediate insulin in the evening
3. Monitor blood glucose (bedside methods) before and after each main meal and at bedtime
4. Aim to maintain fasting blood glucose <8 mmol/l and other values between 4 and 10 mmol/l
5. Check urea, electrolytes, and renal, cardiovascular, and neurological systems

B. Peri-operative

1. Schedule operation for early in the day
2. Check fasting blood glucose level. If >10 mmol/l, delay operation
3. Omit morning insulin and breakfast
4. Start infusion of glucose-insulin-potassium as early as possible and at least one hour pre-operatively
5. If operation delayed more than 2 hrs from onset of infusion, recheck blood glucose; adjust infusion if necessary
6. Recheck blood glucose at end of operation (and during lengthy operations). Modify regimen if necessary
7. Check K^+

C. Postoperative

1. Check blood glucose 2–3 hourly, and K^+ 6-hourly then twice daily.
2. Continue infusion until first meal. Restart S.C. insulin at pre-operative dose 1 hr before infusion stopped
3. Consider total parenteral nutrition if oral refeeding not recommenced within 48 hrs

Table 19.10 The management of Type 2 diabetics during surgery (from Alberti & Hockaday, 1983)

A. Minor operations	
Diet treated	1. If fasting blood glucose (FBG) ≤8 mmol/l treat as non-diabetic 2. If FBG >8 mmol/l treat with insulin infusion regimen during operation
Oral agent	1. Stop biguanides and long-acting sulphonylureas 2–3 days pre-operatively. Stabilize on diet alone or short-acting sulphonylureas. 2. If FBG ≤8 mmol/l on day of operation treat as non-diabetic. If FBG >8 mmol/l treat with insulin infusion regimen during operation.
B. Major operations	
Diet treated	1. If FBG ≤7 mmol/l, treat as Type 1 diabetic on day of surgery 2. If FBG > 7 mmol/l stabilize on short-acting insulin three times a day for two days pre-operatively. Treat as Type 1 diabetic on day of surgery
Oral agent treated	1. Stop all oral agents 2–3 days pre-operatively 2. Stabilize on three times a day short-acting insulin 3. Treat as Type 1 diabetic on day of surgery
Postoperative management	1. Minor surgery: recommence usual therapy with first meal. 2. Major surgery: convert to three times a day S.C. insulin with first oral feeding. Recommence oral agent or diet-alone therapy 24–28 hours later

hyperglycaemia and hyperosmolarity and ketoacidosis may develop in type 1 diabetics. All these changes lead to disturbances in electrolyte balance. The aim of management is to minimize electrolyte disturbances, protein breakdown, and hypoglycaemia or excessive hyperglycaemia. Insulin is essential for normal wound healing and control of blood glucose levels will minimize the risk of infection.

The clinical management of diabetic patients undergoing surgery will vary depending on whether they are type 1 or type 2 diabetics (see Tables 19.9 and 19.10). Clearly nurses have a major role in the care of these patients, through planned care to minimize stress, the accurate monitoring of blood glucose levels and punctual administration of insulin and diet. Exposure to infection must be minimized so scrupulous wound care and attention to hygiene is required, and those nurses with any infection should not come into contact with these patients (Bovington et al, 1983).

Diabetic patients may be particularly anxious about the possibility of their disorder being exacerbated. In addition to the information given to every surgical patient, they should be told about the methods to be used to control blood glucose levels. They should feel confident that the staff involved in their care are competent in the management of diabetes.

HYPOGLYCAEMIA

Hypoglycaemia can result from many causes but the commonest is overdosage of insulin (Marks & Rose, 1981). The acute symptoms are mainly related to cerebral dysfunction due to a fall in the glucose supply to the brain. However, there may be some variation in presentation due to the ability of the brain to adapt to prolonged reduction in glucose supply (Owen et al, 1967). Hypoglycaemia has three main groups of causes, and the presentation and management varies (Wyngaarden & Smith, 1982).

Hypoglycaemia in the fed state

The first group is described as hypoglycaemia in the fed state, and results from a lag between glucose absorption and the secretion of insulin. This leads to reactive hypoglycaemia. Patients may suffer from this after gastric surgery when nutrients reach the intestine rapidly leading to speedy glucose absorption. This stimulates considerable insulin release, and blood glucose levels fall quickly. The excessive insulin secreted is not matched by continuing glucose absorption from the gut and hypoglycaemia develops 2–3 hours after a meal. Reactive hypoglycaemia can also occur in the early stages of diabetes mellitus (type 2) when insulin secretion in response to glucose absorption is sluggish, and the effects continue after the blood glucose level falls. These patients show a diabetic glucose tolerance curve for 3 hours after glucose ingestion and reactive hypoglycaemia in the fourth and fifth hours.

In these patients signs and symptoms develop rapidly and are partly due to the release of catecholamines in response to hypoglycaemia. They consist of tachycardia, sweating, trembling, weakness, hunger and anxiety. Consciousness is not usually lost. Management of this group of patients is concerned with damping down the rapid rise in blood glucose levels after eating, by dietary means. Small, frequent meals and high protein, low carbohydrate meals have both been suggested. A high-fibre, high-complex carbohydrate diet has recently been advocated.

Spontaneous hypoglycaemia in fasting

This type of hypoglycaemia is due to underproduction of glucose during fasting. This may be due to lack of glucose production by the liver, as in specific enzyme deficiency or liver disease. Alternatively, excessive insulin secretion or lack of hormones antagonistic to insulin (as in panhypopituitarism) can result in hypoglycaemia. In this group the low blood sugar levels develop slowly, without stimulating catecholamine secretion, and the signs and symptoms are due to glucose deprivation of the central nervous system. Confusion and disorientation lead to psychotic behaviour. Paraesthesias and transient paralysis develop into convulsions and coma.

The commonest cause of this type is islet cell tumour (or tumours), of which about 10% are malignant. The most usual treatment is surgery. Pre-operative care is directed towards stabilizing blood glucose concentrations, either by infusion of glucose or by the administration of glucagon or hydrocortisone. Postoperative complications are due to either deficiency of pancreatic enzymes or the development of diabetes mellitus, due to a deficiency of islet cells. Enteric coated pancreatic enzyme capsules can be administered to alleviate pancreatic enzyme deficiency and symptoms of diabetes mellitus can be treated as previously described.

Induced hypoglycaemia

Hypoglycaemia externally induced in the fasting state is the third type and is caused by some exogenous substance. This can result from substances which increase insulin levels in the blood (e.g. administered insulin or antidiabetic drugs) or agents which block glucose release quite independently of insulin. Alcohol (ethanol) is probably the commonest cause, but salicylates can also result in hypoglycaemia. The signs and symptoms are similar to those of hypoglycaemia in the fasting state and glucose must be administered to restore blood glucose levels to normal. Difficulties can arise in differentiating between inebriation and hypoglycaemia resulting from ethanol intake, and the first may progress to the second without recognition and with disastrous results.

DISTURBANCES OF ADRENAL FUNCTION

The adrenal glands are composed of two different types of tissue, the cortex and the medulla. The adrenal medulla has a common origin with the ganglion cells of the sympathetic nervous system and is the site of synthesis of the catecholamine hormones, adrenaline (epinephrine) and noradrenaline (norepinephrine). Secretion of these hormones is under direct control of the nervous system.

The adrenal cortex develops from embryonic mesoderm into three layers which synthesize 40 to 50 different steroids. These steroid hormones can be classified into three groups: the mineralocorticoids, the glucocorticoids and the sex hormones. Although these are three functional groups, there is considerable overlap between their activities, as glucocorticoids, which mainly affect the metabolism of carbohydrate, fats and proteins, also have some mineralocorticoid activity and some sex hormone activity.

DISORDERS OF THE ADRENAL MEDULLA

Phaeochromocytoma is a tumour, normally benign, of the adrenal medulla or sympathetic chain which causes hypersecretion of the catecholamines, mainly noradrenaline but also adrenaline. The primary symptom is paroxysms of hypertension associated with pallor, sweating, tachycardia felt as palpitations and sometimes causing chest discomfort, headache and a feeling of anxiety. These are the expected results of excessive activity of the sympathetic nervous system. In acute cases cardiovascular damage, blindness and cerebral haemorrhage may develop. As a result of its intermittent nature, extensive laboratory tests and close observation of the patient are required to confirm the diagnosis. The determination of plasma and urinary catecholamines will require blood samples and accurate 24-hour urine collections. CAT scan or adrenal venography may also be used to aid diagnosis. Surgical removal of the tumour is the mode of treatment (Sanford, 1980).

Neuroblastomas are malignant tumours which occur mainly in the adrenal medulla. These tumours occur primarily in children and if detected early can be treated by excision of the adrenal gland. Subsequent radiotherapy and chemotherapy depends upon the extent of metastatic invasion.

DISORDERS OF THE ADRENAL CORTEX

Hyposecretion

Chronic primary adrenocortical insufficiency is termed Addison's disease. This disease is relatively rare and is believed to have an autoimmune basis, although infective agents such as tuberculosis and fungi are documented causative factors (Irvine & Barnes, 1972). Symptoms do not develop until the disease is well advanced and reflect deficiencies in aldosterone, glucocorticoid and androgen synthesis. Defective aldosterone synthesis results in polyuria, dehydration, hyponatraemia, hypotension and diminished cardiac output. Glucocorticoid deficiency leads to hypoglycaemia, anorexia, weight loss and emotional changes such as depression and irritability. Diminished cortisol secretion with lack of feedback inhibition of the production of melanocyte-stimulating hormone by the pituitary gland, results in increased pigmentation of the skin and mucous membranes. Androgen deficiency only develops in females, the symptoms being loss of axillary and pubic hair.

As the development of the disease is slow, a detailed history and examination is essential for diagnosis (Hamdi, 1971). Muscle weakness, general fatigue and lethargy, nausea, irritability, hypotension, weight loss, salt craving and excess thirst, as well as changes in skin pigmentation, are typical findings. Laboratory evaluation involves serum electrolytes, urea and glucose determination as well as hormonal provocative tests. The intravenous ACTH test measures urinary excretion of 17-ketosteroids in response to ACTH challenge. Normally excretion of these ketosteroids increases at least threefold following ACTH infusion (8 hours), whereas in Addison's disease there is no increase in urinary excretion. The plasma cortisol test measures the increase in plasma cortisol 30 minutes after 25 units of ACTH is injected intramuscularly. If there is no increase in plasma cortisol, Addison's disease is indicated. Other tests include water excretion and haematological profiles. The management of a patient with Addison's disease is focused on strict maintenance of a regime of additive synthetic corticosteroid drugs (Table 19.11).

Hypersecretion

Adrenocortical hyperfunction exhibits in three forms: adrenal glucocorticoid, mineralocorticoid and androgen steroid hypersecretion.

Hypersecretion of glucocorticoids

Cushing's syndrome is due to increased levels of glucocorticoids and may be considered to fall into two main groups as shown in Table 19.12.

Effects. The clinical symptoms of the disease reflect excess glucocorticoid secretion. Hyperglycaemia is a common condition and the metabolism of lipid and protein as gluconeogenic precursors results in abnormal distribution of lipid, and in protein wasting. The abnormal lipid distribution, which is accentuated by oedema, results in a moon face, a buffalo hump on the patient's neck, truncal obesity and pink striae on the breasts, abdomen and legs. Changes in protein metabolism are reflected in muscle weakness, capillary fragility, osteoporosis, skin fragility and poor wound healing and, in children, stunted growth. Persistent hyperglycaemia may result in diabetes mellitus due to excessive stress on the pancreatic beta cells. Fluid and electrolyte imbalances result in sodium retention and oedema, while hypokalaemia also develops. Corticosteroids also lower the ability of T-lymphocytes to combat infection. Hypertension is a common feature which leads to atherosclerosis, ischaemic heart disease and nephrosclerosis. Occasionally increased androgen production can induce mild virilism in women, with acne and hirsutism being common symptoms.

Diagnosis. As the onset of the disease can be either prolonged or precipitate, a detailed history and physical examination are of particular value in diagnosing this condition. Documentation of the onset of the symptoms of hyperglycaemia and the noting of the physical features can aid in diagnosis. Laboratory testing involves determination of serum electrolytes, glucose, protein and lipids as well as haematological examination of lymphocytes and eosinophils. The synthesis of these cells is dramatically inhibited by glucocorticoids. High concentrations of plasma and urinary cortisol supports a diagnosis of Cushing's syndrome. The ACTH stimulation test examines the ability of ACTH to elevate the urinary excretion of 17-ketosteroids and 17-hydroxycorticosteroids. The rate of excretion in patients with Cushing's syndrome is three to four times that in control patients. The cortisone suppression test measures the ability of dexamethasone (a synthetic steroid) to suppress

Table 19.11 Aspects of management for patients with Addison's disease

Purpose of care	Specific actions	Teaching aspects
1. Correct administration of drugs	1. Attempt to achieve optimal drugs dosage before patient is discharged	1. Explain to the patient the role of glucocorticoid and mineralocorticoid drugs 2. Describe to the patient the symptoms of Cushing's syndrome which indicate overdosage 3. Ensure that oral preparations are administered with meals to minimize gastric irritation, and large dose given a.m, small dose given p.m. to mimic normal circadian rhythm 4. Warn the patient that symptoms of fatigue, weight loss, irritability and postural hypotension often indicate insufficient dosage of drugs, and to consult a physician
	2. Enable patient to adapt dosage under conditions of stress	5. Teach patient to double glucocorticoid dose if exposed to stressors e.g. fever over 38°C, infection, accident etc.
	3. Ensure able to take drug even if vomiting	6. Teach patient how to give drugs by injection in case this situation arises
2. Appropriate response to emergency	1. Prepare a kit for the patient containing an emergency supply of hydrocortisone and injection materials	1. Instruct the family and friends of the symptoms of Addisonian crises and how to administer drugs and to get medical help immediately 2. Give information to patient about Medic-Alert identity bracelet/disc 3. Advise patient to see physician to reassess drug protocol if stress situations are encountered 4. Ensure that patient consults a physician twice each year
3. Minimize exposure to infection and minimize risks	1. Keep patient separate from patients with infectious diseases	1. Teach about risks of infection and importance of reducing exposure to infection
	2. Prevent spread of infection within body	2. Educate the patient that glucocorticoid drugs suppress immune and inflammatory reactions. All wounds should be immediately treated and continuously monitored and infections of any sort treated with the appropriate antibiotic

Table 19.12 Causes of Cushing's syndrome

Cushing's syndrome (increased glucocorticoids)	
ACTH — dependent	**Non-ACTH — dependent**
1. Pituitary hypersecretion of ACTH 2. Ectopic ACTH—secreting tumour 3. Iatrogenic — administration of ACTH	1. Glucocorticoid secreting tumour of adrenal cortex (adenoma or carcinoma) 2. Iatrogenic — administration of glucocorticoids

Table 19.13 Aspects of management of patients receiving steroid therapy

Purpose of care	Specific aspects of care	Teaching aspects
To correct endocrine malfunction OR to maintain control of disease process for which steroids are being given	Clinician determines steroid and method of administration	Instruct patient and immediate family on the type of steroid administered and the function of this preparation
	Attempt to optimise management with minimal dosage	Ensure that the patient understands the need for correct dosage at the prescribed times
	To minimize side effects examine alternate-day administration — high morning-low evening dosage	Explain unacceptable side effects and the need to consult a physician if these symptoms develop (see Table 19.14) Ensure patient understands the need for higher doses when stressed
To prevent complications when possible	Minimize risk of infection	Minimize exposure to infection and develop protocol for asepsis
	Regulate diet to maintain Nitrogen balance	Explain how a high protein, high carbohydrate diet rich in calcium is necessary to maintain nitrogen balance and prevent osteoporosis
	Minimize gastric disturbances	Advise the patient to be aware of the signs of gastric haemorrhage due to steroid induced gastric irritation
	Maintain electrolyte balance through high potassium, low sodium intake	Instruct the patient how to estimate a low sodium, high potassium diet, and to be aware of oedema and increase in weight developing
	Minimize stressful situations	Because steroids modulate response to stress instruct the patient and family of the need to live in as quiet an environment as possible
	Carefully monitor the healing of any wounds	Because steroids can interfere with wound healing ensure that wounds which heal slowly are examined by a physician. Reinforce the need for strict hygiene Instruct patient to exercise to promote general wellbeing and prevent stasis e.g. lungs, bladder
To recognise complications if they occur	Patient will know what side effects can be expected and what are exceptional	(see Table 19.14)

Table 19.14 Potential side effects of steroid therapy

Side effects	Reason	Management
Weakness, tiredness, alkalosis	Potassium depletion	Administer prescribed potassium and diuretics
Weight gain, oedema, increased blood pressure	Sodium and water retention	Diuretics, restricted calorie intake modify steroid
Nocturia and increased frequency	Genitourinary infection or steroid induced diabetes mellitus	Urinalysis for glucose and/or infection
Facial mooning	Steroid induced weight gain Redistribution of body fat	Restrict calorie intake
Infection	Steroids decrease eosinophils and lymphocytes	Antimicrobial medication
* Osteoporosis, fractures	Glucocorticoid induced calcium and phosphorus efflux from bone	Calcium supplement. Refer to clinician
* Allergic reactions		Withdraw steroid and refer to clinician
* Hypertension	Steroid disturbance of mineralo-corticoid system	Reduce dosage of steroids
* Eye complications	Water retention	Refer to clinician
* Steroid psychosis		Refer to clinician

* Unacceptable side effects

pituitary secretion of ACTH. Patients with adrenal tumours or ectopic tumours do not respond to this inhibition.

Treatment of hypersecreting tumours. When the cause of the Cushing's syndrome is a hypersecreting tumour, treatment is by surgical removal often followed by chemotherapy. Pituitary hyperfunction is treated by irradiation of the pituitary gland which may be followed by hypophysectomy and bilateral adrenalectomy.

Chemotherapy with drugs and steroids is usually prescribed palliatively in inoperable cancer (Thorn & Lauler, 1972). Dichlorodiphenyldichloroethane (DDD) destroys cortical tissue and thus controls hypersecretion of glucocorticoids. Careful administration of the drug is required in order to prevent complete inhibition of cortisol secretion and to minimize toxic effects which include nausea, lethargy and skin rash. As this drug is stored in adipose tissue and released over a period of time, the toxic effects persist after discontinuation of the drug. Aminoglutethimide and metyrapone are drugs which inhibit cortisol synthesis and produce toxic effects similar to DDD. Subsequent therapy is dependent upon supplementary hormonal therapy depending upon the mode of surgical or chemotherapeutic intervention.

Management of iatrogenic Cushing's syndrome. The relatively wide use of steroid preparations in the management of a variety of disorders results in iatrogenic Cushing's syndrome being of considerable concern to doctors, nurses and patients. It is important to note here, however, that many patients receiving steroids have doses lower than, or for shorter periods than, the prolonged high doses required to cause Cushing's syndrome. The same physiological changes are occurring in these patients as in those on higher doses, but to a lesser extent. Problems of management are therefore inherently similar although less acute, and some aspects of such management are included in Table 19.13.

This section is concerned with those patients who, due to their therapy, have developed Cushing's syndrome.

Management in this situation is fraught with difficulties. Firstly, the administration of hormones depresses the normal function of the relevant gland. This has two results:

- The patient will be unable to respond normally to physiological stress (see Ch. 8). Situations of stress are inevitable. Some are planned, e.g. an operation, others are unanticipated, e.g. emotional upsets or infection. In any such situation an increase in steroid dosage will be required, often intravenously. For this reason, patients on steroids must always carry a steroid warning card.
- The drug cannot be stopped suddenly. If appropriate, the dosage is reduced gradually to allow the gland to regain normal function. It is important during this period of adjustment for the patient to be observed carefully.

Secondly, there is often no alternative form of treatment for conditions treated with the high dosage required to cause Cushing's syndrome. Typically, the diseases are widespread in effect and thought to be autoimmunological in aetiology; for example, systemic lupus erythematosus or systemic sclerosis. Also, this form of treatment is used for patients undergoing transplant surgery where depression of the normal immune response is necessary for successful acceptance of the foreign tissue.

Nursing management. Nursing management of a person with Cushing's syndrome must be particularly carefully planned if the situation is not to be worsened. The state of the body tissues generally is extremely fragile due to the changes in protein metabolism (Sanford, 1980). This is particularly noticeable in relation to the skin; pressure, minor knocks and the ordinary processes of patient handling such as assisting out of bed can cause bruising and skin abrasions. These are extremely difficult to heal and are highly prone to infection. If abrasions occur on the legs, oedema further complicates the situation. Clearly, anticipating such events and taking preventative action is preferable. Careful handling on the nurse's part and informed caution on the part of the person concerned will do much. The selection of equipment such as bed, chair, table and bedside cabinet without knobs, sharp edges or obtrusive handles — and where possible with padded surfaces — also reduces the risk of injury. In addition, if the skin is particularly friable, padding may be required on the areas at risk, usually the arms and legs. The wearing of jumpers and trousers, rather than nightwear, in hospital or the use of padded tube bandage is a valuable precaution. Soft, easy fitting and absorbent material will also reduce the risk of skin breakdown from moisture or constriction. If wounds are present they need to be treated with meticulous care. Non-adherent dressings, strict asepsis and non-adherent methods of securing the dressing are all clearly important.

Back pain from osteoporosis can become an overwhelming problem. Bedrest may be indicated if vertebral collapse is occurring and until the process is stabilized. This will clearly not occur while the blood corticosteroid level remains high. If osteoporosis is severe paraplegia can result, and fractures of long bones occur either spontaneously or due to relatively minor trauma. The management of such bony injury has a twofold purpose: first, to stabilize the collapsed or fractured site; conservative methods such as rest, reduction by skin traction and splinting by light casts will be utilized, as the bony tissue will not support pins and plates. Secondly, to control the associated pain; due to the chronic nature of this problem, pain management requires considerable and imaginative planning (see Ch. 9). The major features to note here are:

- Drugs liable to create dependency are contraindicated due to the non-terminal but longstanding nature of the disease.
- Injections are contraindicated due to the risk of injection site breakdown and infection.
- Gastric irritant drugs such as salicylates and the non-steroid anti-inflammatory

drugs which have an analgesic effect, are contraindicated due to the friability of the gastric mucosa.

The risk of the person succumbing to infection is also great. This has a number of contributory factors:

- Friable skin allows easy entry of microorganisms into the underlying tissues.
- Capillary fragility allows easy entry of microorganisms into the bloodstream.
- The inflammatory reaction to infection is reduced thus microorganisms are not restricted to their point of entry to the body.
- The immune response is depressed thus general response to invasion is reduced.

Effectively, therefore, microorganisms are more able to invade initially and less likely to be localized. The reduction in both localized and generalized response also creates a further problem, that of non-recognition. For example, an abrasion that has been invaded with microorganisms will not produce the signs of inflammatory response, i.e. it will not be red, nor will it be warm, painful or produce pus. Thus local infections may go untreated. Similarly, infections of the lungs or kidneys which normally present with pyrexia may simply make the patient feel extremely unwell without other obvious signs. Clearly in this situation the disease can become rampant before diagnosis. In observing and monitoring the patient's condition constantly, the nurse is in a good position to identify slight deterioration or a lack of general progress — signs that might point to underlying infection. Management is concerned with controlling or destroying the invading microorganism, and assisting the body to cope with the infection. Two specific, high dose bacteriocidal antibiotics are usually used in combination, in order to reduce development of bacterial resistance. Steroids are given or increased to enable the body to respond and cope with the stress (see Ch. 8). This treatment might be confusing to the nurse and of major concern to the patient if the rationale is not understood.

Viral infections are more difficult to manage. It is important for the nurse to realize that, even in the absence of pyrexia, the patient may be gravely ill and will require all the care normally required by patients with acute infections. Rampant infections may present with classical signs such as hyperpyrexia, toxaemia and rigor. It is important to note that they are likely to respond less quickly to treatment, and that the risk of permanent tissue damage is considerable. If the Cushing's syndrome is iatrogenic, death may result from infection rather than from the original disease.

Two other aspects are important, particularly associated with the person with iatrogenic Cushing's syndrome. First, that by reducing the body's natural supply of corticosteroids the fixed dose of the artificial steroid makes it impossible for the circulating amount to vary in response to physiological demand. Physiologically, therefore, the body cannot respond to stresses such as infections (as already discussed), to trauma and to long term stresses such as anxiety. Therefore, when exposed to such situations, an increased amount of corticosteroids must be administered. A Medic-Alert bracelet should be worn to ensure that appropriate doses of steroids are given in emergencies, even if the patient is not sufficiently conscious to give the necessary information.

Secondly, the patient will have observed considerable body changes during the process of the disease or treatment. Indeed, a patient on high dose steroids may be unrecognizable within three months of commencing treatment. Some of these changes, facial 'mooning', pot belly, muscle wasting on arms and legs, and hair loss are reversible once the blood steroid level is reduced. Others, such as osteoporosis, may cause more permanent damage. Some very positive reassurance can therefore be given, but this should be realistic.

In discussing these implications of Cushing's syndrome it is clear that a number of important ethical issues arise in relation to treating patients for any disease with corticosteroids. If high doses are known to be required to control the disease process, the medical staff clearly have to weigh up costs and benefits. In the context of prevalent medical ideology the decision to treat is the more likely outcome. The notion of informed consent to drug therapy, as opposed to operative procedure, is not widespread but is clearly relevant when the effects of treatment might be as, or more, devastating than the disease itself. It may also be a source of conflict between doctor and nurse, and it is therefore important that the nurse work out his or her own position in relation to this issue.

Hypersecretion of mineralocorticoids

Conn's syndrome refers to hyperaldosteronism which is caused by an aldosterone-secreting adrenal tumour (Conn, 1977). This tumour is believed to be a major cause of hypertension and is most common in middle-aged females. Hypertension due to sodium and water accumulation, hypokalaemia with consequent muscle weakness, and loss of neuromuscular response are characteristic symptoms of Conn's syndrome. Polyuria and polydipsia are common features due to impaired reabsorption of sodium and water in the renal tubule due to potassium depletion. Metabolic alkalosis develops because hydrogen ion loss occurs to counteract further potassium loss. Diagnosis is based on serum and urinary electrolyte measurements and serum and urinary aldosterone determinations. Early diagnosis of this disease is important in preventing permanent renal damage. The usual method of treatment is surgical removal of the tumour. Pre- and postoperative care is the same as for patients undergoing adrenalectomy.

Hypersecretion of androgens

Androgen hypersecretion is a rare condition which often has a genetic aetiology. Because of inherited enzyme defects, hyposecretion of cortisol occurs which cannot regulate pituitary synthesis of ACTH, resulting in androgen hypersecretion by the adrenal cortex (Burnett, 1980). In female infants symptoms include pseudohermaphroditism, while older females develop hirsutism, masculine body features, breast atrophy and baldness. Young males become sexually precocious and adult males develop heavier facial hair. Women in particular suffer socially because of their facial appearance, and require guidance and counselling. Elevated urinary and plasma testosterone and 5-dihydrotestosterone, and elevated urinary 17-ketosteroids, confirm the clinical diagnosis. Treatment is directed towards restoring normal cortisol concentrations. This can be achieved by the administration of cortisol preparations, which also inhibit ACTH release. If adrenal tumours are detected they are surgically removed. The return to normal plasma cortisol concentrations usually reverses most of the clinical symptoms of androgen hypersecretion.

Nursing care of the patient undergoing adrenalectomy

Pre-operative care

Pre-operative care is directed towards reducing hypertension, stabilizing blood glucose levels, combating infection and enhancing the general health state of the patient. Psychological support and sedated rest may reduce hypertension. A high protein and potassium, low sodium and carbohydrate diet will reduce oedema and electrolyte imbalance as well as minimizing diabetogenic stress. The urine should be tested daily for glucose and ketone bodies, and the patient should be separated from others with any infection. Particular care should be exercised in handling and bathing these patients to prevent pathological fractures. On the day of surgery an intramuscular injection of a glucocorticoid is administered to minimize acute adrenal insufficiency during surgery, and water soluble steroid preparations should be available for infusion during surgery.

Postoperative care

Much of the postoperative care is similar to that for other surgical patients, but with a number of aspects requiring particular consideration. The general aims of care include maintaining respiratory function, preventing shock, controlling pain, minimizing the risk of postoperative infection, maximizing conditions for wound healing and promoting rehabilitation.

The stress of anaesthesia and surgery is considerable and the normal response includes increased secretion of glucocorticoid hormones. These patients are unable to respond in this way and are at risk of developing shock because of this. Therefore the administration of glucocorticoids such as hydrocortisone or cortisol (usually by intramuscular injection at first, and later orally) is essential, and regular recording of pulse and blood pressure, initially every 15 minutes, is necessary (Melick, 1977).

The site of operation has certain implications. As the adrenal gland is above the kidney, high up on the posterior wall of the abdominal cavity, the surgical incision extends over the lower ribs and results in pain on respiration. These patients, therefore, are at increased risk of developing a respiratory infection and need encouragement to carry out breathing exercises and must receive adequate analgesia. In addition, the pleural cavity is sometimes entered and signs of pneumothorax (chest pain, increased respiratory rate, breathlessness) must be noted. A chest drain will be needed and management of this is discussed in Chapter 24. Particularly when bilateral adrenalectomy is performed, the approach may be through an upper abdominal incision and nasogastric suction may be required until gastrointestinal activity returns to normal. After a unilateral adrenalectomy with a loin incision, the patient is nursed on the affected side of the body in order to promote wound drainage.

As previously discussed, these patients are at increased risk of developing an infection if exposed to pathogenic organisms. Therefore they must be protected from infection as far as possible and carefully observed for any signs. The spread of infection takes place readily and the effects are often masked until it is widespread throughout the body. These patients normally have chest X-rays carried out more frequently than usual, and urine samples and wound swabs are sent for microbiological examination regularly. Minor changes in pulse and respiration rate may be significant and any complaints by the patient of feeling unwell must be taken seriously.

Wound healing tends to be poor because of the metabolic effects of corticosteroid hormones. In order to provide the best attainable conditions for wound healing, a number of aspects of care need consideration. A high protein diet is encouraged and nutritional supplements given if little normal diet is taken. Vitamin and mineral content must be adequate. The circulation should be stimulated by controlled exercise in order to provide oxygen and nutrients to the healing tissues, and the blood volume maintained by a good fluid intake. Minimizing anxiety modifies the physiological changes of stress and is also of great importance. Using a semi-permeable dressing such as OpSite provides the optimum conditions at the incision for healing to take place.

The problems of the patient with Cushing's syndrome previously discussed continue postoperatively, only becoming moderated with time. Therefore rehabilitation takes a considerable period of time and the patient must understand that progress will seem slow. Care must be taken in everyday activities and the patient's abilities must be taken into account when planning a programme of rehabilitation.

If bilateral adrenalectomy is performed, development of a programme of lifetime steroid replacement therapy is required (Blount & Kinney, 1974). The choice and method of administration of steroid will be determined on an individual basis by the physician. It is important that patients are fully aware of the implications of taking steroids. Table 19.13 indicates some aspects of management and teaching. The patient and immediate family will need to be taught about the possible side effects of steroid therapy. They must learn to recognize symptoms of adverse reactions, how to minimize them, and to consult a physician if they persist.

Appendix Guidelines for education of the diabetic patient (select appropriate items from those in [ ])

AIMS

1. Patient will accept condition and importance of good diabetic control and adapt lifestyle accordingly
2. Patient will understand disease and why good control of blood glucose levels is important.
3. Patient will have technical skills needed to monitor blood glucose level and give required drugs safely.
4. Patient will understand contribution of diet, exercise and insulin in maintenance of glucose levels and necessity for achieving and monitoring balance.
5. Patient will recognize disturbances of blood glucose level and development of complications.

ASSESSMENT

* Of knowledge and ability to learn
* Of acceptance and willingness to learn
* Of manual dexterity and sight
* Of resources and support

CONTENT AND TEACHING APPROACHES

1. **Acceptance of condition and importance of control**

Disease is not going to go away, will need life-long adaptations to lifestyle
With good management, risk of development of complications is reduced
With experience and knowledge, lifestyle can continue with relatively minor changes
Will be able to take part in sport and other activities
Will be able to eat normal foods in controlled amounts and go out for meals
[Is unlikely to need injections if sticks to diet]
[Able to have family but good control essential to reduce risk to baby]
Has a hereditary implication

Nursing care

Discussion
Allow patient to talk
Listen
Discuss with family, significant others
Opportunity to discuss with other diabetics
British Diabetic Association booklets and local group contact
Reiteration of material as often as necessary
Counselling

2. **Knowledge of disease**

Major disturbance is loss of control of blood glucose levels due to lack of sufficient insulin
Insulin lowers blood glucose level by allowing use and storage of glucose, secreted in response to food
Blood glucose can be fairly accurately controlled by balancing diet, excercise and insulin
Lack of insulin leads to rise in blood glucose and signs and symptoms of diabetes — thirst, weight loss etc. can lead to hyperglycaemic coma due to fluid loss and electrolyte imbalance [Type 1 diabetes — fat breakdown leads to ketone formation and ketoacidosis]
[Excess insulin leads to fall in blood glucose and hyperglycaemic coma as brain deprived of glucose]
Complications can develop after long period, but risk reduced by accurate control
Normal blood glucose levels

Nursing care

Explanation in small doses with reiteration
Use of diagrams
Answer questions
Relate to experience of patient
Repeat as necessary
Booklets from British Diabetic Association

Appendix continued

3. **Technical skills**

Obtaining capillary blood sample, applying to blood glucose [monitoring stick and reading glucose content with reflectance meter, recording blood glucose levels]
[OR Urine testing for glucose and ketones]

[Storage of insulin, warming to room temperature and mixing before administration
Types of insulin, reason for regime ordered and importance of correct timing in relation to meals
Drawing up insulin accurately and aseptically and reasons why asepsis and accuracy essential
[Select fixed volume syringe if poor sight]
Injection of insulin subcutaneously, using rotation of appropriate sites (Fig. 19.5) to reduce skin changes]

[Oral drugs to be given, how they work, importance of correct dose and time in relation to meals, side effects.]

Nursing care

Demonstration and explanation
Repeat as necessary
Allow patient to do procedure[s] in small sections, gradually building up till able to carry out procedure[s] completely and safely
Answer questions
Reinforce correct techniques, praise
Correct errors
Check correct technique at intervals after learning

4. **Balance between diet, exercise and insulin to regulate blood glucose**

General/Monitoring blood glucose level

Monitoring blood glucose allows patient control by adjusting diet, exercise, insulin.

At first — check before breakfast, lunch, evening meal, 3 am (for hypoglycaemia), then after meals
Later — less frequent checks needed
Maintain pattern of diet, exercise, insulin for 5-7 days before adjusting
Recording and interpreting of blood glucose results.
Gradually — recognising modifications needed at weekends, time of month (women), seasonal changes.

Diet

Nutritional content of foods, including alcohol. Need for balanced diet
Planning sample menus taking account of patient's weight, age, sex, activity pattern, likes/dislikes, income, preparation
Effective use of insulin by food intake divided into several meals, high fibre, high complex-carbohydrate diet [weight loss].

Exercise

Importance of exercise for health
Effect on blood glucose [reducing insulin dose before exercise reduces risk of hypoglycaemia]
Monitor blood glucose at first [to calculate change in insulin needed, later becomes unneccesary]

Insulin

[Dose and type of insulins prescribed, method and length of action, periods of possible hypoglycaemia
Need to modify dose before exercise, in infection or illness (usually needs to be increased)
Must take insulin (smaller dose) if unable to eat — but contact doctor]

[If unable to take oral hypoglycaemic agents — contact doctor]

Nursing care

Explanation
Use charts of blood glucose levels
Give practice in recording, interpreting blood glucose results
Answer questions
Involve dietician
Use lists of nutritional content of foods
Demonstrate sample menus, then patient to work out own menus

Appendix continued

Compile scrapbook of recipes
Explanation and discussion
Controlled exercise with measurement of blood glucose level
Discussion

5. Complications

Events leading to hypoglycaemia or hyperglycaemia, signs and symptoms of both
Recognition of onset of hypoglycaemia and action required
Importance of carrying glucose and wearing Medic-Alert bracelet/disk
Importance of care of feet (see Table 19.6) and immediate treatment of any infection
Possibility of complications developing in eyes, kidneys, blood vessels, nervous system and early indications of these
Importance of control of blood glucose level and regular exercise in minimizing risk of long term complications
Need for regular ophthalmic examination — 2 yearly for first 10 years, annually after 10 years and over 40 years old
Risk of diabetes developing in children

Nursing care

Explanation and discussion
Answering questions
Provide BDA booklets
Allow hypoglycaemia to develop under supervision
Demonstrate care of feet
Refer for genetic counselling

EVALUATION

Blood glucose results recorded — chart examined and results discussed with patient
Glycosylated haemoglobin measured at clinic — gives picture of average control over past 8–10 weeks
Instances of hypoglycaemia and hyperglycaemia noted
Ask patient to explain aspects covered in education programme
Discuss lifestyle and ability to adjust diet, exercise and insulin and maintain blood glucose level within normal limits
Observe carrying out blood glucose testing
[Observe drawing up and injecting insulin: ask about and examine sites used for injection]

REFERENCES

Alberti K G M M, Hockaday T D R 1983 Diabetes mellitus. In: Weatherall D J, Ledingham J G G, Warrell D A (eds) Oxford textbook of medicine. Oxford University Press, Oxford

Alexander S 1982 Skin disorders associated with diabetes. In: Keen H, Jarrett J (eds) Complications of diabetes, 2nd edn. Arnold, London

Blount M, Kinney A B 1974 Chronic steroid therapy. American Journal of Nursing 74:1626–1631

Bovington M M, Spies M E, Troy P J 1983 Management of the patient with diabetes mellitus during surgery or illness. Nursing Clinics of North America 18(4):661–671

Brady L W, Antoiniades J, Fause D S, Ham S H 1979 Radiation therapy in pituitary adenomas. In: Kryston L J, Shaw R A (eds) Endocrinology and diabetes. Grune & Stratton, New York

Burnett J 1980 Congenital adrenocortical hyperplasia — nursing interventions. American Journal of Nursing 80:1309– 1311

Chandler P T 1976 Diabetic foot care. Postgraduate Medicine 60:59–63

Conn J W, 1977 Primary aldosteronism. In: Genest J, Koiw E, Kuchel O (eds) Hypertension. McGraw-Hill, New York

Cranley M S, Frazier S A 1973 Preventative intensive care of the diabetic mother and her fetus. Nursing Clinics of North America 8:489–499

Cryer P E 1984 Glucose counter regulatory mechanisms in normal and diabetic man. In: Nattrass M, Santiago J V (eds) Recent advances in diabetes — 1. Churchill Livingstone, Edinburgh

Deckart T, Poulsen J E, Larsen M 1978 Prognosis of diabetes with diabetes onset before the age of thirty-one. 1: Survival, causes of death and complications. Diabetologia 14:363–370

De Groot L J, Larsen P R 1984 The thyroid and its diseases, 5th edn. Wiley, New York

Dupuis A, 1980 Assessment of the psychological factors and responses in self-managed patients. Diabetes Care 3:117–120

Felig P, 1974 Current concepts, diabetic ketoacidosis. New England Journal of Medicine 290:1360–1362

Felig P, Tyson J, 1975 Diabetes in pregnancy: managing diabetes and pregnancy together. Patient Care 9:56

Fletcher H P, 1976 The oral antidiabetogenic drugs: pro and con. American Journal of Nursing 76:596–599

Gharibe H, 1974 Triiodothyronine — physiological and clinical significance. Journal of the American Medical Association 227:302–304

Giles A M, Ross B D 1983 Normal or reference values for biochemical data. In: Weatherall D J, Ledingham J G G, Warrell D A (eds) Oxford textbook of medicine. Oxford University Press, Oxford

Glick S M 1979, Acromegaly: newer methods of diagnosis and results of therapy. In:Kryston L J, Shaw R A (eds) Endocrinology and diabetes. Grune & Stratton, New York

Goldstein S, Podolsky S 1980 Inheritance of diabetes and genetic counselling. In: Podolsky S (ed) Clinical diabetes: modern management. Appleton-Century-Crofts, New York

Grodsky G M 1981 Chemistry and functions of the hormones: 1. Thyroid, pancreas, adrenal and gastrointestinal tract. In: Martin D W , Mayes P A , Rodwell V W (eds) Harper's review of biochemistry, 18th edn. Lange Medical, Los Altos, California

Guthrie D W, Guthrie R A 1983 The disease process of diabetes mellitus: definition, characteristics, trends and developments. Nursing Clinics of North America 18(4):617–630

Hamdi M E 1971 Nursing intervention for patients receiving corticosteroid therapy. In: Kintzel K C (ed) Advanced concepts in clinical nursing. Lippincott, Philadelphia

Hartman C E 1979 Elements of the teaching program. In: Blevins D R (ed) The diabetic and nursing care. McGraw-Hill, New York

Hayter J 1976 Fine points in diabetic care. American Journal of Nursing 76:594–596

Hoette S J 1983 The adolescent with diabetes mellitus. Nursing Clinics of North America 18(4):763–776

Hoffenberg R 1983 Thyroid disorders. In: Weatherall D J, Ledingham J G G, Warrell D A (eds) Oxford textbook of medicine. Oxford University Press, Oxford

Hoffman J T T, Newby T B 1980 Hypercalcaemia in primary hyperparathyroidism. Nursing Clinics of North America 15(3): 469–480

Horwitz D L 1984 Advances in dietary treatment of diabetes. In: Nattrass M, Santiago J V (eds) Recent advances in diabetes — 1. Churchill Livingstone, Edinburgh

Ireland J T, Viberti G C, Watkins P J 1982 The kidney and renal tract. In: Keen H, Jarrett J (eds) Complications of diabetes, 2nd edn. Arnold, London

Irvine W J, Barnes E W 1972 Adrenocortical insufficiency. Journal of Clinical Endrocrinology and Metabolism 1:549–594

Jarrett R J, Keen H, Chakrabarti R 1982 Diabetes, hyperglycaemia and arterial disease. In: Keen H, Jarrett J (eds) Complications of diabetes, 2nd edn. Arnold, London

Kemmer F W, Berger M 1984 Exercise in diabetes: part of treatment, part of life. In: Nattrass M, Santiago J V (eds) Recent advances in diabetes — 1. Churchill Livingstone, Edinburgh

Kemmer F W et al 1982 Decreased risk of exercise induced hypoglycaemia by reduced insulin dose or increased carbohydrate intake in insulin dependent diabetics. In: Berger M, Christacopoulos P, Wahren J (eds) Diabetes and exercise. Huber, Berne

Keyes M 1977 The Somogyi phenomenon in insulin dependent diabetics. Nursing Clinics of North America 12:439–446

Kiehm T G, Anderson J W, Ward K 1976 Beneficial effects of high carbohydrate, high fibre diet on hyperglycaemic diabetic man. American Journal of Clinical Nutrition. 29:895–899

Klimt C R, Knatterud G L, Meiners C L, Prout T E 1970 The University Group diabetes program. A study of the effects of hypoglycaemic agents on vascular complications in patients with adult-onset diabetes. Part II Mortality results. Diabetes 19 (Suppl 2):789

Kohner E M, McLeod, D, Marshall J 1982 Diabetic eye disease. In: Keen H, Jarrett J (eds) Complications of diabetes, 2nd edn. Arnold, London

Kriss J P 1975 Graves' ophthalmopathy: aetiology and treatment. Hospital Practitioner 10:125–134

Marchesseault L C 1983 Diabetes mellitus and the elderly. Nursing Clinics of North America 18(4):791–798

Marks V, Rose F C 1981 Hypoglycaemia, 2nd edn. Blackwell Scientific, Oxford

Melick M E 1977 Nursing intervention for patients receiving corticosteroid therapy. In: Kintzel K C (ed) Advanced concepts in clinical nursing, 2nd edn. Lippincott, Philadelphia
Miller B K, White N E 1980 Diabetes assessment guide. American Journal of Nursing 80:1314–1316
Miller E, Hare J W, Cloherty J P, Dunn P J, Gleason R E, Soeldner J S, Kitzmiller J L 1981 Elevated maternal haemoglobin A_{IC} in early pregnancy and major congenital anomalies in infants of diabetic mothers. New England Journal of Medicine 304:1331–1334
Miller L V, Goldstein J, Nicholaisen G 1978 Evaluation of patients' knowledge of diabetes self–care. Diabetes Care 1: 275–280
Moorman N H 1983 Acute complications of hyperglycaemia and hypoglycaemia. Nursing Clinics of North America 18(4):707–719
Neumark S R 1976 Hyperthyroid crisis:on the metabolic side. Emergency Medicine 8:63–64
Olefsky J M 1976 Decreased insulin binding to adipocytes and circulating monocytes from obese subjects. Journal of Clinical Investigation 57:1165–1172
Owen O E, Morgan A O, Kemp H G, Sullivan J M, Herrera G, Cahill G F 1967 Brain metabolism during fasting. Journal of Clinical Investigation 46:1589–1595
Peacock I, Hunter J C, Walford S, Allison S P, Davison J, Clarke P, Symonds E M, Tattersall R B 1979 Self-monitoring of blood glucose in diabetic pregnancy. British Medical Journal 2:1333–1336
Podolsky S, Krall L P, Bradley R F 1980 Treatment of diabetics with oral hypoglycaemic agents. In: Podolsky S (ed) Clinical diabetes and modern management. Appleton-Century- Crofts, New York
Rancilio N 1979 When a pregnant woman is diabetic: postpartal care. American Journal of Nursing 79:453–456
Sanford S J 1980 Dysfunction of the adrenal gland: physiologic considerations and nursing problems. Nursing Clinics of North America 15(3):481–498
Scarpello J H B, Ward J D 1984 Diabetic neuropathy. In: Nattrass M, Santiago J V (eds) Recent advances in diabetes — 1. Churchill Livingstone, Edinburgh
Schneeberg N G 1979 Anterior pituitary failure: its recognition and therapy. In: Kryston L J, Shaw R A (eds) Edocrinology and diabetes. Grune & Stratton, New York
Scobie I N, Sönksen P H 1984 Methods of achieving better diabetic control. In: Nattrass M, Santiago J V (eds) Recent advances in diabetes — 1. Churchill Livingstone, Edinburgh
Small D 1976 Special needs of the geriatric diabetic patient. Journal of Practical Nursing 26:23–36
Steel J M, Parboosingh J, Cole R A, Duncan L J P 1980 Pre-pregnancy counselling: a logical prelude to the management of the pregnant woman. Diabetes Care 3:371–373
Sterling K 1975 Diagnosis and treatment of thyroid disease. C R C Press, Ohio
Stowe S W 1973 Hypophysectomy for diabetic retinopathy. American Journal of Nursing 73:632–637
Stubbs S M, Brudenell J M, Pyke D A, Watkins P J 1980 Management of the pregnant diabetic: home or hospital, with or without glucose meters. Lancet 1:1122–1124
Tattersall R B, Walford S, Peacock I, Gale E, Allison S 1980 A critical evaluation of methods of monitoring diabetic control. Diabetes Care 3:150–154
Thomas P K 1976 Diabetes mellitus in elderly persons. Nursing Clinics of North America 11(1) : 157–168
Thomas P K , Ward J D, Watkins P J 1982 Diabetic neuropathy. In: Keen H, Jarrett J (eds) Complications of diabetes, 2nd edn. Arnold, London
Thorn G W, Lauler D P 1972 Clinical therapeutics of adrenal disorders. American Journal of Medicine 53:673–684
Wake M M, Brensinger J F III 1980 The nurse's role in hypothyroidism. Nursing Clinics of North America 15(3):453–468
Ward G M, Simpson R W, Ward E A, Turner R C 1981 Comparison of two twice–daily insulin regimens:ultralente/soluble and soluble/isophane. Diabetologia 21:383–386
Welborn T A 1984 The definition of diabetes. In: Nattrass M, Santiago J V (eds) Recent advances in diabetes -- 1. Churchill Livingstone, Edinburgh
West K M 1980 Recent trends in dietary management. In: Podolsky S (ed) Clinical diabetes and modern management. Appleton-Century-Crofts, New York
West K M 1982 Hyperglycaemia as a cause of long-term complications. In: Keen H, Jarrett J (eds) Complications of diabetes, 2nd edn. Arnold, London
Williamson J R, Vogler N J, Kilo C 1971 Microvascular disease in diabetes. Medical Clinics of North America 55(4):847–860
Wimberly D 1979 When a pregnant woman is diabetic: intrapartal care. American Journal of Nursing 79:451–452
World Health Organization Expert Committee on Diabetes Mellitus Second Report 1980 WHO Technical Report Series No 646
Wright A D 1984 Diabetes in pregnancy. In: Nattrass M, Santiago J V (eds) Recent Advances in Diabetes — 1. Churchill Livingstone, Edinburgh
Wyngaarden J B, Smith L H 1982 Cecil textbook of medicine. Saunders, Philadelphia

20

Disturbances of protective mechanisms — the skin

INTRODUCTION

The skin is an organ with a number of functions which are mainly concerned with protection of the body. Thus damage places the physiological integrity of the individual at risk. It is also the part of the body visible to others and obvious damage may alter the way in which people interact with the person affected and the individual's feelings about him or herself. This is discussed in more detail in later sections of this chapter, particularly in relation to the patient with burns, but this is as applicable to any patient with a disfiguring condition of the skin.

FUNCTIONS OF THE SKIN

A break in the integrity of the skin may affect, to a greater or lesser extent, the efficiency with which this organ carries out its functions.

Temperature regulation

The skin plays an important role in control of body temperature in two ways. The blood flow through the skin is regulated by the autonomic nervous system under the control of the hypothalamus, and the amount of heat radiated from the body is increased or decreased with vasodilatation or vasoconstriction respectively. In addition, sweat that is formed evaporates and cools the body in so doing. Lack of the ability to form sweat, as in the sex-linked disorder hypohidrotic ectodermal dysplasia, means that the individual affected is susceptible to heat stroke (Ryan, 1983). Loss of skin, as in widespread burns, leads to excessive loss of body heat as body fluids evaporate and the insulating 'shell' of the body is lost.

Protection against infection

The skin protects the body against infection through being a physical barrier against the entry of microorganisms and by the presence of bactericidal substances such as lysozyme in the sweat. Damage to the skin, whether large or small in area, will provide a route for the entry of microorganisms and will put the patient at risk of infection. The prevention of infection is a major concern in the care of any patient in whom the physical integrity of the skin is damaged by burns, pressure sores, varicose ulcers or ulcerating disease of the skin.

Protection against fluid loss

The skin is a waterproof barrier which prevents loss of fluid from the body and absorption of water from the environment. In severe burns of large surface area, large volumes of fluid are lost from the body and have to be rapidly replaced. A similar situation can arise in severe blistering disorders of the skin such as pemphigus vulgaris or epidermolysis bullosa (Ryan, 1983).

Protection against physical trauma

The presence of nerve endings in the skin provides information about the environment and potential sources of damage to the body. The loss or absence of this ability is more likely to be a cause, rather than a result, of skin damage, as for example in diabetic patients with neuropathy or those rare individuals with a congenital inability to feel pain (Melzack & Wall, 1982).

Protection against ultraviolet radiation

The presence of melanin in the skin protects against the effects of the ultraviolet rays in sunlight. Thus individuals with smaller amounts of melanin in the skin (the white races) are more prone to burning if exposed to fierce sunlight, and to the development of basal cell carcinoma of the skin (Ryan, 1983). However, the large amounts of melanin in the skin of dark and brown people reduces the absorption of the ultraviolet radiation needed to produce vitamin D. Thus, if living in high latitudes where the sunlight is less, they are particularly at risk of developing rickets due to vitamin D deficiency.

TYPES OF SKIN DISTURBANCES

Disturbances of the skin being discussed in this chapter fall into four major groups:

- Diseases of the skin itself due to a wide variety of causes, for example, immune reactions, genetic causes, infection, malignant change, infestation.
- Burns which may damage the superficial layers of the skin or destroy the full thickness and may be small or large in area.
- Pressure sores in which the integrity of the skin is breached due to prolonged pressure cutting off the circulation.
- Leg ulcers in which the integrity of the skin is impaired as a result of changes in the tissues, possibly initiated by trauma and linked with reduction or stasis of the circulation.

EFFECT ON THE INDIVIDUAL

The effect of disturbances of the skin on the individual affected can range from minor to life-threatening in physiological terms and from a mild irritant to a condition which radically effects one's self-concept and relationships with others.

Life-threatening conditions are those which render the individual unable to maintain homeostasis. This may be with regard to fluid and electrolyte balance and temperature regulation, as in severe burns and certain severe blistering skin diseases. On the other hand, a break in the integrity of the skin exposes the patient to the risk of infection which, in an immunocompromised patient, can result in a widespread dissemination of the infection.

All of the activities of living can be modified in some patients with disruption of the skin. The patient with severe burns or severe skin disease will be bedfast and unable to carry out the physical activities normally, while the respiratory tract may be damaged by inhaled smoke or affected by the skin disease thus affecting breathing. The effect of skin disease on activities related to one's psychological state may be considerable. However, the degree to which these activities are altered may bear little or not relationship to the severity of the skin damage. While a naevus may be of little physiological concern, if it is on the face it may drastically influence the individuals's self-concept, the activities performed in relation to seeking stimulation and reward, and the development of relationships with others.

THE CARE OF THE INDIVIDUAL WITH A SKIN DISEASE

INTRODUCTION

Very few people possess a perfect skin but many seek perfection, as can be seen by the large variety of cosmetics and other skin care products available in chemists and department stores.

Most skin disorders are not sufficiently serious to warrant hospitalization, but the economic costs, in terms of time lost from work, are high. A recent American survey indicated that nearly one-third of 20 749 Americans studied between the ages of 1 and 74 years had one or more skin conditions serious enough to require medical attention (Rook, 1980). A community survey in Lambeth, London, revealed an overall prevalence of skin diseases thought to justify care of 22.3% (Rook, 1980). Some of the commoner skin disorders are allergic skin reactions, acne, warts and moles — consultation for acne is one of the most common reasons for seeking medical attention. Iatrogenic skin disease is becoming an increasingly common and complex problem as the number of pharmaceutical agents available increases. Apart from reactions to systemically administered drugs, reactions to topically administered drugs are becoming more frequent (Wright, 1980).

Skin manifestations of systemic diseases are numerous and may be the first presenting symptoms of the particular disorder. The nurse may be the first person to observe these early symptoms and it is important to have sufficient knowledge and understanding to refer the patient to a medical practitioner.

Patients suffering from dermatological conditions may have many problems, particularly in relationship to altered body image and physical discomfort. Nursing interventions based on an understanding of patient problems can assist the patient and his or her family to deal with the disease experience (Abramovich, 1979; Baum & Jones, 1979; Franklin, 1974).

ASSESSMENT

The first stage in the nursing process involves assessment and it is important that the nurse has an understanding of some of the more common terms used to describe skin lesions (Table 20.1) (Bates, 1974). In the assessment phase of the nursing process it is helpful to obtain a nursing history as part of a data base to identify nursing problems. This will include obtaining information about skin disturbances in the patient and in the patient's family, the circumstances which were involved in the development or exacerbation of the condition, and any self-treatment used. Areas which need to be explored include detail about the diet taken, allergies, possible exposure to exoparasites, psychological stressors in the recent past and the patient's present emotional state.

Physical assessment

Any examination of the skin and its appendages should be conducted under a good light; sunlight is best but white artificial light, preferably fluorescent light, will be adequate (Roach, 1974). The whole skin surface including mucous surfaces, hair and nails should be examined in a systematic and thorough fashion. It is desirable that the skin surface be clean so that details are not obscured. The environmental temperature

Table 20.1 Descriptive terminology of dermatology (Bates, 1974)

Term	Description
Macule	A small circumscribed discoloration of the skin
Papule	An elevated pathologic formation of the skin not larger than a split pea.
Vesicle	An elevated pathologic formation of the skin not larger than a split pea and containing free clear fluid
Bulla	Similar to a vesicle but larger; blisterlike
Pustule	A vesicle or bulla containing pus
Nodule	A circumscribed, elevated area of the skin larger than 1 cm in diameter, and usually rounded or dome-shaped
Tumour	A solid pathologic formation larger than a peanut
Wheal	A transitory, circumscribed elevation of the skin produced by swelling of the dermis
Scale	A mass of exfoliated epidermis
Crust	A mass formed upon the surface of the skin by dried exudate
Excoriation	A superficial break in the skin, produced by scratching
Fissure	A deeper break in the skin
Ulcer	A circumscribed loss of the epidermis, exposing the dermis to the surface — may extend to subcutaneous layer or even bone
Comedo	A plug of secretion contained in a follicle because of closure of its opening by excessive hardening
Atrophy	Thinning of the skin with loss of normal skin workings
Sclerosis	Localized or diffuse hardening of subcutaneous tissue which may also involve the dermis

should be comfortable for the patient to prevent redness due to excessive warmth or pallor because of cold. An examination involves visual inspection to determine the exact size and shape of lesions, measurement to determine the exact size of lesions, and palpation to determine skin texture and elasticity. The condition of the skin is considered in relation to what is accepted as normal for a person of the particular age, sex, occupation, etc.

Age results in skin changes. Degenerative changes in elastic and collagen tissues produce a wrinkled appearance, and sebaceous and sweat glands become less active due to decreased hormonal activity causing the skin to become dry. Melanocyte areas may increase pigment production resulting in the appearance of 'brown spots'.

The occupation followed will also influence skin condition. Working outside will cause tanning of the skin while a manual worker will have callouses and rougher hands than an office worker. Particular occupations may expose people to substances, such as chemicals, which may lead to allergic changes.

Table 20.2 summarizes the features of a physical assessment of the skin.

Table 20.2 Physical assessment

Site	Assessment
Skin of face, neck, scalp Skin of posterior and anterior thorax Skin of abdomen, genitalia Skin of arms, hands, fingers Skin of thighs, legs and feet	Colour Texture Elasticity/turgor Temperature Moisture Lesions colour size shape description
Hair	Colour Distribution normal abnormal Texture
Finger nails	Colour Shape Texture

Skin colour

Skin colour is not always easy to assess and in fair skinned people, variations in colour may be caused by exposure to changes in temperature or to sunlight. Certain physiological factors also influence skin tones — colour of blood in

Table 20.3 Causes of abnormal skin colour

Colour	Possible causes	Distribution
Pallor	1. Anaemia	Face, mouth, conjunctiva, nails
	2. Shock — decreased perfusion of superficial skin layers	
	3. Renal impairment	Oedema masks colour of haemoglobin
	4. Fungal infections	Chest, upper arms, back
	5. Albinism	All skin surfaces
Yellow	1. Liver disease — increase in bilrubin	Generalized jaundice, most in sclera of eyes
	2. Chronic renal disease	General
	3. Diabetes, hypopituitarism — increase in carotenoid pigments	Face, palms, soles
Red	1. Fever, alcohol–dilatation of superficial blood vessels	Face, upper chest
	2. Inflammation	Area of inflammation
Reddish-blue	1. Polycythaemia vera — increased red cell count	Face, mouth, conjunctiva, hands, feet
Blue (Cyanosis)	1. Cardiac & respiratory disorders — reduced oxygen in blood	Mouth, lips, nails, earlobes, fingers
Brown	1. Suntanned	Exposed areas
	2. Addison's disease	Generalized, particularly in areas where pressure or friction
	3. Pregnancy	Face, nipples, alveolae, linea alba

superfical capillaries and the amount of pigments (melanin and carotene) in the superficial layers. Skin that is protected by clothing is usually more pallid than skin that is exposed. Thus it can be seen that there is considerable variation in colour of normal healthy skin. In brown or black skinned people, normal, healthy skin has a healthy glow due to the underlying red tones. If the underlying red tones are absent due to anaemia or other disease process, brown skin takes on a yellowish brown hue and black skin an ashen appearance. The palms of the hands are a good site for assessing the degree of pallor. Table 20.3 indicates the distribution and possible causes of various skin colours.

Skin texture

The assessment of skin texture is done by touch and refers to the 'feel' of the skin. The finger pads provide the best method of tactile discrimination. Skin that is normally protected by clothing should feel smoother than usually exposed skin surfaces. A rougher than normal texture may indicate clothing friction or some other form of irritation. The presence of lesions such as scabs, plaques or papules will give the skin a characteristic roughness or hardness (Berbeu, 1973). Hardness of the skin may also be caused by the presence of oedema.

Skin temperature

Temperature assessment also is performed by touch and it is important for the nurse to ensure that her/his hands are at normal temperature. The temperature of the skin is influenced by both external and internal factors, and in order to assess temperature accurately the environmental temperature must be normal. The dorsal finger surfaces should be used as these are more sensitive to temperature than the palmer surface. Blood vessel dilatation increases blood flow and raises skin surface temperature; vasoconstriction produces the opposite effect. An elevated skin temperature may indicate inflammatory skin disease or a systemic disease process. Oedema lowers skin temperature due to an increase in the distance of blood vessels from the skin surface (Roberts, 1975).

Skin turgor (tissue tension)

The elasticity of the skin and skin turgor is ascertained by pinching the skin between the thumb and forefinger and raising the skinfold slightly. If the skin returns promptly to its original contour, the elasticity and turgor are normal. Age and skin atrophy due to loss of subcutaneous tissue reduces skin elasticity. Turgor reflects the hydrational status of the skin cells.

Skin moisture

Skin moisture is measured in much the same manner as skin texture. Skin moisture is the result of sweat gland secretion which can be affected by psychic or physiological factors. Moist palms, soles and forehead may be indications of fear, anxiety or tension. Generalized skin moisture can result from physical activity or external heat. Excessive skin dryness may be caused by a deficiency of sebum production or by excessive removal of sebum by cleansing agents. Excessive dryness may result in skin scaling.

Skin lesions

Skin lesions involve any abnormal tissue formation in the epidermis, dermis or other underlying tissues and may be classified as primary or secondary. Primary lesions occur in the early stages of a skin disorder and are characteristic of it. These primary lesions include macules, vesicles, bullae, pustules, papules, wheals and tumours (see Table 20.1). The secondary lesions are the result of the primary lesions and occur in the later stages of the skin disorder; they include crust formation, excoriations, fissures, scales, sores and ulcers. Observations and recording of lesion description should include colour, texture, shape, size and distribution.

Hair and nails

Hair conditions can be indicative of a dermatological disorder, systemic disorder and the general health status. Distribution and colour of hair varies amongst individuals — age, sex and genetic factors produce this variation. Abnormal loss of hair can be chemically induced by such things as hair dyes, bleach, certain drugs, or may be indicative of systemic disease. Dull and brittle hair may be caused by inadequate nutrition.

The condition of fingernails and toenails can provide valuable information regarding the presence of certain systemic diseases and the general state of health. The nails are normally pink in colour, smooth and reasonably thick and flexible. Colourless nails may indicate reduced oxygen in haemoglobin as a result of smoking or systemic disorders. Dark discoloration of the nail bed may be a reaction to certain drugs. Transverse white lines, ridging or abnormal nail thickness may be indicative of metabolic disorders. Brittleness may indicate dietary deficiency or hypothyroidism. Clubbing of the nail or a bulb-like enlargement of the nail is present in patients with chronic cardiac and pulmonary disorders.

TYPES OF SKIN DISEASES

The main groups of skin diseases with examples of each type are shown in Tables 20.4 — 20.10.

NURSING CARE

Any nursing care plan should include the listing of patient problems (sometimes called a nursing diagnosis) as the final stage of assessing the patient with a skin disorder, as well as possible interventions related to those problems (Marriner, 1975).

Skin disorders often cause a change in appearance, may be slow in resolving and are often made worse by stress. These factors may cause the patient to feel a lowering of self-esteem and a sense of isolation, depression and frustration — all of which can cause serious delay in the healing process.

The nursing care must be sensitive and based upon knowledge and understanding of each individual patient. Careful observation of the patient's behaviour may provide useful clues to the nurse's understanding of the patient's perception of his/her illness as well as the means of providing realistic encouragement and support. Patients have a need for information about their disease in order for them to integrate their illness experience within a framework of life experience and also as a realistic basis for making decisions about their disease and the involved treatment. Numerous studies have indicated that informed patients experience a significant reduction in anxiety, have fewer days in hospital and are more willing and equipped to comply with medical regimes (Redman, 1980; Skipper & Leonard, 1965; Wilson-Barnett, 1979). Any plan of nursing care must include a teaching plan, designed by members of the health team with the patient and based upon each individual patient's learning needs and abilities.

A teaching plan should include the importance of good skin care; importance of avoiding factors in the environment (including stress) which may exacerbate the condition and the benefits of adequate rest. The dangers of self treatment of a skin disorder should be stressed, including the fact that inappropriate self treatment may cause a violent skin reaction. Good nutrition is essential for the patient with a skin disorder, as well as the avoidance of food that may aggravate the condition.

The patient's need for rest, sleep and comfort is often disrupted by some of the symptoms of skin disorders — the most distressing often being pruritus.

Pruritus

The aetiology of pruritus or itching is obscure but it is thought to be associated with a disruption in the skin nerve endings. The patient's natural response to pruritus is to scratch (an action which seems to be unconsciously designed to destroy these nerve endings and relieve the symptom). Scratching can cause further discomfort and result in tissue damage and infection. Application of appropriate topical creams or ointments, as well as the administration of prescribed systemic drugs, may relieve itching but the ultimate goal of care is to remove or give some relief to the cause of the disorder.

There are certain nursing measures which can be employed to provide some relief to itching.

Cool temperatures tend to promote vasoconstriction and often result in varying degrees of relief from itching. Soothing tepid baths (without soap which may irritate skin) containing sodium bicarbonate, starch, oatmeal or bland oils may be helpful. The patient's room should be cool and bedclothing kept at a comfortable minimum. The patient's nails should be kept short and clean to prevent tissue trauma and infection from scratching. If possible the patient should not scratch but be instructed to apply gentle pressure on involved skin surfaces.

It is important for the nurse to record not only the presence or absence of pruritus in patients with skin disorders (this symptom may be diagnostic) but also the frequency, duration and extent of itching. Diversions such as reading or television may also be helpful.

TREATMENT OF SKIN DISORDERS

Treatment of skin disorders can be divided into the following categories: local treatment by chemical or physical means and systemic treatment.

The local treatment by chemical means is accomplished by using an appropriate medium to apply medication to the skin. The most common mediums used are as follows:

- Creams — may have an oil or water base and tend to have a soothing effect on inflamed skin.
- Lotions — usually a powder in suspension and have a drying and cooling effect on moist inflamed skin.
- Ointments and pastes — greasy base and have a softening and lubricating effect on dry thickened skin: pastes tend to be thicker in consistency.
- Powders — absorb moisture and have a drying effect on moist skin.

Table 20.4 Examples of the papulosquamous group of disorders

Condition	Signs and symptoms	Sites affected	Treatment
1. **Psoriasis** — a chronic, conspicuous disease. Lasts a few months to a lifetime Exacerbated by infection, stress, trauma	The initial lesion is a bright red, sharply outlined pinhead to pea-sized papule that is elevated, round or oval shaped with a flattened surface. The papule is covered with a dry, shiny, silvery scale which covers all but the margins of the papule. The scales become heaped up layer on layer and if scraped off, leave a bright red surface with one or two bleeding points. This is a characteristic finding of psoriasis. Papules usually coalesce with adjacent papules to form patches that vary in size and shape. The patches are sharply demarcated from surrounding skin.	Usual sites: extensor surface of knees and elbows, scalp, nails The disease may also involve: — palms and soles, axilla, behind the ears, ano-genital region, sternum, trunk, face, extremities	Crude coal tar ointment Ultraviolet light Dithranol ointment Topical steroids Methotrexate and other cytotoxins (severe cases)
2. **Lichen planus** — acute or chronic — mainly in adults — more common in women Aetiology — unknown Incidence seems to be related to stress	Lesions are purplish with a flat top Primary lesion is purplish papule — the surface of the papules shows a faint pattern of white lines Coalescence of papules can occur giving a wart-like appearance. Intense pruritus	Wrists and ankles. penis, lips, tongue vaginal mucosa, mouth May occur, however, on any part of the body	
3. **Pityriasis rosea** — a self-limiting disease lasting 6–10 weeks. Seldom experienced more than once, usually in spring or autumn Aetiology unknown - ? viral	There is usually a herald patch of dermatitis which precedes the general eruption by 1 or 2 weeks. This patch is pinkish salmon coloured, varying in size. The generalized eruption appears from 1–2 weeks after a herald patch. The individual lesions are much smaller than the herald patch. they are flat, covered by a thin, dry scale which is adherent, and crinkly much like cigarette paper. The lesions are oval with their long axis in the direction of the lines of cleavage of the skin. The eruption usually does not itch.	Trunk or thigh Limited to trunk, thighs and arms	
4. **Seborrhoeic dermatitis** — a common disease, rarely disabling. Affects areas rich in sebaceous glands. Aetiology — unknown — neurogenic factors — diet of fats, carbohydrates and spices — endocrine disturbances	Primary lesions are closely grouped, small papules which occur as pinkish patches which are not well demarcated from normal skin. The scale has a yellowish, dirty colour and is greasy to feel and easily removed by scratching. The lesions are only occasionally pruritic.	Usual sites: scalp, naso-labial fold, behind ears, mid-line of chest, axillae, genital region, nasal cleft	Sulphur and salicylic acid ointments and lotions Hydrocortisone ointments Vioform

Table 20.5 Bullous eruption group of diseases

Condition	Signs and symptoms	Sites	Treatment
1. **Pemphigus vulgaris** — an acute, fulminating skin disorder. May be fatal if untreated. Cause unknown Patient usually middle-aged	Generalized formation of large bullae containing clear fluid. Bullae may be easily ruptured. Bullae appear on apparently normal skin. Certain areas of apparently normal skin exhibit Nikolsky's sign (if firm pressure is applied with a finger to the skin, the superficial layers of the epidermis will slide over deeper layers, causing a permanent wrinkling). When the roof of the bullae is removed, there remains a raw, red denuded surface. Cause of death often due to loss of blood protein and/or secondary bacterial infection.		Systemic cortico-steroids
2. **Erythema multiforme** Cause unknown — ? viral Sudden onset — lasts a few weeks. Recurrences common in spring and autumn	Lesions may occur in many forms in same patient at any one time, e.g. papules, vesicles, urticarial wheals (like hives). Bullae may form on top of the urticarial lesions.	Extensor surface of the arms and legs Face	Steroids Antihistamines

Table 20.6 Diseases of the pilosebaceous follicles

Condition	Signs and symptoms	Sites	Treatment
1. **Acne** The familiar bad complexion of adolescence. It is a chronic inflammatory infection involving the sebaceous glands and the pilosebaceous follicles, particularly of the face and upper trunk where the glands are largest and most numerous Aetiology: — hormonal — bacterial sensitization — dietary — hereditary influence.	The primary lesion is the comedo (blackhead) The comedo is a plug which closes the opening of the sebaceous gland. The latter becomes involved with infection that is unable to drain to the surface. As a result of this, an inflammatory papule forms and still later, a pustule forms. The pustule is finally opened (either spontaneously or by the patient) and a scar forms in the site of the inflammatory reaction.	Face Upper trunk	Acne diet; avoid milk, chocolate, nuts, fried fat foods, pastries etc. Tetracycline Ultraviolet light Careful removal of black heads Astringent lotions by day Peeling and antiseptic or antibiotic cream at night Frequent washing
2. **Rosacea** Rosacea is a chronic disease affecting the flush area of the face, the central area which includes the nose and adjacent portions of the cheeks, the chin and the centre area of the forehead. The familiar red nose of alcoholics, depicted so frequently by old time artists, is due to rosacea. Aetiology (in predisposed people: adults over 40 years usually) — gastric irritants: spicy foods, alcohol, emotional disturbances, menopausal flushing	The faces of persons with rosacea are constantly red and congested Tiny dilated blood vessels are visible in the flush area. Dilated and enlarged pores. Greasy skin. Acne type papules and pustules. In men, there is atrophy of sebaceous glands and connective tissue of the nose giving rise to large bulbous noses. This is called rhinophyma.	Butterfly area of the face (nose, cheeks) Forehead Chin	Related to relief of factors producing vasodilatation

Table 20.7 Contagious and infectious diseases of skin

Condition	Signs and symptoms	Sites	Treatment
A. THOSE CAUSED BY ANIMAL PARASITES			
1. **Scabies** Familiarly known as the 'itch'. Aetiological agent — *Acarus scabiei*. The female mite produces the disease. After the female mites are impregnated, they bore their way through the skin of the host, producing at the site a small vesicle. From the point of entrance (vesicle), the mite burrows from ⅛ to ¼ inch through the skin, leaving a red streak in its path. This gives rise to the typical comet lesion, the vesicle being the head of the comet. At the lower horny layer of the skin she leaves a trail of eggs and faeces.	Pruritus (maximal when person is warm). The primary lesion of scabies is a tiny vesicle or papule surrounded by a red halo from which there extends a small blackish red streak. Excoriations of the skin from scratching. Mode of transmission: dirty towels bed linens wearing apparel of infected persons sexual intercourse or sleeping in the same bed.	Thin skinned areas: webs of fingers (diagnostic) breasts flexural surface of wrist axilla penis inner aspect of thigh	Softening of horny layer then application of an acaricidal preparation.
2. **Pediculosis** The skin becomes infected with lice. Important in the spread of typhus.			
(a) *Pediculosis capitis* seen frequently in children of school age who live in crowded areas. The presence of pediculosis is often due to neglect and the disease is seen in children with thick, unkempt hair. It is rare in adults. Rare in those who apply grease to their hair.	The lice (insects) with moving legs can easily be seen with naked eye or hand lens. Nits (eggs) can be seen as pear-shaped bodies attached to hairs near the scalp. Mousy odour. Secondary infection of the scalp from scratching. Crust formation resulting from infection which in turn causes hair to mat together. Enlarged lymph nodes in the back of the neck (caused by infection of the scalp).	The scalp	Lorexane or Dicophane
(b) *Pediculosis pubis* attacks pubic hair, eyebrows. Attacks any race, sex and social group.	Same as pediculosis capita except there is inguinal adenopathy — commonly called the crab.	The pubic region	Lorexane or Dicophane
(c) *Pediculosis corporis* prevalent among indigent old men and alcoholics who seldom bathe or change their underwear, a hardy organism and can live for several weeks in clothing, as do its nits (eggs). Lives in the seams of underwear and attacks the skin only for nourishment	It attacks skin that is in constant contact with underwear. Primary lesions are red, oedematous papules, the top of which are crusted from scratching. Pustules may form due to secondary infection.	The body	Cold cream for the body Disinfectant for clothing and bedding

Table 20.7 continued

Condition	Signs and symptoms	Sites	Treatment
B. THE PYODERMAS (caused by bacteria of streptococcus or staphylococcus group)			
1. **Erysipelas**			
Acute inflammation of the skin and subcutaneous tissue caused by streptococci, generally seen in persons with poor resistance to infection. It may occur from a scratch or pulling out hairs.	The skin of the involved areas is bright red, oedematous, shiny and tense with a sharply defined advancing border. Prognosis — formerly erysipelas was a very serious disease because it attacked persons with lowered resistance and the mortality rate was high. Since the introduction of antibiotics, the prognosis is good.		Internal antibiotics Topical antibiotics
2. **Other conditions caused by bacteria**			
(a) *Folliculitis* simple, relatively non-contagious pustular eruption involving the hair follicles, caused by staphylococci.			
(b) *Furunculosis* the common boil, an infection caused by staphylococci or streptococci. Involves the entire hair follicle and adjacent subcutaneous tissue. Starts as a painful, hard induration situated in the deeper layers of corium; overlying skin is red and hot. The indurated area becomes soft and opens spontaneously to discharge a core of necrotic tissue and pus			
(c) *Carbunculosis* condition exists when furuncles develop in adjoining hair follicles and coalesce to form a conglomerate mass. Usually has more than one core.	It begins as a small red spot, which changes into a vesicle. The vesicle ruptures forming a yellow gummy crust. When the fluid from the vesicle escapes and is carried to uninfected areas, new vesicles are formed.	Face — around mouth, nose, chin, cheeks, arms and legs	Systemic antibiotics Local antibiotics
(d) *Paronychia* a painful, inflammatory bacterial infection of the tissue around the nails. Frequently caused by careless manicuring.			
3. **Impetigo** An acute contagious disease of the superficial layers of the skin due to streptococcus and staphylococcus. There are several types of impetigo, the most common being impetigo contagiosa.			

Table 20.7 continued

Condition	Signs and symptoms	Sites	Treatment
Other clinical types of impetigo. (a) *Ecthyma* — same as impetigo contagiosa except that the process is deeper causing ulceration and scarring. (b) *Secondary* — to an itching moist rash such as occurs with scabies or impetigo. (c) *Impetigo neonatum* — a highly contagious pustular eruption which occurs in newborn infants. Will spread rapidly through the nursery, causing many deaths.			
C DISEASES CAUSED BY FUNGI (TINEA)			
1. **Ringworm of the scalp** Occurs only before puberty. Extremely contagious, responds slowly to treatment. Diagnosis by: wood lamp examination direct examination of hair under microscope	Greyish, scaly, round patches appear on the scalp. These areas appear to be devoid of hair Closer examination will reveal that these areas are not devoid of hair but the hairs have broken off close to the scalp (not to be confused with hair loss of alopecia areata, a non-contagious disorder characterized by hair loss often related to stress). Certain types of fungi may cause pustular eruptions of the scalp. *Kerion* is a well-defined, elevated, boggy mass in the scalp which appears in some types of ringworm infection, caused by a violent pustular involvement of the hair follicles.	The scalp	Local application of fungicides Treatment of source
2. **Ringworm of the feet** *(tinea pedis)*, **athlete's foot** Common in warm climates. Flat feet, ill-fitting shoes, moisture and warmth are predisposing factors.	Maceration and exfoliation of skin between the toes (usually between the 4th and 5th toe.) There may be breaks (fissures) between the toes. Blisters (vesicles) may form on the soles of feet. Fungi may be found in the skin over the roof of the blisters. Chronic scaling dermatitis of the soles of the feet. Complications of ringworm of the feet: (a) secondary infection with bacteria causing cellulitis (b) lymphangitis (spread by lymphatics of a bacterial infection on skin) (c)lymphadenitis — enlarged infected lymph nodes.		Treatment of fungal conditions Local: salicylic acid benzoic acid permanganate soaks Internal: Griseofulvin therapy

Table 20.7 continued

Condition	Signs and symptoms	Sites	Treatment
3. **Other fungal conditions**			
(a) *Ringworm of the hands (tinea manus)* All manifestations of ringworm of the feet are also found on the hands with one exception. Fungi rarely attack the web of the fingers because the webs of the fingers do not become as moist as the webs of the toes. There is one exception to this latter statement – Monilia (the cause of thrush in babies) has as a site of predilection the webs of the fingers. Monilia is not a fungus, but a yeast (closely related to fungi).			
(b) *Ringworm of the body (tinea corporis)* takes the form of circular lesions with clearing centres. These start as a small, slightly erythematous scaly spot which spreads peripherally with a scaly border. As the lesion enlarges, the centre clears, forming a perfect circle in most cases.			
(c) *Tinea axillaris* infection of the skin of the axillae with fungi. The involved skin is brownish, red, scaly with a well-demarcated border.			
(d) *Onychomycosis* infection of the nails with fungi. The involved nails become lustreless, pitted, discoloured, brittle. The undersurface of the distal end of the nail is packed with keratin material. It must be carefully differentiated from psoriasis of the nails.			

Table 20.7 continued

Condition	Signs and symptoms	Sites	Treatment
(e) *Tinea cruris* fungal involvement of the groin. Similar to tinea axillaris. It is more resistant to treatment because of increased moisture.			
(f) *Ringworm of the beard (tinea barbae, tinea sycosis)* organisms attack the hair of the beard, forming follicular pustules.			
(g) *Paronychia due to fungus* infection of the nail folds by fungus. Usually caused by Monilia (a yeast).			
(h) *Thrush* involvement of mucous membranes by Monilia (a yeast). Produces white (curd-like) plaques on the mucous membranes. These look like particles of clotted milk but cannot be removed by scaping. If they are removed, a bleeding surface remains.			
D. DISEASES CAUSED BY VIRUS			
1. **Verrucae** (warts) (a) *Verruca vulgaris (common wart)*	Lesions are brownish to flesh coloured, firm, rough surfaced, elevated.	Occur commonly on the hands, elbows, knees and sites of minor traumas	Salicylic acid Freezing
(b) *Verruca planus (flat wart)(juvenile wart)*		Occur commonly on hands and face	
(c) *Venereal wart (acuminate wart)*	These warts are usually larger than common warts and have a moist, soft, rough surface	Occur in the ano-genital region	
2. **Herpes zoster (shingles)** attacks an area of the skin (unilateral), supplied by one of the nerve root ganglia of the spinal cord or brain. Caused by invasion of the involved sensory ganglia with the herpes virus.	The area of skin which the ganglia supplies is involved with a *painful* vesicular eruption. The condition may last several weeks and the pain may last for years.		Treatment is of the symptoms

Table 20.8 The eczema-dermatitis group of diseases

Condition	Signs and symptoms	Sites	Treatment
1. **Contact dermatitis** *(dermatitis venenata)* This is caused by some specific substance which is in external contact with the skin.	Pruritus Redness Papule and vesicle formation, weeping, crust formation	Distribution variable, depending upon where the offending agent comes into contact with the skin Forehead and behind the ears: frequently caused by hair dyes, shampoos, etc. Eyelids: frequently from fingernail polish. Dorsal aspect of fingers and hands: frequently caused by soaps and detergent cleansers. Dorsum of toes and feet: frequently caused by sensitivity to fabric or leather in shoes.	
2. **Atopic dermatitis** It usually occurs in families where there is a history of asthma and hayfever. These people take life very seriously, are constantly competing with their environment. Usually a history of childhood eczema (infantile eczema) or asthma in patients, or a history of these diseases in patient's family.	Pruritus Redness and later hyperpigmentation of skin Papules Thickening of skin (lichenification)	Face Neck Cubital fossae Behind the knees Wrists Back of hands	Treatment of eczematous and dermatitic eruptions Internal treatment: antihistamines, steroids, sedatives, bacterial vaccines, desensitization with allergens Soaks, lotions, ointments. Protection from environment (gloves)
3. **Other conditions** (a) *Nummular eczema* This is a true eczema, which may occur on any part of the body and almost always in coin-shaped patches (b) *Stasis dermatitis* Associated with venous stasis in the legs and frequently associated with varicose veins. Caused by poor venous return from the legs. The most common site is the inner aspect of the leg just above the ankle. (c) *Eczematous dermatitis* A large group of skin diseases which has many forms and many causes. Usually there is more than one factor involved in any one case: bacterial infection, bacterial allergy, external irritation (soaps, detergents, etc.), food allergy, etc. Eczematous dermatitis is more or less a waste paper basket diagnosis to name eczematous eruptions which cannot be placed in one of the above categories.			

Table 20.9 The collagen diseases

Condition	Clinical manifestation	Treatment
1. **Lupus erythematosus** Unknown cause, associated with varying degrees of degeneration of collagen fibres. Chronic, sub-acute and acute forms: may involve almost every organ system in the human body. Many different manifestations lead to wide distribution within medical specialities. More commonly occurs in young women with fair complexion, blond or red-haired; may occur in either sex. Aetiology: unknown. Onset or exacerbation may be related to stress, sun's rays, infection and certain drugs.	(a) *Chronic discoid* Skin manifestations only. The patient is not sick and usually consults a physician because of skin eruptions. (Face and forearms and hands, but usually only the face.) This is fortunately the most common type. There are many manifestations which vary greatly in their appearance and are most often diagnosed by the dermatologist. The eruption occurs as sharply demarcated plaques in the butterfly area of the face (cheeks and bridge of the nose), but may occasionally involve the ears, forehead, chin, neck, chest and extremities. These patches vary from pink to purplish-brown and may or may not be covered with a scale. When a scale is present, it is usually adherent to the skin and frequently presents a carpet tack appearance: a tough projection from the under-surface of the scale projects into the opening of dilated hair follicle, thus the name, carpet tack scale. These patients seem to be sensitive to sunlight and their lesions are usually more active during the summer months. (b) *Sub-acute* In addition to skin manifestation, various degrees of involvement of internal organs; kidneys, heart, reticulo-endothelial system (blood-forming and antibody-forming systems). (c) *Acute (disseminated)* The patients are acutely ill and ususally die from the disease. Skin manifestations vary from marked involvement to no involvement at all. When skin manifestations do occur, they are very distintive and, to the experienced observer, leave no doubt as to the correct diagnosis. In this form of the disease, almost any organ in the human organism may be involved. This is a very serious systemic disease that is usually fatal. The classical clinical picture is one of over-whelming toxaemia beginning with vague abdominal symptoms, high fever, migratory arthritis, sub-acute nephritis (when present carries a very grave prognosis), cardiac and nervous symptoms. There appears on the face (in the butterfly area), a flushed, oedematous area which resembles erysipelas. With the advent of modern diagnostic methods, many relatively mild and relatively early cases are being	The course of disseminated lupus erythematosis has been altered since the introduction of ACTH and cortisone. These drugs must be continued indefinitely since the disease promptly recurs when they are discontinued. In milder cases, treatment may be quite conservative and not employ much drug therapy but rely on rest and general measures.

Table 20.9 continued

Condition	Clinical manifestation	Treatment
	detected. In addition, many cases of bizarre LE are being found, for instance those displaying only epilepsy or hepatitis, etc. Laboratory findings: anaemia leukopenia increased sedimentation rate ECG changes changes in protein of the blood (reversal of A/G ratio) false positive tests for syphilis positive LE test (not present in the chronic discoid type) definite diagnostic pathological picture in biopsy specimens	
2. **Scleroderma** Relatively rare chronic disease; in early stages, strongly resembles systemic lupus erythematosis in clinical appearance. Resemblance disappears as the skin becomes immobile, firm, thickened, smooth and shiny in appearance Cause of both types unknown. Attacks mostly females. Prognosis: diffuse type is serious; for the localized type, the prognosis is excellent.	(a) *Diffuse* Involves the connective tissue of the skin and various internal organs. The involved parts become thickened, hard and immobile. The oesophagus is sometimes involved, making it impossible for the patients to swallow food. (b) *Localized* — called Morphoea Characterized by the development of one or more circumscribed discrete, persistent areas of infiltration, yellowish or ivory in colour with faint lilac or violaceous borders. The skin is smooth, shiny and atrophic with loss of normal skin markings.	Corticosteroids may be of some benefit in early cases

Table 20.10 Neoplasms of the skin

Condition	Signs and symptoms	Usual sites	Treatment
1. **Basal cell carcinoma**			
— occurs usually over the age of fifty in either sex. Spread involves local invasion without metastases.	A shallow, scabbed ulcer with a raised, well defined edge.	Usual location — face, most commonly found in light-skinned individuals	Destruction of lesion by either surgery or radiotherapy. Prognosis excellent if treatment is started early.
2. **Squamous cell carcinoma**			
— occurs usually in outdoor workers with fair complexions.	Elevated tumour, volcano-like in shape.	Usual location — areas most often exposed to ultraviolet rays	Destruction of lesion by either surgery or radiotherapy. Prognosis excellent if treatment is started early
3. **Intra-epidermal carcinoma**			
(Bowen's disease) squamous cell carcinoma which remains in the epidermis, spreading laterally.	Erythematous scaling lesion that grows slowly. Edges may be irregular.	Not confined to a particular area	Surgery or radiotherapy
4. **Melanoma**			
— a malignant tumour involving the melanocytes. Metastatic dissemination is relatively common. The incidence seems to be related to prolonged exposure to the sun by fair-skinned people. The incidence in Queensland, Australia is greater than in any other areas of that country. (Little et al, 1980; Norris, 1980)	Premalignant — flat irregularly pigmented macule Malignant — preinvasive nodular thickening with decreased pigmentation Invasive — nodules may be jet black	Most commonly found in areas of the skin exposed to sunlight	Surgical excision Cytotoxic therapy

The most common medications used in the treatment of skin disorders mixed with the appropriate medium and applied locally are as follows:

- for infected skin, antiseptic and/or antibiotics are used (e.g. neomycin, phenol)
- for pruritus an anti-pruritic agent such as tar or a corticosteroid may be used
- for inflamed skin an anti-inflammatory drug such as a corticosteroid may be used.

Dressings

An essential part of the local treatment of skin disorders by chemical means is the use of dressings. There are many different types of dressings that may be ordered by the physician, the most common being a polythene occlusive dressing.

Polythene occlusive dressings applied over the appropriate local medication have been found to promote rapid healing of non-infective skin disorders. The polythene causes the retention of sweat causing maceration of the horny layer of the skin thus promoting easier drug penetration into the epidermis.

Wet dressings are commonly used for patients suffering from acute inflammatory skin disorders (Hawkins, 1978). Wet dressings help to relieve itching, reduce redness by promoting vasoconstriction and help the removal of skin exudates. Fine mesh gauze is preferable for use as a wet dressing — cotton-filled material can leave fibres on the skin surface. Solutions for soaking the dressing should be at body temperature and excess moisture wrung out of the dressing. After the dressing is applied, a flannelette covering is secured around the dressing to prevent evaporation of the moist dressing. It is important to explain to the patient what you are doing so that he/she has the opportunity to participate in his/her care (Redman, 1980; Skiper & Leonard, 1965). If gloves are used during any procedures the nurse must realize that the patient may feel further isolation and must explain why gloves are necessary. Baths or soaks may also be used in the treatment of skin disorders as a means of rehydrating the skin, soothing, applying medications and preventing infection. The bath should be at a comfortable temperature and the water should not be allowed to cool. If oils are used in the bath, care should be taken to see that the patient does not fall.

After any plan of care is implemented it is important that the nurse evaluates the results of care, and makes adjustments to the care based on that evaluation.

CARE OF THE INDIVIDUAL WITH BURNS

This section of the chapter concerns itself with the consequences of thermal injury upon the functions of the skin, upon the adult patient as a whole and the resulting implications for nursing thermally injured patients.

INTRODUCTION

Over 100 000 people per year are burned or scalded, comprising approximately 6% of all accident and emergency cases; between 10–20% of these patients require hospital treatment (Lawrence, 1985). Therefore, severe thermal injuries are relatively infrequent in occurrence, but they are uniquely devastating both physically and psychologically. For this reason the prevention of burns, and the treatment and aftercare of burned patients, deserves every effort of those involved.

Thermal injuries are not merely caused by accidents, for they are not random and inevitable as the word 'accident' implies (Feck et al, 1979). Instead, there is a discernible pattern to their occurrence, and many researchers have identified factors which predispose people to thermal injuries (MacLeod, 1970; Martin, 1970; McNeill, 1976; Learmonth, 1980). Bowden et al (1979) have discussed both personal and environmental factors which affect the occurrence of a burning injury (Table 20.11).

The aetiological factors shown in Table 20.11 are significant in that they are likely to be exacerbated by the burn injury they cause and by the protracted hospital stay that may follow. The length of hospitalization for a thermal injury is longer than for other types of injury. A survey of 1100 patients with domestic thermal injuries admitted to specialized centres (Department of Trade, 1983) noted that 26% of the patients were hospitalized for more than 30 days and only 13% for less than 5 days. 8.5% of cases (82 patients) died and these were mainly elderly patients.

A comprehensive nursing history will alert the nurse to various stresses and she/he should involve the specific skills of the whole caring team (social worker, doctor, psychologist, occupational therapist, physiotherapist, chaplain, etc.) in order to provide for the whole range of patient needs.

THE NATURE OF THERMAL INJURY

Thermodynamic laws govern the transfer of heat from one object to another and, whilst all thermal injuries obey these laws, most burns are confined to relatively few types, i.e. scalds, flame burns, flash burns, contact burns, electrical injuries and chemical burns.

Knowledge of the physics governing these injuries is useful in three ways:

- it aids estimation of the severity of the injury
- it may confirm or refute the patient's account of the injury
- it may aid in anticipating other

Table 20.11 Summary of important factors affecting the occurrence of a thermal injury

Personal factors	
Age	Children under 4 years of age most liable to thermal injuries
Sex	More males than females burned in age group under 65 years old
Premorbid psychopathology	'Behaviour problems', a psychiatric diagnosis or previous psychiatric hospitalization, alcoholism and drug abuse, suicide attempts and self-destructive behaviours all predispose to thermal injuries
Previous physical disability	Neurological disorders and cardiovascular disease understandably contribute to burn injuries; more unexpectedly, so does obesity
Environmental factors	
Socio-economic	Crowded and poor quality housing; unemployment, or the wage earner in an unskilled or semi-skilled job, increase risks for all occupants
Family stress	Thermal injury often coincident with one or more other major life events in the family such as physical, emotional, financial and housing problems, or with conflict in the family, pregnancy, a move of house and social isolation, amongst other stresses

clinical conditions (for example, inhalational or blast injuries, fractures, etc.).

When a hot object contacts a cooler one, the heat transfer, which causes structural damage, is governed by the temperature difference and the time in contact. An unconscious patient lying against a domestic radiator for 3 minutes may sustain a similar injury to someone only briefly touching a stove surface.

Flame burns are often the result of clothing catching fire and are rarely insignificant. The high temperatures generated, the close contact and prolonged exposure (which may continue even after the burning clothes are extinguished) cause severe thermal injuries by conduction and radiation. The latter mechanism may operate during housefires when no direct contact with hot objects or flames occurs. This was seen in the Bradford football disaster of 1985, when many victims were burned at a distance by radiant heat.

Flame burns carry another special significance, namely the risk of lung and airway injury. This may either be the result of inhaled hot air burning, or of irritant particles and chemical gases damaging the respiratory epithelium. Burning compounds such as PVC may give off noxious chemicals (e.g. cyanide) which poison other systems of the body when inhaled.

Another sort of radiant heat causes the flash burn which accompanies explosions (e.g. gas) or high tension electrical discharges. These injuries may be severe, particularly if clothing catches fire.

Chemical 'burns' are usually caused by industrial accidents. They destroy tissue by denaturing protein, by vascular thrombosis or through cellular toxicity. Chemicals pose special problems in that they may continue to injure so long as there is any of the chemical remaining on the skin; also, systemic damage may result from absorption of the chemical. For example, chromic acid used in the plating industry not only can produce necrosis of the skin and subcutaneous tissues, but may also damage the kidneys, causing renal failure.

The final common type of burn is an indirect thermal injury caused by electricity. Here, the current passing through tissues generates heat, which, in UK domestic voltage, coagulates skin and deeper tissues. In higher voltage supplies, such as high tension (15 000 V) overhead railway cables, deep tissue damage may be extensive but not immediately obvious, as necrosed muscle may lie beneath unburnt skin in the part of the body affected.

First aid treatment

The principles of first aid treatment for all thermal injuries are to remove the source of heat and to cool the affected area as quickly as possible. If this is carried out within one minute of burning, heat conducted to the deeper tissues will be reduced, thus limiting the depth of burn (Harvey Kemble & Lamb, 1984).

Flame burns

Smother flaming clothing with the victim made to lie prone (the horizontal position avoids flames licking upwards to the face and chest; also air is expelled from the undersurface making it less likely to be burned). Remove patient to an area free from smoke gases and the risk of inhalation injury. Douse clothes with cold water to disperse the thermal effect on the tissues. Leave clothing to be removed at hospital in a clean environment, carefully, with analgesia.

Scalds

Quickly remove soaked clothing and run cold water onto the wound. The affected area should be cooled for at least 10 minutes in this way, as this has been shown to minimize injury to the deeper layers of the skin.

Chemical burns

Immediately wash away chemicals with copious quantities of running water. Wasting time searching for the appropriate antidote permits unnecessary tissue damage. There are a few exceptions to this treatment, notably burns by metallic sodium or potassium which ignite on contact with water; instead, these metals, which stick to the skin, should be picked off with forceps after covering the wound with petroleum jelly. Cement and lime become hot when mixed with small quantities of water and therefore require copious amounts, for several minutes, until cleared from the skin.

Electrical burns

Remove the current by switching off the electrical supply or levering the victim off the appliance using a non-conductor, such as a piece of wood. Electrical current can result in cardiac arrest which requires external cardiac massage and mouth-to-mouth resuscitation.

In addition to the above, the first aider should maintain the victim's airway (e.g. place in the recovery position, remove false teeth or any vomit from the mouth and extend the neck of an unconscious patient). Medical help should be sought and urgent transfer to hospital effected if damage is extensive. The burn should be wrapped in a clean sheet or pillowcase and no topical agent applied as this may mask the burn depth and extent.

CONSEQUENCES OF SKIN DESTRUCTION FROM THERMAL INJURY

The obvious consequence of thermal injury is seen in the wound, but in the extensive burn all systems of the body may be affected, causing serious physical illness and threat to life.

The local effects will be described first and then the systemic consequences.

Local effects

The depth of a burn is related to the amount of thermal energy dissipated in the skin. It influences the systemic effects of the burn, the residual ability of the wound to heal, and therefore the nursing and surgical management of the wound and the patient.

Severity of the burn

Traditional classification of burns has been by degrees of severity, first degree being simple erythema and fourth degree being destruction deep to the skin. This classification has widely been replaced by a more anatomical description of the level of injury within the skin. Thus a burn is described as superficial (epidermis alone injured), partial thickness (extending into, but not through, the dermis), or full thickness (Harvey Kemble & Lamb, 1984). In practice, the partial thickness injury is commonly split into 'dermal' and 'deep dermal', the boundary between the two being indistinct and the significance being that, although the latter wound will heal, it will do so only slowly and with poor cosmetic result.

Superficial burns. In superficial injuries the basal layer of the epithelium remains intact. The skin is dry, red, oedematous and is not blistered. The affected area is tender and blanches on compression, the capillaries refilling immediately the pressure is removed. In these respects the injury resembles a mild sunburn and healing is equally rapid. The only treatment needed is analgesia and a soothing emollient cream until sebum production returns.

Partial thickness burns. When the burn extends into the superficial dermis (which, unlike the thin epidermis, contains vascular plexi), the injury to the vessels allows exudation of fluid, thus raising the epidermis to form blisters. If the blister is removed, a swollen, pink, wet surface, which blanches and refills on light pressure, is revealed. Sensation is intact. In this superficial dermal wound healing occurs within 10 days; the raw area is resurfaced with epithelium growing and migrating outward from the undamaged walls of 'skin appendages' such as creases, sweat glands and hair follicles.

As the depth of the dermis affected is increased, so other trends occur: sensation is diminished as the dermal nerve endings are killed. Most blood vessels are destroyed and so less exudation occurs, and blanching and refilling on pressure is not as evident. In fact, fixed, coagulated capillaries may be seen in the wound. As more skin appendages are destroyed re-epithelialization becomes slower.

In the deep thermal burn, very few uninjured skin appendages remain. Re-epithelialization is therefore slow, and granulation and scar formation occur which, in conjunction with the loss of dermis, produce a poor cosmetic result. In addition, the exposed and injured dermis is fragile, its survival hanging in the balance. Desiccation, infection and circulatory stasis may destroy the remaining dermis and it is a tenet of contemporary surgery that early skin grafting, and perhaps certain dressings, may prevent this destruction, so reducing scarring.

Full thickness burns. In full thickness burns all the skin layers are destroyed and involvement may include the underlying fat, muscle and bone. The appearance can vary and may be white, waxy, tan coloured, charred or red (from haemoglobin following haemolysis fixing in the tissues). Thrombosed subcutaneous veins may be seen under the translucent tissue. The coagulated wound is dry and feels hard. Sensation is absent. No skin appendages remain and so spontaneous re-surfacing and healing is only possible by epithelial proliferation from the wound edges. Surgery to heal the wound is necessary in all but the smallest of full thickness burns.

Nurses should be aware of the depth of the patient's injury, as this influences the treatment received as well as the patient's final appearance.

Oedema and contraction of eschar

Apart from tissue damage, other local effects results from oedema. Coagulated protein shrinks and in circumferential deep burns oedema, together with the contraction of burnt skin (eschar), causes increased tissue pressure which may impair circulation and lead to ischaemia of areas supplied by the affected vessels. Similarly, contraction of deep circumferential burns to the chest can produce respiratory embarrassment. To relieve pressure, escharotomies are performed. These longitudinal incisions through the insensitive eschar into the underlying fat allow the constricting tissue to relax. The eschar does not contain live nerve endings and so the procedure is painless; however, gaping wounds result which make a portal for infection and may bleed considerably. For these reasons escharotomies are only performed if strongly indicated. Dressings should be applied and limbs elevated to reduce peripheral oedema. The circulatory status of all circumferentially or near-circumferentially burnt limbs should be monitored for at least the first 48 hours following injury. Limb warmth and the presence of a pulse should be noted; some units use Doppler ultrasonic flow monitors to determine the need for escharotomy.

Oedema develops rapidly in the lax tissues of

the burnt face. Eyelids often become so swollen that they cannot be opened and, if ocular damage is suspected, eyes should be examined as soon as possible following injury. Nurses should warn patients that this swelling will develop but will only be temporary and will begin to subside some 48 hours after the injury. During the period that the patient is 'blind', nurses should explain smells, sounds and other sensations to him/her to avoid fear and panic, and provide diversions such as conversation and music to reduce boredom.

General effects

Body fluid loss

Following a thermal injury, fluid is lost from the intravascular space as capillaries become more permeable. The greatest loss occurs at the site of the burn, but loss occurs throughout the body — a process probably mediated by kinins and other products of tissue injury. The loss of this fluid, which resembles plasma, is maximal during the first 12 hours and tails off over the first 48 hours (the so-called 'shock period'). The rate of fluid loss is proportional to the size of burnt surface area, and may be so extensive as to threaten life. Settle (1974) writes: 'The insidious leak of plasma from the patient's circulation is less dramatic than when bright red blood is spurting out onto the floor, but it can kill him just the same'.

As the intravascular fluid volume declines, so venous return and cardiac output fall. This reduces tissue perfusion, leading to tissue hypoxia. This effect may be exacerbated by a reduction in cardiac contractility (again as a result of products of tissue injury) and by poor oxygen exchange in patients with inhalational injuries.

As plasma-like fluid loss continues, peripheral vasoconstriction and the increase in haematocrit (and therefore blood viscosity) demand increased cardiac work to maintain blood pressure. The clinical signs of 'shock' (see Ch. 10) become apparent, and tissue hypoxia threatens those organs with a high metabolic demand, such as the kidney. Lack of perfusion may result in acute tubular necrosis if not rapidly corrected. Renal damage may be further exacerbated by the haemoglobin released from red cells, which become excessively fragile in extensive burns.

Many more changes occur, in organ function (e.g. lung, liver), in electrolyte levels (particularly in calcium, sodium and phosphate ions), in hormonal secretions (e.g. catecholamines, insulin, antidiuretic hormone, mineralo-corticoids) and in metabolic function. These are discussed in several texts and are outside the scope of this brief review (Artz et al, 1979; Cason, 1981; Davies, 1982).

Settle (1974) has drawn attention to how rapidly the shock phase develops and emphasizes the need for prompt fluid replacement.

Treatment of the patient during the 'shock period'. *Care of airway.* Clinical signs and a history of inhalational injury (including arterial hypoxia and carbon monoxide poisoning) or upper airway obstruction from progressing oedema (e.g. from extensive facial burns) may demand airway protection (e.g. intubation) and ventilatory support.

Replacement of fluid loss. If the burnt surface area is not too great, the body will compensate adequately for the fluid loss and the patient may overcome the 'shock phase' with no other help than the provision of extra fluid to drink. The approximate dividing line between whether or not a patient requires intravenous fluid resuscitation to replace the lost body fluid is 15% (or over) area of body burn in an adult and 10% in a child. To accurately assess the size of burn, the area covered should be drawn on a surface area chart (see Fig. 20.1) which takes into account the age and therefore the bodily proportions of the patient. The calculation of fluid loss in the burned patient is made difficult by oedema, burnt limbs (which make blood pressure readings impracticable) and the complexity of the injury, which add to the unreliability of central venous pressure (CVP) measurement as an index of blood volume. Therefore since the Second World War, various 'formulae' have been proposed to estimate fluid requirement, which is governed by these factors:

BURN RECORD (Birth — Adult)

Name: ______________________ Age: __________ Unit No: __________

Date of observation: ______________________ Total % burn __________

% deep dermal __________

% full thickness __________

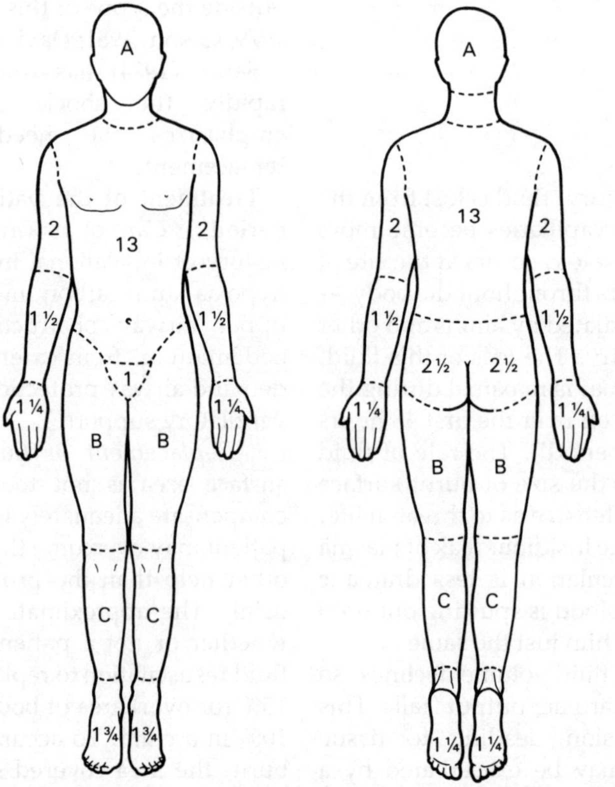

Relative percentage of areas affected by growth

Area	Age 0	1	5	10	15	Adult
A = ½ of head	9½	8½	6½	5½	4½	3½
B = ½ of one thigh	2¾	3¼	4	4½	4½	4¾
C = ½ of one leg	2½	2½	2¾	3	3¼	3½

Fig. 20.1 Burn record

- burnt surface area
- body weight
- time since injury.

The most commonly used formula in the UK is that of Muir & Barclay (1974) which uses plasma as the replacement fluid and allows for the fact that most fluid is lost over the first 12 hours and then gradually declines. The formula is therefore divided to give equal volumes of fluid in six successive 'periods' of 4, 4, 4, 6, 6, and 12 hours.

Muir & Barclay formula:

$$\frac{\text{Total percentage area of body burn} \times \text{Weight in kg}}{2} = \text{Amount of plasma (in ml) to be given in each period}$$

In practice, human plasma protein fraction (human albumin solution) is usually administered rather than fresh frozen plasma (which would prove too expensive and too difficult to obtain for such large quantities). When human plasma protein fraction is given, it has been found that for each 'period', an extra 30% of the calculated volume is required. The regimen is calculated from the time of injury. Therefore, if the infusion is set up two hours after injury (as if often the case), the first 4 hour fluid volume should be delivered in 2 hours, to catch up with fluid loss.

In addition to the replacement fluids, maintenance fluids are usually also given intravenously for at least the first 12 hours, or until bowel sounds can be heard. (Paralytic ileus is common following a major burn as peristalsis is often reduced due to splanchnic vasoconstriction.) 'Hartmann's solution' is usually the maintenance fluid and is given at a rate of approximately 100 ml/h (2400 ml/24 h).

In extensive burns, blood transfusion may be required as a result of reduction in red cell mass (due to direct loss of erythrocytes in the burn wound and their increased fragility in the circulation). Some establishments calculate the loss by isotope dilution methods. Blood transfusion is usually deferred until the end of the 'shock' phase.

Often two intravenous sites are needed to cope with the large volumes of fluid and if the patient is shocked a 'cutdown' to deeper vessels may be necessary. The patient's life may depend upon the intravenous infusion and therefore its maintenance should be a nursing priority. The cannula must be securely fastened and the site should be frequently inspected for signs of infection and phlebitis. (Venous cannulation increases the possibility of sepsis from the often heavily colonized body surface.)

Monitoring of replacement fluids. The formulae only serve as guides to the fluid requirements in the first 36 hours. The adequacy of therapy needs continual assessment using the patient's clinical condition, haematocrit and urine output measurements and, to a lesser degree, other monitoring techniques.

Haematocrit measurement acts as a guide to intravascular fluid deficit because increased vascular permeability allows plasma to leak from the vessels, but erythrocytes are retained, causing a rise in haematocrit, (ignoring the possibility of haemolysis, which, if extensive, will be identified by red coloured urine and a red supernatant on centrifuging blood). Intravascular fluid deficit may be calculated as follows:

$$\text{Fluid deficit} = \text{Blood volume expected} - \frac{\text{Blood volume expected} \times \text{Normal haematocrit}}{\text{Observed haematocrit}}$$

In this way, using the haematocrit, the hourly fluid requirements can be calculated and constantly adjusted.

Urine output is a useful guide to renal perfusion and so to intravascular volume and, of course, warns of the first major consequence of shock, renal failure. Therefore all major burn patients are catheterized to enable hourly monitoring of the urine output and also for patient convenience. Fluid replacement should aim to maintain an unaided urine flow of 30–50 ml/hour in an adult. If renal failure is already incipient on arrival, or is threatened by extensive myoglobinuria from muscle damage in high tension electrical injury, a diuresis may be induced whilst restoring intravascular volume in order to maintain renal function.

Twenty four hour urine collections will also be

used to monitor the kidneys' ability to concentrate and differentially excrete electrolytes; daily osmolality and ion concentrations are measured and compared to the plasma values. Creatinine clearance is also measured to provide a guide to glomerular filtration rates.

Further monitoring and procedures in the shock phase. Some patients with existing renal or myocardial disease, or in whom circumstances have greatly delayed or confused resuscitation, may require more direct measurement of intravascular volume. This is best obtained (where the expertise is available) by the use of a pulmonary wedge catheter to measure left atrial filling pressure. In combination with a thermodilution catheter, cardiac output can be directly measured and the relative roles of low intravascular volume, poor myocardial performance and raised systemic vascular resistance assessed, before appropriate treatment is given.

It has been found that simple central venous pressure measurement in major thermal injuries is not a helpful guide to fluid replacement.

In summary (see Table 20.12), monitoring in the shock phase aims to detect and arrest inadequate vascular volume, insufficient oxygenation and incipient renal damage. Other procedures are performed in the shock phase and these are included in the admission procedures for severely burned patients in Table 20.13, whilst further care of the thermally injured patient is discussed in the following sections.

Catabolism

Apart from the protein rich fluid and erythrocyte loss, the hypermetabolic response of the body to a thermal injury results in a marked negative nitrogen balance proportional to the extent of the injury. This catabolism, which may continue for weeks and be increased by infection, often occurs in patients who are already poorly nourished and can lead to the impairment of wound healing and a lowering of immunological competence and resistance to infection.

It is therefore vital to provide dietary protein and calories to aid early recovery and healing. Sutherland (1976) advocates the following energy and protein requirements for burned adults:

- Energy — 83.6J (20 Cal)/kg of body weight + 292.7J (70 Cal)/1% of burn
- Protein — 1g/kg + 3g/1% of burn

A 60 kg man with a 40% burn will require 16 728 kJ (4000 Calories) and 180g protein/day. These large requirements will not be achieved on the average hospital diet and burned patients require energy and protein-rich augmentation, often by naso-enteric feeding tubes.

Dietary advice should be sought to provide nourishing, tempting food, rich in iron and vitamins and containing enough fibre to prevent constipation. Meals should be presented at appropriate times, that is, not immediately after a dressing or when the patient is recently sedated.

Despite such preparations, it is unlikely that a seriously ill patient will voluntarily ingest adequate nutrition and naso-enteric feeds may be used. Commercial preparations are available and should be introduced gradually in dilute form. Nurses need to be aware of complications such as diarrhoea and nausea, or more seriously, gastric dilatation and aspiration of gastric contents (heralded by discomfort, bloating, nausea, pallor, clamminess, tachycardia and loss of bowel sounds). Naso-enteric feeding should be used with extreme caution in obtunded or demented patients and the tube should always be aspirated prior to the administration of a feed to check that the gastric contents are not accumulating.

Immobility

Patient immobility is the bane of those nursing adult burned patients. Often the patient is obese, may be demented, psychiatrically ill or just plain obstinate. Swathed in dressings, perhaps in pain, often sedated and listless, these patients are prone to all the complications of immobility, such as pressure sores, venous thrombosis and pneumonia. In addition, the problems are often exacerbated by incontinence, burns on pressure areas and extensive infection, even before the surgical insult of skin grafting.

Table 20.12 Summary of the monitoring of burned patients in the shock phase

Condition assessed	Clinical observation and measurement	Investigation
Intravascular volume	Clinical signs of shock Urine output Pulse Blood pressure Direct arterial pressure Left atrial pressure (rare)	Haematocrit — after each 'period' or more frequently
Oxygen exchange	Respiratory rate Soot in nose/mouth Colour/cyanosis Intraoral swelling/stridor/hoarseness Inspired oxygen concentration Ventilator parameters	Arterial gas analysis Arterial pH Arterial/venous carboxyhaemoglobin Chest X-rays (perhaps daily)
Renal function	Urine output Urine colour (myoglobin, haemoglobin, concentration) Urine specific gravity	Urine and plasma osmolality Urine 24 hour electrolytes Creatinine clearance

Table 20.13 Admission procedures for severely burned patients

Reason for procedures	Procedures	Comments
Assessment of fluid requirements	Weigh patient Ascertain time of injury Calculate % of burn	Fluid resuscitation required if burn is greater than 15–20 % of body surface area Formulae to guide fluid resuscitation (see text)
Assessment of respiratory status	Ensure adequate airway (? intubation/ ventilation) Observe for signs of smoke inhalation Arterial blood gas sampling Arterial/venous carboxyhaemoglobin Chest X-ray	See text and Table 20.12 Repeated arterial sampling is easier than from an arterial line
Administer fluid	Site intravenous infusions Care of infusion site	May need more than one cannula, as large as possible (as fluid requirements usually great) May need 'cut down' (if shocked)
Continual assessment of fluid needs and renal functions	Catheterize Hourly urine measurement 24 hour urine collection Blood samples for grouping and cross-matching, haematocrit & electrolytes	See text and Table 20.12
Pain	Administer intravenous morphine PRN	See text
Prevent aspiration of gastric contents	Pass nasogastric tube Nil by mouth till bowel sounds heard	Paralytic ileus common Acid antagonists given to prevent gastric bleeds
Prevent limb ischaemia/ease respiration	Limb/trunk escharotomies Elevation of burnt limbs	Infection risk from escharotomies Elevation reduces peripheral oedema
Prevent/monitor infection	Tetanus toxoid administered PRN Throat and wound swabs daily Dressing of wound	See text
Maintenance of clear airways (particularly in patients with smoke inhalation injury)	Chest physiotherapy ('bagging', 'suctioning', 'turning', 'clapping', 'shaking', etc) Provision of humidification Care of ventilator Regular chest X-rays	Pulmonary oedema usually peaks at 24–28 hours after injury Physiotherapy for short periods, frequently (1–2 hourly) Suctioning may be required every 10–15 minutes

Whilst some benefit is derived from equipment such as low loss air beds, there is no substitute for regular, frequent turning and pressure area care, and intensive physiotherapy. These needs, together with dressing and feeding requirements, make these truly high-dependency patients. Burns units should be staffed day and night to a level where these requirements need not be neglected, and strong, willing ancillary staff play an invaluable role in nursing the burned patient.

A further problem, apart from that of plain immobility, is that of positioning the patient. Often, the position of comfort is that of contracture and attention to correct positioning is required to prevent future disability. Splints for limbs and hands and rolls of foam and towels to extend the neck are all employed to improve positioning and, therefore, future functioning.

Infection

The burn wound represents an ideal culture medium for a wide range of microorganisms and for a variety of reasons. There is a large amount of necrotic tissue, oedema and transudate, making an excellent nutrient medium for bacteria. Other factors such as shock, anaemia, hypoproteinaemia, loss of immunoglobins, electrolyte disturbances and high levels of corticosteroids, reduce resistance to infection (Cason, 1981).

Infection can be considered at two levels. Firstly, there is contamination of the burn wound alone. This is usually detected by wound and body swabs taken on admission and whenever the wound is dressed. Secondly, there is bacterial invasion of the tissues and the blood stream; the latter is usually detected clinically from the condition of the patient and the wound. Blood cultures may show a negative growth despite obvious clinical sepsis, and waiting for a result before treatment is commenced may prove fatal. Septicaemia is a major cause of death in severely burned patients.

Lowbury (1973) has outlined methods of preventing infection in burns in keeping with the two levels of infection already outlined.

The 'first line of defence' (against contamination) includes:

- wound excision and skin grafting
- aseptic measures — isolation measures, aseptic dressing techniques, the wearing of plastic gowns and gloves for certain procedures, and especially the washing of hands before and after coming into contact with all burns patients
- antiseptic measures — topical antiseptic applications in dressings.

The 'second line of defence' (against invasion) consists of:

- systemic antibiotic therapy — where clinically indicated
- immunoprophylaxis
- methods of supporting the natural defences — high protein/calorie diet, blood transfusions for anaemia, control of diabetes, etc.

Many pathogens colonize the burned patient, but one in particular which causes concern is *Streptococcus pyogenes* (Beta-haemolytic streptococcus, Lancefield group A) which extends the tissue injury and may destroy skin grafts. Therefore, if this is found on a wound or throat swab, the patient is treated with antibiotics (usually penicillin) and nursed in strict isolation until subsequent swabs become clear. Usually this is the only bacteria to be treated at the contamination level, in order to prevent antibiotic resistance developing on the unit.

The Infection Control Nurse and staff in the bacteriology and virology departments play an important role in the control of infection, and the burns team should liaise closely with them.

Pain

Surprisingly, not all burned patients experience pain in the early stages of care since in deeper burns the sensory nerve endings are destroyed. However, in most superficial injuries pain can be severe, constituting a major problem for the patient.

The perception of pain has physical, psychological and social origins and its management is complex (see Ch. 9). The pain of an anxious patient will not be adequately treated by analgesia alone, since anxiety heightens perception of pain (Hayward, 1979). To help such patients, nurses should discuss with them the origin of their anxiety and take practical steps (explanation, assurance, social help) to alleviate it.

It has been found that '. . . compared with patients' own estimates nurses tended to underestimate the patient's pain level, and overestimate the amount of relief obtained from analgesics' (Hunt, 1979). In addition, '. . . exposure to pain on one occasion heightens a person's expectations and sensitivity to pain on subsequent occasions' (Hayward, 1979). These views emphasize the nurse's duty in pain management to heed guidance from the patient on the level of analgesia required, and to administer it regularly to prevent pain (and so anxiety) building up and reinforcing each other.

Morphine with its analgesic and anxiolytic qualities is a suitable preparation for these patients, provided respiratory depression and nausea are avoided.

For brief painful procedures (e.g. small dressings) Entonox (50% oxygen and 50% nitrous oxide) inhalation may be effective. In more extensive procedures, it may supplement morphine. Its effect is enhanced by self administration and it has proved effective in making dressing procedures less distressing for both patients and staff (Diggory, 1979).

Psychological effects

Feller et al (1973) described three phases of the treatment for seriously burned patients:

- the Emergent phase (the period of physiological shock 2 to 3 days post-burn)
- the Acute phase (the time required to resurface all areas of skin loss, which may take several months)
- the Rehabilitation phase which is concerned with returning the patient to a 'useful' place in society (during this phase, re-hospitalization for cosmetic and functional reconstruction may be necessary).

At each of these stages, the patient and relatives will experience various emotional conflicts and these may be exacerbated by stresses which existed prior to the injury.

Fear of dying. During the Emergent and Acute phases, patients often speak of their fear of impending death, as do relatives.

The risk of death from burns can be calculated in various ways (Bull, 1971; Roi et al, 1981; Harvey Kemble & Lamb, 1984). An estimate of the probability of death is obtained by adding the patient's age in years to the percentage of body surface area burnt; this gives the probability of dying as a percentage. The estimate will be altered by the presence of pre-existing disease, inhalational injury and extensive, full thickness burns, nor does it apply to children under 10 years of age. The very elderly and the very young have a high burns mortality.

Death from burns is usually delayed and due to organ failure or septicaemia, so producing an unique situation in that it is possible to predict that a presently alert patient will shortly die. The management of such a sitution is intricate and the role of the nurse is central. The severely burned patient is often not in great pain yet there is a temptation to obtund him/her with drugs and not to resuscitate. This risks treating the staff and not the patient, who may prefer to remain alert in order to say goodbyes, make reparations and prepare for death (Imbus & Zawacki, 1977).

Three common fears of the dying are the fear of pain, the fear of loneliness, and the fear of meaninglessness (Blake et al, 1976). Adequate analgesia given regularly and frequently enough to prevent pain mounting up, comfortable positioning and attentive care will help alleviate the first fear. The latter two fears can be helped by permitting the patient to maintain self-determination and by encouraging relatives and staff to tell the patient what he/she means to them. In addition, staff and relatives, by being always readily available to just listen or to provide for physical needs, will give support to the patient, and thus help alleviate each of these fears.

Stages of grief. Both patients and relatives pass through stages of grief and, to provide support, nurses need to be aware of these. Engel (1964) has described three stages of grief in relatives who have lost a loved one and Kübler-Ross (1970) has reported five stages of grief in patients who learn that they have a fatal illness.

The initial response described by Engel is that of 'shock and disbelief' which is similar to the 'shock and denial' stage of Kübler-Ross. This state may be accompanied by the physiological responses of tachycardia, nausea, sweating, gastrointestinal disturbances, etc.

For the relative, the second stage is that of 'developing awareness' in which the reality begins to dawn on the consciousness of the griever. The person will feel sad, guilty, hopeless and helpless. There is a strong urge to cry. Alongside this stage, Kübler-Ross describes for the patient stages of 'anger,' 'bargaining' and 'depression' through which the patient works to become aware of his/her condition (from 'No, not me!' to 'Yes, me, but' to 'Yes, me'). People react differently in these middle phases of awareness in the grief process. An understanding nurse will allow people to express their feelings, from explosive anger to silent anger or continual criticism of care. This acceptance and understanding will provide immeasurable comfort to patients and relatives alike.

The final stage of grief is described by Engel as that of 'restitution and recovery', and Kübler-Ross's similar stage is that of 'acceptance'. This stage is one of peace of mind, and will only be reached if the preceding stages have been traversed.

These stages have been described in detail elsewhere, as have the ways in which nurses can provide support for the dying (Glaser & Strauss, 1965; Blake at al, 1976; Hinton, 1976). However, in order to care for the dying, nurses should first come to terms with their own feelings about death and dying, and to do this they will need support from other members of the team who all have the need to talk about their feelings and express their emotions. Essentially, a gentle, caring, understanding approach, an empathetic outlook and, above all, an ability and a willingness to listen, will help patients and relatives (and also colleagues) work through the grief process of shock, anger and finally acceptance.

It is important for burns nurses to understand the stages of grief, because it concerns not only the dying, but all patients who have suffered a burn with resultant scarring. Both the patient and relatives will grieve at the change in body image, for the loss of the former self.

Other behavioural changes. Many research studies have reported changes in the psychological state of patients who have been severely burned (Hamburg et al, 1953; Miller et al, 1976; Andreasen et al, 1971; Andreasen et al, 1972; Bowden et al, 1979). The three most frequently mentioned behavioural states are delirium, depression and regression:

- Delirium — the occurrence of delirium is affected by both physical and psychological factors. It occurs more frequently in the elderly, those with a history of pre-morbid psychopathology (see introduction) or alcoholism.
- Depression — severe depression with symptoms of crying, loss of hope, feelings of worthlessness, decreased appetite and insomnia have been described.
- Regression — regressive behaviour may produce a demanding attitude, dependence, intolerance and anger.

Pennisi et al (1970) observed two opposing types of behaviour in 25% of their patients. The first of anxiety/depression/regression and the second of rebellion/hostility. They have labelled this behaviour the 'Dependency—Rebellion Syndrome' and believe that it results from 'psychological conflicts in the area of independent versus dependent needs'.

Reasons for psychological responses. The reasons for this variety of psychological responses to burn trauma are:

Pre-existing psychiatric and behavioural abnormalities (including alcoholism). These abnormalities have predisposed the patient to the injury in the first place.

Physical complications (e.g. septicaemia). These often result in delirium and require urgent medical diagnosis and treatment (Jackson, 1974).

Sensory deprivation. Sensory deprivation can result from lying alone in a strange environment. Nurses should provide company, explanation, temporal indicators (e.g. clocks) and patient involvement in care to help combat this.

Fear of dying. This may be well founded in severe injuries, but may also result from the patient's awareness of his/her vulnerability which is impressed on him/her by the initial treatment, monitoring equipment and intensive care setting. To reduce patient fear, nurses should explain all equipment and procedures in a manner suitable for the understanding of the patient and relatives. A confident manner will reinforce the belief that the team is competent.

Fear of disability. This occurs particularly if the limbs are badly injured. Patients wonder if they will be able to keep their jobs and continue to support their families. Here the social worker, physiotherapist and occupational therapist will have an important role to play. Employers should be contacted to receive assurance about future employment or, if this is impossible, alternative employment may be arranged. Physiotherapy, though painful, will often be tolerated if encouragement is given that improved functioning will facilitate employment prospects or the continuation of a cherished hobby. In addition, involvement in self-care will enhance self-esteem and self-determination.

Fear of disfigurement. Patients can be helped by being given opportunity to express their emotions. If the patient is going to be scarred, they should not be told otherwise. However, the patients' psychological defences, e.g. denial, regression, depression, or anger, should be permitted for as long as they are needed (unless these reactions are abnormally protracted or severe, when psychological or psychiatric advice should be sought). Patients with facial burns tend only to ask to see their faces when they are psychologically ready. Each patient differs in his/her reaction to a change in body image. They will have to grieve for their loss. The burn team can help by not being unrealistically optimistic about the patient's appearance, as this will betray trust and confidence; however, they should preserve hope and encourage the patient, allowing him/her to come to terms with the new situation in his/her own way, by permitting the expression of the grieving emotions and showing a caring, understanding and non-rejecting attitude.

Fear of the loss of loved ones. The continuation of the patient's closest and significant relationships should be encouraged. Visitors may need assistance from the social work department concerning travelling expenses and this should be offered, as some people may be too proud to mention financial difficulties.

Nurses and doctors should explain the injury and disfigurement to visitors to help them accept and understand these more easily. Weekly meetings attended by relatives and patients, together with team members (e.g. nurse, social worker, psychologist) will allow open discussion of worries and encourage frank communication between all parties.

Relatives may be embarrassed and worried about the patient's behaviour and will be reassured by explanations that such behavioural reactions are a normal occurrence following a burn injury and will improve along with the physical state. Similarly, the offensive smell of burn patients which results from infected wounds is also distressing to patients and relatives alike. Regular dressing changes, antibiotics, ventilation and the removal of the sealed, dirty dressing bags from the unit at frequent intervals will help, but will not remove the smells. Again, explanations about the cause will help to prevent misconceptions and to foster understanding.

Physical dependency on staff. Patients often find this difficult to accept at first, but dependency will persist if the patient becomes behaviourly regressive. Independence should be fostered by encouraging the patient to care for him/herself in any way possible, e.g. cleaning his/her own teeth. Patient autonomy should be encouraged, allowing the patient to make choices in his/her own care where possible.

Emotions arising from the accident. A patient may feel guilt if he/she caused the accident and survived whilst another died. Anger and resentment may be felt at a person blamed for causing the accident or because the accident has obstructed a goal in life. Patients can be helped with these feelings by giving them the opportunity to express them and permit them to come to terms with the accident.

Management of behavioural changes. The variety of psychological responses resulting from a burn injury is a demanding challenge for the burn team. One way to view the behaviour of burned patients is in the context of the grieving process of shock, anger and finally acceptance. Similarly, patients can be helped through the same interactional approaches as those used for dying patients and their relatives.

Steiner & Clarke (1977) looked at the burn experience as involving many losses. They identified three stages through which the burned patient must pass in order to adapt: stage one, physiological emergency; stage two, psychological emergency; stage three, social emergency. Similarly, Brodland & Andreasen (1974) have described an adjustment process for the relatives; the first stage of acute shock and grief and the second (or convalescent stage) when relatives begin to accept the injury and support the patient in his/her recovery.

Management of the behavioural changes involves the whole burn team — nurses, surgeons, psychologist, psychiatrist, priest, social worker, physiotherapist, occupational therapist, etc. No one person can provide every facet of care and therefore the burn team need to work together, supporting each other, in order to provide care for the patient. Communication between members of the team is important and frequent liaison, including weekly team meetings, is necessary to achieve adequate support for patients, relatives and staff.

HEALING AND REPAIR

Surgical management

The following paragraphs summarize the current attitudes in burns surgery.

The objective in almost all burns surgery is to provide intact skin cover for three reasons:

- appearance
- function
- protection.

In smaller wounds the former two may predominate, but in a large, life-threatening burn, extensive skin cover to protect the body is essential.

Traditional treatment has been to treat even deep dermal wounds conservatively, allowing some to heal (albeit after weeks and with contracted hypertrophic scars), and others to slough and granulate, later to accept skin grafts. This regimen caused prolonged hospital stays, high infection rates and fibrotic, contracted wounds. There is now a trend to early skin cover on partial thickness and full thickness injuries.

Partial thickness injuries

Janzekovic (1970) has pioneered the 'early tangential excision' of burn wounds at the deep dermal level. These wounds, if left, would heal slowly and patchily, with considerable scarring. However, if within the first few days the burnt tissue is shaved off, layer by layer, until healthy dermis is reached and then the wound grafted with split skin, early healing can be achieved. In addition, further death of dermal cells (see earlier) is prevented leading to a less scarred, more supple and functional result. Hospital stay and infection are also greatly reduced with early tangential excision in wounds of less than 20%.

Early tangential excision presents its own drawbacks however, in that operative blood loss is extensive. Also, the differentiation between a dermal and deep dermal injury is difficult and may only be resolved at surgery, so that some patients may have unnecessary operations.

Extensive or deep burns

After the 'shock' phase, the common cause of death in extensive burns (over 20%) is sepsis and, in these patients, the burn surgeon will strive to reduce the burnt surface area to less than 20% as early as possible. In patients with burns of over 80%, this may necessitate early extensive excision of wounds (perhaps to deep fascia, to reduce blood loss and ensure graft take) and expedient graft cover (see below). Where appropriate, early attention with tangential excision and grafting may still be given to functional areas, such as eyelids and hands, but not at the expense of early extensive skin cover.

Skin grafting

In scalds and partial thickness burns, where early tangential excision is employed to preserve dermis, enhance the healed appearance and conserve function, the wound will be resurfaced, where possible, with sheets of split skin of a thickness roughly corresponding to the depth of skin lost.

Split skin is obtained by tangentially removing the epidermis and part of the dermis as a sheet, leaving the donor site to re-epithelialize from skin pits, which takes approximately 10 days (Lendrum, 1981).

In extensive burns, these sheets of skin can be 'meshed' by machine, to give them a net-like appearance and, by stretching the net, they can then cover a greater area. The interstices of such a net epithelialize secondarily from the edges. This technique is valuable in patients where the burnt surface area exceeds the donor area available. It also prevents blood being trapped under the graft (as this escapes through the holes in the net) and, therefore, vascularization of the graft is not hindered. However, these benefits should be weighed against the fact that, where significant expansion is achieved in meshed skin, the resulting cosmetic appearance may be poor. Therefore this technique is reserved for patients with major burns and only small donor areas, for whom urgent skin cover is required to reduce the burnt surface area to a level where the risk of life-threatening infection is almost eradicated.

Post-operative care. Postoperatively, thermally injured patients resemble other surgical patients with some major exceptions.

Pain. Following split skin grafting, the pain from the donor site is often severe and exceeds that of the grafted wound. Considerable analgesia may be required for several days.

Blood loss. Donor sites and some grafted areas will continue to bleed considerably into dressings (which will need frequent repadding) for approximately 36 hours postoperatively. This loss is hard to assess directly and so reliance is placed on signs of hypovolaemia and anaemia.

Graft and donor site care. Grafts may be exposed or dressed, but either way they require care and attention (Lendrum, 1981; Harvey Kemble & Lamb, 1984) to ensure a successful 'take'. This is usually carried out by specially trained nursing or medical staff.

Thermal injury. It is important to rem-ember that the patient is still suffering from a thermal injury with all the psychological, nutritional, bacteriological and metabolic problems that entails.

LONG-TERM CONSEQUENCES

Physical

Soon after healing, many patients have a 'satisfactory' scar appearance. However, within weeks hypertrophic scarring results in itchy, red, raised, unsightly scars which are hard to the touch, and the shortening of which causes contracture across joints. These consequences of deep dermal and full thickness thermal injuries may be reduced by early tangential excision, but nevertheless can lead to severe disfigurement and disability unless treated. For these reasons the aftercare of burned patients is equally as important as the treatment received in hospital and is undertaken by a team which includes the occupational therapist, physiotherapist, burns aftercare nurse and doctor.

The severity of hypertrophic scarring and contractures can be reduced and even prevented by three measures:

- by frequent greasing and firm massaging (which replaces absent sebaceous excretions)
- by the application of continuous and controlled pressure to the scars through the use of tailored elastic pressure garments

- by splinting joints against contracting forces.

Pressure garments may have to be worn for between 6 months and 2 years following healing to ensure a flat, smooth, pale and supple scar and a good range of joint movement. This lengthy and often uncomfortable treatment has been found so greatly to improve scar appearance and mobility, that the need for re-hospitalization and reconstructive surgery has been reduced (Larson et al, 1973).

Psychological

Many burned patients have higher expectations of their final physical appearance than the health care team (even if they have been given honest accounts of what residual scarring will occur). Often it takes a while before patients realize how badly scarred they are going to remain and, therefore, before they can begin to adjust to their change in body image.

The reported prevalence of psycho-social maladjustment in burned adults varies in the literature (10% in Browne et al, 1985, 15–30% in Bowden et al, 1979, and not less than 30% in Malt, 1980).

Malt (1980) categorizes the types of long-term emotional problems into four groups:

- depression
- anxiety syndromes
- reduced social interaction without special mental problems
- possible psychotic syndrome.

Other writers report similar emotional problems following a severe thermal injury. However, the fact that many of these patients had pre-injury psycho-social problems should be borne in mind when considering the effects of burns in the long-term.

Browne et al (1985) report that the variability in psycho-social adjustment is related to unemployment, loss of occupational status, avoidance coping, and little involvement in recreational activities. Unlike other writers, they did not find that adjustment was related to the severity of the burn or to the time since injury. In other words, they suggest that psycho-social adjustment is 'a function of both coping responses and social resources' rather than burn severity.

Therefore to help patients adjust to a burn injury the aftercare team should be aware of these emotional effects, and patients and their families should be encouraged to talk through their feelings and fears. Referral should be made to a psychologist or psychiatrist if needed, and there should be liaison with employers to allow the patient appropriate work. Patients should be helped to keep active and thus able to continue in employment or with their recreational activities, and encouraged to continue and make new friendships to allow easier adjustment to their drastic change in body image.

A severe thermal injury affects all the human activities. Thermally injured patients therefore require specialized nursing skills to deal with the physical, psychological and social disturbances which occur. It is demanding, but nevertheless, rewarding work.

CARE OF THE INDIVIDUAL WITH PRESSURE SORES

INTRODUCTION

Pressure sores are wounds which result from the death of the skin and its underlying tissue. In the past they were called bedsores and more recently decubitus ulcers, pressure ulcers or pressure sores. The changes in name indicate firstly a change in nursing care, in that there are now as many patients with sores up in chairs as in bed (Jordan & Clark, 1977). They cannot therefore be termed 'bed' sores or decubitus ulcers (Latin 'decumbere' — to lie down). Secondly, the link with pressure as a cause, either direct or indirect, in the term 'pressure sore' enables us to encompass by the one name a great variety of lesions. Because of this wide variation most workers in the field attempt to grade sores according to the tissues involved (Lowthian, 1979a; Morden & Bayne, 1976; Barbenel et al, 1977), and hence the severity. Four grades are generally recognized:

- where the skin is permanently discoloured, raised by blisters containing blood or clear fluid, but still intact
- where the epidermis is broken
- where there is complete destruction of the skin, but where no other tissue is involved
- where both skin and underlying tissues are involved and a cavity is formed.

In addition, sores may also be divided into those which develop when the capillaries are occluded by excessive pressure, Type I (direct), and those which result from disruptive (indirect) pressure or shear, Type II. Type I is associated with immobility, while Type II is related to friction between the body and its supporting surface (Crow et al, 1981).

Pressure sores are not in themselves a disease; they develop where pressure exceeds that which the tissue can tolerate. In the healthy individual excessive pressure results in blisters, and the management of these lesions is to remove the cause (e.g. new shoes) which allows the body to repair the damage caused. If the insult is repeated before healing is fully complete, more damage and slower healing will result.

Where a patient is seriously ill, has some degree of immobility or loss of sensation, the normal response to discomfort (to move) is impaired or lost. In this situation the resulting sores will develop as a 'side-effect' of illness, in the same way that drug 'side effects' accompany some therapeutic regimes. In both cases the severity of the side-effects can range from being a minor irritation to being life threatening; their development may be a necessary risk of treatment and it is realistic to accept that in some cases prevention will not be possible.

PREVENTION OF PRESSURE SORES

In order to prevent sores the nurse must be able to recognize those patients who are at risk, know how pressure causes damage, be aware of the equipment available for the care of the vulnerable patient and the principles upon which it works.

Patients at risk

Surveys in recent years (Petersen & Bittmann, 1971; Barbenel et al, 1977; Lowthian, 1979a) have shown that the number of patients with sores at any one time (prevalence) ranges from 2–8.8% of hospital patients. The lower figure comes from Denmark where all patients in the district of Arhus were included, the upper figure comes from the Greater Glasgow Health Board Area where two low-prevalence groups of patients (maternity and psychiatry) were excluded from the figure. Of more interest to nurses than the actual numbers found, was the distribution of sores according to variations in the patient:

- Age — in all surveys there was a direct correlation between the increase in prevalence of sores and an increase in age
- Mobility — sore prevalence increases with the degree of paralysis
- Continence — incontinent patients are more likely to develop sores (Lowthian, 1976)
- Diseases — patients diagnosed as suffering from diseases of the vascular system, neurological and orthopaedic disorders show a higher prevalence of pressure sores.

The association of these factors, together with the general physical state of the patient, are the basis of the clinical assessment of risk. As an aid to those still developing skills in assessment, the risk calculation score developed by Norton et al (1975) for use in geriatric nursing is of considerable value. Patients are assessed in five areas:

- physical condition
- mental condition
- activity
- mobility
- continence.

Each area is given up to 4 points for most satisfactory (e.g. fully continent) down to 1 point for worst possible (e.g. doubly incontinent). When points for all five assessments are added together any patient with a total of 14 or below is at risk.

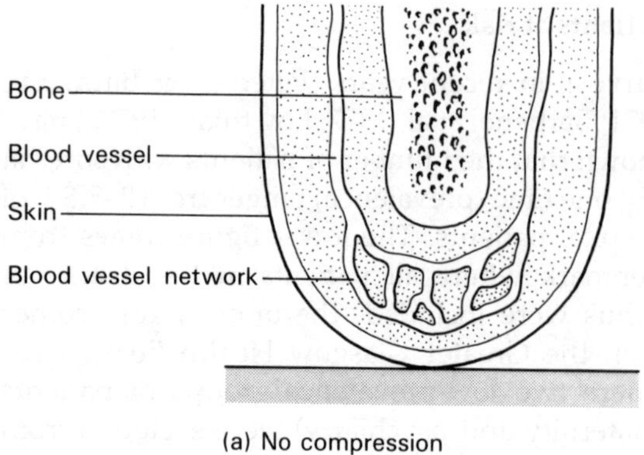

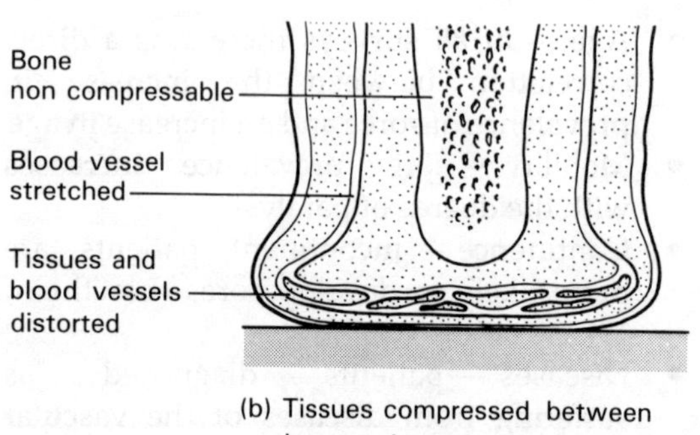

Fig. 20.2 The effects of tissue compression.

The assessment of risk therefore depends on the nurse's judgement rather than any physical measure. Risk can also change either slowly or dramatically; the fit pre-operative patient becoming a risk when immobilized by post-operative restraints, deprived of food and sedated. Changes like these are the signal for additional care.

Pressure as a cause of damage

In a multicellular organism the cells within a tissue depend on the extracellular fluid for the transport of nutrients, oxygen and waste materials to and from the cell. In some tissues the distance between the cell and the blood vessels, which act as the main transport system, is short. These tissues (such as muscles) are generally active, demanding large amounts of nutrients and oxygen and, consequently, suffer rapidly when deprived. Less metabolically active tissues (e.g. adipose) demand less and survive longer, in particular the epidermis which relies upon the underlying dermis for all transport of nutrients is relatively inactive. As such it is able to survive without nutrients for up to two weeks.

Compression of the body tissues results in distortion (Fig. 20.2), the blood vessels will be kinked or stretched, both effects leading to disruption of the transport system. A compressed area will appear white (blanched) because fluid, mainly blood, is squeezed out of the area. When pressure is relieved blood rushes back into the area producing a reactive hyperaemia. Prolonged pressure will lead to death of cells from anoxia, while excess pressure or shear causes damage to the vessels themselves which also results in cellular anoxia following vessel thrombosis. Pressure is in effect squeezing, it can only take place therefore when there are two opposed forces with a compressible tissue sandwiched between. Pressure sores develop mainly over bony prominences because the bony skeleton within acts as one force, while the supporting surface acts as the other. The smaller the bony prominence the greater the pressure exerted; it is more comfortable to lie flat on a hard surface than to sit up straight on the ischial tuberosities (Fig. 20.3).

Shear occurs when the pressure is directed at an angle to the support surface, as when a patient slides in a bed or chair. The movement of the body surface is retarded by the friction between it and the supporting surface (Fig. 20.4). This causes not only superficial grazing of the skin, but tearing and disruption deep within the tissue which may eventually break down to form a crater. The danger of shear increases when the surfaces are damp from urine or sweat, are rough, or where weight on the point of contact is increased (bedclothes pressing on feet). When tissues are damaged by pressure the ability to repair that damage depends on:

- the extent of the damage
- the body's ability to repair the damage
- the prevention of further damage.

These in turn are the very things that must be assessed as risk factors. Where the patient is ill,

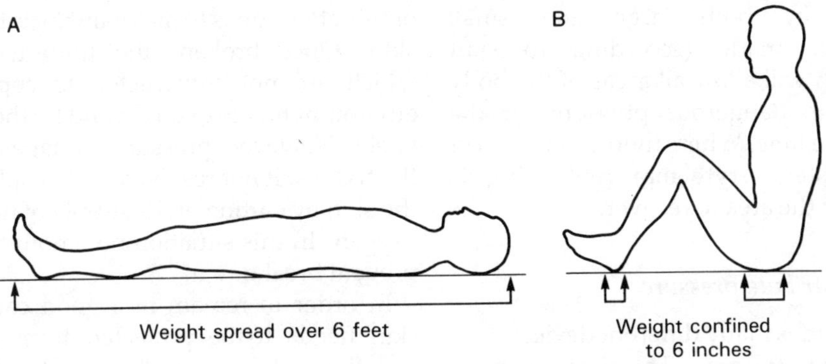

Fig.20.3 Differences in support surface according to position.

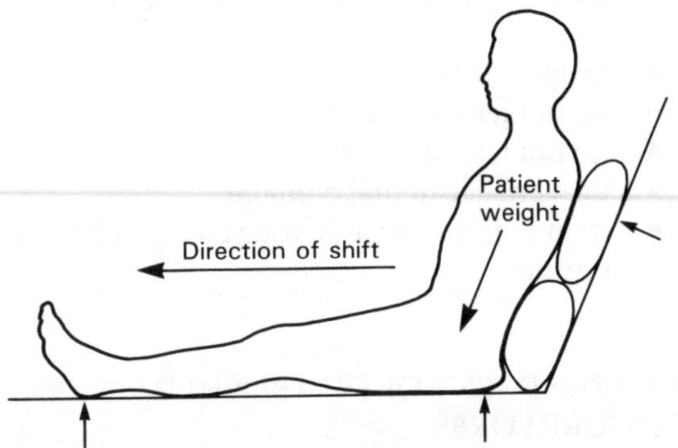

Fig. 20.4 Areas subject to damage by shearing.

immobile or incontinent, the damage will be large and the possibility of repeated damage will increase. Their illness, poor physical state, and lack of nutrition will reduce their ability to repair the damage caused. The prevention of sores, therefore, depends upon removing the cause (pressure) and reducing the risk to the patient (improving his/her status).

The relief of pressure

Pressure relief can be divided into two mechanisms:

- that which aids natural behaviour
- that which uses devices which redistribute pressure.

Aiding natural behaviour

As stated above, one of the major predisposing causes of pressure sores is the lack of movement in response to discomfort. The nurse can restore this activity either by moving the patient or by teaching the patient to move and ensuring that he/she does so. The effect of movement is to relieve pressure from one area and transfer it to another. It is therefore an activity which must continue throughout both day and night, as well as when the patient is undergoing investigations (X-ray) or being transported from one place to another. The general principles to be borne in mind when devising a routine for any patient are:

- The routine needs to be individualized, no two patients are the same.
- Low pressure can be tolerated for a longer period than high pressure (pressure is always lower when more of the body rests on the supporting surface – see Fig. 20.3).
- Damaging high pressure should not be repeated in the same area within 24 hours. To prevent this it is essential to record the position at each move and plan movements so that the patient is able to feed easily (i.e. not prone at meal times) (Lowthian, 1979b).
- The use of mechanical devices does not mean that the patient need not be moved.

With these principles in mind a plan can be devised whereby both large and small movements are made (according to staff available) which will allow all areas of the body to be subject to dangerous pressure for the shortest possible time. Where there is any sign of damage (persistent erythema) replanning is needed to allow the area to recover.

Devices to redistribute pressure

This group includes many different devices.

Beds and mattresses. The mechanism of action of special beds and mattresses is discussed by Torrance (1981) and Lowthian (1977) and it is important that the nurse should understand the principles by which these devices work and be sure that they are working properly (Bliss, 1978). Instructions should be supplied with the bed and advice is always available from the manufacturer. Beds and mattresses can be divided into three main groups, shown in Table 20.14.

Cushions. Cushions are used for patients who need to sit for long periods. These can be divided into the same groups as mattresses and beds (Table 20.15). The principles upon which they work are similar, in addition there is now a trend for bioengineers to be involved in the individual tailoring of cushions using pressure gauges to enable them to equalize pressure under the ischial tuberosities (Ferguson-Pell et al, 1980). These do not and should not include sorbo air or water rings which only improve comfort for patients who have to sit, and may even increase pressure under the ischia.

Equipment to improve the local environment. Within this group come a vast number of different devices which only marginally relieve pressure, but do protect vulnerable areas from friction, contamination by urine, or a dangerous micro-environment (hot and damp from sweat) (Table 20.16). Alone these devices cannot prevent pressure damage, but in conjunction with other devices or movement they are of great value.

Care of the skin

The skin over pressure areas has been the subject of much nursing attention; the object of this attention is to maintain the integrity of the skin. Once broken, the underlying tissues, which are not constructed to cope with the environment, are exposed and further damage is likely. However, pressure damage deep within the tissues, if not resolved, will result in death of the skin by cutting off its supply of nutrients and oxygen. In this situation no amount of care will prevent breakdown.

In order to remain in a good condition, the skin needs to be protected from maceration, irritation, the removal of natural oils, and accidental damage. Treatment therefore depends on the state in which the skin is found, rather than any routine set down for care:

- keep it clean
- do not let it remain wet
- do not let it dry out
- prevent accidental damage
- treat it as you would your face or a baby's bottom.

THE TREATMENT OF ESTABLISHED PRESSURE SORES

Much is said about, and many things are claimed to be effective treatment for, pressure sores. However, the general justification for choosing any one preparation as being of use is that it has worked in the past. In making a choice, the nurse needs to look at these preparations as chemicals which produce an action, rather than as magic potions. The choice is difficult because few studies exist which demonstrate useful actions, and the number of preparations available for use is considerable (the author has listed more than 80). The intention of this section is to discuss what action the nurse can take to encourage the healing process in pressure sores, look at what is required of the preparations used in relation to the state of the sore, and discuss the properties of some of the preparations at present in use. This, it is hoped, will give some basis for choice until more scientific information becomes available.

The nurse has to decide what she/he hopes to

Table 20.14 Examples of beds and mattresses

Action	Equipment	Manufacturer
1. Equalize pressure over the support surface	Flotation (water) bed Low air loss bed Net suspension bed Fluidized air bed (Clinitron) Roho mattress	Beaufort-Winchester Mediscus Egerton Astec Raymer
2. Spread the supporting surface	Low pressure air bed Water mattress Water bed Slit foam mattress (Clinifloat, Polyfloat)	Kellie Lotus, Lyco Western Medical Astec, Tally Medical Equipment
3. Alter the area subject to pressure	Alternating pressure beds Ripple bed Pulsair bed Rippling bed Airwave system Alternating Pressure bed	 Tally Medical Equipment Tally Medical Equipment Hawksley Dermalex Astec

Table 20.15 Examples of cushions

Action	Equipment	Manufacturer
1. Equalize pressure over the support surface	Roho cushion Specially tailored foam	Raymar Custom made in bioengineering Department Clinics
2. Spread the supporting surface	Water cushion Reston pad Nuclear foam pad Cubex (polystyrene beads) Silicone gel cushion	Western Medical, Lyco, Lotus 3M Kennick Medical Nottingham Handcraft Spenco
3. Alter the area subject to pressure	Ripple seat	Tally Medical Equipment

Table 20.16 Examples of equipment to improve the local environment

Action	Equipment	Manufacturer
1. Prevent contamination with urine	Kylie sheet	Kylie
2. Absorb moisture	Cubex bead pad Sheepskin (lamb pad) Artificial sheepskin Decipad Mullipel Silicore pads Foam pads	Nottingham Handcraft Dermalex Domex Bayer Spenco, Parkhouse, Tendercare
3. Protect bony prominences	Boots, elbow pads sheepskin (lamb pad) synthetic sheepskin (Posey) foam (QB2000) Nuclear foam pad Silicore pads	 Dermalex Martin Creasey Rehabilitation Roussel Kennick Medical Spenco

achieve by treatment. Healing is a natural process essential to survival. In the healthy individual, damage to the skin and underlying tissues will be repaired quickly, for example a surgical wound will heal in 14–21 days. The process is demanding on the body, requiring energy, nutrients, oxygen, vitamins and trace elements, all of which must be brought to the site by the circulation. During illness the same demands are made for the repair of the damage caused by disease. It is realistic therefore to believe that healing will be delayed in patients, particularly where the ability to take in or circulate the raw materials for repair is restricted. In addition, the presence locally of healthy tissue, particularly epithelial cells (Schilling, 1976) is essential. The absence of an inflammatory response to injury will delay the rejection of infective material and consequently delay healing (Ryan, 1976). The nurse's aim should therefore be to assess the sore and decide where intervention is necessary.

Intervention

Remove the cause

The essential first step to treatment is to remove the predisposing cause or causes of the pressure sore. This means taking all the measures discussed in the section on prevention above.

Remove dead tissue

Some surgeons advocate the complete debridement of pressure sores and plastic surgery as treatment for sores (Agris & Spira, 1979). This is, however, beyond the brief of nurses and will not be discussed here. The removal of dead tissue must therefore be achieved by a gradual process by which successive layers are removed during each dressing session.

Mechanically. This is achieved either by careful dissection with sharp scissors or using 'wet to dry' dressings. These dressings of gauze applied wet are allowed to dry; necrotic tissue which adheres to them is then removed with the dressing. Hydrogen peroxide is sometimes advocated in the undercut wound or sinus, dislodging and washing out debris by its effervescent action. New osmotic agents such as Debrisan draw damp or liquid debris away from the wound surface by capillary action (McClemont et al, 1979).

Proteolytic enzyme preparations (Varidase, Santyl, Collagenase). These have been demonstrated as being useful in denaturing necrotic tissue. Again action is only at the surface and application needs to be repeated over a period of time to achieve complete debridement. Where the slough is hard it will need careful scoring or injection to allow penetration; here it is best to obtain medical assistance.

Softening agents. Agents of many descriptions have traditionally been used, these range from antiseptics to oils and many combinations of chemicals. These are time-honoured but generally untested.

Remove pathogenic organisms

Pressure sores are chronically contaminated wounds. Any swab taken will grow many types of bacteria. The best guides to pathogenic infection are the smell and appearance of the sore; where these are apparent a swab should be taken to identify the pathogen so that the appropriate antibiotic can be employed. Until recently the penetration of systemic antibiotics into the wound area was doubted. However, clindamycin has been measured in adequate concentrations in the wound exudate (Berger et al, 1978). It is hoped that other relevant antibiotics will be similarly tested in the future. In infection frequent dressings with the removal of contaminated material are needed. However, the over-zealous use of bactericidal agents in wounds should be avoided as they may be detrimental to healing (Agris & Spira, 1979).

Provide an environment in which healing can progress

These measures are those which the nurse can employ to rectify delay and allow the natural process of healing to progress uninhibited. The extent to which any application made locally can enhance healing is debatable, indeed it is just as likely that repeated intervention may in fact delay healing. Local requirements are for oxygen, nutrients and moisture. The extent to which these can be beneficially applied to the sore are discussed briefly.

Oxygen. There is some evidence (Torelli, 1973) that oxygen directed at the damaged area is absorbed and that a lack of oxygen will inhibit the activity of fibroblasts. It is probable that absorption only occurs to any appreciable extent when oxygen is applied at above atmospheric (hyperbaric) pressure. The difficulty with the application of oxygen is that it will cause drying of the tissue, a property for which it is often employed but which is detrimental to healing.

Nutrients. Locally applied nutrients have not been demonstrated to be of value, although some nurses do still consider the possibility of feeding the sore. The raw materials for body building are the products of digestive breakdown, foodstuffs as we know them are therefore obviously useless. However, experiments are being made with amino acid solutions infused into deep craters and this does appear to have some effect (Calver & Stanley, 1980). In the absence of any real evidence it is best to use foods as they are intended and give nutritious supplements to the patient to eat.

Moisture. Although wet wounds have been generally considered to be dangerous, the idea of protecting the wound surface with a semi-occlusive dressing is not new. In the past gold leaf has been used (Williams & Hysick, 1974) and more recently synthetic skins (OpSite, Synthaderm) and treated animal skin (porcine dermis) have been used. It has been shown (Winter, 1976) that in a moist environment, epithelial growth is faster than under a dry scab. This also allows for the free movement of macrophages in bacterial surveillance. It is logical to extrapolate from this that a moist environment will be beneficial to the regrowth of any tissue, as in a culture where the cells are bathed in a nutritious medium. Infection could be a problem if pathogens were contained in the medium. Because disruption of the occlusive dressing causes damage, sterile aspiration of the wound fluid for laboratory examination should be performed if infection is suspected, rather than prematurely removing the dressing.

Having decided what, if any, intervention is required to enable the healing process to proceed, patience is necessary. Progress will be slow. Encouragement can be gained by keeping records of the sore assessments, grade, size and state, at regular intervals of about one week. When keeping such records it must be appreciated that the progress will not always consist of the sore getting smaller. The early appearance of any sore is generally much less extensive than the damage incurred. As dead tissue is removed the full extent will be revealed; only then can healing commence. As yet there is no answer to the many questions associated with pressure sore treatment. This does not mean that the nurse should be contented to continue in the use of the traditional methods without question. Rather she/he should make use of the scientific knowledge available to assess both sore and preparation before deciding what to use.

THE CARE OF THE INDIVIDUAL WITH A LEG ULCER

THE LEG ULCER AS A WOUND

A wound may be defined as a disruption of tissue continuity with or without opening of the skin (Chelgren, 1979). There are essentially two types of wound, those which do not involve tissue loss and those which do (Westaby, 1981a) and the leg ulcer falls into the second of these categories. Wounds which involve tissue loss may result from surgical and traumatic intervention or, as in the case of leg ulcers, because the individual lacks the ability to recover tissue vitality for a variety of reasons. Marks (1985) states that the healing of wounds of skin represent a complex series of interrelated events in the various tissue components of that organ. Healing of such wounds starts soon after the wounding stimulus, unfolds in a regular and orderly manner and stops after restoration of structure and function.

Before discussing the methods by which nursing intervention may support a person with a leg ulcer due to impaired healing ability, it will be necessary briefly to review the process of wound healing and the factors necessary for its completion. It will then be possible to identify the factors underlying the development of leg ulcers which are characteristically persistent and slow to heal and, even when improving, may break down again suddenly (Hazarika & Wright, 1981).

The wound repair process

Wound repair is a continuous process, but for ease of description may be described as including four stages of healing (Westaby, 1981b).

Traumatic inflammation

This commences at the time of wounding and may last for as long as three days. It involves a localized inflammatory response which is not due to infection but is the body's defence mechanism and results in the formation of a clot (later a scab) which affects temporary closure of the skin.

The destructive phase

This occurs between the first and sixth day following wounding. The polymorphonuclear leucocytes and macrophages which invaded the wound during phase one clean the wound by engulfing and ingesting devitalized and unwanted tissue. Macrophages are probably the key cells in the initiation and maintenance of connective tissue repair, and interact with a very wide range of other cells such as fibroblasts and endothelium. They are also the primary agents in debridement. The process is primarily oxygen dependent.

The proliferative phase

This occurs between the third and twenty-fourth days. The fibroblasts promote collagen and capillary formation known as angiogenesis which is dependent on a critical oxygen gradient easily disturbed by vascular insufficiency (Silver, 1985). Collagen is the principal structural protein of the body and the main constituent of skin, tendons, ligaments and bones, cartilage, fascia and scar tissue. Collagen synthesis depends to a critical degree on the vascularity and the degree of perfusion by the circulatory system; fibroblasts require nutrients to produce collagen, the most prominent being vitamin C, without which collagen synthesis is inhibited and tissue breakdown continues. It is also well established that fibroblasts are aerobic cells and require oxygenation for collagen synthesis (Pikkareinen & Kulonen, 1973). The considerable cellular and chemical activity during this phase results in the formation of new capillary loops supported on a fragile framework of collagen fibres — known as granulation tissue.

The maturation phase

This is the stage of contraction and epithelialization — the final tissue reorganization which may last up to a year. Contraction is the process by which open wounds are facilitated in healing by specialist cells at the wound edges, the myofibroblasts, which provide the motive force of contraction. Myofibroblasts have attributes of both the fibroblast and smooth muscle cells, and together with epithelialization cause the free wound edges to come together. This process of contraction does not occur in wounds of the lower leg that are fixed closely to the tibia (Westaby, 1981c). Epithelialization is the process by which the outer covering of the skin, the squamous epithelial cells, migrate over live granulation tissue to complete skin closure. These cells will burrow beneath the debris of clot and scab formation in their efforts to seal the invasion to skin integrity. In wounds with tissue loss the protective influence of a scab (or surgical dressing) prevents physical trauma, drying, haemorrhage and contact with foreign materials while the delicate epithelial cells cut their path over the viable granulation tissue beneath. However, successful epithelialization cannot occur in the presence of infection or absence of adequate oxygenation, which in turn depends on a good blood supply to the area.

Epidermal cell movement is an energy dependent process and cells near the wound edge accumulate glycogen stores before they start moving from their site of attachment on the basement membrane. The glycogen disappears during mitosis and migration, and the amount of energy derived from it is directly dependent on oxygen availability (Silver, 1985). Epidermal healing is accelerated when a wound surface is moist but relatively free of exudate; where exudate is present it is frequently contaminated by bacteria which are oxygen-consuming (Silver, 1985) and in such circumstances the oxygen supply to the epidermis (and the granulation tissue) must be derived almost exclusively from the underlying circulation.

Requirements for wound healing

From the foregoing resumé of the normal wound healing process, it is clear that there are two major requirements if wounds are to heal — first a healthy circulation and secondly the nutritional state of the individual, of which the first is the most important fact, as clearly it matters little how well nourished the patient is if essential factors cannot reach the wound because of impaired vascularity. White (1982) has demonstrated that vascular insufficiency, from whatever cause, inevitably results in infected lesions, especially in the lower limbs.

Nutritional requirements

The importance of diet cannot be ignored, and Westaby (1981c) highlights the need for adequate protein and vitamins A and C in the diet for collagen formation, and also the presence of the trace elements zinc and copper. The absence of one or all of these factors will retard healing. Conditions which are particularly associated with the predisposition to a poor nutritional state are:

- inadequate food intake for social/financial reasons
- malignancy
- protein losing enteropathy
- hepatic failure
- inflammatory bowel disease
- renal failure
- autoimmune disorders
- chronic infection
- diabetes
- drug therapy:
  steroids (fibroblast suppression);
  cytotoxic drugs (cell proliferation suppression).

In turn, these factors may result in the individual's decreased resistance to infection, both endogenous and exogenous. Stephenson (1984) in a small study of three individuals relates nutritional needs to the healing of leg ulcers. The importance of a high fibre/low fat diet should also be recognized as persons with ulceration of the limb, with or without nutritional disorders, will have vascular insufficiency. The relationship between high fat/low fibre diets and disease of the circulatory system is well known and Cornwall & Lewis (1983) have demonstrated the high incidence of arterial involvement in leg ulcers, even those considered to be primarily venous in origin.

CIRCULATION RELATED TO LEG ULCERS

While the aetiology of leg ulcers is multifactorial, malfunctioning of the circulatory system is the underlying cause. Two evolutionary influences are involved. Seville & Martin (1981) note that the human race has been at risk of circulatory impairment of the lower limbs since adopting the upright position, thus increasing the venous pressure in the lower limbs and rendering 0.5% of the British population at risk of developing leg ulceration. Camp (1977) and Kaisary (1982) claim that venous insufficiency is the cause of between 85–95% of all causes of leg ulceration, but it is necessary to be aware of the other likely possibilities in order that the correct treatment be given in individual cases. Kaisary (1982) and Cornwall (1985a) agree on the list of other predisposing factors in Table 20.17. Heredity has been suggested as a major predisposing factor

Table 20.17 Predisposing factors in the development of ulceration of the lower limb

Venous disease
Arterial disease
Trauma
Infection
Other systemic diseases (e.g. rheumatoid arthritis, diabetes)
Neoplasia
Factitious (self-mutilation)

(Wright, 1982; Seville & Martin, 1981) in that some patients can recall a relative who has also had leg ulcers, indicating that a proportion of individuals may be genetically predisposed to impairment of the venous and arterial blood circulation.

Venous disease

A knowledge of the anatomy of the veins of the leg is important in understanding venous leg ulcers. The veins of the leg are divided into three main systems:

- the superficial veins
- the deep veins
- the perforating veins.

Venous blood drains from the superficial system (long and short saphenous veins and tributaries) through the deep fascia via the perforating veins to the deep veins (anterior tibial, posterior tibial and peroneal) which in turn drain into the deep femoral vein and vena cava. Valves throughout the system ensure one way flow, and this is especially important in the perforators. The number and location of the valves are a genetic variable.

The return of blood to the heart is assisted by the muscular action of the calf supported by the tight fibrous fascia of the leg. Any damage to the valves in the system (as a result of thrombophlebitis, DVT, thickening with age or congenital absence) results in an increase of hydrostatic pressure resulting in leakage of fluid into the tissues and the development of oedema. In turn the pressure of oedema fluid disturbs the circulation, impairing the blood supply to the tissues resulting in tissue death which triggers the body's wound repair mechanism.

The onset of oedema is usually insidious, appearing first after long periods of standing and during periods of warmer weather. If the oedema is allowed to persist, the leakage of red blood cells into the tissue with the oedema fluid will result in the development of varicose eczema. The clinical manifestation is superseded by a diffuse area of redness (inflammatory phase) and a brown pigmentation resulting from the destruction of the red cells by macrophage activity (the destructive phase of the wound repair process) and the release of haemosiderin. The staining is darker in men and becomes calcified over time to give the characteristic elephant hide appearance. Minor trauma (a knock, or scratching of the eczema) may then produce an ulcer, which as a result of poor circulation remains in the destructive phase, growing larger and predisposed to infection which in turn causes pain and immobility.

The resultant loss of calf muscle pump action reinforces the circulatory inactivity in the area thus exacerbating the condition.

The elderly person, who may already be incapacitated and immobile as a result of normal ageing with or without arthritis, paralysis, congestive cardiac failure, or tumours of the pelvis, all of which further impair venous return to the heart, is clearly at greater risk of developing venous ulcers. Dale et al (1983a) estimated that while chronic leg ulcers occur in 8 per thousand of the total population of Scotland, there is an incidence of 36 per thousand in those over the age of 65.

Arterial disease

Arterial ulcers are caused by occlusion of large and small vessels resulting in ischaemia of the surrounding tissues. Large vessel occlusion is a medical emergency — characterized by sudden pain, pallor, pulselessness, coolness — and is frequently the culmination of chronically progressive intermittent claudication (Cobey & Cobey, 1974).

The intermittent claudication characteristic of large vessel atherosclerosis is usually found in conjunction with small vessel arterial disease

Table 20.18 Clinical factors to consider when assessing leg ulcers

Feature	Venous	Arterial
Site	Commonly commences on the medial aspect of leg or above the malleolus	Commonly on the toes, side and sole of the foot (as in diabetes), and the lateral aspect of the leg over and around the malleolus
Size	May be large and shallow, very moist	Small and deep and dry
Duration	Progresses slowly	Progresses rapidly
Skin appearance	Reddish brown staining Irritable eczema	White when elevated Bright red or bluish (or a mixture) on dependency
	Warm to touch Oedema	Cold to touch Wasting, skin and tissue atrophy, thickened nails
Pain	Not painful except when oedema severe and in the presence of infection when the pain is intermittent	Extremely painful/unremitting, especially on exercise, elevation at night, and when warm
Sleep	Little disturbance	Frequent disturbance due to pain
Foot pulses	Present (if oedema minimal)	Absent

which is the chronic occlusion of small arteries and arterioles — it is most frequently seen as a long-term complication in individuals with diabetes.

The clinical manifestations are a pale cool leg with loss of hair and atrophy of the skin. Any pressure will further diminish the incompetent circulation with the result that an arterial ulcer frequently occurs on the feet where even slight pressure from contact with a shoe has acted as a trigger.

Diagnosis

Cornwall (1985b) highlights the importance of differentiating between arterial and venous ulcers prior to implementation of treatment, and the necessity for assessment of arterial circulation using continuous wave ultrasound where the diagnosis is in doubt. Venous circulation may also be assessed using continuous wave ultrasound photoplethysmography. Differential diagnosis between a venous and arterial ulcer (Table 20.18) is straightforward, but the difficulty arises when there is both venous and arterial involvement and the plethora of symptoms confuses the issue. The importance of the nurse's observations cannot be over-emphasized, as she/he is likely to spend more time with the affected individual than the doctor, who may diagnose one variety or the other as a result of one consultation. It may then fall to the nurse to act as the person's advocate in reporting the observations made during continuous assessment. It is especially important to remember that anyone reporting sleeplessness due to pain and the need to hang the limb over the side of the bed at night to gain relief almost certainly has some arterial involvement, however varicose the initial appearance may be. It is equally important to remember that individuals with diabetes and associated neuropathy may not report pain or sleep disturbance until the limb is pre-gangrenous. The Harrow Study (Cornwall & Lewis, 1983) found a surprisingly high number of ulcers associated with an ischaemic element, the majority of which were being treated as venous in origin. This reinforces the importance of the need for accurate assessment prior to the commencement of treatment.

Assessment

It has been demonstrated that the majority

of day to day management of the ulcerated limb is performed by the district nurse (Cornwall & Lewis, 1983). Dale (1984) found that 87% of people with leg ulceration were reported from community services and 13% from hospitals. 50% of those in hospitals were in long-stay wards.

The nursing assessment of the person with a leg ulcer will nevertheless involve the same principles regardless of whether a hospital-based nurse or a district nursing colleague carries it out. Assessment involves the formation of the relationship between the nurse and patient and the conscious gathering of information to be weighed against existing knowledge. The purpose of the assessment is to make a diagnosis about the needs of the patient, who in this instance will have a leg ulcer, in his or her unique circumstances.

A chronic leg ulcer has been defined as 'an open sore below the knee, anywhere on the leg or foot which takes more than 6 weeks to heal' (Dale et al, 1983a). In a later work Dale (1984) found that 40% of a sample of 600 patients with leg ulcers were between the ages of 50 and 70 years and of these, the female/male ratio was 3.26:1. 53% of the sample were over 70 years old when the sex ratio rose to 3.68:1. Clearly, these facts need to be borne in mind when the nurse is assessing a patient with a leg ulcer. She/he will need to draw on her/his knowledge of psychosocial development and expectations of the elderly person as well as their particular health needs. The nurse may choose to use a specific model for nursing or other framework for gathering information. Factors to be considered in the general nursing assessment are to be found in Table 20.19.

Following general assessment of the individual, specific assessment of the ulcerated limb will be made. The condition of the legs should be noted, with particular reference to the presence or absence of oedema, eczema and skin pigmentation, pallor, hairlessness, and skin atrophy. The shape and severity of the ulcer should also be assessed. A diagram can be made by placing a thin polythene bag onto the ulcer and gently tracing the outline with a felt pen. The soiled underside of the bag is then discarded, which enables the tracing to be used for evaluating future progress of the ulcer. Alternatively, a photographic record may be kept.

Table 20.19 Particular factors to note when making the general assessment

Influencing factors:
- Age
- Sex
- Height
- Weight
- The number of pregnancies in women (? silent DVT)

Past history of surgery (? silent DVT)

Ability of individual to communicate and express feelings

Physical health
- Absence/presence of disease, especially diabetes, rheumatoid arthritis or allergies
- Presence or absence of pain and stiffness

Ability to care for self
- Shop
- Cook
- Move about

Social conditions and general lifestyle

Knowledge and understanding of own condition
Feelings about the leg ulcer, and expectations of healing
Desire or otherwise for nursing intervention

Time of onset of ulcer, previous treatments and their results

Sleep patterns — does leg pain awaken at night?

Smoking habits

Urinalysis to detect diabetes and recording of blood pressure to detect hypertension will have formed part of the routine general assessment. The collection of a wound swab for culture may also be necessary when there is a suggestion of either local or spreading infection. Routine blood tests may also be indicated if anaemia or vitamin deficiency is suspected.

If there is doubt about the exact diagnosis, specialized studies with the continuous wave ultrasound and photoplethysmography will also be necessary (Cornwall, 1985c). From this assessment the exact nature of the type of leg ulcer will be determined and a care plan for the particular individual in his/her unique circumstances formulated.

NURSING MANAGEMENT OF LEG ULCERS — GENERAL DISCUSSION

The treatment of leg ulcers should be the result of a team approach involving the patient and his family, the nursing team and the doctor. Members of the wider care team may also be involved, e.g. the physiotherapist, occupational therapist and social worker. It is essential that the person with the leg ulcer should understand the rationale for treatment if any success is to be achieved. The aim of ulcer management may be to heal the ulcer, but must always be realistic. It has been reported that, of the individuals with leg ulcers surveyed, 55% had had open ulcers for more than 6 months, 40% for more than one year and 10% for more than 6 years. One patient had had his ulcer for 42 years (Dale, 1984). In the latter instance it might be unrealizable for the nurse to aim to heal the ulcer as part of the management programme, and in such circumstances a more appropriate aim might be to improve the quality of life, and return the individual to independence and self-caring as soon as possible.

However, Cornwall (1985a) demonstrated that, in the absence of ischaemia, ambulatory compression therapy healed 80% of leg ulcers with deep vein damage in eleven weeks and 90% with superficial vein damage in 10 weeks of commencement of treatment, following accurate diagnosis. The ulcers that failed to heal were those with ischaemic involvement and where the degree of severity was such as to render the individual immobile with fixed ankle joints and muscle wasting. It is worth noting here that the incidence of squamous cell carcinoma and basal cell carcinoma in venous and ischaemic leg ulcers of long standing may be a complicating factor (Ackroyd & Young, 1983) and it is recommended that any ulcer on the lower leg that fails to heal within four months be biopsied to exclude malignancy.

Venous ulcers

Management of the limb with a venous ulcer will involve:

- eliminating oedema and improving venous drainage
- restoring the action of the venous pump function of the leg muscle and the flexibility of the legs (exercise)
- controlling the micro-environment of the wound to promote optimum wound healing.

Eliminating oedema and improving venous drainage

It has been claimed that all purely venous ulcers will heal when the individual is prescribed a course of bedrest, however they may recur as soon as ambulatory activities are resumed (Kaisary, 1982). Raising the foot of the bed is an effective method of draining the limb providing the patient does not have congestive heart failure, in which case the ulcer may heal but the individual may be considerably more ill as a result. Advice to drain the limb by resting with the legs elevated at an angle of 45° will be useful for those individuals with leg ulcers who may be fit enough to achieve this, but for the remainder ambulatory treatment should be advocated with compression bandaging to control oedema and aid venous return. Compression must be applied evenly from the base of the toes to below the knee with the greatest pressure aimed at the ankle, graduating to a lower pressure at the calf. This graduated compression may be achieved using roller bandages or the tubular variety or a combination of the two. Where impregnated paste bandages are used to improve the micro-environment these will form part of the compression agent. Dale et al (1983b) revealed that bandages lose much of their compression in a relatively short time, especially after washing; indeed a single washing reduced the pressures attained by a cotton stretch bandage by 20%. Bandages that slip and wrinkle not only fail to achieve compression, they also indent the skin with resultant tourniquet action, leading to further oedema, impairment of the circulation and worsening ulceration. Fox (1983) advocates the irregular application of the bandage to prevent slippage and the use of a combination of roller and tubular bandages for optimum compression.

Schraibman et al (1982) in comparing the

available elastic supports of the lower limb found that the best results were to be obtained when using Elset roller bandaging and shaped support bandaging together. Cornwall (1985d) suggests using either shaped support bandage over roller bandaging — in which case two layers are required — or the use of support stockings over roller bandaging. Straight tubular bandage may be used (as a double layer over roller bandaging) but will not compress to the shape of the leg as effectively as the shaped variety. Cornwall reinforces Dale's findings and claims that the tubular bandaging should be renewed every 3–4 weeks if sufficient elasticity is to be maintained.

While correctly fitting support stockings provide the optimum pressure gradients (Cornwall, 1985d) they are also the most difficult compression to apply, requiring considerable agility and physical strength — precisely the attributes likely to be lacking in the ageing and/or diseased person. The nurse and leg ulcer sufferer must appraise the available options when planning the application of pressure, and together arrive at a mutually agreeable solution. Where there is no arterial involvement, all compression layers may remain in situ overnight, but some individuals find this intolerable in which case removal of the tubular layers is acceptable, but they should be replaced prior to getting up in the morning. Availability of carers to assist in this activity, where necessary, will be another individual variable to be considered when the affected person is living at home. If necessary the doctor will prescribe diuretics to assist in eliminating oedema, but these are not a substitute for compression, merely an adjunct.

Exercise

Exercise of the leg muscles is another important feature in the promotion of limb drainage. Walking 2–3 miles a day is advocated, and standing should be positively discouraged, but for many people walking this distance is not possible due to age, disease, or the severity of the ulcer. In this case foot and toe exercises — to be carried out while sitting — will greatly improve venous return and prevent the ankle joint from becoming fixed.

Other factors affecting venous return from the limb to be considered when planning care, and upon which the nurse can have a positive influence, are the wearing of tight clothing or garters, the occurrence of constipation, or a propensity to sit with the legs crossed. The presence of obesity may also hinder venous return and increase immobility.

Microenvironment of the wound

The dressing. Earlier in this chapter a brief examination of wound healing indicated the optimum micro-environment necessary for wound healing. The management of the ulcer should neither retard nor inhibit the process. There are two factors involved in wound management — the dressing and the cleansing agent. Turner (1985) lists general performance parameters which a dressing must possess if the optimum micro-environment is to be produced.

The optimum dressing should:

- remove excess exudate and toxic components
- maintain high humidity at wound/dressing interface
- allow gaseous exchange
- provide thermal insulation
- afford protection from secondary infection
- be free from particulate and toxic contaminants
- allow removal without trauma (to granulation tissue and surrounding skin) at dressing change.

An infinite variety of dressings is available for care of leg ulcers, some of which fulfil these criteria more effectively than others. The traditional gauze squares, sleeve dressing pads and multilayered pads are effective in providing varying degrees of absorbency (Turner & Coombs, 1982), but are no barrier to infection, cause trauma on removal and are poor insulators. Modern developments such as the addition of non-adherent layers or semi-permeable adhesive backing have improved this type of dressing marginally, but they are inferior in comparison with the modern occlusive dressings. Eaglstein (1985) states that occlusive dressings allow moist wound healing by:

- spreading epithelialization
- inducing granulation tissue in chronic wounds
- reducing pain.

Semi-permeable films (e.g. OpSite), polymeric materials (e.g. Debrisan), hydrogels (e.g. Scherisorb) and occlusive hydrocolloids (e.g. Granuflex) have particular application to the various stages of wound healing.

The semi-permeable, transparent, auto-adhesive polyurethane film such as OpSite, simulates lost epithelium, is permeable to water vapour and air and impermeable to bacteria, particulate matter and water. It encourages rapid epithelialization and rapid increase in vascular supply, and is useful in the management of shallow, clean leg ulcers.

Polymeric materials, such as Debrisan, are hydrophilic, spherical beads with an absorption capacity of four to five times its own weight. In the absorption of this liquid a gel is produced. The osmotic gradient which occurs reduces inflammation, oedema and bacterial contamination. Its basic property is one of debridement and once granulation commences its use should be discontinued.

The semi-permeable hydrogels such as Scherisorb, Vigilon and Geliperm are described by Turner (1985) as combining the properties of the films and polymeric materials, but are contraindicated where anaerobic infection is suspected and may support the growth of microorganisms.

The occlusive hydrocolloids, such as Granuflex and Comfeel, combine hydrogels with elastomeric and adhesive components and are available as an adhesive sheet with waterproof backing and as granules. The hydrogels swell in a linear fashion expanding into the cavity of the wound, resulting in their recommended use in the management of venous ulcers. The compression produced by the expansion of the hydrocolloid between the wound floor and the outer waterproof layer is an added benefit. In the presence of excess wound exudate, however, the absorption ability of the hydrocolloid is rapidly exceeded, necessitating frequent change of the dressing — sometimes more than once a day — and in these circumstances an unpleasant smell often accompanies the excess exudate and hydrocolloid mixture (Stevanovic, 1985). As Silver (1985) states, it is important to appreciate that whatever the properties of an occlusive dressing, its oxygen permeability is likely to have little influence at the wound surface unless that surface is kept relatively free of exudate. In the selection of an appropriate dressing, the nurse and doctor will have to decide when a desirable moist area becomes excessively swamped with exudate. Paste bandages are useful for all types of venous ulcers (Harkiss, 1985) as they are soothing and protect the eczematous skin. As has already been noted, their contribution to the compression ratio is considerable. However, sensitization may occur (Gawkrodger, 1984) and bandages may set hard on some patients, limiting patient comfort and mobility. The nurse should consider it part of the duty of care to patch test paste bandages prior to applying them for the first time to the whole leg, lest an allergic/intolerant reaction occur. The use of compound dressings containing charcoal (Actisorb) have no therapeutic properties, but absorb offensive exudate resulting in reduction/elimination of wound odour, which is of immense comfort to the individual.

The increasing evidence is that in selected use the modern occlusive dressings can heal persistent ulcers by promoting epithelialization and granulation tissue, and also result in a marked reduction in the incidence of allergenic sensitivity reactions.

The cleaning agent. Antiseptics are used routinely by hospital and community nurses to debride and disinfect chronic ulcers (Stewart et al, 1985) but there is some evidence to suggest that antiseptics may have toxic effects on healing tissues and may delay the healing process (Harkiss, 1985). Far from there being any evidence to suggest that ulcer surface cleaning enhances healing, Eriksson (1985) demonstrates that the presence of bacteria in ulcers was not found to influence the healing process. Leaper (1984) supports this view and shows that superficial infection, other than with pseudomonal organisms, does not significantly delay healing. In a survey into the use of cleansing agents when managing chronic lower limb ulceration, Stewart et al (1985) found the substances most commonly used were:

- normal saline
- Eusol and paraffin
- Savlodil
- Betadine, and
- hydrogen peroxide

of which normal saline was the only innocuous substance. The others were at best ineffective and at worst harmful to granulation tissue (hydrogen peroxide), hyperallergenic (Betadine) or with detrimental systemic effects (uraemia associated with long-term use of Eusol).

This evidence suggests that irrigation of the ulcer with normal saline prior to applying the dressing of choice is to be advocated. Where a debriding agent is necessary, an appropriate dressing (Debrisan) is indicated rather than the use of corrosive antiseptics. As swabbing can damage granulation tissue, irrigation is to be preferred.

Ischaemic ulcers

Ulcers associated with ischaemia due to arterial disease, either in isolation or in combination with venous disease, are more difficult to manage.

Intermittent claudication, painful cold extremities and atrophied limb tissues may accompany the ulcerated area which has developed as a result of ischaemia. Conservative management of the micro-environment will not differ from that outlined for venous ulcers, occlusive hydrocolloid having been found to be particularly suitable in certain trials (Stevanovic, 1985). Compression bandaging has no place in the management of ischaemic ulcers, and where a combination of venous and ischaemic factors are involved it is crucial that the ischaemic element is identified, because compression of any sort rapidly causes deterioration. Dressings may be held in place with a loosely applied bandage, but in the case of Granuflex no such fixative will be necessary. The use of compression during the day may be advocated where the venous element predominates (Cornwall, 1985d) but only after careful assessment, investigation and expert advice.

Arteriography and continuous wave ultrasound may indicate the need for arterial reconstruction. Regrettably, such reconstruction may be impossible or may merely provide temporary respite, and eventually amputation of the limb becomes inevitable. Every year approximately 5000 new individuals are referred to DHSS artificial limb and appliance centres following amputation of the lower limb. Of these, 70% are over the age of 60 years and 70% have lost their legs due to ischaemic disease, with or without diabetes (DHSS, 1980).

A painful ischaemic limb restricts mobility. If the individual has been immobile, diffuse muscle atrophy and restricted movement at the synovial joints may be present, resulting in dependence on others to perform and assist with activities of daily living. In addition, prolonged pain and anxiety lead to:

- depression
- debilitation
- anorexia
- sleep disturbance.

All these problems may be identified in a nursing assessment. Relief of pain, maintenance and improvement of circulation to the limb by wearing light layers of clothing (e.g. several soft, loose, woollen leg warmers), improved sleep patterns and relief of anxiety are all within the province of the caring team. Time should be given to allow for expression of fear and anxieties. Individuals with diabetes may know of family members and friends with the condition in whom the development of an ischaemic ulcer led to the loss of a limb soon afterwards. The district nurse in particular will be in a position to form a relationship of trust with the individual in order that she/he may be helped to make the decision to have the limb removed should it become necessary.

HEALTH PROMOTION

Individuals with leg ulcers of whatever cause, those identified as being at risk of developing

Table 20.20 Guidelines for foot care

Wash and dry the feet daily. Do not rub fiercely or use excessive amounts of powder.
Ischaemic feet are prone to fungal infections with rapid progression to cellulitis. Placing a thin layer of absorbent cotton wool between the toes will help this — but care should be taken not to use too thick a layer, thus constricting an already precarious circulation.
Any lesion or discolouration should be reported to the doctor or nurse immediately.
Professional chiropody should be sought for nail cutting.
Shoes should not have tight laces, should be large enough to avoid pressure, and where possible should be removed several times a day and pairs alternated to prevent them becoming damp.
Removal of shoes while lying or sitting down is acceptable, but going barefoot is to be avoided if the risk of trauma is to be minimized.
Feet should be kept warm, with several light loose layers of cotton/woollen socks and stockings. Woollen leg warmers are especially useful. Synthetic fibres are less warming and promote perspiration.

them and those whose ulcers have healed will all benefit from information about health maximizing behaviour. Poor circulation can be improved by encouraging as much exercise as possible, if only the regular performance of the ankle and toe exercises already described. Family members can be involved in group exercises, and health education initiatives at day centres, residential homes, and wherever groups meet together can do much to encourage the taking of regular, moderate but effective exercise which will improve not only the individual's circulation but also his/her sense of control over his/her own destiny and self esteem.

An imaginative nurse may devise games, pictures or charts to promote suitable exercise in individual cases, and modify them in accordance with the varying sociocultural backgrounds of the person. A similar strategy may be employed when promoting healthier dietary habits, encouraging the individual to stop smoking, and in foot care.

For people with ischaemic peripheral vascular disease, with or without the presence of ulcers, regular foot care is vital. If possible the person should wash and inspect his/her own feet daily, but if immobility and/or eyesight are problems a relative or other carer may help. Guidelines for footcare are shown in Table 20.20.

Psychological aspects

Nursing management of an individual with leg ulcers must involve careful psycho-social assessment and aim to maximize self-care and autonomy and encourage normal living. The tendency to adopt the sick role in individuals with long standing leg ulcers has been reported (Seville & Martin, 1981). This is understandable, as for some the self-perception is of being chronically sick and disabled.

Impairment has been defined as 'having a defective limb or organ', while handicap is 'the disadvantage or restriction of activity' and disablement 'the loss or reduction of functional ability' (Harris, 1977). Disease, disorder or injury lead to physical impairment, functional limitation and activity restriction and, as a result of a change in self-perception of the individual involved and the behaviour of others towards him/her, social handicap may result. Such social handicap is observable in people with chronic leg ulcers.

The fact that some people have leg ulcers for a long period of time, enduring many forms of treatment with only variable success, has already been highlighted (Dale, 1984). Such people have low levels of energy, pain, sleeplessness and limitations of physical mobility. Many are housebound, are unable to use the stairs or stand for any length of time, are limited in their ability to carry out household tasks and endure curtailment of social life, holidays, hobbies and interests (Hunt et al, 1982).

Another study (Moody, 1984) highlighted the social isolation in an individual case where the continued presence of painful leg ulcers resulted in a woman becoming immobile and isolated, not least because of the offensive smell from the constantly damp bandages and resultant loss of self-esteem. Even with daily or twice daily dressing changes and the use of mild diuretics and compression bandaging, the almost constant presence of damp bandages can, in the author's experience, be a most distressing factor for people with large, chronic venous ulceration. The result may lead to the individual having a sense of powerlessness.

A study of seven patients with long standing leg ulcers (Smith, 1982) resulted in the following psycho-social problems being identified at nursing assessment:

- low morale owing to the prolonged duration of the ulcer and the loss of the left leg owing to ulceration
- lack of self-care due to lack of understanding of condition
- poor emotional state owing to prolonged ulceration and associated pain
- boredom and loneliness because of debilitating condition and being housebound
- inability to perform self-care due to prolonged debilitating condition
- poor emotional state caused by prolonged ulceration and associated pain
- boredom and loneliness because of debilitating condition and being housebound
- inability to perform self-care due to prolonged debilitating condition
- poor emotional state caused by prolonged period of leg ulceration.

In each case, management was carefully planned and was aimed at involving the individual and his/her spouse in care.

Each was encouraged to learn to care for the ulcer him/herself, and to learn the rationale for the treatment chosen. Attention was paid to improved exercise/rest routines, diet and smoking habits and foot care and hygiene. Encouragement was given to socializing outside the home and taking responsibility for decision making. Even where the individual had already lost one limb due to ulceration, improvement was demonstrated after 6 months and four out of seven of the ulcers had healed. More importantly the seven individuals had assumed responsibility for their own care which resulted in a greater feeling of control of their own lives.

CONCLUSION

This section has examined the nature of leg ulcers in relation to wound healing, the causes and specific nursing management. It has also explored the psycho-social aspects of caring for a person with a chronic leg ulcer and the preventative and health educative roles of the nurse in caring for individuals with this condition.

REFERENCES

Abramovich F E 1979 A study of some ophthalmic patients' knowledge and understanding of the information given concerning the disease. Unpublished thesis, University of Manchester

Ackroyd J S, Young A E 1983 Leg ulcers that do not heal. British Medical Journal 286:207–208

Agris J, Spira M 1979 Pressure ulcers: prevention and treatment. Ciba Clinical Symposia 31(5)

Andreasen N J C, Norris A S, Hartford C E 1971 Incidence of long–term psychiatric complications in severely burned adults. Annals of Surgery 174(5):785–793

Andreasen N J C, Noyes R, Hartford C E 1972 Factors influencing adjustment of burn patients during hospitalization. Psychosomatic Medicine 34(6):517–525

Artz C P, Moncrief J A, Pruitt B A 1979 Burns — a team approach. W B Saunders, Philadelphia

Barbenel J C, Jordon M M, Nicol S M, Clark M O 1977 Incidence of pressure sores in the Greater Glasgow Health Board Area. Lancet 2:548–550

Bates B 1974 A guide to physical examination. J B Lippincott, Philadelphia

Baum M, Jones G M 1979 Counselling removes patient's fears. Nursing Mirror 148(10):38–40

Berbeu V J 1973 Skin rashes: recognition and management. Nursing (Horsham) 73(3):44–49

Berger S A, Barza M, Haher J, McFarland J J, Louie S, Kane A 1978 Penetration of clindamycin into decubitus ulcers. Antimicrobial Agents and Chemotherapy 14(3):489–499

Blake S L, Brimigion J, O'Keefe Diran M et al 1976 Dealing with death and dying. Ravenswood Publications, Beckenham

Bliss M 1978 The use of ripple beds in hospitals. Hospital and Health Services Review 74:190–193

Bowden M L, Jones C A, Feller I 1979 Psychosocial aspects of

a severe burn — a review of the literature. National Institute for Burn Medicine, Ann Arbor
Brodland G A, Andreasen N J C 1974 Adjustment problems of the family of the burn patient. Social Casework January, 13–18
Browne G, Byrne C, Brown B et al 1985 Psychosocial adjustment of burn survivors. Burns 12:28–35
Bull J P 1971 Revised analysis of mortality due to burns. Lancet 2:1133–1134
Calver R F, Stanley J K 1980 Enhancement of secondary wound healing by local tissue nutrition. Clinical Trials Journal 17(4):144–158
Camp R 1977 Leg ulcers. Nursing Times: 73 (suppl):25–28
Cason J S 1981 Treatment of burns. Chapman & Hall, London
Chelgren M 1979 Caring for persons with wounds. In: Sorensen K, Luckman J (eds) Basic nursing: a psychophysiologic approach. W B Saunders, Philadelphia
Cobey J C, Cobey J H 1974 Chronic leg ulcers. American Journal of Nursing 74:258–259
Cornwall J V 1985a Leg ulcers: fact sheet. Community Outlook January:37
Cornwall J 1985b Leg ulcer specialist. Journal of District Nursing, 4(3):9–10
Cornwall J V 1985c Diagnosis of leg ulcers. Journal of Community Nursing 4(3):4–11
Cornwall J V 1985d Treating leg ulcers. Journal of District Nursing 4(4):4–6
Cornwall J V, Lewis J D 1983 Leg ulcers revisited. British Journal of Surgery 70:681
Crow R, David J A, Cooper E J 1981 Pressure sores and their prevention. Nursing (Oxford) 26:1139–1142
Dale J 1984 Leg Work: research. Nursing Mirror 159(20):22-25
Dale J J, Callam M J, Ruckley C V, Harper D R, Berr P N 1983a Chronic ulcers of the leg: a study of prevalence in a Scottish community. Health Bulletin (Edinburgh) 41(6):310–314
Dale J J, Callam M, Ruckley C V 1983b How efficient is a compression bandage? Nursing Times 79(46):49–51
Davies J W L 1982 Physiological responses to burning injury. Academic Press, London
Department of Trade 1983 Domestic thermal injuries: a study of 1100 accidents admitted to specialised treatment centres. Department of Trade, London
DHSS Statistics and Research Division 1980 Amputation Statistics in England, Wales and Northern Ireland 1979. Blackpool, DHSS
Diggory G 1979 Entonox and its role in nursing care. Nursing (Oxford) 1(1):28–31
Eaglstein W H 1985 The effect of occlusive dressings on collagen synthesis and re-epithelialisation in superficial wounds. In: Ryan T (Ed) An environment for healing: the role of occlusion. Royal Society of Medicine Congres and Symposium Series No. 88
Engel G 1964 Grief and grieving. American Journal of Nursing 64(Sept):93–98
Eriksson Gunnel 1985 Bacterial growth in venous leg ulcers — its clinical significance in the healing process. In: Ryan T (Ed) An environment for healing: the role of occlusion. Royal Society of Medicine Congress and Symposium Series No. 88
Feck G, Baptiste M S, Tate C L 1979 Burn injuries: epidemiology and prevention. Accident Analysis and Prevention 11:129–136
Feller I, Koepke G, Richards K E et al 1973 Rehabilitation of the burned patient. In: Lynch J B, Lewis S R (eds) Symposium on the treatment of burns. CV Mosby, St Louis
Ferguson-Pell M W, Wilkie I C, Reswick J B, Barbenel J C 1980 Pressure sore prevention for wheelchair-bound spinal injury patients. Paraplegia 18:42–51
Fox J A 1983 A method of venous ulcer therapy used in the UK In: Cadaxomer iodine: Symposium in Munich. Schattauer Verlag, New York
Franklin B L 1974 Patient anxiety on admission to hospital. Royal College of Nursing, London
Gawkrodger D J 1984 The Treatment of venous ulcers. The Practitioner 228(1388):211–216
Glaser B G, Strauss A L 1965 Awareness of dying. Aldine, Chicago
Hamburg D A, Hamburg B, deGoza S 1953 Adaptive problems and mechanisms in severely burned patients. Psychiatry 16(1):1–20
Harkiss K 1985 Leg ulcers — cheaper in the long run. Community Outlook August:19–22
Harris A 1977 Physical impairment: social handicap. Office of Health Economics
Harvey Kemble J V, Lamb B E 1984 Plastic surgical and burns nursing. Baillière Tindall, London
Hawkins, K 1978 Wet dressings: putting the damper on dermatitis. Nursing (Horsham) 78(8):64–67
Hayward J 1979 Pain — psychological and social aspects. Nursing (Oxford) 1(1):21–27
Hazarika E Z, Wright D E 1981 Chronic leg ulcers: the effect of pneumatic interrmittent compression. The Practitioner 255(1352):189–192
Hinton J 1976 Dying. Penguin, Harmondsworth
Hunt J M 1979 Protracted pain and nursing care. Nursing (Oxford) 1(2):56–64
Hunt S M, McEwen J, McKenna S P, Backett E M, Pope C 1982 Subjective health of patients with peripheral vascular disease. The Practitioner 226(1363):133–136
Imbus S H, Zawacki B E 1977 Autonomy for burned patients when survival is unprecedented. The New England Journal of Medicine 297(6):308–311
Jackson D M 1974 The psychological effects of burns. Burns 1(1):70–74
Janzekovic Z 1970 A new concept in the excision and immediate grafting of burns. Journal of Trauma 10:1103
Jordon M M, Clark M O 1977 Incidence of pressure sores in the patient community of the Greater Glasgow Health Board Area on Janauray 21st 1976. The Bioengineering Unit, University of Strathclyde and Greater Glasgow Health Board.
Kaisary A V 1982 Treatment of venous ulcers of the leg and Aetiology and pathogenesis of venous leg ulcers. In: Leg ulcers: a practical guide to treatment. Nursing (Oxford) (suppl August):1–5
Kübler-Ross E 1970 On death and dying. Tavistock Publications, London
Larson D L, Abston S, Dobrkovsky M et al 1973 The prevention and correction of burn scar contracture and hypertrophy. Shriners Burn Institute, Texas
Lawrence J C 1985 The bacteriology of burns. The Journal of Hospital Infection 6(suppl B):3–17
Leaper D J 1984 Experimental infection and hydrogel dressings. Journal of Hospital Infection 5:69–73
Learmonth A 1980 Factors in child burn and scald accidents: a review of the literature. School of Science and Society, Bradford University

Lendrum J 1981 In: Keen G (ed) Operative surgery and management. John Wright, Dorchester
Little J H, Holt J, Davis N 1980 Changing epidemiology of malignant melanoma in Queensland. The Medical Journal of Australia 1:66–69
Lowbury E J L 1973 Burn disease. In: Urbaschek B, Urbaschek R, Neter E (eds) Gram-negative bacterial infections. Springer Verlag, Vienna
Lowthian P T 1976 Underpads in the prevention of decubiti. In: Kenedi R M, Cowden J M, Scales J T (eds) Bedsore biomechanics. Macmillan, London
Lowthian P T 1977 A review of pressure sore prophylaxis. Nursing Mirror Supplement 144(11):vii, ix, xi, xiii, xv
Lowthian P T 1979a Pressure sore prevalence : a survey of sores in orthopaedic patients. Nursing Times 75(9):358–360
Lowthian P T 1979b Practical nursing. Turning clock system to prevent pressure sores. Nursing Mirror 148(21):30–31
McClemont E J W, Shand I G, Ramsay B 1979 Pressure sores: a new method of treatment. British Journal of Clinical Practice 33(1):21–25
MacLeod A 1970 Adult burns in Melbourne: a five–year survey. Medical Journal of Australia 2:772–777
McNeill D C 1976 A survey of 1,600 admissions to a regional burns unit. In: Calnan T (ed) Recent advances in plastic surgery. Churchill Livingstone, Edinburgh
Malt U 1980 Long-term psychosocial follow-up studies of burned adults: review of the literature. Burns 6(3):190–197
Marks R 1985 The use of models for the study of wound healing. In: Ryan T J (ed) An environment for healing: the role of occlusion. Royal Society of Medicine Congress and Symposium Series No 88
Marriner A 1975 The nursing process: a scientific approach to nursing care. C V Mosby, St Louis
Martin H L 1970 Antecedents of burns and scalds in children. British Journal of Medical Psychology 43:39–47
Melzack R, Wall P 1982 The challenge of pain. Penguin, Harmondsworth
Miller W C, Gardner N, Mlott S R 1976 Psychosocial support in the treatment of severely burned patients. Journal of Trauma 16:722–725
Moody M 1984 A new lease of life. Nursing Times 80(26):46
Morden P, Bayne R 1976 Prevention, assessment and treatment of decubitus ulcers. Canadian Family Physician 22(1301):111–113
Muir I F K, Barclay T L 1974 Burns and their treatment. Lloyd-Luke (Medical Books), London
Norris W 1980 A pioneer in the study of melanoma. The Medical Journal of Australia 1:52–54
Norton D, McLaren R, Exton-Smith A N 1975 An investigation of geriatric nursing problems in hospital. Churchill Livingstone, Edinburgh
Pennisi V R, Deatherage J, Templeton J, Capozzi A 1970 The psychogenic dependency of the acute burn patient. In: Matter P, Barclay T L, Konickova Z (eds) Research in burns. Transactions of the Third International Congress on Research in Burns. Hans Huber, Bern
Petersen N C, Bittmann S 1971 Epidemiology of pressure sores. Scandinavian Journal of Plastic and Reconstructive Surgery 5:62– 66
Pikkareinen J, Kulonen E (eds) 1973 The biology of the fibroblast. Academic Press, London
Redman B K 1980 The process of patient teaching in nursing, 4th edn. C V Mosby, St Louis
Roach L B 1974 Assessing skin changes: the subtle and the obvious. Nursing (Horsham) 74(4):64–67
Roberts S 1975 Skin assessment for colour and temperature. American Journal of Nursing 75:610–615
Roi L D, Flora J D, Davis T M, Cornell R G, Feller I 1981 A severity grading chart for the burned patient. Annals of Emergency Medicine 10(3):161–163
Rook A 1980 Symposium: dermatology. The Practitioner 224:469
Ryan G B 1976 Inflammation and localisation of infection. Surgical Clinics of North America 56(4):831–845
Ryan J J 1983 Diseases of the skin. In: Weatherall D J, Ledingham J G G, Warrell D A (eds) Oxford Textbook of Medicine. Oxford University Press, Oxford
Schilling J A 1976 Wound healing. Surgical Clinics of North America 56(4):859–874
Schraibman I G, Lewis B, Parmar J R 1982 Clinical comparison of elastic supports in venous diseases of the lower leg and thrombosis prevention. Phlébologie Année 35(1):61–71
Settle J A D 1974 Burns — the first 48 hours. Smith and Nephew Pharmaceuticals, Romford
Seville R H, Martin E 1981 Leg ulcers. Nursing Times 77:1249–1253
Silver I A 1985 Oxygen and tissue repair. In: Ryan T (ed) An environment for healing: the role of occlusion. Royal Society of Medicine Congress and Symposium Series No 88
Skipper J K, Leonard R C (eds) 1965 Social interaction and patient care. Lippincott, Philadelphia
Smith M 1982 Nursing Management of the leg ulcer in the Community. Nursing Times 78:1228–1232
Steiner H, Clarke W R 1977 Psychiatric complications of burned adults: a classification. Journal of Trauma 17(2):134–143
Stephenson V 1984 An alternative treatment: Leg ulcers one, Nursing Times 80(26):40–44
Stevanovic D V 1985 Effect of hydrocolloid dressing on the healing of ulcers of various origins. In: Ryan T (ed) An environment for healing: the role of occlusion. Royal Society of Medicine Congress and Symposium Series No. 88
Stewart A, Foster M, Leaper D 1985 Cleaning v. healing. Community Outlook August:22–85
Sutherland A B 1976 Nitrogen balance and nutritional requirements in the burn patient. Burns 2(4):238–244
Torelli M 1973 Topical hyperbaric oxygen for decubitus ulcers. American Journal of Nursing 73(3):494–496
Torrance C 1981 Pressure sores: Parts 3 and 4. Nursing Times 77: Occasional Papers 9–16
Turner T D 1985 Semiocclusive and occlusive dressings. In: Ryan T (ed) An environment for healing: the role of occlusion. Royal Society of Medicine Congress and Symposium Series No 88
Turner T, Coombs T 1982 Which dressing and why — 2. Wound Care No 12, Nursing Times Supplement August 18
Westaby S 1981a The classification of wounds. Wound Care No 1, Nursing Times Supplement September 24
Westaby S 1981b Healing: the normal mechanism — 1. Wound Care No 3, Nursing Times Supplement November 18
Westaby S 1981c Healing: the normal mechanism — 2. Wound Care No 4, Nursing Times Supplement December 16
White S 1982 Wound infection — cause and prevention. Wound Care No 8, Nursing Times Supplement April 21
Williams E, Hysick R M 1974 Gold leaf treatment for decubitus ulcers. Journal of Psychiatric Nursing and

Mental Services 12:42–44
Wilson-Barnett J 1979 Stress in hospital. Patients' psychological reactions to illness and health care. Churchill Livingstone, Edinburgh
Winter G D 1976 Some factors affecting skin and wound healing. In: Kenedi R M, Cowden J M (eds) Bedsore biomechanics. Macmillan, London
Wright J T 1980 Some cutaneous manifestations of systemic disease. The Practitioner 224:489–496
Wright P 1982 The nursing of leg ulcer patients. In: Leg ulcers: a practical guide to treatment. Nursing (Oxford) Supplement August, p 6–7

21

Disturbances of protective mechanisms — the musculoskeletal system

INTRODUCTION

The broad term 'Musculoskeletal' refers to the skeletal and muscular systems which serve to give the body structure, static stability, and voluntary and involuntary movement. Patients who have some sort of disturbance in either of these systems are usually referred to as 'orthopaedic' patients (although some will be found in medical or other units), and the speciality of orthopaedics is a well established field in acute health care services.

The skeletal system is a rigid framework which gives shape and support to the body and is jointed to allow movement. The individual bones of the skeleton are categorized into three types — flat bones which protect delicate organs, long bones which act as levers, and short bones which confer strength. All of the bones give attachment to muscles.

The skeletal muscles contract and lengthen under the control of nerve impulses arising in the cerebral cortex. They are attached by tendons to the long bones, which act as levers when the muscles contract and relax. Two bones articulate at a joint and the opposing surfaces are covered with a layer of smooth cartilage. Synovial joints are those encapsulated by a synovial membrane which secretes the lubricating fluid synovium. The musculoskeletal system is, as other systems, closely allied to the nervous system and disturbances in the nervous system inevitably affect motor activity.

Disturbances to the musculoskeletal system embrace medical conditions, injuries, and malformed bones and muscles. The range of disturbances can be summarized into five groups:

- disturbances which arise as a result of trauma
- degenerative conditions of the bones, muscles and tendons
- inflammatory conditions
- congenital malformation of the bones, muscles, or joints
- malignant conditions.

Whilst nursing management is often specific to each of these groups, a number of basic principles can be applied to any patients who are suffering from musculoskeletal disturbance.

BASIC PRINCIPLES OF NURSING MANAGEMENT

As the musculoskeletal system is concerned with body movement and posture, a number of basic problems common to all orthopaedic patients are often present.

- First, mobility, and thus independence, is frequently affected. Often the medical treatment for the disturbance also demands enforced, continuous and prolonged immobilization of the affected part.
- Secondly, the internal damage or malfunction of bone or muscle very often can be seen externally. In other words, deformity of the body may be obvious.
- Thirdly, most patients with diseases and injuries to bones, muscles and joints experience pain. Bone pain is often thought of as being very difficult to control and is described as 'aching and boring in nature' whilst muscular pain is 'sore and aching' (Keele, 1972).
- Finally, if the goal is to assist the patient to become independent, or to cope with dependence, nursing is charged with planning a logical programme of initially doing things for the individual, teaching the individual to do them him/herself, and eventually supporting the move towards independence. The concept of rehabilitation is of primary importance in the management of patients with disturbances due to musculoskeletal disorders.

Because orthopaedic conditions often need long periods of treatment and some form of immobilization, nursing is of particular importance. These common problems give rise to the basic principles of nursing management.

THE PROBLEMS ASSOCIATED WITH ENFORCED, CONTINUOUS AND PROLONGED IMMOBILIZATION

Murray (1976) defines immobilization as 'any prescribed or unavoidable restriction of movement in any area of a person's life. The source of immobilization may be physical, emotional, intellectual or social'. Any patient may experience these four types of immobilization to a greater or lesser degree, especially if the condition means admission to hospital. In orthopaedics, physical immobilization is common and may vary from the full body cast to the immobilization of a finger in a metal splint. Between these two are such things as traction, splints and enforced bed rest.

The prolonged inactivity imposed on people who have an orthopaedic complaint can give rise to specific problems and complications, not least a progressive loss of function in otherwise normal organs. For example, the knee immobilized in a plaster cast to rest the joint may recover to the detriment of the previously healthy quadriceps muscles in the thigh which will rapidly waste if they remain inactive.

Musculoskeletal function

Musculoskeletal function can rapidly deteriorate in prolonged inactivity. Nursing aims at preventing contracture deformities and at maintaining as much normal function as possible. Prolonged immobility affects the resting length of the muscle and the patient may easily develop a flexion deformity if the limbs are placed in non-functional positions. Muscular strength declines quickly if the muscles are not used, and wasting begins within 48 hours of inactivity (Murray, 1976). Nursing management to avoid these problems revolves around positioning and exercise. The patient's trunk and limbs must be positioned in accordance with correct principles of body alignment. Elhart (1978) defines body alignment or posture 'as the position in which the various parts of the body are held while sitting, standing, walking, and lying and good posture is then inferred to be efficient posture, which will vary with the individual and the activity'. In general, the patient's joints should be positioned in a neutral, functional position as far as possible, preventing prolonged hyperextension or flexion of opposing muscle groups.

Changes in position to prevent prolonged pressure on vulnerable tissues, stimulate circulation, facilitate lung expansion, and to permit joint movement are as important as actual positioning. Creativity in using and devising supportive equipment is important, so that pillows, sand bags, foam wedges, etc., can be effectively placed to support functional positions. Muscle exercises can help to maintain or improve muscle strength, restore optimal joint function, prevent deformities, and stimulate circulation. In association with the physiotherapist, passive, isometric and active exercise of the muscles and joints is an essential part of any nursing care plan in an orthopaedic area (see Ch. 13).

Cardiovascular function

Cardiovascular function is affected in a number of ways by inactivity. If the patient is confined to lying in bed, it is especially difficult for the heart to cope with the resulting sluggish venous return and orthostatic hypotension may occur (a drop in blood pressure on standing due to a failure of the autonomic nervous system to balance blood supply after prolonged bed rest) (Guyton, 1974). Inactivity may also give rise to stasis of the venous blood and changes in blood composition which precipitate venous thrombosis. This is even more likely to occur when the lower limbs are specifically immobilized in splints or traction. Close monitoring of the patient to detect signs of these problems occurring is an important aspect of nursing management and planned exercise within the limits of the patient's capabilities is fundamental to orthopaedic nursing.

The skin

The skin can break down easily when the patient is nursed in a fairly fixed position for a prolonged period. This risk is heightened when appliances to ensure immobility are in place, for example splints and casts. Motor paralysis with associated muscular wasting reduces the 'thickness' of tissue between the skin and bones, which may precipitate the occurrence of pressure sores. The risk is heightened further by the tendency of the paralysed patient to lie in one position for prolonged periods. With the body weight concentrated on small areas of skin, blood vessels may collapse and blood flow be reduced (Agris & Spira, 1979). Splints, traction equipment, and casts often rub against the skin, and increase perspiration. Friction was found directly to cause sores by Reichel (1958), and Dinsdale (1974) concluded from his study into pressure sore formation that friction played a major role. Cooney & Reuler (1983) suggest that the presence of moisture, either urine or perspiration, increases the risk of sore development fivefold.

The relief of pressure, stimulation of circulation, and general care and hygiene of the skin, common to all fields of nursing, therefore take on added importance in caring for the patient suffering from a disorder of the musculoskeletal system.

Relieving pressure on parts of the body by frequent position change and regular checks of splints and appliances may prevent the occurence of pressure and friction sores. The prolonged ischaemia which precipitates the formation of a pressure sore usually arises as a result of pressure on the tissue which exceeds the capillary pressure of 15–30 mmHg and thus occludes capillary circulation (Dinsdale, 1974, Kosiak et al, 1958, Agris & Spira, 1979). A constant pressure of 70 mmHg applied for longer than 2 hours was found by Dinsdale (1974) to produce irreversible damage, but little change occurred up to pressures of 240 mmHg if this pressure was regularly relieved. Norton et al (1962) found that regular position change was the only action which effectively reduced the incidence of pressure lesions, and Goldstone & Roberts (1980) report how the mobility and activity of orthopaedic patients, and thus their ability to change position frequently, is indicative of pressure sore risk.

Although actual repositioning of many patients immobilized because of an orthopaedic condition is often impossible, regular relief of pressure, for example by lifting the patient free from the bed surface for two or three minutes every two hours, will allow perfusion of the tissues and removal of toxic byproducts in the area subject to pressure. Judson (1983) describes how this process takes place fairly rapidly when pressure is relieved and capillary circulation is facilitated.

Whilst regular, careful checking of skin surfaces in contact with appliances and ensuring that they are kept clean and dry is of much value, some splints and tractions may inevitably produce sores in areas not visible or accessible. Any complaints of pain, burning, or loss of sensation in areas not accessible should be investigated carefully.

Psycho-social problems

The psycho-social well-being of the patient facing immobility at any level can be adversely affected. The immobilization of one limb alone will present previously unfaced barriers to independence for the patient. Patients who have had a below-knee walking cast applied to a leg as an outpatient report major difficulties in carrying out many of the activities of living, and often experience long periods of depression because they are unable to carry on with their usual living patterns for the relatively short period of 6 weeks (Pearson, 1981). Olsen (1967) says that restricted activity affects intellectual ability and the patient's sense of identity as an individual and social being is disturbed. These feelings may manifest themselves as anger, apathy, aggression or withdrawal.

Nursing management must be based on an understanding of the effects of immobilization and on an energetic attempt to involve the patient in his/her own care. In the case of immobility of a limb, Pearson (1981) found that giving written information on how to carry out the activities whilst wearing a cast increased self care ability and thus lessened the effects of immobilization. Teaching the patient self care techniques which are tenable, given the immobilization, and then allowing him/her to take responsibility for his/her own care can lessen some of the psycho-social problems. Patients who are immobilized and in hospital can be helped by the provision of an environment which enables them to pursue a daily living pattern similar to home. Brunner & Suddarth (1984) suggest that 'action absorbs anxiety' and Geis (1972) reports on how the patient's emotional needs can partly be met by making meaningful activity possible. A regular programme of activity, constructed together with the patient, can be incorporated into the nursing care plan and may also involve the occupational therapist and voluntary workers. Such an activity programme often gives enough stimulation to prevent intellectual stagnation and may help to preserve the patient's self image and worth.

PHYSICAL DEFORMITY AND DISABILITY

A disorder of bones, joints, or muscles often gives rise to obvious physical deformity, and there is much evidence which suggests that society treats the physically disabled person as a social reject (Miller & Gwynne, 1974). Deformity is stigmatizing (Goffman, 1963) and its bearers are often deprived of the usual privileges and obligations to which 'normal' people are entitled. It may affect the person's physical attractiveness, sexuality, ability to get a job, and the chance to take part in the social events of the community around him. Depending on the extent of the disability, many places of entertainment and interest may be denied because of difficulty with access, and the right to independence may not be a feasible option. In the young adult these difficulties may be heightened and in those who have previously been well and independent, for example the young paraplegic, adjusting may seem to be impossible to the patient.

Whilst the help of social workers and sometimes psychologists and psychiatrists is invaluable, the nurse alone of the professional health carers stays next to the patient as he/she progresses through daily life and begins to make sense of, and adjust to, his/her predicament. Hall et al (1975) report on the favourable outcomes of care which arise when the nurse becomes involved with the patient and takes on the leadership role within the multi-disciplinary clinical team as the central care giver, and Lynch (1978) describes how the 'simple act of touching' has observable therapeutic effects. Acceptance of the disability by both the patient and the nurse is a crucial element of nursing management. The patient's reaction may be apparently flippant, or may be manifested by mild tension and depression, withdrawal and apathy, or anxiety and anger. The disability may have a direct impact on the individual's body image with the realization that his/her body has deteriorated, his/her shape and appearance may have changed, and his/her position in society may be altered. The patient needs to be allowed to work through his/her own feelings until a realistic acceptance seems to be reached. The nurse may find it difficult to accept patients with gross physical deformities and it is often necessary to come to terms with oneself about feelings towards the disabled and to acknowledge fears and prejudices before acceptance is real. In cases of long-term handicap, Miller & Gwynne (1974) describe how those who care for such patients seem to exhibit the feeling towards them that 'you are normal, but not really'. They report that some nurses re-interpret the cure-goal of the medical model to mean postponement of death as long as possible and expect patients to be dependent. Others see the patient as having unrealized potential and try to develop abilities, rather than care for disabilities. This latter approach is a basic principle of nursing management for those with disability, of a long term or short term nature.

PAIN

Because orthopaedic conditions require long periods of treatment, the management of the patient with pain is important. Pain is a subjective experience and cannot be objectively assessed. Alderman (1983) and Punton (1983) both report on the use of the 'pain thermometer' used by Hayward (1975) to measure the patient's subjective perception of pain and to establish and monitor analgesia administration. If the patient feels pain, then sleep, comfort, and morale will be in jeopardy and exhaustion a likely result (Johnson & Rice, 1974). Nursing management aims to reduce the pain experience to a level acceptable to the patient, if not altogether resolving it. This is achieved both by adhering to the medical prescription (and evaluating its effectiveness with a view to altering analgesia regimes if necessary) and by systematically identifying factors associated with the pain and utilizing care techniques that minimize the pain experience. The position of the patient should ensure correct alignment of joints and limbs, and painful areas of the body should be supported. Moving the patient should be done gently; sharp, sudden movements should be avoided. Establishing any acts or factors which aggravate the pain may give direction to planning strategies to resolve it, either by avoiding specific acts, or by seeking medical prescription of analgesia before essential, painful procedures are to take place.

Whilst the general approaches to any patient with pain, discussed in Chapter 9, are relevant to the orthopaedic patient, specific measures — such as applying heat to muscles in spasm, and cold to inflamed and swollen joints – have a special relevance in orthopaedic nursing. Chronic pain is evident in many of the degenerative and inflammatory bone and joint conditions, as is bone pain in trauma and orthopaedic surgery. An understanding of pain is a crucial prerequisite to effective nursing management.

REHABILITATION

The concept of rehabilitation is a component of nursing management in any disturbance. However, it is especially important in disturbances of the musculoskeletal system since this system is crucial to functional activity. An initial dependence on the nurse in the activities of living progresses on to growing independence — a basic description of rehabilitation. Murray (1976) defines rehabilitation as

> . . . the continuing, co-operative process of restoring the individual to optimal functioning in all areas of his life. Its goal is to maintain, as far as possible, the person's ability to live a productive, ego-satisfying life in his home and community environment.

In orthopaedics, rehabilitation in nursing management refers to:

- the prevention of deformities and complications
- initiating, teaching and supporting the patient and his/her family in the activities of daily living leading to self care
- referring patients to the appropriate people who can help them, with the nurse, to pursue the goal of self care.

Atrophy of tissues which make up the musculoskeletal system can be prevented by the following nursing actions:

- assisting the patient to carry out a planned programme of exercise
- assisting and encouraging the patient to maintain independence in his/her acts of daily living
- preventing and relieving pressure on any part of the body
- assisting the patient to maintain a desirable posture and positioning of limbs, etc.
- providing adequate nutritional intake.

Planned exercise programme

A planned exercise programme is usually formulated by the physiotherapist, but regular repetition of the exercises often relies on the encouragement of the nurse. Four basic types of exercises are described by many authors (e.g. Elhart, 1978). A more comprehensive discussion of these exercises is contained in Chapter 13.

Passive exercises

Passive exercises are those carried out for the patient, but without his/her assistance, by the physiotherapist, nurse or relative, either because the patient is unable to move the part unaided or because the movement needs to be controlled. The purpose of passive exercise is to maintain joint movements and muscular activity, and to maintain circulation. Passive limb exercises are carried out by holding the proximal part of the limb firmly and moving the joint smoothly and slowly through its full range of movements or holding the distal part and moving it.

Assisted active exercise and active exercise

Both of these involve the patient carrying out exercises, the former requiring assistance by the nurse, and the latter carried out independently. The purpose of active exercise is to increase or maintain muscle strength. The joint is moved through its full range of movements, against gravity.

Resistive exercise

This is active exercise carried out by the patient against some manual or mechanical force. The purpose of resisting the movement is to increase muscle power. The patient moves the joint through its range of movements whilst the nurse or physiotherapist resists slightly at first, and then with greater power. Alternatively, sandbags or weights can be lifted, or springs can be pulled or compressed.

Isometric or muscle setting exercises

These are active and resistive exercises carried out by the patient, the purpose being to maintain strength whilst a joint is immobilized. The muscle is 'tightened' without moving the joint; it

Table 21.1 A guide to teaching acts of daily living (after Brunner & Suddarth, 1984)

1. Establish that mehods can be used to carry out the task (e.g. there are several ways of putting on a given garment).
2. Establish what the patient can do by watching him/her do it.
3. Establish what specific movements are needed to carry out the task.
4. Encourage the patient to exercise those muscles needed to carry out the task.
5. Start off with those activities which encourage gross functional movements of the limbs (e.g. bathing, holding large objects).
6. Gradually introduce tasks which require finer movements (e.g. buttoning clothes, using cutlery).
7. Increase the period of activity as rapidly as the patient can tolerate.
8. Perform and practise the activity in a real life situation.
9. Encourage the patient to do every activity within his/her capabilities.
10. Support the patient by giving justifiable praise.

is held tight for several seconds and then relaxed.

The programme of exercise

The exercise programme should be incorporated into the patient's care plan and particular strategies made explicit. Continuity of the plan is important if atrophy is to be averted, and clarity and specificity of the written care plan assists in continuity. The patient's fears and pain levels may also mitigate against continuity of exercises and need to be considered in care planning. Pain may lead the patient to hold his limbs in a fixed position and result in stiffness and disinclination to persist in exercising. Similarly, fear may make the patient assume protective positions, as well as leading to a reluctance to exercise. A clear understanding of the purpose of the exercises often reduces fear.

Independence in activities of daily living

The overall goal of rehabilitation is independence in the activities of living and this is also seen by Roper et al (1980) as the overall goal of nursing. The capacity of the patient to carry out the activities of daily living will be dependent on the nature of the disability. All orthopaedic patients, however, experience some degree of impairment in their ability to be independent. Brunner & Suddarth (1984) suggest that each activity be analysed with each patient, and offer a guide to teaching each task (Table 21.1).

In addition, setting realistic goals, both short and long term, together with the patient will both promote a partnership and encourage motivation. Whilst such a systematic and specific approach may demand extra nursing time in the short term, and will sometimes conflict with the method of care organization within many hospital settings, it is essential if the goal of independence is to be achieved. In the longer term nursing time should therefore be saved.

Patient support and teaching

Patient support and teaching takes on an added dimension of importance because the activities of living are always affected to some degree. Orthopaedic nursing is a multi-faceted speciality in that it embraces, at one end of the spectrum, the totally immobile patient with multiple injuries, and at the other, the patient needing non-life-threatening correction of deformity or with internal derangements of joints. Overall, the ability to engage in self care in the activities of living, or to cope with dependence, the prevention of further disability and the maintenance of good posture are the goals of any patient teaching initiative. Many disorders arise out of accidents, such as road traffic accidents or sporting activities, leading to the educational role of the nurse becoming wider to include such things as the correct lift techniques, the wearing of seat belts, use of protective apparatus and so on. The comparatively brief encounter between patient and nurse in an accident unit when a plaster cast is applied demands a systematic teaching approach to ensure that the cast remains intact for as long as it should, that the muscles do not waste, circulation is maintained, and daily living acts are carried out during the period of immobilization.

The team approach

The involvement of other health care workers and a multi-disciplinary team approach to patient care is now common in most orthopaedic settings. A typical team may include doctors, nurses, physiotherapists, occupational therapists, social workers, and splint/appliance makers. Each specialist brings his/her unique contribution to the total care of the patient, and one of the 'unique' aspects of care by the nurse is the co-ordination of the efforts of the other team members. Similarly, the fact that nursing continues 24 hours a day, 7 days a week, often means that those activities prescribed by the team members may need to be pursued by the nurse during the 'unsocial hours' when nursing is the only service readily available. For example, the quadriceps exercises taught to the patient suffering from a sports injury to the knee may need to be encouraged and supervised by the nurse at the weekend; the support needed by the elderly lady with a fracture of the neck of the femur who uses a walking frame will need to take place first thing in the morning when she wishes to go to the toilet. The overlapping of roles and patient directed approaches to care, rather than professional role-delineated approaches, is one of the fundamental principles of orthopaedic nursing (Alfano, 1969). A full and accurate initial patient assessment, either on admission to the ward or during attendance at the outpatient or accident department, should lead to the nurse making appropriate referrals to other team members according to the individual patient's needs.

THE EMPHASIS IN NURSING ON ACTING FOR, TEACHING AND SUPPORTING THE PATIENT

Orem (1980) suggests that nursing uses five helping methods:

- acting for, or doing for the patient
- guiding the patient
- supporting the patient
- providing a developmental environment for the patient
- teaching the patient.

Such a broad description of the acts of nursing transcends the boundaries of specialities, and of course these five methods of helping are not unique to orthopaedic nursing. However, caring for patients who have some restriction in functional ability requires that these helping methods be the focus of nursing to a stronger degree than in some other specialities.

Prolonged immobilization of one or more of the limbs often demands that the carer acts for the patient in some activities; the prevention of contractures and muscle wasting, and the gradual progression to full mobility demands a systematic application of the guiding, supporting and teaching methods of help. The enforced mobility demands the provision of a developmental environment. Discharging a patient wearing a cast or splint demands a comprehensive teaching strategy to help him cope with his daily life until the cast or splint is removed.

Because nursing is often described as being concerned with the activities of living and musculoskeletal disturbance usually has obvious effects on these activities, therapeutic nursing becomes a major contributor to the patient's eventual recovery. Alfano (1969) asserts that nursing in itself is a therapeutic act:

> ... the nurse takes advantage of her unique opportunity of working with the patient in a learning process. It is she who assists the patient through his first activities and as he moves into each new phase. She is there not to direct or enforce, but to guide and give assistance. It is our firm belief that in this way nursing becomes a therapeutic force in assisting patients to achieve rehabilitation.

She differentiates between this 'therapeutic' style of nursing, which focuses on bringing about an acceptable change, and 'caretaking' nursing which concentrates on safeguarding and maintaining patients. Thus, the nursing input to care for patients with a musculoskeletal disturbance needs to be a 'healing' force in itself (Pearson, 1983).

The function with which all people are concerned thus provides a focus for nursing assessment and intervention. Disturbances to muscles and bones inevitably lead to restrictions in the carrying out of these functions. Table 21.2 identifies problems common to orthopaedic patients and suggests some nursing interventions.

Orem's nursing systems

Orem's (1980) description of nursing, again, helps to clarify the broad principles of nursing care for orthopaedic patients when her 'nursing systems' are considered. Orem suggests that nurses utilize one of three nursing systems when giving care:

- wholly compensatory system: where the nurse acts for the patient who is totally incapacitated (e.g. the unconscious patient with multiple injuries, the quadraplegic patient, the patient in a full body cast, etc.)
- partly compensatory system: where the nurse and patient perform care measures together, allowing for patient limitations
- educative-developmental system: where the patient is able to carry out self care, or can do so with assistance, often by the nurse acting in a consultative role.

These three nursing systems can be used to group together the general types of problems encountered by patients whose disturbances are subsumed under the extremely broad umbrella of 'orthopaedics'.

Examples of disturbances of the musculoskeletal system which demand a wholly compensatory nursing system:

- debilitating conditions at an advanced stage such as rheumatoid arthritis, cancer of the bones
- conditions which require prolonged immobilization, such as fractures of the spine
- permanent paralysis such as para- or quadriplegia
- initial care of patients who have undergone orthopaedic surgery, on a temporary basis in the immediate postoperative period.

Examples of disturbances of the musculoskeletal system which demand a partly compensatory nursing system:

- conditions which demand prolonged immobilization of a limb but do not prevent patient participation in care, e.g. patients with a fracture of the shaft of the femur being treated by fixed traction on a Thomas splint
- patients recovering from an orthopaedic operation, after the immediate postoperative period
- Long term patients who have themselves adapted to permanent paralysis.

Examples of disturbances of the musculoskeletal system which demand an educative-developmental nursing system:

- patients who are discharged from hospital with a cast or splint in position
- patients in the later stages of recovery from an orthopaedic operation
- patients treated as outpatients in an outpatient or accident unit.

The nursing management of patients with specific disturbances of the musculoskeletal system will now be discussed.

DISTURBANCES DUE TO TRAUMA

A large proportion of disturbances of the muscles or bones arise out of unexpected injury as a result of an accident. This may range from the major road traffic accident to the slip of a hammer onto the thumb when putting a picture hook on the wall. Thus, the consideration of trauma in this chapter must be limited to generalizations. Further in-depth study of the subject can be pursued through specialized texts.

Injury to any part of this system inevitably involves injury to other parts, particularly the surrounding structures. A fracture affects the movement of the muscles attached to that particular bone and often injures the surrounding soft tissues. Furthermore, blood vessels near the fracture site may be torn and

Table 21.2 Problems common to orthopaedic patients

Usual problems	Possible interventions
Breathing	
Inability to expand lungs adequately, potentially leading to chest infection e.g. — when patient is immobilized in bed or in full body cast — fracture of ribs, when breathing is painful	Regular chest physiotherapy Patient teaching about need for physiotherapy, and how to carry out deep breathing Assessment of pain associated with breathing Giving prescribed analgesics at planned intervals, e.g. 20 minutes before physiotherapy
Eating and drinking	
Inability to eat or drink unaided e.g. — when patient must lie flat — injuries to arms and hands — paralysis	Use of aids to eating and drinking which are appropriate e.g. feeding cups, straws, non-slip mats, plate walls Assistance with feeding by the nurse
Inadequate intake or utilization of calcium e.g. — Osteomalacia	Dietetic advice and provision of diet rich in calcium
Loss of appetite e.g. — because food does not match patient's taste — timing of meals does not meet with patient's past experience	Planning and arranging for appealing meals Planning to serve meals at acceptable times
Potential dehydration and renal stones	Monitoring and recording of fluid intake and output and balance Planning for specific daily intake of fluid
Elimination	
Constipation because of immobility	Daily recording of bowel actions High fibre diet Muscle tone and maintenance exercises
Inability to attend to own toilet needs	Sensitive provision of bedpans, urinals, commodes etc. Providing privacy Providing handwashing facilities
Potential retention of urine	Assistance with acceptable positioning Planning for, and monitoring, specific daily fluid intake (e.g. 1 litre per day)
Movement and protection potential	
Muscular atrophy	Developing specific plans with physiotherapist which will subject muscles to activity, e.g. isometric exercises to quadriceps muscles x 10 four times per day at 10am, 2pm, 6pm and 10pm for a patient in a plaster of Paris cylinder
Joint stiffness	Developing specific plans with physiotherapist for regular exercise programme which will subject joint to full range of movement, e.g. active/passive flexion and extension of knee joint x 10 four times per day at 10am, 2pm, 6pm and 10pm
Circulatory stasis or restriction	Stimulation of circulation through planning a regular muscle exercise programme Daily observation and recording of skin colour and sensation of toes in patients in cast splint or traction to lower limb and of fingers to upper limb Rapid reporting to medical staff when tightness of appliance or pressure from it connotes impairment to circulation

Table 21.2 continued

Usual problems	Possible interventions
Potential pressure sores	Assessment of risk Frequent position change when possible e.g. 2-hourly lift of patient to relieve pressure : Teach patient to move regularly, if possible Daily check of specific pressure points especially when splints or traction are in place Provision of suitable position changing equipment where appropriate e.g. Stryker frame to turn patients who have spinal conditions, circular turning beds, net suspension beds Provision of suitable bed surfaces, e.g. firm foam mattresses with polythene-coated knitted covers Use of pressure-relieving devices/skin protecting surfaces, e.g. ripple mattresses, water beds, foam blocks and wedges, flotation pads, heel pads and sheepskins
Pain on movement	Encouragement and support to pursue planned exercise Assessment and development of plan to give prescribed analgesics, e.g. give prescribed PRN analgesia 30 minutes prior to physiotherapy
Inability to maintain personal hygiene	Planned assistance with hygiene without loss of dignity Providing opportunities, facilities and privacy for patient to make decisions about his/her personal hygiene and to continue as far as possible with past habits
Inability to meet own safety needs in mobility	Planned supervision, e.g. involve patient in developing a plan where the nurse is summoned whenever he/she wishes to walk to bathroom etc. Provision of walking aids in association with physiotherapist, e.g. Zimmer frame, crutches, walking sticks, etc.
Rest and sleep	
Pain	Use of strategies to avoid painful situations. e.g. support of joints and limbs, gentle, smooth and slow movement in lifting Applications of pain-relieving strategies, e.g. heat via hot water bags, electric pads, infra-red lamps; cold via ice packs Assessment of pain to establish if a pattern exists e.g.2-hourly assessment by nurse, or measurement of patient's subjective perception of pain through use of pain thermometer Planning, with patient, criteria for giving and timing of PRN analgesia, e.g.give PRN analgesia before physiotherapist attends in the morning and whenever patient records a pain level of 6 or more on the pain thermometer, according to medical prescription
Cramp	Adherence to planned exercise programme; gentle massage of tense muscles
Discomfort caused by position splintage, bed, etc	Assistance with position change Checking and adjusting splintage Ensuring comfortable environment for sleep, e.g.pillow arrangement, body position, lighting, etc.

Table 21.2 continued

Usual problems	Possible interventions
Stimulation and motivation	Providing informal and relaxed environment
Boredom because of restricted activity	Playing and talking with the patient Facilitating and encouraging visitors to spend time with patient Providing a range of diversional activities Referral to occupational therapists, disablement resettlement officers, social workers Involve patient in goal setting and in planning to meet goals Introducing patient to those with similar interests
Self concept	Offering opportunity to discuss such feelings
Feeling of being stigmatized e.g. – long term disability – physical disfigurement	Introduction to self help groups, e.g. Paraplegic Society, sections disabled living foundation: 'SHAPE', Riding for the Disabled, etc.
Feeling of loss of worth to society	Referral to Disablement Resettlement Officer
Relating to others	Include family/friends in care
Social isolation because of disability or immobility	Introduction to self help groups Providing social activities
Restricted sexual expression because of – Hospitalization	Providing opportunities for privacy For patients who are to be in hospital for a long period, attempting to minimize disruption to normal sexual expression by encouraging patient's partner to visit and ensuring privacy
–Disability	Teaching how to resume sexual activity within the limits of the disability Helping the patient to come to terms with his/her own sexuality and the limits imposed on it by disability; offering opportunities to discuss feelings Providing facilities needed by the patient to outwardly express sexuality, e.g. hairdressers, beauticians, opportunity to wear desired clothing, etc.

nerves severed. The ensuing treatment regimes therefore depend upon the total effects of the injury. Usually, injuries to the musculoskeletal system require support to the injured part so that the natural healing processes can begin and continue until the damage is resolved. This support may take the form of

- bandages
- adhesive strapping
- splints
- plaster of Paris (or casts of new materials)
- traction
- special shoes or appliances
- internal fixation of bones in the form of plates, screws or pins.

Initially, pain and swelling are major problems, and often the sheer shock or fright of having sustained an accident needs to be understood and accepted. The execution of the medical prescription and its evaluation, together with appropriate positioning of the affected part, aim at the resolution of pain, as does the specific method of support. Swelling may be reduced through using the principles of gravity so that the swollen part is elevated to help the circulatory processes remove excess tissue fluid. The psychological effects of an accident need to be considered individually, but allowing the patient to express and talk through his/her feelings, and sorting out practical problems such as arranging help in the home until recovery is complete, are as important as the physical aspects of care.

When these immediate problems are identified and the crisis is over, fibrosis and stiffness in the affected muscles, bones and tissues must be prevented. A rapid return to active function by the patient serves best to prevent these possible complications, but the physiotherapist may prescribe isometric exercises or planned passive exercises which will exercise the muscles or joints without demanding active function or disturbing the supporting measures applied.

TRAUMA TO SOFT TISSUES

This may be caused by a blow or fall, or by twisting or wrenching a part of the body. Some damage to blood vessels is usual, giving rise to haematoma (or bruising), rapid swelling and pain due to the pressure of such swelling. For example, in sprains of the ankle following a twisting injury the patient often experiences severe pain, gross swelling, and marked bruising. Walking is greatly limited — if not impossible — in the first stages of recovery. In relatively minor sprains, a crepe bandage or elastic adhesive strapping may give enough support, whilst in more severe sprains, immobilization of the ankle joint in a below-knee walking cast may be prescribed by the doctor. Nursing care would focus on encouraging the patient to keep the limb elevated as much as possible and on teaching specific strategies for coping with the activities of living whilst mobility is impaired. Sometimes the application of moist heat to the affected part accelerates absorption of the haematoma. At an earlier stage the application of cold has a vasoconstricting effect which will slow down the extravasation of fluid into the tissues and thus prevent further swelling and pain (Nursing Update, 1971).

Although soft tissue injuries are traditionally regarded as passing and somewhat trivial, the recovery period, from 2–6 weeks, will not appear trivial to the patient. Nursing therefore must take account of such injuries and actively assist the patient in reducing the discomfort and inconvenience caused.

TRAUMA TO JOINTS

Trauma to joints may lead to some derangement of the internal structure of the joint, with dislocation occurring if the articulating bones are involved in the damage. The patient experiences severe pain, the joint looks 'out of alignment' and normal mobility is not possible. In some joints, the associated limb becomes shorter in length and the axis of the articulation is changed. Medical action consists of manipulating the joint into correct alignment again — reduction of the dislocation. Specific nursing management after reduction involves the maintenance of immobilization of the joint to allow the ligaments and other joint structures to heal. Splints and casts are often used and the ability to maintain personal hygiene may be restricted. For example, in dislocations of the shoulder the splintage applied may make it difficult for the patient to keep the axilla clean and dry or to manage normal activities such as dressing and undressing. Assistance may need to be given by the nurse, or the injured person or the carer at home may need guidance and suggestions as to how to manage.

Internal derangement of joints is usually associated with the knee and hip because of the internal structures involved. In the knee the half moon shaped cartilages frequently tear in twisting injuries of the knee, particularly in football and rugby players. The cruciate ligaments in this joint are sometimes torn or bruised. The ligamentum teres in the hip joint can be damaged due to trauma and thus constitute a derangement within the joint. In all synovial joints, effusion may occur and this excessive amount of fluid within the joint space would represent a derangement. Medical intervention may take the form of aspirating this excess fluid, operating on the joint to remove or repair damaged structures or resting the joint to enable the natural healing mechanisms to occur.

In all of these approaches the specific nursing management concentrates on the maintenance of pressure over the joint, through the use of pressure bandages to prevent further swelling and immobilization of the joint to allow healing.

FRACTURES

Fractures of the bones are common sequelae of falls, blows, and road traffic accidents. A fracture is a break in the continuity of the bone and a number of different types are described according to the extent of damage to the bone (Fig. 21.1).

Whilst most fractures occur as a result of trauma, pathological fractures occur when the bone structure is weakened, for example in old age when osteoporosis is present, in cases of bone carcinoma and in gross mineral deficiency. Other systems and structures are often damaged

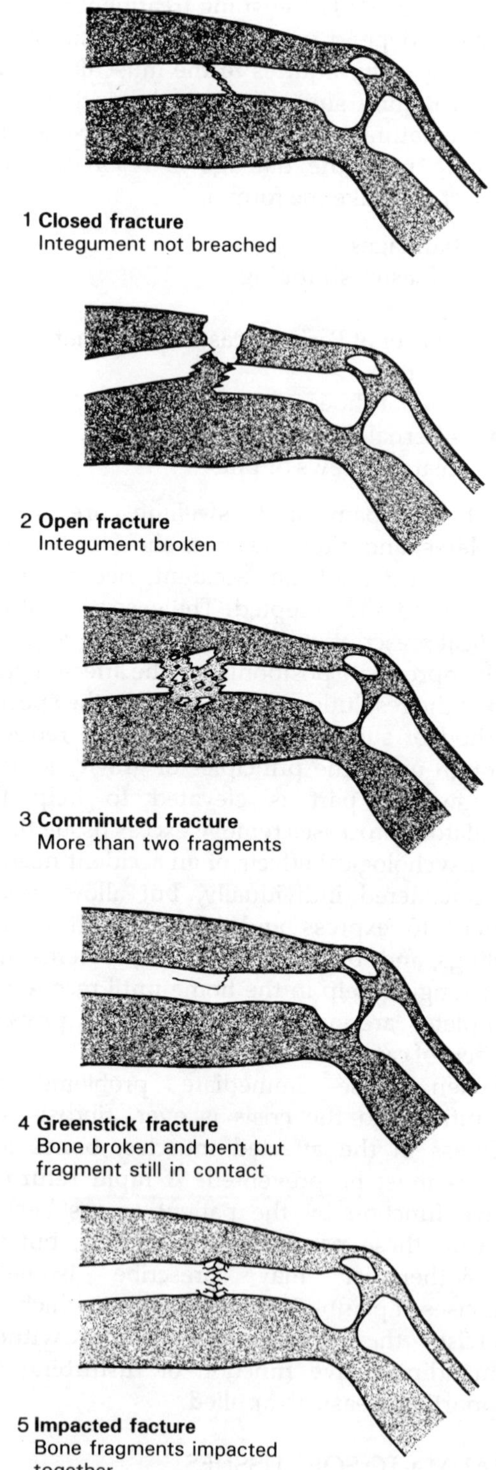

Fig. 21.1 Types of fractures

by the bones involved in the fracture, for example the bladder in fractures of the pelvis, the lungs in fractures of the ribs, and nerves and blood vessels in any fracture.

Medical management

Medical management consists of reducing the fracture and maintaining this reduction until healing has occurred. Nursing management supports this and assists, educates, rehabilitates and meets the basic needs in those activities of living beyond the capability of the patient.

The fracture may be reduced by manipulation, usually in association with a local or general anaesthetic, and the application of a plaster cast or a splint (often called closed reduction). Open reduction may be used, whereby the surgeon operates and fixes the bone fragments together with an internal fixation device such as plates, pins, screws, wires or rods. A third form of reduction is the use of traction. This is the application of force in two directions and needs to be continuous and prolonged. Because the maintenance of traction has major implications on nursing management it is considered in some depth later in this chapter.

Regardless of the method of reduction or type of fracture, the basic principle of care is to allow the re-aligned fragments to re-unite through the process of bone healing. Within 24 hours a blood clot develops at the fracture site and the healing process centres on this clot. Around it cells proliferate and the callus forms. The callus is a complex structure composed of fibrous connective tissue and cartilage. The callus then ossifies and unites the fracture ends together. Finally, the union strengthens and the 'lump' around the fracture site created by the callus is levelled out in a process of remodelling (Fig. 21.2).

Immobilization of the affected part is crucial if the injured bone is to heal and, although the method of immobilization is a medical choice, care of the specific splint, cast or equipment becomes a part of nursing care. The nursing support of the patient in his/her activities of living is determined very often by the form of immobilization used.

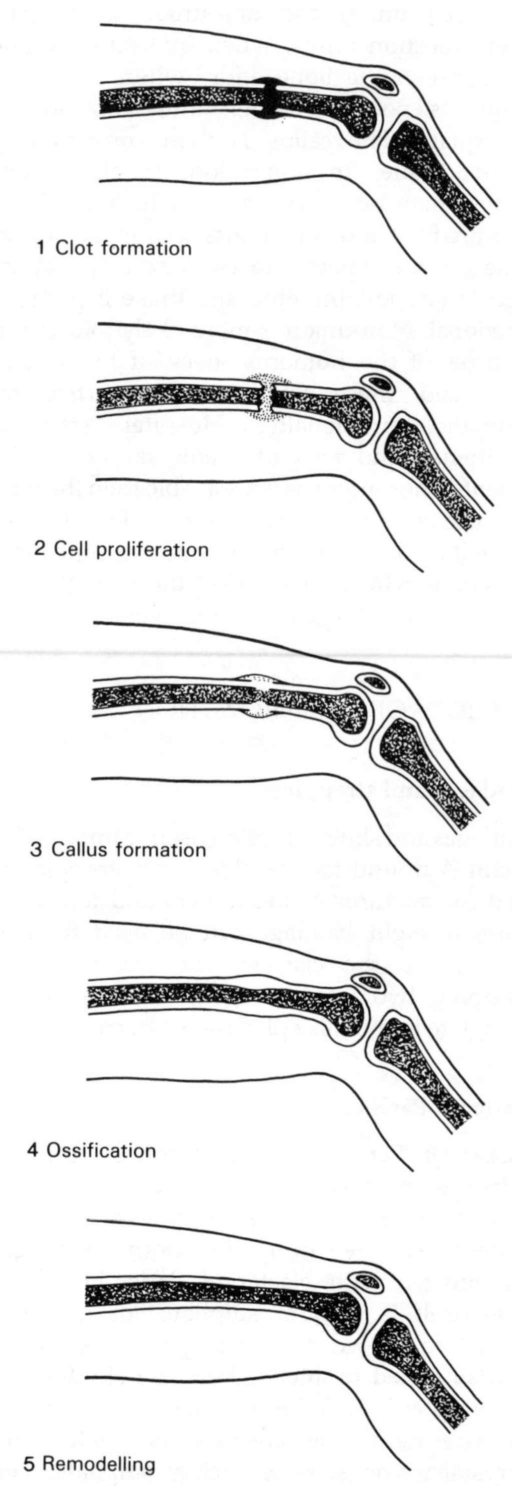

Fig. 21.2 Stages in the healing of bone

Delayed union and non-union may occur when infection arises, when interposed tissue lies between the bone ends, when the blood supply is poor, or when immobilization is inadequate. The callus is then converted to fibrous tissue. In non-union, surgical intervention may be necessary, in which the bone ends are filed and bone grafts are carried out. In some cases callipers, braces or splints may be used to support the limb and make it partially functional. Non-union is more likely to occur in fractures of the humerus, neck of femur and tibia, and these fractures are particularly traumatic emotionally. Hospital stay is lengthened and an end seems far off to the patient. If non-union is irresolvable then the long term use of callipers has the same effect as other disabilities on body image, and the functional limitations which result affect the patient's self concept and feelings of personal worth.

METHODS OF IMMOBILIZATION

Bandages and strapping

Bandages and slings are often used to immobilize fractures around the shoulder, and strapping is used for fractures of the fingers and toes. The figure of eight bandage can be used to treat fractures of the clavicle, for example, and strapping two fingers together is sometimes enough to immobilize phalangeal fractures.

Plaster of Paris casts

Plaster of Paris is the commonest form of splintage and has been widely used since the early 1800s because of its cheapness. Casts are applied in the form of cloth bandages impregnated with plaster of Paris. Plaster of Paris itself is calcium sulphate, or gypsum, reduced to a powder to break up the crystals and then subjected to intense heat to dehydrate it. When water is added to the plaster, the calcium sulphate dehydrate absorbs the water and recrystalizes or 'sets' as calcium sulphate. The result is a rigid cast. Soft wool and tubular stockinette are usually applied around the part before applying the plaster to protect the skin and soft tissue and, in fractures, some form of traction is maintained until the cast is applied and becomes rigid. The plaster bandages are immersed in warm water and then applied as in bandaging. Before drying the surface is smoothed by the hands and moulded into the contours of the part. The skin above and below the plaster is cleaned because any of the remaining splashes may dry and fall down between the skin and cast, causing friction and possible sores. In most patients the cast must remain in position, and effectively immobilize the part, for some time — weeks or months. There are a number of deficiences in plaster of Paris which make this period one of difficulty for the wearer, particularly if he/she is discharged home in the cast and is expected to become mobile whilst wearing it. Fennimore (1979) describes the major deficiencies of plaster of Paris as 'very poor water resistance, poor strength to weight ratio, and slow attainment of load bearing properties'. Plaster of Paris casts are heavy and they take 48 hours to dry before weight-bearing can be attempted. In carrying out the activities of living, patients often find themselves limited. The poor water resistance may mean that outdoor mobility is restricted during bad weather and toileting and bathing are difficult (Lane, 1971). The heaviness of the cast often affects mobility and the 'normal' living processes may be extremely difficult for patients who are treated in accident departments and sent home in a plaster cast.

Nursing care of the patient in a plaster of Paris cast

Drying the cast. For drying to take place evenly, without cracking or weakening, it is essential that the cast is exposed to the circulating air and that it is well supported. Drying usually takes up to 48 hours and any weight bearing or pressure on the cast before it is fully dry will damage it. Casts on the upper limbs should be supported in a sling when the patient is upright and on pillows when sitting or lying down. The patient with a cast on the lower limb should rest it in an elevated position on pillows and must walk with crutches to avoid weight bearing at all costs until the cast is dry. The patient with a full body cast or hip spica should be nursed on a firm mattress and the curves of the cast supported with plastic covered pillows. Even drying demands 2-hourly repositioning to expose the total surface of the cast to the air; this turning requires careful lifting.

Prevention of complications. The two major complications which may occur are the development of pressure sores under the cast and circulatory impairment due to constriction by the cast.

Any complaint of pain under the cast may indicate that a pressure sore is developing and should be reported and action taken. The action may include splitting or 'windowing' the plaster. Patients at home should be advised to contact the hospital or local doctor should pain develop.

Swelling of the parts encased in the plaster is a particular danger within the first 48 hours after injury and may lead to impairment of the circulation, eventually to the point of onset of tissue necrosis. Toes or fingers of the extremities involved should be regularly observed for cyanosis and loss of sensation. If this occurs the limb should be elevated and if this does not lead to restoration of normal skin colour and sensation, this should be reported and action taken as above.

Patients with arm casts should be encouraged to move the fingers and to remove the arm from the sling and exercise the shoulder regularly. Similarly, those with leg casts should move the toes and exercise the hip. Patients in a body cast are susceptible to the further complication of 'cast syndrome' which leads to acute intestinal obstruction and is due to compression of the mesenteric artery.

Finally, stiffness and muscle atrophy may occur in cast wearers. This can be averted by the patient carrying out planned exercises of the involved limb, as well as active exercises of those joints which he/she can move.

Patients discharged home in a cast. Very often, the nurse/patient contact in an out-patient or accident department is brief and takes place whilst the patient is still somewhat shocked and shaken. This situation demands a painstakingly thorough approach to teaching the patient and ensuring he/she has sufficient understanding in detecting possible complications, caring for the cast and carrying out the activities of daily living. Many hospitals issue written instructions about complications and cast care so that the patients have a ready reference source should they forget the verbal instructions. Few hospitals have considered constructing written notes on how patients can carry out the activities of living.

Alternative casting materials

Meredith (1979) states that 'until about five years ago a cast was, by definition, made of plaster. Now, however, there are several new cast materials on the market that provide immobilization and support without some of the discomfort and disadvantages of plaster'. A number of these alternatives are in sporadic use and warrant consideration in individual cases.

- Lightcast is an open weave fibreglass tape impregnated with a light sensitive resin. Exposure to a lamp radiating near-ultraviolet light in a range of 3200–4000 angstroms hardens the cast within approximately three minutes, at which time it is fit for weight bearing.
- Hexcelite consists of rigid rolls of open weave cotton impregnated with a thermoplastic resin. It must be softened with heat before it is applied by immersing each roll in hot (170°F) water until it becomes pliable. The cast hardens as it cools, and is usually weight bearing within fifteen minutes.
- Cutter cast casting tape is a polyester and cotton open weave fabric impregnated with water-activated polyurethane. When it is immersed in cold water a chemical reaction occurs and the cast begins to set. It sets in about seven minutes and is weight bearing within fifteen minutes after setting.
- Crystona is open weave cotton impregnated with a water soluble polymer and a specifically formulated glass. In the presence of water, the glass

releases calcium and aluminium ions at a controlled rate; weight bearing can begin one hour after application.

A number of other alternatives to plaster of Paris exist, all having advantages such as resistance to water once set, lightness of weight and quick drying, but they are all more expensive than plaster of Paris. If nursing assessment should reveal that the patient is likely to face more than the usual difficulties in functional ability, for example the very elderly frail person, then it is sometimes appropriate for the nurse to advise the doctor that plaster of Paris may adversely affect progress.

Splints

A wide range of splints and appliances are available for the treatment of fractures and for the correction of deformity, relief of pain and for the general support of weak joints. Scrutton (1974) suggests that the purpose of splinting can be considered in several ways:

- to replace or supplement the function of bone, muscles, or ligaments
- to correct or maintain alignment or to receive or reduce weight bearing loads
- to improve or to maintain mobility; to improve stability of joints; to prevent or to lessen deformity; and to protect parts of the body.

Kennedy (1974) describes a wide range of splints in detail, and stresses how they must be worn correctly. Nursing management of patients wearing splints therefore aims at their correct use and fitting, as well as the general principles of care of the immobilized.

Traction

Traction is frequently used in fractures of the lower extremities, the spine and the pelvis. It involves the use of a pulling force which overcomes muscle spasm and thus fracture reduction or maintenance is achieved. Traction basically involves:

- a grip and subsequent pull on the body

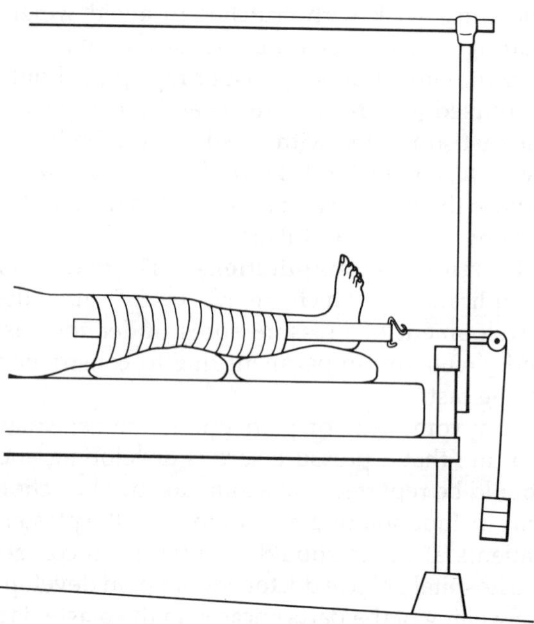

Fig. 21.3 Simple or 'Pugh's' traction

- an opposing pull, or countertraction, of sufficient magnitude to prevent the patient's body moving with the traction pull
- uninterrupted line of pull.

For example, the patient with a fracture of the lower limb may require a type of traction known as Pugh's or simple traction (Fig. 21.3). The extensions fixed to the skin and the cord and weight attached to them represent the grip and pull on the body. The patient's body lying on the bed with the foot elevated pulls against the traction because of gravity and this represents the countertraction. For healing of this fracture to take place, the traction will probably need to be maintained for at least eight weeks.

Traction can be classified both by the way in which it is applied to the skin (i.e. how it 'grips') and by how the pull is exerted.

Skin traction

Skin traction can be applied to the skin through the use of extensions made of spongy rubber, adhesive strapping or plastic materials. The

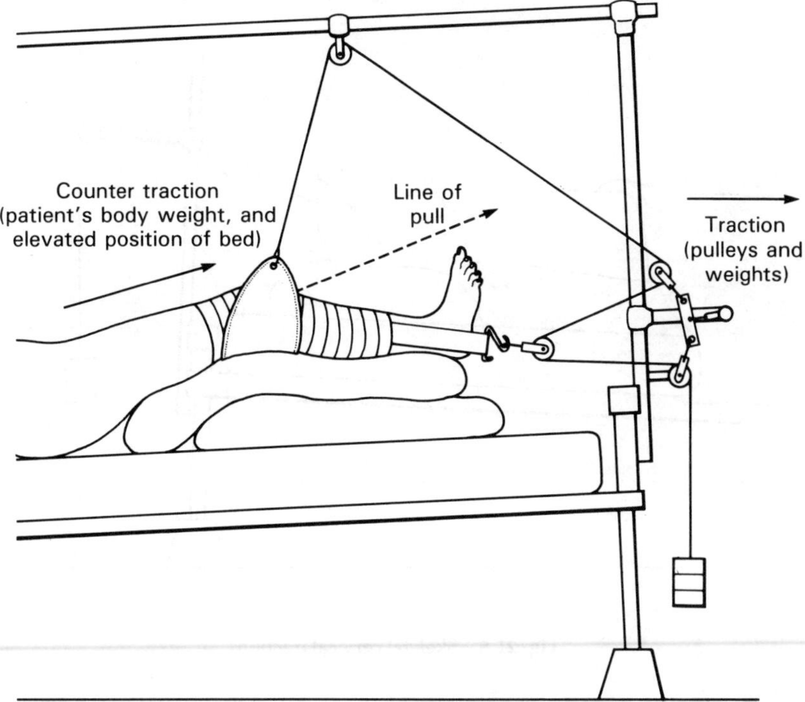

Fig. 21.4 Hamilton-Russell traction

extensions are applied to the skin on either side of the limb, and the material of which they are made is such that they will not slip off when weight is applied. Whilst skin traction is useful in that application is simple, its greatest disadvantage is that only a small amount of weight can be exerted before the extensions become detached from the skin. Adhesive extensions may give rise to allergic reactions and other extensions may place shearing forces on the skin and lead to sores and skin breakdown. Common types of skin traction used are Pugh's traction and Hamilton-Russell traction (Figs. 21.3 and 4).

Skeletal traction

Skeletal traction is applied to the bones via metal pins or wires. These are usually inserted into the bone through a small incision in the skin, using aseptic operative techniques. Skeletal traction is, on the whole, much more stable than skin traction and more pull can be exerted. Its disadvantages stem from the fact that application is invasive and the possibility of infection arises. Common types of skeletal traction are cervical traction and the balanced traction applied for management of a fractured femur using a Thomas splint with a Pearson's extension piece (Figs. 21.5 and 6).

Fixed traction

Fixed traction maintains traction and countertraction between two fixed points and does not depend on gravity. For example, the Thomas splint forms a complete traction unit in itself (Fig. 21.7). Traction is exerted on the leg by the pull of the extensions fixed to the foot of the splint. Countertraction is exerted by the splint ring in the groin.

Balanced traction

Balanced traction maintains traction through the use of weights and pulleys and countertraction

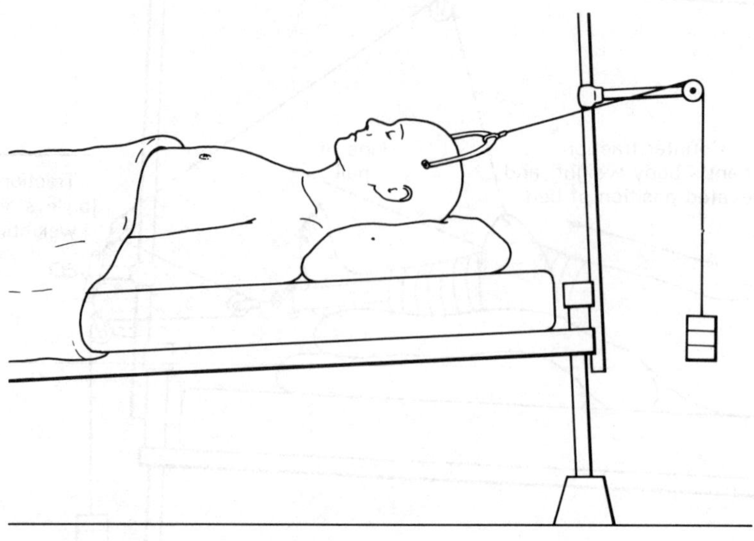

Fig. 21.5 Skeletal cervical traction

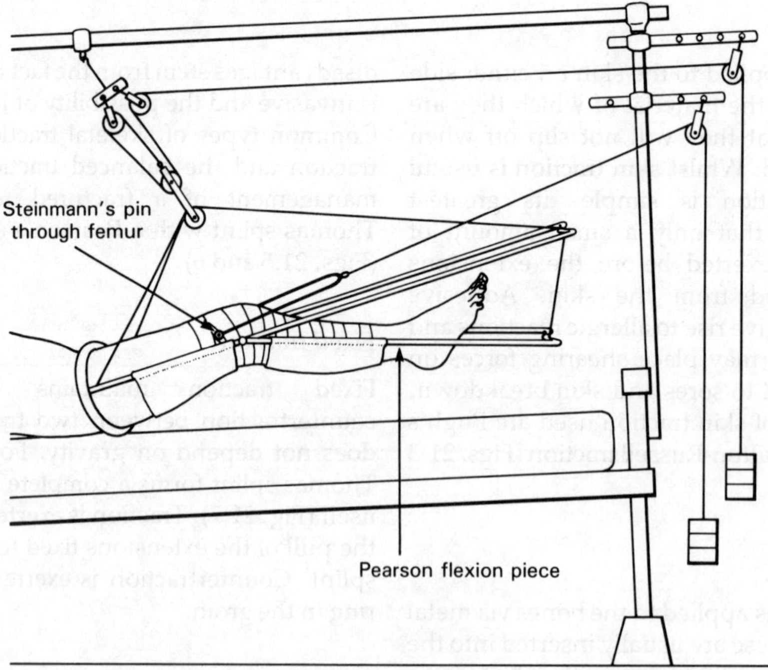

Fig. 21.6 Skeletal traction in Thomas splint, with balanced traction

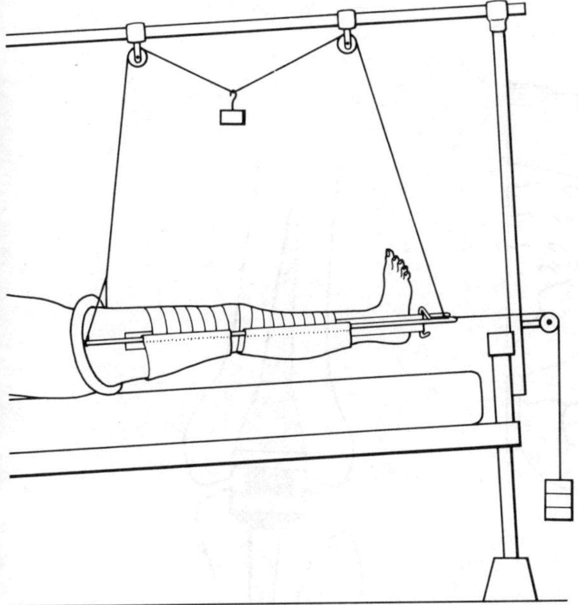

Fig. 21.7 Fixed traction in Thomas splint, with balanced traction

through the body weight and the gravity pull exerted through elevating the foot of the bed. Pugh's traction (Fig. 21.3) is an example of this.

In all forms of traction, suspension methods may be employed to lift the leg off the bed and thus help the patient in the activities of living. As such, suspension does not have direct bearing on the treatment of the fracture itself. For example, the leg in Figure 21.7 is on fixed traction in a Thomas splint. The 'M' suspension arrangement fixed to the splint allows for easy movement and promotes comfort but does not exert any influence on the fixed traction.

Nursing management of the patient in traction

As far as is possible, the overall goals of nursing such patients are to support the activities of living whilst the traction is in position, to ensure that the traction and countertraction are satisfactory, to prevent complications during the process of rehabilitation and to promote independence in the activities of living as far as possible.

Specifically, the traction and countertraction need to be regularly checked. Cords should be in alignment, weights free of obstruction, and the foot of the bed adequately elevated. The enforced immobility related to the traction affects the breathing, eating and drinking and hygiene activities. The risks of pressure sores, venous stasis and thrombosis and muscle atrophy are heightened, and the patient's need for stimulation, creativity and social interaction become important. Generally, pain gradually becomes less of a problem as the patient adapts to being on traction.

PSYCHO-SOCIAL EFFECTS OF TRAUMA

Disturbances in the musculoskeletal system due to trauma cover a wide range of functional disabilities, and there is an even wider range of possible courses of action which may need to be considered. The unifying principle of care for patients with such disturbances is that each individual has experienced trauma to a greater or lesser degree, and the psycho-social effects of this event pose nursing problems equally as important as the physical results. Pashley & Wahlstrom (1981) describe how the victims of trauma and their families experience multiple emotional crises, and how the designation of a primary nurse can work towards overcoming these, through co-ordinating care and follow-up. The incidence of multiple injuries is rising and Pashley & Wahlstrom (1981), in discussing 'polytrauma', assert that nurses caring for such patients 'must have an understanding of the significant impact of trauma on the patient, the patient's family and society'.

DISTURBANCES DUE TO DEGENERATIVE PROCESSES

OSTEOARTHRITIS

Degenerative conditions of the muscles and bones are equally as frequent as traumatic conditions in orthopaedic care. By far the most common of these is degenerative joint disease, commonly referred to as osteoarthritis but more

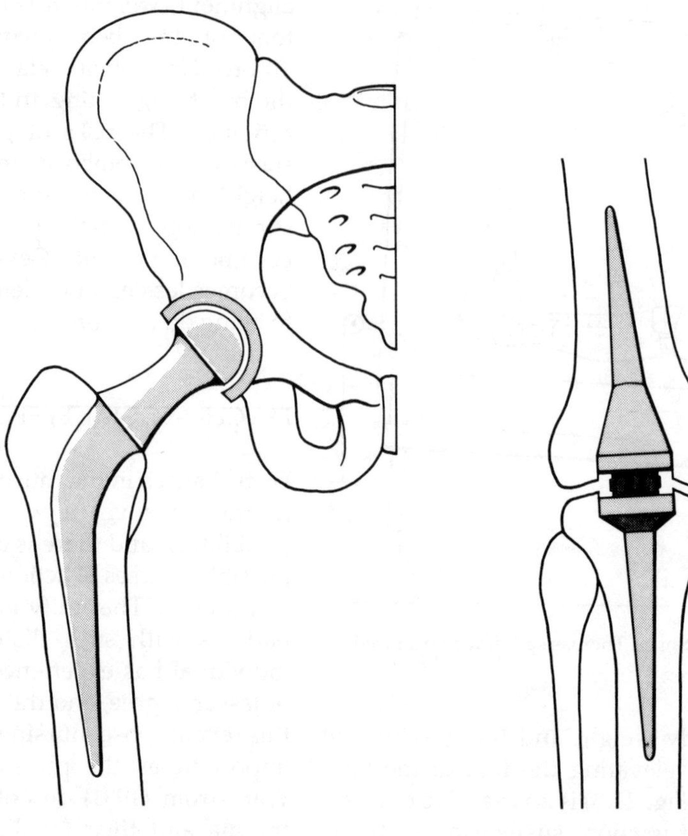

Fig. 21.8 Joint replacement

accurately described as osteoarthrosis. The 'itis' of the former term implies inflammation, whereas the condition is really a degeneration of the articular cartilages in joints, progressing to erosion of the bone ends. Although trauma, excessive joint use and obesity often contribute to osteoarthrosis, it is typically a condition which results from the general wear and tear of living and as such mainly affects those over 60. The hips, knees and spine are most frequently affected and the patient suffers from pain, stiffness and immobility. Medical objectives are concerned with pain relief and maintenance of function. Numerous surgical procedures have been developed, the most effective of which are total joint replacement with prostheses. The hip and knee joints are particularly suitable for replacement and a number of prostheses have evolved (Fig. 21.8).

Prostheses

In general, replacement prostheses are made of inert materials and usually consist of a pseudo ball-and-socket joint for the hip, or a hinge-type joint for the knee. Because a certain degree of rotation also takes place in the knee joints, the earlier pure hinge joints had only a moderate success rate and later prostheses now allow for rotation as well as flexion. The principles of prostheses for both joints are much the same and the following discussion of hip prostheses, by far the most frequent intervention, illustrates these principles.

Adams (1975) states that 'the successful development of total replacement arthroplasty of the hip might well be acclaimed as the most important achievement of the century so far as reconstructive surgery is concerned. It has brought inestimable benefit to countless victims of degenerative and rheumatoid arthritis'. The procedure entails the replacement of the femoral head and the enlarged acetabular lining with a prosthesis (Fig. 21.8). The Journal of the American Medical Association (1982) reported 'numerous' approaches to hip replacement. There are three types of hip replacement in common use:

- the McKee-Farrer prosthesis
- the Charnley prosthesis
- the Ring prosthesis.

All are composed of inert materials, and both the McKee-Farrer and the Charnley rely on the use of methylmethacrylate as a fixative cement. All consist of a femoral component, comprising a stem with a spherical pseudo femoral head, and an acetabular lining shaped like a cup.

The Charnley prosthesis is characterized by a relatively small pseudo femoral head on a stem composed of vitallium, and an acetabular component lined with high density polyethylene. The operative procedure he describes utilizes a lateral approach to the hip joint and requires removal and then re-attachment of the greater trochanter. The femoral head is excised and the acetabular socket enlarged. The stem of the femoral component of the prosthesis is inserted into the medullary canal of the femoral shaft and fixed with methylmethacrylate. The acetabular component of the prosthesis is fixed with the same substance and the removed greater trochanter is re-attached and then held in place with a metal clip (Fig. 21.9). Many modifications have, of course, been made to the classical procedure and removal and re-attachment of the greater trochanter is being used less by surgeons. The characteristically small pseudofemoral head increases the potential risk of dislocation, although it later increases potential joint movement. Thus, some surgeons regard it as necessary to maintain the hip in a position of abduction for a few days postoperatively, varying from 48 hours to 10 days. Occasionally, plaster of Paris hip spicas are applied, whilst a number of surgeons request the use of a triangular abduction frame placed in between the legs or foam rubber moulds in which the legs are placed (Fig. 21.10). The McKee-Farrer prosthesis and the Ring prosthesis are less prone to dislocation because the acetabular component is larger than that of the Charnley prosthesis.

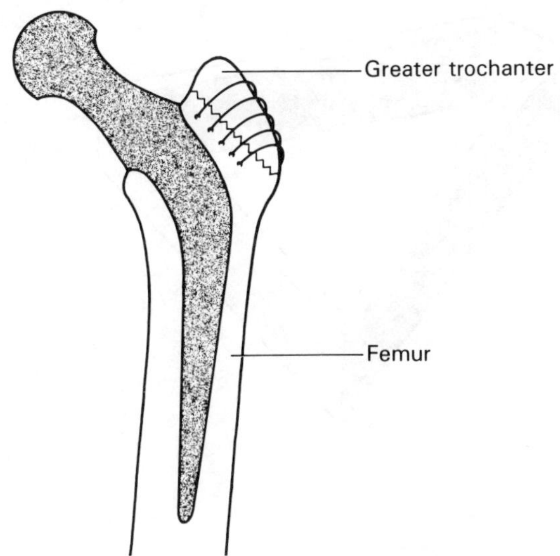

Fig. 21.9 Femoral part of Charnley arthroplasty

Immediately postoperatively, a free running drainage system from the operation site must be maintained for 24–48 hours to prevent the formation of a haematoma. Isometric muscle exercises must commence early after operation to prevent any muscle wasting. The success rate of total joint replacement, especially for the hip, is impressive. A 92% success rate for hip replacements in osteoarthrosis and 85% in rheumatoid arthritis have been reported, and occurrence of complications is low. The greatest benefit appears to be the relief of pain.

Nursing management of patients with osteoarthrosis

Pain relief

Pain is exacerbated by excess activity and regular rest periods help to lessen this, as does the use of splints, collars and pillows. Good posture also serves to reduce pain, and teaching the patient the rudiments of body mechanics and posture is

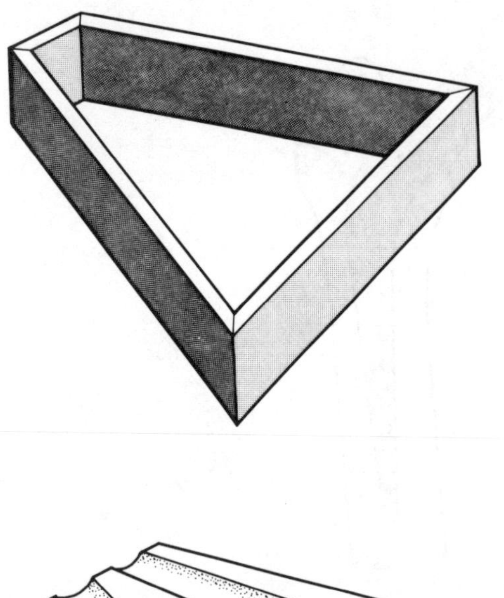

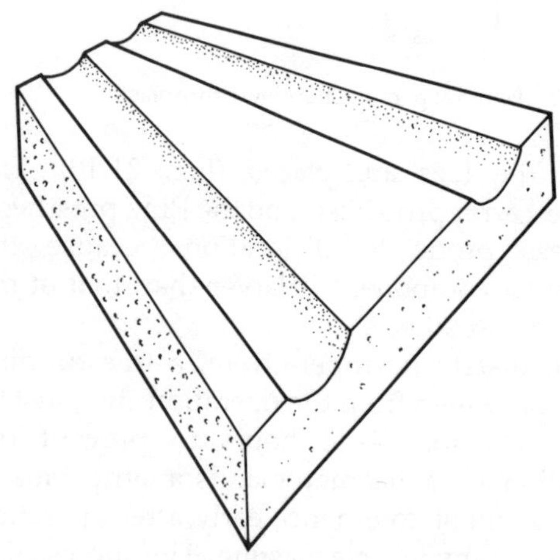

Fig. 21.10 Wooden and foam rubber hip abduction wedges

a helpful nursing intervention. Supporting mobility aids such as walking sticks, crutches etc. reduce the strain of weight bearing on the hips and knees, and may be supplied, and correct usage taught, in conjunction with the physiotherapist. All such aids are initially difficult to use, and the patient requires instruction and supervised practice before assuming correct use. For example, crutches depend on the user assuming a 'tripod' stance i.e. the two crutches and the 'good' leg of the user form a tripod. Following this stance, the user moves using a 'crutch gait' appropriate to the person and the injury.

Stiffness can be lessened, and muscle spasm controlled, by applying heat and cold. Isometric exercises help to preserve muscle tone. Finally, carrying out the medical prescription of analgesics, antispasmodics and other drugs is an important nursing function, especially as the former are often prescribed 'PRN', and thus sensitive assessment and planning is essential.

Prevention of further trauma and deterioration in the joints

The patient may be prepared to accept support in modifying his/her lifestyle and activities to prevent further deterioration. In the obese patient, advice on weight reduction, and the necessary support, may be appropriate, while those who are usually excessively physically active may need to restrict such activities and divert their energies elsewhere.

Maintenance and restoration of joint function

A planned exercise programme devised by the physiotherapist may prevent any further restrictions in function and often improves existing function. Muscular atrophy and flexion deformities are potential problems and these too may be prevented by regular exercise.

Nursing management of patients who have undergone reconstructive surgery of the joints

Pre-operative care

Prior to surgery a multi-disciplinary team including the patient assesses the patient's physical, emotional and social capabilities. This creates a framework for the setting of future goals with the patient. An explanation of the operation itself and the expected pain has had observable effects on pain reduction (Hayward, 1975). Pre-operative preparation also includes intensive active physiotherapy and instruction in the re-mobilization regime for the period following the operation. Because of the increased risk of severe infection involved with bone surgery, some surgeons advocate elaborate skin preparation 24–48 hours before the operation and prescribe an 'antibiotic cover' for the peri-operative period.

Postoperative care

After surgery, specific management relates to positioning of the joint and re-mobilization. For example, hip replacement may demand that the hip is abducted and externally rotated in the early postoperative days. Postoperative care principles are notoriously variable according to individual medical beliefs, but the general principles discussed earlier in rehabilitation are generally applicable. Early mobilization is increasingly becoming the norm to avert the danger of thrombophlebitis, pulmonary embolism and dislocation of the joint.

OTHER DEGENERATIVE CONDITIONS

A number of degenerative processes in bone give rise to symptoms, functional disability and pathological fractures.

Osteoporosis

This is a condition in which decreased density of the bone is found, thought to arise out of hormonal disturbances. These disturbances relate to:

- age
- hyperthyroidism
- Cushing's syndrome
- hypogonadism
- myelomatosis
- metastatic carcinoma
- drugs such as corticosteroids
- immobility (Stevenson & Whitehead, 1982).

The resulting brittle bones are susceptible to fractures and collapse, presenting particularly as Colles fractures, femoral neck fractures and collapse of the vertebrae (Frost, 1981). Various medical approaches to the condition are described. The use of oestrogen in post-menopausal osteoporosis has little evidence to support it as a treatment, but has been found to be effective as a prophylactic measure (Lyndsay et al, 1980). Calcium has been found to minimize bone loss and has few side effects, but it is questionable whether or not vitamin D has any value although vitamin D deficiency must be resolved. Jowsey et al (1972) record increases in bone density when combined doses of calcium fluoride and vitamin D are given. Calcitonin levels are known to decline with age (Deftos et al, 1980) and deficiencies in post-menopausal women are notable. Zanzi et al (1981) found that 'prolonged calcitonin administration increases bone mass in post menopausal osteoporosis', and it is becoming a popular medical regime.

The brittle bones arising in osteoporosis are susceptible to fractures and collapse. Immobilization can lead to osteoporosis, as can a deficiency of calcium or protein in the diet. Various medical approaches to the condition are described, and nursing management focuses on the maintenance of physical activity to prevent further decreases in the mass of bone tissue, as well as the application of the general principles of orthopaedic nursing care, and principles specific to any functional disability present.

Osteomalacia

Osteomalacia is weakening in bone strength due to a disturbance in the metabolism of calcium and phosphorus caused by vitamin D deficiency. Nursing care supports the medical regime of dietary control, or the correction of malabsorption syndromes if they are found to be the cause, as well as the application of the principles of rehabilitation. Paget's disease is both a thickening of the bulk of bone tissue and a weakening in its strength, and no specific medical treatment is yet available although calcitonin may afford some pain relief. The large bones tend to bow, there is often gross physical deformity, and general deterioration in the cardiovascular, respiratory and nervous systems may develop. Specific nursing management is largely related to psycho-social support.

Other disorders

A number of other degenerative processes are becoming common and relate to specific structures. For example, Dupuytren's contracture is a common deformity caused by

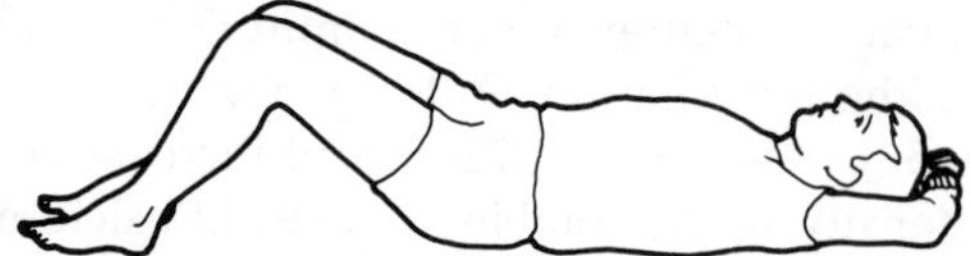

1 Lie flat on back with knees bent and tighten abdominal muscles and buttocks to press small of back into the floor

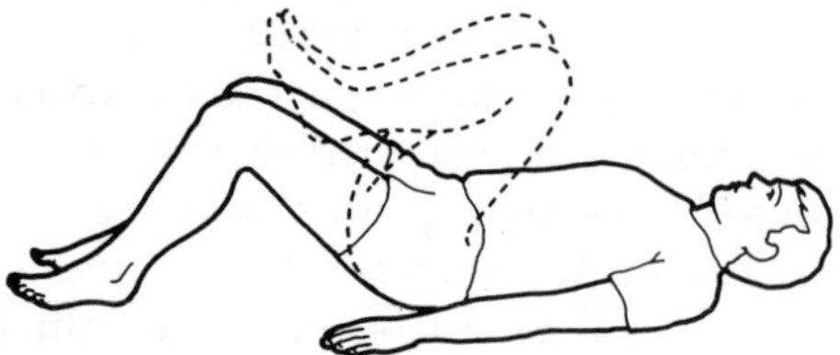

2 Lift legs to chest (a) alternately
(b) together

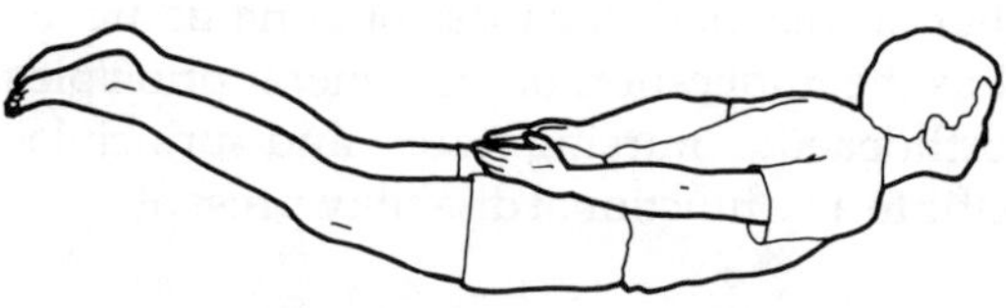

3 Lie on stomach, and raise head and feet together to extend spine

Fig. 21.11 Back extension exercises

contracture of the palma fascia of the palm of the hand leading to flexion of the fingers. Medical management usually involves operative correction and nursing supports this.

Low back pain is an even more common problem, particularly in Western societies, and is generally due to the degeneration in the spine caused by wear and tear. Whilst traction and the use of plaster casts may be prescribed by the doctor, the eventual goal of care is to improve the elasticity of the back muscles and to prevent muscle spasm. Symptomatic medical treatment is supported by the teaching of good posture and simple exercises (Fig. 21.11).

Although many of the degenerative conditions can be partially improved through medical treatment, many patients face the prospect of having to tolerate the condition and the possibility of some further deterioration. An acceptance of this by the patient and motivation to reach his/her full potential with these limitations are often the major goals of nursing.

DISTURBANCES DUE TO INFLAMMATORY PROCESSES

Such disturbances can be broadly divided into those which present as inflammation due to injury, strain, or unknown causes, and those which arise because of infection.

RHEUMATOID ARTHRITIS

Rheumatoid arthritis is idiopathic — that is, its causes as yet are not fully understood. It is, however, one of the most debilitating conditions in orthopaedics and its incidence is widespread. The condition can be defined as a chronic, non-bacterial inflammation of joints, often associated with mild constitutional symptoms. It affects both men and women, predominantly the latter, with a ratio of approximately three women to one man. Various theories of causation are advanced. Some postulate that the disease is one of a group of diseases caused by prolonged or severe stress, and the influence of this on hormone secretion and the immune system. Much research suggests that the disease has its origins in a disorder of autoimmunity (Williams et al, 1979). The characteristic presence of abnormal antibodies in the blood of patients suffering from the disease (rheumatoid factor) in some ways supports this theory. Ziff (1971) states that the proposal of an autoimmune response based on genetic susceptibility as the cause has not been adequately demonstrated and suggests that an immunological response initiated by an exogenous agent is worthy of serious consideration. In particular, he cites findings of various studies which would support the theory that the exogenous agent giving rise to the immunological response is a virus. In recent years, the suspicion that the cause may be viral has become more generally accepted (Ginsberg, 1977). There is thus evidence to support infection, autoimmune disorder and stress as the causes of the disease (Kean & Buchanan, 1983). It remains the task of those involved in research into the aetiology of rheumatoid arthritis to identify the major cause.

Symptoms

In this condition, the synovial joints become grossly swollen, painful and stiff. The fingers and upper limbs and the knees are often the most severely affected, and general systemic symptoms are associated with this localized pain. The joints become progressively destroyed and gross deformity is common.

Medical management

Medical management utilizes a wide range of drug therapies and surgical intervention. Drugs used in the treatment of rheumatoid arthritis can be loosely grouped into the categories of analgesics, anti-inflammatory agents and corticosteroids. Aspirin, phenylbutazone, indomethacin, ibuprofen, flufenamic acid, gold, penicillamine, chloroquine and a vast and increasing array of related drugs are frequently used as analgesics and anti-inflammatory drugs. Some of these, e.g. phenylbutazones, have been found to have diverse side-effects and are being withdrawn. The use of corticosteroids is controversial and becoming less acceptable, although they are still undergoing trials. In severe episodes they give rapid relief from symptoms. Intra-articular injection of corticosteroids produces worthwhile relief, but their many disadvantages restrict their use (Chandler & Wright, 1958; Stevens, 1982).

No drug seems to be effective for all patients, and many are excessively toxic. Wright & Amos (1980) report that no evidence exists to suggest that drug therapy can do more than temporarily reduce the rate of the progression of the disease.

Nursing care

Specific nursing management aims at the prevention of crippling deformities, pain relief, rehabilitation and pyscho-social adjustment for the patient and the family. In the acute stages the joints need supporting in splints or casts, and a programme of passive exercises is important to prevent the muscular spasm and atrophy, as well as joint stiffness. A rapid resumption of normal daily living is desirable and, once the acute phase is lessening, the occupational therapist may be consulted for help in assessing the need for, and supplying, aids to daily living.

Pain relief centres on a range of drugs discussed earlier which are often potentially toxic. An awareness of, and observation for, side-effects is important in nursing care. Discrete structures within the system may become inflamed, such as the synovial membrane in joints and tendons. Specific nursing management usually focuses on pain relief through support, hot and cold applications and exercise.

Many patients face major psychological and social adjustments and understanding, patience and an open honest approach are fundamental to effective care. Because the progress of the condition is long term, community nurses are integrally involved and the whole team becomes vitally important in future management. A major lifestyle change is usually demanded of the patient and too much help and support can never be given. The educative and supporting role of the nurse comes to the fore for such patients, and a systematic individually planned teaching programme related to the achievement of relative independency must be incorporated into the nursing care plan.

INFECTIONS

Infections in the system may affect the bone, the joints, or soft tissue. Tuberculosis may affect all of these structures, but fortunately this condition responds to anti-tubercular treatment. In some cases long periods of immobilization are required and the general principles of care of the immobilized patient are applicable.

Osteomyelitis is an infection of the bone, usually caused by *Staphylococcus aureus.* Patients suffer the symptoms associated with acute systemic infections and are acutely ill. The bone involved is usually a long bone and an abscess develops, with consequent breakdown of bone tissue. Usually a disease of youth and childhood, early detection of the condition is sometimes masked by a suspicion of generalized infection. Medical management includes antibiotics and often the abscess is drained operatively. Patients experience very acute pain and the discharge from the abscess is sometimes foul smelling. Nursing management supports the prescribed immobilization of the body. As the wound itself is very painful, the dressing technique needs to be gentle and appropriate analgesia should be given an effective time before it is carried out. Good air fresheners help to reduce the smell which may be a cause of embarrassment to the patient. Immobilization of young people limits their opportunities for adventure and stimulation and a creative, informal atmosphere with diversional activities may help to lessen their frustration.

CONGENITAL ABNORMALITIES

A number of deformities are present at birth, for example congenital dislocation of the hip, curvatures of the spine and extra digits on the feet or hands. Many foot deformities, such as flatfeet or hammer toe, are also congenital. Nursing management depends on the medical approaches and corrective surgery is often carried out. More gross deformities, such as dislocation of the hips, necessitates the application of bulky casts and repeated re-admissions. Parents of such children require both sensitive teaching in the care of the child and prolonged support to help them to cope with the problems of care over a long period. Sometimes the obvious deformity is distressing to parents and the nurse can help them to overcome their feelings either by listening and reassuring, or by referral to other members of the team. The enormous burden on the parents of children with cystic fibrosis found in a study by Harrison (1977) is similar to that borne by parents of children with congenital deformities.

DISTURBANCES DUE TO MALIGNANCY

Malignancy in the bone tissue is a particularly serious condition and the prognosis is often poor. As in all malignant diseases, much psycho-social support is needed and pain relief is a major goal. The bone pain present is particularly severe.

CONCLUSION

Nursing patients with disturbances of the musculoskeletal system demands both skill and creativity. It is a field which relies heavily on expert therapeutic nursing and the efforts of the multi-disciplinary team. Nursing itself incorporates an almost unique amalgam of knowledge including physics, anatomy, physiology and functional activity. A serious application of such a body of knowledge through the nursing process, based on the principles of rehabilitation, makes a crucial contribution to patient recovery and is therapeutic in itself, rather than simply a supporting activity to the medical and paramedical contributions.

Acknowledgement

Grateful thanks are expressed to Anne Footner, Nuffield Orthopaedic Centre, Oxford for Figures 21.1-6, 21.8, 21.10 and 21.11.

REFERENCES

Adams J C 1975 Standard orthopaedic operations. Churchill Livingstone, Edinburgh

Agris J, Spira M 1979 Pressure ulcers: prevention and treatment. Clinical Symposia 31(95):1–32

Alderman C 1983 Individual care in action. Nursing Times 79(3): 15–17

Alfano G J 1969 A professional approach to nursing practice. Nursing Clinics of North America 4(3):487–494

Alfano G J 1971 Healing or caretaking — which will it be? Nursing Clinics of North America 6(2):237–280

Brunner L S, Suddarth D S 1984 Textbook of medical surgical nursing. Lippincott, Philadelphia

Chandler G N, Wright V 1958 Deleterious effect of intra-articular hydrocortisone. Lancet 2:661–663

Cooney T C, Reuler J B 1983 Protecting the elderly patient from pressure sores. Geriatrics 38(2):125–134

Deftos L J, Weisman M H, Williams G W, Karpf D B, Frumar A M, Davidson B J, Parthemore J G, Judd H L 1980 Influence of age and sex on plasma calcitonin in human beings. New England Journal of Medicine 302(24):1351–1353

Dinsdale S M 1974 Decubitus ulcers:role of pressure and

friction in causation. Archives of Physical Medical Rehabilitation 55: 147–152
Elhart D 1978 Scientific principles in nursing, 8th edn. CV Mosby, St Louis
Fennimore J 1979 Development and laboratory evaluation of Crystona. In: Symposium on a new strength, water resistant splinting system. Smith and Nephew, Welwyn Garden City
Frost H M 1981 Clinical management of the symptomatic osteoporotic patient. The Orthopaedic Clinics of North America 12(3):671–682
Geis H J 1972 The problem of personal worth in the physically disabled patient. Rehabilitation Literature 33:34–39
Ginsberg I 1977 Can chronic and self perpetuating arthritis in the human be caused by arthrotrophic undegraded microbial cell wall constituents? A working hypothesis. Rheumatology and Rehabilitation 16:141–149
Goffman E 1963 Stigma. Penguin, Harmondsworth
Goldstone L A, Roberts B V 1980 A preliminary discriminant function analysis of elderly orthopaedic patients who will or will not contract a pressure sore. International Journal of Nursing Studies 17:17–23
Guyton A C 1974 Function of the human body, 3rd edn. W B Saunders, Philadelphia
Hall L E, Alsand G J, Rifkin E, Levine H F 1975 Longitudinal effects of an experimental nursing process. Loeb Center for Nursing, New York
Harrison S 1977 Families in stress. Royal College of Nursing, London
Hayward J 1975 Information — a prescription against pain. Royal College of Nursing, London
Johnson J E, Rice V H 1974 Sensory and distress components of pain. Nursing Research 23:203–209
Jowsey J, Rigg B L, Kelly P J 1972 Effect of combined therapy with sodium fluoride, vitamin D and calcium in osteoporosis. American Journal of Medicine 53:43–49
Journal of the Americal Medical Association 1982 Consensus Conferences — Total hip-joint replacement in the United States. Journal of the American Medical Association 248(5):1818–1821
Judson R 1983 Pressure sores. Medical Journal of Australia 9: 417–422
Kean W F, Buchanan W W 1983 Rheumatoid arthritis. Some personal considerations on aetiology and treatment Part 1. British Journal of Clinical Practice 37(1):4–15
Keele K D 1972 Pain: how it varies from person to person. Nursing Times 68:890–892
Kennedy J M 1974 Orthopaedic splints and appliances. Bailliere Tindall, London
Kosiak M, Kubicek W G, Olson M, Danz J M, Kottke F J 1958 Evaluation of pressure as a factor in the production of ischaemic ulcers. Archives of Physical Medicine and Rehabilitation 39: 623–629
Lane P A 1971 A mother's confession — home care of a toddler in a spica cast — what it's really like. American Journal of Nursing 71:2141–2143
Lynch J J 1978 The simple act of touching. Nursing (Horsham) 8(6):32–36
Lyndsay R, Hart D M, Forrest C, Baird C 1980 Prevention of spinal osteoporosis in oophorectomised women. Lancet 2:1151– 1153
Meredith S 1979 Preparing your patient to live with his cast. R.N. 42(7):34–43
Miller E J, Gwynne G V 1974 A life apart. Tavistock, London
Murray M 1976 Fundamentals of nursing. Prentice Hall, New Jersey
Norton D, McLaren R, Exton-Smith A N 1962, reprinted 1975 An investigation of geriatric nursing problems in hospital. Churchill Livingstone, Edinburgh
Nursing Update 1971 For that you use ice ... or is it heat? Nursing Update 2(1):11–15
Olsen E V 1967 The hazards to immobility. American Journal of Nursing 67(4):780–796
Orem D 1980 Nursing: concepts of practice. McGraw-Hill, New York
Pashley J, Wahlstrom M L 1981 Polytrauma — the patient, the family, the nurse, and the health team. Nursing Clinics of North America 16(4):721–727
Pearson A 1981 A study examining the effects of preparation and a new casting material on patients wearing a below knee cast. Unpublished MSc Thesis, University of Manchester
Pearson A 1983 The clinical nursing unit. Heinemann Medical, London
Punton S 1983 The struggle for independence. Nursing Times 79(9):29–32
Reichel S M 1958 Shearing force as a factor in decubitus ulcers in paraplegics. Journal of the American Medical Association 166:762–763
Roper N, Logan W, Tierney A 1980 The elements of nursing. Churchill Livingstone, Edinburgh
Scrutton D 1974 Orthopaedic splints and appliances. Nursing Mirror 139(18):73–75
Stevens M B 1982 Rheumatoid arthritis VI: Corticosteroid therapy. Maryland State Medical Journal 31(10):31–33
Stevenson J C, Whitehead M I 1982 Postmenopausal osteoporosis. British Medical Journal 285:585–588
Williams B D, Lockwood C M, Russell B A, Cotton C 1979 Defective reticulo-endothelial system function in rheumatoid arthritis. Lancet 1:1311–1314
Wright V, Amos R 1980 Do drugs change the course of rheumatoid arthritis? British Medical Journal 280:964–966
Zanzi I et al 1981 In:Cohn D V, Talmage R G, Matthews J L (eds) Endocrine control of bone and calcium metabolism. International Conference Proceedings, Amsterdam. Excerpta Medical
Ziff 1971 Viruses and the connective tissue diseases. Annals of Internal Medicine 75:951–958

22

Disturbances of physical and chemical transport mechanisms

INTRODUCTION

All functions of the human body are dependent upon an efficient transport system whereby nutrients are supplied to all tissues, waste products of metabolism are removed for disposal and hormonal influences are transmitted.

Effectively the mechanisms of the transport system comprise:

- the pump — the heart
- the transporting substances — blood, lymph, tissue fluid
- transport tubes — arteries, veins, lymph ducts
- systems of interchange within tissues — capillary networks,
- sinusoids.

Other systems of the body are involved in transporting substances, but only within the particular system, e.g. gastrointestinal, respiratory, and genitourinary systems. They are not concerned with tissue nutrition and excretion in general and are therefore not the focus of this chapter.

This chapter is concerned with exploring the effect of disturbances of the major transporting network, the cardiovascular system. Due to the nature of the system, disturbances may be either general — as in pump failure or inadequacy of nutrient intake — or local as in restriction of flow to or from a body part.

The material in this chapter is examined in the following order:

- Disturbances of the transporting substances
- Disturbances of the flow within the vessels and heart
- Disturbances of the pump mechanism or efficiency.

The most common disease of the heart — coronary heart disease — is therefore discussed within the section on vessels. This allows commonality of cause and effect in respect of all arterial disruption to be emphasized and principles of management to be drawn out more clearly.

The widespread nature of disorders of transporting mechanisms, the specific nature of some of the diseases and the increasing life expectancy within Western societies, results in diseases discussed in this chapter being particularly prevalent. Where data is available, incidence will be indicated and discussed. Some disorders that are predominant in our so called 'developed' society — coronary heart disease being the obvious example — appear to be related to lifestyle patterns. Others, such as rheumatic fever and consequently rheumatic heart valve disease appear to be related to the increasing urbanization and poor housing conditions in the 'developing' countries. The message of some of these class and ethnic differences in disease incidence is clearly political. However, the focus of the chapter is on the nature of the disease, the effect on the person and on health promoting and screening measures, on care during illness and on rehabilitative and educative programmes. There is no assumption that the person with a particular disorder will be in hospital. Indeed, the majority of persons with hypertension, coronary heart disease, a degree of heart failure or anaemia will be coping with their usual lifestyle or one adapted to their reduced capacity. For those persons the fact of their disorder, the regular visit to their family doctor for a check up or a repeat prescription and the intermittent visit to, or stay in, hospital for reassessment, adjustment of therapy or treatment during an acute phase, will become a part of their lives.

There are few disorders of transport mechanisms that are transient and curable. Most are controllable, many gradually and permanently reduce the health state of the person and result in varying levels of disability. If nursing is to enhance, rather than diminish, the person's ability to cope with their incapacity, the nurse must take cognisance of their current perceptions and beliefs about their illness, their previous experience of health care — health centre, hospital or alternative form — and of ways that they have found of coping with activities of daily living. The person who is the patient and others important to him or her then become central to any plan of care the nurse may develop (with the exception perhaps of an acute crisis). The care given is then more likely to meet the expressed needs of the person.

Finally, the nature of the problems with which patients with cardiovascular disease present, create dilemmas for nursing and medical staff of an ethical nature — those inherent in health education, those of resuscitation, continuance of active medical treatment when prognosis is poor, medical intervention versus lifestlye change, and so on. It is not the intention in this chapter to discuss these dilemmas, simply at this point to identify that dilemmas exist and should be recognized and considered as such.

ASSESSMENT OF CARDIOVASCULAR AND HAEMATOLOGICAL FUNCTION

THE NURSE'S ROLE IN ASSESSMENT

Persons presenting with symptoms suggestive of cardiovascular or haematological disturbance will be assessed in a number of ways ranging from fundamental history-taking and observation through to the most technologically advanced investigation. The individual person, the patient, will experience them all. The doctor will undertake some aspects and will order other investigations. The nurse has a primary responsibility for ongoing 'routine' monitoring of cardiovascular function including that of response to drug therapy, to increasing or decreasing activity levels, to dietary changes and so on. In addition the nurse both prepares a patient for certain investigations and is involved in care during and after such investigations. In summary, the nurse's function in relation to a person's cardiovascular and haematological status can be seen to include:

- Accurate monitoring of function, in particular:
  - level of awareness, alertness, consistency of conscious level
  - pulse(s), apex beat, blood pressure, colour and warmth of skin and membranes
  - respiratory rate and pattern, particularly related to activity level, presence of cough, sputum
  - presence of pain and in relation to rest and activity pattern.

Clearly other functions may be involved, for example appetite, but the four listed are of fundamental importance to the assessment of cardiovascular and haematological state.

- preparation of the patient for an investigation, care of the patient during and after the procedure. This will involve:
  - knowledge of the procedure itself, its purpose and what it is likely to feel like
  - understanding the principles underlying the investigation and ensuring, in the preparation and organization, that essential requirements are met
  - understanding or anticipating the specific patient's fears, anxieties and needs in relation to physical care and support
  - understanding the potential problems and complications of the procedure in order to institute preventive care and a rational programme of observation and monitoring
  - on the basis of the above, instituting and co-ordinating a plan of care to ensure that the patient's need for knowledge and understanding of the procedure, for physical preparation and for support is met, and that complications are prevented if at all possible and identified early if they occur.

In this section only those techniques requiring special instrumentation are described, including blood pressure recording. Aspects of assessment indicative of diagnosis and progress are included in the relevant sections of the chapter.

BLOOD PRESSURE

Recording a person's blood pressure is regarded as a routine observation. The implications for that person if the recording reveals hypertension, however, are considerable in that 'hypertension' is diagnosed on blood pressure recordings alone. Indeed the condition is often asymptomatic, in spite of carrying a considerably increased morbidity and mortality if not treated (see section on hypertension). Thus a diagnosis and treatment decision might be made primarily on the blood pressure recording.

In spite of its importance, recording of blood pressure is generally found to be improperly undertaken (Thompson DR, 1981). With care it can give systolic and diastolic recordings within 4mmHg of intra-arterial pressure (Holland & Humerfelt, 1964).

Blood pressure is recorded by exerting a measured pressure on an artery. Sounds, assumed to relate in some way to changes in blood flow or resultant vibrations in surrounding tissues, are identified by means of a stethoscope placed over the artery distal to the regulated pressure. The sounds were first described by Korotkoff and take his name. They consist of:

- Phase 1 Clear tapping 'systolic'
- Phase 2 Softening
- Phase 3 Return of sharper sound
- Phase 4 Abrupt muffling 'diastolic 4'
- Phase 5 Disappearance 'diastolic 5'

There is considerable debate as to whether 4 or 5 are recorded as the diastolic pressure (O'Brien & O'Malley, 1981a). Traditionally UK practitioners have used 4, whereas USA practitioners have used 5. There may indeed be as little as 5 mmHg between the two but in high cardiac output states the difference is much greater, and sometimes the sound may not disappear at all — hence the UK's traditional use of 4. Most research work appears to use 5. Both O'Brien & O'Malley (1981a) and Thompson DR (1981) suggest recording all three significant points — 1, 4 and 5. If any two of the three are being used, the sound not recorded should be indicated '—' in the appropriate slot. Thus a typical recording might read 130/85/75 or 130/—/75.

'Normal' blood pressure is immensely variable on a minute to minute basis. It is all the more important therefore that the conditions in which blood pressure is recorded are as stable and relaxing as possible (unless measures of exercise tolerance or stress are being made). The definition of 'hypertension' is discussed elsewhere. Sufficient to say here that the diagnosis of hypertension would not be made on a single recording.

There is no clear definition of hypotension, as the significance of a blood pressure level can only be assessed reliably in the knowledge of previous levels and in relation to the person's current health state. Thus a person admitted to hospital showing clinical signs of shock but with a blood pressure of, say, 130/90 may well have had pressures far exceeding this prior to his admission. Conversely, a person with blood pressure of 95/60 may be perfectly healthy.

Errors in blood pressure recording

Errors in recording patients' blood pressure may arise from each aspect of the recording:

- the observer
- the patient
- the apparatus
- the technique.

The observer

Clearly the observer's hearing will affect the accuracy of recordings. However, there are a number of less obvious sources of error. The distance of the observer both from the sphygmomanometer and above or below the level of the meniscus can result in either high or low recordings. Nurses frequently demonstrate a preference for the terminal digits of '0' and '5' (Choi et al, 1978) thus over- or underestimating pressures. An observer who is in a hurry will decompress too quickly or make other technical errors. Finally, observers have been known to demonstrate patient bias, for example, favourably in the case of young men, unfavourably if a patient is obese (O'Brien & O'Malley, 1981b). Additionally, bias has been shown to occur if a particular value is believed to differentiate between normal and abnormal states — the unfavourable value being avoided (Oldham et al, 1960). Doctors' recordings have also been found to be higher than those of nurses (Richardson & Robinson, 1971).

The patient

Blood pressure demonstrates enormous variation — through the lifespan; during naturally occuring cycles, e.g. menstrual cycle, diurnal cycle; and during wakefulness, varying with physical activity, mental or emotional stimulation, food, drink, cigarette smoking and so on. Continuous recording intra-arterially in a normal subject demonstrated variation during the day from 120–160 mmHg systolic and 85–118 mmHg diastolic(5) (O'Brien & O'Malley, 1981e). Control of those factors amenable to immediate regulation, i.e. activity, ingestion of food or drink (particularly alcoholic or stimulant beverages such as tea or coffee), smoking and a degree of stress within the half hour prior to recording, is particularly important if a high degree of accuracy is required. For example, if the person has a full bladder this not only creates stress but also raises intra-abdominal pressure, thus raising the blood pressure.

Not only does general activity affect blood pressure but the muscle tension in the arm from which the recording is being made also affects the pressure. An unsupported arm is effectively in a state of isometric exercise and this may raise the diastolic pressure by as much as 10 mmHg (Thompson D R, 1981). This effect is greater in persons who are hypertensive and those who are taking adrenergic-blocking agents (O'Brien & O'Malley, 1981c).

There may be pressure differences between

the right and left arm. Normally these are slight. However, they may be considerably more than 10 mmHg, thus providing a source of apparent variation if different arms are used for successive recordings. In situations where this is found to be so, recording from an agreed arm is important, normally the arm presenting the highest pressure.

Normally there is no significant difference in the blood pressure lying supine, sitting or standing. However, persons receiving anti-hypertensive therapy may well demonstrate a marked drop when moving from lying to standing. In this situation, both values need to be recorded.

If the patient is obese, a cuff with a larger bladder will need to be used in order to achieve even decompression. This is important, as a cuff that is too small will result in high readings (O'Brien & O'Malley, 1981d). While hypertension is more likely in obese patients, overestimating the blood pressure may result in treating patients unnecessarily or too vigorously.

The irregularity of pulse waves in persons with atrial fibrillation suggests accuracy should be achieved by taking the mean of three successive blood pressure recordings.

The apparatus

A number of sphygmomanometers are available but the mercury type is the most commonly used and, if maintained properly, the most accurate. However, surveys of those in hospital use demonstrate about 50% to be inaccurate (Conceicao et al, 1976; North, 1979). Functionally, the top of the meniscus of the mercury should be at zero prior to use and the manometer glass should be clean of mercury. O'Brien & O'Malley (1981d) recommend annual checking and cleaning.

Aneroid sphygmomanometers have been found to be less accurate, 30–35% having a deviation of some 3 mmHg and 6–13% of some 7 mmHg or more.

A major source of problems is the tubing, cuffs and pump bulbs. Clearly those should be free of leaks, i.e. capable of maintaining a pressure within 3 mmHg over a 5 minute period, and be capable of a slow controlled release of air. Blocking of the air vent of the bulb by fluff creates a stiff bulb and is easily rectified. Tubing can be replaced. Whilst velcro fastening appears to be taking over from the tuck-in cuff, it is likely to become inefficient over time and should then be discarded.

The size of the bladder in the cuff in relation to the patient's arm size is an important issue. Readings from bladders that completely encircle the arm correlate best with intra-arterial pressures (O'Brien & O'Malley, 1981c). If the bladder is too short or too narrow in relation to the arm, readings will be falsely high. This can create ongoing inaccuracies in relation to obese patients which could potentially lead to inappropriate treatment. Conversely, a bladder that is too large will give falsely low readings. O'Brien & O'Malley (1981d) recommend that the bladder width be not less than 40% of the circumference of the arm. The length of the bladder should encircle the arm, but failing that the centre of the bladder should be placed over the artery being occluded.

Some apparatus has been developed for self-monitoring of blood pressure. At the moment no model appears to be very satisfactory but it is likely that compact and reliable instruments will emerge for home and ambulatory monitoring. The possible effect that anxiety in relation to self-monitoring might have on blood pressure level needs to be considered in recommending self monitoring.

The technique

Some aspects related to technique have already been mentioned within the previous sections. These will be indicated here, but not further discussed. Aspects totally related to technique will be explained further.

Errors may arise from the patient's immediate state. These have been discussed. It is clear that the patient should be as relaxed as possible and have the arm supported. Problems will occur if the patient has tight clothing proximal to the cuff as this may reduce blood flow or create venous congestion in the arm. The size of the cuff in relation to the size of the patient's arm has been mentioned. Application of the cuff should be smooth and firm with the bladder over the relevant artery. If the cuff is applied loosely the pressure recording will be falsely high, if very tight, too low (Thompson DR, 1981). The sphygmomanometer should be placed level as substantial errors arise if the manometer is not vertical (O'Brien & O'Malley, 1981d).

Two major sources of error relate to auscultation of the sound phases. Firstly, due to the nature of phase 2, the beat is sometimes absent. It is therefore possible to miss phase 1 — the systolic pressure — if the stethoscope is applied immediately to the chosen arterial point (usually over the brachial artery) and the cuff pumped up to a notional 150 mmHg. It is strongly recommended that the pulse be palpated first and the cuff pumped up until the palpated pulse disappears. Experienced observers may then rapidly pump the cuff a further 30 mmHg and apply the stethoscope over the artery. Inexperienced observers will need to let the cuff down between these two operations.

Secondly, the cuff may be let down too rapidly. This will result in the systolic pressure being recorded below its real level, and the diastolic pressure being recorded above its level. The slower the person's pulse, the greater will be the inaccuracy.

A final source of error in technique occurs if the cuff is kept inflated for a long time or is repeatedly inflated causing venous congestion. O'Brien & O'Malley (1981d) report deviations of as much as +30 mmHg to −14 mmHg in the systolic pressure and +20 mmHg to −10 mmHg in the diastolic in relation to intra-arterial pressure. As a result they emphasize that the cuff should be inflated rapidly, deflated slowly and deflated completely between inflations.

What is clear from the research available is that the average blood pressure recording is inaccurate. Nurses who are knowledgeable of the potential sources of inaccuracies are clearly in a better situation to make accurate recordings, to encourage and educate others to record accurately and to take steps to ensure efficient equipment. Increasing awareness of the role of treatment of hypertension in reducing morbidity and mortality rates, and the importance of careful monitoring of those persons identified as 'borderline' hypertensive, indicate that high priority should be given to accurate recordings.

Blood pressure as an indicator of cardiovascular and haematological functions

As indicated, blood pressure is immensely variable in normal persons without cardiovascular or haematological disturbance. Hypertension and hypotension refer to pressures that are considered to be high or low in relation to the population at large, or high or low in relation to the individual's normal.

Hypertension as a primary disorder ('essential' hypertension) is discussed elsewhere. In a small proportion of persons a high blood pressure will be associated with other diseases. In relation to the transport system the most likely cause is generalized arteriosclerosis. Polycythaemia, by increasing blood viscosity without volume reduction, is also associated with increased pressure. Renal artery occlusion or partial occlusion, due to agglutination of blood cells resulting from an antibody response to foreign blood cells introduced in transfusion, results in a rapid rise in blood pressure.

Hypotension is associated with low cardiac output states, such as left ventricular failure, and with hypovolaemic and cardiogenic shock. Short term hypotension also occurs in the no-output state of temporary asystole in some forms of heart block. This also results in syncope and is termed Stokes-Adams attacks.

An inability to increase systolic blood pressure significantly during exercise is indicative of considerable myocardial damage and may be a useful prognostic tool 3 – 4 weeks post infarction.

ELECTROCARDIOGRAPH (ECG)

An ECG records the pattern of electrical activity in the heart and is a standard investigation for the majority of persons admitted to hospital. In addition it is increasingly used in health centres, homes and occupational settings for the purposes of health checks, screening and for persons presenting with cardiac symptoms.

The procedure involves no tissue invasion and the person experiences no sensation. However, although the health care practitioner understands this, the patient may have concerns about feeling an electrical stimulus and needs to be reassured on this point. The full ECG recording will utilize arm and leg leads and a 'roving' chest lead which is repositioned between each recording. In this way the electrical activity between any two electrodes is recorded and a three dimensional pattern of heart electrical activity is built up. This enables tissues not transmitting electrical activity to be identified with reasonable precision.

Normally the ECG is recorded when the person is resting. Increasingly, however, the ECG is also being used to record problems that might occur intermittently in the course of everyday activity and to identify a person's cardiac tolerance of exercise. In the former situation an ambulatory ECG recording is made using a portable machine strapped to the person. In the latter a recording is made while the person is exercising on a treadmill or exercise bike.

The ECG is therefore used:

- to identify arrhythmias and disorders of conduction
- to help to establish if myocardial ischaemia exists
- to help to establish the presence, size and position of myocardial infarction.

Arrhythmias and disorders of conduction

Since the advent of ambulatory ECG, much has been learned about normal heart rhythm and conduction which sheds a somewhat cautionary light on what had been assumed to be abnormal. Petch (1985) points out that 'bradycardias are common in young people, sinus pauses, first degree atrioventricular block and modal escape rhythms are not unusual and may be regarded as normal in youth, and atrial extrasystoles are common'.

With this in mind, however, abnormalities of rhythm on ECG accompanied by other signs of cardiac disease should be assumed to be pathogenic.

Myocardial ischaemia and infarction

The ECG changes associated with ischaemia are due to the alteration in the cell membrane as a result of hypoxia or anoxia (Watson, 1983). If infarction has occurred, the necrosed tissue will be incapable of impulse transmission with resultant deflection of the wave of activity.

The earliest sign of severe ischaemia is seen in elevation or depression of the ST segment. It is assumed that the severity of ST depression correlates with the amount of ischaemic myocardium. Patients with an ST depression of 3mm or more on exercise testing are likely to have severe left main artery stenosis and 69% will have disease in all three major coronary vessels. If infarction has occurred, this will be followed by the development of significant Q waves, which persist after the return of the ST segment to isoelectrical level, and the inversion of the T wave over the infarcted area. Thus the presence of ST changes is indicative of current ischaemia but is not diagnostic of infarction or of previous episodes of ischaemia.

ECG tracing during exercise is increasingly being used to pace rehabilitation programmes and to identify persons at risk from ischaemia. In the latter, changes in the ST segment during exercise have been found to be significant indicators of coronary heart disease although they are no more reliable than a thorough history-taking (MacDonald, 1979). Indeed, angina, even in the absence of ST change, is as predictive of multi-vessel disease as ST change alone.

Increased use of computers for storing, comparing and analysing ECG patterns may provide further understanding of normal and abnormal patterns, but at the moment, advances in investigation are focused on other techniques (Burchell, 1981).

Other abnormalities

Other patterns indicate abnormalities of conduction or abnormalities in the origin of the impulse — ectopic beats. Common patterns include:

- Atrial fibrillation. This is frequently

associated with mitral valve disease. The sinoatrial node is dysfunctional showing erratic rapid 'P' waves of which only some are transmitted via the atrioventricular node. The ventricular rate is irregular, as is the pulse, and they may not be in synchrony, the output in some beats being too weak to initiate a pulse wave to the radial artery.

- Ventricular fibrillation. This is an erratic pattern of activity of the ventricles and results in no cardiac output. It is a common cause of death linked with myocardial ischaemia.
- Heart block. This occurs in varying degrees demonstrating delay of conduction across the A-V node, bundle of His or Purkinje fibres. It may result from myocardial infarction and if not corrected may lead to periods of asystole with syncope known as Stokes-Adams attacks.

For a more detailed understanding of ECGs the reader is referred to any of the many specialized texts available.

X-RAY

Plain

Chest X-rays are an important part of assessment of cardiovascular function. The most commonly used X-ray is the 'straight' or posterior — anterior chest X-ray which demonstrates the size and shape of the heart, the position of the great vessels and the vascularity of the lung fields. In addition it will reveal pulmonary problems and the presence of pleural effusion which may be associated with cardiac problems.

Whilst of immense value, however, plain X-rays are limited by their inability to differentiate soft tissues. For example, it is not possible to identify if an 'enlarged heart' is due to dilatation or myocardial hypertrophy (Watson, 1983).

Fluoroscopy or screening

Fluoroscopy is the observation of body parts continuously via a fluorescent X-ray screen — hence the name screening. In relation to the cardiovascular system, it is of limited value but is used to identify calcification of valves and prosthetic valve function.

Computerized tomography (CT scan)

This is a well-established radiographic imaging technique for visualizing the distribution of X-ray attenuation in the body. The attenuation is achieved by using a collimated X-ray tube which produces a fan of radiation rather than a beam. A series of X-rays are produced, the X-ray tube and detector having been moved through a small angle each time. It may be used in conjunction with a contrast medium.

Technological advance on computerized scanners now enables a dynamic three-dimensional picture to be presented which may replace the use of cardiac catheterization (Burchell, 1981; Lipton et al, 1983).

Angiography, venography and angiocardiography

Angiography, venography and angiocardiography are specialized X-rays involving the injection of a radio-opaque dye into an artery or vein in order to demonstrate the lumen of the specific artery, vein or the chambers of the heart. The procedure for coronary angiography and angiocardiography is generally termed 'cardiac catheterization'. It involves feeding a specially designed fine catheter along the brachial or femoral artery for left sided cardiac and coronary investigation, and via an arm or leg vein for right-sided cardiac investigation. In addition to contrast medium X-rays being taken, the pressure at various points of the heart and great vessels is also recorded and blood samples may be taken for estimation of oxygen saturation.

The procedures, whilst now relatively safe, are invasive and do carry a degree of risk. This is estimated to be as low as 2–2.5 per 1000 for coronary angiography (Davis et al, 1979). The primary complications are:

- induced ventricular arrhythmias (in cardiac catheterization)

- introduction of infection
- haematoma
- thrombosis or embolism.

It is for this reason that medical staff are increasingly using alternative non-invasive techniques such as Doppler waveform analysis, CT scanning and radionuclide techniques.

However, these procedures are still developing and large numbers of patients are still undergoing angiography, venography and angiocardiography. These patients will fall into one of four diagnostic groups:

- coronary heart disease
- congenital or acquired heart valve disease
- arterial disease (ischaemic or occlusive disease, aneurysms)
- deep vein insufficiency.

The procedure is used to assess the nature and extent of the disruption to blood flow and may therefore be used both prior to treatment and to evaluate the progress of the disease or the effect of the treatment. Individual patients may therefore experience the procedure on more than one occasion.

Care of the person

Due to the potential complications, the person is usually admitted to hospital as a day or overnight patient. This leaves limited time for full explanation and preparation and it may be advisable to arrange an educative preparation programme in the context of a cardiac or vascular outpatient clinic.

The procedure is carried out with the patient slightly sedated.

Normal pre-operative precautions regarding general hygiene, the wearing of a clean open-backed gown, bladder and bowel comfort, fasting for four hours prior to the procedure and labelling the patient are carried out. The patient is taken to the appropriate department on a trolley and the procedure carried out aseptically under local anaesthetic.

In this way the procedure equates with an operation and the principles of pre-operative education and preparation apply. However, the evidence for the effectiveness of psychological preparation pre-procedure is equivocal. Rice et al (1986) found patients prepared for cardiac catheterization through an educative/relaxative programme had more understanding of the procedure but experienced no less anxiety or distress than those not so prepared. However, Watkins et al (1986), in a larger study, found that patients who had been prepared with a tape-slide programme giving information about the procedure and the sensations involved were significantly less anxious than those who had information on the procedure only or who had gained their information from health care professionals alone. In addition, using a scale to differentiate patients on their coping style, they found that those who prefer to blunt their response (a 'head in the sand' approach = 'blunters') were not only more likely to be women and to have higher anxiety scores in general but in addition responded better to having information about the procedure only, rather than information about the sensations involved. The majority of the blunters also said that they would rather not have known about the risks involved and that this knowledge heightened their anxiety. In contrast, those who preferred to monitor their response ('know what's going on' = 'monitors') responded better to having information about the procedure and the associated sensations and said they preferred to have the information about the risks. The highest pulse and blood pressure recordings were found in the blunters who were in the control group. If these findings were validated by replication of the study, use of the scale would assist significantly in tailoring pre-procedure information to the needs of specific patients.

The procedure itself involves unpleasant sensations, particularly when the dye is injected. Patients report a flushing and bursting sensation. If the catheter or the dye evokes vasospasm the patient will experience searing pain in the affected vessel and the procedure may have to be abandoned.

During the procedure, the primary risks are those of ventricular arrhythmias (in cardiac catheterization) and the dislodging of atheroma or loose clots which then form emboli which may lodge in the pulmonary or systemic circulations. Both of these complications are clearly life-threatening.

Postoperatively the patient may require analgesic medication and should remain resting in bed for 4–6 hours to reduce the risk of haemorrhage or haematoma at the site of the insertion of the catheter. Observations of the vital signs and of the puncture site are maintained during this time.

ECHOCARDIOGRAPHY OR ULTRASOUND, DOPPLER WAVE-FORM ANALYSIS

This is a safe non-invasive investigation relying on the differential reflection of an ultrasonic beam by tissues of varying density. It has been used as an adjunct to X-ray and ECG for some time, in particular to study valve function and heart wall function. However, the development of the Doppler beam has 'rejuvenated' echocardiography and it is now used extensively in the investigation of arterial disease (Burchell, 1981). Its particular contribution is likely to be in the early diagnosis of arterial disease before ischaemic symptoms have appeared but as yet it remains unreliable in this field (Campbell et al, 1985).

SCINTIGRAPHY OR RADIONUCLIDE SCANNING

This is the most rapidly expanding field in cardiovascular investigation (Burchell, 1981) and is particularly valuable in the assessment of myocardial perfusion, metabolism and left ventricular function. It is therefore used extensively in the screening of patients for coronary artery disease with myocardial ischaemia and in the assessment of operative results.

It involves the injection of a radio-labeled substance (radiopharmaceutical) that will be selectively taken up by specific tissues. In relation to myocardial perfusion, for example, recent myocardial damage may be identified by using a radiopharmaceutical (e.g. Technetium tagged pyrophosphate) which concentrates in acutely injured cells — 'hot-spot' scanning. More commonly 'cold spot' scanning is used, involving the use of ionic tracers that have similar physiological behaviour to potassium and will therefore accumulate in viable perfused myocardium. The infarcted or ischaemic area will therefore appear as a region of diminished or absent uptake. Thallium 201 is frequently used, as it is rapidly cleared from the blood (50% within 5 minutes) (Rowlands et al, 1981). However, cold spot scanning cannot differentiate between new and old areas of infarction and is of no value in the initial 24 hours post-infarction diagnostic period.

Radionuclides are also of value in the estimation of the degree of myocardial ischaemia in patients presenting with angina. The perfusion defect is induced on exercise and usually relates to the size of coronary artery stenosis.

In scintigraphic ventriculography the ventricular performance is assessed by estimating the ratio of blood ejected from the left ventricle in relation to the blood remaining in the ventricle — the ejection fraction. As the radioactivity is required within the blood rather than within tissues a non-diffusable radiopharmaceutical is used.

The patient's experience of radionuclide scanning consists of the intravenous injection, which normally does not result in any adverse sensations. The speed of tissue uptake determines how rapidly the scan will follow the injection. In ventriculography it is clearly simultaneous. The majority of radioisotopes used are rapidly excreted so that no precautions regarding exposure to radioactivity need be taken outside of the investigation room. Some radiopharmaceuticals may be taken up by tissues that are not the focus of investigation (e.g. spleen, thyroid gland). Dependent on the tissue involved this uptake can be blocked by, for example, saturating the tissue with a similar substance that has not been radio-tagged. The patient may need to be fasted for 12 hours. In the case of myocardial perfusion assessment, drugs affecting cell membrane transport (e.g. nifedipine) will need to be discontinued for as long as it takes for them to be cleared from active function.

PROBLEMS OF OXYGEN TRANSPORT AND RED CELL ABNORMALITIES

As the primary mode of oxygen transport from the lungs to the tissues is by being loosely attached to the haemoglobin molecule in the red blood cells, it follows that a reduction in the haemoglobin or red cells will result in a reduced oxygen carrying capacity. Thus the anaemias are the main group of disorders considered under this heading.

An additional disorder, that of displacement of the oxygen molecule by carbon monoxide, is also briefly discussed.

The excessive production of red cells — polycythaemia — is also discussed here although the problems created by this disorder are primarily those of increased viscosity of the blood.

ANAEMIA

Definition

The definition of anaemia is complicated in that it relates to 'normal' values of red cells, haemoglobin and oxygen-carrying power rather than being a disease entity of itself. Thus a usual definition might be 'a reduction in the haemoglobin concentration, red cell count or haematocrit to below normal levels' (Wickramasinghe & Weatherall, 1982) or a 'level of haemoglobin in the blood below that which is expected, taking into account both age and sex' (MacLeod, 1984). The World Health Organization defines anaemia in terms of specific haemoglobin values — below 13g/dl for adult males, below 12g/dl for adult females (Wickramasinghe & Weatherall, 1982). However, there is wide variation in haemoglobin values within the population and most laboratories now consider that a level within the range of values within two standard deviations of the mean to be normal. Because of this wide variation, individuals with haemoglobin values within the normal range may well have subclinical, latent anaemia whilst 2.5% of 'normal' individuals with adequate iron stores and utilization and no clinical signs of anaemia will have levels below the normal range (Wickramasinghe & Weatherall, 1982). In view of this it is suggested that, functionally, anaemia is the state in which the number of circulating red cells is insufficient to meet the oxygen requirements of the tissues.

Prevalence

The prevalence of anaemia is difficult to estimate due to the problems of definition. However, there is agreement as to the general trend. It is much more common in women during their menstrual years than in men, one estimate being 14% women as opposed to 3% men. It is also more common in both sexes after the age of 75 years (Wickramasinghe & Weatherall, 1982). In developing countries the incidence is probably higher and fluctuates markedly with the incidence of diseases such as malaria.

Cause

Causes of anaemia are numerous and can be related directly to the production and destruction of red blood cells and to blood loss. Figure 22.1 indicates some of the causes of anaemia related to these processes. They are further discussed in subsequent sections.

Effects of anaemia

As the oxygen-carrying power of the red cells far exceeds the normal demand of the tissues, the effects of a decreased carrying power will not be felt by the individual for some time, unless the cause of the reduction is sudden as in acute haemorrhage.

In mild to moderate anaemia, the body compensates in two ways:

- the oxygen dissociation curve shifts to the right
- there is a redistribution in tissue perfusion to vital centres.

The shift of oxygen dissociation results from

Tissue	Time	Red cell life cycle	Cause of anaemia	Disorder
Tissues		Oxygen supply reduced ↓		
Kidney	1–2 days	Production of erythropoietin ↓	Lack of erythropoietin production	Renal failure
Bone marrow	4–5 days	Production of haemocytoblasts ↓	Reduced or disordered blood cell production	Bone marrow disordered — toxins — drugs — irradiation — leukaemia
		Differentiation and Proliferation of basophil erythroblasts ↓	Failure of nuclear maturation and division (megaloblastic)	Folate deficiency — lack in diet — gut disorder B_{12} deficiency — lack in diet — lack of intrinsic factor — gut disorder — parasites or bacteria
	Synthesis of haemoglobin	Polychromatophil erythroblast ↓ Normoblasts ↓ Reticulocytes ↓	Cells low in haemoglobin	Iron deficiency — lack in diet — chronic blood loss
Circulation	120 days	Erythrocytes ↓	Excess loss from system	Blood loss
		Ageing changes in cell wall density and spleen ↓	Early destruction	Early cell wall rupture — toxins — drugs — infections
Circulation Spleen		Phagocytosis		Immune destruction — incompatible blood transfusion — rhesus incompatibility Excess cell wall fragility — sickle cell

Fig. 22.1 Red cell production and anaemia

an increase in a byproduct of glucose metabolism, 2–3 diphosphoglycerate (2-3-DPG), within the red cells. An increase in 2-3-DPG results in a decrease in the oxygen affinity of haemoglobin, thus more is released to the tissues. The redistribution of tissue perfusion results in vasoconstriction in the skin and kidneys, the latter not affecting function, thus conserving oxygen supplies for the brain, myocardium and skeletal muscle (MacLeod, 1981; Wickramasinghe & Weatherall, 1982). Thus the person who is anaemic may initially simply be rather pale and lethargic.

In severe anaemia (e.g. Hb levels below 7–8g/dl) the effects are likely to produce more marked symptoms as the initial compensatory mechanisms are no longer adequate. Cardiac output is increased both at rest and in exercise. The healthy heart can tolerate this demand for a considerable time but in the presence of a degree of coronary artery disease, angina results with signs of left ventricular failure — cardiomegaly, pulmonary oedema and ultimately ascites and peripheral oedema.

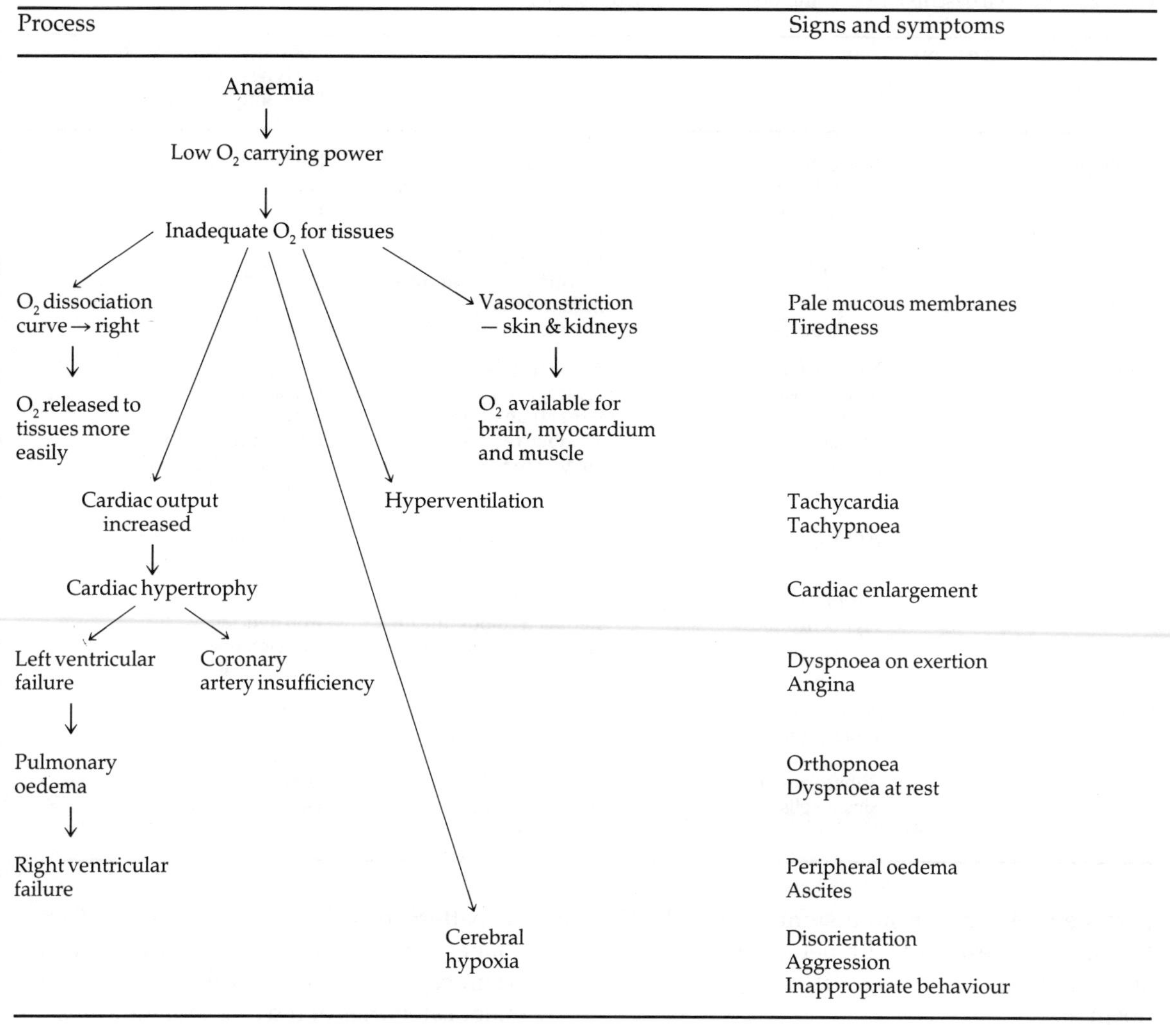

Fig. 22.2 Progressive effects of anaemia

In addition dyspnoea develops, irrespective of signs of heart failure. Wickramasinghe & Weatherall (1982) describe this as an 'inappropriate mechanism' in that it will not result in an increased uptake by the red cells of oxygen from the alveoli because the haemoglobin is normally fully saturated.

Figure 22.2 illustrates the progressive effects of chronic anaemia. Of note in terms of the symptoms of severe anaemia is the absence of cyanosis, although the person will appear dyspnoeic and their tissues are short of oxygen. Whilst oxygen exchange is unimpaired in the lungs the circulating haemoglobin will be fully saturated, thus cyanosis will not develop in spite of lack of oxygen.

In addition, if the onset of anaemia is particularly insidious, the individual may become grossly anaemic before compensatory mechanisms fail and the person notices anything more than tiredness. The author has nursed one middle-aged lady who suffered irreversible brain damage due to cerebral hypoxia. This resulted from gross iron deficiency anaemia due to

Table 22.1 Red cell descriptions in common use and related disorders

Nature of descriptive term	Term	Definition	Conditions with which cell type is most frequently associated
Developmental	Nucleated normoblast	Premature cell not normally in circulation	Megaloblastic anaemias
	Reticulocyte	Early red cell with fragments of nuclear material. Normally small number in circulation	Blood loss
	Erythrocyte	Normal mature red cell	Normal
Size	Normocyte	Normal cell size	Normal
	Macroytosis	Average red cell larger than normal	Megaloblastic anaemias
	Microcytosis	Average red cell smaller than normal	Iron deficiency and other disorders of haemoglobin synthesis
	Anisocytosis	Cells are unequal in size	Megaloblastic anaemias
Colour	Normochromic	Normal cell colour	Normal
	Hypochromic	Reduced colour due to reduced haemoglobin	Iron deficiency, associated with microcytosis
Shape	Biconcave	Normal shape	Normal
	Poikilocytosis	Irregularity of shape	Always associated with anisocytosis
	Spherocytosis	Rounded cells	Genetic disorders
	Sickle-cells	Sickle or scythe-shaped cells	Genetic disorder

persistent bleeding from a symptomless hiatus hernia. She presented with behavioural disturbances and was admitted initially to a psychiatric hospital.

Types of anaemia

There are numerous classifications of anaemia.

However, at it simplest, anaemia may be considered to be due to:

- an impaired red blood cell production (haemopoietic)
- an increased rate of red cell destruction (haemolytic)
- an excess loss of cells (haemorrhagic).

However, histologically, and prior to the cause of the anaemia being established, the anaemia may be described by the shape, size and colour of the red cells, these being the result in changes in the pattern of cell production. Thus certain cell shapes, sizes or degrees of colour are typical of certain types of anaemia. Table 22.1 indicates the major categories of red cells and indicates the type of condition with which abnormal cells are commonly linked.

Excess loss of red cells (haemorrhagic)

Normally the body is extremely efficient in its reprocessing of materials salvaged from red cell breakdown. In particular, although it is estimated that total body iron amounts to about 4g in the adult, only 1mg is lost from the body per day, thus needing replacement from the diet (Jacobs, 1982). Absorption of iron from the intestine appears to be regulated by the state of the iron stores in the cells within the intestinal wall and is normally very low, matching the 1mg requirement.

Absorption is normally facilitated when the stores are depleted. However, if blood is lost from the body the stores are used up and, unless intake of iron is increased, iron deficiency anaemia will result.

Chronic blood loss. This is a common cause of anaemia and is insidious in onset. The most frequent causes of blood loss are:

- menorrhagia in females
- gastro-intestinal bleeding
  - hiatus hernia
  - peptic ulceration
  - regional ileitis
  - ulcerative colitis
  - haemorrhoids.

Treatment of the cause and of the iron deficiency corrects the anaemia.

Acute blood loss. Acute haemorrhage will cause immediate anxiety and hypovolaemic shock rather than problems related to anaemia. In treating the haemorrhage, whole blood is normally used if it is required and available. As this serves not only to correct the hypovolaemia but also the red cell loss, anaemia may not develop. If it is less dramatic and untreated, a degree of anaemia will develop over 24–48 hours as the extracellular fluid level returns to normal, and the reticulocyte count will be raised to 5–10% as the erythropoietic bone marrow responds. As iron stores are normal, the anaemia will be self-correcting, more iron being absorbed from the diet until haemoglobin and storage levels are returned to normal. A balanced diet and iron supplements are recommended at this stage (Woodliff & Herrmann, 1979).

Increased rate of red cell destruction (haemolytic)

The normal life span of erythrocytes is 120 days. Destruction in excess before this time results in depletion of the bone marrow and body iron stores, hence the anaemia. Due to the excess destruction, the haemolytic anaemias may also be associated with a mild non-obstructive jaundice.

Causes of haemolytic anaemia. These anaemias are caused by a number of factors:

- toxins such as
  - infections
  - drugs
- genetic abnormalities of cell shape or fragility such as
  - sickle-cell disease
  - spheroidosis
- immune response
  - to mismatched blood (or in the newborn to maternal antibodies to fetal blood being in the fetal circulation, i.e. rhesus incompatability)
  - autoimmunity.

In the genetic forms splenomegaly is common and splenectomy to reduce red cell breakdown is sometimes performed. In other forms the treatment will be specific to the cause, the problem of anaemia often being of secondary importance to other life-threatening occurrences such as agglutination of cells blocking capillaries and causing widespread minute infarctions.

Two genetic disorders of red cell production inherited in a Mendelian fashion and associated with a reduced erythrocyte life span are of particular note:

- sickle-cell disease
- thalassaemia.

Sickle cell disease. Sickle-cell disease is relatively common in negros in Africa, America and the UK. Sickle-cell trait occurs in the heterozygote and is found in 10–20% of the negro population (Woodliff & Herrmann, 1979). It is normally asymptomatic, although if exposed to low oxygen tension or low atmospheric pressure sickling may occur causing minute tissue infarctions.

Sickle cell anaemia occurs in the homozygous condition. The haemoglobin in the sickle or scythe-shaped cells is abnormal and the red cells are more susceptible to haemolysis and are more viscous than normal cells. At low oxygen tensions the abnormal haemoglobin forms insoluble bonds.

The condition is thereafter characterized by two features:

- anaemia due to excessive destruction of red cells

- widespread vascular problems due to thrombosis and infarction.

Vascular problems may affect any body tissue. Thus infarctions may present in bone, spleen and lungs. Leg ulceration is common. Renal infarction causes a reduced ability to concentrate urine and may lead to renal failure. Pain will occur when new infarctions occur.

Treatments aimed at increasing oxygen tension, altering the blood pH, or in other ways trying to reduce the cells' ability to agglutinate have been proved largely ineffective (Woodliff & Herrmann, 1979). Currently there is no satisfactory form of treatment and persons with sickle-cell disease are treated symptomatically.

Thalassaemia. The thalassaemias are a group of disorders in which there is an inherited defect of haemoglobin synthesis. This results in the red cells having a reduced life span. It is found mostly in individuals of Mediterranean origin. The homozygous form, termed thalassaemia major, creates profound anaemia, children failing to thrive and seldom reaching adulthood (Woodliff & Herrmann, 1979).

In the heterozygous form, thalassaemia minor, the anaemia is much less profound and presents as a mild hypochromic anaemia not of iron deficiency.

Autoimmune haemolytic anaemias. These are not common. In the absence of other identifiable causes of haemolytic anaemia, idiopathic autoimmunity is assumed. The anaemia runs an acute or chronic course, treatment including corticosteroids, splenectomy and immunosuppressants. A secondary autoimmune haemolytic anaemia is associated with leukaemias and lymphomas, disseminated lupus erythematosus and some infections during the acute phase.

Nursing considerations. The nurse will most commonly meet patients with sickle-cell disease amongst those with this group of anaemias, with the exception of autoimmune haemolytic anaemia associated with leukaemia (discussed elsewhere). Acute sickling crisis presenting as diffuse organ and tissue infarction will cause the person to be in pain, often with dyspnoea. Symptomatic relief is currently all that is available, although other treatments may be attempted. Patients become extremely distressed and nurses and other health carers feel helpless. Patience, support and attention to symptomatic relief is nevertheless crucial if the patient's distress is to be relieved in any way.

Those with sickle-cell trait must be warned to ensure that the anaesthetist is informed of the trait if they undergo surgery.

Impaired red cell production

Impaired red cell production accounts for a very wide variety of anaemias but they can be logically divided into further subgroups:

- reduced erythropoietin production
- disordered bone marrow function
- disorders resulting from deficiency of essential components.

Reduced erythropoietin production. This is associated, primarily, with renal failure, the kidney responding inadequately to tissue hypoxia. This results in reduced erythropoiesis but as the bone marrow is functioning normally red cells produced will also be normal.

Disordered bone marrow function. This may result from a number of disorders:

- temporary or permanent depression of bone marrow function by drugs or irradiation
- primary idiopathic aplastic or hypoplastic anaemia
- bone marrow disorders such as leukaemia, myeloma

Leukaemia is discussed elsewhere.

Primary aplastic or hypoplastic anaemia. In about half of the patients presenting with hypo- or aplastic anaemia the cause cannot be traced and the diagnosis of primary or idiopathic aplastic anaemia is made. There is a reduction in the total amount of erythroid tissue and granulocytes, and platelets are usually also reduced. Thus the patient may present with symptoms of anaemia, infection or bleeding. Treatment with transfusion and corticosteroids may bring about remission and about 50% of the patients recover completely (Woodliff &

Herrmann, 1979).

Secondary aplastic anaemia. This is due to drugs such as chloramphenicol and some drugs used in the treatment of epilepsy and rheumatism. Cytotoxic drugs also depress bone marrow function but the effect is usually reversible. Treatment and prognosis is similar to that of primary aplastic anaemia.

Nursing considerations. These individuals will be relatively frequent visitors to medical short stay in-patient facilities (whether day unit or ward) as blood transfusion is required intermittently. Particular care needs to be taken with observations as transfusion reactions increase in frequency due to antibody formation following repeated exposure to foreign antigens in the blood. Packed cells are usually used to decrease the additional volume loading on the heart. Patients taking corticosteroids are particularly at risk of a transfusion reaction not being recognized due to the masking of pyrexia and other normal signals.

Patients with aplastic anaemia have normally adjusted their lifestyle to their lowered oxygen availability but may be reassured by being given the opportunity to discuss this during their hospital stay.

Disorders resulting from deficiency of essential components. The most common anaemia of all, the iron deficiency type, falls into this group. In addition the megaloblastic anaemias, due to vitamin B_{12} or folate deficiency type, are also relatively common.

Vitamin B_{12} deficiency. Vitamin B_{12} is essential for DNA production, and deficiency therefore affects cells other than red cells. However, as red cells are being produced constantly and in large numbers, vitamin B_{12} deficiency results in severely disordered and reduced red cell proliferation. Typically the cells are large — macrocytic — because the cells have continued growing as cell division is reduced (MacLeod, 1981). There is no inhibition of haemoglobin formation so that the cells are normochromic. In very severe forms of the disease the cells fail to mature and massive destruction takes place within the bone marrow eventually leading to bone marrow failure. In addition, vitamin B_{12} deficiency can result in neurological complications, not discussed in this chapter.

There are four main causes of vitamin B_{12} deficiency:

- inadequate intake of vitamin B_{12}
- deficiency of intrinsic factor in the gastric mucosa (pernicious anaemia)
- disease or resection of the terminal ileum
- bacterial proliferation or parasitic invasion of the ileum.

The diet is normally adequate in B_{12} but vegetarians who restrict their diet totally to plant products (vegans) will develop vitamin B_{12} deficiency unless they take artificial oral supplements.

The normal gastric mucosa produces the 'intrinsic factor' which is essential for absorption of vitamin B_{12} taken in the diet. Persons with an atrophic gastric mucosa will therefore not be able to absorb dietary vitamin B_{12} and will present with symptoms of anaemia. Investigations to determine the nature of the problem will include radionuclide uptake tests and possible endoscopy. Treatment by intramuscular injections of cyanocobalamin or hydroxocobalamin is highly successful. These are initially given daily or on alternate days and decrease to monthly injections for lifelong maintenance. Investigation, diagnosis and initial treatment may all be undertaken as an outpatient or in a short stay ward. Treatment is maintained by self-administered injections or, more commonly, injections given by a health centre practice nurse or a visiting district nurse.

Vitamin B_{12} is absorbed at very specific points in the terminal ileum (MacLeod, 1981). Severe disease such as regional ileitis (Crohn's disease) or resection of the terminal ileum for inflammatory or neoplastic disease usually results in megaloblastic anaemia, although this may take 1–3 years to develop. Treatment is by vitamin B_{12} injection as previously indicated.

Proliferation of bacteria in blind loops in the intestine, such as in diverticulosis, and the invasion of the intestine by parasites such as tapeworm will deprive the individual of nutrients, including vitamin B_{12}. Treatment clearly involves treating the cause in addition to temporary treatment with vitamin B_{12} injections.

NURSING CONSIDERATIONS. Apart from caring for persons during investigation, the major contribution nursing makes to patients in this group is the administration of cyanocobalamin injections to those with pernicious anaemia. This normally falls to the community nurse and may provide opportunity for wider discussion of the individual's health problems and health promotion.

If patients receiving regular cyanocobalamin are admitted to hospital for reasons other than their anaemia, the date the injection is due should be noted and the treatment maintained.

Folate deficiency. Folate is found in both vegetable and animal sources but is readily destroyed by cooking. It is essential for normal nuclear maturation and cell division, so lack of folate results in megaloblastic anaemia as in vitamin B_{12} deficiency. It is distinguished from B_{12} deficiency by estimation of serum and red cell folate levels which will be low.

It is caused primarily by dietary inadequacy — lack of fresh vegetables and over cooked, highly processed foods — but also by extensive disease of the upper part of the small intestine where folate is absorbed, and at times when the body's demands exceed a normal supply. The latter situation arises from the relatively small stores of folate in the body so that at times of cell proliferation — during pregnancy and in such diseases as leukaemia — the demand outweighs the normal dietary intake. In addition certain drugs interfere with folate utilization, notably methotrexate and some anticonvulsant drugs, phenytoin and primidone.

Folic acid may be given in tablet form orally. If given to patients who also have a vitamin B_{12} deficiency, it can aggravate or precipitate the neurological consequences of that deficiency. For this reason, accurate diagnosis of the precise deficiency is essential.

NURSING CONSIDERATIONS. Whilst folic acid is available in tablet form, dietary modification may make medication unnecessary after initial treatment in those patients in whom there is no pathological cause. Fresh vegetables and foods and a review of cooking times should be the focus of dietary advice.

Iron deficiency anaemia. Although iron deficiency anaemia has a variety of causes, the two most common being chronic blood loss (from the gastrointestinal tract or female reproductive system for example) and dietary insufficiency, it is a term often used as a diagnostic label. Investigating the cause is clearly important. However, that apart, treatment of the iron deficiency will involve two major aspects:

- iron therapy
- dietary review.

In addition, in the rare situation that a person with iron deficiency anaemia is given a blood transfusion, the nurse must be fully aware of the implications of this for a person without volume depletion and potentially on the edge of cardiac failure. This is more fully discussed in the section on blood transfusion.

MANAGEMENT AND NURSING CONSIDERATIONS. There are four main areas of concern:

- care related to iron therapy
- dietary review
- review of activity levels while haemoglobin levels are low
- care of persons receiving blood transfusion.

IRON THERAPY. Iron is normally given orally in the form of ferrous sulphate 200mg up to 3 times daily. This may cause gastrointestinal disturbance and there are numerous proprietary brands of ferrous iron available, some combined with vitamins or folic acid, which attempt to overcome these problems. The majority of persons develop some degree of constipation but 'indigestion' and diarrhoea may also be experienced. As iron is poorly absorbed much will be excreted in the faeces. All persons taking oral iron, therefore, will develop black stools and should be warned of this.

If there is evidence that iron will not be absorbed from the intestine or the deficiency is very profound, the iron may be administered by deep intramuscular injection or intravenously. In both instances it is important that iron does not leak into subcutaneous tissues as it causes staining. Apart from scrupulous care in administration, a needle change after drawing up the solution will reduce the risk of a trace of iron staining developing at the injection site. Iron therapy is normally continued for up to a year after the haemoglobin levels have returned to normal, as repletion of body iron stores is a slow process (MacLeod, 1981).

DIETARY REVIEW. Dietary review is advisable in all persons presenting with iron deficiency anaemia. Normally the intake of iron per day is about 16.0mg of which about 5–10% may be absorbed (Ministry of Agriculture, Fisheries & Food, 1985). As indicated, more can be absorbed at times of relative depletion. In addition, iron is more readily absorbed from meat, up to 25%, than from other foods such as eggs and cereals, perhaps 5%. The primary sources of iron in the diet are meat, bread, flour and other cereals, potatoes and vegetables. Wholegrain cereals contain larger quantities than more refined products. Milk contains very little iron, liver and kidneys contain more than beef and much more than chicken or fish. Thus a 'light diet' of milk foods, chicken and fish will contain relatively little iron. It is also important to realize that vegetarians — while their diet can be sufficient in iron to meet normal requirements — are considerably more at risk than meat-eaters if iron stores are depleted or they are not eating a balanced diet.

REVIEW OF ACTIVITY LEVELS. During periods when the haemoglobin is low, individuals with anaemia will need to adjust their activity levels to reduce oxygen utilization. This will usually happen without special planning as the person experiences weakness and tiredness. However, some individuals are impatient with themselves and will try to retain normal patterns of activity. This will precipitate cardiac problems and will not have any beneficial effect as the haemoglobin present in the red cells is already fully oxygen-saturated. Discussion about activity is therefore of value and should be geared towards sustaining activity below levels that induce dyspnoea or tachycardia.

CARE OF PERSONS RECEIVING BLOOD TRANSFUSION. Blood transfusions are commonly given to individuals with disorders of the blood. The reasons for the transfusion as well as the nature of the disorder are important as both have implications for nursing.

The most usual reasons for transfusion are:

- low haemoglobin level incompatible with normal activity and/or requiring urgent rectification
- low blood volume due to haemorrhage

The first of these arises from a number of disorders but particularly:

- iron deficiency anaemia
- megaloblastic anaemia
- aplastic anaemia
- leukaemia.

Of these, blood transfusion should only be given in the initial stages of treatment of iron deficiency and megaloblastic anaemia, as treatment of the cause or replacement of vitamin B_{12} will result in a cure.

Repeated transfusion, however, is normally required in both aplastic anaemia and leukaemia.

Problems with transfusion are of three different types:

- Problems related to any intravenous infusion including venospasm, leakage, reduction in self care ability.
- Problems related to antibody reaction to the foreign protein. This problem is minimal with first transfusions unless the person has a history of allergy. However, it is an increasing problem with each transfusion for patients with aplastic anaemia or leukaemia.
- Problems of circulation overload precipitating acute cardiac failure. This is a danger in all patients who have not lost fluid, but particularly so if the person is elderly and has incipient or actual heart failure. It is therefore a particular risk with the elderly person with iron deficiency anaemia.

The nursing care planned for the individual patient should take account of the relative risk of these problems occurring. In particular, the more at risk the patient, the more frequent should be the observation of TPR, blood pressure and the general condition of the patient. In general, all transfusions given to patients without volume deficit will be relatively slow, packed cells and slower rates being used if the risk of heart failure is high. Diuretics may also be given to ensure rapid removal of the extra fluid load.

CARBON MONOXIDE POISONING

The ready combination of carbon monoxide with haemoglobin results in carboxyhaemoglobin being formed in preference to oxyhaemoglobin. It follows that relatively small amounts of carbon monoxide will have severe consequences in terms of the availability of oxygen for essential tissue function.

Smokers have a carboxyhaemoglobin level of 2–5% (Greenhalgh, 1984). The precise physiological effects of this are not known except to postulate that of a deleterious effect on vulnerable tissues and additional myocardial demand.

The more dramatic and potentially fatal effect is that of deliberate or accidental inhalation of carbon monoxide from car exhaust or coal gas. At only 0.2% of inhaled air, that is with nearly 20% oxygen still present in air, the concentration is such that the tenacious affinity of the carbon monoxide for haemoglobin can result in death within a matter of minutes (Guyton, 1984).

Nursing considerations. Immediate attention to removing the individual from the carbon monoxide source and ensuring the airway is maintained is clearly of prime importance.

Administration of pure oxygen increases the chances of survival. Pure oxygen produces an alveolar oxygen pressure six times that of normal. At this pressure the force at which oxygen can combine with haemoglobin is sixfold thus speeding up the process of replacing carbon monoxide molecules (Guyton, 1984).

POLYCYTHAEMIA (ERYTHRAEMIA OR POLYCYTHAEMIA VERA)

In this condition there is an increase in red cells and frequently in leucocytes and platelets. It is more common in men than women and the individual appears plethoric and, due to increased amounts of reduced haemoglobin, slightly cyanosed. It is considered to be a benign neoplastic condition and is of unknown aetiology.

Symptoms relate to the increased blood viscosity. This leads to relative stagnation of blood and the risk of thrombosis. Breathlessness and palpitations also occur, and haemorrhage from the nasal or gastrointestinal mucosa is not uncommon. The patient in hospital with polycythaemia will therefore normally present with haemorrhage or thrombosis.

Treatment of the polycythaemia includes:

- venesection
- depression of bone marrow activity.

Venesection of 500ml of blood is a useful initial treatment and will help to reduce symptoms in the short term. In the longer term, however, bone marrow depression by radioactive phosphorus or cytotoxic drugs is more satisfactory and may bring about a remission that may last from six months to several years. Uric acid levels, sometimes high due to the increased nucleoprotein turnover, are further increased by cytotoxic agents so that monitoring of uric acid levels and the administration of the xanthine oxidase inhibitor, allopurinal, are important measures if gout and renal failure are to be avoided.

Nursing considerations. Apart from care relating to the presenting problem, nursing support consists primarily of observation so that problems can be identified early. In addition assistance and support may be required during venesection. Due to the high risk of thrombosis it is important that the person remains mobile.

PROBLEMS OF WHITE CELL PRODUCTION

LEUKAEMIA

The leukaemias (together with lymphomas) are neoplastic conditions in which there is an abnormal proliferation of the leucopoietic tissue. There may be excessive multiplication of cells although not necessarily, but the immature cells usually fail to develop into those capable of carrying out their function and have abnormal life expectancies (Taylor, 1980).

Table 22.2 Leukaemias — incidence and prognosis

Type	Incidence/mortality	Age group, prognosis and other comments
Acute lymphoblastic Null cell (80%) B cell (2–3%) T cell (15–20%)	Mid 1970s–12% of total leukaemic mortality 15% of incidence 0.5 per 100 000	Most common childhood leukaemia. Incidence very low in young to middle-aged adults, rising again at 60+ years. B cell prognosis poor. Complete remission possible in 80–90% of children — 5 yr survival 50%. Girls respond better than boys. Complete remission 21–58% in adults. Survival 1–8 years, most die within 18 months.
Acute myeloblastic Granulocytic Progranulocytic Myelomonocytic Monocytic Erythraemic myelosis	40–50% of leukaemic mortality 0.25:100 000 in mid years 1:100 000 in elderly	Most common adult leukaemia. Except for progranulogic, prognosis relatively poor. Some preceded by other diseases — poorer prognosis. Prognosis poor over 50yr as difficult to bring into remission. Without remission — survival less than 3 mth. Complete remission in 20–80%. Survival 1 wk–5+ yr, 80% less than 2 yr.
Chronic myeloid Philadelphia positive (95%) Philadelphia negative Juvenile	15-20% of leukaemic mortality 1:100 000	Chronic phase 3 mth–3 yr, treatment improves quality of life but no true remission. Acute phase inevitably terminal 2–12 mth. Disease of middle and old age, peak incidence mid-50s.
Chronic lymphoblastic B cell (90%) T cell Other	25% of leukaemic mortality Increase quadrupled in past 20 yr to 1:100 000	Survival 1–15 yr. Most die within 5 yr. Only occurs over 35 yr, primarily a disease of older persons Male to female ratio 2:1.

The term itself is confusing being a Greek term literally meaning 'white blood' and first used by Virchow in 1847 to describe the disease characterized by splenic enlargement and yellowish-white blood on post-mortem examination (Taylor, 1980). The term leukaemia includes widely differing conditions, from those with large numbers of leucocytes to those where leucocytes are not increased, those with and without abnormal circulating cells, those arising from myeloid tissue and from lymphoid tissue and running a rapid and more chronic course. The latter two categories give rise to the four main groups of leukaemias:

- Acute myeloid (AML)
- Chronic myeloblastic (CML)
- Acute lymphoblastic (ALL)
- Chronic lymphocytic (CLL)

Other terms used are:

- *leukaemic leukaemia* — high concentration of leucocytes in blood, including abnormalities
- *subleukaemic leukaemia* — normal or low leucocyte concentration in blood but recognizable abnormalities
- *aleukaemic leukaemia* — normal leucocyte concentration in blood and no abnormal cells in blood
- *leukosis* — an alternative term to leukaemia (Woodliff & Herrmann, 1979).

Although the four terms indicated are in general use these are subdivided further on the basis of the precise type of cell involved. These subdivisions are indicated in Table 22.2.

Incidence and prognosis

The incidence in the UK and some other countries appears to have risen in the last three decades and, although part of this rise is due to better diagnosis, it is generally accepted that the rise is real. Woodliff & Herrmann (1979) report an overall incidence of about 5 per 100 000 of the population. In the 1960s leukaemia accounted for nearly 10% of the child mortality, this being nearly half the child cancer deaths. However, the huge advances in treatment have resulted in an 80%+ chance of 5 year survival in some childhood leukaemias, especially in girls (Taylor, 1980). In adults the picture is less promising and remissions are difficult to bring about in the over 50s. Acute adult leukaemias are now the commonest form of leukaemia in the Western world, the incidence being 0.25 per 100 000 for middle aged adults and 1 per 100 000 in the elderly (Woodliff & Herrmann, 1979). Table 22.2 summarizes the incidence and prognosis in the four main groups, including age and sex distribution where relevant.

Overall, males have a higher incidence than females. Previous differences in social class, north/south and urban/rural leukaemia mortality rates have evened out in the last two decades, probably due to better access to medical care of the disadvantaged groups (Taylor, 1980). The rising incidence of the later age onset chronic lymphocytic leukaemia suggests that long term exposure to leukaemogens within the environment may be a factor in causation. Some studies have reported an increase in childhood acute lymphoblastic leukaemia in the Manchester area and an increase in myeloid leukaemia in Lancashire (Taylor, 1980). At present the interpretation of the available statistics is open to question and the link with environmental radiation levels disputed.

There is wide variation in incidence internationally which is apparent despite problems of comparison. For example, the incidence of chronic myeloblastic leukaemia in Japan is very low, whereas the overall incidence in the USA is higher than in the UK, although it is lower for black persons and particularly high for white persons in California (Taylor, 1980).

Causes

Chromosome abnormality

While the aetiology of leukaemia is unknown, chromosome abnormalities are clearly implicated. Over 50% of people in a pre-leukaemic state show chromosome abnormalities (Taylor, 1980) and in the blastic (acute) stage of chronic myeloblastic leukaemia, 80% of patients have been found to have the 'Philadelphia' chromosome (Hellriegel, 1984). Children with Down's syndrome have 10–20 times the normal risk level of developing acute lymphoblastic leukaemia. Heredity does not appear to be implicated. It is possible that the chromosomal abnormalities arise due to a failure of ability to repair genetic material which then makes the person vulnerable to environmental factors which damage that material, e.g. radiation, cytotoxic drugs, certain viruses and benzene (Taylor, 1980).

Radiation

Exposure to ionizing radiation is clearly related to leukaemia incidence. This was most obviously demonstrated with the explosion of the nuclear bombs on Hiroshima and Nagasaki. The incidence of leukaemia is positively correlated with estimated radiation dose. For example, in Hiroshima the annual mortality rate at 100 rads exposure was 20 per 100 000, at 300 rads it was 65 per 100 000, and at 450 rads 118 per 100 000 (Taylor, 1980).

The more contentious question however is the dose of irradiation that can be considered 'safe'. For example, X-ray in late pregnancy has been linked with an increased incidence of leukaemia in the child – probably the cause in 1–2% of cases. In adults about 10% may be caused by man-made radiation utilized for industrial or medical purposes. As Taylor (1980) points out, however, over half the radiation to which people are exposed comes from natural sources, the amount in some areas being significantly higher. In these 'high risk' areas the incidence of leukaemia is no different than in areas with lower levels of natural radiation.

Infection and immunity

The role of infection and immunity in causation of leukaemia is unclear. Positive links emerge from reported success in treatment with BCG vaccination and with the clear value of immunosuppressants in the initial phase of treatment. The BCG success, however, is in some doubt, as is the reported link between maternal influenza during pregnancy and increased incidence of leukaemia in the children (Taylor, 1980).

Other factors

Acute myeloid leukaemia is associated with precedent disorders in as many as a third of patients (Moloney & Rosenthal, 1980). The disorders are primarily of haemopoietic tissue. Those with precedent disorders tend to be older and more resistant to remit than those without a precedent disorder.

Presentation and diagnosis

While the varying forms of leukaemia present in differing ways there is commonality in the nature of the signs and symptoms.

- Anaemia and the presence of malignancy
  General:
    Lethargy
    General feeling of illness
    Dyspnoea
    Pallor
    Anorexia
  Blood:
    Normocytic normochromic anaemia — severe in late chronic forms

- Abnormality of white cells and leucopoietic tissue
  General:
    Recurrent infections
    Splenic enlargement particularly in chronic forms
    Lymphadenopathy
    Bone pain
  Blood:
    Leucocytosis in varying degrees
    Presence of leukaemic leucocytes in peripheral blood
    Bone marrow infiltrated with leukaemic cells

- Altered platelets
  General:
    Purpura
    Bleeding gums
    Haemorrhage
  Blood:
    Usually thrombocytopenia

The diagnosis is usually tentative on the basis of the person's health history and the physical examination. Examination of the blood and bone marrow offers rapid and reliable confirmation.

Disease progression

Progression is more rapid in the acute forms, death from infection or haemorrhage occurring within 3 months in untreated patients (Woodliff & Herrmann, 1979; Moloney & Rosenthal, 1980). However, with treatment it is possible to bring the disease into a state of remission. Complete remission occurs when leukaemic cells are no longer present in either peripheral blood or bone marrow. However, because these cells recur even if treatment is maintained the term 'cure' is not used — 5 or 10 year survival rates being reported. Treatment success with the childhood acute lymphoblastic leukamia would suggest that 'cure' is an appropriate word in some situations.

Remission rates in acute leukaemia vary between 20% for persons over 50 years who have acute myeloid leukaemia associated with a precedent disorder (Moloney & Rosenthal, 1980) to 85% for younger persons (Foon & Gale, 1984). Remission rates and the duration of remission are steadily improving with developments in treatment patterns. Patients with acute leukaemia achieving remission may expect to remain in remission for 9–16 months, many will continue for 2 years and some for as long as 5 years (Foon & Gale, 1984).

The chronic leukaemias run a more benign

course but many patients will die within 5 years. Some persons with chronic lymphocytic leukaemia will survive 15–20 years, some of these without treatment (Theml & Ziegler-Heitbrock, 1984). As these patients also tend to be older they frequently die of diseases other than leukaemia. Chronic myeloid leukaemia, however, has two distinct phases, the first being relatively benign but inexorably leading to an acceleration and a highly malignant terminal blastic phase. Treatment has little effect on the course of the disease, remission never being achieved. However, treatment is valuable in symptom control (Hellriegel, 1984). The chronic phase might last about 3 years, the blastic phase 8–12 months.

Death in leukaemia (apart from those with chronic lymphocytic leukaemia who die of other causes) is invariably due to haemorrhage or infection.

Treatment

Again, the principles of therapy are common to all forms, as is the range of therapies available. The treatment regimes, however, differ between the forms of the disease and with ongoing experimentation with drug combinations and other modes of therapy.

The primary aim of therapy is to bring about remission. This is the first distinct phase of treatment and is called the induction phase. Effectively the intention is to depress leucopoietic tissue function to the extent that the abnormal proliferation of leukaemic cells is reduced and, if complete remission is to be achieved, leukaemic cells disappear from bone marrow and peripheral blood. This is an aggressive phase of treatment, particularly in acute leukaemia, with combinations of two or three cytotoxic drugs being given consistently or in a pattern of combination and/or timing. Daily checks are kept on the level of the patient's blood cells, drugs being withdrawn if the levels fall too low. Blood transfusion, platelet transfusion and antibiotics are given if required. It is at this stage of treatment that the experience of the effects of the drugs is often worse than the effects of the disease in the short term.

Due to the aggressive nature of the therapy, persons with chronic lymphocytic leukaemia are not treated if their disease is causing them few problems and if the lymphocyte doubling time indicates that the disease is not progressing rapidly. The time taken for the lymphocytes to double correlates well with both disease progression and survival time (Theml & Ziegler-Heitbrock, 1984).

Once remission is achieved the second phase of treatment is entered, that of maintenance of remission. Again, combinations of drugs are used, often including corticosteroids. The side-effects, however, are much less drastic and the person concerned will be out of hospital and may be leading a relatively normal life.

The leukaemic therapy comprises a choice of cytotoxic drugs (alkylating agents, antimetabolites, antineoplastic antibiotics and plant alkaloids), corticosteroids, immunoglobulins, radiation and bone marrow transplantation. Table 22.3 gives a summary of some of the commonly-used cytotoxics. These are normally used in combination and will vary between those used to bring about remission and those to maintain remission. The drug regimes used so successfully with children with acute leukaemia are not as effective in adults (Hoelzer, 1984). Total body irradiation is being used with some success in those with chronic myeloblastic leukaemia in its chronic phase (Taylor, 1980). Bone marrow transplantation appears to have considerable potential in children but its use with adults is controversial (Powles et al, 1980; Hoelzer, 1984).

The nature of the treatments inevitably brings unpleasant side-effects, indeed the therapeutic goal of reducing leucopoietic function itself causes increased risk of haemorrhage and infection. In addition nausea and vomiting are usual as is alopecia. These are indicated in Table 22.3 and discussed more fully in the nursing considerations.

Nursing considerations

During the acute phases, individuals with leukaemia will require treatment as an in-patient in hospital. For some who do not gain remission

Table 22.3 Cytotoxic drugs used in the treatment of leukaemia (Sources: Taylor, 1980; BNF, 1986)

Group and example	Mode of action and other aspects	Side-effects
All cytoxics	Interfere with cell division Absorption, metabolism and excretion vary widely	Damages all rapidly dividing cells whether normal or neoplastic: 1. cause bone marrow depression, therefore reduced erythrocytes, granulocytes and platelets, therefore infection and haemorrhage 2. gastrointestinal disturbance — nausea and vomiting 3. alopecia
1. **Alkylating agents**	Damage DNA and interfere with cell replication	Problems with prolonged use: gametogenesis is impaired — sterility during therapy permanent if long-term.
Busulphan	Selective depression of bone marrow Used for chronic myeloid	Excessive myelosuppression leading to aplasia Hyperpigmentation of skin Rare — interstitial pulmonary fibrosis
Chlorambucil	Chronic lymphocytic	Few side-effects
Cyclophosphamide	Widely used Inactive until metabolised in liver Fluid intake needs to be increased to avoid haemorrhagic cystisis	
2. **Cytotoxic antibiotics**	Interfere with DNA and RNA replication, also protein synthesis	Tend to increase tissue sensitivity to radiotherapy
Actinomycin	Given as IV bolus — important not to allow leak — would cause severe reaction	
Daunorubicin Doxorubicin	Fast running IV — important not to allow leak — would cause inflammation and necrosis	Cardiac toxicity — supraventricular arrhythmias may occur immediately after administration. High dose tends to cause cumulative irreversible cardiomyopathy.
3. **Antimetabolites**	Acts by incorporation into new nuclear material or by irreversible combination with vital cellular enzymes	
Cytarabine	Interferes with pyramidine synthesis Used for induction and maintenance in acute leukaemias	
Mercaptopurine	Analogue of adenine Used for maintenance in acute leukaemias	
Methotrexate	Inhibits an enzyme essential for synthesis of purines and pyramidines Oral, IM, IV or Intrathecal Mainly used for children for CNS involvement or maintenance of remission	
Thioguanine	Used solely for acute leukaemias	
4. **Vinca alkaloids**	Plant alkaloids which disrupt mitosis	
Vinblastine Vincristine	Particularly used for induction of remission Given IV	Neuropathy — usually sensorimotor peripheral with paraesthesia, loss of tendon reflexes and muscular weakness Autonomic neuropathy not uncommon in causing constipation, ileus and abdominal pain.
5. **Other cytotoxics** Razoxane	Has some effect in acute myeloid May increase response to radiotherapy.	

this will be the totality of their experience of leukaemia. Others will return to their homes, to be readmitted when remission ceases to be maintained. Due to the life-threatening and debilitating nature of both the illness and the treatment, staff on the haematological ward become particularly important to patients and others significant to them. A relaxed partnership between the health carers and the patient and family based on confidence, understanding and competence should be the aim.

From an examination of the nature of the disease, the aims of nursing management can be seen to fall into four groups

- Protection of the patient from unnecessary risks
  - infection
  - bleeding
  - necrosis at IVI sites used for the administration of bolus or fast-flow cytotoxics
  - crystallizing effects of uric acid
  - nutritional deficit
- Rapid identification and control of symptoms arising from the disease or treatment
  - infection
  - bleeding
  - nausea and vomiting, diarrhoea
  - pain
- Support and physical care during periods of dependency
  - hygiene and grooming
  - nutrition and hydration
  - elimination
  - rest and sleep
  - expression of anger, hopelessness
- Education of the patient and others significant to them
  - the disease
  - treatment regime and implications
  - self care.

These are discussed under common headings in approximate order of priority.

Haemorrhage/bleeding

Together with infection, haemorrhage is a major cause of death in leukaemia. Massive bleeding can occur in the gastrointestinal tract and epistaxis can also cause severe blood loss. Less life threatening, but contributing to general discomfort, debility and anaemia are repeated small bleeds from the gums, nose or gastrointestinal tract. Severe bruising, petechial haemorrhages and purpura also occur. Bleeding into joints causes acute pain and reduced mobility in the joint concerned. These effects are due primarily to the reduction in platelets brought about by displacement of production by leukaemic cell proliferation, or to bone marrow depression during therapy. In addition, corticosteroids increase cell friability, and even without platelet reduction are associated with gastrointestinal and petechial bleeding. In relation to haemorrhage therefore, the aims of nursing care may be identified as follows:

- to protect the patient from tissue damage
- to monitor the extent of small bleeds and identify any increase or signs of acute haemorrhage as early as possible
- to administer prescribed antacids, blood and platelet transfusions safely
- to give care to promote comfort and minimize the risk of infection when bruising, tissue damage, or intra-articular haemorrhage has occurred.

Care related to these aims is indicated in Table 22.4.

Infection

Both the disease and the treatment make the patient extremely vulnerable to infection. With the exception of the chronic myeloblastic type in its chronic phase, the abnormal leucocytes do not respond to invasion by microorganisms so are incapable of localizing or phagocytosing. In addition, treatment depresses bone marrow production, reducing the total circulating numbers of leucocytes and preventing the leucocytosis which would normally occur in response to infection. The immuno-suppressant

Table 22.4 Possible care plan related to bleeding

Nursing aim	Nursing approach
To protect the patient from tissue damage	Careful handling of dependent patient. Regular position change. Remove or pad furniture with obtruding knobs, handles, cot sides, handles for winding bed up. Position furniture to allow patient easy access to personal belongings, call bell, etc. Ensure furniture is not in a position to cause stumbling. Non-slip floor. Restriction of access during cleaning. Non-slip firm footwear, dressing gown cords not trailing. Protect mouth and gums from damage as indicated under infection. Avoid overinflation of BP cuff and minimise duration cuff is inflated.
To monitor the extent of small bleeds and identify increase or signs of acute haemorrhage as early as possible	4 hourly observation of P and BP. At least daily enquiry and observation of — mouth for signs of bleeding, ulcers — skin for bruising, tissue damage, purpura, especially of arms, legs and pressure areas — movement for signs of intra-articular bleeding — abdominal discomfort for signs of gastrointestinal bleeding — faeces for obvious blood, change in consistency or colour. Daily urine testing for blood. Weekly laboratory testing of faeces for occult blood.
To administer safely prescribed antacids, blood and platelet transfusions	Antacids to be taken before and after meals, may be left by the bedside for patient self-administration if possible Scrupulous checking of blood and platelets. 1 hourly observations throughout transfusion of temperature, pulse and general condition. Hourly blood pressure recording.
To give care to promote comfort and minimise risk of infection when bruising, tissue damage or intra-articular haemorrhage has occurred	Protect damaged areas by generous, supportive but non-restrictive padding. If the skin of arms and legs is very friable, padding may be applied before tissue damage occurs. Scrupulous asepsis. Restrict use of damaged joint, warmth or cold may be applied. The joint may be elevated. Request or administer analgesia and monitor effectiveness.

action of corticosteroids reduces the overall response to infection. The cumulative result is that the person with leukaemia is more vulnerable to infection, made even more so by initial treatment, and will demonstrate signs of infection only when the infection has got a considerable hold. Thus the aims of nursing care may be expressed as follows:

- to reduce to a minimum the risk of the patient acquiring an infection
- to identify the signs of infection at the earliest opportunity and ensure treatment is prescribed
- to administer prescribed antibiotics and antifungal agents strictly to time to optimize effectiveness
- to give care that facilitates infection control and patient comfort.

Care related to these aims is indicated in Table 22.5.

Nutrition and hydration

Problems with nutrition and hydration arise from a number of sources in patients with leukaemia. The disease itself, in common with most malignant disorders, tends to result in loss of weight and loss of appetite (the weight loss not being solely food-intake dependent). Even without treatment, oral and gastrointestinal ulceration may cause discomfort and pain in relation to food intake. Cytotoxic and

Table 22.5 Possible care plan related to infection

Nursing aim	Nursing approach
To reduce to a minimum the risk of the patient acquiring an infection	Patient nursed in an environment relatively or completely free of infection. This may include isolation with reverse barrier nursing or isolation in a sterile environment in those at very high risk Nurses with colds, boils or other infections should not handle the patient. Skin abrasions or IV sites should be protected by an occlusive dressing. Strapping should not be adherent to the patient's skin, risk of skin abrasion high. Scrupulous aseptic technique with wound dressings or attention to IV sites. Careful technique for bolus injections of cytotoxics to avoid leakages. Care in handling a dependent patient to avoid abrasions. Immaculate toilet hygiene — cleansing of toilet seat, in females wiping vulval area from front to back to reduce risk of enteral bacteria infecting urethra. Optimal mobility to reduce risk of pulmonary and urinary stasis. Great care with mouth and teeth cleaning — use of antibacterial mouth washes 2 hrly (e.g. chlorhexidine). Toothbrushes to be avoided. Remove and replace dentures with great care. Gentle swabbing with soft disposable cloth or cotton buds if food adherent to teeth or gums. Avoid abrasive food such as toast. Thermometer placement underarm.
To identify the signs of infection at the earliest opportunity and ensure treatment is prescribed	4 hrly observation of TPR. At least daily enquiry and observation regarding — skin abrasions, spots, boils — urinary symptoms such as burning, abnormal small, proteinuria — symptoms of colds, chestiness — IV site. Daily–weekly swabbing of body orifices for microbiological examination and if symptoms appear. Rapid contact with medical staff if symptoms appear.
To administer prescribed antibiotics and antifungal agents strictly to time to optimize effectiveness	This is self-explanatory. If the patient is able and reliable he/she may administer his/her own antibiotics. If oral drugs are prescribed and the patient is vomiting, a prescription for intramuscular or intravenous administration must be obtained. Oral antifungal agents such as amphotericin lozenges should be taken after the chlorhexidine mouthwash after food.
To give care that facilitates infection control and patient comfort	This will be variable dependent on symptoms. For example urinary infection — high fluid intake to 3000 ml in 24 hours to reduce stasis and dilute the infection Pyrexia — tepid sponging and/or fanning may be required.

corticosteroid therapy increase this problem. In addition, cytotoxic drugs cause major gastro-intestinal problems resulting in severe nausea and, frequently, vomiting. A separate problem due to cytotoxics is the rise in uric acid resulting from leucocyte destruction. Crystallization in the kidneys results unless a high urinary dilution is maintained. Possible nursing aims may therefore be defined as follows:

- to control nausea and vomiting
- to maintain a high fluid intake (3000 ml minimum in 24 hours)
- to minimize discomfort associated with eating
- to maintain an adequate level of nutrition.

Table 22.6 indicates a possible care plan related to this area.

Elimination

Urinary elimination is potentially affected by four factors. Firstly, the risk of uric acid crystal formation due to cytotoxic agents. This causes glomerular destruction, pain and eventually suppression of urine formation. Secondly, dehydration related to lack of fluid intake and profuse sweating during pyrexial episodes results in reduced and concentrated urine output. Thirdly, lack of mobility due to periods of illness or the restriction of IVIs increases the risk of urinary stasis. Fourthly, being required to

Table 22.6 Possible care plan related to nutrition and hydration

Nursing aim	Nursing approach
To control nausea and vomiting	Identify and modify particular stimulants in environment, food or drink that trigger nausea. Regulate food intake to avoid times when nausea or vomiting is known to be worse. Offer small meals or liquid supplements of type and temperature that patient prefers. Administer prescribed anti-emetics at optimal time in relation to food intake.
To maintain a high fluid intake (3000 ml minimum in 24 hr)	Plan schedule of favourite and varied drinks with patient. If at all possible the patient should take over the responsibility for achieving the fluid intake including preparation and charting.
To minimise discomfort associated with eating	Control of mouth infections. Avoid abrasive foods. Soft ice-cold foods are often preferred. Local anaesthetic lozenges or mouthwashes may be used if pain from ulceration is severe but can cause problems in reducing sensitivity of swallowing. Edentulous patients may prefer not to wear dentures.
To maintain an adequate level of nutrition	Monitor patient's weight weekly and relate to pre-illness weight, height and body build. Plan meals and fluids with patient, focusing on high nutrient fluids such as 'Build-up', 'Hi cal' and egg flips if dietary intake is a problem. Serve attractively and hot/warm/cold as intended. Monitor intake, recording daily. Offer nutrient fluids if meal not eaten. Encourage significant others to bring in favourite foods.

use bedpans or commodes unnecessarily, without adequate privacy or without guarantee of reasonably immediate response from the nurses, may result in a reluctance to drink adequately.

Some of these factors clearly relate to faecal elimination as well. In addition, gastrointestinal disturbance from the drug regime and gastrointestinal bleeding due to the disease or treatment results in diarrhoea and abdominal pain being frequent problems.

The aims of nursing care in relation to elimination may therefore be defined as follows:

- to maintain a high urinary output, 2500 ml minimum
- to control faecal elimination so that abdominal, rectal and anal discomfort is avoided
- to identify early deviations from the normal pattern of elimination
- to optimize privacy, dignity, comfort and independence in relation to toilet needs.

Measures related to reducing the risk of infection and to monitoring the patient for signs of infection and haemorrhage have been noted. Table 22.7 indicates an approach to care related to elimination.

Pain

Pain in leukaemia has a variety of sources. Enlargement of reticuloendothelial tissues causes bone pain and discomfort related to splenomegaly and lymphadenopathy. Bleeding into joints or tissues creates further problems. Ulceration of the mouth and gastrointestinal system cause yet more pain. Friable skin tissue may be knocked or torn if adhesive tape has been used, leaving subcutaneous tissues exposed. Control of pain is complicated by a reluctance to use narcotics which may create dependence and the danger of using aspirin and non-steroidal anti-inflammatory agents due to their gastrointestinal effects. Effectively, therefore, the aim of nursing is to control pain to a level acceptable to the patient and commensurate with the patient's prognosis.

Suggested approaches are indicated in Table 22.8.

Prevention or control of infection, tissue damage, nausea, vomiting and diarrhoea also

Table 22.7 Possible care plan related to elimination

Nursing aim	Nursing approach
To maintain a high urinary output (2500 ml+)	Basically this relies on a high fluid intake, especially if the patient is pyrexial and sweating or has diarrhoea. While on induction therapy IV fluids assist oral intake. Fluid output chart essential.
To control faecal elimination so that abdominal, rectal and anal discomfort is avoided	Control of diarrhoea may be achieved via constipating antacids. Water absorbent gels such as isogel are not usually tolerated. Kaolin and morphine may be required. Acid fruits are best avoided. If constipation occurs high fibre foods and stool softeners are preferable. Aperients causing increased peristalsis should be avoided.
To identify early, deviations from the normal pattern of elimination	Monitor as indicated under infection and haemorrhage. Daily record of elimination pattern.
To optimize privacy, dignity, comfort and independence in relation to toilet needs	Wherever possible site the patient near a toilet suitable for his/her use with available materials to cleanse toilet seat and themselves. Otherwise prompt attention when required. Commodes are always preferable to bedpans unless the patient opts for bedpan. Pleasant deodorant sprays (or perfume sprays) and attention to personal hygiene after toileting reduce potential embarrassment and transmission of infection.

Table 22.8 Possible care plan in relation to pain

Nursing aim	Nursing approach
To control pain to a level acceptable to the patient and commensurate with the patient's prognosis	Full pain assessment especially if pain is clearly persistent and not amenable to measures taken. Identification and modification of pain triggers if evident. Use of topical anaesthetic lozenges and sprays. Limb support. Meticulous care when giving IV bolus or rapid infusion of cytotoxics to prevent leakage causing inflammation, pain and tissue necrosis. Maintenance of optimal body position individual to that person, altering position 2 hrly if dependent to avoid stiffness and decubitus ulceration. If required, regular anticipatory analgesia as prescribed. Narcotics appropriate to terminal phase. Salicylates and other gastric irritants to be avoided. Careful monitoring of both pain and the effect of positioning and analgesia. At least daily reporting.

help to achieve this aim, as does the suggested approach for encouraging nutrient intake.

Rest, sleep and general comfort

Rest and sleep may become severely compromised by the symptoms associated with the disease and treatment. Management of the symptoms mentioned is therefore the most important factor. Other aspects such as the frequency and timing of care giving, treatments, observations, meals and visitors can equally compromise a patient's rest. The overall nursing plan should take account of this and allow specific times for undisturbed rest. Observations and treatment at night should be cut to a minimum and scheduled to coincide.

Every attempt should be made to promote the person's comfort, including the provision of comfortable chairs, self care facilities for preparation of drinks, privacy when required and with visitors, and other facilities that enhance the individual's sense of value and dignity.

Support

Although many patients with leukaemia will be

familiar with hospital routines, the majority of persons newly admitted with symptoms of acute leukaemia will be relatively young and are unlikely to have previous illness or hospital experience. Almost certainly they will not have had experience of such a devastating nature. Unlike many malignancies, the diagnosis of leukaemia is difficult to conceal (even if this were desirable) due both to the nature and progression of the disease and the aggressive nature of the treatment. Disbelief, anger, hostility and depression can all be anticipated. Continued support by listening and showing empathy; by managing symptoms in partnership with the patient; by allowing anger and hostility without platitudes or reciprocal aggression; and by allowing expression of fear, hopelessness and self-pity in the context of realistic expectation of prognosis, is the least a nurse can do but is not easy to achieve. Group support of both patients and nursing staff is an additional support strategy.

Information and education

If partnership in care between the patient, others significant to them and the health carers is to be achieved, information needs to be free-flowing in both directions. To comply with treatment regimes and to anticipate, prevent or promptly treat problems as they arise, the patient needs to know what he or she might expect. To manage symptom control and treat the disease effectively the health care team need to know how the patient is experiencing his or her illness and what he/she has found helpful. Individual and group discussions while the patient is in hospital and after discharge can be used both to promote information sharing and as a support mechanism.

Conclusion

The nature of leukaemia, particularly in its acute and blastic form, and the aggressive nature of the treatment regime affects the individual sufferer in the most fundamental of ways. His/her life is threatened, the illness and treatment create wretched and personally disintegrating symptoms of pain, vomiting, bleeding, mouth ulceration and diarrhoea, and prognosis is unsure and frequently limited. Knowledgeable and sensitive planning, execution and monitoring of care in partnership with the patient would appear to be best achieved in the context of primary nursing. In this way continuity of planning, education and support, and effective symptom control may be achieved.

DISORDERS OF PLATELETS (THROMBOCYTES)

Primary disorders presenting as platelet increase, decrease or malfunction are uncommon. However platelet increase (thrombocythaemia) and platelet decrease (thrombocytopenia) occur frequently in association with other disorders.

THROMBOCYTHAEMIA

This accompanies some myeloproliferative disorders such as chronic myeloid leukaemia and polycythaemia. In the absence of other relationships it is termed idiopathic. The thrombocytes are increased but malfunctional, giving rise both to thrombosis and haemorrhage, the latter gastrointestinal. Radioactive phosphorus or cytotoxic therapy may be effective, and aspirin in small doses may help to counteract the tendency to thrombosis (MacLeod, 1984).

THROMBOCYTOPENIA

This may be primary (idiopathic) or secondary to other factors. General depression of bone marrow due to hypo- or aplasia or to bone marrow disease such as leukaemia or secondary carcinoma result in thrombocytopenia. Excessive or chronic alcohol consumption also causes a temporary thrombocytopenia.

Thrombocytopenia also occurs with excessive production of platelets and may be due to toxic reactions to drugs, after severe infections or in an idiopathic form.

The primary problem with thrombocytopenia from whatever cause is bleeding. This may be in the form of acute haemorrhage usually from nasal or gastrointestinal mucosa, haematoma in joints or tissues or capillary bleeds causing purpura. As haemorrhage is life-threatening, persons with low platelet counts are usually admitted to hospital for close observation even though 'treatment' may be to wait for natural resolution of the problem.

If the disease is idiopathic, splenectomy and short term steroids may bring about a remission. Platelets given by transfusion are usually rapidly destroyed so are ineffective as a mode of therapy except for very short term action to reduce an immediate risk of haemorrhage.

Nursing considerations with the thrombocytopenic patient are those included under the care related to the risk of haemorrhage in the previous section on nursing considerations.

DISORDERS OF PLASMA COAGULATION FACTORS

While there are a number of disorders of platelet coagulation factors, the incidence of the majority of diseases is small. The major disease in this group, haemophilia A, is discussed briefly.

HAEMOPHILIA A

Haemophilia A is due to a genetic disorder of the coagulant part of antihaemophilic globulin (AHG) or Factor VIII — one of the complex chain of factors essential to normal haemostasis. The incidence varies but is quoted as 1–10 per 100 000 population, 75% of which are inherited and 25% being due to spontaneous mutation (Woodliff & Herrman, 1979). It is a sex-linked recessive defect carried on the X chromosome and predominantly affects males although, rarely, girls inheriting the abnormal X chromosomes (one from each parent) will develop haemophilia. The defect varies in severity from absence to 20% of normal AHG levels, the latter being compatible with normal lifestyle. Clearly the more severe the disorder, the higher the risk of haemorrhage.

There is no long-term treatment of haemophilia, but acute episodes of haemorrhage, usually intra-articular or gastro-intestinal, can be treated with intravenous injections of cryoprecipitate containing AHG. The short half-life of AHG means that injections have to be given 12 hourly unless the injury or bleeding is minimal. Individuals who have haemophilia and are scheduled for surgical operation need to have higher doses of AHG 12 hourly for a 3 day postoperative period to reduce the risk of haemorrhage.

Nursing considerations

The precautions that pertain to caring for individuals with an increased haemorrhagic risk become part of the way of life of people with haemophilia. Adults admitted to hospital for other reasons, e.g. surgery, or for a 2–3 day course of cryoprecipitate because of injury, are very much more used to their condition than the nursing staff. Clearly they should be facilitated in their self-care by the staff. In addition the patient may well be concerned that nursing staff will not understand his needs. Listening and learning from the patient therefore becomes central, and pre- and postoperative management should include great care with patient handling during periods of dependancy and meticulous and frequent observations of vital signs and of the wound.

DISTURBANCE OF FLOW WITHIN THE ARTERIAL AND VENOUS SYSTEM AND THE HEART

This section includes some of today's major health problems — hypertension, coronary heart disease, acquired heart valve disease. Many of the disorders are interrelated. For example, atheroma is implicated in coronary heart disease, peripheral arterial disease and aneurysm. Hypertension is an accepted 'risk factor' with coronary heart disease but in the majority of persons is not caused by atheroma. For this reason hypertension is discussed first. This is followed by an explanation of atheroma, which precedes the section on coronary artery disease, central arterial disease and peripheral arterial disease. Subsequently, acquired heart valve disease is discussed and the section is completed by focusing on the effect of disorders of peripheral venous blood flow.

HYPERTENSION

The term 'hypertension' means high arterial pressure, that is, pressure within the arterial system that is higher than ' normal'. Given that morbidity and mortality rises with rising blood pressure, the definition of 'hypertension' in terms of what is considered to be 'pathological' and worthy of treatment, and what is considered to be 'normal' becomes an important issue.

In addition, while hypertension is a feature of many diseases the aetiology in 90–95% of all hypertensive persons is unclear (Cowley, 1978; Guyton, 1984). In these individuals the condition is currently described as 'primary' or 'essential' hypertension and the treatment is primarily directed towards lowering the blood pressure.

Definition and 'incidence'

Burt et al (1982a) define mild to moderate hypertension as a diastolic pressure (phase 5) over 95mmHg and severe hypertension as over 100mmHg. By this definition 26% of the male population between 45 and 64 years is hypertensive (Wells, 1982). 4% of the middle-aged population have a diastolic pressure between 110 and 129mmHg, 5% a pressure of over 130mmHg (Bannan et al, 1981a). Hamer (1981) suggests that a diastolic pressure of 105mmHg should be considered as indicative of moderate hypertension worthy of treatment, on the basis that this level marks the point at which the mortality curve begins to rise more steeply. The term 'borderline hypertension' is increasingly being used for those with mild hypertension, variously defined as having a diastolic pressure of over 90 or 95mmHg (dependent on age). The debate about the efficacy of treatment is particularly related to this group (Julius, 1978). The mortality for these persons is raised, but it is known that not all will develop moderate or severe hypertension and the treatment itself may precipitate other problems, particularly those related to myocardial or peripheral ischaemia. The definition of hypertension cited by Bannan et al (1981a) appears particularly apt: 'that level of blood pressure above which investigation and treatment do more good than harm'.

Systolic hypertension

The traditional focus of measurement has been on the diastolic pressure as the important criterion for hypertensive status. However the Framingham study (Kannel & Gordon, 1970) confirmed earlier impressions that the incidence of cardiac enlargement, heart failure, coronary artery disease and strokes all correlated more closely with systolic pressures than diastolic. More serious attention therefore is now paid to the systolic pressure, and 'systolic hypertension' is recognized as a clinical entity and treated accordingly. Tarazi and Gifford (1978) suggest a 'rule of thumb' definition of systolic hypertension as a systolic blood pressure of more than 150mmHg with a diastolic blood pressure of less than 90mmHg.

Prognosis

The causes of morbidity and mortality related to hypertension are associated with cerebral, renal or cardiac conditions, the primary ones being stroke, cardiac failure and coronary heart disease.

The risk of problems rises with rising blood pressure. Of those with moderate hypertension, cardiovascular problems are likely to ensue within 3 years in 26% of untreated persons. This risk reduces to 15% if treatment results in poor control (diastolic BP above 90mmHg) and to 10% if treatment results in the diastolic pressure being maintained below 80mmHg (Taguchi & Freis, 1974). Thus control of hypertension is important if morbidity is to be reduced.

The mortality for those with a diastolic pressure of 110–129mmHg is 20% within 5 years if untreated. 35% of those with a diastolic pressure of over 130mmHg will die within

2 years. In those with a diastolic pressure of over 150mmHg, 50% will die within 2 years (Bannan et al, 1981a). These figures again illustrate the importance of reducing hypertension.

Nature of the disturbance and associated factors

While the precise nature of the problem is not known, in over 90% of persons with hypertension there is general agreement that hypertension is a disease of physiologic regulation (Dustan, 1981). Many regulation systems have been identified involving for example, cardiovascular, neurological, endocrine and renal systems, but the way in which they interrelate to control blood pressure in both normotensive and hypertensive states is less clear.

Research into causation/aetiology focuses around a number of the factors controlling blood pressure, e.g. neural control of the circulation; the importance of vasopressin; the mechanisms of vascular smooth muscle contraction and the relative importance of structural versus functional changes responsible for increased vascular resistance; the role of sodium in determining vascular resistance; the role of vascular smooth muscle calcium; the question whether the kidney is a dominant controlling factor, and renal-neural interrelationships. Genetic predisposition is a constant theme (Dustan, 1981).

For example, sodium levels are significantly related to blood pressure levels in hypertensive persons but not in normotensive. Renal vascular reactivity is abnormally high during neurogenic stimulation and the average renal resting blood flow is higher in young normotensive persons with hypertensive parents than in those with normotensive parents. Similarly there is an exaggerated increase in blood pressure to sympathetic stimulation in normotensive adolescents of hypertensive parents (WHO, 1983).

Typically individuals with established hypertension have the following physiological characteristics:

- normal cardiac output
- decreased stroke volume
- increased heart rate
- elevated peripheral resistance
- plasma volume is decreased
- plasma renin may be normal or low
- resistance to vasodilatation is raised
- responsiveness to vasoconstrictors is increased

These latter characteristics are indicative of structural change in the arterioles (WHO, 1983).

The majority of those with borderline hypertension follow the above pattern, although some people present with a raised cardiac output, raised heart rate, raised cardio-pulmonary blood volume, raised stroke volume and raised peripheral resistance.

Course of the disease

The course of the disease does not follow an inevitable pattern, and for the most part is asymptomatic until cardiovascular events intervene. Adolescents with blood pressures higher than normal are at greater risk. Of those with established hypertension at 40 years the frequency of borderline hypertension at the age of 20 years is 20%, three times higher than the general population (WHO, 1983). The majority with moderate hypertension do not progress to malignant hypertension. The morbidity and mortality has already been indicated. Symptoms of hypertension other than its presentation through cardiovascular disease and strokes are unusual except in malignant hypertension where severe headache may be a persistent and uncontrollable symptom.

Factors associated with hypertension

A number of factors, genetic, environmental and personal are associated with hypertension. These will be reviewed briefly as they form the basis of primary prevention.

Genetic factors

The evidence for a genetic contribution to essential hypertension comes from studies of both humans and animals (Nora & Nora, 1983). There are, for example, specific ethnic groups who have a high incidence of hypertension, the most notable being men of negro origin (Hamer, 1981). In addition the blood pressure distribution curve of relatives of hypertensive persons is slightly shifted to the right (Nora & Nora, 1983). The effects of hypertension can also be seen to be genetically influenced, black people having fewer heart attacks than white and Asian people (Cruikshank & Beevers, 1980).

Cross-cultural studies also show a statistically positive relationship between estimated salt intake and blood pressure levels between communities, but within any one community there is little evidence of such a relationship (DHSS, 1984). The genetically determined ability to handle salt appears to be a crucial factor in studies of the response of rats to salt excess; some animals remain normotensive no matter how high the salt loading, whereas those with hypertension demonstrate an abnormal salt handling (Nora & Nora, 1983). Such evidence may be of relevance to furthering the understanding of human responses.

Dietary intake

The influence of salt intake on blood pressure has already been mentioned. Essentially it would appear that only those who are genetically susceptible are at particular risk from a high salt intake (Nora & Nora, 1983).

Other minerals such as potassium and calcium have been implicated, as has the ratio of sodium to potassium, calcium and magnesium (WHO, 1983).

There is some evidence that reducing the intake of fats will reduce blood pressure, but this effect is not marked and it has no effect on normotensive young adults (WHO, 1983). This may relate to a reduction in other disease processes such as atheroma rather than to the hypertensive process (Hamer, 1981), although this link is equally suspect.

Obesity

There is an increased incidence of hypertension with obesity (DHSS, 1984). To an extent this may be due to the artefact of fat-arm high blood pressure recordings (O'Brien & O'Malley, 1981d) or to dietary factors. For example it is known that obese people have a higher salt intake and that the sodium pump is impaired in some obese people (WHO, 1983). However by careful blood pressure recording, use of intra-arterial measurement and variate analysis of the data these confounding variables can be controlled and the consensus view is that obesity is an independent factor (Reisin, 1983; WHO, 1983). The obese and those who gain weight are six times as likely to develop hypertension as those who remain thin; in those whose weight is variable the blood pressure rises with weight gain and falls with weight loss (WHO, 1983). Shifting the population weight distribution curve to the left has been estimated to have the potential to reduce prevalence of hypertension by as much as 25% (WHO, 1983).

Alcohol

Alcohol appears to raise the systolic pressure but not the diastolic, the blood pressure falling following alcohol withdrawal and rising again if intake is restarted. The rise in heavy drinkers may be as much as 10mmHg systolic and 6mmHg diastolic (WHO, 1983). The way in which this effect is mediated is in some doubt, blood cortisol, catecholamines and the effect on renin-angiotensin being possible mechanisms.

Cigarette smoking

Cigarette smoking does exert a brief pressor effect especially if taken with coffee but, in the long term, smokers do not have higher blood pressure levels than non-smokers. However, smoking greatly increases the adverse vascular effects of hypertension (Isles et al, 1979).

Physical exertion

Physical exertion appears to have no relationship with the development of hypertension, although some hypertensive persons have shown a reduction of diastolic pressure when increasing their regular exercise level (WHO, 1983).

Psycho-social factors

There is considerable evidence that blood pressure varies for any one individual within a 24 hour period dependent on the activity and 'stress' involved in the situation (O'Brien & O'Malley, 1981e). Low job satisfaction with high role conflict at work and demanding occupations have also been associated with higher blood pressure levels (WHO, 1983). Studies of people from so-called 'primitive' communities who display normally low blood pressures but have been transferred to an alien society show that the blood pressure subsequently rises (Prior, 1979). The findings of Masterton et al (1981), that patients in a long term psychiatric unit have lower blood pressures than the general population, might suggest that this environment is protective from outside pressures. The relative reduction of hypertension in the black population in the United States (mortality from strokes in black people was 6 fold before 1950, 2 fold since 1950 compared with the white population) and the levelling of incidence of hypertension between black, Asian and white people within the same social class grouping (Cruikshank & Beavers, 1980) would also point to a social, rather than ethnic, origin of hypertension in this instance. This is supported by the clear evidence that groups that are disadvantaged socially or educationally have a higher incidence of hypertension than more advantaged groups (WHO, 1983).

While it is clear that personal, social and environmental factors do influence blood pressure, Steptoe (1981) concludes that the contribution of these factors can best be seen in the context of an interactional framework. In this way, the social, cultural and economic climate can be seen to influence individuals, individual behaviour can be seen to influence choice of diet, individuals respond physiologically to food intake and, via emotional response, to environmental situations in part on the basis of genetic predisposition. Age and pathophysiological factors further influence the cardiovascular dynamics that result in blood pressure level.

Secondary hypertension

Hypertension is secondary to identified disease or drugs in about 5% of patients. Renal, vascular, endocrine and neurological mechanisms are usually involved. The following is a brief list of these associated disorders:

- coarctation (narrowing) of the aorta
- renal and renal artery disease
- adrenocortical and adrenomedullary lesions
- expanding intracranial lesions
- drugs
  - oral contraceptives
  - corticosteriods
  - carbenoxolone
  - monoamine oxidase inhibitors
  - tricyclic antidepressants
  - non-steroidal anti-inflammatory agents (Robertson, 1983).

Primary prevention

While it is clear that there are associated and modifiable risk factors in hypertension, the situation is not one of clear causation. For this reason the World Health Organization Scientific Group (WHO, 1983) recommend that primary prevention of hypertension utilize both mass intervention and a 'high risk' approach and define the aims as:

- in high risk individuals, to prevent attainment of levels of blood pressure at which the institution of management and treatment would be considered
- in the general population, to delay or arrest further progression of blood pressure levels beyond those attained upon reaching adulthood.

Those at risk can be identified from the associated factors previously discussed:

- those with a family history of hypertension
- racial background
- obesity
- increased heart rate (WHO, 1983).

The advice both to high risk individuals and to

populations at large is two fold:

- avoid obesity
- reduce salt intake.

Other measures that might have some influence in preventing hypertension include:

- alcohol moderation
- relaxation
- social and educational improvement (WHO, 1983; Robertson, 1983).

The effect of these measures, however, can only be estimated as no long term investigations have been undertaken to study the feasibility or effect of such programmes.

Early detection of those at risk

Early detection can focus on those groups already identified above and can involve screening the general population. Study of such mass screening programmes indicates that about 80% of the population can be reached in this way. The World Health Organization Expert Committee (WHO, 1978), however, identified that 80% of the population see their family doctor approximately once in 3 years. A cost-effective method of screening therefore would be for general practitioners to record the blood pressure of each of their visiting patients at least once in 3 years. In addition the argument for blood pressure measurement to become part of routine health checks in schools is overwhelming and would enable those displaying higher than normal blood pressures, particularly teenagers, to be followed up systematically (Robertson, 1983).

Treatment

Treatment regimes primarily include:

- dietary restriction, modification or moderation
- drug regimes.

In addition there is some evidence that exercise and relaxation may be beneficial.

Two other issues however are also of concern in relation to treatment. Firstly, the selection of those who should be treated by drugs. The significance of this has already been discussed in the initial section on definition and incidence and will not be further discussed here. Secondly, due to the asymptomatic nature of the disease, most persons with hypertension are going about their everyday life quite normally. In this situation compliance with treatment is a major issue. This is therefore discussed further.

Overall, the efficiency of the health care system in treating persons with hypertension is poor. Non-identification of persons with asymptomatic hypertension continues to be high in the absence of planned screening programmes, in the absence of routine blood pressure measurement in school medical examinations and visits to the family doctor, and in the absence of reliable follow-up schemes. The debate about the efficacy of drug therapy in borderline hypertension results in more persons not being treated than is desirable. Of those who are treated, non-compliance and lack of real evaluation of treatment leads to a high percentage in whom control is poor. Bannan et al (1981b) illustrated this with the 'rule of halves' illustrated in Figure 22.3.

Dietary therapy

Dietary advice primarily revolves around:

- weight reduction (if required)
- salt intake reduction
- reduction in intake of saturated fats
- alcohol moderation.

The evidence for these factors being implicated in hypertension has already been reviewed. The only factor with a known positive outcome is that of weight reduction. This will be accompanied by a lowering of the blood pressure. The evidence for the role of the remaining three substances is equivocal, although on balance it appears that reduction or modification will be beneficial in terms of lowering the blood pressure.

A small study by Margetts et al (1985) investigated the effect of a vegetarian diet. While the results demonstrated an average 5mmHg

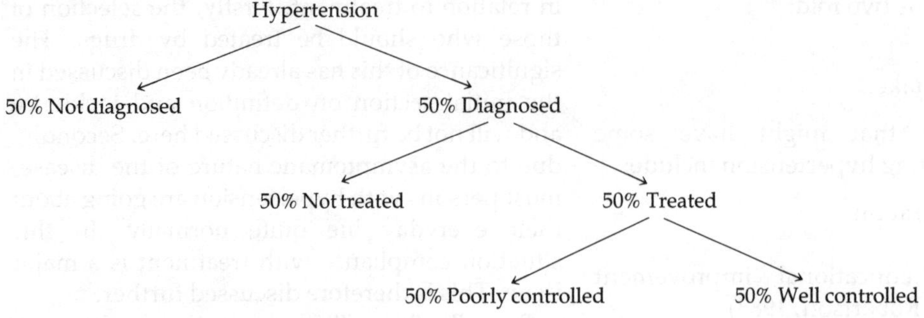

Fig. 22.3 Rule of halves applied to hypertension control (Bannan et al 1981b)

reduction in diastolic pressures, the elements contributing to this could not be identified. Certainly if dietary modification is found to be effective the need for drug therapy in borderline hypertension might well be reduced.

Relaxation

There is some evidence that regular periods of meditative relaxation reduce diastolic and systolic pressures by 5–10mmHg. In reviewing the literature and undertaking a small study on stress and hypertension, Benson et al (1978) concluded that a 20 minute period of relaxation twice a day will be beneficial regardless of whether or not the person is on drug therapy. They recommend that the relaxation period should include the following features:

- a quiet environment
- relaxation, decreased muscle tone
- a passive attitude
- a mental device or constant mental stimulus (such as a repeated word) to reduce extraneous thinking.

It is thought that such relaxation measures are effective via a decrease in catecholamines.

Hamer (1981), however, doubts that individuals would maintain such a programme over a period of time and points out that there is no evidence that it would remain effective in the long-term.

Again, the potential for this mode of therapy is considerable and deserves rigorous and long-term evaluation.

In evaluating another aspect of stress reduction — knowledge and understanding — Tanner & Noury (1981) found that a teaching programme had no significant effect on blood pressure levels, although the level of knowledge was increased.

Exercise

While physical activity does not seem to be related to the incidence of hypertension there is some evidence that exercise training can reduce the diastolic, but not the systolic, blood pressure by 6mmHg at rest, 10mmHg on exercise. Heart rate is also reduced by exercise training (Westheim et al, 1985). On the training programme within the research, exercise consisted of 45 minute periods three times a week for 12 weeks. How well this relates to general levels of physical activity at home or work, or to shorter more frequent periods is not known.

Drug therapy

The drugs used for hypertension control fall into three groups:

- thiazides or alternative diuretics
- beta-adrenergic blocking agents
- vasodilators or other potent drugs.

Thiazides are usually tried first, beta blockers being utilized if thiazides are ineffective. The two may then be combined. Vasodilators and other potent drugs are used by themselves or in combination as a last resort. There appears to be reasonable agreement as to this strategy (Bannan et al, 1981c; Hamer, 1981). There is no place for sedatives in the treatment of hypertension (Hamer, 1981). Table 22.9 lists some of the drugs commonly used in treating hypertension.

The value of drug therapy with good control is unquestioned in those with moderate to severe hypertension. For example, in a major international study of over 6000 individuals with an initial diastolic (phase 5) pressure of 110–125mmHg who were followed up over a five year period, the risk of stroke and cardiac events was halved with a reduction of 5mmHg in the diastolic or 20mmHg in the systolic (IPPPSH, 1985).

Considerable attention is now focused on those with borderline hypertension and on the elderly with hypertension. Non-drug intervention and careful follow up would seem to be the safe course of action with the former group (Julius, 1978). In a recent report of the European Working Party on High Blood Pressure in the Elderly (EWPHE, 1985) it would appear that treatment of hypertension in the elderly with diuretic therapy significantly reduces cardiovascular mortality.

Compliance with therapy

Bannan et al's (1981b) rule of halves applied to hypertension suggests that in approximately 50% of persons treated for hypertension the therapy results in poor control. Compared with some studies this percentage appears generous (Wilber & McCombs, 1975). However, apart from the efficacy of the treatment itself, compliance with treatment is identified as a major problem (Vidt, 1978). Three aspects contribute to compliance:

- the nature and effect of the therapy
- the location of the monitoring clinic
- the nature of the personnel involved.

The nature of the studies, however, does not enable firm conclusions to be drawn as to the specific contribution the three factors may have. For example Wilber & McCombs (1975) report a study in which 81% of patients returned to a nurse's clinic compared with 55% to a hospital clinic and 41% to a private doctor's office. This resulted in good control being achieved in 50%, 23% and 26% respectively. Whether the professional role, the place, the individual or the time and approach taken was the significant feature here is impossible to say. Bannan et al (1981d) conclude from their literature review that as good control can be achieved in health centres as in hospital clinics. In a recent investigation of non-compliance, Silverberg et al (1985), in a study in Israel, found that a significant factor was the waiting time involved in clinic attendance. By concentrating effort nationally on family clinics, the drop-out rate has been reduced to 2.1% (startling compared with the Wilber & McCombs 1975 study) and the waiting time from 105 minutes to 7 minutes. This seems a notable achievement and an example worth following.

In reviewing the evidence, Vidt (1978) identifies the following features as contributory to achieving compliance:

- the treatment regime is relatively simple — for example once daily drugs
- drugs do not have unpleasant side-effects
- the treatment regime does not interfere with lifestyle, restrict behaviour or involve dietary modification
- there is a good supportive relationship with the doctor
  - no fundamental disagreements
  - expectations are met
  - explanations are given
  - there is consistency of personnel.

Nursing considerations

Clearly, as the majority of hypertensive patients are asymptomatic and leading normal lives the contact nurses have with them is minimal. However, that contact may be highly significant in that the nurse is frequently recording blood pressures and is in a good position to discuss weight, diet and lifestyle with individuals. Nurses in health centres, in schools and in industry potentially have a vital role in screening and detecting early those persons in whom

Table 22.9 Drugs commonly used in hypertension (sources BNF, 1985; Robertson, 1983; Bannan et al, 1981c)

Type	Action	Side effects and comments
Thiazides and diuretics Bendrofluazide Chlorthiazide Clopamide Cyclopenthiazide Hydrochlorothiazide Hydroflumethiazide	Diuretic, blocks sodium reabsorption in distal tubule. Therefore reduces blood volume Also has a direct peripheral vasodilatory effect so reducing peripheral resistance	Cheap and effective in mild hypertension, however they tend to increase blood viscosity by their diuretic action, increase platelet aggregation and increase plasma catecholamines, cholesterol and triglycerides. They are therefore not of benefit in preventing coronary heart disease. Used in conjunction with potassium supplements or with potassium sparing diuretics — Amiloride hydrochloride, Triamterene
Beta-adrenergic blocking agents Propanolol hydrochloride Acebutolol Atenolol Labetalol hydrochloride Metoprolol tartrate	Competitively inhibit the action of catecholamines on the beta-adrenergic receptors. Some block both β_1 and β_2 receptors, those that block only β_1 are relatively cardioselective. Overall they are therefore thought to lower the blood pressure by decreasing the heart rate, decreasing conductivity and having a central effect on the vaso-motor centre. They lower peripheral resistance by vasodilation and block the release of renin from the renal juxtaglomerular apparatus.	Increasingly common in use and may be superior in reducing cardiac morbidity. However they sometimes cause problems due to a fall in cardiac output reducing coronary and peripheral perfusion. Not given to asthmatics or in congestive cardiac failure unless the latter is caused by hypertension.
Vasodilator antihypertensives Hydralazine hydro-chloride Prazozin hydrochloride	Cause peripheral dilation reducing peripheral resistance	Used for moderate to severe hypertension and in hypertensive crises. Some cause tachycardia — reduced by combining with beta-blocking agent.
Centrally acting antihypertensives Methylodopa Clonidine	Act on vasomotor centre	Less frequently used since introduction of Beta blockers. Inadvisable if person has a history of depression
Adrenergic neurone block agents Bethanidine sulphate Guanethidine monosulphate	Block the release of noradrenaline from post-ganglionic neurones Action is potentiated by diuretics	Cause large degree of postural hypotension
Alpha-adrenergic blocking agents Indoramin	Used in conjunction with diuretic or beta-adrenergic blocker.	
Angiotensin — converting enzyme inhibitors Captopril	Inhibits conversion of angiotensin I to angiotensin II. Used in severe hypertension not otherwise controlled	Rashes and loss of taste. Proteinuria

hypertension has not been identified. 'Well person' clinics in this respect are particularly useful.

In the hospital situation, apart from the identification of hypertension in routine blood pressure monitoring, the nurse will be caring for those who have been admitted specifically for hypertension control. In addition a great many patients will be admitted with cardiovascular disease such as heart failure, coronary heart disease or strokes, with hypertension as a contributory factor. For those with severe or malignant hypertension a quiet, unstressed environment is recommended, but the person is normally self-caring. The nurse's role becomes one of monitoring, of rapid action should hypertensive crisis occur and of general support, dietary and other advice.

In summary the nurse's role can be seen to involve:

- accurate blood pressure monitoring (see above)
- weight and dietary advice
- promoting exercise and relaxation
- administering and teaching self administration of drugs
- support.

ATHEROMA

Atheroma is a widespread disorder of the arterial system generally associated with increasing age. While its precise pathogenesis is unclear (Fuster et al, 1985; Lewis, 1985; Smith, 1985) the early stages are believed to begin with mild damage or deterioration of the very thin endothelial cells lining the inner wall of the artery (Guyton, 1984). Thus, atherosclerotic tissues are more commonly seen in areas of high pressure or turbulence, such as the arch of the aorta or the point of bifurcation where arteries divide (Long & Phipps, 1985). This appears to lead to platelets adhering to the lining and subendothelial tissue. Subsequent to this, there is debate about the sequence of events. Traditionally it was thought that platelets and lipids (primarily cholesterol) infiltrated the intima. More recently, however, attention has been focused on the role of growth factors released from the platelets and possibly the endothelial cells and macrophages (Lewis, 1985). These factors are capable of stimulating growth of smooth muscle cells, endothelial cells and fibroblasts. In addition, arterial smooth muscle cells themselves appear capable of producing collagen and other substances associated with growth (Fuster et al, 1985). Whether lipids or growth factors are responsible for initiating the process, they are both implicated in the progression (Lewis, 1985; Smith 1985). Smooth muscle cells from the media migrate towards the endothelium, possibly using a fibrin network (Smith, 1985). They then multiply and protrude against the endothelial cell lining. Lipids are deposited in and around the smooth muscle, these largely being derived from cholesterol from the low density lipoproteins in the plasma (Smith, 1985). Ultimately the lesion becomes fibrosed and may calcify, the mature lesion being described as occlusive, inelastic and incapable of dilating (Burt et al, 1982b).

Figure 22.4A illustrates the probable course of events, and Figure 22.4B illustrates a cross-section of an artery showing the mature atherosclerotic lesion.

Implications of atheroma

As the major vessels involved are those which have a high amount of elastic tissue in the media, i.e. the aorta, coronary and cerebral arteries, the implications of the loss of elasticity are considerable. For example, the aorta will no longer be able to adjust to accommodate the increase in blood volume during systole. This increases peripheral resistance, presenting an increased pressure load (afterload) to the left ventricle which eventually fails.

In the coronary vessels the loss of elasticity results in a diminished coronary reserve. This reserve is necessary to maintain continuous myocardial perfusion during systole, when coronary artery perfusion is diminished. Loss of elasticity in coronary and peripheral vessels reduces autoregulation, causing reduced ability to vasodilate in response to tissue oxygen

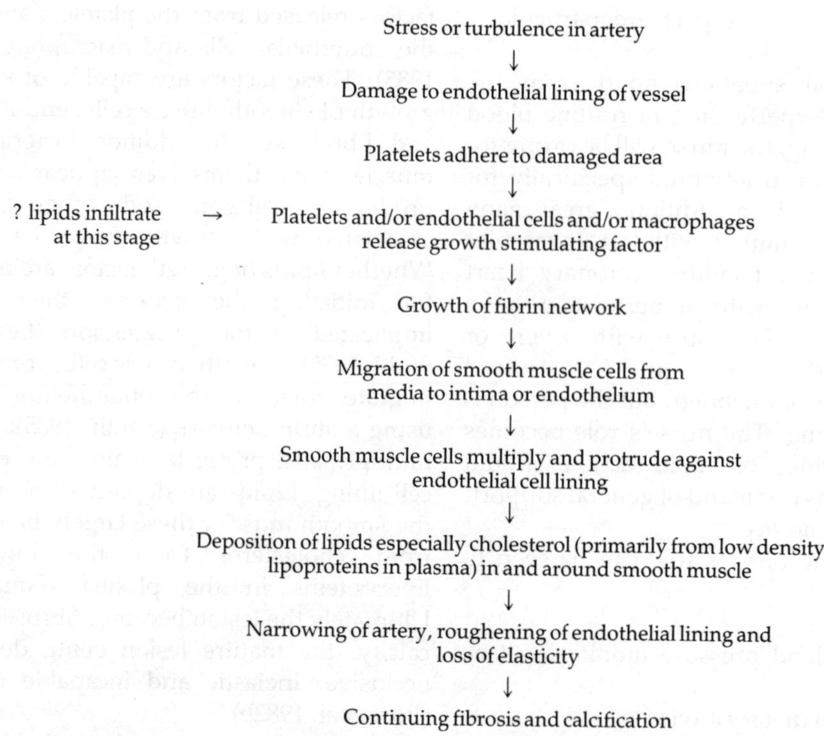
Stress or turbulence in artery
Damage to endothelial lining of vessel
Platelets adhere to damaged area
? lipids infiltrate at this stage
Platelets and/or endothelial cells and/or macrophages release growth stimulating factor
Growth of fibrin network
Migration of smooth muscle cells from media to intima or endothelium
Smooth muscle cells multiply and protrude against endothelial cell lining
Deposition of lipids especially cholesterol (primarily from low density lipoproteins in plasma) in and around smooth muscle
Narrowing of artery, roughening of endothelial lining and loss of elasticity
Continuing fibrosis and calcification

Fig. 22.4 A Probable course of events in the development of atheroma

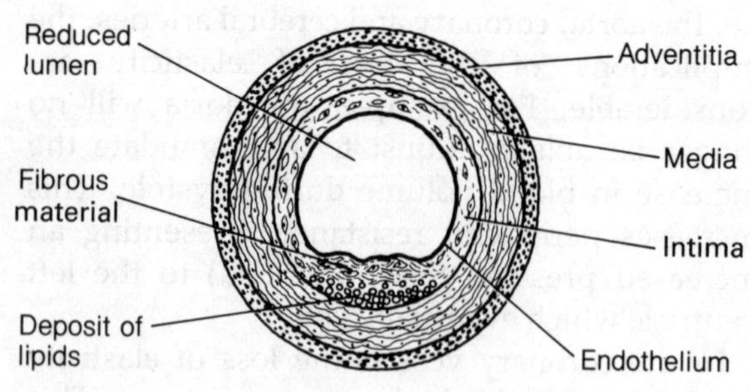
Reduced lumen
Adventitia
Media
Fibrous material
Intima
Deposit of lipids
Endothelium

Fig. 22.4 B Cross-section of artery

demand during activity. Thus, the ischaemic pain of angina and intermittent claudication is experienced during periods of exercise or increased tissue demand.

The occlusive effects of atheroma are of more concern in vessels of smaller lumen than the aorta. Occlusion of any artery threatens the survival of the tissue supplied. Thus, coronary artery occlusion leads to myocardial ischaemia and infarction, cerebral artery occlusion results in strokes or transient ischaemic attacks, and femoral-popliteal artery occlusion leads to ischaemic or gangrenous legs.

A third presentation of atheroma is that of vessel wall weakening — aneurysm. This occurs in areas of high pressure such as the arch of the aorta.

It is important to realize, however, that atheroma is asymptomatic in many instances as it affects the large arteries primarily and does not usually lead to occlusion of these (Lewis, 1985).

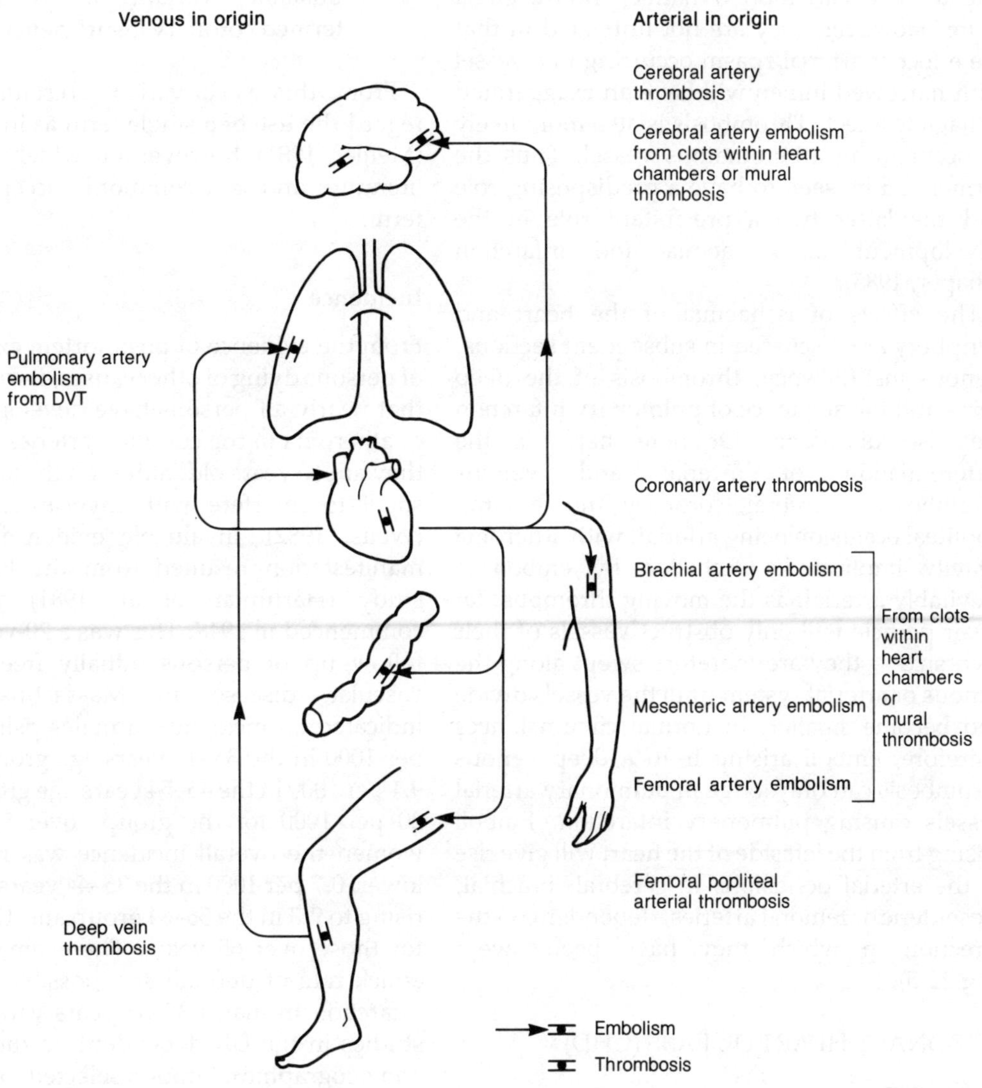

Fig. 22.5 Embolism and thrombosis

It is also important to recognize that each of the disorders in which atheroma is heavily implicated is also caused by pathogenic processes other than atheroma.

Ischaemia, thrombosis and embolism

Ischaemia occurs when the blood supply to a tissue is inadequate to meet its oxygen and nutritional needs. Apart from the severing of an artery or the deliberate occlusion by a tourniquet there are four major causes of ischaemia.

- fibrosis of arterioles associated with collagen disorders
- atherosclerosis
- arterial spasm
- thromboembolism.

The first two of these present a relatively stable but slowly progressive pattern of symptoms leading to gradual loss of function and disability.

The latter two are more dynamic, and the effect acute. However, they are not unrelated in that the effect of arterial spasm occurring in a vessel with narrowed lumen will have an exaggerated ischaemic effect. Thrombosis is also more likely to occur in an atheromatous vessel. Thus the former can be seen to have a predisposing role and the latter two a precipitant role in the development of ischaemia and infarction (Shaper, 1985).

The effects of ischaemia of the heart and periphery are discussed in subsequent sections. Venous insufficiency, thrombosis of the deep veins and the sequence of pulmonary infarction are also discussed. Of note here, is the differentiation of arterial and venous thrombosis — cerebral, coronary and femoral-popliteal occlusion being arterial, with atheroma heavily implicated. Occlusion by emboli is inevitably arterial, as the moving thrombus, fat or air particle will only obstruct vessels of their own size — they are therefore swept along the venous or arterial system until the vessels divide and become smaller. In normal circumstances therefore, emboli arising from a deep venous thrombosis can only lodge in pulmonary arterial vessels causing pulmonary infarction. Emboli arising from the left side of the heart will give rise to the arterial occlusions in cerebral, brachial, mesenteric or femoral arteries, dependent on the direction in which they have been swept (Fig.22.5).

CORONARY HEART DISEASE (CHD)

Definition

Coronary Heart Disease (CHD), also termed Ischaemic Heart Disease or IHD, is a collective term for disturbances of blood flow within the coronary arteries giving rise to altered myocardial perfusion and disruption of the normal electrical cycle controlling heart rhythm. It presents in a number of forms, the main groups of which are:

- sudden death
- myocardial infarction (MI)
- angina pectoris
  - — stable
  - — unstable, variant or crescendo, also termed coronary insufficiency.

From this very varied presentation some regard the use of a single term as inappropriate (Meijler, 1981), however it is widely used in the literature and is a commonly accepted clinical term.

Incidence

From the evidence of postmortem examinations of persons dying of other causes, it would appear that nearly all persons have developed patches of atheroma in the coronary arteries by the time they are 40 years old, although these may be too small to interfere with myocardial perfusion (Wells, 1982). Invaluable evidence of clinical manifestation resulted from the Framingham study (Hartunian et al, 1981) which was commenced in 1948. This was a 20-year biennial follow up of persons initially free of cardiovascular disease in Massachusetts. This indicated an incidence in males rising from 3.9 per 1000 in the 35–44 years age group, through 9.1 per 1000 in the 45–54 years age group, to over 20 per 1000 for the groups over 55 years. In women the overall incidence was found to be lower; 0.7 per 1000 in the 35–44 years age group, rising to 9.3 in the 55–64 group and 12.4 per 1000 for those over 65 years. The estimated annual attack rate of definite and possible myocardial infarction in males 35–65 years varies between studies in the UK dependent on the age range and geographical location selected, but averages 6.2 per 1000 (Shaper et al, 1985). About half will have had a previous history of CHD, the annual attack rate being 4 per 1000 for those with no previous history.

The mortality statistics indicate that 1 in 4 persons in England and Wales die of CHD. It accounts for 38% of male deaths between the ages of 30 and 65 years, and 41% if this is focused on the male age group 45–54 years (Wells, 1982). It is therefore a major contributor to 'premature' death. Contrary to popular belief the mortality is higher for unskilled groups than for professional groups, a trend which has reversed since the 1950s. There are also regional differences, the

North of England, Wales and Scotland having higher rates than the South (Wells, 1982).

The incidence in some countries, for example Australia and the USA, has been declining since the late 60s; in the latter by as much as 20% in the 10-year period from 1968 (Wells, 1982; Rose, 1981). The incidence in Great Britain is relatively high and is not decreasing. The incidence in Japan, by contrast, is very low and appears stable (Wells, 1982). Possible explanations of these differences is included in the discussion of risk factors.

Factors associated with coronary heart disease — 'risk factors'

There is considerable debate and controversy about the causation of atheroma, coronary heart disease and related disorders. It is not the purpose here to reflect the vast amount of research available, simply to highlight the main issues as these are crucial both to the understanding of preventative measures and to the development of realistic and rational rehabilitative programmes.

In spite of the controversy over the contribution of specific factors there is general agreement that the cause is multifactorial, genetic factors interacting with environmental, social and occupational factors and lifestyle. Thus the term 'risk factor' is more commonly used in the literature than 'cause'. However, in itself the term is controversial as the assumption behind its use is that of preventative measures being taken in order to reduce 'the risk' (Julian & Humphries, 1983). Herein lies the debate! As Meijler (1981) points out, the majority of 'risks' in relation to coronary heart disease are genetic — having close relatives who have the disease and being male — and are thus non-modifiable by the individual. Meijler (1981) contends that the emphasis on risk factors has detracted from efforts to investigate cause. Cigarette smoking emerges as the only risk factor positively associated with coronary heart disease that is, in a real sense, modifiable by the individual; that is, when consumption is lowered, the risk of coronary heart disease is reduced for that individual.

Table 22.10 Factors associated with coronary heart disease and related disorders

Type of factor	Factor
Genetic endowment	Race Sex Disorders of fat metabolism Inability to 'handle' salt
Genetic/disease	Hypertension Diabetes mellitus Hypothyroidism Gout
Social/environmental/ work	Urban living Occupation, e.g. mining Stress 'Type A' behaviour
Personal behaviour	Cigarette smoking Diet – fat consumption – fibre consumption – salt consumption – obesity Lack of physical activity Lack of relaxation Contraceptive method

That the majority of factors identified as 'risk', even if modifiable by the individual, have not been proved to reduce the personal risk is of importance to the individual concerned. It is nevertheless true that longer-term national modification of behaviour is likely to lead to a reduced incidence of coronary heart disease in the population.

An indication of the factors demonstrated or thought to be associated with coronary heart disease are noted in Table 22.10. The subsequent discussion focuses on the nature of this association.

Genetic factors

There are undoubtedly genetic factors operating in coronary heart disease and related disorders. As already pointed out, being a male and having a close relative with the disease constitutes a very high risk. Three areas are briefly discussed here — ethnic group, sex and other factors.

Ethnic group. There is some evidence that the incidence of coronary heart disease is higher in persons who are not white. This may be related to the high incidence of essential hypertension in the black population (Long & Phipps, 1985). It may also be attributed to high fat diets, smoking and other socioeconomic and environmental factors associated with immigrant populations (Silman et al, 1985). Much research effort is directed towards teasing out the relative contribution of socioeconomic factors, diet, smoking and ethnic group.

Sex. Men have an incidence of coronary heart disease more than eleven times that of women below the age of 65 years, after which the difference diminishes (Wells, 1982). This suggests a hormonal protecting influence, possibly that of oestrogens reducing the levels of blood lipids (Long & Phipps, 1985). The increased risk of thrombosis formation with the contraceptive pill, however, would suggest alternative explanations have to be sought.

Other genetic factors. There are undoubtedly other genetic factors implicated in atheroma-related disorders. The highest risk factor for having a myocardial infarction early in life is having a first degree relative who has had one before the age of 55 years, and the second highest is having a first degree relative who has had one before the age of 65 years (Nora, 1983). The heritability of early onset coronary disease is 56% (excluding monogenic lipid disorders).

The majority of genetic research in relation to atheroma has focused on specified populations and family groups. In particular the focus has been on lipid and lipoprotein abnormalities. These abnormalities divide into those that are single gene or monogenic in origin and those that are polygenic. Some early onset forms of atheroma and arteriosclerosis are associated with single mutant genes. However, this only explains a tiny number of those who have a family history of atheroma-related disorders. In the absence of a single gene being found responsible, the problem then becomes one of separating the contribution of several genes from the contribution of the familial pattern and lifestyle, in particular diet and environment.

Nora & Nora (1983) suggest the concept of multifactorial inheritance'. By this they mean a genetic predisposition, usually produced by the small effect of many genes, interacting with an environmental 'trigger'. This means that a member of a family with a strong genetic predisposition to cardiovascular disease will only require a minimal environmental trigger, for example a high fat diet, to develop problems. By contrast, members of families with little predisposition will only develop problems if they have overwhelming environmental triggers.

Thus, for a small proportion of persons the chances of developing cardiovascular disease are very high and their opportunities for reducing the risk are limited in their effect. For example, individuals with monogenic hyperlipoproteinaemia have a high genetic risk and have to exist on a very low or no-fat diet.

The majority of persons, however, are at lower genetic risk and might be able to increase or decrease their risk of cardiovascular disease by modifying (over a long period) their lifestyle and diet.

Hypertension

Hypertension is one of the three primary risk factors in coronary heart disease identified by the DHSS (1981). The nature of hypertension and its relationship with general morbidity and mortality has already been discussed above. Its primary sequelae are cardiovascular — coronary heart disease, heart failure and cerebrovascular disease. For coronary heart disease the risk increases with rising blood pressure. Estimates of the risk vary slightly between studies. Kannel & Gordon (1970) for example, found that the risk increased by some 20% for each rise of 10mmHg in the diastolic (phase 5) pressure above 110mmHg. Since the Framingham study demonstrated that the systolic pressure was, if anything, a better predictor of coronary heart disease than the diastolic (Wells, 1982) and the current British Regional Heart Study has demonstrated both pressures of equal predictive value (Shaper et al, 1985) the focus has been on both values rather than diastolic alone. In the prospective phase of the latter study, Shaper et al report a doubling of the risk of coronary heart disease for the top 40% of men who have a systolic pressure of more than 148 mmHg and a threefold risk for the top 20% of men who have a diastolic pressure of above 93mmHg compared with the bottom 20% with a diastolic of below 72mmHg.

Theoretically the indications are that the earlier the intervention in hypertension, the greater the risk reduction (Nora, 1983). However, possibly due to the nature of the earlier drug therapy available this did not occur as clearly in relation to coronary heart disease as in preventing strokes, cardiac failure and deterioriation of renal function (Robertson, 1983). Recent reports on an extensive controlled trial of beta-adrenergic blocking agents appear to have confirmed the 'cardio-protective' function of those drugs, possibly mediated by their action in reducing myocardial contractility and heart rate (IPPPSH, 1985).

Diet and blood lipids

By far the most attention in relation to 'risk' factors has been focused on diet and blood lipids and their relationship with cardiovascular disease. The widespread concern is not only reflected in the popular media and advertising but in a variety of Health Education Council endeavours and in a series of reports of national significance. The most recent of these, the National Advisory Committee on Nutrition Education report (NACNE, 1983) and the DHSS report on Diet and Cardiovascular Disease (DHSS, 1984) both provide a series of recommendations on nutritional intake based on available research evidence. In this section the major issues in relation to diet and cardiovascular disease only will be highlighted. Recommendations regarding diet are included in primary prevention in Chapter 14.

A number of dietary factors have come under review in addition to total energy consumption and the interaction of fat consumption and blood levels. As the latter is the focus of considerable debate it will be discussed last.

Total energy intake. Men with the greatest calorie intake appear less likely to develop cardiovascular disease. This may be a result of their greater level of physical activity (Shaper, 1985).

Alcohol. Non-drinkers appear to have a higher mortality rate from coronary heart disease than moderate drinkers (Wells, 1982; Shaper, 1985). However Shaper (1985) questions the validity of the assumption that might be made from that association, suggesting that a number of non-drinkers have given up alcohol due to health problems. He cites work indicating that high density lipoprotein levels are raised only slightly in those who drink moderately (6 drinks a day). While this might be perceived as 'protective', the same research shows that these same individuals demonstrate significant hepatic enzyme disturbance!

Salt. Individuals genetically unable to handle salt appropriately have an increased risk of hypertension. It is the hypertension that is likely to be the 'risk' factor in other cardiovascular disease (DHSS, 1984).

Dietary fibre. Low fibre intake has been associated with an increased risk of coronary heart disease. However, as most dietary fibre is obtained from cereals which are also high in starch it is difficult to separate the two factors (Shaper, 1985). Its mechanism — if it is an independent factor — has yet to be identified. While its importance in the prevention of cardiovascular disease is uncertain, its importance in reducing the risk of gastro-intestinal problems is undisputed.

Hardness of water. The cardiovascular mortality has been found to be higher by 10–15% in very soft water areas compared to medium to hard water areas (Pocock et al, 1980). The question remains whether this is due to a 'protective' factor in the hard water or a 'risk' factor in the soft water (Wells, 1982).

Fats. The basic contention in relation to dietary fats and cardiovascular disease is as follows:

- dietary intake of saturated fats is positively correlated with serum cholesterol levels
- serum cholesterol levels are positively correlated with coronary heart disease.

While this is a simplification of the very complex work ongoing on dietary and blood lipids, there is general agreement as to these two positive relationships (Wells, 1982; Shaper, 1985). There is, however, very serious debate as to whether or not it is appropriate to label dietary intake of fats as a 'risk factor' in the absence of clear evidence demonstrating that the incidence of cardiac mortality can be reduced with appropriate dietary modification (Meijler, 1981; Wells, 1982).

Evidence for the two relationships abound. For example, in Japan the median plasma cholesterol for 35-year-old men is 3.7–4.5 mmol/l (Lewis, 1981) compared with 6.0–6.4 mmol/l for middle-aged men in Britain (Shaper et al, 1985). The Japanese have a diet low in saturated fats and relatively high in polyunsaturates compared with an average UK diet. In spite of having a high incidence of hypertension and smoking, Japan has one of the lowest rates of coronary heart disease in developed countries (Lewis, 1981).

Those with familial hypercholesterolaemia, who have a plasma cholesterol level 2–3 times higher than average (9–18 mmol/l) have a 10-fold increase in risk of coronary heart disease (Lewis, 1981). Sugrue et al (1981) found that 60% of males and 30% of females with familial hypercholesterolaemia develop coronary heart disease before the age of 50 years.

The findings of the prospective phase of the British Regional Heart Study (Shaper et al, 1985) confirm earlier findings (e.g. Pooling Project Research Group, 1978) that in normal, initially healthy males, the association of total serum cholesterol with risk from coronary heart disease is highly significant. Those with a total serum cholesterol in the middle range (6.0–6.4 mmol/l) had twice the risk compared with those with lower levels. However, Shaper et al (1985) are at pains to point out that those in the lower two-fifths of the range of total cholesterol values are not at zero risk. 22% of those who developed coronary heart disease were in this lower band. Overall, therefore, Shaper and his colleagues 'confirmed total serum cholesterol as an independent risk factor whose predictive performance is of a similar order to that of smoking and blood pressure'.

However, the study does not support the view that high levels of high density lipoprotein (HDL) cholesterol are 'protective' against coronary heart disease. The findings of other studies with respect to the role of HDL cholesterol are contentious (Shaper et al, 1985). Serum triglycerides are not implicated in coronary heart disease (Grundy, 1981; Shaper et al, 1985).

The evidence that change in dietary fat intake in the middle years of life will effect a change in risk is insubstantial (Wells, 1982). The data for recommendations of dietary change come primarily from cross-cultural studies where dietary patterns are established from childhood (Meijler, 1981). The consistent recommendation, however, is for a change in dietary fat intake with a decrease in saturated fat intake and a partial substitution with polyunsaturates (NACNE, 1983; DHSS, 1984; Shaper et al, 1985). It is likely that this will be of long term benefit to the population as a whole rather than to the individual or of immediate, consequence.

Obesity

The link between obesity and coronary heart disease is contentious and may be associated with other factors such as diabetes mellitus, hypertension or hyperlipidaemia.

In developing countries obesity is consistent with low levels of plasma lipids and although hypertension and diabetes are common, coronary heart disease is uncommon (Shaper, 1985). In view of the positive relationship between 'body mass' and known independent risk factors, such as those mentioned above, and the easy detectability of obesity, Shaper and his colleagues (1985) suggest that its lack of independence of effect is clinically irrelevant.

Exercise

The contribution of lack of exercise to cardiovascular diseases is as yet unproven (Wells, 1982) but there appears to be a general acceptance that the less one does, the greater the risk (Long & Phipps, 1985). Overstrenuous or sudden activity, however, is possibly harmful.

There is considerable evidence from occupational studies that high activity occupations have a lower risk of heart disease than low activity occupations (Wells, 1982). In particular, high levels of physical activity appear to be highly protective against coronary deaths and sudden death (Nora, 1983). In a recent study, Menolti & Saccareccia (1985) found that the highest mortality in Italian railroad workers was amongst those who had low physical activity and high job responsibility.

In relation to leisure activity, it again appears that regular exercise lowers the risk of coronary heart disease by about half. Taking smoking into account, regular exercisers who do not smoke lower their risk by four-fifths in comparison to their inactive smoking colleagues (Wells, 1982).

However Professor Morris, a significant proponent of exercise in the UK, points out that exercise, needs to be 'vigorous enough for the possibility of a 'training' effect for the individual: mere expenditure of energy without some overload, does not appear to affect coronary incidence' (Morris, 1985).

There are a variety of theories as to why exercise should be 'protective' in this way. They include factors such as a redistribution of cholesterol in favour of high density lipoproteins, augmentation of the fibrolytic response and lowered heart rate (Wells, 1982; Nora, 1983).

Cigarette smoking

Repeated studies have shown the positive association between cigarette smoking and coronary heart disease. The greater the number of cigarettes smoked the greater the risk (Alderson et al, 1985), particularly in the younger age group. American studies for example, suggest that 1 in 3 of 40-year-old men who smoke 20 or more cigarettes a day will have a heart attack before they reach 65 years of age compared with 1 in 7 non-smokers (Pooling Project Research Group, 1978). Overall the mortality rate would appear to be double in smokers than that of non-smokers (Wells, 1982), increasing to fourfold if more than 40 cigarettes are smoked per day (Kannel, 1981). The proportionate risk decreases with age despite continuation of smoking (Kannel, 1981) which may indicate the decreasing influence of genetic susceptibility.

Specifically related to women, the incidence of heart attack in women who smoke and use contraceptives is reported to be 10 times greater than in those who have neither exposure (Nora, 1983). It is also postulated that the changes in the intima of umbilical arteries of neonates whose mothers smoke may reflect changes in arteries elsewhere in the body which may form the focus for atheromatous changes in later life (Asmussen, 1980). The babies of mothers who smoke tend to be smaller than those of mothers who do not, the placentae demonstrating the gritty appearance typical of multiple minute infarctions.

The association of smoking with atherosclerosis affecting the lower limbs is similar to that of smoking with coronary heart disease. This is also the case for aortic aneurysm and occlusion of vascular grafts (Lewis, 1981).

Persons who give up smoking appear to decrease their risk of coronary heart disease proportionately with each year of their abstinence (Alderson et al, 1985). After ten years their risks are as those of non-smokers (Lewis, 1981). Some evidence, however, contradicts this comparatively welcome finding!

The pathological processes resulting from smoking are less clear than the relationship. They are likely to involve vasoconstrictive, clotting effects and other effects (Long & Phipps, 1985). Nicotine, for example, stimulates the sympathetic system leading to the release of noradrenaline and adrenaline. These increase platelet adhesion and aggregation. It may therefore serve to accelerate the formation of atheromatous plaques (Lewis, 1981). The sympathetic trigger also serves to cause vasoconstriction and increase myocardial contractility, thus increasing myocardial workload and oxygen demand. Carbon monoxide interferes with oxygen transport thus aggravating the effects of coronary narrowing. It is also reported to impair the catabolism of lipoprotein remnants in the liver (Lewis, 1981).

Personality and behaviour

In spite of considerable scepticism on the part of the medical profession and a comparative scarcity of literature, there does appear to be some genuine acceptance that persons displaying particular behaviour patterns are at higher risk of coronary heart disease than others. The initial thesis was put forward by two cardiologists, Friedman and Rosenman (1974). Their 'Type A' person is characterized by an excessive competitive drive, a sense of time urgency and a free floating but well-rationalized hostility. In a prospective study of over 3000 healthy men aged 35–60 years, classified into personality Types A and B at the beginning of the study and followed up for 10 years, they found that Type A men were 3 times as likely to develop coronary heart disease as Type B. They concluded that 'in the absence of Type A behaviour pattern, coronary heart disease almost never occurs before seventy years of age, regardless of the fatty foods eaten, the cigarettes smoked or the lack of exercise' (Friedman & Rosenman, 1974). Nora (1983) reports a 1.5 increase in risk with Type A behaviour but accepts that this is still statistically significant. Lewis (1981) sees Type A behaviour as a 'well-defined independent CHD risk factor'.

Friedman & Rosenman postulate that the influence of Type A behaviour is mediated via sympathetic arousal and catecholamine increase. This is commensurate with the rise in blood pressure found in times of stress (O'Brien & O'Malley, 1981e). Friedman & Rosenman found that some cholesterol levels rose at times when Type A behaviour was exhibited whereas these levels did not change with smoking or exercise.

In terms of modification, whereas the authors suggest that Type A individuals are able to modify their behaviour others see it as immutable (Lewis, 1981). Sir Peter Medawar in his foreword to Friedman & Rosenmans' book points out that Type A behaviour is now the expected behaviour of the successful person in society, excessive competitiveness, drive and working beyond work hours being the assumption of many job descriptions. Thus, whether or not Type A behaviour can be modified by the individual is questionable.

Stress

Stress is a concept not clearly defined in relation to cardiovascular disease. If defined by its physiological link with a rise in catecholamines, it can be seen that the vascular and cardiac responses would exacerbate existing problems as indicated in the discussion of personality and behaviour. Nora (1983) sees stress, or the handling of stress, as contributing to the vulnerability of individuals to coronary events. Certainly there is some evidence that the onset of clinical symptoms is related to stressful life events such as bereavement, work change, house moving and unemployment (Wells, 1982).

Environment

The effects of environment are difficult to differentiate from other potential factors such as race, lifestyle and diet. However, it is of note that the incidence of coronary heart disease is seven times higher in North America, Australia, New Zealand and Europe in comparison with Japan, Africa and South America (Luckmann & Sorensen, 1980). It is also of note that there is a higher incidence in urban areas than in rural populations and in the North of England than the South.

Oral contraceptives

Oral contraceptives are associated with an increased blood pressure and also predispose to thrombus formation (Long & Phipps, 1985). The risk of death from coronary heart disease is four times as great in those who take oral contraceptives compared with those who do not. As already mentioned, smoking increases this risk enormously, as does age. Thus the death rate from cardiovascular disease for women aged 35–44 who smoke and use oral contraceptives is 63.4 per 100 000 compared with the non-smoking, non-users of 15.2 per 100 000 (Royal College of General Practitioners, 1979).

Metabolic/endocrine disorders

Diabetes mellitus. The risk of coronary heart disease is 2–3 times as high in those who have diabetes mellitus compared with those that have not (Nora, 1983). This is regardless of blood lipids. However, as diabetes is also associated with hypertension and obesity the problem is one of differentiating the contributing factors. Those with diabetes also have a high incidence of peripheral vascular disease.

Although there is some evidence that careful regulation of the blood glucose level reduces the incidence of 'complications', Nora (1983) concludes that atherosclerotic manifestations are unrelated to the duration and severity of hyperglycaemia. The question, as always, is whether or not the many manifestations of diabetes mellitus have a common metabolic mechanism of genetic origin.

Gout. There is some evidence that those who suffer gout or who have uric acid levels above 7.5 mg/dl are more at risk of coronary heart disease (Luckmann & Sorensen, 1980).

Other factors

Hypothyroidism has also been implicated in increasing the risk of coronary heart disease, as has coffee drinking (Beland & Passos, 1975).

Primary prevention of coronary heart disease

It is clear from the startling statistics of premature death and disabling disease associated with coronary heart disease that primary prevention should be taken seriously. However, as the discussion of 'risk' factors indicates, genetic factors are strongly influential and, apart from reducing smoking, there is little evidence that altering a lifestyle mid-life will reduce morbidity. However, this is not a strong argument for ignoring primary prevention on the following bases:

- lifelong lifestyle does appear to influence morbidity
- reducing 'risk' factors has no demonstrable harmful effects
- available evidence for the impact of lifestyle change is limited to relatively small, short term studies.

On this basis therefore, and on the evidence of factors associated with CHD, the following key aspects of lifestyle form the basis for primary prevention:

- avoid cigarette smoking
- take a diet
  - low in saturated fats and relatively high in polyunsaturates
  - low in salt
  - high in fibre
  - moderate in alcohol
- exercise vigorously regularly
- practise relaxation-meditation daily
- maintain weight within recommendations for height/build

Health education programmes such as the 'look after yourself' and 'look after your heart' illustrate the type of scheme which is undifferentiated in its target group. Media attention to general health issues, activity and diet may arise from such campaigns or from other influences. Other approaches have specific target groups, e.g. children, who may be the target for posters or more complete programmes encouraging them not to smoke, to develop 'healthy' eating patterns, to take exercise and so on. Individual persons may be identified as genetically at high risk. This occurs via the primary care team and will be related to what is known of family health profiles. In this way information specific to that individual's 'risk' can be offered on which the person concerned or their family can make an informed decision about, for example, dietary modification. This form of intervention is one with considerable potential for development (McCance, 1983).

The impact of such programmes may be measured in the short term by altered food consumption patterns, cigarette sales, attendance figures for health or sporting clubs or events. The long term effect may be measured in CHD incidence. The figures from North America are encouraging but by no means conclusive.

The role of the nurse in primary prevention has traditionally been linked in the UK with that of the health educators, the health visitors, and, to a lesser extent, the school nurse and the occupational health nurse. However, it would be to avoid the issue not to at least raise the question in relation to nurses working with those who are physically ill.

Three aspects are identified:

- the health behaviour of the nurse him/herself
- the role of the nurse in relation to his/her input to health-awareness of the general public
- the role of the nurse in relation to general health education of the physically ill persons and their families with whom he/she is involved.

These aspects raise many questions as to the nature of health education and the relationship between one's behaviour as an individual and information or advice given in a professional capacity. They are beyond the scope of this book to develop further.

Prognosis

The prognosis of CHD varies with the presentation of the disorder. It would appear that the extent of atherosclerosis increases over time, at any rate in those who have identified coronary artery disease (Kramer et al, 1981), and that it rarely regresses (Bruschke et al, 1981). Those with stable angina have double the probability of death within 5 years than those without the condition (Sorlie, 1977), and have double the risk of myocardial infarction, that is 50% of men over 45 with stable angina will have a myocardial infarction within 8 years (Kannel & Feinleib, 1972).

The prognosis following myocardial infarction is not good. Studies invariably report a 40–50% mortality within 28 days of diagnosis (Wells, 1982; Sloman et al, 1981). Of those who die, 50% do so within 15 minutes, 60% within one hour and 70% within 4 hours (Sloman et al, 1981). Of those who are discharged from hospital, 7–25% will die within the year (Lau et al, 1980). Lau and his colleagues found that this varied significantly between those who were discharged 'early' from hospital (5–7 days post MI) who were by definition 'uncomplicated' and those who had a delayed discharge for medical reasons (13+ days). 50% of the survivors of an infarct can expect to have angina, of whom 60% will have it for the first time (Kannel & Sorlie, 1977); 50% of those who do not recover completely will die within 5 years, 75% will die within 10 years (Luckmann & Sorensen, 1980).

Table 22.11 Causes of death in myocardial infarction (MI) (Luckmann & Sorensen 1980)

Cause of death	% of MI deaths
Arrhythmia (especially ventricular fibrillation	40–50
Shock	9
Congestive cardiac failure	40
Rupture at the heart wall	5–10
Recurrent myocardial infarction	5

Rupture of the myocardium is a complication resulting in 10–17% of the infarct mortality. While the statistical evidence is limited it would appear that those persons who are experiencing their first infarct, or are females, or who have sustained chest pain are more likely to have a ruptured myocardium, whether fatal or otherwise, than others (Dellborg et al, 1985).

The causes of death are indicated in Table 22.11.

Presentation of coronary heart disease

In this section, secondary prevention and intervention are discussed in relation to each form of the presentation of the disease.

Sudden death

Sudden death is estimated to account for 15–25% of persons with coronary heart disease (McDonald, 1979). Infarction, however, is not usually the cause of death, being found in only 8–27% of coronary deaths. Severe atheroma (Julian & Campbell, 1981) with perhaps 85% stenosis of the vessels, however, is usually present. Death is normally due to spontaneous ventricular fibrillation, the myocardium rarely showing signs of infarction at postmortem (Petch, 1985). However rupture of the myocardium is also a significant cause of sudden death, being found in 10–17% of persons who die of coronary heart disease (Julian & Campbell, 1981; Dellborg et al, 1985).

There is considerable controversy as to whether there is anything significant in the history of persons who die suddenly that would differentiate them from others at risk. There does appear to be general agreement that there is little to differentiate them from those who sustain a myocardial infarction without sudden death (Kannel et al, 1975). In a retrospective study Madsen (1980) found that 75% of a sample of 166, 50–66 year old men who had suffered a sudden cardiac death had had previous coronary heart disease or hypertension. In addition, about twice as many of those with previous CHD had prodromes prior to death compared to those without previous CHD; half had consulted their doctor within a month of death compared to only a quarter of those without CHD. Having said that, a fifth of those that died had neither prodromes nor a suspect medical history.

In reviewing all the evidence then available, Julian & Campbell (1981) concluded that, of the risk factors investigated, hyperlipidaemia and hypertension do not appear to carry any greater risk of sudden death than other manifestations of coronary heart disease. However they did find that smoking and low activity levels appeared to predispose to sudden death.

Nursing considerations. Sudden death presents the nurse with two major considerations:

- resuscitation
- support of significant persons.

Resuscitation. Whether or not resuscitation is considered when sudden death occurs will clearly depend on the situation. In public situations such as recreational or work places and in hospitals, resuscitation is likely to be initiated. The techniques used will vary in sophistication from external cardiac massage with mouth to mouth breathing to defibrillation and full mechanical stimulation and ventilation. The nurse, as an individual or in the role of nurse, may be initiating and participating at any level. Sudden death at home is less likely to be treated heroically and indeed may occur 'during sleep' although there is some doubt as to whether it occurs without any premonition, however transient.

The principles of resuscitation are:

- restoration of an adequate cardiac output to support vital organ perfusion (heart, lungs, kidneys, brain)
- ventilation of lungs sufficient to allow oxygen diffusion.

In medical or paramedical care two further principles apply:

- correction of acidosis
- stabilization of arrhythmias.

Support of significant persons. Clearly if death occurs the need for support lies in the persons close to the individual who has died. Empathetic undemanding support allowing the individuals to express their grief or shock is most helpful at this time. A barrage of questions regarding the death or instructions regarding property or death certificates is unlikely to facilitate the grieving persons.

Angina pectoris

Angina is the classic symptom of ischaemic heart disease reflecting a transient situation with no permanent damage to the myocardium. The pain experienced is episodic, usually central chest pain which often radiates down the medial aspect of the left arm. It may occur in the arm, wrist or jaw, sometimes without accompanying chest pain. The pain is typically described as 'dull' or 'aching' and occurs retrosternally, there being no sensation of cutaneous pain. It gives rise to anything from mild discomfort, sometimes mistaken for indigestion, to severe crushing pain and feelings of impending death.

'Stable' angina describes the condition in which the pain experience has a known pattern and is brought about by consistent triggers such as a known amount of exercise, emotion, etc.

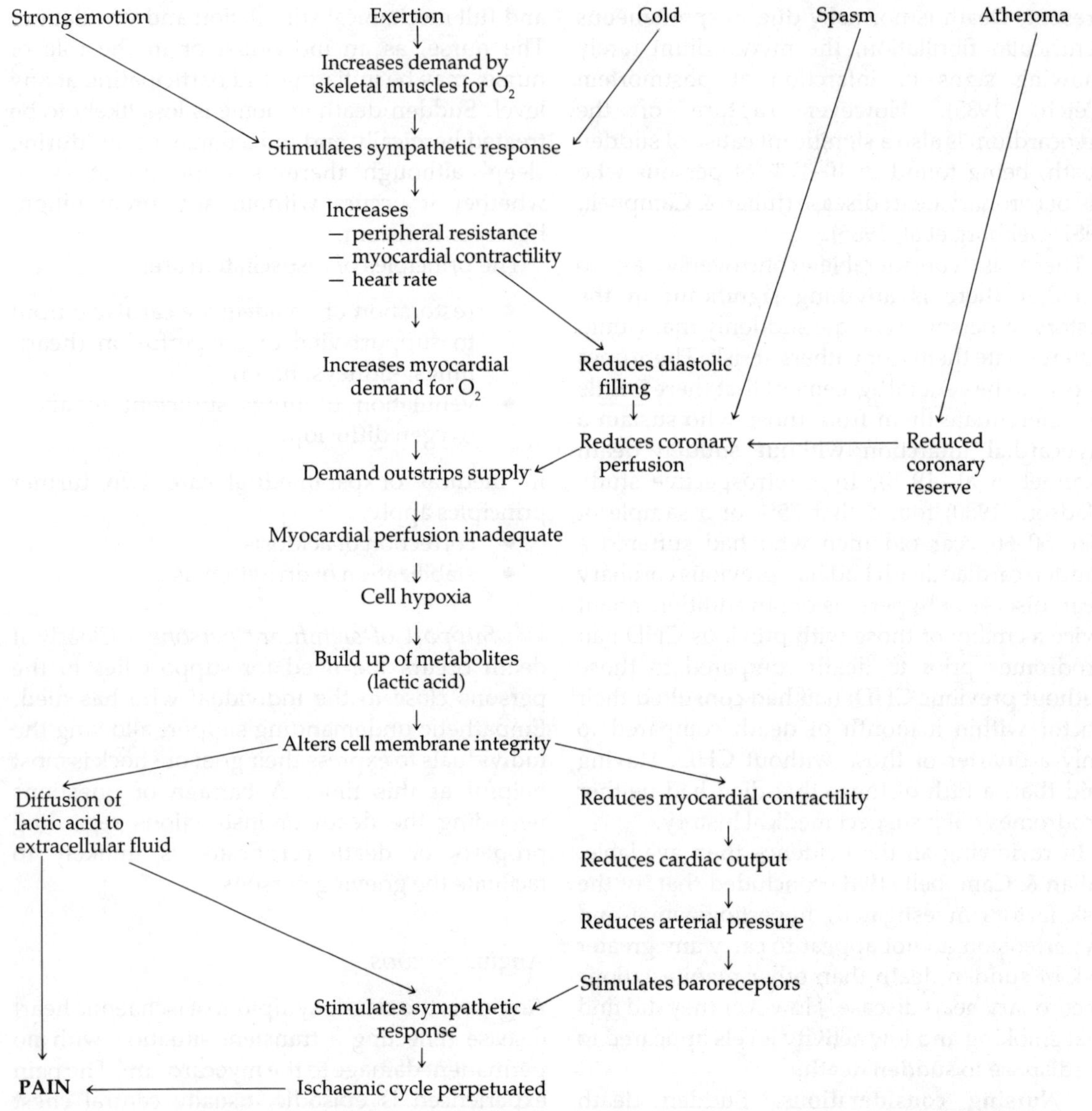

Fig. 22.6 Classic sequence of events in angina

'Unstable', 'variant' or 'crescendo' angina describes the condition in which the pain experience does not conform to a common pattern and is not necessarily precipitated by an identified trigger. It may be more persistent in nature and can be much more resistant to satisfactory pain control.

The pain experience is assumed to relate in some way to a degree of myocardial ischaemia, although ECG changes associated with ischaemia such as alteration in the ST segment do not always occur with attacks of pain (Petch, 1985; Quyyumi et al, 1985). The ischaemia may be caused by atheroma. However, it is increasingly recognized that the presence of atheromatous plaques is not synonymous with a degree of ischaemia or of angina (McDonald, 1979). Conversely, angina does occur in the absence of atheroma. It appears that coronary vasospasm is also a significant factor in ischaemic heart disease and may be responsible for the 'unstable' type of angina (Maseri et al, 1978; Weintraub & Helfant, 1983).

The cycle of events in angina is essentially one of the myocardial demand for oxygen outstripping the supply. This will occur in any circumstances which increase the demands of the myocardium in the context of a coronary supply reduced in quantity or quality. The latter will be affected by reduced elasticity or patency of coronary vessels as occurs in atheroma and spasm, and by reduced perfusion of the coronary vessels as occurs during tachycardia as a result of shortened diastole. Figure 22.6 illustrates this sequence.

Diagnosis. The diagnosis of angina pectoris will be made on the basis of:

- history and description of chest pain
- ECG, particularly on exercise.

Depending on the severity and progression of the angina, other investigations such as coronary angiogram (via cardiac catheterization) or radioscanning may be undertaken. These are described more fully under the section headed 'assessment of cardiovascular function'.

Management. Management of angina involves both longer term management in order to prevent anginal attacks and the management of the attack itself. As the doctor or nurse will not witness the majority of anginal attacks, the onus of management of the acute attack rests on the individuals themselves and on those close to them. It is therefore particularly important that they understand how to avoid and cope with their own attacks. Both medical and nursing staff have a responsibility to ensure that all aspects of the attack have been adequately explored and that the individuals involved are fully conversant with measures aimed at prevention and effective management of an attack.

Management may be considered as having three aims:

- decreasing myocardial demand
- optimizing or increasing myocardial perfusion
- adjusting activity to the capacity of the myocardium.

Any one aspect of management is likely to contribute to more than one of these aims.

Acute attack. Acute attacks may be the result of specific and identifiable precipitating events, such as exercise or severe emotional stress, or may be unheralded, such as occurs with variant or unstable angina.

Management involves:

- physical inactivity and rest
- administration of sublingual glyceryl trinitrate.

The first of these will bring about a reduction of demand on the heart. The pain will normally bring about this physical inactivity, although some exercise-minded individuals are reported to have deliberately gone out jogging during an angina attack. This is clearly inappropriate and may account for some of the sudden deaths reported during jogging. If the physical inactivity is accompanied by a deliberate attempt to relax this will theoretically reduce sympathetic stimulation. Deep breathing, however, should be avoided as this enhances venous return and thus increases cardiac pre-load.

Glyceryl trinitrate is taken sublingually from where it is absorbed directly into the systemic (as opposed to the portal) system. It is thought to act as much by venous dilatation, thus reducing cardiac pre-load, as by arterial dilatation reducing peripheral resistance (afterload) and increasing myocardial perfusion. During an acute attack up to 3 tablets may be taken at 5 minute intervals. If the pain is not considerably reduced after this time medical services should be contacted without delay.

An outline of the mechanism of management during an acute attack is indicated in Figure 22.7.

Long-term management. This is discussed together with the long- term management of post-myocardial infarction on page 676.

Myocardial infarction

Myocardial infarction is the death or necrosis of part of the myocardium as a result of severe or

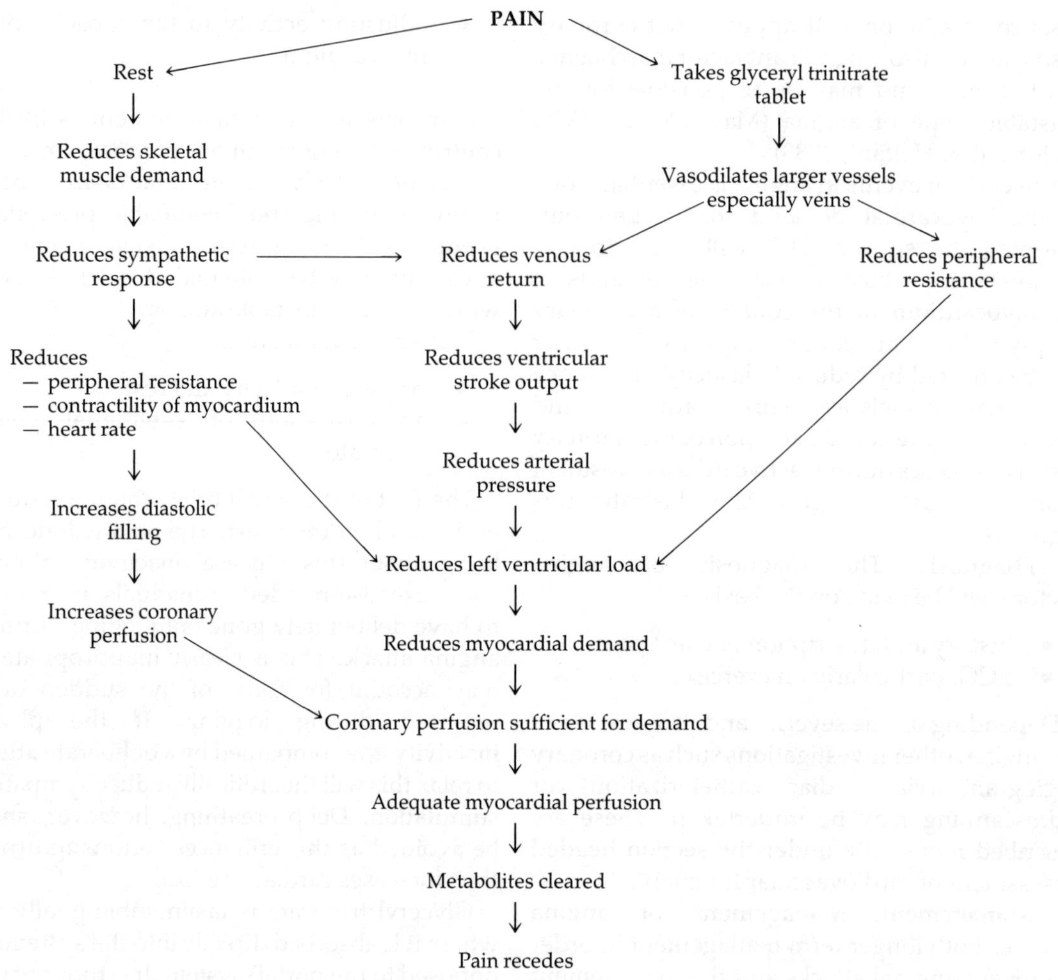

Fig. 22.7 Typical sequence of events in the management of an anginal attack

complete deprivation of the blood supply. Whether or not the deprivation is due to thrombus formation within an atheromatous artery, due to the atheroma itself or due to other pathologies is a subject of debate (Wells, 1982). In atheroma-related myocardial infarction the central controversy is whether the thrombus that is formed (as found in postmortem examination) is the cause of, or the result of the process of infarction (Brest & Goldberg, 1983). On balance, it seems likely that thrombosis of the relevant artery is a primary causative factor in fatal transmural myocardial infarction but may not be so in the smaller subendocardial infarcts. It is also likely that some recanalization of the affected vessels by the body's intrinsic fibrinolytic system occurs (Brest & Goldberg, 1983).

The prognosis for persons having had a myocardial infarction has already been discussed. The essential message of the statistics is that the first few hours constitute the greatest risk, the risk of death decreasing with each hour, day and week of survival. In addition it is clear that those whose initial hours post-infarction are uncomplicated by arrhythmia or ventricular failure have a much better chance of survival than those who experience those complications (Lau et al, 1980; Wells, 1982).

The life threat is primarily from two causes:

Table 22.12 Common sites of myocardial infarction

Artery occluded	Part of heart wall	Name of infarct
Left anterior descending coronary artery	Anterior surface of left ventricle near the apex	Anterior
	Involving the septum	Anterospetal
Circumflex coronary artery	Lateral or posterior surface of left ventricle	Lateral Posterior
Right coronary artery	Inferior surface of left ventricle	Inferior

- left ventricular failure
- arrhythmia particularly ventricular fibrillation

These two conditions account for 80–90% of deaths after myocardial infarction (Luckmann & Sorensen, 1980). There is a close correlation between the amount of myocardial damage and the development of left ventricular failure in the early stages. Similarly the total non-contractile area will determine subsequent left ventricular function (Brest & Goldberg, 1983). Infarct size may also be an important determinant of the occurrence of ventricular arrhythmias although the site of infarction is also of importance (Brest & Goldberg, 1983).

The most common site of infarction is the anterior surface of the left ventricle implicating the left coronary artery. Infarction of the right ventricle occurs in only 5% of persons (Luckmann & Sorensen, 1980). Infarcts are classified according to the section of the myocardium involved. Table 22.12 illustrates the artery implicated together with the aspect of the myocardium affected.

In addition, infarcts may affect all or some of the layers of the heart. Thus the following terms may be used:

- transmural — involving pericardium, myocardium and endocardium
- subendocardial — involving myocardium and pericardium only.

All infarcts result in thinning of the myocardium (Becker, 1981). This may reult in aneurysm or rupture of the myocardium. This need not result in a fatal outcome if treated promptly (Dellborg et al, 1985).

The effect and prognosis of myocardial infarction will therefore depend on:

- site of the infarct
  - ventricular infarcts result in less effective muscle action
  - those involving the A-V node or septum are likely to cause arrhythmias
- size of the infarct
  - the larger it is the poorer the prognosis
- extent of reperfusion of the injured area.

The latter is a feature not only of the ability of the myocardial tissue to develop a collateral blood supply but of the treatment initiated at the crucial early phase post-infarction. There is histological evidence that a zone of tissue exists between the definitely infarcted or necrosed area and the healthy tissue (Becker, 1981). This zone is considered to be potentially retrievable, dependent in part, on early treatment. Beland & Passos (1975) talk of three zones — that of necrosis, injury and ischaemia. Whether areas of tissue can be differentiated to this extent is questionable, nevertheless if the areas — represented as separate zones — are seen as a continuum, the concept is a useful framework for considering cellular and electrical processes. These are represented in Figure 22.8 and Table 22.13.

The precise sequence of events post-infarction is also the subject of debate (Becker, 1981). However, what is clear is that at the core of the infarct, the cell walls disintegrate discharging their contents into the extracellular fluid. Thus

Table 22.13 Zones of tissue damage following coronary artery occlusion (adapted from Beland & Passos, 1975)

Zone	Cellular effect	Electrical effect	Outcome
Zone of infarction	Cellular death	Pathological Q waves	Permanent scar tissue
Zone of injury	Moderately deprived of O_2 but cells still partially viable and functional	Elevation or depression of ST segment	Usually succumbs to infarction — termed 'extension'
Zone of ischaemia	Minimally O_2 deprived Potentially dysfunctional	Inversion or flattening of T waves. Possibly origin of arrhythmias	Reduced function, probable cause of continuing angina

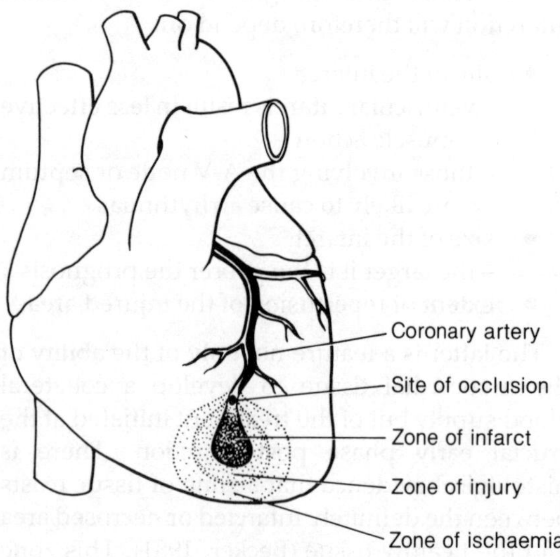

Fig.22.8 Diagram of heart showing site of occlusion

there is an area of tissue not capable of conducting electrical impulses, hence the typical ECG changes, and not capable of contraction, hence the danger of left ventricular failure. The metabolites from the cell are likely to be the cause of the acute, crushing, retrosternal chest pain experienced by the person. Subsequently a process of repair ensues, either by the normal process of granulation or by collagenization from the remaining sarcolemmal components of pre-existent tissue (Becker, 1981). Invasion by capillaries or reperfusion of pre-existing capillaries enables the fibrous collagen tissue to form a relatively strong but inelastic scar.

Within the 'zone of injury' there appears even less certainty as to the processes involved. However, there is general agreement that this area has the potential to recover (Becker, 1981). Tissue that has been ischaemic, however, and is then perfused appears to be subject to 'contraction band necrosis' (Becker, 1981). These are cuffs of swollen cells which exhibit abnormal transverse bands in their cytoplasm. Contraction band necrosis has been demonstrated not only in the zone of injury post-infarction but also in myocardial necrosis after coronary artery bypass graft in the absence of a blocked graft. The number of collateral vessels increase with the severity of the destruction of the coronary arteries, but in view of the increased risk of contraction band necrosis it seems likely that there is a critical stage at which collaterals become dysfunctional rather than restorative (Becker, 1981). The timing of intervention related to reperfusion thus becomes critical; the longer the time between infarction and reperfusion the more likely the development of contraction band necrosis.

The probable sequence of events subsequent to infarction are shown in Table 22.14.

Presentation and diagnosis. Individuals suffering a myocardial infarction will experience severe retrosternal chest pain during which they may feel that they are going to die. The infarction may occur at any time and is not related to exercise. Typically the person is woken by the

Table 22.14 Postulated sequence of events subsequent to myocardial infarction.

Time post-occlusion	Zone of infarction	Zone of injury	Zone of ischaemia
0–5 hours	Cell walls disintegrate Electrical impulses not conducted	Reduced function Source of electrical problems	
5–6 hours	Necrosis	Function still reduced	
24 hours	Area infiltrated by polymorphonuclear leucocyte - phagocytosis		
4–5 days	Infiltrated by fibroblasts macrophages and capillaries	Collagenous tissues generated from remnants of sarcolemmal components of pre-existent tissue Reperfusion of pre-existent capillaries	Collateral vessels enlarge May succumb to infarction due to enlarging collateral vessels outstripping ability of coronary artery to supply blood or due to contraction band necrosis
2–3 weeks	Fibrosis, collagen tissue formed		Collateral system continuing to enlarge
2–3 months	Scar formed		Function restored

pain during the night. They may clench their fist and clutch their chest. Depending on the severity of the pain they may become acutely agitated and collapse in cardiogenic shock. They may have pulse irregularities and develop the no-cardiac output state of ventricular fibrillation. 50% of deaths from myocardial infarction occur in this first 15 minutes. Delay in obtaining expert medical supervision is therefore potentially critical to survival.

Diagnosis is confirmed by ECG recordings demonstrating typical changes (Fig. 22.9). Serum enzymes from 6 hours and over the period of 2–3 days show patterns typical of infarction (Table 22.15). Additional techniques of scintigraphy to demonstrate areas of non-perfusion are also of value in diagnosis. The importance of diagnosis is emphasized by the fact that 60% of patients admitted to Coronary Care Units are found not to have had a myocardial infarction (Julian & Humphries, 1983).

Management of the person with a myocardial infarction. Death in the early hours post-infarction is largely due to ventricular fibrillation. Subsequent recovery is dependent on the size of the infarction. On the basis that fatal arrhythmias can be corrected and that early treatment can reduce the eventual size of the infarct, it follows that early treatment can have a substantial effect on outcome both short- and long-term.

The nature of care falls under two headings:

- the care environment and personnel involved in the care
- the physical treatment given to the patient, e.g. drugs, defibrillation, etc.

To an extent these are interdependent — the individual requiring defibrillation and intravenous drugs inevitably needs the urgent services of highly qualified staff. However, a large proportion of the patients who will survive have uncomplicated recovery patterns and the need for the stressful drama of hospital admission and 'hi-tech' care has been questioned.

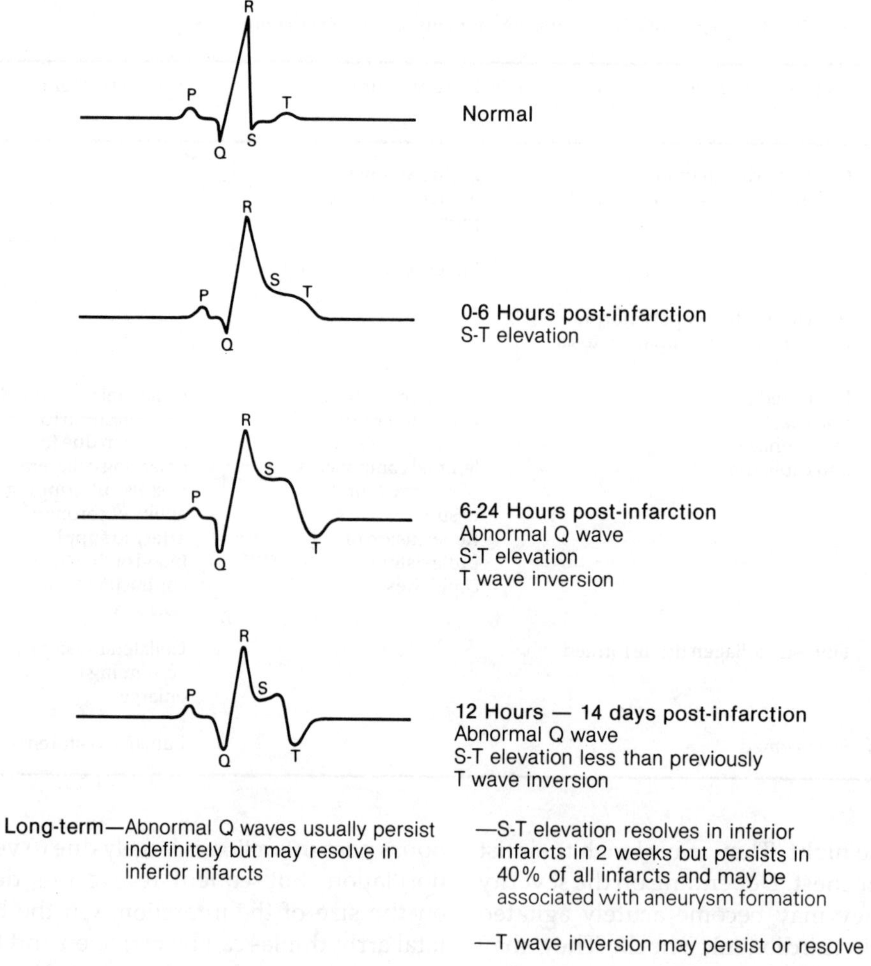

Fig. 22.9 ECG changes indicating myocardial infarction (adapted from Watson, 1983).

The care environment and care personnel. General public awareness and skill in cardiopulmonary resuscitation (CPR). There appears to be general agreement that public awareness of resuscitation procedures such as external cardiac massage and mouth-to-mouth respiration has had a significant impact on mortality (Sloman et al, 1981; Julian & Humphries, 1983) although the estimated numbers are not quoted . The current mass education programme in CPR is indicative of a central concern with its effectiveness.

CORONARY CARE UNITS (CCU). With the developed techniques, both electrical and chemical, for controlling arrhythmias in the early stages post-infarct, the 1960s saw the development of coronary care units. The initial assumption that these units would reduce mortality dramatically, however, was soon seen to be false, as the expected fall did not take place. Indeed it is now estimated that, realistically, the maximum potential improvement in mortality with CCUs is between 4–5% (Wells, 1982).

MOBILE CORONARY CARE AMBULANCES (MCCA). A critical element in reducing this early mortality appears to be the time lapse between the onset of symptoms and treatment received. Further to the development of CCUs, therefore, the 1970s saw the development of Mobile Coronary Care Ambulances. These are equipped to a high level

Table 22.15 Enzyme release post myocardial infarction (Beland & Passos, 1975; Watson, 1983; Oostenbroek et al, 1985)

Enzyme	Found in circulation post-infarct			Range		Other features
	Initial	Peak	Fall	Normal	Infarct	
Creatinine phosphokinase (CPK) Catalyses the conversion of creatine phosphate to adenosine diphosphate – precursor to adenosine triphosphate, the biochemical necessary for cellular function	6 hr	18–36 hr	2–3 days if no extension	100u/ml	200u–1000u	Rises also if IM injections are being given as skeletal muscle has high concentration. Also rises in pulmonary infarct. Not raised in liver damage. If in doubt, cardiac specific enzyme is measured CPK(MB)
Serum aspartate transferase (previously glutamic oxaloacetic transaminase SGOT) Serum alanine transferase (previously glutamic pyruvic transaminase SGPT) precipitates synthesis of oxaloacetic acid, critical point of entry into Krebs cycle of catabolism	12–24 hr	36–48 hr	3–4 days	50u/ml	Above 100u	Also found in liver but SGOT higher in cardiac muscle so SGOT 2–3 times higher than SGPT in myocardial infarction SGOT also raised with anabolic steroids, morphine sulphate and Aldomet
Lactic acid dehydrogenase (LDH) and P-hydroxybutyric dehydrogenase (HDB) catalyses the conversion of lactic acid to pyruvic acid during glycolysis	2–3 days		7 days			LDH also raised in liver disease but isoenzymes can be differentiated

and staffed by specially trained ambulance personnel, paramedics, medical or nursing staff.

Their role, however, has been questioned as studies vary in their estimate of 'success'. In Australia for example, there is a reported decrease in mortality in the early post-myocardial infarction stage from 35% to 15%. The introduction of CCUs and MCCAs is seen as being responsible for 20–55% of this reduction (Sloman et al, 1981). In the UK a study in Brighton of the effect of MCCAs showed a positive benefit but one in Nottingham did not.

In a well-conducted trial in Ireland comparing mortality from CHD in two similar communities, one served by an MCCA and a CCU and one with a CCU alone, the evidence of the value of the MCCA was convincing, the 28-day mortality for those below 65 years being 34% as opposed to 55% (Mathewson et al, 1985). It must be noted however that the control group mortality was considerably higher than that reported elsewhere. On balance it appears that MCCAs are beneficial.

ADMISSIONS PROCEDURE. Two further features of care that are consistently reported as delaying the time between the onset of symptoms and treatment within a CCU are delays due to general practitioners and delays due to the hospital admissions procedure (Callan & Irving, 1986). The recommended practice therefore now bypasses both of these routes, the public being enabled to call for an MCCA directly and the MCCA team being able to admit a person directly to the CCU. In this way the ideal of patients being in CCU within an hour of the onset of symptoms may be achieved (Sloman et al, 1981). This does not mean it is achieved in practice. In Dundee where this system operates, the public still call the GP and the GPs still delay admission. In 1982 the average referral time to the GP was 1h 45 m, and to the MCCA, 2h 30m. This compared unfavourably with 1978 mean referral times and is in stark contrast to the 1h referral time when the public call the MCCA directly (Callan & Irving, 1986). Clearly public and general practitioner education is required if the system is to be effective.

HOME CARE. As indicated, the development of CCUs in the 1960s did not bring about the expected reduction in mortality. Throughout the 1970s a number of doctors developed and evaluated alternative patterns. The earliest of these, the results of which were published in 1971, showed no difference in mortality rates between hospital care and care at home (Mather et al, 1971). However there were a number of methodological problems associated with the study, not the least of which were differences in the sample population in factors known to affect mortality, such as age. Nevertheless, subsequent studies have failed to show any benefit of hospital care in terms of mortality for large groups of patients with myocardial infarction (Mather et al, 1976; Colling et al, 1976) although the hi-tech facilities are certainly life-saving for some (Wells, 1982).

The high mortality in the first hour post-infarct before referral to GP or MCCA might account for some of the lack of difference between home and hospital mortality. However, the lack of the stress that is related to emergency hospital admission and hi-tech care environments is given as the probable reason for the success of home care.

Clearly some patients are unsuitable for home care. The indicators for maintaining a person in their own home would appear to be:

- absence of complications such as arrhythmia, cardiogenic shock, signs of heart failure
- adequate facilities for being cared for
- over 3 hours from onset of symptoms
- over 65 years of age.

The principles of management and care wherever it takes place are similar. Care of the person in their own home, however, is unlikely to involve 'critical care' elements and 'rehabilitation' can usually commence sooner and without the trauma of transfer from coronary care unit to ward and of discharge home. Relatives or significant others including neighbours are central to the observation, support and care of the person at home. A clear line and pattern of communication needs to be established so that medical or nursing support is quickly available if the need arises and the care required is understood by all concerned.

Care and treatment. **CARE DURING THE INITIAL PHASE.** Initial management of the person who has had a myocardial infarction involves:

- Maintenance of cardiac output adequate to maintain vital functions, involving:
  - control of arrhythmias
  - management of shock
  - management of left ventricular failure.
- Reduction in demand on and by the myocardium and maintenance or increase in myocardial perfusion, involving:
  - reduction in activity
  - management of pain
  - improvement in myocardial perfusion
  - management of anxiety.

These will be discussed briefly here but the reader is referred to the many specialist texts on coronary care for more detailed study.

MAINTENANCE OF CARDIAC OUTPUT ADEQUATE TO MAINTAIN VITAL FUNCTIONS. In order that the facility to give drugs intravenously to achieve rapid action is available as soon as possible, an infusion is set up immediately (via a cut down if necessary), as is an ECG monitor.

CONTROL OF ARRHYTHMIAS. A number of arrhythmias may arise, the most common being ventricular extrasystoles which occur in 90% of patients (Watson, 1983). Life-threatening ventricular fibrillation occurs in 10% of patients. Bradycardias and degrees of heart block may also arise dependent on the site of the infarction and parasympathetic activity. Ectopic beats are controlled primarily by lignocaine. There is no evidence that giving lignocaine routinely is of any value in preventing ectopic beats so that use should be restricted to treatment as they occur (Watson, 1983). In the event of ventricular fibrillation not responding to lignocaine, electrical defibrillation is both safe and effective and is increasingly used by trained paramedical and nursing staff.

Heart block occurs in 10–15% of patients and may resolve spontaneously, especially if it accompanies an inferior infarction. Heart block with an anterior infarction indicates much greater damage. Temporary pacing is indicated if cardiac output is not sufficient and may be regulated to stimulate only on demand.

MANAGEMENT OF SHOCK. This is discussed more fully in Chapter 10. Cardiogenic shock is presumed to be caused by the profound disruption of the myocardium. It is important that the blood pressure is raised as rapidly as is possible without inducing cardiac failure, as myocardial perfusion as well as renal and cerebral perfusion are dependant on systolic pressure. Prognosis is poor if the degree of shock is profound.

Treatment regimes are not particularly successful and include catecholamines to stimulate myocardial contractility, vasodilators to reduce peripheral resistance and volume expanders such as dextran. Intra-aortic balloon counterpulsation may be used to reduce left ventricular work and improve coronary blood flow. This is brought about by providing a pulsation opposite to that of the circulatory system during ventricular diastole. It results in an increase in arterial diastolic pressure and a decrease in arterial systolic pressure. Thus the afterload (pressure load) is reduced, reducing myocardial work. The improved diastolic pressure results in increased coronary perfusion.

MANAGEMENT OF LEFT VENTRICULAR FAILURE. This will present as systemic collapse and pulmonary oedema. Management includes oxygen administration, loop diuretics intravenously, morphine and digoxin as in any other patient with ventricular failure.

This group of potential complications presents few problems for specialized coronary care units with highly qualified staff constantly in attendance and equipment and drugs to hand. However, management of these problems can create real difficulties and anxieties for general ward staff and, in the absence of CCU facilities, constant observation and 'specialling' is advised. Management at home is virtually impossible. Monitoring ventricular rhythm (via leads and a cardiac monitor), pulse, respiratory rate, blood pressure (and central venous pressure if required, via CVP line) are critical in these early hours. A low BP is a poor prognostic sign.

REDUCTION IN DEMAND ON AND BY THE MYOCARDIUM AND MAINTENANCE OR INCREASE IN MYOCARDIAL PERFUSION. This is an area of increasing interest and is of vital importance to the health potential of the individual concerned.

REDUCTION IN ACTIVITY. This is the clearest and simplest form of reduction in demand. If the patient has or is experiencing pain, inactivity will not be difficult to achieve. However, patients who do not continue to experience pain and those who deny that anything is wrong may need considerable explanation, tact and firmness to persuade them to comply. Bed rest is advisable initially, partially propped up. Lying flat increases venous return (pre-load) and therefore the work of the heart. Patients who do not have complications may be allowed up in a chair the day after the infarction. There is no evidence that undue activity restriction, e.g. washing the patient's hands and face, feeding the patient, is less stressful than allowing the patient to do these things for him or herself.

MANAGEMENT OF PAIN. Morphine is the drug of choice for pain and should be given intramuscularly rather than subcutaneously to enhance absorption. Reduction in pain reduces the risk of shock. Pain and anxiety are linked and as anxiety provokes a physiological sympathetic response it should be minimized. This is discussed in some detail subsequently because of its importance to nursing management of the patient.

IMPROVEMENT OF MYOCARDIAL PERFUSION. Drug therapy aimed at optimizing myocardial perfusion in the ischaemic zone, salvaging it from infarction, is an area of current interest. There is some evidence that beta-adrenergic blocking agents are of value here. In addition there is a lowered incidence of ectopic beats so that overall function is improved. Anticoagulants and antiplatelet drugs have also been evaluated, but the evidence of their effectiveness is equivocal.

Intracoronary thrombolysis via cardiac catherization is a technique used more in the USA than the UK. It is undertaken 3–5 hours after the onset of symptoms and before necrosis sets in. Streptokinase is infused over a period of 4–6 hours. This activates plasminogen to speed up the formation of the proteolytic enzyme plasmin. This digests the fibrin strands of clot and allows the blood flow to re-establish. There is said to be a 70–80% success rate for reperfusion although less than a third of the results are classified as 'good', others going on to bypass surgery or continuing to have significant problems (Bouman, 1984). The basis of the care is that which is given to any patient undergoing cardiac catherization with three additional significant aspects:

- The infusion takes time, so prolonging the period of stress, increasing the risk of introducing infection and prolonging separation from relatives.
- Streptokinase is a naturally occurring protein of beta-haemolytic streptococcus. It is therefore antigenic in nature and may provoke an allergic reaction.
- The person is in an acute phase of illness and is therefore particularly stressed, may be experiencing severe ischaemic pain and will be prone to arrythmias.

MANAGEMENT OF ANXIETY. Early studies of patients nursed in coronary care units (CCU) demonstrated considerable problems created by the environment, in addition to the threats imposed by the nature of their illness and the fact of hospitalization. For example, the presence of cardiac monitors, the severity of the illness of other patients, feelings of being closed in and lack of sleep due to frequent disturbance were commonly reported (Goh, 1977). As Ashworth (1984) points out, the conditions of patients within CCUs may represent any or all of the six features identified by Lazarus (1966) as stimulating psychological stress:

- disruption or danger to life-values and goals
- threat to physical survival
- threat to personal identity
- inability to control one's environment
- inability to avoid pain and privation
- separation from community and significant persons

Such psychological stress has been linked not only with physiological indicators of stress, such as raised catecholamines, raised BP and raised pulse rate — reactions creating greater demands on an already compromised myocardium – but also with high levels of anxiety and hopelessness, reactions associated with high death rates in CCUs (Ashworth, 1984). Denial is also a frequently reported, though contentious, 'coping mechanism' (Thomas et al, 1983). This has been linked with unfavourable consequences such as high stress levels and to poorer rehabilitation prospects, as well as with more positive consequences such as giving 'psychological time' for adjustment to the new situation.

The nature and management of stress in general is discussed fully in Chapters 8 and 12. There are, however, specific areas for consideration in relation to the care given in CCUs that may affect the quality of the patients' stay in the unit and their subsequent progress:

- the overall environment — layout, lighting, noise, routine
- nurse-patient communication
- involvement of relatives/significant others
- management of transfer to the general medical ward.

These will be discussed very briefly.

With an increasing public awareness and understanding of 'hi-tech' medical care, some of the aspects of CCUs that were stressful to patients (and relatives) in the early days are now widely accepted. For example, in a recent small study by Thompson et al (1986) 99% of patients said that they did not mind being attached to monitors although 61% felt that its purpose had not been adequately explained. However, this lack of patients' anxiety about their own monitors does not appear to be recognized by nurses (Wallace et al, 1985). Nurses' awareness of anxiety caused by watching other people's monitors can result in more careful positioning of the monitors. Judicial use of screens and curtains can protect patients from exposure to very ill patients. Other aspects of routine and timetabling also need to be considered, such as the maintenance of day-night rhythms by varying the lighting level, maintaining settling down and waking up habits and reducing intrusive observations at night when possible; maintaining mealtimes; providing a clock visible to all and encouraging the companionship of visitors. A very deliberate nursing focus on the needs of patients and visitors in conjunction with attention to medical staff, monitors and other apparatus and charts may enable the individual patient to view the environment as supportive to him/her rather than as overwhelming.

Ashworth (1984), utilizing her work on patient-nurse communication in Intensive Care Units, suggests that the aims of nurse-patient, nurse-family communication in CCUs may be seen as:

- to establish a relationship in which the patient perceives the nurse as friendly, helpful, competent, reliable and as recognizing the patient's worth and individuality
- to try to determine the patient's needs as perceived by him/her and when necessary to help him/her to recognize other needs as perceived by the nurses
- to provide factual information on which the patient can structure his/her expectations
- to assist the patient to use his/her own resources and those offered to him (e.g. information) to meet his/her own needs.

This framework may be useful in all patient care situations and, if used, might result in a better 'matching' of nurse perceptions with those of the patient. Currently there is little evidence that nurses' perceptions of patient anxieties concur with the patients' own concerns or that the information received by patients is considered by them to be adequate (Ashworth, 1984; Wallace et al, 1985).

Relatives or others of significance to the patient still tend to be restrained from being with the patient for any length of time. Three possible explanations may account for this — interference with essential medical and nursing care; tiring for the patient; anxiety-provoking for the relatives. However, not only are these readily challenged but there is evidence that separation during this critical period leads to variance of patients' and relatives' perceptions of progress, prognosis and management (such as level of activity desirable) which reduces the effectiveness of support relatives are able to give both at the time and subsequently. At the least it would appear beneficial to facilitate the relatives being with patients and receiving information with them from medical and nursing personnel. A more structured approach would involve family assessment and inclusion in the care plan (Gaglione, 1984) with the aim of maximizing the use of their patient supportive role from the acute phase of illness through to rehabilitation.

Transfer to the general medical ward is a period of potential stress and is associated with increased anxiety (Mayberry & Kent, 1983). On the basis of the small scale studies available it would appear that recommended practice would involve:

- an indication to the patient (and relatives) as soon as his/her condition is nearing stable that transfer will take place at some time
- if possible, 12 hours notice (to patient and relatives) of when transfer is to take place and to which ward, including information as to where it is, how to get there and other information such as visiting times (if applicable)
- clear information as to the reason for transfer
- a planned reduction in monitoring/ observation prior to transfer
- a pre-transfer visit from a nurse of the receiving ward
- accompaniment of the patient on transfer by the nurse who visited from the receiving ward

- initial placement in receiving ward in ready view of nursing staff
- continuity of care regime on transfer.

Table 22.16 is a suggested basic care plan for a patient in the initial stages of post-infarction and without complications and is suitable for modification to the home environment.

POST-CRISIS CARE AND REHABILITATION. Subsequent management after the inital crisis is over relies on continuing observation of the patient for signs of cardiac failure and arrythmias, continuing management of ischaemic pain and anxiety, and the development of a planned programme of rehabilitation. The latter should commence as soon as the patient's physical state is stable, with the aim of minimizing the impact of the infarction on the patient's lifestyle and self-concept and optimising his/her health potential. Rehabilitation is discussed further in the subsequent section on tertiary prevention.

During this period the patient will gradually regain self care and may be discharged from hospital after 5–7 days. At this stage they should be able to tolerate mild exertion such as walking on the flat without experiencing pain or any other unpleasant sensation. It is of note that the physiological demand of bathing is 3 times that of resting but is considered to be 'light exertion' by patients. There is no difference in demand between washing at a basin, in a shower or in a bath (Winslow et al, 1985). Those who have had recoveries complicated by arrhythmias or other problems will normally have a slower rehabilitation pattern and will be discharged from hospital later. Their overall prognosis is poorer.

Tertiary prevention in relation to coronary heart disease

Adequate rehabilitation and the development of effective long-term strategies for the maintenance of optimal health and function are the central areas of concern in tertiary prevention.

Three areas of intervention are discussed:

- drug therapy
- operative intervention
- rehabilitation/adaptation.

Drug therapy (see Table 22.17)

Three major groups of drugs are involved:

- longer-term nitrates
- beta-adrenergic blocking agents (β-blockers)
- calcium antagonists.

Longer term nitrates. Longer-term nitrates such as isosorbide mononitrate are thought to act in the same way as glyceryl trinitrate by selective vasodilatation, reducing venous return as well as reducing peripheral resistance and increasing myocardial perfusion.

Beta-adrenergic blocking agents. The beta-adrenergic blocking agents include those that have a general vasodilatory effect and those that are more cardioselective. The latter action is particularly important in that it reduces both the contractility of the myocardium and the heart rate. It also acts as a 'protection' against sympathetic provocation thus reducing the sympathetic response to exercise and emotion.

Calcium antagonists. This newer group of drugs, such as nifedipine, block the inward displacement of calcium ions across the cell membrane. Thus they reduce the excitability and contractility of the myocardium, effectively reducing cardiac demand for oxygen.

The use of these drugs enable many persons to maintain an active life relatively or completely free of disabling symptoms. Others may have to reduce their activities to a level commensurate with their energy levels and their tolerance of ischaemic pain or dyspnoea. Activity may also be diminishing for other reasons associated, for example, with ageing, such as movement limitation.

Operative intervention

Three operative procedures are currently available, all of which have been developed in the last 10–20 years. As a result the techniques are still in a phase of rapid development. These are:

- coronary angioplasty
- coronary artery bypass grafting
- cardiac transplantation.

Table 22.16 Suggested basis for an initial care plan for a patient with an uncomplicated infarction (0–48 hrs)

Problem	Goal	Nursing intervention	Method of evaluation
Myocardial necrosis and ischaemia causing: 1. **Pain**— crushing retrosternal chest pain radiating down left arm	Pain reduced to a level of mild discomfort or less as demonstrated by expressed feelings of patient and absence of identified pain behaviour	Analgesia as prescribed and required Information and support as in (2) Reduce environmental stressors to optimum level for individual Assist to adopt the most comfortable position commensurate with heart function	Enquire of patient ½ hr post analgesia and at 2 hrly intervals initially changing to 4 hrly when pain controlled Observe for pain behaviours Record × 3 in 24 hours
2. **Anxiety** — feeling of impending death — unbelief as to what has happened — role change — potential occupational threat — disruption of current ventures and activities — worry for partner — admission to hospital — technology of CCU/or — lack of expertise at home	Anxiety levels within the ability of the person to cope — expressing fears — demonstrating trust in staff to make appropriate decisions — understanding and acceptance of monitoring and treatment regimes	Maintain contact of patient with person of significance Describe what is happening within the environment and in relation to the illness. Explain procedures, treatments, monitoring. Repeat explanations as events occur. Involve in decision-making whenever possible commensurate with medical condition and expressed wishes. Listen to queries and take action as appropriate. Allay expression of fears and give realistic reassurance.	Enquire of person Observe for behavioural indications of anxiety Record x 3 in 24 hours
3. **The need to reduce demand on and by myocardium**	Demand on myocardium is minimal. Optimal salvage of myocardium — demonstrated on ECG Cardiac output maintained	Maintain comfortable position supported by 3–4 pillows. Maintain IVI and drug regime as prescribed. Inform medical staff of any change and institute treatment within scope of nurse.	Observations of vital signs ¼–½ hrly until stable then 4 hrly and continued
4. **Potential complications** — arrhythmias — shock — ventricular failure	Early detection and treatment of complications	Reduce extraneous stimulation and activity allowing essential self-care — feed self; wash hands & face — assist to commode — avoid straining (Valsalva manoeuvre). Maintain quiet restful environment.	
5. **Inability to maintain self-care or mobility** **Potential problems of bedrest:** — venous thrombosis — respiratory stasin — constipation — urinary stasis — pressure sores	Patient — clean and groomed in accordance with wishes — skin intact — comfortable, resting — hydrated — taking 1000–2500Cals per day — micturating without discomfort — defaecating without any strain — breathing quietly — venous circulation maintained	Wash patient as required, offer facilities for teeth cleaning/mouthcare/mouthwash hair combed, clothed acceptably to patient Re-position 2 hourly Allow undisturbed period of rest. Lights dimmed at night. Maintain fluid intake to total of 2–2500 ml. Offer light frequent meals or drinks supplement. Stool softener if required, up to commode. Gentle active exercise of legs and controlled deep breathing Up in chair after 24 hr for 1 hour period	Observation and enquiry of patient Fluid balance chart Weight when up × 1

Table 22.17 Drugs in common use in the management of coronary heart disease

Type	Action	Comments
Nitrates	Widely used for symptomatic relief and control of angina	Side-effects are those related to vasodilation — flushing, headaches and hypotension.
Glyceryl trinitrate (GTN)	Vasodilation of major vessels including veins — reduce volume load (pre-load), stroke output and systolic BP. With reduction in peripheral resistance left ventricular work is reduced and therefore the demand on the myocardium. Possibly some coronary vasodilatation	GTN taken sublingually-aiding rapid absorption. Effective within 5 minutes and lasts 20–30 minutes. Ideal during angina attack and safe to repeat every 5 minutes up to 3 tablets. In stable angina, of use in preventing attack if taken prior to exercise. Tablets kept by patient including in hospital for rapid self-administration. Deteriorate in light so dark container required, replenished after 6 months.
Isosorbide dinitrate		Regular oral administration as a longer term control. Rapidly metabolised in liver so that little is found in circulation — efficiency therefore in doubt.
Isosorbide mononitrate		Recent compound largely replacing dinitrate. Not metabolised by liver so is more predictable in effect.
Beta-adrenergic blocking agents (see pages 650 & 676 for further detail)	Increasingly used. May optimise myocardial salvage Block response of beta adrenergic receptors to sympathetic stimulation — slow heart, reduced liability to arrhythmias therefore decreases myocardial O_2 requirement therefore protects from physical/psychic overstimulation	Not given if atrio-ventricular block is evident Caution with asthmatic patients or if hypotension present Useful in management of atrio-ventricular tachycardias
Calcium antagonists Verapamil	Interferes with inward displacement of calcium ions across cardiac cell membrane, therefore inhibits excitation–contraction coupling. Decreases cardiac contractility therefore decreases myocardial O_2 requirement. Does not block beta-adrenergic receptors.	Not to be given within 8 hours after beta blockers. May precipitate heart failure Used previously in control of atrioventricular tachycardias
Nifedipine	More potent peripheral and coronary vasodilator than verapamil	Does not have any anti-arrhythmic activity. Minor side-effects — flushing, headache, gastrointestinal intolerance Used in long-term control of angina
Other anti-arrhythmic drugs		
Ventricular arrhythmias — Lignocaine		Drug of choice to treat ventricular extra systoles and tachycardia but effect in prevention in some doubt
Mexiletine		
Procainamide		
Disopyramide		
Supraventricular dysrhythmias — Digoxin		Slows ventricular response — used in atrial fibrillation/flutter
Quinidine		Suppresses atrial ectopics
Atropine		Bradycardia post-infarction or caused by beta-blockers
Analgesics		
Morphine	Narcotic analgesic	Causes nausea and vomiting, constipation, respiratory depression. May be combined with antiemetic such as prochlorperazine or cyclizine

These are discussed briefly individually and are followed by a general section on cardiac surgery.

Percutaneous transluminal coronary angioplasty (PTCA). This is a technique of increasing importance. It involves the dilatation of stenosed coronary arteries by means of a balloon catheter inserted via cardiac catherization.

It is thought that the dilatation may result in an increase in the vessel's outer diameter, compression of the fluid portion of the atheroma and intimal splitting, tearing or dissection. Reabsorption of the atheroma is thought to occur. It is estimated that it offers an alternative to by-pass grafting in about 10%–20% of patients (Loan, 1986).

Clearly the technique is only suitable where the atheroma is still pliable and is not calcified. Realistically therefore it may only be offered to persons whose onset of angina is recent, who are not responding to medical treatment and whose angina is disabling (O'Neil, 1986). A 60% success rate is reported, success being identified as a 20% decrease in stenosis. However, a small number will require emergency by-pass grafting as occlusion occurs during the procedure (Bouman, 1984). More recently laser assisted angioplasty has been introduced, whereby the laser is used to disintegrate the clot allowing for the passage of the balloon catheter (Rutter & Ellis, 1986). Electronic pacing wires may be introduced to manage arrhythmias should they occur (Loan, 1986).

Nursing considerations are as for cardiac catherization with the additional precaution of having the patient, relatives and staff prepared for emergency by-pass surgery. Many patients will experience anginal pain during the inflation of the balloon and should be warned of and supported during this experience. Nitroglycerine and nifedipine may be administered to control these effects (Loan, 1986).

Coronary artery bypass grafting. Coronary artery bypass grafting is now routinely performed for persons whose angina is seriously disrupting to life but whose myocardial function remains reasonable. Although common, however, the surgery constitutes a major event for the patient. The heart is approached via a sternal split. The graft normally used is the saphenous vein, in which case the patient will have an additional wound site, which may cause considerable problems postoperatively. A third of patients followed up in one study had delayed leg-wound healing and a quarter still experienced gross leg swelling and pain 1 year after surgery (Wilson-Barnett, 1981). An alternative graft is the internal mammary artery which, although it creates a greater propensity for bleeding due to more tissue damage and is a challenge in terms of pulmonary management because of its proximity to the lungs, shows superior patency both in the short and long term due to a reduced propensity to develop atheroma (Jansen & McFaddon, 1986). The 5-year survival rate is 70–85%.

Cardiac transplantation. Cardiac transplantation is undoubtedly the most dramatic therapeutic development for cardiovascular disease that has emerged in the last decade.

Any person currently considered for cardiac transplantation has terminal cardiac disease for which there is no alternative medical or surgical therapy. In writing up the experience of one hospital, Reitz & Stinson (1981) report the following. The majority of recipients are relatively young — the mean age for those with coronary artery disease being given as 45 years, for those with idopathic cardiomyopathy, 39 years. Only 15–20% of those referred are accepted and 20% of the accepted potential recipients die before a suitable donor heart is available in spite of the average 'wait' for a heart being only 38 days. The 5 year survival rate post transplant is now 50–60% compared with 15–20% in the first years of operating. At 1 year post-transplant the majority of the 91% who survive have returned to a normal level of exercise tolerance and lifestyle. Infection is the major cause of death. In spite of the small numbers to have undergone this operation, impressive progress has been made and it seems likely to become an accepted part of the range of therapeutic modes available, albeit one of 'last resort'.

Currently donor hearts are human, the person having suffered irreversible brain death, normally due to road traffic accident. Reitz &

Stinson (1981) report the average age of the donors as 25 years. When the heart donor's age is over 35 years the incidence of late graft coronary atherosclerosis occurring post-transplant increases. The hearts are either transferred direct or transported from one centre to the transplant centre. In this situation the heart is perfused with a mildly hyperkalaemic electrolyte solution and packed in sterile cold saline with the container in ice. Hearts have been satisfactorily maintained for 2½–3 hours in this way.

Contraindications for selection of recipients for cardiac transplantation include the existence of active infection, insulin dependent diabetes (due to the problems of control with immunosuppressant therapy), advanced age, elevated pulmonary vascular resistance, multiple organ failure and pulmonary embolism. Persons who do not comply with medical regimes and who do not appear motivated to rehabilitate or have a poor support system are also not considered suitable (Reitz & Stinson, 1981).

Suitability or matching of hearts is based on ABO blood group compatibility, body size and lymphocyte crossmatch. The latter must be compatible as any mismatch is predictive of graft rejection.

The operation is carried out via a medial sternotomy and requires cardiopulmonary bypass. Simple topical hypothermia is maintained and the donor heart is anastomosed at mid-atrial level. Temporary pacing may be required for up to 3 days postoperatively.

Pre- and postoperative care is similar to that discussed in the general section on cardiac surgery. The exception is the need for immunosuppression. The problem of avoiding graft rejection while retaining a degree of resistance to infection is the most difficult aspect of management. Immunosuppression will commence pre-operatively and be maintained indefinitely. Acute rejection episodes normally occur between 10 and 30 days, the majority being reversed by temporarily increasing the immunosuppressant drugs. Drug regimes are constantly developing, current examples being azathioprine and methylpresdnisolone, with Rabbit Antihuman Thymocyte Globulin (RATG) being used over the operative period. Graft rejection is indicated by the patient becoming lethargic, a change in heart sounds suggesting a change in ventricular compliance and ECG and haematological changes. Endomyocardial biopsy via the internal jugular vein may be carried out safely and may be confirmatory of early graft rejection enabling prompt action to be taken.

Cardiac surgery. Surgery on the heart is increasingly common and broadly comprises the following groups of operations:

- surgery on the valves
  - valvotomy
  - valve replacement
- surgery on the coronary vessels
  - bypass grafting
  - angioplasty
- heart transplantation.

Persons with previously undetected small septal defects may also require surgery during adulthood, as will those with other acquired defects such as ventricular aneurysm or rupture.

The purpose of this section is to highlight general issues of nursing concern related to the specific requirements of patients undergoing cardiac surgery. The reader is also referred to the standard pre- and postoperative care plans included in the chapter on surgery (Ch. 17), the sections about specific operative procedures in this chapter and the chapters on shock and disorders of oxygenation and carbon dioxide exchange. Students working within specialized cardio-thoracic and intensive care units will require the more detailed exploration contained within the specialist books and journals.

The decision to operate. The problems of any patient undergoing surgery are present for the person undergoing cardiac surgery, and in many areas are increased. The connotations of 'heart surgery' are emotive in the extreme and such surgery is not undertaken lightly by surgeons or patients. Patients will have experienced a wide range of investigatory procedures which will have demonstrated the nature and/or the extent of the structural and physiological problem. This information, taken together with the functional deficit experienced by the patient, is the basis of the decision regarding operative intervention.

Occasionally a life-threatening situation such as ventricular rupture or massive coronary artery occlusion will result in such a crisis that the decision to operate is the only alternative to inevitable death.

Aspects specific to care of persons undergoing cardiac surgery. The following aspects are identified as important to take into acount in caring for persons undergoing cardiac surgery. These will modify all aspects of usual pre- and postoperative care based on a standard plan.

- The patient is actually or potentially in a critical physiological condition pre- and postoperatively.
- The thoracic cavity will be entered.
- The heart cavity or major blood vessels may be entered.
- Cardiopulmonary bypass may be necessary.

The implications of these will be discussed briefly.

IMPLICATIONS OF THE PERSON'S CRITICAL OR POTENTIALLY CRITICAL CONDITION. The clear implication of this situation is the need for close monitoring. The mechanical aids now available to assist medical and nursing staff in observing the patient's state and in the management of the person adds to the complexity of the environment in which the patient finds him/herself and to the demands made on the nurses' knowledge and skill. It is not unusual to find the patient post-cardiac surgery with the following:

- intravenous infusion/transfusion
- Central Venous Pressure line and manometer
- intravenous or intrathecal drug pump (heparin, analgesic)
- cardiac monitor
- endotracheal tube/ventilator
- oxygen — humidified
- suction
- chest drainage tubes — low pressure vacuum.

This need for close monitoring together with the specialized knowledge and skill required for the effective care of these persons results in their care taking place in intensive care units. These units as care environments, in addition to the critical nature of the illness and the equipment required specific to each patient, raise additional nursing concerns. Most of these issues have been discussed in the context of coronary care units (p. 674). As a reminder here it is useful to restate the areas for consideration:

- the overall environment — layout, lighting, noise, routine
- nurse-patient communication
- involvement of relatives/significant others
- management of transfer from the intensive care unit.

These aspects will be in addition to those of:

- pain control and patient comfort
- maintenance of vital functions
  - — circulatory state
  - — respiration
  - — fluid and electrolyte balance
- maintenance of other body functions.

IMPLICATIONS OF ENTERING THE THORACIC CAVITY. The thoracic cavity is entered normally via a sternal split into the mediastinum. Alternately a thoracotomy may be performed. Very rarely the approach will be via the abdominal cavity and diaphragm. The pleural cavity therefore may or may not be entered. However, due to the position of the wound and the proximity of the heart and great vessels to the lungs, interference with respiration is inevitable. Mechanical ventilation via an endotracheal tube for a limited period postoperatively is common. The problems of establishing an effective communication system must be anticipated in the pre-operative phase of care. Frequent chest physiotherapy is essential and requires adequate pain control to be effective. Closed chest tubes with water-seal drainage to allow for fluid and air to escape and thereby to promote full lung expansion are usually in situ. Particular care needs to be taken in moving and positioning the patient in order that the system remains sealed and is effective.

In the rehabilitation phase the sternotomy wound may be a cause of major discomfort, taking up to 3 months to heal and causing severe pain. Wilson-Barnett (1981) found that nearly a third of the patients followed up after coronary artery bypass grafting with sternotomy wounds had severe pain one year postoperatively.

IMPLICATIONS OF ENTERING THE HEART CHAMBERS OR MAJOR VESSELS. Clearly where incisions have been made into the heart cavity or through major vessels there is a potential for leakage at the incision site. In the context of other haemodynamic changes it may be difficult to identify such leakage early. An increase in local pain, in blood draining into dressings or sealed drainage systems, or in the level of shock with which the patient is presenting, are all indicators.

A second complication to arise from incising the heart or vessels is that of coagulation at the incision site. Thus mural thromboses (and resultant obstruction to blood flow) or emboli formation are hazards. The signs will be those associated with occlusion of the coronary, plumonary, peripheral or cerebral arteries.

Finally, heart wall incision inevitably threatens cardiac rhythm, as will interference with coronary blood flow.

IMPLICATIONS OF CARDIOPULMONARY BYPASS (CPB). Cardiopulmonary bypass has significant effects on cardiovascular physiology of itself and as a result of concomitant management techniques such as haemodilution, hypothermia and anticoagulation. These are fully explained by Weiland & Walker (1986), for example, but are summarized here.

DIRECT EFFECTS. The direct effects of CPB are:

- Attachment of CPB to patient's arterial and venous system — potential site for bleeding and thrombus formation.
- Interface between blood and the plastic and metal surfaces of the CPB system — potential for haemolysis due to the shearing force, the risk increasing with the length of time blood is exposed to the surfaces.
- Non-pulsatile blood flow — causes an increased sympathetic response and therefore hypertension.

HAEMODILUTION. This results from the use of autologous blood diluted with an isotonic solution (such as Ringer's Solution) with 5% Dextrose to prime the extracorporeal circuit. Such haemodilution reduces the risk of a number of clinical problems (e.g. coagulation) and is more feasible in terms of availability and cost.

HYPOTHERMIA. This is used to reduce the tissue oxygen requirements thereby reducing the risk of ischaemia of the vital organs such as the brain and heart. In addition the lowered temperature enables lower flow rates to be utilized, thus decreasing the shear of blood cells against the surfaces of the CPB apparatus and reducing haemolysis.

ANTICOAGULATION. Anticoagulation with heparin is used to reduce the extravascular coagulation which is inevitable within the CPB apparatus if such precautions are not taken.

These, together with the direct effects of CPB, result in the clinical effects indicated in Table 22.18.

Rehabilitation/adaptation. The experience of angina or myocardial infarction involves the individual in a process of reappraisal of self, of relationships and of role and function. It may result in a dramatically reduced functional capacity and/or in frequent experience of pain. For many it can mean little change in lifestyle once the initial phase of illness has passed. Some, however, may change their pattern of living with the intention of reducing the risks of recurrence or of improving their general health status.

In recent years much attention has been given by nurses and other health care professionals to develop and evaluate rehabilitation programmes to support individuals and their families in the post-infarction phase. Such programmes may commence in, or be linked with, the coronary care unit, the general medical or cardiology ward or the outpatients clinic. In general they are individually planned within a broad framework, being based on the person's

- age and previous health state
- previous activity and lifestyle
- cardiac response to increasing mobility and exercise testing.

There are many examples of rehabilitation programmes available, particularly in the North

Table 22.18 Summary of some of the clinical effects of cardio-pulmonary bypass (CPB)

Clinical effect	Cause	Comment
Blood pressure fluctuation	Hypothermia lowers BP as a result of reduced cardiac output The non-pulsatile flow causes a sympathetic response which raises BP Haemodilution lowers the plasma colloidal osmotic pressure, which together with the Blood–CPB interface which causes platelet damage, causes Extravasation of fluid into the interstitial compartment	Severe hypotension threatens vital organ function Hypertension increases the stress on suture lines Fluid replacement difficult to estimate Intravascular fluid depletion increases risk of coagulation
Oedema including pulmonary oedema		O_2/CO_2 exchange compromised Adds to existing lung expansion problems
Polyuria/oliguria	Haemodilution may cause diuresis Hypotension and extravasation of fluid into interstitial compartment may cause oliguria	Potential renal failure
Bradycardia	Hypothermia depresses cardiac functions	
Increased risk of bruising/bleeding	Anticoagulation and the effects of CPB surface — blood interface causing haemolysis and an increase in capillary permeability	Internal bleeding somtimes difficult to identify due to BP fluctuation
Risk of blood vessel occlusion	Platelet damage causing thrombus formation	
Cerebral dysfunction		
Disorientation	Hypotension, poor oxygenation	
Stroke	Blood vessel occlusion	
Hyperglycaemia	The non-pulsatile flow causes a sympathetic response Hypothermia reduces Islet function	

American literature. The key aspects of these programmes include:

- resumption of self-care and a graduated increase in activity level
- acceptance of self and of the infarction
- compliance with drug therapy and other medical regimes such as
  - cessation or reduction in smoking
  - alteration in dietary regime
  - regular exercising.

They therefore focus around

- imparting knowledge of coronary heart disease, influencing factors and preventive strategies
- providing a support group
- supervising exercise and other regimes
- achieving compliance with medical regimes.

While the concept of such programmes appears logical and sound the reality is somewhat different. There are two major questions:

- What is the evidence that the content of such programmes is valid, i.e. that if compliance occurs the risk of further ischaemic attacks or infarction is reduced or that the quality of life is enhanced?
- What is the evidence that such programmes achieve their aims in terms of compliance with medical regimes?

Clearly the necessity of asking the second question is dependent on the answer to the first. Much of the evidence has already been reviewed within the earlier section on primary prevention of coronary heart disease. For example, there is clear evidence that a reduction in smoking is beneficial in reducing risk of further attack, but the evidence for promoting changes in dietary pattern is disputed. The evidence for the effectiveness of a graduated exercise programme post-infarction is controversial. The primary purpose of the exercise is to improve myocardial function. This function can be said to improve if exercise tolerance is increased — that is, an increase in the amount of exercise (e.g. exercise bike/treadmill) taken before signs or symptoms of ischaemia occur (e.g. ECG changes, angina). However, whilst exercise tolerance does improve in the weeks following myocardial infarction there is little evidence that structured exercise facilitates this. What does emerge is that the person gains a sense of well-being by taking regular exercise.

By contrast, there is considerable evidence that those who have been involved in rehabilitation programmes which include information-giving and discussion are better informed about the nature of their disorder and its management. Similarly, there is evidence that such programmes are seen as supportive in the same way as self-help groups — enabling those persons who have had myocardial infarctions, and others significant to them, to air their fears and to share experiences.

The evidence that rehabilitation programmes are effective in terms of their influence on the person's behaviour is fairly negative, although not wholly so. A large number of studies report poor compliance despite increased knowledge (Mayberry & Kent, 1983). A recent small study by Hentinen (1986) showed that some patients did reduce their butter intake and increase their exercise at initial follow-up. However this did not necessarily last and alcohol consumption and cigarette smoking habits did not change. From the results of a study of indicators of medical regime adherence, Miller et al (1984) suggest that greater compliance may be achieved by intervention later in the post-hospital phase, when the nature of adjustments in lifestyle are known rather than anticipated.

In conclusion it must be stated that so long as the evidence for lifestyle change is controversial in terms of effectiveness in reducing risk of further infarction, the validity of the aim of rehabilitation programmes as behaviour change is questionable. The value of such programmes in providing a human support and information service is less in dispute, but in times of economic constraint is vulnerable in terms of resource priorities. Further development and evaluation of programmes in a UK context and utilizing home-based community health care facilities has considerable potential.

PROBLEMS OF FLOW WITHIN THE CENTRAL ARTERIES

ANEURYSM

The major problem of flow within the central arteries of the body is that caused by aneurysms. These are bulges in the arterial wall due to weakening and as they develop they are felt to be pulsatile and may cause pressure symptoms.

Incidence, prognosis and cause

Abdominal aortic aneurysm is responsible for 1.2% of male and 0.6% of female deaths in the USA, the incidence at postmortem being found to be 1–3%, 10% in men over 60 years (Joyce, 1983). 98% of aneurysms develop below the renal arteries, and 95% are atherosclerotic in origin. It is not surprising therefore that 40% of patients also have coronary heart disease, peripheral arterial disease, hypertension or obstructive lung disease. The life expectancy of individuals who have developed symptoms from the aneurysm is 6 months. Rupture of the aneurysm inevitably causes death unless surgical repair is undertaken. There is a 40-60% success rate if surgery is undertaken as an emergency. Elective surgery carries a 0–5% mortality and is considered to be extremely effective (Joyce, 1983).

Presentation and diagnosis

Aneurysm is frequently asymptomatic, the arterial wall gradually distending over a period of years. The aneurysm may therefore be identified during physical examination related to cardiovascular or other disorders. Compression of abdominal organs or veins, however, may occur, as may arteriovenous fistulae. On examination typically a pulsatile epigastric mass is felt.

If the aneurysm is in the process of rupture it may do so into the peritoneum, gastrointestinal tract or vein. This may occur suddenly or more gradually as when the walls of the artery become separated and the aneurysm 'dissects'. Severe pain with hypotension and a tender epigastric mass are classic symptoms of a ruptured aneurysm. The situation is critical and surgery essential (Joyce, 1983).

Treatment

Reconstructive surgery, using Teflon grafts, has revolutionized the prognosis.

Pre- and postoperative care

There is no care specific to the operation except that of careful monitoring for haemorrhage and observation of leg and pedal pulses, feet colour and warmth. Mobilization is rapid and the postoperative period normally uneventful.

PROBLEMS OF FLOW WITHIN THE PERIPHERAL ARTERIAL SYSTEM

PERIPHERAL OCCLUSIVE DISORDERS

Peripheral arterial disease of the lower limb is primarily a manifestation of atherosclerosis, which results in ischaemia of the lower limbs. This presents as intermittent claudication (ischaemic pain in the legs on exercise), rest pain and gangrene.

Associated factors

It is clear that in the majority of cases, peripheral arterial disease is associated with atheroma and therefore shares 'risk' factors in common with both coronary heart disease and hypertension. For example, in a small study of 183 patients presenting with peripheral arterial disease Greenhalgh (1984) found that the mean age of the patients was just over 58 years and the male to female ratio was 4:1; 18% had a history of myocardial infarction and 13.6% had diabetes mellitus; 90% of the group were heavy smokers (more than 20 cigarettes a day for 20 years or more); 30% had hypertension (resting diastolic more than 90 mmHg, systolic more than 160 mmHg).

From this it can been seen that the characteristics of persons who presented with peripheral arterial disease were very similar to those presenting with coronary heart disease. In addition, blood analysis demonstrated that the average serum cholesterol levels of those with arterial disease were significantly higher than that of controls (237mg/100ml compared with 197 mg/100ml) as were the serum triglyceride and uric acid levels. The carbon monoxide haemoglobin levels were also found to be higher than in controls (mean 3.3% as opposed to 0.9%).

Disease progression and success of reconstructive surgery was also found to be dependent on smoking — the mean carbon monoxide haemoglobin level being 5.6% in those for whom the surgery had failed, compared with 2.88% in those whose surgery was successful. However serum cholesterol, triglycerides and uric acid levels, while found to be higher in those with the disease, did not appear to make any difference to the outcome of reconstructive surgery. While the effect of control of diabetes mellitus and hypertension has not been demonstrated to affect the atherosclerotic process, nevertheless the risk of serious sequelae such as gangrene and mortality from other vascular disorders has been shown to decrease if the manifestations of these disorders (blood glucose and blood pressure) are well controlled (Greenhalgh, 1984).

Cause and disease presentation

The cause in the majority of persons with peripheral arterial disease is atheroma. However, excessive vasoconstruction or fibrosis of arterioles can also cause ischaemic disorders. Sudden arterial occlusion occurs with emboli dislodging from a mural thrombosis or from loose thrombi in the chambers of the heart associated with atrial fibrillation. In this situation emergency embolectomy or bypass surgery is required if the leg is to remain viable.

Atherosclerosis both reduces the lumen size and the elasticity of the arterial wall and causes occlusion, due to the atheromatous plaques themselves obstructing flow or being the focal point for thrombus formation.

It presents in three forms:

- intermittent claudication — 50%
- rest pain — 40%
- gangrene — 10%

These are not necessarily progressive. For example elderly persons with diabetes appear to present with gangrenous toes more frequently than with intermittent claudication. Intermittent claudication usually occurs in the calf muscle during exercise, the pain being due to metabolite release during ischaemia. Rest pain may involve part or most of the leg and is particularly troublesome at night when the circulation is diminished.

Effect on individual and diagnosis

The ischaemic pain at rest or on exercise is experienced as an excruciating cramp which, if severe, is exhausting and debilitating. By contrast, gangrene is not necessarily painful, particularly in those persons with diabetes who also have peripheral neuropathy. A toe is usually first affected and will appear red, possibly developing an ulcerated tip before becoming necrotic. If the individual has associated eye problems, the process of ischaemia and necrosis may not be noticed. The chiropodist or the district nurse visiting the person may be the first to observe that circulation is reduced. The diagnosis of peripheral artery disease is usually therefore not in doubt, either from the patient's account of the pain or by observation of the foot. The appearance and temperature of the ischaemic limb may differ from its counterpart, unless that too is ischaemic. Pulses below the point of occlusion will be absent or weak. Diagnosis is confirmed and the extent and location of atheroma identified by two investigations — doppler ultrasound and angiogram.

Treatment

Treatment is really restricted to physical dilatation of the artery or reconstructive surgery, as drugs that act as peripheral dilators are relatively ineffective on diseased, atheromatous arteries. The decision to reconstruct the arteries is a serious one and every attempt is made to reduce the progression of the disease or to modify lifestyle to live within its limitations. Advice will include:

- reduce or cease smoking
- maintain activity at a level below that which produces ischaemic pain in order to maintain optimum arterial flow
- avoid elevating legs to level of body as this reduces arterial flow
- avoid excessive warmth to feet — this stimulates superficial vasodilatation and diverts blood flow from deeper vessels
- avoid excessive cold as this leads to peripheral vasoconstriction
- meticulous foot care.

Compliance with medical recommendation, however, is poor. For example Greenhalgh (1984) reports a relatively high incidence of deception regarding cigarette smoking and relies on measurement of haemoglobin carbon-monoxide levels, although these too can be manipulated by short-term cessation.

The nurse has an important role in helping the patient understand the reasons for the advice given and in developing a realistic plan of campaign to help him/her achieve mutually agreed goals. Visits to outpatient clinics, to day or short term care for investigations or for a longer stay in a general ward can be used to advantage. Care regimes on the ward should include education and discussion sessions and support the preventative measures.

Surgical intervention

Three surgical procedures are available:

- transluminal dilatation
- reconstructive surgery
- amputation.

Clearly these increase in order of severity, the third requiring major personal adjustment. They are unfortunately not interchangeable.

Transluminal dilation

This is a method of treating occlusive athero-

Table 22.19 Drugs used in the prevention and treatment of arterial and venous thromboembolism

Type	Effect	Comment
Anticoagulants	Prevents development or extension of venous thrombosis	Bleeding is an inevitable risk
Heparin sodium	? acts on fibrin	Intravenous rapid action, initiates anticoagulation and is best given continuously. Protamine sulphate is the specific antidote
Heparin calcium		Low dose heparin for prophylaxis. Given subcutaneously
Warfarin sodium	Antagonises effects of Vit. K	Taken orally, not effective for 36–48 hours therefore commenced during heparinisation Prothrombin time maintained 2–3 times normal Not used in arterial occlusion Contraindicated in pregnancy as it crosses the placental barrier and is weakly teratogenic
Antiplatelet drugs Dipyridamole Aspirin	Decreases platelet adhesiveness — useful for arterial thromboembolism	Aspirin is effective used in very small doses over a prolonged period of time

sclerosis by insertion of a catheter, with or without laser, and inflation of a balloon within the affected artery.

It is thought to be effective by fracturing the atherosclerotic plaque and separating it from the media. The inflammatory process is initiated and results in subsequent fibrosis, re-endothelialization and remodelling (Johnson, 1984).

As a procedure it is currently relatively limited in its application. Johnson (1984) identifies lesions most suitable for treatment in this way as having the following characteristics:

- being localized (i.e. the adjacent arteries being patent) and minimally diseased
- the stenosis or occlusion being less than 10 cm in length
- the lesion being accessible.

As the procedure does not carry the same operative risk as reconstructive surgery and does not require a general anaesthetic it is particularly suitable for elderly persons or for those at high risk with general anaesthetic. It is also of value in those whose saphenous vein is not suitable for use as an arterial graft.

The success rate is reported as 55–65%, the results being shorter term and less dramatic than surgery. Post-dilatation angiograms are performed immediately after the procedure utilizing the same catheter.

Pre- and postoperative nursing care therefore is that of any person who has had an aortic or femoral angiogram. Particular attention, however, should be paid to the catheter insertion site. Oozing should not occur as a cut down will normally have been performed. Distal blood flow should be noticeably improved as demonstrated by moderate to strong pedal pulses and a warm foot.

Anticoagulants may be given over the operative period and for 1 month afterwards. Early mobilization, regular exercise and a reduction or cessation of smoking is advised.

Reconstruction surgery. Reconstructive surgery is the most common operative procedure for severe peripheral artery disease. Essentially it consists of bypassing the occluded artery by an artificially created alternative route. The reconstruction normally consists of the saphenous vein. Teflon, an artificial alternative, is seldom used due to an increased incidence in thromboembolic problems.

The most commonly used procedure involves removing the saphenous vein from the leg and reversing it so that the valves do not obstruct arterial flow. More recently, however, interest has been shown in using the saphenous vein in situ (Karmody & Leather, 1984). This technique has the clear advantage of reducing tissue damage as the vein does not have to be stripped out. The valves, however, have to be made impotent. Early methods of achieving this were not successful. The more recent technique involves incising the valve leaflets with valvotomy scissors or a valvulotome (similar to a tiny stitch cutter on a long handle). This appears to result in reasonable success, the valve leaflet remnants retracting into the valve sinus.

The overall success rate of reconstructive surgery appears to vary from 93– 63% at 1 year postoperative to 70–30% 4–5 years post-surgery (Karmody & Leather, 1984; Greenhalgh, 1984) The wide range appears to be due to a number of factors of which the operative centre, the operative technique and smoking are three. In situ reconstruction appears to be superior to reverse vein grafts (Karmody & Leather, 1984) and smoking has a deleterious effect (Greenhalgh, 1984). Many surgeons will not undertake surgery unless the patient contracts to give up smoking because of the poor success rate if smoking is continued.

Nursing implications. Care related to any person with peripheral artery disease also applies to the operative patient. Due to the high failure rate of surgery in some situations, some patients will be having second reconstructions and need particularly supportive care.

SPECIFIC PRE-OPERATIVE CARE. Sites of planned incision or the route of a vessel may be marked on the person's skin.

The strength and position of all leg pulses should be noted on the nursing records, as should the colour and warmth of the skin at specific points on the foot and leg. These are essential if postoperative comparisons are to be meaningful. Anticoagulants may be given.

SPECIFIC POSTOPERATIVE CARE. Meticulous observation of blood flow to the affected leg is undertaken.

Isometric and active leg exercises are carried out under supervision and rapid mobilization all helps to optimize tissue perfusion.

Anti-embolic stockings are used to promote venous return.

Non-compliance with postoperative instructions on discharge is again reported as being relatively high. In a small study Ronayne (1985) found the greatest non-compliance amongst those undergoing repeat surgery. Support stockings amd smoking caused the greatest problems, the former being 'uncomfortable and too tight'.

Amputation. Amputation is the surgical procedure only undertaken if all else fails. It is clearly a drastic step but results in a reduction in pain and discomfort. Even in the elderly, mobility may be regained with an artificial limb or in a wheelchair.

It is essentially an orthopaedic procedure although undertaken for vascular reasons, and is further discussed in the appropriate chapter.

PERIPHERAL VASOSPASTIC DISORDERS

The most common vasospastic disorder is that of Raynaud's disease. This is a primary disorder generally affecting the upper limbs. Vasospasm, secondary to identified pathologies such as occlusive arterial disease, collagen disorders such as scleroderma, neurological, traumatic or allergic conditions, is termed Raynaud's phenomenon.

Raynaud's disease is five times as common in women than men, and usually develops in young adults (Spittell, 1983). It is characterized by changes in skin colour and temperature due to excessive vasoconstriction of the arterioles and small arteries. It is thought to be due to a faulty mechanism within the vessels, no changes occuring with sympathetic stimulation (Fagius & Blumberg, 1985). In the absence of an identified cause, the management is based on symptomatic relief. This includes:

- avoidance of triggers (if present)
- avoidance of smoking
- vasodilator drugs
- calcium antagonists
- sympathectomy.

DISTURBANCE OF BLOOD FLOW THROUGH THE HEART

Heart valve disease is the major cause of altered flow within the heart, the other cause being defects of the septum. The latter are congenital. Major problems with the heart valves may also occur as part of a congenital defect. However as care of infants with congenital defects is largely the province of neonatal and paediatric health care personnel, the defects and their sequelae are not discussed further here.

ACQUIRED HEART VALVE DISEASE

Acquired heart valve disease presents as:

- stenosis of valves creating restriction of blood flow
- incompetence of valves creating regurgitation of blood
- a combination of stenosis with incompetence.

It may affect any of the four major valves of the heart but the mitral valve is most commonly affected (Gorlin, 1985).

Traditionally, acquired cardiac valvular disease has been termed 'rheumatic heart disease'. While this may continue to be so, in fact only 55% of those presenting with disorders of the most commonly affected valve — the mitral valve — have a history of rheumatic fever (Davies, 1985). Further, there are serological, clinical and epidemiological differences between those with and without a history of rheumatic fever, indicating that it should be appropriate to discuss rheumatic and other post-inflammatory heart disease as separate entities (Davies, 1985). However, the literature tends to handle all acquired valvular disorders together and it could be argued that, in the context of adults presenting with valvular disturbance, this is totally appropriate. In this section therefore the term rheumatic heart disease (RHD) will be used throughout to include all acquired cardiac valve disorders. As rheumatic fever is heavily implicated in the cause of RHD and is the only cause widely explored, a discussion of rheumatic fever is integral to the discussion of RHD.

Rheumatic fever and rheumatic heart disease

Rheumatic fever is associated with infection of the Type A β-haemolytic streptococcus and is assumed to be immunological in origin — the streptococcus and cardiac antigens evoking a tissue response. This response is characterized by mitral valve lesions, although other valves may be affected (Gorlin, 1985).

Incidence

Although the statistics available are incomplete it is nevertheless apparent that both rheumatic fever and RHD have dramatically decreased in the Westernized world. In Denmark, the incidence of rheumatic fever has fallen from over 200 per 100 000 in 1860, to 11 per 100 000 in 1962 (DiSciascio & Taranta, 1980). In Nashville, Tennessee the incidence in 1969 was found to be 6.4 per 100 000 (Quinn & Federspiel, 1974). Similarly with RHD the incidence in America fell from 4–5 per 1000 schoolchildren in 1920, to 0.5 per 1000 in 1980 (Markowitz, 1983); and in Japan the incidence has fallen even further, from 4.6 per 1000 in 1958 to 0.1 per 1000 in 1971 (Shiokawa & Yamada, 1977).

The picture in developing countries presents a stark contrast. In Sri Lanka for example, the incidence of rheumatic fever in 1978 was 142 per 100 000 for the 5–19 year old group and 47 per 100 000 for the general population (WHO, 1980), figures similar to those of the Westernized world 50 years previously (Markowitz, 1983). In relation to RHD, in India there is a 2–11% prevalence amongst school age children, in Thailand it is 21%. Of persons admitted to hospital with cardiac disease 25–50% have RHD, varying between different developing countries (WHO, 1980). From the very flimsy evidence available of incidence in previous decades in developing countries it would appear that the 1970–1980 figures indicate a dramatic rise in the problem, as dramatic as the fallen incidence in the West. Thus, an editorial in the Lancet in 1982 could state 'rheumatic heart disease is today the commonest form of acquired cardiac disease in children and young adults and one of the most common cardiovascular disorders in adults' (Lancet, 1982).

Examination of the incidence, beyond differentiating between the developed and developing worlds, indicates that the incidence is higher in females than males, has no ethnic predilection and appears to be accelerated in countries near the equator where the onset is earlier (Gorlin, 1985). The incidence amongst the poor in urban comunities is higher than in other groups. An example illustrating this in the context of an industrialized country, the USA, is that of Baltimore where the incidence in selected poor populations of black persons was 26.8 per 100 000, compared with 8.1 per 100 000 in the remainder of the city (Gordis, 1973).

Prognosis

Approximately 85% of those who have an attack of rheumatic fever will have a recurrence within 8 years (Lancet, 1982). With each recurrence the risk of rheumatic heart disease rises. An international study demonstrated that, of those with active rheumatic fever, 64% had suspected or definite carditis and 19% had cardiac failure usually associated with valvular disease (Strasser et al, 1981). The condition is seen in a more severe form in developing countries than in Westernized nations (Perloff, 1985).

From the initial attack of rheumatic fever it may take 7–10 years for signs of valvular disease such as heart murmur to develop, but 25% will die within this period. Two-thirds of the remainder will have RHD. 39% will die within 10 years of RHD being diagnosed, 79% within 20 years (Gorlin, 1985). Death is due to cardiac failure, respiratory problems or systemic (usually cerebral) embolism.

Stenosis due to fusion of the commissures (attached edges) of the valve is more common in younger people, whereas stenosis due to fibrosis and calcification of the valve leaf is more common in older persons (Perloff, 1985). As already mentioned the mitral valve is the most common valve to be affected (Strasser et al, 1981). Atrial fibrillation develops in 50% of persons with mitral stenosis and increases the already high risk of pulmonary oedema and systemic embolism, two-thirds of the latter being cerebral. Epilepsy is also more common in those with mitral valve disease, presumably due to undiagnosed micro-emboli causing cerebral infarction (Gorlin, 1985).

The influence of prophylaxis on prognosis. In areas where secondary prevention has been introduced in the form of long-term prophylactic antibiotics, the 7–10 year mortality rate has dropped to 1% with two-thirds of those who have had rheumatic fever having no residual RHD (Markowitz, 1983).

Causes

As already mentioned, the link between rheumatic fever and RHD is evident although this only accounts for 55% of those presenting with RHD (Davies, 1985).

Other identified causes of valve disorders include myocardial infarction leading to papillary muscle dysfunction, bacterial endocarditis and syphilis. Congenital heart abnormalities may continue to cause valve dysfunction in adult life.

The cause of rheumatic fever would appear to be an interaction of the following factors:

- group A β-haemolytic streptococcus
- poor living conditions, particularly high density housing
- possible genetic susceptibility.

Group A β-haemolytic streptococcus. The implication of streptococcus in causation is undisputed. The early evidence came from the reduction in cases of streptococcal throat infections and recurrent attacks of rheumatic fever when daily prophylactic doses of sulphonamides were introduced (Coburn & Moore, 1939; Thomas & France, 1939). Later it was shown that persons with a group A β-haemolytic streptococcal pharyngitis treated with sufficient penicillin to eradicate organisms were less likely to develop RHD (Denny et al, 1950). More recently, Gordis (1973) demonstrated a decrease of 60% in the incidence of rheumatic fever following the introduction of a comprehensive health programme including prophylactic antibiotics. Without doubt therefore, group A β-haemolytic streptococcus can be seen as a major cause of rheumatic fever and thus RHD.

The exact nature of the link, however, is more in doubt. Almost certainly there is an immunological response to the streptococcus resulting in carditis affecting both myo- and endocardium (Davies, 1985).

Poor housing conditions. Equally, however, it is apparent that other factors must be implicated in the cause. For example, the incidence of rheumatic fever started dropping before specific anti-streptococcal therapy became available (Markowitz, 1983). The incidence within a city varies between the areas of poor housing and the remainder of the population (Gordis, 1973). The incidence in the developing countries has risen with the growth of urbanization (Markowitz, 1983). Thus it would appear that poor living conditions, and in particular overcrowding, are also implicated in causation. This suggests that rheumatic fever attacks high risk populations (Markowitz, 1983).

Genetic considerations. Identifying an hereditary susceptibility is fraught with problems in a disease with clear social and environmental links, because the poor social conditions implicated are frequently linked with particular ethnic groups (Nora & Nora, 1983). Indeed, the incidence was so linked with particular social/ethnic groups that much of the early research focused on hereditary susceptibility (e.g. Wilson & Schweitzer, 1937). Now the question is more 'why do some individuals who are infected with group A β-haemolytic streptococcus, whether treated or not, develop rheumatic fever whilst others do not?' (Nora & Nora, 1983). Current work is exploring a genetic immunological basis for susceptibility, for example the possibility of auto-antibodies in rheumatic fever or a shared antigen between β-haemolytic streptococcus and cardiac tissue (Nora & Nora, 1983).

Rheumatic heart disease progression

In the initial stages RHD is characterized by areas of inflammation. These occur at particular sites on the heart valves:

- at the edges of the valves, especially the commissures
- at the point of contact where the chordae tendinae insert
- within the valve leaflets themselves (Gorlin, 1985).

The inflammation gives rise to progressive thickening and fibrosis of the affected valve, with calcification in some instances (Davies, 1985; Gorlin, 1985). The cause of the progression is thought to be due to one or other, or a combination of the two, factors:

- continuing subclinical rheumatic activity indicated by the presence of Aschoff bodies (see below), i.e. primary progression
- the increased turbulence caused by the disordered valve causing a secondary progression

The progression may also involve subvalvular destruction (Gorlin, 1985).

'Aschoff bodies' are indicative of active rheumatic disease. They are acute lesions in the myocardium, with a central zone of necrotic collagen surrounded by a collection of histiocytotic cells (scavenging cells derived from reticuloendothelial cells) including the specific cells — Aschoff bodies (Davies, 1985).

Stenosis and incompetence. The end result of the disease progression is a stiffened valve with a reduced opening, stenosis, and/or an inability to close properly, and incompetence, which leads to regurgitation of blood through the valve during systole.

The primary effects of stenosis and/or incompetence will clearly be:

- a reduction in forward pressure (pre-load or stroke volume) beyond the disordered valve
- an increase in backpressure (afterload) behind the disordered valve.

In addition, regurgitation will further reduce the volume of blood ejected from that chamber.

Thus the effects are largely those described in the sequence of events in cardiac failure. As mitral stenosis is the most commonly occurring problem, the effect of this particular problem and the treatment will be discussed more fully here.

Figure 22.10 illustrates the cycle of events in mitral stenosis.

The patient will thus present with symptoms as of left ventricular failure, except that the cardiac output may not be so severely reduced. The initial symptom is likely to be dyspnoea on

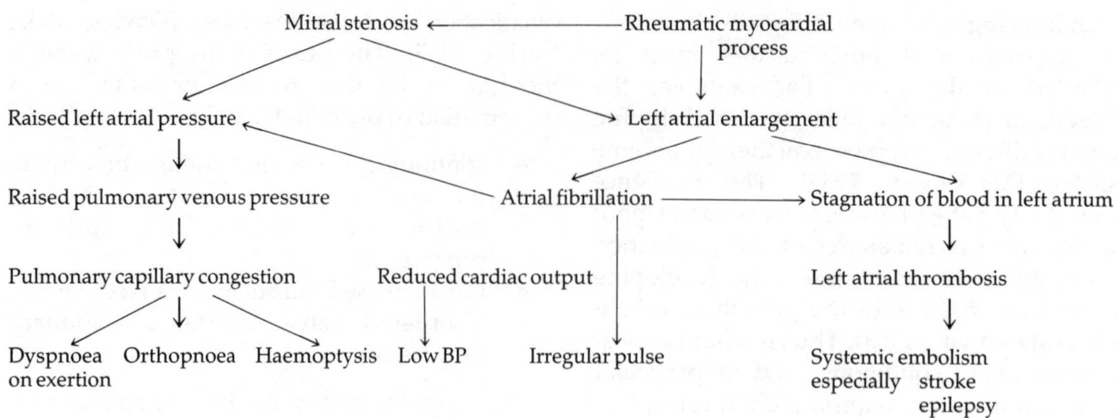

Fig. 22.10 Initial sequence of events in mitral stenosis

exertion. On examination, auscultation will reveal a heart murmur typical of mitral stenosis.

Subsequently the chronically raised pulmonary capillary pressure results in pulmonary artery vasoconstriction which, in the long-term, leads to hypertrophy of smooth muscle, intimal changes and fibrosis. This, in turn, leads to loss of lung substance, intrapulmonary shunts right to left (enabling blood to bypass the oxygenating surface) and disturbed pulmonary perfusion, the increased pulmonary resistance leading to right ventricular failure (Gorlin, 1985).

Primary prevention

The implications for prevention of the links between streptococcal infection, rheumatic fever and rheumatic heart disease are clear. Primary prevention of rheumatic fever involves modification or eradication of the causes listed previously:

- group A β-haemolytic streptococcal infections
- poor living conditions
- genetic factors.

As the genetic link is, as yet, not clear this is not a cause open to control of any sort.

Eradicating or treating all group A β-haemolytic streptococcal infections would involve, firstly, identifying all those with such infections and secondly, treating them. Large numbers of children and young people would therefore have to be treated in order to prevent RHD in those that are susceptible. In the context of the developing countries this is not considered to be feasible given the huge resource implications, nor, necessarily to be desirable (Lancet, 1982).

The two drugs of choice are:

- penicillin
- sulphadiazine.

It is recommended that these should be given for a minimum period of 5 years after the first attack and ideally into adulthood. Penicillin has the slight problem of the development of resistance. There are also non-compliance problems with oral administration. Monthly injections of benzylpenicillin are therefore recommended, having a high compliance rate and being 99% effective (Markowitz, 1983).

Presentation and diagnosis of acquired heart valve disease

The person with acquired cardiac valvular disease will present with symptoms dependent both on the valve affected and on the degree and nature of the disordered valve function. Thus both aortic stenosis and mitral stenosis are likely to create problems related to raised pulmonary venous pressures initially, although this will happen more rapidly in mitral valve disease than aortic. Differentially, left ventricular hypertrophy will be an early sign in aortic stenosis, but not in mitral stenosis where left atrial enlargement will occur. Signs of right ventricular hypertrophy and failure will occur with both pulmonary stenosis and mitral stenosis but more rapidly with the former and accompanied by signs of severe pulmonary disturbance in the latter.

Both the medical history and the physical examination are important in the initial identification of heart valve problems. Of particular note will be:

- signs of reduced cardiac output such as:
  - low BP
  - cold periphery
- signs of pulmonary congestion such as:
  - dyspnoea with or without exertion
  - orthopnoea
  - haemoptysis
  - cyanosis
  - abnormal respiratory sounds
- signs of cardiac enlargement such as:
  - deviation of apex
- signs of right ventricular failure such as:
  - raised jugular venous pressure
  - enlarged liver
  - peripheral oedema
- specific signs of cardiac valve disorder such as:
  - heart murmurs.

Further investigations will be directed at:

- confirming that the suspect valve is dysfunctional
- identifying the nature of the dysfunction:
  - stenosis
  - incompetence
- identifying the extent of the dysfunction
  - nature and extent of tissue damage
  - blood flow pattern
  - pressure pattern
- identifying the extent of the effect on general cardiac function.

These investigations may include the invasive technique of cardiac catheterization in addition to non-invasive techniques such as chest X-ray, ECG, echocardiography, Doppler ultrasound and nuclear techniques.

Medical management

Medical management will involve:

- management of the heart failure:
  - drug therapy, e.g. diuretics
  - possible dietary restriction
  - possible activity restriction
- management of arrhythmias and the sequelae
  - cardiac glycosides
  - anticoagulants
- consideration of surgery.

The latter involves valve repair or more commonly valve replacement.

Valve replacement. Pluth (1981) states that the ideal artificial valve will have the following attributes:

- durability
- assurance of function
- physiological haemodynamic features
- low thromboembolic incidence
- improved survival over diseased natural valve.

To date, however, the ideal valve has not been developed and the three major types available all fall short in some respect. In addition they all result in a mild to moderate stenosis relative to normal valve function. Because of these features persons with minimal problems arising from their valve disease are not offered surgical intervention. Valve replacement in patients whose left ventricle is markedly hypertrophied due to aortic stenosis or due to mitral incompetence is less successful than in others whose left ventricular function is unimpaired (Pluth, 1981).

Three types of valve are currently available:

- ball and cage valves
- disc prostheses
- biological valves.

The first two of these are very durable but thromboembolism is a problem, the rate per year being reported as 2.9 for aortic valves and 5.2 for mitral valves (Pluth, 1981). Biological valves may be homo- or heterografts, the latter most commonly porcine. They have a low incidence of thromboembolism but a shorter valve life than artificial valves, an average durability being 10–12 years. The choice of valve therefore depends on a number of factors including the age and sex of the patient, his or her access to medical supervision and the surgeon's preference. The relatively short life, low thromboembolitic valve, for example, is likely to be most suitable for older persons. It may also be essential for young women as the anticoagulant therapy utilized with the artificial valves causes problems during pregnancy and childbirth. The more durable valve is probably more suitable for young and middle-aged adults who would have to contemplate repeated major surgery at intervals, if a shorter life valve was inserted. In developing countries many will not have good access to health care and anticoagulant therapy could not be supervised adequately.

The operative procedure is carried out with cardiopulmonary bypass and hypothermia either with coronary perfusion of the empty beating heart or cardioplegia. The approach may be right or left thoracotomy or medial sternotomy. An atrial pressure catheter may be left in situ for immediate postoperative monitoring of valve function, and temporary pacing may also be required. Pluth (1981) reports an overall hospital mortality of 4% for aortic valve replacement and 6% for mitral valve replacement. The five year survival rate is good — 80–90%.

The nursing considerations for patients undergoing cardiac valve surgery are those already discussed in the section on care of patients undergoing cardiac surgery.

PROBLEMS OF FLOW WITHIN THE VENOUS SYSTEM

While problems within the venous system may not appear as dramatic or life-threatening as arterial problems, they nevertheless cause an enormous amount of life-long discomfort to those who suffer. Dodd (1971) estimated, for example, that in terms of disability and work days lost in England and Wales, problems of venous stasis were second only to the common cold.

The term 'chronic venous insufficiency' is the term used to describe problems of venous flow (Lofgren, 1983). It is primarily a problem of the leg veins due to the gravitational pressure exerted on these dependent parts. Problems fall into two main groups dependent on the leg veins involved:

- superficial — primarily varicose veins
- deep venous insufficiency — primarily presenting as deep venous thrombosis and leg ulceration.

INCIDENCE AND PROGNOSIS

It is estimated that over 16% of the population have chronic venous insufficiency (Lofgren, 1983), 12% being superficial, 4% deep. In the UK about 500 000 persons have leg ulcers of venous origin and about 250 000 will have a deep venous thrombosis in a year, 90% of which result in longer term post-phlebotic sequelae for the patient (Lofgren, 1983).

Estimates of the incidence of pulmonary embolism — the major life threatening consequence of deep venous thrombosis — vary but the incidence appears to be rising. Embolism is fatal in 18–35% of instances if untreated, this being reduced to 8% if treated (Sharma et al, 1983).

CAUSATION

There appear to be genetic factors influencing the development of superficial venous insufficiency as 50% of persons with problems have family members who also have varicose veins (Lofgren, 1983).

The primary cause of deep venous insufficiency is a direct result of venous thrombosis, 90% of persons with chronic problems having a history of deep venous thrombosis (Lofgren, 1983).

Four other reasons seem to aggravate the condition:

- obstruction to flow, either extrinsic or intrinsic to the veins
- excessive gravitational pressure in the absence of muscle pumping
- lowered venous tone
- trauma.

Thus factors such as abdominal neoplasms, fibroids and pregnancy can create pressure on the iliac veins, as can constricting garments.

Intrinsic obstruction is more likely to be through acute thrombosis but may also be due to primary tumours or ligation.

Occupational standing is the most likely cause of long-term excess gravitational pressure in the absence of muscle pumping. The high level of oestrogens circulating in pregnancy create lowered venous tone. This, together with the pressure of a gravid uterus accounts for the high incidence of varicose veins in women who have borne children, particularly those who are multiparous.

Trauma can set up an inflammatory process involving the veins both superficial and deep, and may result in thrombophlebitis.

DISEASE PROCESS

The valves of both deep and superficial leg veins play a highly significant part in maintaining the blood flow and are able to withstand a pressure of 300 mmHg without yielding (Lofgren, 1983). The more distal the vein, the more muscular it is and the closer together the valves. If the valve leaflets fail to close, venous flow is reduced and venous insufficiency develops. Failure to close may be due to dilatation of the vein, in which case the valve leaflets are unable to come into apposition. Alternatively it may be due to damage or destruction to the valves from previous thrombophlebitis. It is likely that the former is the mechanism in superficial venous insufficiency presenting as varicose veins (Watts, 1986) and that the latter is the mechanism in deep venous insufficiency arising from deep venous thrombosis (Lofgren, 1983)

Presentation and diagnosis

Both superficial and deep venous insufficiency cause the following uncomfortable symptoms in the affected leg:

- aching
- heaviness
- swelling
- nocturnal leg cramps.

In addition the skin may show discolouration.

Superficial venous insufficiency is also characterized by varicose veins — the tortuous congested vein with incompetent valves being apparent under the skin. Ulcers are rare and tend to be small but bleeding into the subcutaneous tissue (ecchymosis) is not uncommon. External haemorrhage can occur and may be fatal if not treated by direct pressure and elevation (Lofgren, 1983).

In deep venous insufficiency the symptoms tend to be more severe, these veins normally carrying over 85% of the total venous return from the legs. The aching and swelling are disabling and the limb appears cyanosed due to the venous stasis. The nutrition of the subcutaneous tissue is compromised by increased interstitial pressure. This sets up the inflammatory process that frequently leads to skin breakdown.

'Varicose ulcers' are therefore indicative of deep venous insufficiency and occur most commonly in the lower third of the leg. At this point the leg musculature is weakest so the muscle pump action has the least effect on venous return. In addition the gravitational venous pressure is highest.

Diagnosis is usually apparent on leg examination but in some instances deep venous thrombosis may be difficult to identify. Blood flow studies by Doppler ultrasound will confirm diagnosis. This has largely replaced the more risky contrast-phlebography, although if the contrast medium is diluted post-phlebography inflammation is markedly reduced (Bettman & Salzman, 1981).

TREATMENT

Treatment is aimed at reducing venous stasis. It consists primarily of:

- graduated pressure stockings (anti-embolic)
- periodic elevation of legs (both of these measures enhance venous return)
- moderate exercise (this promotes blood flow)
- avoidance of standing.

Venous pressure is at its greatest during standing, 22% of the blood volume being contained within the leg veins when standing as opposed to 12% when lying down. The muscle pump of the legs reduces normal hydrostatic venous pressure of 80 mmHg by about a third.

Thus the basic treatment does not rely on drugs or surgery, but falls very much within the province of the nurse. A thorough discussion of the rationale of the treatment and joint planning of a realistic schedule in terms of rest and exercise should potentially increase compliance.

Varicose veins

If superficial varicose veins do not respond to treatment, or cause increasing discomfort or bleeding, the surgical operation of 'stripping' is usual. Although the results appear to be good (Lofgren, 1983), if the pathogenesis of the varicosities is dilatation of the vein, diverting the 10–15% of the venous blood in the legs to the deep veins might be seen to create worse problems in the long term (Watts, 1986). Sclerotherapy — using an inflammatory solution (phenol) to induce closure of the vein — is now seldom used.

Three surgical techniques for occluding varicose veins are used, often in combination:

- ligation, i.e. tying off
- dissection, i.e. cutting out
- stripping, i.e. pulling out by threading a blunt ended instrument through the vein and pulling.

Whilst they are all considered relatively 'minor' operations they result in either numerous small wounds (dissection) or considerable bruising (stripping). Patients are usually treated in a day or short-stay ward.

Pre- and postoperative care

There is no particular pre-operative care except to ensure that the patient remains on his or her normal treatment schedule of support stockings, elevation of legs and exercise.

Postoperatively the leg tends to be and feel very bruised and this is a particular problem at the groin, especially if the support stocking ends over a bruise. Essentially the pre-operative schedule should be regained as soon as possible, initially with more rest but rapidly graduating to one mile walks.

Deep vein thrombosis

Deep vein thrombosis is a major problem as already indicated. Its occurrence is associated with a number of factors:

- increased blood viscosity
  - dehydration
  - polycythaemia
- increased platelet activity
  - trauma
  - surgery
- decreased blood velocity
  - hypotensive states
  - immobility
  - incompetence of vein valves
  - peripheral arterial disease
  - increased hydrostatic pressure
  - direct external pressure

As the incidence is high amongst patients in hospital whose mobility is restricted and/or who have had surgery, prevention is a major concern of both medical and nursing staff. Prevention has four elements which are universally applicable:

- maintenance of mobility, the use of isometric and active exercise whenever possible to maintain blood flow
- elevation of the legs of persons at high risk to facilitate venous return
- avoidance of pressure on the leg veins, e.g. avoid crossing of legs
- maintenance of hydration and blood pressure.

Three other preventive measures are utilised:

- application of anti-embolic stockings
- use of prophylactic anticoagulation (calcium heparin subcutaneously)
- use of antiplatelet drugs (aspirin).

Deep venous thrombosis is suspected if the patient complains of calf pain and leg swelling. If Homan's sign is positive (calf pain experienced on passive dorsiflexion of the foot) and if the patient's temperature shows a low grade pyrexia, diagnosis may be confirmed by Doppler ultrasound or diluted contrast phlebography.

Treatment essentially is that indicated for

prevention, with two alterations:

- complete rest, legs to be elevated at all times
- anticoagulation with a loading dose of sodium heparin intravenously followed with continuous injection via a heparin pump. This is usually maintained for 3–5 days followed by oral warfarin, the amount being controlled by blood clotting rates (BCR).

Rest is maintained until the calf is no longer tender and the leg swelling is decreasing, indicated by leg measurements.

The long-term sequelae of deep vein thrombosis is deep venous insufficiency.

The short-term risk of pulmonary embolism is life threatening.

CARDIAC FAILURE

Failure to maintain an output of blood sufficient to meet the body's requirements is termed heart failure or cardiac failure.

It may vary in severity from a mild degree, as when a person with mitral stenosis becomes breathless on exertion, through acute forms as demonstrated by the sudden onset of severe cyanosis, wheezing and dyspnoea with circulatory collapse associated with acute left ventricular failure, to the disabling chronic congestive form with widespread peripheral oedema. The term congestive heart failure is commonly associated with the latter form. The terms right or left ventricular failure are used when the primary source of failure is restricted to one side of the heart. It is important to realize however, that due to the complex renal, endocrine and sympathetic responses that occur with changes in cardiac output, primary failure of one side inevitably affects performance of the other. An older term 'cor-pulmonale' is occasionally used to indicate the heart failure (initially right sided) that occurs as a result of chronic obstructive lung disease.

INCIDENCE AND PROGNOSIS

The incidence of heart failure is not well documented due to its multivariate causes. However, in the Framingham study overt evidence of congestive cardiac failure developed in about 3% of the cohort within the 16 years of the commencement of the study. In spite of treatment the mortality rate is between 35–62%. Death occurs due to progressive failure or presents as sudden death, the incidence of the latter being estimated variously as 11–90% (Dollery & Carr, 1985). In the Framingham study hypertension preceded the development of heart failure in 75% of cases. This is now likely to have changed due to the vast improvement in the control of hypertension.

CAUSES OF HEART FAILURE

Heart failure essentially develops due to:

- diminished efficiency of the myocardium
- excessive workload due to:
  - an increased pressure load (increased afterload or resistance)
  - an increased volume load (increased pre-load).

Due to the effects of failure, however, these cannot be seen as discrete, mutually exclusive categories.

Diminished efficiency of the myocardium.

The heart muscle itself may be impaired due to myopathy, to inflammation, and to hypoxia and ischaemia or a part of the muscle may be dysfunctional due to infarction (Watson, 1983). Overall this has the effect of diminishing myocardial contractility.

The efficiency of the myocardium may also be reduced by constriction due to pericardial effusion or pericarditis.

Increased pressure load (afterload)

This occurs whenever there is resistance to the outflow of blood from the ventricles. Thus chronic obstructive lung disease and pulmonary hypertension create an increase in afterload for the right ventricle, whereas hypertension, aortic stenosis, coarctation of the aorta and increased blood viscosity cause problems for the left ventricle (MacLeod, 1981).

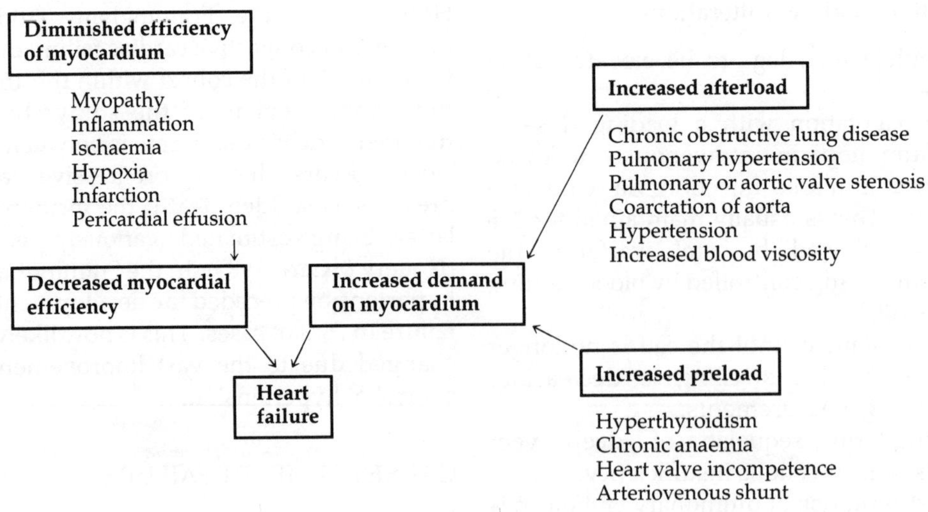

Fig. 22.11 Causes of heart failure

Increased afterload causes hypertrophy of the myocardium which eventually both reduces the cavity of the ventricle and outstrips the ability of the coronary vessels to maintain adequate myocardial perfusion.

Increased volume load (pre-load)

This occurs when the heart must expel more blood than normal due to increased tissue demand. Conditions such as hyperthyroidism, with its resultant increase in metabolic rate, and chronic anaemia, with its reduced oxygen carrying ability of the blood, result in increased volume load. In these situations, cardiac output is high and the term 'high output state' is used (Watson, 1983).

Alternatively, the increased volume load can be due to structural changes in the valves or chambers of the heart or the pulmonary vessels resulting in regurgitation of blood back into the pumping chamber, or in the shunting of blood from the left to right or from arteries to veins — arteriovenous shunts (Watson, 1983). In this case the effort of the myocardium can be seen to be 'wasted', the cardiac output being normal or low. If arterial blood oxygen saturation is low due to arteriovenous shunts, tissue hypoxia also increases demand.

Over time an increased volume load will result in the ventricles dilating. This, however, has the effect of increasing the work of the heart, as the more a ventricle is stretched the more it has to contract to expel a given amount of blood (MacLeod , 1981).

These effects are summarized in Figure 22.11.

As already mentioned the effects are not discrete entities and in reality the mechanisms interrelate. For example, with aortic stenosis there is clearly an increased resistance to output flow causing increased afterload. In addition the low output results in poor coronary perfusion which reduces the efficiency of the myocardium. Chronic obstructive lung disease not only causes an increased afterload for the right ventricle, but poor oxygen saturation of arterial blood increasing the output demand on the left ventricle.

As the heart increasingly fails to meet the body's requirement, compensatory responses occur in order to improve cardiac output and maintain the blood pressure. These responses modify the three key factors on which pump performance depends and which are already implicated in causation of failure, i.e.:

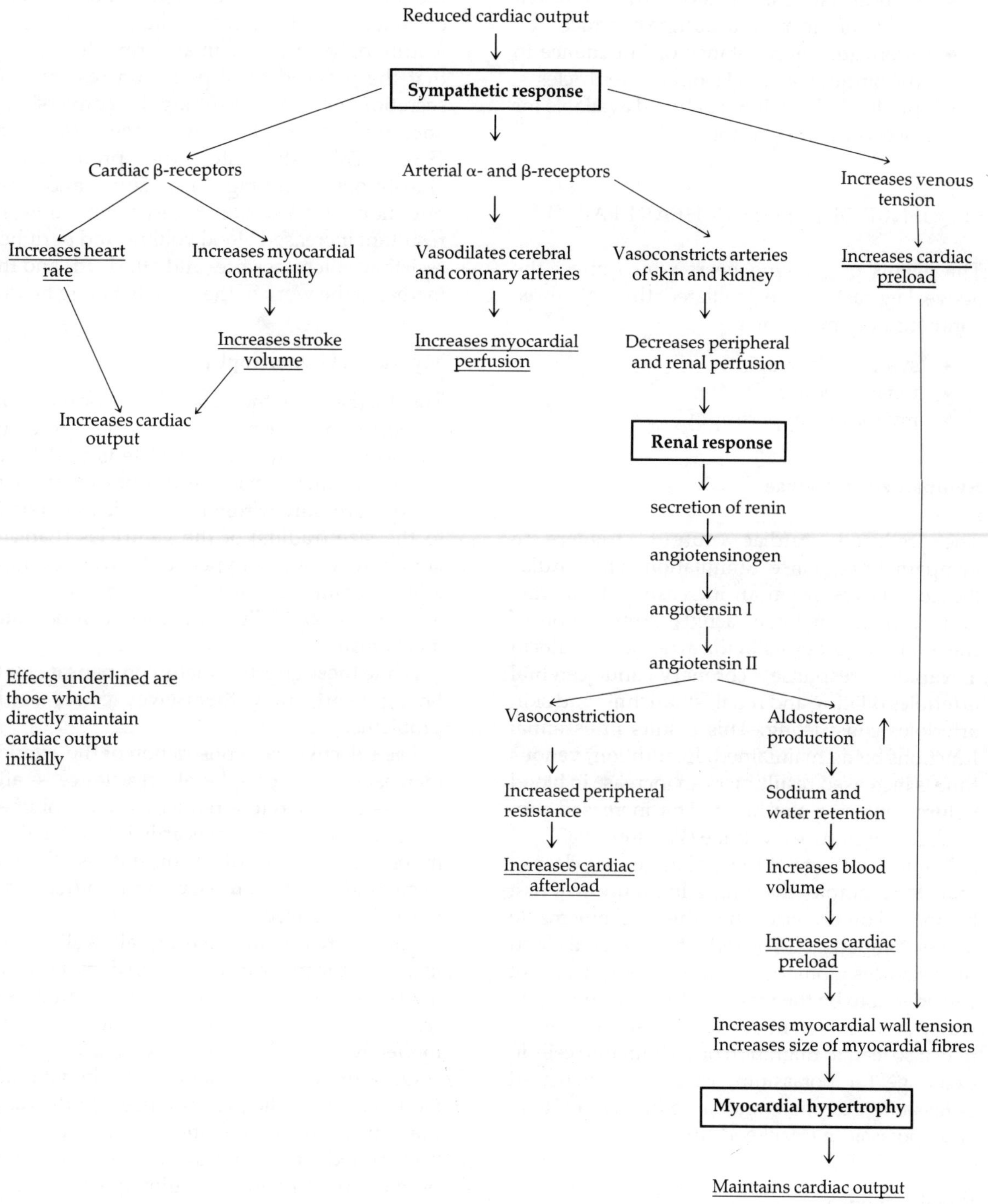

Fig.22.12 Compensatory mechanisms in heart failure

- myocardial contractility: the inherent ability of the myocardium to contract
- afterload: the resistance or impedence to the outflow of blood from the ventricles
- pre-load: the volume of blood available for ejection during systole.

SEQUENCE OF EVENTS IN HEART FAILURE

The events of a failing heart which affect the above key factors are mediated through three compensatory mechanisms:

- sympathetic response
- renal response
- myocardial hypertrophy.

Sympathetic response

The reduced cardiac output triggers a sympathetic response. Stimulation of the cardiac β-receptors results in an increase in heart rate and in myocardial contractility. Stimulation of the α- and β-receptors in the arterioles results in a variable response, coronary and cerebral arterioles dilating and renal, splanchnic and skin arterioles constricting. This results in essential functions being maintained. In addition, venous tone is increased resulting in an increase in blood volume entering the heart. The increased pre-load increases stroke volume (Watson, 1983).

The implications of these changes are clear in that, for example, the effects in failure will first be noticed on exercise when the mechanisms no longer compensate. The reduction in renal blood flow reduces glomerular filtration but this is not considered to be the major factor contributing to water and salt retention. Poor tissue perfusion may also lead to migration of sodium into cells in exchange for potassium, leading to increased potassium excretion and a reduction in total body potassium (MacLeod, 1981).

Renal response

The reduced glomerular filtration has already been mentioned. Another mechanism which is still not fully understood and which emerges 2–3 days after the onset of heart failure results i considerable retention of sodium and water — feature of heart failure in all forms. It is though that the reduced renal perfusion results in th secretion of renin resulting in conversion c angiotensinogen to angiotensin (MacLeod 1981). This stimulates the production c aldosterone resulting in sodium and wate retention, and also causes vasoconstriction. Th resultant increased blood volume and periphera resistance increases pre- and afterload, and thu increases the work of the already failing heart.

Myocardial hypertrophy

The increase in the size of myocardial fibre (hypertrophy) results from the prolonge increase in the myocardial wall tension (Watsor 1983). As this tension is proportional to th systolic pressure within the ventricles in relatio to the size (radius) of the ventricles (Laplace' law), it follows that hypertrophy will develop a a result of an increase in both afterload and pre load. Figure 22.12 illustrates these compensator mechanisms.

While these effects initially compensate for th failing heart, they themselves create furthe problems.

The selective vasoconstriction of the arteriole increases the peripheral resistance — afte load — and therefore reduces stroke volume. there is co-existent myocardial disease this i more marked. Cardiac output is therefor decreased and coronary and other tissu perfusion reduced.

The increase in myocardial wall tensio increases the myocardial oxygen demand which if it is not met, reduces contractility and thus th response to an increased preload become ineffective.

Once the ventricles fail to clear the volume c blood entering, the pressure rises. In the case c the left ventricle, the increase in pressure i transmitted via the mitral valve, left atrium an pulmonary vein to the pulmonary capillaries causing congestion. Once the hydrostat pressure in the capillaries exceeds the osmot pressure of the plasma proteins, fluid exude from the capillaries into the interstitial space

Table 22.20 Causes of left and right ventricular failure

Effect	Left ventricular failure	Right ventricular failure
Diminished myocardial efficiency	All causes as listed below	
Increased afterload	Hypertension Aortic stenosis Coarctation of the aorta Increased blood viscosity	Chronic obstructive lung disease Pulmonary hypertension, e.g. from mitral stenosis
Increased preload	Hyperthyroidism Chronic anaemia Arteriovenous shunt Mitral incompetence	Tricuspid incompetence

causing pulmonary oedema.

If the right ventricle fails, the increase in pressure is transmitted to the systemic veins with resultant congestion of the liver and gastrointestinal tract. Oedema develops in the dependent parts — ankles and sacrum; ascites and pleural effusion may also develop.

The clinical effects of this decompensatory phase are indicated in Figure 23.13.

RIGHT AND LEFT VENTRICULAR FAILURE

These decompensatory effects can be seen to be due to:

- forward failure causing:
  - generalized hypoperfusion
- backward failure causing:
  - pulmonary oedema
  - engorged liver and gastrointestinal system
  - ankle and sacral oedema.
  - ascites and pleural effusion.

(generalized hypoperfusion and pulmonary oedema: left ventricular failure; engorged liver and gastrointestinal system, ankle and sacral oedema, ascites and pleural effusion: right ventricular failure)

While right and left ventricular failure are, to an extent, interdependent, the various causes of heart failure may initially create symptoms characteristic of failure of one side or the other. Thus the terms right and left ventricular failure are used and the causes discussed earlier can be regrouped as indicated in the Table 22.20.

Acute left ventricular failure

Most conditions develop gradually due to the slow build up of demand or the reduced cardiac capacity. However acute left ventricular failure (LVF) may occur if the volume load is suddenly increased or the myocardium is acutely embarassed. Thus acute LVF may occur in the following situations.

- myocardial infarction
- venous overload due to
  - overinfusion
  - reabsorption of oedema from dependent parts
  - action of beta-adrenergic blocking agents.

The symptoms of acute LVF therefore develop suddenly, the patient presenting in a collapsed state with poor peripheral perfusion, rapid often irregular pulse and low or unrecordable blood pressure. If conscious the person will be extremely distressed and will have severe dyspnoea with wheezing and will be coughing up copious frothy sputum. In the person with chronic heart failure this typically occurs at night, when the oedema that has developed in dependent parts in the day is reabsorbed, creating volume overload. The patient wakes fighting for breath, hence the term paroxysmal nocturnal dyspnoea (PND) or cardiac asthma.

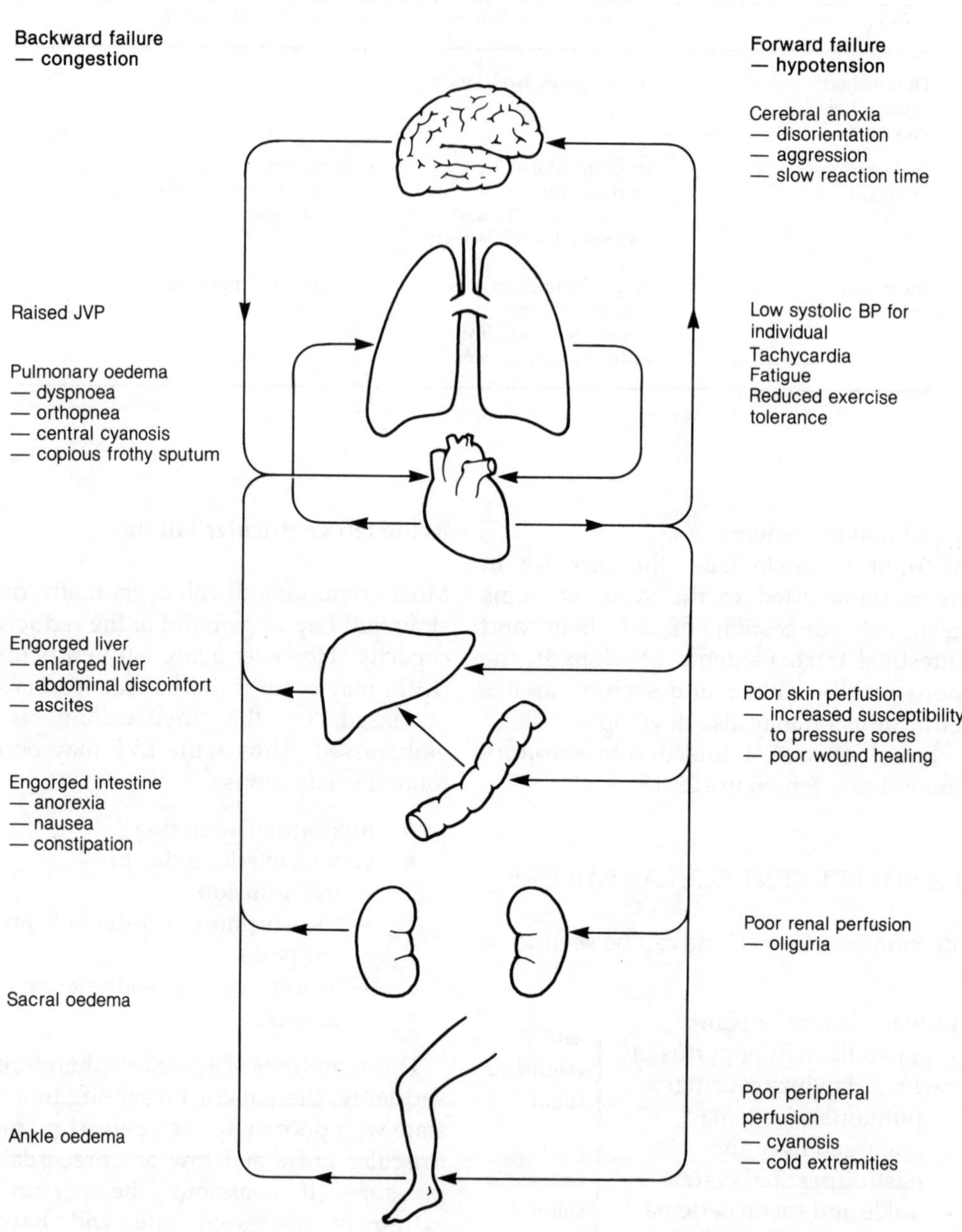

Fig.22.13 Clinical effects of decompensatory phase of ventricular failure.

DIAGNOSIS OF HEART FAILURE

Diagnosis is made primarily on the history and physical examination. Chest X-ray is helpful in confirming the nature of pulmonary congestion.

Treatment

Treatment has four primary aims:

- treatment of the cause if possible
- reduction in cardiac workload
  - rest
  - reduction in weight if required
- reduction in salt and water retention
  - diuretics
  - restricted salt intake
- improved cardiac efficiency
  - digoxin.

Cardiac failure resistant to the above treatment may be treated with vasodilators such as the nitrates and the α-adrenoreceptor blocking agent, prazosin. These are thought to be effective by reducing venous tone and allowing venous pooling. A similar principle is effected by morphine in the treatment of acute LVF, morphine having the additional benefit in this situation of allaying anxiety (MacLeod, 1981).

MANAGEMENT OF THERAPY AND NURSING IMPLICATIONS

Drug therapy (see also Table 22.21)

Diuretics

Due to the toxic effect of digoxin, diuretics are usually given first, thiazides and loop diuretics both increasing sodium (and also potassium) loss from the renal tubule. The weaker potassium-sparing diuretics and the aldosterone-anatagonist, spironolactone, may be used to potentiate the action of thiazides or loop diuretics.

The nurse's responsibility falls into four discrete areas (see also Table 22.22):

- administration of the drugs
- ensuring appropriate toilet facilities are readily at hand
- measuring fluid output in relation to input, monitoring weight lost/gained, observing status of oedema and dyspnoea
- observing the patient for signs of dehydration or hypokalaemia, e.g. muscle weakness or arrhythmias, and for other side-effects of drug treatment.

Digoxin

Digoxin is nevertheless freqently used, although in smaller doses than in previous years. In addition, loading doses — digitalization — are now reserved for those demonstrating severe atrial fibrillation (MacLeod, 1981). Its precise mode of action is unclear but it increases the controlling effect of the vagus, delays conduction over the atrio-ventricular node and strengthens myocardial contraction.

Nausea and vomiting are not uncommon unwanted effects of digoxin administration, normally resolving if the dose is decreased. As conduction delay can result in heart block, digoxin is not normally given if the ventricular rate falls below 60 or the pulse beat is coupled. It is important to note that in atrial fibrillation the pulse rate may not be synchronous with its ventricular rate due to variability in stroke volume. In this situation weak pulse waves may not extend to the radial artery and will therefore not be felt as a pulse. The decision to omit digoxin should therefore be made on the estimate of the ventricular apex rate.

Dietary and weight modification

Dietary modification will almost certainly involve a reduction in salt intake although the unpalatable 'no salt' diet is not now recommended. Not adding salt to cooked food and the avoidance of high salt foods such as Bovril, Marmite, kippers, ham and flavoured or salted potato crisps, usually reduces salt intake sufficiently. Reducing salt in cooking and using unsalted butter or margarine, particularly if the latter is low in saturated fats, may be of further benefit and is in line with current nutritional advice (NACNE, 1985; DHSS, 1984).

Restricted calorie intake is advised if the

Table 22.21 Drugs commonly used in the treatment of heart failure(Sources: MacLeod, 1981; BNF, 1985; Chamberlain, 1985)

Type	Effect	Comment
Cardiac Glycosides Digoxin Digitoxin	Increases vagal activity and sensitizes sinoatrial and atrio-ventricular nodes to this activity thus depressing nodal function and delaying conduction. Stimulates myocardium probably by altering intracellular environment and increasing accumulation and availability of calcium ions. Effects change in peripheral venomotor tone.	Used in atrial fibrillation and heart failure. Causes side effects of nausea, vomiting, arrhythmias and heartblock, muscle weakness, visual disturbances, e.g. Scotoma (blind spots), abnormalities of red/green discrimination, hazy vision Not advised if ventricular rate drops below 60 — pulse or apex beat check before administration.
Diuretics – Thiazides Bendrofluazide Chlorothiazide Clopamide Cyclopenthiazide Hydrochlorothiazide Hydroflumethiazide	Increases urinary output Acts on beginning of the distal tube	Potential dehydration Side-effects: hypokalaemia — particularly dangerous if patient being treated with digoxin Often given with potassium supplements or potassium-sparing diuretics
Loop diuretics Frusemide Bumetanide Ethacrynic acid	Inhibits resorption from the ascending loop of Henle in renal tubule	Powerful. Effective IV or orally — effective up to 6 hours. Side-effects: hypokalaemia — given with potassium supplements or potassium sparing diuretics Useful in patients who have become refractory to other diuretics
Potassium-sparing diuretics Amiloride hydrochloride Triamterene	Causes retention of potassium therefore used as alternative to potassium supplements	Weak diuretics usually used in combination with thiazide or loop diuretic
Spironolactone	Antagonises aldosterone	Weak diuretic but potentiates thiazide or loop diuretic Potassium retained therefore potassium supplements not used
Morphine	Narcotic — allays anxiety reducing catecholamine output and causing systemic veno-dilation thus reducing venous return and cardiac preload	Drug of choice in acute left ventricular failure unless hypotension is severe

individual is overweight. This not only reduces total body weight and therefore cardiac workload, but also enables more exercise to be taken thus improving cardiac function.

As always, dietary modification is one of the most difficult aspects of treatment to achieve. An authoritarian restrictive approach might serve to maintain compliance in hospital but is likely to result in an angry, bitter or depressed individual who will revert to his or her normal eating pattern as soon as he/she gets a chance. Sensible and rational compromise resulting in a mutually agreed and understood regime appears the most useful approach, especially when overall prognosis is kept in mind (MacLeod, 1981). Fluid restriction is not normally necessary but excessive intake should be avoided.

Rest and exercise

If the degree of heart failure does not cause undue problems to the person concerned, regular periods of steady activity is preferable to prolonged rest with its attentive problems.

Table 22.22 Specific problems and suggested nursing approaches for a person with heart failure

Problem/potential problems	Possible nursing approaches
Dyspnoea due to pulmonary oedema, possible chronic lung disease and pleural effusion	Sit well propped up to allow maximal lung expansion and enable fluid to collect in lung bases. Encourage deep breathing. Encourage expectoration and provide sputum pot and tissues. Minimise distress by responding promptly to requests Give medication and oxygen as prescribed (the latter normally at low concentrations and humidified) and observe and give care related to these.
Slow reaction time, disorientation and aggression due to cerebral hypoxia	Approach from the front in an unhurried and friendly manner. Address by name and identify self. Discuss routines or procedure to be performed and describe each step prior to undertaking. Position in ward in a relatively stable atmosphere. Ensure person is safe in immediate bed/chair environment. Provide clear evidence of location in time and place.
Distress and discomfort due to dyspnoea, oedema, and diuresis	Position in whatever way is most comfortable, including using a chair all the time if necessary. Ensure toilet facilities at hand or promptly offered.
Loss of appetite due to congestion of gastrointestinal tract, ascites, digoxin and reduced salt and possibly reduced calorie intake	Offer favourite allowable foods in small quantities and frequently. Nutritious drinks may replace solids if sodium and calorie intake are not exceeded.
Constipation due to immobility and gastrointestinal stasis	Avoid by giving stool softeners prophylactically and encourage high fibre intake
Potential Damage to skin — pressure sores due to immobility, loss of skin elasticity if aged, oedematous areas and poorly perfused periphery	Avoid by gentle handling and 2 hourly position change. Skin on legs may be protected by stockings or light weight stockinette.
Potential Venous stasis causing deep venous thrombosis	Encourage exercise as soon as patient is able. Active leg exercises 2 hourly while resting

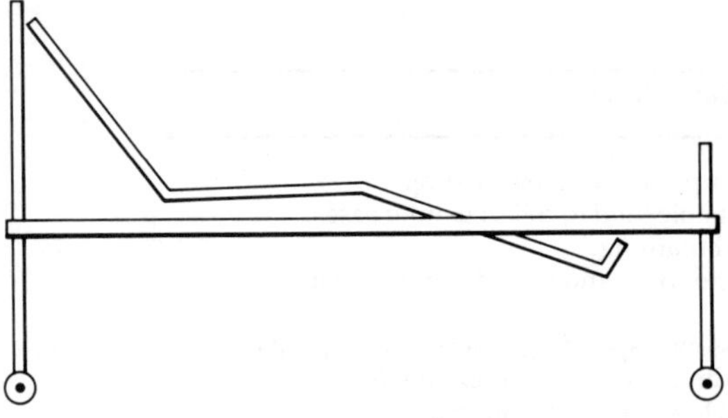

Fig. 22.14 Cardiac bed.

However complete rest may be appropriate for the severely dyspnoeic patient. Sitting well propped up with legs in a relatively dependent position may be found to be the most comfortable. Raising the legs may result in reabsorption of oedema and precipitate acute left ventricular failure. 'Cardiac' beds (see Fig. 22.14) or a chair may be more suitable for use than a standard bed.

REFERENCES

Alderson M R, Lee P N, Wang R 1985 Risk of lung cancer, chronic bronchitis, ischaemic heart disease and stroke in relation to type of cigarette smoked. Journal of Epidemiology and Community Health 39:286–293

Ashworth P M 1984 Staff-patient communication in coronary care units. Journal of Advanced Nursing 9(1):35–42

Asmussen I 1980 Effects of maternal smoking on the fetal cardiovascular system in childhood. In: Lauer R M, Skekalle R B (eds) childhood prevention of atherosclerosis. Raven Press, New York

Bannan L T, Beevers D G, Wright N 1981a a blood pressure reduction: the size of the problem. In: Lock S (ed) A B C of hypertension. British Medical Journal Publication, London

Bannan L T, Beevers D G, Jackson S M D 1981b Detecting hypertensive patients. In: Lock S (ed) A B C of hypertension. British Medical Journal Publication, London

Bannan L T, Beevers D G, Wright N 1981c Blood pressure reduction: drug treatment. In: Lock S (ed) A B C of hypertension. British Medical Journal Publication, London

Bannan L T, Beevers D G, Jackson S M D, Wright N 1981d Blood pressure reduction: difficulties and developments in treating hypertension. In: Lock S (ed) A B C of hypertension. British Medical Journal Publication, London

Becker A E 1981 The pathology of ischaemic myocardial necrosis. In: Hamer J, Rowlands D J (eds) Recent advances in cardiology. Churchill Livingstone, Edinburgh

Beland I L, Passos J Y 1975 Clinical Nursing: pathophysiological and psychosocial approaches. 3rd edn. Macmillan, New York

Benson H, Kotch J B, Crassweller K D 1978 Stress and hypertension : interrelations and management. In: Onest G, Brest A N (eds) Hypertension; mechanisms, diagnosis and treatment. F A Davis, Philadelphia

Bettman M A, Salzman E W 1981 Recent advances in the diagnosis of deep vein thrombosis and pulmonary embolus. In: Poller L (ed) Recent advances in blood coagulation. Churchill Livingstone, Edinburgh

Bouman C C 1984 Intracoronary thrombolysis and percutaneous transluminal coronary angioplasty: nursing implications. Nursing Clinics of North America 19(3):397–409

Brest A N, Goldberg S 1983 Coronary thrombosis: historic aspects. In: Goldberg S (ed) Coronary artery spasm and thrombosis. FA Davis Co., Philadelphia

British National Formulary 1986 British Medical Association and the Pharmaceutical Society of Great Britain, London

Bruschke A V G, Wijers T S, Kolsters W, Landmann J 1981 The anatomic evolution of coronary artery disease demonstrated by coronary arteriography in 256 nonoperated patients. Circulation 63(3)527–536

Burchell H D 1981 Future trends in academic cardiology. In: Yu P N, Goodwin J F (eds) Progress in cardiology. Lea & Febiger, Philadelphia

Burt B W, Greene R J, Harris N D 1982a Cardiovascular system, part 3, hypertension. Chemist and Druggist 137–151

Burt B W, Greene R J, Harris N D 1982b Cardiovascular system, part 4; ischaemic heart disease. Chemist and Druggist 866–877. Cited by Wells N 1982 Coronary heart disease: the scope for prevention. Office of Health Economics, London

Callan E, Irving M 1986 Mobile coronary care units: the Dundee experience. Intensive Care Nursing 1:119–122

Campbell W B, Skidmore R, Woodcock J P, Baird R N 1985 Detection of early arterial disease: a study using Doppler wave form analysis. Cardiovascular Research 19(9):206–211

Chamberlain D A 1985 Digitalis: where are we now? British Heart Journal 54:227–233

Choi S C, Boxerman S B, Steinburg L 1978 Nurses' preference of terminal digits in data reading. Journal of Nursing Education 17(9):38–41. Cited by Thompson D R 1981 Recording patients' blood pressure: a review. Journal of Advanced Nursing 6:283–290

Coburn A F, Moore L V 1939 The prophylactic use of sulfanilamide in streptococcal respiratory infections with especial reference to rheumatic fever. Journal of Clinical Investigation 18:147–155. Cited by Markowitz M 1983 Prevention of acute rheumatic fever and rheumatic heart disease. In: Julian D G, Humphries J O'N (eds) Preventive Cardiology. Butterworths, London

Colling A, Dellipiani A W, Donaldson R J, MacCormack P 1976 Teeside coronary survey: an epidemiological study of acute attacks of myocardial infarction. British Medical Journal 2:1169–1172 Cited by Wells N 1982 Coronary heart disease: scope for prevention. Office of Health Economics, London

Conceicao S, Ward M K, Kerr D N S 1976 Defects in

sphygmomanometers: an important source of error in blood pressure recording. British Medical Journal 2:886–888
Cowley A W 1978 Perspectives on the physiology of hypertension. In: Onesti G, Brest A N (eds) Hypertension: mechanisms, diagnosis and treatment. F A Davis, Philadelphia
Cruikshank J K, Beevers D G 1980 Is blood pressure really 'worse' in black people? Lancet I, 371
Davies M J 1985 The pathology of the mitral valve. In: Ionescu M I, Cohn L H (eds) Mitral valve disease 1: diagnosis and treatment. Butterworths, London
Davis K, Kennedy J W, Kemp H G Jn, Judkins M P, Gosselin A J, Killip T 1979 Complications of coronary arteriography from the collaborative study of Coronary Artery Surgery (CASS) Circulation 59(6):1105–1112
Dellborg M, Held P, Swedberg K, Vedin A 1985 Rupture of the myocardium; occurrence and risk factors. British Heart Journal 54(1):11–16
Denny E W Jr, Wannamaker L W, Brink W R, Rammelkamp C H Jr, Custer E A 1950 Prevention of rheumatic fever: treatment of the preceding streptococcal infection. Journal of the American Medical Association 143:151–153. Cited by Markowitz M 1983 Prevention of acute rheumatic fever and rheumatic heart disease. In: Julian D G, Humphries J O'N (eds) Preventive cardiology. Butterworths, London
DHSS 1981 Prevention and health: avoiding heart attacks. HMSO, London
DHSS 1984 Report on health and social subjects 28: diet and cardiovascular disease. HMSO, London
DiSciascio G, Taranta A 1980 Rheumatic fever in children American Heart Journal 99:635–658. Cited by Markowitz M 1983 Prevention of acute rheumatic fever and rheumatic heart disease. In: Julian D G, Humphries J O'N (eds) Preventive cardiology. Butterworths, London
Dodd H 1971 Varicose veins and venous disorders of the lower limb Part 1: anatomy, physiology and physiopathology. British Journal of Clinical Practice 25:19–22
Dollery C T, Carr L 1985 Drug treatment of heart failure. British Heart Journal 54:234–242
Dustan H P 1981 Understanding hypertension — a look into the future. In: Yu P N, Goodwin J F (eds) Progress in cardiology. Lea & Febiger, Philadelphia
EWPHE (European Working Party on High Blood Pressure in the Elderly) 1985 Influence of hypotensive drug treatment in elderly hypertensives. Journal of Hypertension 3(suppl 3):5501–5508
Fagius J, Blumberg H 1985 Sympathetic outflow to the hand in patients with Raynaud's phenomenon. Cardiovascular Research 9(9):249–253
Foon K A, Gale R P 1984 Acute myelogenous leukaemia — current status of therapy in adults. In: Thiel E, Thierfeider S (eds) Leukaemia: recent developments in diagnosis and therapy. Springer-Verlag, Berlin
Friedman M, Rosenman R H 1974 Type A behaviour and your heart. Wildwood House, London
Fuster V, Badimon L, Chesebro J H 1985 Coronary artery bypass grafting — a model for the understanding of the progression of atherosclerotic disease and the role of platelet inhibitor drugs. In: Kakker V V (ed) Atheroma and thrombosis. Pitman, London
Gaglione K M 1984 Assessing and intervening with families of CCU patients. Nursing Clinics of North America 19(3):427–432
Goh T K 1977 Patient's anxiety in the coronary care unit. The Nursing Journal of Singapore 17:58–64. Cited by Mayberry J, Kent S V 1983 Recent progress in cardiac nursing and rehabilitation programmes. Journal of Advanced Nursing 8:329–333
Gordis L 1973 Effectiveness of comprehensive care program in preventing rheumatic fever. New England Journal of Medicine 289:331–335. Cited by Markowitz M 1983 Prevention of acute rheumatic fever and rheumatic heart disease. In: Julian D G, Humphries J O'N (eds) Preventive cardiology. Butterworths, London
Gorlin R 1985 Natural history, medical therapy and indications for surgery in mitral valve disease. In: Ionescu M I, Cohn L H (eds) Mitral valve disease 1: diagnosis and treatment. Butterworths, London
Greenhalgh R M 1984 Management of risk factors in patients undergoing arterial surgery. In: Bergan J J (ed) Arterial surgery. Churchill Livingstone, Edinburgh
Grundy S M 1981 Can dietary change prevent coronary heart disease? In: Yu P N, Goodwin W I (eds) Progress in cardiology. Lea & Febiger, Philadelphia
Guyton A C 1984 The physiology of the human body, 6th edn. Saunders, Philadelphia
Hamer J 1981 Modern treatment of hypertension. In: Hamer J, Rowlands D J (eds) Recent advances in cardiology. Churchill Livingstone, Edinburgh
Hartunian N S, Smart C N, Thompson M S 1981 The incidence and economic costs of major health impairments. Lexington Books, D C Heath & Co, Massachusetts. Cited by Wells N 1982 Coronary heart disease: the scope for prevention. Office of Health Economics, London
Hellriegel K P 1984 Management of chronic myelogenous leukaemia and blastic crisis. In: Thiel E, Thierfelder S (eds) Leukaemia: recent developments in diagnosis and therapy. Springer-Verlag, Berlin
Hentinen M 1986 Teaching and adaptation of patients with myocardial infarction. International Journal of Nursing Studies 23(2):125–138
Hoelzer D 1984 Current status of ALL/AUL therapy in adults. In: Thiel E, Thierfelder S (eds) Leukaemia: recent developments in diagnosis and therapy. Springer-Verlag, Berlin
Holland W N, Humerfelt S 1964 Measurement of blood pressure: comparison of intra-arterial and cuff values. British Medical Journal 2:1241–1243
IPPPSH (International Prospective Primary Prevention Study in Hypertension) Collaborative Group 1985 Myocardial infarction and cerebrovascular accident in relation to blood pressure control. Journal of Hypertension 3(suppl 3):S513– S516
Isles C, Brown J J, Cumming A M M, Lever A F, McAreavey D, Robertson J I S 1979 Excess smoking in malignant phase hypertension. British Medical Journal 1:579–581. Cited by Robertson J 1983 Hypertension: primary and secondary prevention. In: Julian D G, Humphries J O'N (eds) Preventive cardiology. Butterworths, London
Jacobs A 1982 Disorders of iron metabolism. In: Hoffbrand A V (ed) Recent advances in haematology. Churchill Livingstone, Edinburgh
Jansen K J, McFaddon P M 1986 Postoperative nursing management in patients undergoing myocardial revascularization with the internal mammary artery bypass. Heart and Lung 15(1):48–54

Johnson K W 1984 A surgeon's view of peripheral arterial transluminal dilation. In: Bergen J J (ed) Arterial surgery. Churchill Livingstone, Edinburgh

Joyce J W 1983 Aneurysmal disease. In: Spittell J A Jn (ed) Clinical vascular disease. F A Davis, Philadelphia

Julian D G, Campbell R W F 1981 Sudden coronary death. In: Hamer J, Rowlands D J (eds) Recent advances in cardiology. Churchill Livingstone, Edinburgh

Julian D G, Humphries J O'N 1983 Preventive cardiology. Butterworths, London

Julius S 1978 Borderline hypertension: significance and management. In: Onesti G, Brest A N (eds) Hypertension: mechanisms, diagnosis and treatment. F A Davis, Philadelphia

Kannel W B 1981 Update on the role of cigarette smoking in coronary artery disease. American Heart Journal 101(3):319–328

Kannel W B, Gordon T 1970 The Framingham study. U S Government Printing Office, Washington D C

Kannel W B, Feinleib M 1972 Natural history of angina pectoris in the Framingham study. Prognosis and survival. American Journal of Cardiology 29:154- -163. Cited by Wells N 1982 Coronary heart disease: scope for prevention. Office of Health Economics, London

Kannel W B, Doyle J T, McNamara P M, Quickenton P, Gordon T 1975 Precursors of sudden coronary death. Circulation 51:606–613. Cited by Julian D G, Campbell R W F, 1981 Sudden coronary death. In: Hamer J, Rowlands D J (eds) Recent advances in cardiology. Churchill Livingstone, Edinburgh

Kannel W B, Sorlie P 1977 Utility of conventional risk factors in evaluation of patients with coronary disease. In: Syllabus: the first decade of bypass graft surgery for coronary artery disease. Cited by Wells N 1982 Coronary heart disease: the scope for prevention. Office of Health Economics, London

Karmody A M, Leather R P 1984 The saphenous vein used 'in situ' for infra-inguinal arterial bypass. In: Bergan J J (ed) Arterial surgery. Churchill Livingstone, Edinburgh

Kramer J R, Matsuda Y, Mulligan J , Aronow M, Proudfit W L 1981 Progression of coronary atherosclerosis. Circulation 63(3):519–526

Lancet 1982 Editorial: prevention of rheumatic heart disease. Lancet 1:143– 144

Lau Y K, Smith J, Morrison S L, Chamberlain D A 1980 Policy for early discharge after acute myocardial infarction. British Medical Journal 280:1489– 1492

Lazarus R S 1966 Psychological stress and the coping process. McGraw-Hill, New York

Lewis B 1981 Ischaemic heart disease: the scientific bases of prevention. In: Yu P N, Goodwin J F (eds) Progress in cardiology. Lea & Febiger, Philadelphia

Lewis G P 1985 Chairman's introduction, Part II. In: Kakkar V V Atheroma and thrombosis. Pitman, London

Lipton M J, Brundage B H, Higgins C B, Boyd D P 1983 CT scanning of the heart. In: Fowler N O (ed) Noninvasive diagnostic methods in cardiology. F A Davis, Philadelphia

Loan T 1986 Nursing interaction with patients undergoing coronary angioplasty. Heart & Lung 15:(4):368–375

Lofgren E P 1983 Chronic venous insufficiency. In: Spittell J A Jn (ed) Clinical vascular disease. F A Davis, Philadelphia

Long B C, Phipps W J (eds) 1985 Essentials of medical-surgical nursing: a nursing process approach. C V Mosby, St Louis

Luckmann J, Sorensen K C 1980 Medical-surgical nursing — a psychophysiologic approach, 2nd edn. Saunders, Philadelphia

McCance K L 1983 Genetics: implications for preventative nursing practice. Journal of Advanced Nursing 8:359–364

McDonald L 1979 Very early recognition of coronary heart disease. In: Yu P N, Goodwin J F (eds) Progress in cardiology. Lea & Febiger, Philadelphia

MacLeod J 1981, 1984 Davidson's principles and practice of medicine, 13, 14th edn. Churchill Livingstone, Edinburgh

Madsen J K 1980 Ischaemic heart disease and prodromes of sudden cardiac death: is it possible to identify high risk groups for sudden cardiac death? British Heart Journal 54(1):27–32

Margetts B M, Beilin L J, Armstrong B K, Vandongen R 1985 Vegetarian diet in the treatment of mild hypertension. Journal of Hypertension 3(suppl 3):5429– 5431

Markowitz M 1983 Prevention of acute rheumatic fever and rheumatic heart disease. In: Julian P G, Humphries J O'N (eds) Preventive cardiology. Butterworths, London

Maseri A, Klassen G A, Lesch M (eds) 1978 Primary and secondary angina pectoris. Grune & Stratton, New York

Masterton G, Main C J, Lever A F, Lever R S 1981 Low blood pressure in psychiatric inpatients. British Heart Journal 45:442–446. Cited by Robertson J 1983 Hypertension: primary and secondary prevention. In: Julian D G, Humphries J O'N (eds) Preventive cardiology. Butterworths, London

Mather H G, Pearson N G, Read K L Q, Shaw D B, Steed G R, Thorne M G et al 1971 Acute myocardial infarction: home and hospital treatment. British Medical Journal 3:334–338

Mather H G, Morgan D C, Pearson N G, Read K L Q, Shaw D W, Steed G R, Thorne M G et al 1976 Myocardial infarction: a comparison between home and hospital care for patients. British Medical Journal 1:925–929

Mathewson Z M, McCloskey B G, Evans A E, Russell C J, Wilson C 1985 Mobile coronary care and community mortality from myocardial infarction. Lancet 1:441– 444

Mayberry J, Kent S V 1983 Recent progress in cardiac nursing and rehabilitation programmes. Journal of Advanced Nursing 8:329–333

Meijler F L 1981 Prevention of coronary heart disease: a cardiologist's view. In: Yu P N, Goodwin J, F (eds) Progress in cardiology 10. Lea & Febiger, Philadelphia

Menolti A, Saccareccia F 1985 Physical activity of work and job responsibility as risk factors in fatal coronary heart disease and other causes of death. Journal of Epidemiology and Community Health 39:325–329

Miller P, Wikoff R L, McMahon M, Garrett M J, Ringel K 1984 Indicators of medical regimen adherence for myocardial infarction patients. Nursing Research 34:268-272

Ministry of Agriculture, Fisheries and Food 1985 Manual of Nutrition. HMSO London

Moloney W C, Rosenthal D S 1980 Acute leukaemia in adults secondary to other disorders. In: Roath S Topical reviews in haematology. John Wright & Sons, Bristol

Morris J N 1985 Exercise: the implications for health. In: Kakkar V V Atheroma and thrombosis. Pitman, London

NACNE (National Advisory Committee on Nutrition Education) 1983 Proposals for nutrition guidelines for health education in Britain. Health Education Council, London

Nora J J 1983 Primary prevention of atherosclerosis. In: Julian D G, Humphries J O'N (ed) Preventive cardiology. Butterworths, London

Nora J J, Nora A H 1983 Genetic aspects of preventive cardiology. In: Julian D G, Humphries J O'N (eds) Preventive cardiology. Butterworths, London
North L W 1979 Accuracy of sphygmomanometers. Association of Operating Room Nurses Journal 30:996–1000
O'Brien E T, O'Malley K 1981 Blood pressure measurement (a) Technique; (b) The Observer; (c) The patient; (d) The sphygmomanometer; (e) Future Trends. In: Lock S (ed) A B C of hypertension. British Medical Journal, London
Oldham P D, Pickering G W, Roberts J A F, Sowry G S C 1960 The nature of essential hypertension. Lancet ii:1085–1093. Cited by Thompson D R 1981 Recording patients' blood pressure: a review. Journal of Advanced Nursing 6:283–290
O'Neil H 1986 Percutaneous transluminal coronary angioplasty — the alternative treatment. Intensive Care Nursing 1:23–29
Oostenbroek R J, Willems G M, Boumans M L L, Soeters P B, Hermens W T 1985 Liver damage as a potential source of error in the estimation of myocardial infarct size from plasma creatine kinase activity. Cardiovascular Research 19(9):113–119
Perloff J K 1985 Overview of long term results of medical and surgical treatment of mitral valve disease. In: Ionescu M I, Cohn L H (eds) Mitral valve disease 1: diagnosis and treatment. Butterworths, London
Petch M C 1985 Lessons from ambulatory electrocardiology. British Medical Journal 291:617–618
Pluth J R 1981 Prosthetic valve replacement. In: Hamer J, Rowlands D J (eds) Recent advances in cardiology. Churchill Livingstone, Edinburgh
Pocock S J, Shaper A G, Cook D G, Packham R F, Lacey R F, Powell P, Russel P F 1980 British regional heart study: geographic variations in cardiovascular mortality, and the role of water quality. British Medical Journal 280:1243–1249
Pooling Project Research Group 1978. Relationship of blood pressure, serum cholesterol, smoking habits, relative weight and ECG abnormalities to incidence of major coronary events; final report of Pooling Project. Journal of Chronic Diseases 31:203–306. Cited by Wells N 1982 Coronary heart disease: the scope for prevention. Office of Health Economics, London
Powles R L, Palú G, Raghavan D 1980 Curability of acute leukaemia. In: Roath S (ed) Topical reviews in haematology. John Wright & Sons, Bristol
Prior I 1979 Primary prevention of hypertension. In: Gross F J, Robertson J I S (eds) Arterial hypertension. Pitman Medical, Tunbridge Wells
Quinn R W, Federspiel C 1974 The incidence of rheumatic fever in Metropolitan Nashville. American Journal of Epidemiology 99:273–280. Cited by Markowitz M 1983 Prevention of acute rheumatic fever and rheumatic heart disease. In: Julian D G, Humphries J O'N (eds) Preventive cardiology. Butterworths, London
Quyyumi A A, Wright C M, Mockus L J, Fox K M 1985 How important is a history of chest pain in determining the degree of ischaemia in patients with angina pectoris? British Heart Journal 54(1):22–26
Reisin E 1983 Obesity and hypertension. In: Robertson J I S Handbook of hypertension Vol 1: clinical hypertension. Excerpta Medica, Amsterdam. Cited by Robertson J I S 1983 Hypertension: primary and secondary prevention. In: Julian D G, Humphries J O'N (eds) Preventive cardiology. Butterworths, London
Reitz B A, Stinson E B 1981 Cardiac transplantation. In: Hamer J, Rowlands D J (eds) Recent advances in cardiology. Churchill Livingstone, Edinburgh
Rice V H, Caldwell M, Butler S, Robinson J 1986 Relaxation training and response to cardiac catheterisation: a pilot study. Nursing Research 35(1):39–43
Richardson J E, Robinson D 1971 Variations in the measurement of blood pressure between doctors and nurses: an observational study. Journal of the Royal College of General Practitioners 21:698–704
Robertson J I S 1983 Hypertension: primary and secondary prevention. In: Julian D G, Humphries J O'N (eds) Preventive cardiology. Butterworths, London
Ronayne R A 1985 Feelings and attitudes during early convalescence following vascular surgery. Journal of Advanced Nursing 10(4):435–441
Rose G 1981 Impact of primary prevention programmes on ischaemic heart disease. In: Hamer J, Rowlands D J (eds) Recent advances in cardiology. Churchill Livingstone, Edinburgh
Rowlands D J, Sheilds R A, Testa H J 1981 Radionuclides in cardiology. In: Hamer J, Rowlands D J (eds) Recent advances in cardiology. Churchill Livingstone, Edinburgh
Royal College of General Practitioners 1979 Morbidity statistics from general practice 1971–72 second national study. Studies on Medical and Population Subjects No 36, HMSO
Rutter S, Ellis R 1986 Laser-assisted angioplasty. Nursing Times/Mirror 82(33):40–41
Shaper A G 1985 Diet, atherosclerosis and coronary heart disease. In: Kakkar V V (ed) Atheroma and thrombosis. Pitman, London
Shaper A G, Pocock S J, Walker M, Phillips A N, Whitehead T P, Macfarlane P W 1985 Risk factors for ischaemic heart disease: the prospective phase of the British Regional Heart Study. Journal of Epidemiology and Community Health 39:197–209
Sharma G V R K, Barsamian E M, Parisi A F, Cella G, Sasahara A A 1983 Pulmonary embolism. In: Spittell J A Jn (ed) Clinical vascular disease. F A Davis, Philadelphia
Shiokawa Y, Yamada T 1977 Epidemiology of rheumatic fever and rheumatic heart disease with surveillance of hemolytic streptococcus. Japanese Circulation Journal 41:167–173. Cited by Markowitz M 1983 Prevention of acute rheumatic fever and rheumatic heart disease. In: Julian P G, Humphries J O'N (ed) Preventive cardiology. Butterworths, London
Silman A, Loysen E, DeGraaf W, Sramek M 1985 High dietary fat intake and cigarette smoking as risk factors for ischaemic heart disease in Bangladeshi male immigrants in East London. Journal of Epidemiology and Community Health 39:301–303
Silverberg D S, Baltuch L, Hermoni Y, Eyal P 1985 A national programme of hypertension control using a doctor-nurse team approach: the Israeli experience. Journal of Hypertension 3(suppl 3):5453–5455
Sloman J G, Hunt D, Sutton L D 1981 Management of myocardial infarction. In: Hamer J, Rowlands D J (eds) Recent advances in cardiology. Churchill Livingstone, Edinburgh
Smith E B 1985 Lipoproteins and atheroma. In: Kakkar V V (ed) Atheroma and thrombosis. Pitman, London

Sorlie P 1977 Cardiovascular disease and death following myocardial infarction and angina pectoris. Cited by Wells N 1982 Coronary heart disease: the scope for prevention. Office of Health Economics, London

Spittell J A Jr 1983 Vasospastic disorders. In: Spittell J A Jr (ed) Clinical vascular disease. F A Davis, Philadelphia

Steptoe A 1981 Psychological factors in cardiovascular disorder. Academic Press, London

Strasser T, Dondog N, El Kholy A, Garagozloo R, Kalbian V V, Ogundi U, Padmavati S, Stuart K, David E, Bekessy A 1981 The community control of rheumatic fever and rheumatic heart disease. Report of a WHO international co-operative project. Bulletin of the World Health Organisation 59:285–294

Sugrue D D, Thompson G R, Oakley G M, Trayner I M, Steiner R E 1981 Contrasting patterns of coronary atherosclerosis in normocholesterolaemic smokers and patients with familial hypercholesterolaemia. British Medical Journal 2:1358–1360

Taguchi J, Freis E D 1974 Partial reduction of blood pressure and prevention of complications in hypertension. New England Journal of Medicine 291:329–331

Tanner G A, Noury D 1981 The effect of instruction on control of blood pressure in individuals with essential hypertension. Journal of Advanced Nursing 6:99–106

Tarazi R G, Gifford R W 1978 Clinical significance and management of systolic hypertension. In: Onesti G, Brest A N (eds) Hypertension: mechanisms, diagnosis and treatment. F A Davis, Philadelphia

Taylor D 1980 Leukaemia: towards control. Office of Health Economics, London

Theml H, Ziegler-Heitbrock H W L 1984 Management of CLL and allied disorders with reference to their immunology and proliferation kinetics. In: Thiel E, Thierfelder S (eds) Leukaemia: recent developments in diagnosis and therapy. Springer-Verlag, Berlin

Thomas C B, France R 1939 A preliminary report on the prophylactic use of sulfonamide in patients susceptible to rheumatic fever. Bulletin of the John Hopkins Hospital 64:67–77. Cited by Markowitz M 1983 Prevention of acute rheumatic fever and rheumatic heart disease. In: Julian D G, Humphries J O'N (eds) Preventive cardiology. Butterworths, London

Thomas S A, Sappington E, Gross H S et al 1983 Denial in coronary care patients — an objective assessment. Heart and Lung 12:74–80

Thompson D R 1981 Recording patients' blood pressure: a review. Journal of Advanced Nursing 6:283–290

Thompson D, Bailey S, Webster R 1986 Patients' views on cardiac monitoring. Nursing Times 82(9):54–55

Vidt D G 1978 The struggle for drug compliance in hypertension. In: Onesti G, Brest A N (eds) Hypertension: mechanisms, diagnosis and treatment. F A Davis, Philadelphia

Wallace L M, Joshi M, Wingett C, Wilson C, Spellman D 1985 Nurses' perceptions of patients' needs for information and their concerns in an English coronary care unit. Intensive Care Nursing 1:84–91

Watkins L O, Weaver L, Odegaard V 1986 Preparation for cardiac catheterisation: tailoring the content of instruction to coping styles. Heart and Lung 15(4):382–389

Watson H (ed) 1983 Cardiology. MTP Press, Boston

Watts G T 1986 Fallacies: varicose veins are caused by defective valves in the veins. The Lancet 1:31–32

Weiland A P, Walker W 1986 Physiologic principles and clinical sequelae of cardiopulmonary bypass. Heart and Lung 15(1):34–39

Weintraub W S, Helfant R H 1983 Coronary artery spasm: historic aspects. In: Goldberg S (ed) Coronary artery spasm and thrombosis. F A Davis, Philadelphia

Wells N 1982 Coronary heart disease: the scope for prevention. Office of Health Economics, London

Westheim A, Simonsen K, Schamaun O, Müller O, Stokke O, Teisberg P 1985 Effect of exercise training in patients with essential hypertension. Journal of Hypertension 3(suppl 3):5479–5481

Wickramasinghe S N, Weatherall D J 1982 The pathophysiology of erythropoiesis. In: Hardisty R M, Weatherall D J (eds) Blood and its disorders, 2nd edn. Blackwell Scientific, Oxford

Wilber J A, McCombs N G 1975 Hypertension 1975: The allied health professionals role. Drug Therapy May/June, p 56

Wilson M G, Schweitzer M D 1937 Rheumatic fever as a familial disease — environment, communicability and heredity in their relation to observed familial incidence of disease. Journal of Clinical Investigation 16:555–570. Cited by Nora J J, Nora A H 1983 Genetic aspects of preventive cardiology. In: Julian D G, Humphries J O'N Preventive cardiology. Butterworths, London

Wilson-Barnett J 1981 Assessment of recovery: with special reference to a study of post-operative cardiac patients. Journal of Advanced Nursing 6:435– 445

Winslow E H, Lane L D, Gaffney F A 1985 Oxygen uptake and cardiovascular responses in control adults and acute myocardial infarction patients during bathing. Nursing Research 34(3):164–169

Woodliff H J, Herrmann R P 1979 Concise haematology, 2nd edn. Edward Arnold, London

WHO 1978 Arterial hypertension: Report of a WHO Expert Committee. Technical Report Series No. 628. World Health Organization, Geneva

WHO 1983 Primary prevention of essential hypertension: report of a WHO scientific group. Technical Report Series No. 686. World Health Organization, Geneva

WHO 1980, Community control of rheumatic fever in developing countries 1: a major public health problem. World Health Organization Chronicle 34:336–345

23

Disturbances of nutrient supply

INTRODUCTION

Deficiency of nutrient supply to the cells of the body can arise from disturbances at a number of points in the process of obtaining, ingesting, digesting, absorbing and metabolizing nutrients. It can also arise from disorders of transport around the body or utilization in the cells. Disturbances of transportation are dealt with elsewhere (Ch. 22). A major disorder of nutrient utilization is diabetes mellitus discussed in Chapter 19. Other conditions of genetic origin are primarily important during childhood, when conditions such as phenylketonurea are diagnosed and the appropriate diet prescribed. Although these children may live into adult life the diet is managed by the individual and is not particularly relevant to the subject of this book.

The material in this chapter falls into two major sections.The first part concentrates specifically on nutritional disorders and examines causation and principles of management of such disorders. The second section deals with disorders of the structures involved in the digestion and absorption of nutrients, although the effect on nutritional status of the individual may be relatively slight.

NUTRITIONAL DISORDERS

INTRODUCTION

The body is made up of many materials, all of which are supplied by the diet; it is, broadly speaking, the product of its nutrition. The ability to react to changes depends almost totally on nutritional status and, therefore, on the nutrients available.

Optimal nutritional status is achieved when all essential nutrients are supplied to the tissues requiring them for normal function. Poor nutritional status results when an inadequate amount of these nutrients is available over an extended period although, as body stores of some nutrients are greater than others, this is a relative situation.

Nutritional deficiencies may be primary or secondary. Primary deficiencies arise when the diet lacks one or more essential nutrients; secondary deficiencies occur in conditions interfering with digestion, absorption or utilization of nutrients or which increase requirements, destruction or excretion.

To obtain the necessary nutrients the body primarily depends on a wise selection of foods as, if these are not properly chosen, there may be an inadequacy of one or more essential nutrients. Nutrient supply also depends on normal control of feeding behaviour, normal functioning of the gastrointestinal tract and on the ability to metabolize and utilize the nutrients available.

DISTURBANCES OF FEEDING BEHAVIOUR

Determinants of feeding behaviour

People eat in certain ways or eat only certain kinds of food for many reasons, the most important being habit influenced by convention and upbringing. Personal likes and dislikes also play their part and religious beliefs are important to some individuals. Food habits, influenced by social, cultural and economic factors, play a major role in food selection (Ch. 14)

Feeding behaviour is a motor activity largely controlled by the ventromedial and lateral nucleii of the hypothalamus — the satiety and hunger centres. The amygdala and cortical areas of the limbic system, closely coupled with the hypothalamus, play a role in controlling the appetite; stimulation of these regions may increase or decrease feeding activity. Surgical section of the brain between the hypothalamus and mesencephalon allows the mechanical acts of feeding to continue indicating that these are controlled by the brain stem (Guyton, 1981). Table 23.1 illustrates those factors believed to control feeding behaviour.

The chemical senses, particularly taste and smell, are often responsible for guiding the individual to palatable and nutritious foodstuffs thus making the selection of food possible. Taste is determined by both the sensory properties of the food and by bodily requirements. For example, Mayer-Gross & Walker (1946) asked subjects to choose between 5% or 30% sucrose solutions as a drink. All chose the 5% solution, finding the 30% too sweet. However, following an injection of insulin and a fall in blood glucose concentration the 30% sucrose was no longer sickeningly sweet and was chosen by all, i.e. the taste of sucrose was modified by the action of insulin on blood glucose levels.

Sensory stimuli created by food increase the flow of saliva (Sharon, 1965), gastric juice (Lepkovsky, 1977), pancreatic juice (Janowitz et al, 1950) and bile, thus indirectly contributing to the digestion and absorption of nutrients.

Obesity

The rate of feeding, normally regulated in proportion to body stores, is usually reduced to prevent overstorage, but in many obese people this is not the case and body weight continues to rise to a level well above normal. In effect, therefore, obesity may result from an abnormality of the regulatory mechanisms, which may arise from psychogenic factors or from actual abnormalities of the hypothalamus, although the latter are rare in the normal obese subject (Guyton, 1981). Lesions of the ventromedial nucleii or stimulation of the lateral nucleii can result in voracious eating (Larsson, 1954) and hypophyseal tumours may encroach

Table 23.1 Factors believed to control the activity of the feeding centre

Nutritional regulation — Principally concerned with the maintenance of normal nutrient status	
Glucostatic theory (Mayer et al, 1965)	A decrease in blood glucose concentration is associated with hunger. Glucoreceptors in the hypothalamic nuclei are sensitive to the rate of glucose utilization measured as an arteriovenous (AV) ratio. Feeding inhibited when this ratio is high; feeding stimulated when this ratio is low
Lipostatic theory (Edholm et al, 1970)	This is concerned with control of long term feeding behaviour. The overall degree of feeding varies inversely with the amount of adipose tissue in the body. Thus, as the quantity of adipose tissue increases the rate of feeding is decreased.
Thermostatic theory (Brobeck, 1948)	This is thought to result from an interaction between the temperature regulating system and that regulating food intake within the hypothalamus. ? due to the pre-optic anterior hypothalamus (POAH), the heat responsive centre, and may be related to the specific dynamic action of food which causes an increase in metabolic rate and in heat production following eating. This may be the satiety signal and be mediated by the POAH.
Increase in blood amino acid concentration (Harper et al, 1970)	An increase in amino acid concentration results in inhibition of the food intake, whereas a decrease stimulates feeding. This is believed to be mediated by brain neurotransmitters as many of these are affected by the supply of amino acids which is dependent on the dietary intake
Alimentary regulation — Primarily concerned with the immediate short term effects of feeding on the gastrointestinal tract	
Distension of GI tract	Stretch and chemoreceptors are present in oropharynx, stomach and intestines. Distension therefore relayed to the brain causing inhibition of the lateral nucleii reducing desire for food

on the hypothalamus producing progressive obesity.

Definition

Obesity, the most prevalent form of body weight imbalance, is a medical problem of growing importance (Royal College of Physicians, 1983). It is defined as excess adipose tissue exceeding socially accepted norms or in excess of that consistent with good health and, in adults, is based on actuarial analyses indicating a weight range for each height category (Metropolitan Life Insurance Co., 1960). Obesity is regarded as exceeding these limits by 10% (Royal College of Physicians, 1983) although other workers regard a 10% excess as representing overweight and 20% excess as obesity (Krause & Mahan, 1984). Morbid obesity (i.e. obesity sufficient to prevent normal activity (Stedman, 1982)) represents a weight 45.4 kg (100 lb) above ideal body weight.

Causes of obesity

In principle, obesity may arise from either a high food intake or a low level of activity (energy expenditure), although it is now recognized that not all obese individuals eat more or exercise less than those of normal weight (Royal College of Physicians, 1983). However, within any group of individuals, there will be some in whom gluttony is the prime cause. Two forms of obesity are recognized — exogenous and endogenous. The former arises from an excessive food intake combined with a low activity level and the latter from a metabolic, physiological or psychological disorder.

In recent years there has been a growing interest in the search for a metabolic basis for the condition and in the significance of low energy expenditure in its development. This owes much to the work of Miller & Payne (1962) who argued that a reduction in one component of energy expenditure — adaptive thermogenesis — was a key factor, particularly that related to food intake (dietary thermogenesis). Although this function has been attributed to one organ, brown adipose tissue, direct evidence has not yet implicated this as a heat producer in man. However, it seems increasingly likely that the effectiveness of the brown adipose tissue in adapting to increased food intake by increasing the rate of heat formation plays an important role in determining whether an individual remains lean or becomes fat (Trayhurn & James, 1981).

A large proportion of obesity arises from psychological effects; overindulgence in food compensating or substituting for disagreeable affective elements (Simon, 1963). Thus food may represent love, security or satisfaction; it may provide a means of relieving nervous tension and enable a pattern of compulsive eating to become established. A vicious cycle of low self esteem, depression and overeating for consolation develops; obesity increases and creates further lowering of self esteem (Flack & Grayer, 1975).

Effects of obesity

The mechanical trauma of excess body weight may aggravate or create other ailments such as osteoarthritis, varicose veins and ventral arc diaphragmatic hernias. Gall bladder disease and maturity onset diabetes mellitus occur more commonly in the obese. Hypertension is common, blood pressure falling when weight is reduced (Flack & Grayer, 1975). The extra mechanical work required to move an overweight body combined with increased peripheral resistance in patients with hypertension results in an increased cardiac load which, together with the tendency to atherosclerosis, contributes to the development of angina pectoris and cardiac failure.

The 'Pickwickian syndrome' is characterized by hypoventilation, somnolence and carbon dioxide retention. It arises, in some very obese individuals, from decreased compliance of the thoracic wall and the resultant increased work of respiration combined with a failure to make the necessary increased respiratory effort (Albrink, 1975).

In view of these many complications, life expectancy is reduced.

Treatment and implications for nursing care

Weight reduction cannot be achieved unless the patient is motivated and understands why weight loss is necessary or desirable. Thus the nurse should help the patient to understand and accept this and to enhance their self-esteem. However, for some people it may be healthier in terms of psychological, emotional and social well being to maintain their weight and learn to accept it, rather than attempt to lose weight and have to cope with the guilt of failure.

Treatment consists of a reduction in energy intake, and no successful slimming diet exists which does not depend on a reduction of food intake. Patients must be involved in planning their dietary regime and allowed to evaluate the possible solutions to their problems so that the dietary plan may be individualized to meet their specific needs. A trial period will indicate whether or not this plan is satisfactory and will enable adjustments to be made. Weight loss cannot be achieved rapidly, and effective changes occur gradually. Patients will require continuous psychological support, although weight loss itself will provide encouragement. They should be taught the role of food and food habits in relation to obesity, and during the treatment programme the nurse should guide the process of change so that good habits are acquired which can continue, once the diet is completed, to maintain the weight loss.

Whilst dietary therapy is seen as the most important treatment of obesity this may be supplemented by exercise programmes. In some cases behaviour modification may be used to break obsessive eating patterns and create healthier ones. If a contributory cause of the obesity is hormonal, e.g. hypothyroidism or Cushing's syndrome, appropriate management of this disturbance will help to ameliorate the problem. Surgery is a drastic measure in the treatment of obesity and is only undertaken if the obesity has become life threatening and dietary regimes have proved impossible to implement or maintain. Such surgery includes wiring the jaws to restrict food intake to fluids only, a procedure sometimes accompanied by long term parenteral nutrition or intragastric feeding. Ileal bypass surgery on a temporary or permanent basis may also be performed to reduce absorption of nutrients and occasionally a gut resection is undertaken.

Anorexia nervosa

Possible causes

Anorexia nervosa (AN) was first described by Gull (1874) as 'the want of appetite due to a morbid mental state' which he attributed to the 'wiles' of young women whom he considered 'specially obnoxious to mental perversity'. The cause is unknown although it is believed to be of psychological origin and to arise from conflicts occurring during puberty and adolescence (Russell, 1975). An alternative view regards this as a disorder of the feeding and endocrine functions controlled by the hypothalamus, and an atypical, secondary form may be associated with a hypothalamic tumour (Warren & Van de Wiele, 1973).

As destruction of the feeding centre is known to cause food refusal, the pathogenesis of the disorder may involve a change of hypothalamic function (Russell, 1975) although studies have failed to demonstrate any primary disorder in the control of food intake and there is often no true loss of appetite. There is, however, specific failure of the hypothalamic-anterior pituitary-gonadal axis, thus gonadotropins are not secreted by the anterior pituitary, oestrogens are not produced by the ovaries and ovulation does not occur (Mecklenberg et al, 1974). Amenorrhoea may precede weight loss suggesting that the endocrine disorder is not only a sequela of malnutrition (Russell, 1975). The precise nature of any hypothalamic disorder is not known.

Presentation

Typically AN presents in girls aged 14–17 years (i.e. after the age of puberty) from apparently stable, upper middle class families but it has, rarely, been seen in men and older women. The essential criteria forming the basis of diagnosis depend on a triad of clinical disturbances:

- There is significant weight loss, which may be the first noticeable symptom, in which the loss of subcutaneous fat sharply delineates the underlying muscles. The patient commonly deprives herself of foods which she considers 'fattening' (i.e. high carbohydrate foods) and exists on a diet of fruit and vegetables. Weight loss may be very rapid and is often accentuated by devices such as purgative abuse, self-induced vomiting and violent exercise.
- There is a specific psychopathology in which there is a relentless pursuit for excessive thinness accompanied by a distortion of body image. These patients commonly overestimate their body size, believing themselves fat when they are obviously emaciated (Bruch, 1977). There is also a distorted perception of the physiological stimuli of hunger, appetite and satiety so that they eat less whenever they feel that their body is too large. There is often a change in temperament, the patient becoming irritable, impatient or depressed and withdrawing from their usual social life, becoming preoccupied with school work or exercise. As a result family relationships become strained as parents react to this behaviour and, as a result, the patient becomes more unhappy.
- The endocrine disorder differs according to sex. In the female, amenorrhoea occurs following significant weight loss but may also occur at an early stage of the illness. In the male there is a loss of sexual interest and potency.

Treatment and implications for nursing care

The patient with severe AN denies that she is ill and requires prompt attention. There is no specific treatment and the approach is usually empirical, relying on those treatments found to be effective in practice.

There are three main aims in the treatment:

- to gain the patient's confidence and, at least, some measure of co-operation
- to restore the patient's weight to its previously healthy level and to correct malnutrition resulting from continued food refusal
- to shorten the duration of the disorder whilst minimizing any residual disability.

The treatment of 'cause' is contentious and dependent on the perspective of the medical practitioner. For example, a physician may be concerned with the threat to life posed by severe malnutrition and the emphasis in treatment would be physical, primarily concentrating on food intake; a behavioural therapist may introduce a programme to modify the patient's behaviour in relation to food intake; a therapist using a psychoanalytic approach may attempt to identify root causes of the psychological disturbance.

Treatment is best administered in a psychiatric unit but it is essential that there are good nursing facilities. A good relationship must be built with the patient and her family; several out-patient interviews may be required before this is achieved and the patient can be persuaded to accept admission voluntarily. Most patients require in-patient treatment for a minimum of 6 weeks (Russell, 1982) during which time the principal aim is to restore the patient's weight and to treat the malnutrition. Refeeding is best achieved by skilled nurses who are able to build a good relationship with the patient, which is based on trust but which is not dependent on giving in to her wishes to avoid weight gain by refusing food.

The nurse must be aware of the psychopathology of AN, including the distress experienced by the patient, and she must make it clear that she is aware of the temptation to be deceitful about eating, vomiting or purgative abuse. At first, close supervision is required to reduce this. Observation is required throughout every meal and the patient must be persuaded to eat all the food on her plate. By sympathizing with the patient about her preoccupation with her body weight and size, the nurse may be able to offer to take responsibility for choosing and supplying food, particularly if she promises not to induce 'fatness' whilst not defining the limits of any weight gain. This relieves the patient of decision-making regarding food and, by providing a protective and non-punitive environment, the hospital may provide a setting in which the patient feels able to eat (Bruch, 1977). However, many patients will continue to refuse to eat solid foods but will agree to take liquids. In this case high calorie, high protein liquids should be given. In general, special diets are not required as long as carbohydrate foods are not excluded. Initially 6300 – 8400 kJ (1500 – 2000kcal) should be provided daily, but within 7–10 days 12.6 – 21.0MJ (3000 – 5000 kcal) should be given which will lead to a daily weight gain of 200–400 g (Russell, 1982).

Psychotherapeutic support. During hospitalization psychotherapeutic support should be initiated, and it should be continued following discharge. Removal of the patient from family stresses forms part of the value of in-patient treatment, as parental pressure may be the basis of the psychological and behavioural changes. Psychotherapy may begin with determining the underlying psychological reasons for this behaviour, thus it is vital to obtain as much co-operation as possible from the patient. Some therapists feel that it is necessary to treat the family as a whole in order to promote healthy patterns of family interaction (Minuchin et al, 1978).

The nursing care required during the in-patient period is demanding and can be seen both as a contribution to the psychotherapy and as a form of behaviour modification. Denial of privileges unless a certain daily weight gain is achieved can provide motivation; particularly valuable is the denial of any kind of activity as this may be of great importance to these patients. As weight gain continues more activity is allowed. However, Bruch (1974) has identified some serious repercussions from these techniques in some patients, as 'its very efficacy increases the inner turmoil in those who feel that they have been tricked into relinquishing control of their bodies and lives'. Short term weight gain may be excellent but relapses are frequent and the illness itself may last 2–3 years or even longer; treatment results in a return to normal weight accompanied by a marked improvement in mental state. Poor prognostic signs include a late age of onset or illness lasting longer than 5 years but, in the majority, health returns to normal and they may marry and bear children. There is however a small but definite mortality rate, mainly as a result of suicide (5%) (Morgan & Russell, 1975).

Whilst the majority of patients suffering from anorexia nervosa are treated in a psychiatric ward, a number will be admitted to medical wards for intensive nutritional therapy. In these situations sympathetic but firm understanding of the principles of management will result in consistency of treatment.

Bulimia nervosa

Bulimia nervosa is a condition characterized by:

- an exaggerated dread of becoming fat and a self imposed weight threshhold
- severe cravings for food and recurrent bouts of gross overeating
- self induced vomiting, purgative abuse or both (Russell, 1982).

Treatment and nursing care follow a similar pattern to that of anorexia nervosa but results are often disappointing unless the patient's attitudes and way of life change and she can be persuaded to accept a higher body weight.

THE GASTROINTESTINAL TRACT

The gastrointestinal tract, a long hollow 'tube' extending from the mouth to the anus, is divided into 5 main areas — the mouth, oesophagus, stomach, small and large intestines. Its primary functions are to provide the body cells with nutrients and to provide a means of elimination of residue and waste products.

Nutrients contained in foodstuffs sustain life, their availability determining the individual's nutritional status which is reflected in his or her state of health, level of activity and ability to resist disease or respond to its treatment. However, nutrients contained within the tract are essentially 'outside' the body and must be 'processed' and assimilated before they can be utilized by the body, i.e. the processes of digestion and absorption must occur. Disorders within the tract may, therefore, threaten survival by interfering with ingestion, digestion or absorption of food or with the elimination of waste products. Disturbance of gastrointestinal function may be secondary to disease in another part of the body, to fatigue or to emotional stress, the manifestations depending largely on the area affected and the nature of the causative factor.

Many gastrointestinal symptoms result from disturbances of gut motility and are associated with no recognizable morphologic or biochemical lesions. On the other hand, disturbances can result from physiological and clinical effects of morphologically definable disease processes.

Peristalsis (rhythmic contractility), an intrinsic property of the intestinal wall is, in the absence of extrinsic nerves or humoral influences, maintained by local reflexes for which afferent fibres arise in the mucosa and the efferents include the myenteric ganglia.

Extrinsic neural and humoral mechanisms regulate and adapt gut motility to the needs of the total organism, i.e. to the normal patterns of activity — eating, working, sleeping and defaecating. This is referred to as normal intestinal function.

Many of the common, clinically important disorders occur during periods of stress and emotional tension; in contrast, disorders such as achalasia result from permanent defects of integrative mechanisms.

Common symptoms associated with disorders of the tract

Pain

Pain may occur in any portion of the abdomen or be referred to a site distant from its origin. It may result from contraction of muscle tissue, chemical or mechanical irritation of the mucosa, direct irritation or pressure on associated nerves or inflammation of the peritoneum. Characteristics of the pain may prove valuable in confirming the diagnosis. Thus nursing care should include close observation and discrete questioning to establish any related factors. There is considerable individual variation in the response to pain but pertinent observations include:

- the nature, onset and duration of the pain
- any contributory factors (e.g. taking food, emotional stress)

- nausea, vomiting or flatulence occurring in association with the pain
- pallor, diaphoresis (perspiration) or changes in vital signs.

General pain management is dealt with in Chapter 9, while pain in relation to this system is discussed in the appropriate sections of this chapter.

Anorexia

Anorexia is associated with many disorders and is not exclusive to those of the gastrointestinal tract, although it is a common complaint. Causative factors are many and varied and may be functional in origin, resulting from the response to emotional stress. Anorexia should receive special attention from the nurse and every effort made to persuade the patient to eat. This condition must be clearly differentiated from anorexia nervosa.

Nausea and vomiting

Nausea and vomiting are both unpleasant sensations. Nausea describes a feeling of discomfort in the region of the stomach and the inclination to vomit. Vomiting involves the ejection of the stomach contents through the mouth, preceded by nausea and hypersalivation. This results from stimulation of the emetic centre in the medulla oblongata arising in response to excitation by sensory impulses originating in the tract, by impulses arising in response to fright, unpleasant sights or odours, severe pain or by impulses arising from the area postrema, a chemoreceptor zone of the 4th ventricle (Cockel, 1971). This zone responds to certain chemicals and impulses originating in the inner ear, hence the vomiting which occurs in response to motion sickness, radiation therapy and certain drugs.

Whatever the cause these symptoms interfere with normal nutrition and, if prolonged, lead to malnutrition and weight loss, and may lead to dehydration (fluid loss) and to fluid and electrolyte imbalance.

The care required includes supportive measures and medication to reduce the symptoms and enable normal nutrition to be resumed. Close observation may be valuable in preventing further nausea and vomiting which may, for example, be associated with ingestion of specific foods or drugs, which may be withheld. Rest and quiet may minimize the extent of vomiting and movement should be kept to a minimum. An accurate fluid balance chart must be maintained and the patient carefully observed for signs of dehydration and electrolyte imbalance (see Ch. 26)

Oral intake is normally withheld at first, being introduced gradually and the patient being offered frequent small meals. Stressful stimuli may be decreased by manipulation of the external environment as some sights, smells or sounds may contribute to the condition. Intravenous fluids may be necessary to replace electrolytes or to prevent or correct dehydration. Total parenteral nutrition may be required.

Changes in bowel habits

An intestinal disorder may either accelerate or retard the movement of the intestinal contents.

Diarrhoea. Diarrhoea may be classified as either functional or organic. The former may result from simple overeating or eating the wrong foods, fermentation of the intestinal contents due to incomplete digestion, habitual use of cathartics, nervous irritability or endocrine disorders. Periods of stress may also promote diarrhoea.

Organic diarrhoea results from a demonstrable lesion of the mucosa which is not present in functional diarrhoea. This may result from external poisoning (such as food poisoning) or parasitic infection. It may accompany certain diseases such as tuberculosis, viral hepatitis or ulcerative colitis and may also arise from intestinal enzyme deficiencies.

Any patient suffering an attack of diarrhoea lasting more than a day or two should be advised to seek medical attention, as this may be an early manifestation of serious disease.

The aim of treatment is to correct the physiological effects of the condition whilst identifying the cause and minimizing the diarrhoea. Various drugs may be given:

examples include diphenoxylate hydrochloride (Lomotil) which reduces intestinal spasm and motility and Kaolin which provides a protective coating to the mucosa and is an adsorbent which binds irritating substances. An antibacterial agent may be prescribed for diarrhoea of microbial origin.

During an acute attack, bedrest is recommended to help to reduce peristalsis. Fluids and electrolytes are replaced by the intravenous route and oral intake withheld for 24–48 hours to allow the gastrointestinal tract to rest. Once oral fluids can be tolerated clear fluids are given, avoiding those likely to stimulate peristalsis (carbonated beverages, iced drinks, whole milk).

Large amounts of fluid may be lost causing dehydration and electrolyte imbalance, thus accurate records of fluid intake and output must be maintained and the patient closely observed for signs of toxicity and dehydration. Comprehensive supportive care is required as such a symptom may significantly alter the patient's pattern of activity. Mucosal irritation should be carefully assessed and treated with meticulous perianal care to minimize the risks of secondary infection (Golden, 1975).

Constipation. The slow movement of faeces through the intestine is associated with large quantities of hard, dry faeces which accumulate in the descending colon because of the length of time available for absorption of fluid. It may be associated with organic disease or with any condition in which there is a reduced food or fluid intake or when the diet lacks fibre. Insufficient food fails to stimulate peristalsis, and dehydration results in the production of small, dry, hard stools which irritate the colon causing spasm and failure to stimulate normal colonic motility. This may create considerable discomfort, abdominal pain and distension or a feeling of fullness. Headache accompanied by anorexia and nausea and vomiting is common. Such symptoms in turn create nutritional problems.

Care consists of the alleviation of the condition which may require the use of laxatives or enemas, although the regular use of these should be discouraged. Dietary modification may be all that is needed. Encouraging the intake of whole grain cereals and bread, fruit and vegetables results in an increased dietary fibre intake. A daily fluid intake of approximately 2 litres should be ensured (Bass, 1977).

DISORDERS OF THE GASTROINTESTINAL TRACT

Disorders of chewing and lubrication of food — the mouth

Whilst food is in the mouth it is being moistened by saliva and ground into small particles by the teeth, both of which are important preliminaries to swallowing.

The teeth reflect the faults of the previous diet, and two closely associated pathological processes play a vital part in the role played by the teeth and gums in the maintenance of health. These are dental caries (decay of the enamel) and periodontal disease (disease of the gums; pyorrhoea alveolaris). Caries is the usual cause of loss of teeth up to the age of about 45 years, after which periodontal disease is the prime cause. Inadequate dentition or ill-fitting dentures often lead an individual to choose soft foods comprised mainly of carbohydrate, at the expense of more nutritious foodstuffs which require chewing. Masticatory studies (Neill, 1972) have shown the relationship between denture quality and masticatory performance; subjects with few teeth remaining performed as well as those wearing ill-fitting dentures.

The two types of saliva combine to begin starch digestion (due to the presence of alpha (α) amylase) and to cause adherence of the food particles, lubrication of the bolus and facilitation of swallowing. Saliva also facilitates movement of the tongue and lips — drying of the mouth inhibits speech as well as swallowing. Saliva prevents dessication of the oral mucosa and helps to keep the mouth and teeth clean, the bactericidal action of lysosyme contributing to this effect. When salivary secretion is suppressed the lips, teeth and mouth become coated with a mixture of food particles, dried mucus and dead epithelium which may become the site of bacterial or fungal infection. The absence of saliva (for example in patients undergoing radio-erapy to the oropharyngeal region) can have sigifi-cant effects on swallowing ability, and the maintenance of oral hygiene is essential to the prevention of secondary infection. The condition of the patient's mouth is one of the best indices of the quality of nursing care (Henderson, 1960). Salivation can be stimulated by sucking acid drops or lemon wedges and the mouth moistened with glycerin and lemon swabs or by artificial saliva sprays (e.g. Glandosane).

Stomatitis

Stomatitis (inflammation of the mouth) may result from a local cause such as trauma from the teeth or from alterations of the bacterial flora during antibiotic therapy. It may arise from nutritional deficiency or because immuno-competence has been lowered by disease or immunosuppressive drugs. Finally, it may be due to bacterial or viral infection. Severe stomatitis with ulceration and bleeding is often seen in acute leukaemia. Mucosal irritation can occur subsequent to radiation therapy to the mouth or oesophagus and indicates levels of radiation toxicity. Initially an inflammatory response is seen followed by the formation of a white or yellow glistening membrane (radio-epithelite) which should not be confused with that formed by Candida albicans (thrush) and must not be removed due to the risk of bleeding (Leahy et al, 1979).

These conditions may affect talking and eating and be extremely uncomfortable for the patient, creating direct effects such as pain and indirect effects such as nutritional and fluid imbalances. All substances which may irritate the condition should be avoided (e.g. tobacco, alcohol) and treatment is by improving oral hygiene by the use of frequent, gentle mouth irrigations. When an infecting organism has been isolated the appropriate antibacterial/antifungal agent should be prescribed. Dentures may create additional pain yet their omission can contribute to further deterioration of nutritional status. The use of local anaesthetic sprays or mouthwashes, in addition to analgesic relief of pain, may help to overcome some of the difficulties, thus enhancing the desire to eat, although these substances may create changes in taste sensation. Nutritious but bland, soft foods should be given; spicy or highly seasoned foods are best avoided. These patients often prefer their food at room temperature.

Disorders of swallowing mechanisms

Partial or total paralysis of the swallowing mechanisms may result from damage to the trigeminal, glossopharyngeal or vagus nerves and can result in:

- complete inhibition of swallowing
- uncontrolled passage of food into both the trachea and the oesophagus as the glottis fails to close
- reflux of food into the nose as the posterior nares fail to close
- failure of the cricopharyngeal sphincter to remain closed during breathing; air is drawn into the oesophagus.

Disease states can lead to the malfunction of swallowing muscles (as in muscular dystrophy), failure of neuromuscular transmission (as in myaesthenia gravis) or damage to swallowing centres in the brain stem (as in poliomyelitis).

Disorders of the oesophagus

The oesophagus, a fibromuscular tube, is about 25cm long and 2cm in diameter and joins the pharynx to the stomach at the cardiac sphincter. It is related anteriorly first to the trachea and then to the left main bronchus and the pulmonary artery. It is separated from the left atrium by the pericardium; rarely, enlargement of the atrium may compress the oesophagus. Posteriorly it is closely related to the lower cervical bodies, thus disease of the latter may cause dysphagia. In the mediastinum the oesophagus is surrounded by loose connective tissue which allows it to distend during swallowing. Perforation of the oesophagus may lead to spreading infection of the media-stinum, which is commonly fatal. The symptoms of oesophageal disease are dysphagia, heartburn, oesophageal pain, belching and regurgitation.

Table 23.2 Categories of dysphagia

Type of dysphagia	Causative factors include
Oropharyngeal dysphagia	1. Interference with mucosal sensations, e.g. from inflammation due to acute pharyngitis, candidiasis or iron deficiency (Plummer Vinson syndrome) 2. Pharyngeal paralysis, e.g. from lesions of the central or peripheral nervous system as in poliomyelitis, toxic drugs or lesions of the eleventh (accessory) cranial nerve (as in myasthenia gravis)
Oesophageal dysphagia	1. Oesophageal obstruction a. Intrinsic e.g. foreign body, spasm, stricture or carcinoma b. Extrinsic e.g. mediastinal tumour, aortic aneurysm or goitre 2. Neuromuscular disorders, e.g. achalasia or progressive systemic sclerosis
Globus hystericus	The sensation of a 'lump in the throat' which rarely interferes with swallowing. Sometimes a feature of anxiety states.

Dysphagia is the most serious and its cause must be elucidated.

Dysphagia. Painful or difficult swallowing of food may arise from a number of benign or malignant conditions and may be divided into two main categories as shown in Table 23.2.

Achalasia, the failure of the lower portion of the oesophagus to relax during swallowing, results from either a damaged or absent myenteric plexus. The oesophageal musculature is still capable of contracting but has lost the ability to conduct a peristaltic wave, and the passage of food is impeded or prevented. Dysphagia can be mild and infrequent or become more severe and painful as the condition worsens.

During eating, the oesophagus fills with food until either the pressure forces the opening of the cardiac sphincter, allowing small amounts to pass into the stomach, or the patient is forced to vomit. By the time the patient seeks medical advice he is usually eating very little due to the physical and social problems involved and significant weight loss has occurred.

Dysphagia may result from inflammation of the mucosa arising as a result of radiation therapy and may be severe enough to limit food and fluid intake. This usually occurs 2–3 weeks after the start of treatment and lasts until several weeks after treatment is completed. The late effects of radiation may cause strictures and stenosis.

Treatment and implications for nursing care. Forceful dilatation of the oesophagus results in permanent opening of the oesophagus, which then functions by means of gravity and oropharyngeal pressure. This, however, allows gastro-oesophageal reflux to occur which in turn creates oesophagitis, the commonest symptom of which is heartburn. If this is a chronic condition an inflammatory stricture and subsequent dysphagia may develop.

Care is aimed at preventing irritation of the oesophageal mucosa by preventing or reducing reflux of gastric contents and decreasing the irritating ability of the gastric juice. Thus analgesics should be given prior to meals and frequent irrigations may aid patient comfort. In the acute phase a liquid diet is advised as this is less abrasive to the inflamed area. When solids can be tolerated foods given should be bland and soothing, and small frequent meals should be given to help prevent gastric distension and to reduce gastric acid secretion. A patient may find food from home more appetizing. However, high protein foods should not be given as these stimulate gastrin production and increase cardiac sphincter pressure. A nurse should be present at mealtimes when the patient is having swallowing difficulties (Dietz, 1979).

Antacids will help to reduce the acidity of gastric juice thus reducing its irritant effect on the mucosa. Gaviscon, a mixture of alginic acid and aluminium hydroxide, is a useful addition to treatment as it floats on the surface of the gastric acid pool reducing the movement of acid into the oesophagus.

When the condition is severe, tube feeding or parenteral feeding may be necessary.

General measures which should be adopted when caring for patients with dysphagia include:

- raising the head of the bed to reduce the risk of regurgitation and inhalation and, to reduce this risk still further, no food should be taken within 2–3 hours of going to bed
- a high energy, moderate protein, pureed or liquid diet should be provided and should make adequate provision for trace nutrients (both water and fat soluble vitamins and minerals)
- stagnating contents should be removed by lavage with a wide bore tube to prevent inhalation during sleep, to reduce mucosal inflammation and to improve swallowing.

Disorders of gastroduodenal motility

As the stomach and duodenum share the common function of mixing food with digestive juices it is logical to consider these together. Following ingestion a small amount of food is propelled into the duodenum, after which the pylorus closes as the body of the stomach progessively dilates. Under normal circumstances a series of peristaltic waves follows a period of churning movements and propels small amounts of chyme into the duodenum at a rate consistent with proper digestion and absorption.

Instillation of fat, hypertonic solutions of sodium chloride or glucose, amino acids or hydrochloric acid into the duodenum stimulates contraction of the pyloric sphincter and delays gastric emptying time. These effects are believed to be mediated by secretin and cholecystokinin which stimulate the pylorus when given intravenously. Their action is opposed by that of gastrin, thus a form of regulatory mechanism exists which normally limits regurgitation of duodenal content into the stomach.

A number of important digestive symptoms are related to the disturbances of this pattern and may limit the food intake. These include dyspepsia, vomiting, haematemesis and malaena. Dyspepsia results from the devel-opment of a pressure gradient between the duodenum and stomach which leads to duodenogastric regurgitation and the exposure of the gastric and, on occasions, oesophageal mucosa to the irritant effects of the bile acids and pancreatic enzymes. Nausea is accompanied by a marked reduction of gastric contraction and an associated, sustained contraction of the duo-denum — it is this which creates the pressure gradient initiating the condition.

When vomiting occurs the fundus and body of the stomach are relaxed and the antrum and duodenum strongly contracted. The cardiac sphincter is relaxed. During vomiting, con-traction of the abdominal wall combined with forcible descent of the diaphragm squeeze the flaccid stomach, ejecting its contents.

Haematemesis and malaena following prolonged vomiting are commonly due to laceration of the gastric mucosa which may extend through the mucosa to rupture the submucosal blood vessels. It is thought such lacerations result from the forcible distension of the cardia whilst the lower portion remains contracted.

Disorders of gastric function

Disorders of the stomach may have a considerable effect on the nutrient supply. The reasons for this become clear when the major functions of the organ are considered.

- It stores large quantities of food and controls the rate at which this enters the small intestine.
- It liquifies and mixes food with gastric secretions to form the semifluid chyme.
- By secreting hydrochloric acid, pepsin, gastrin and the intrinsic factor it commences digestion.
- It provides a means of protection against infective and toxic agents ingested in association with foodstuffs.

Absorption from the stomach is slight for two main reasons: first, it is lined with highly resistant mucosal cells; second, it has very tight junctions between adjacent epithelial cells. This barrier is normally highly resistant even to diffusion, but in gastritis it becomes inflamed and its permeability is greatly increased. Hydrogen ions can then diffuse into the stomach wall creating progressive mucosal damage and gastric atrophy. The mucosa simultaneously becomes susceptible to peptic digestion and, frequently, peptic ulceration.

Gastric atrophy

Gastric atrophy, a common sequelae of chronic gastritis, may also in some individuals arise from an autoimmunity against the gastric mucosa which may result in a failure of gastric gland activity. Loss of the stomach's secretions leads to hypochlorhydria, achlorhydria and, on occasions, pernicious anaemia.

Achlorhydria simply means a failure of the parietal cells to secrete gastric acid; hypochlorhydria means diminished acid secretion. When acid secretion fails, the action of pepsin is inhibited as this requires an acid medium for normal activity. Thus essentially all digestive functions are lost, carbohydrates ferment rapidly and the mucosa becomes hypersensitive. However, overall digestion throughout the entire GI tract remains comparatively normal, as trypsin and other pancreatic enzymes are able to digest most dietary proteins, particularly if these are well chewed so that no part of the protein is protected by collagen fibres which depend on pepsin for their digestion.

Gastric acid is, however, necessary to facilitate the absorption of non-haem iron by converting ferric to ferrous iron. Thus achlorhydria may reduce the absorption of ferric iron by approximately 50% (Jacobs et al, 1964).

Pernicious anaemia (see Ch. 22) commonly accompanies gastric atrophy arising from the failure of the parietal cells to secrete the intrinsic factor, a mucopolypeptide, which is essential to vitamin B_{12} absorption. Pernicious anaemia may also arise when large portions of the stomach or ileum are removed.

Treatment. Care must be taken to prevent the introduction of bacteria into the gastrointestinal tract and to avoid foods favouring their growth, thus a low fibre diet is advised as fibrous foods tend to prolong gastric emptying time favouring bacterial activity (Royal College of Physicians, 1980). The diet should also be low in fat as this also prolongs emptying time and inhibits acid secretion (maximum daily intake 70–90 g). Starchy carbohydrates are preferred to sugars as these are least likely to ferment, thus fruit and vegetables are recommended provided that they are low in fibre.

Disturbances of digestion and absorption

The majority of digestion and absorption occurs in the small intestine, which starts at the pylorus and ends at the ileocaecal junction where it joins the large intestine, and consists of the duodenum, jejunum and ileum. Absorption depends on many factors including the area of the absorptive surface, osmotic and intraluminal pressures and concentration gradients. Most nutrients are actively transported from the lumen to the portal blood, two important exceptions being ethanol and water which cross the cells by passive diffusion and may be absorbed from all parts of the intestine including the colon.

Despite the extent of the small intestine, disorders here are surprisingly less common than are those of the stomach and colon. Nonetheless they may cause severe disturbances of digestion, absorption and movement of the content along the tract. Prolonged dysfunction seriously threatens nutritional status.

Malabsorption syndrome

This is a collection of signs and symptoms which indicate the presence of a defect in the absorption of one or more essential nutrients. It is associated with one or more of the following symptoms:

- diarrhoea
- abdominal distension
- anorexia
- muscle wasting

- weight loss
- signs of vitamin and mineral deficiencies.

Steatorrhoea is the most common feature which is diagnosed on the basis of faecal fat estimations in stools collected over at least a 3-day period. In this condition the daily output exceeds 7g when the intake is 50-100g (Baron, 1973). The stools are pale, bulky and offensive, float in water and flush away with difficulty and, when the condition is severe, diarrhoea may be present.

Excess loss of fat in the stools deprives the body of a considerable amount of energy, thus body tissue is used as an energy source and muscle wasting follows. Diarrhoea is associated with considerable losses of water and electrolytes as well as other nutrients. Fatty acids, present in the stools, bind calcium, forming soaps which are excreted thus causing hypocalcaemia. Malabsorption of fat is accompanied by malabsorption of the fat soluble vitamins, which results in a variety of symptoms such as bleeding, ecchymosis and haematuria (vitamin K), osteomalacia, bone pain and fractures (vitamin D), and hyperkeratosis follicularis (vitamin A). A glucose tolerance test may distinguish between the steatorrhoea of pancreatic disease and that of intestinal malabsorption.

The symptoms of the syndrome may be mild and low grade so that medical attention is not sought, hence many patients escape diagnosis. Others with severe malabsorption may present with bleeding or bone pain, or anaemia and fatigue arising from secondary effects of the disease. As there is a wide range of possible defects the treatment must be preceded by an accurate diagnosis (Tables 23.3 and 23.4).

Impaired protein absorption. Impaired protein absorption may depress protein metabolism which is reflected by a decrease in muscle mass and lowered serum proteins. Protein catabolism may be accelerated as a result of an inadequate intake or absorption of carbohydrate. Serum proteins, particularly albumin, may be

Table 23.3 Causes of malabsorption

Defect	Possible causative factors	Examples
Reduction of absorptive area	Villus atrophy	Coeliac disease (gluten-sensitive enteropathy), Radiotherapy
	Intestinal resection Intestinal fistulae	Crohn's disease, malignancy
	Damage by drugs or radiation	Colchichine toxicity
Intraluminal causes	Deficiency of conjugated bile salts	Hepatic disease Extrahepatic biliary tract obstruction
	Failure of pancreatic secretion	Pancreatic insufficiency following chronic relapsing pancreatitis Cystic fibrosis
	Failure of co-ordination between the rate of gastric emptying and secretion of bile and pancreatic enzymes.	Following gastric surgery
	Inappropriate H^+ concentration	Achlorhydria (gastric atrophy) Hyperchlorhydria (as in Zollinger-Ellison syndrome)
	Drugs impairing absorption	Neomycin precipitates bile acids
Mucosal defects	Enzyme deficiency	Disaccharidase deficiency
	Deficiency/failure of transport mechanisms	Cystinuria (amino acids)
Failure of clearance	Lymphatic obstruction	Primary intestinal lymphoma Intestinal tuberculosis
	Venous congestion	Congestive cardiac failure
Infection	Bacterial contamination	Tropical sprue
	Bacterial overgrowth	Gastrocolic fistulae

Table 23.4 Laboratory tests used in the diagnosis of malabsorption

Test	Normal values	In malabsorption
Serum		
Albumin	4.0 g/l	Decreased
Calcium	2.25 mmol/l	Decreased, particularly in small bowel disease
Potassium	4.0 mmol/l	Decreased
Magnesium	0.8 mmol/l	Decreased
Cholesterol	5.2 mmol/l	Decreased
Plasma		
Vitamin B_{12}	200–960 pg/l	Decreased, particularly in tropical sprue
Folic acid	6–20 μg/l	Decreased, particularly in small bowel disease
Prothrombin time	Control value	Prolonged
Tolerance tests		
D-xylose (25 g orally)	4.5–8 g excreted in 5 hours	Diminished in mucosal disease
Glucose (50 g orally)	10 mmol/l at 1 hour	Flat curve in coeliac disease, disease of intestinal wall and in monosaccharide malabsorption
Faecal fat (80–100 g daily)	< 7 g daily (up to 18 mmol/24 h)	Increased (> 18 mmol/24 h)
Urinary excretion 5-hydroxyindole-aceticacid	31 μmol/24 h	> 130 μmol/24 h is diagnostic of carcinoid

decreased by abnormal protein losses into the intestine (protein losing enteropathy) which may be secondary to many diseases particularly those causing malabsorption. Four possible mechanisms have been proposed to explain such abnormal protein losses:

- the passage of plasma proteins into the gastrointestinal tract resulting from inflammation or ulceration of the mucosa (as in Crohn's disease or ulcerative colitis)
- rupture of dilated lymphatic vessels in the mucosa resulting in discharge of their content into the intestine (idiopathic intestinal lymphangiectasis)
- increased lymphatic pressure resulting in increased movement of plasma proteins into the lumen through spaces between mucosal and epithelial cells
- disordered structure of mucosal cells permitting plasma protein loss (as in non-tropical sprue) (Greenberger & Isselbacher, 1977).

Emaciation and weakness may be extreme. Treatment consists of providing large amounts of calories and protein (150g or more daily) to offset the protein loss and is achieved by use of a high protein diet together with protein supplements. Nutritional status must be maintained if these patients are to respond to medical treatment.

Abnormal carbohydrate absorption. This results in reduced glycogen stores in the liver and muscles. Intraluminal fermentation of sugars creates flatulence and abdominal distension and results in chronic watery diarrhoea. The condition most commonly arises from a failure to hydrolyze disaccharides due to disaccharidase deficiencies, the clinical features of which are discussed in detail by McMichael (1975).

Impaired absorption of vitamins and minerals. Absorption of these substances may be affected in disorders resulting in malabsorption and will result in specific clinical conditions.

Impaired absorption of water and electrolytes Dehydration, hypotension and generalized weakness commonly follow malabsorption, when they result from losses of large amounts of water and electrolytes which occur when diarrhoea is severe. Hypokalaemia may cause cardiac arrythmias and muscle flaccidity; hyponatraemia leads to weakness, lethargy, nausea and muscle cramps which rapidly disappear once sodium is given.

Diagnosis and management. Clinical examination can, simply, confirm the diagnosis, but if subsequent treatment is to be successful, precise information regarding which absorptive defects are present is essential. Laboratory tests commonly used to diagnose malabsorption are shown in Table 23.4 and, when used in conjunction with routine haematological studies (blood counts, electrolyte levels and prothrombin time), small intestinal biopsy and radiological studies will enable effective diagnosis to be made.

As there are many conditions which may create malabsorption, both treatment and care must be prescribed on an individual basis dependent upon the symptoms which are present.

Disorders of the pancreas

The endocrine functions of the pancreas are dealt with in Chapter 19.

The exocrine secretions of the pancreas can be affected by a variety of disorders which may influence the quality or quantity of pancreatic secretions:

- abnormalities in the enzymes secreted as a result of genetic disorder, e.g. trypsinogen deficiency
- obstruction to secretion of enzymes through blockage of pancreatic ducts by:
  - extrinsic conditions such as carcinoma of the head of the pancreas
  - intrinsic blockage by, for example, viscid mucus secreted in fibrocystic disease
- inflammation of the pancreas which may involve obstruction as well as diminished function of the cells, e.g. acute pancreatitis
- destruction of pancreatic tissue by carcinoma or chronic pancreatitis
- secondary to other disturbances such as Zollinger-Ellison syndrome (a gastrin-secreting tumour (gastrinoma) of the pancreas).

Pancreatic exocrine insufficiency may be confirmed by measurement of the volume, bicarbonate and enzyme content of pancreatic juice obtained by duodenal intubation. An increased volume of juice with a high bicarbonate content is obtained following administration of secretin; pancreozymin increases the enzyme content. Thus, in the presence of widespread pancreatic damage, secretin and pancreozymin produce a juice of normal volume but with reduced enzyme and bicarbonate content; in the presence of duct obstruction the volume of secretion is reduced whilst the enzyme and bicarbonate content remains within the normal range. However, this is not suitable for routine use due to the difficulty of positioning the duodenal tube correctly (Zilva & Pannall, 1979).

Elevation of serum enzymes — amylase and lipase — indicates obstruction of the pancreatic ducts, and measurement before and after injection of secretin and pancreozymin will help to differentiate the nature of the damage. Total destruction results in a failure to respond to secretin or pancreozymin as measured by either serum enzymes or duodenal intubation.

Effects of pancreatic insuffficiency. Pancreatic insufficiency, whatever the cause, will result in inadequate digestion and absorption of nutrients. This will result in two main groups of problems:

- Disorders resulting from the lack of nutrients entering the body. Weight loss and malnutrition can develop if the condition is prolonged. These disorders may result in a loss of some 30% of the energy supplied by ingested foods (Keele et al, 1982). In addition, specific nutritional deficiencies may result (e.g. hypocalaemia, deficiency of fat-soluble vitamins).
- Disorders resulting from the retention of undigested nutrients in the gut. The osmotic effect of these substances may attract fluid into the gut resulting in diarrhoea while the unabsorbed fat produces steatorrhoea (light, greasy, bulky stools which float on water and have a foul odour). Nausea and vomiting may occur. The loss of fluid from the circulation may lead to dehydration.

Slight impairment may be controlled by simple

dietary modification and avoidance of emotional stress, fatigue and infection. A low fat, high protein, high energy diet divided into 4–5 small meals is recommended. Alcohol should be avoided.

The patient's fear of pain (particularly in chronic pancreatitis) often leads to reluctance to eat and a resultant weight loss. Regular analgesia will help to overcome this but, nevertheless, the nurse may need to exercise considerable skill in persuading the patient to eat.

Secondary pancreatic deficiency resulting from hypersecretion of gastric acid (as in Zollinger-Ellison syndrome) responds well to total gastrectomy.

Disorders of the biliary system

In adults, biliary disease may be of congenital, metabolic, infectious or parasitic origin and causes considerable morbidity. Such diseases interfere with the normal flow of bile into the duodenum. They may be acute or chronic, the intensity of the signs and symptoms paralleling the severity of the condition. Pain, ranging from a persistent dull ache to severe and disabling, may be felt in the right upper abdomen or the mid-epigastric region and it may be referred to the right scapular area. It most commonly follows ingestion of fatty foods. Anorexia, nausea and vomiting occur in many cases although vomiting is rarely severe unless biliary colic or obstructive jaundice are present. Digestive disturbances are usual, the patient experiencing pain or flatulence as well as a feeling of fullness and nausea particularly after fatty or fried foods. Jaundice follows obstruction of the hepatic or common bile duct; pyrexia accompanies infection in the gall bladder or the bile ducts. Obstruction to the flow of bile into the intestine decreases absorption of vitamin K, and thus a reduction in prothrombin level and failure of normal haemostatic mechanisms occurs. Thus, bleeding disorders are common.

Biliary obstruction creates impaired digestion and reduced absorption of fat and, consequently results in faecal changes. Plasma prothrombin falls; haemoglobin formation becomes defective leading to anaemia of obscure origin. The retention of bile in the blood stream and tissue fluids results in jaundice and anorexia. Duodenal ulcer is common, resulting from mucosal damage; this may be responsible for death from haemorrhage or perforation. Blood levels of bile pigments, bile salts and cholesterol are elevated and bile pigments and salts appear in the urine.

Management. An acute attack is almost invariably associated with an obstructive disorder during which the gall bladder should be kept as inactive as possible. This is achieved by omitting all visible dietary fat. In some cases it may be necessary to give a liquid diet of 2–3 litres daily which supplies protein from skimmed milk and carbohydrate from sweetened fruit juices and vegetables. Limited amounts of fat and solid food are added as tolerated. A low fat diet is maintained until it is clear whether surgical removal of the gall bladder is indicated. In rare cases total parenteral nutrition is required.

In chronic cases a low fat diet must be adhered to. This supplies about 25% of the total calories as fat. It is undesirable to insist on too strict a limitation as some fat is important in allowing some gall bladder drainage into the intestine. As many patients with gall bladder disease are overweight attention should be given to weight reduction.

Disorders of the liver

Clearly hepatic disease may significantly affect the functions of the liver (Table 23.5) which are discussed later in this chapter. Only the nutritional and metabolic consequences are discussed here.

Table 23.5 Functions of the liver

Excretion of bile salts and cholesterol
Excretion of bilirubin
Synthesis and storage of glycogen
Synthesis of albumin
Synthesis of urea
Storage of vitamins A, D and B_{12}
Detoxication of hormones (e.g. aldosterone, oestrogens, ADH)
Detoxication of drugs

Weight loss may be a significant problem arising from a reduced food intake (anorexia), malabsorption or increased tissue catabolism in acutely ill patients. A chronic alcoholic with cirrhosis derives most of his calories from alcohol and may, therefore, consume a diet deficient in many nutrients notably protein, folic acid, B group vitamins, ascorbic acid and many minerals. Body weight may be maintained by the energy from alcohol and carbohydrate yet significant muscle wasting may occur to meet the need for available protein. Hypokalaemia and magnesium deficiency may accentuate muscle weakness.

Protein metabolism. The liver cells contain enzymes which enable synthesis of non-essential amino acids, synthesis and catabolism of plasma and cellular proteins, catabolism of amino acids and synthesis of urea.

Amino acids, derived from dietary proteins, are absorbed from the small intestine and transported, by the portal venous blood, to the liver where they are catabolised or used in protein synthesis. Failure of protein synthesis leads to a decrease in plasma protein concentration which may have far reaching effects. Plasma proteins maintain colloidal osmotic pressure in the plasma and play a vital role in the transport of many substances including iron, vitamin B_{12}, hormones, haemoglobin and bilirubin in addition to maintaining normal homeostasis. Hepatic synthesis of plasma proteins may be impaired by hepatocellular failure and is accompanied by increased urinary excretion and elevated plasma levels of amino acids. A reduction in the rate of plasma protein catabolism may, in part, compensate for the reduction in synthesis, but hypoproteinaemia persists and contributes to the development of ascites and oedema.

The effect of reduced ability to deal with ammonia and other toxins is discussed in the section on hepatic encephalopathy later in this chapter.

Carbohydrate metabolism. The liver plays a central role in the regulation of blood sugar concentration. Following absorption the monosaccharides, glucose, fructose and galactose are taken up from the portal blood by the hepatocytes, where they are metabolized to provide energy through the tricarboxylic acid (Kreb's) cycle or converted to glycogen which, during periods of fasting, can be used through glycogenolysis to maintain or increase blood sugar levels. Amino acids are converted to pyruvate and other Kreb's cycle intermediates to support gluconeogenesis. These provide a source of glucose for the brain.

In the fasting state glucose levels are maintained from endogenous energy stores and reflect the balance between endogenous glucose and that derived from gluconeogenesis. The dependence of the brain on glucose for its energy needs means that normal blood sugar levels are maintained whilst utilization of glucose is restricted to prevent excessive catabolism of structural protein for gluconeogenesis. Fatty acids are substituted as energy sources in extracerebral tissues, and hepatic ketogenesis produces ketone bodies which can cross the blood-brain barrier and replace glucose in some oxidative processes in the brain once ketosis becomes established. Tissues reliant on glucose (e.g. erythrocytes) are supported by hepatic gluconeogenesis which recovers lactic acid and prevents a net loss of glucose. Hypoglycaemia, in this case, represents the underproduction of glucose by the liver resulting from hepatic abnormalities which restrict its productive capacity.

When the normal liver is unable to keep pace with the normal rate of glucose utilization, failure of glucose production results either because of functional restraints on the glucose output or because of inadequate availability of gluconeogenic substrates. Absolute failure of glucose production is rare, occurring only when hepatic abnormalities restrict productive capability. Extensive parenchymal damage, hepatic necrosis or congestion secondary to cardiac failures are examples of disease states which may cause hypoglycaemia.

Hypoglycaemia. Such hypoglycaemia develops slowly, the clinical picture reflecting prolonged, severe glucose deprivation. The diagnosis should be suspected whenever a psychiatric disorder occurs regularly before breakfast, or after missed meals, which is rapidly reversed once food is taken. Symptoms include confusion and disorientation, memory lapses, paraesthesiae, convulsions or coma. Focal abnormalities may result in monoplegia or hemiplegia. When hypoglycaemic episodes have no well-defined pattern, induced insulin excess should be considered in which an endogenous agent has blocked normal homeostatic mechanisms. This should be suspected in any individual having access to hypoglycaemic agents.

Hypoglycaemia may also occur in the fed state. Concentration of plasma insulin normally parallels that of the blood sugar and increased amounts of insulin are present in the circulation within a few minutes of eating. At this stage hepatic glucose production is inhibited, inhibition being removed when blood sugar returns to normal and insulin secretion falls. There is a lag phase, even in normal individuals, between the return of blood sugar to normal and the cessation of insulin secretion and a transient hypoglycaemia may occur. In some cases this may be prolonged and, in adults, results from a disturbance of the interaction between glucose and insulin during feeding. Diagnosis is made on the basis of a prolonged (5–6 hr) glucose tolerance test when patients show a lag storage glucose tolerance curve (Zilva & Pannall, 1979) and excessive insulin secretion.

'Reactive hypoglycaemia' may be seen after gastric surgery, when rapid emptying of the stomach allows the entry of hyperosmolar liquid into the small intestine and ingested glucose has rapid access to the absorptive sites, stimulating a rapid insulin secretion (Irving et al, 1975). An abnormally rapid rise of both serum glucose and insulin concentration occurs which later results in a reactive hypoglycaemia as glucose levels fall, whilst the insulin level remains elevated and is not buffered by a continuing absorption of carbohydrates.

When glycogen stores are depleted, alcohol ingestion may precipitate hypoglycaemia by inhibiting gluconeogenesis. Massive hepatic necrosis or a deficiency of the enzymes essential to glycogenolysis may also result in hypoglycaemia (glycogen storage diseases).

Patients with cirrhosis may develop diabetes mellitus either as a result of hepatic dysfunction or from associated pancreatic disease (chronic alcoholic pancreatitis). Such patients often display an abnormal glucose tolerance level due to either a reduced rate of glucose uptake or impaired release from a damaged liver. Characteristically, fasting blood sugar levels are normal, hyperglycaemia following a glucose load is prolonged and a late hypoglycaemia follows (Irving et al, 1975).

Fat metabolism. Dietary triglycerides pass directly into the portal venous blood or enter the circulation as a lipid emulsion (chyle) via the thoracic duct. During fasting, free fatty acids (FFA) are mobilized, entering the circulation as albumin-FFA complexes which are taken up by the hepatocytes where the FFA are stored in triglyceride droplets, incorporated into plasma lipoproteins or catabolized to provide energy.

When peripheral fat mobilization is excessive or when hepatic injury prevents normal triglyceride metabolism, these accumulate in the liver and a 'fatty liver' develops. This is common in diabetics, in normal patients during starvation and in alcoholics.

Endogenous cholesterol synthesized in the liver is incorporated into plasma lipoproteins, excreted in the bile or converted to primary bile acids. Dietary cholesterol is absorbed into the lymphatic system in the presence of bile salts following partial esterification with fatty acids. Cholesterol is involved in the metabolism of lipids and is a source of the steroid hormones. In the liver, cholesterol is esterified with fatty acids and, when parenchymal damage is present, plasma cholesterol ester levels are reduced. Plasma cholesterol concentration is raised in many conditions associated with a secondary lipaemia (e.g. diabetes mellitus, myxoedema, biliary cirrhosis), cholestasis (when it is associated with an increase in high density lipoproteins) and during the late stages of pregnancy. Liver failure depresses serum levels of both lipoprotein and cholesterol, particularly when hepatic synthesis is impaired. A lowered plasma cholesterol is commonly found when severe infection or anaemia is present.

Cholesterol is excreted into the bile together with conjugated bile salts and phospholipids. Two primary bile acids — cholic and chenodeoxycholic acids — are synthesized from cholesterol and secreted in the bile as their taurine or glycine salts. These conjugated bile salts undergo active reabsorption from the small intestine (enterohepatic circulation) and between 20–30g are secreted and reabsorbed daily (Way, 1975). Faecal losses (about 0.5g) are balanced by resynthesis from cholesterol (Davidson et al, 1979).

Cirrhosis creates considerable diminution in the total bile acid pool and is accompanied by a decrease in cholesterol excretion. Thus serum cholesterol levels rise (Jefferies, 1975).

Malabsorption is a common accompaniment to liver disease as the secretion of conjugated bile salts falls and is insufficient to allow the formation of lipid micelles, necessary for absorption. This is commonly manifested by hypoprothrombinaemia owing to malabsorption of vitamin K.

Patients suffering from primary or secondary biliary cirrhosis may develop diarrhoea or steatorrhoea and subsequent weight loss together with symptoms of fat soluble vitamin deficiencies.

DISORDERS DUE TO LACK OF NUTRIENTS

Throughout the previous section a number of conditions have been mentioned which result from inadequate intake of nutrients into the body. This inadequate intake may be due to an inadequate or inappropriate diet or to disturbances of absorption, but the effect will be the same.

Malnutrition

Undernutrition affects the life and health of more people throughout the world than does any disease state. It represents not only dietary inadequacy but a tissue deficiency of one or more essential nutrients and may, therefore, arise from the intake of too few calories, too little high quality protein and/or multiple deficiencies of minerals and vitamins. The most important cause of tissue deficiency is the failure to eat an adequate diet as a result of poor food habits, lack of knowledge or poor economic status (Ch. 14). An adequate diet relies not only on eating enough food to satisfy the appetite but also eating the right kinds of foods to provide the essential nutrients.

Factors interfering with the absorption or utilization of nutrients, or which increase the rate of destruction, excretion or requirement for specific nutrients, mean that a normally adequate diet becomes inadequate and malnutrition develops. Many individuals do not eat an adequate diet every day and yet appear healthy. This is because their diet is generally good or because their requirement is reduced during the short period of inadequacy. If their diet was inadequate for many or protracted periods they would, eventually, develop signs of deficiency.

Malnutrition is no longer synonymous with underweight, and an overweight person may also be malnourished. Body weight alone is not an accurate parameter by which to assess nutritional status (see Ch. 14).

Malnutrition is frequently associated with chronic illness and aggressive or long-term medical or surgical treatment and surveys indicate that about half the medical and surgical in-patients are protein energy malnourished (Jung, 1981). The incidence of malnutrition is believed to be greater in surgical patients. Bistrian et al (1974) and Hill et al (1977) have found that the incidence increased to 55% one week after major surgery, a serious fact recognized in very few hospitals despite the clearly defined metabolic response to surgery or trauma.

Some causes of malnutrition and clinical consequences are shown in Figure 23.1

Protein calorie malnutrition (protein energy malnutrition: PEM)

This term covers a wide range of clinical disorders which are particularly devastating in children and result from an inadequate dietary intake of calories and high quality protein. The condition ranges from marasmus, a continued restriction of both energy and protein in addition to other nutrients, to kwashiorkor, a qualitative

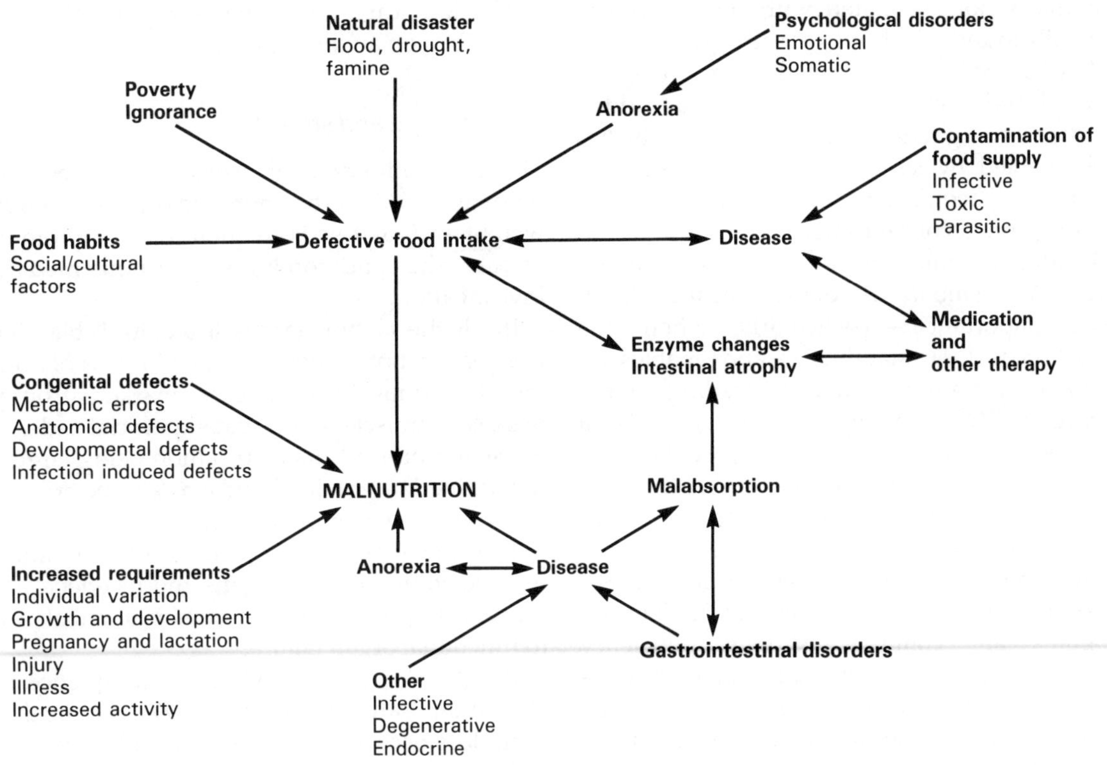

Fig. 23.1 The development of malnutrition (based on Williams, 1962)

and quantitative deficiency of protein when energy intake is adequate. Between these two extremes are clinical forms resulting from varying combinations of protein and energy deficiencies, combined with deficiencies of other trace nutrients.

PEM is less common, and usually less severe, in adults than in children and usually occurs as a sequelae to other diseases. Serious energy deficiency may result from chronic fever (as in tuberculosis), in malignancy or in diseases of the intestinal tract. Protein may be lost in many pathological conditions including diarrhoea, malabsorption syndrome or in the urine in the course of some renal disorders. It is, therefore, easy to see why Jung (1981) suggests that about half of the hospital population suffers from protein energy malnutrition. This is compounded by the effects of many treatment modalities. For example, radiation therapy and cancer chemotherapy can result in malabsorption, increased requirements and a subsequent protein energy deficiency state.

Causes and effects of PEM. The most obvious cause of protein deficiency is the combination of inadequate protein and calorie intake. Other, secondary causes are:

- impaired digestion or absorption of proteins (e.g. diarrhoea)
- inadequate plasma protein synthesis (e.g. hepatic disease)
- increased breakdown of body protein stores (e.g. prolonged fever, raised basal metabolic rate)
- excessive loss of protein (e.g. nephrotic syndrome, ascites, haemorrhage).

An inadequacy of protein and energy leads to the need to use body protein as an energy source and, if this is prolonged, to hypoproteinaemia and oedema. Oedema is one of the first clinical signs of a deficiency; in mild cases it is restricted to the lower limbs but, when the condition is severe, may extend to all parts of the body. Such oedema is not associated with the symptoms normally found which suggest other causes such as cardiac or renal disease. Weight change is marked and there may, in fact, be a sudden increase in weight due to fluid retention which is accompanied by lassitude and weakness. The diagnosis is confirmed by estimation of the plasma protein concentration.

Treatment and implications for nursing care. *Assessment.* A dietary history is of great importance – particularly when the condition is long standing – and enables an evaluation of possible deficits leading to the condition. Of particular importance is a consideration of protein content, quality and utilization as well as other factors of the diet, such as the energy, mineral and vitamin content, as the clinical manifestations of PEM are often complicated by other nutritional deficiencies. For example, concurrent deficiencies of the B group vitamins are common. Protein deficiency typically results in a mild normocytic, normochromic anaemia which is often complicated by simultaneous deficiencies of iron, vitamin B_{12}, folic acid and other haemopoietic factors.

Management. Dehydration and serious electrolyte imbalance often arise from a coexistent diarrhoea – in this case correction of these effects forms the basis of the immediate management.

The major requirement, however, is a diet providing all essential nutrients as it is important that these are all supplied, in addition to protein and an energy intake adequate to replace and maintain body weight and to spare body protein. For example, protein replacement without vitamin A can precipitate vitamin A deficiency, as the protein carrier now available depletes the liver of the stores which were present. Depletion of magnesium and potassium accompanies protein depletion; these must be replaced at the same time.

The return to normal serum protein concentrations is slow – approximately 30g protein must be deposited in the tissues before 1g is retained in the circulation. Nonetheless the treatment of any form of undernutrition must be undertaken with caution and refeeding must be instituted slowly (Scrimshaw, 1975).

Nursing care must be symptomatic and prescribed on an individual basis.

Underweight and starvation

The term underweight applies to individuals who are 15–20% or more below ideal body weight and, as this is frequently a symptom of disease, the condition always warrants medical investigation.

In all the circumstances listed in Table 23.6 there is wasting of body tissue with loss of both muscle and fat. In severe cases marked atrophy of skeletal muscle occurs and superficial oedema is usually present, its distribution being largely determined by gravity. Fluid may also be present in the peritoneal or pleural cavities.

The metabolic consequences of starvation involve all tissues and organs and its effects are far reaching, ranging from metabolic imbalance to functional organ failure.

Weight loss is an inevitable consequence of starvation. Van Itallie & Yang (1977) indicate that rapid loss occurs on the first day and up to 11% of body weight in 24 days, water representing 70% and fat 25% of this weight loss. However, in prolonged starvation a decrease of 24.2% was noted over a 24 week period, in which water contributed 48%, fat 40% and protein 12% during the first 12 weeks (Keys et al, 1950). In the later stages fat contributed up to 54% of the loss of body mass.

Thus, the major effect of starvation is progressive depletion of tissue fat as the sources of energy change as fasting progresses. Protein stores are depleted rapidly at first to provide glucose (through gluconeogenesis) and to supply energy to the brain which, under normal circumstances, utilizes no other energy source. Felig et al (1969) have shown that, if protein catabolism was to continue at the rate found in acute starvation, death would occur by the 10th day. However, protein depletion is greatly slowed as the brain adapts to ketone oxidation, and enzymatic adjustments occur in the liver and kidney (Cahill et al, 1966) which combine to reduce gluconeogenesis. Increased amounts of energy are derived from fat until eventually more than 95% comes from this source (Grande,

Table 23.6 Development of undernutrition

Nutritional disturbance	Possible causative factors
Inadequate intake Affecting both quality and quantity of food consumed	1. Inadequate food selection 2. Disease states leading to anorexia, nausea and vomiting 3. Social or economic factors 4. Ignorance 5. Natural disasters, e.g. famine
Inadequate absorption or utilization	1. Gastrointestinal disease leading to malabsorption or inability to eat, e.g. dysphagia in carcinoma of the oesophagus 2. Congenital defects and inborn errors of metabolism
Alteration of requirements – increased metabolic rate	1. Presence of wasting disease such as tuberculosis or hyperthyroidism 2. Prolonged infection
Disturbance of appetite *or* Disturbance of normal tissue metabolism	1. May be metabolic in origin, e.g. renal or hepatic failure 2. Psychological or emotional stress 3. Psychological abnormality, e.g. anorexia nervosa

1968). Thus the body protein mass is spared until the stage is reached where fat stores are depleted and the only remaining energy source is protein; at that point protein stores are again rapidly depleted. Death follows when body proteins have been reduced to approximately half their normal level (Davidson et al, 1979).

Clinical features. Patients are thin and the skin is loose, confirming recent weight loss. The hair is dull and dry, the eyes dull and sunken, although due to wasting of the orbital tissues they may appear prominent; the skin is dry and thin, its elasticity reduced. Patches of brown pigmentation may be present on the face and trunk. Hypotension is common — the diastolic pressure is often difficult to estimate and the pulse falls progressively as the condition worsens. Hydraemia and mild anaemia are common, but severe anaemia is not a feature of simple starvation; it is, rather, indicative of other, coexistent disease. Amenorrhoea is common, puberty is often delayed, men lose their libido and may develop gynaecomastia.

Severe personality changes are common and, in the final stages, the personality may totally disintegrate. The ability to concentrate is markedly reduced and mental restlessness combines with physical apathy. The patient often becomes self-centred and hypochondriacal.

Secondary infection is common, often presenting in unusual ways; pyrexia is rare. Intractable diarrhoea is usually the terminal occurrence.

Treatment and implications for nursing care. The basic cause of underweight or starvation must be established before any programme of treatment is started as, if a disease state has initiated the condition, then its treatment forms part of the care and diet forms just one part of that treatment.

In conditions of simple undernutrition and underweight all that is required is adequate food. Foods selected must stimulate the appetite; meals should be given at scheduled times and mealtimes should be relaxed and unhurried. It must be recognized that it is often as difficult for an underweight individual to gain weight as it is for an obese person to lose it and it is not always easy to increase the food intake. The patient must be involved in planning his refeeding programme and will often make suggestions as to what will tempt him. If the cause is inadequate food selection, counselling and advice on budgeting, meal planning and preparation will be required and its success relies on the knowledge of staff proffering such advice.

In severe starvation the patient is seriously ill and intravenous (parenteral) nutrition may be necessary, as dysfunction of the gastrointestinal tract may mean that he or she is unable to cope with the large quantities of food required. The desire for food is often immense but provides no guide as to digestive capacity, thus oral food intake may have to be limited, particularly if diarrhoea is present.

Reduced levels of the intestinal enzymes mean that only bland foods can be tolerated and frequent, small meals should be offered as often as the patient is able to tolerate them. Skimmed milk is a suitable food to start the programme; flavouring may be added to provide variety and stimulate the appetite. Some patients may, however, have lactose intolerance and it may be necessary to use dilute milk solutions, 10–15% being a suitable starting strength; in some cases a lactose free diet may be required. As refeeding may result in a temporary increase in oedema, sodium should be restricted in the initial stages.

Some patients may refuse all foods, in which case nasogastric or parenteral feeding provide the only alternatives.

Constant attention is required and nursing staff should observe patients carefully in order to assess tolerance to feeding solutions. However, despite thoughtful care and a well-planned diet some patients show little improvement, and hypotension and diarrhoea persist. This suggests irreversible changes in the small intestinal wall or the myocardium and the prognosis is poor.

Vitamin and mineral deficiencies

Optimal mental and physical status depends on an adequate supply of all the required vitamins (see Ch. 14). The actions of the vitamins are closely interrelated and a deficiency of one may affect the metabolism of others.

Except in specific circumstances (such as severe injury or illness) vitamin deficiencies usually arise from a deficiency of the water soluble vitamins. Secondary deficiencies may be found in alcoholics, patients with gastro-intestinal or mental illness and, occasionally, as a result of drug therapy.

As with all nutritional deficiencies these conditions are most commonly seen amongst the poor, the uneducated and the neglected and, as Youmans (1964) points out, there is a likelihood of their being missed due to a low index of suspicion, unfamiliarity and a lack of experience with them on the part of the health care workers in this country. It is assumed that these conditions no longer occur and many of the diagnostic features are overlooked.

Water soluble vitamins

Vitamin C. A deficiency of vitamin C results in scurvy, a disease manifested by malaise, weakness and lassitude during the early stages followed by dyspnoea and aching in the bones and joints. Perifollicular haemorrhages and petechiae are characteristic features of fully developed scurvy and, as the condition becomes more advanced, ecchymoses develop and larger haemorrhages occur in the subcutaneous tissue, the muscles or the joints. The gums become swollen and spongy, tend to bleed easily and are usually infected. Anaemia may occur, wounds fail to heal and the scars of previous wounds may break down.

Frank scurvy is rare but a deficiency may be seen in individuals consuming a diet lacking in fruit and vegetables or in those who are under a considerable degree of physiological stress. However, it is occasionally found in the elderly, especially in men (Exton-Smith, 1978).

The treatment is administration of the vitamin, combined with a diet containing foods high in ascorbic acid. As vitamin C is heat labile and there fore destroyed by cooking, fresh and raw foods are recommended. Due to soreness of the mouth, liquid foods may be required at first followed by a gradual introduction of solids. 'Miraculous' cures follow administration of the vitamin.

The 'B' complex. *Thiamin.* Beriberi is a metabolic disease resulting from a continued deficiency of thiamin (vitamin B_1) which may arise from a faulty diet, faulty utilization or poor absorption. It occurs primarily in countries where polished rice is the staple food, providing a diet rich in carbohydrate but low in thiamin. It is also possible that the elderly utilize thiamin less efficiently and are at an increased risk of deficiency. Beriberi is the most important of the B vitamin deficiencies found in alcoholism.

The majority of cases of the condition are mild; subacute paraesthesia and altered reflexes being the most common characteristics. Tachycardia and cardiomyopathy are found in well-developed cases and are associated with oedema which may be generalized or limited in its distribution (wet beriberi). Foot and wrist drop are common and are associated with muscle tenderness and disturbances of sensation in the outer aspects of the thighs, chest and forearms.

A chronic, dry form of beriberi with foot and wrist drop may be found (generally in older adults). An infantile form of the disease may also be found.

The treatment of beriberi consists of intake of a balanced diet together with administration of the vitamin. In severe cases parenteral administration may be required for the first few days. A multivitamin supplement is advisable as other B vitamin deficiencies often occur concurrently.

Improvement is rapid but complete cure requires a long period of treatment, particularly with regard to any structural defects.

Riboflavin (vitamin B_2). Riboflavin deficiency is usually found in individuals who consume a marginal diet devoid of animal protein and leafy vegetables. The intake must be low for many months before symptoms become evident.

Early symptoms of ariboflavinosis are soreness and burning of the lips, mouth and tongue which lead to angular stomatitis and cheilosis. Photophobia, lacrimation and burning or itching of the eyes are common and dermatitis is usually present. This has a characteristic scaly, greasy appearance and is associated with erythema. The tongue is, characteristically, purplish red and often has deep fissures.

Riboflavin deficiency rarely occurs alone and its symptoms are not specific to this alone, thus diagnosis is difficult.

Riboflavin is widespread in foods of plant and animal origin; milk and milk products, eggs, meat, and liver in particular, are the best dietary sources. Thus the diet should include liberal amounts of these foods, and a supplement of 5mg twice daily is given. Lesions disappear within a few days.

Nicotinic acid (vitamin B_3). Pellagra is caused by a primary dietary deficiency of nicotinic acid, but the adequacy of the dietary supply is also influenced by the quantity and quality of dietary protein and, particularly, the availability of the amino acid tryptophan, the metabolic precursor of nicotinic acid.

Pellagra is primarily associated with maize (corn) diets, as maize has a low tryptophan and nicotinic acid content. An excessive leucine content in the diet also seems to be associated with the occurrence of pellagra (Krishnaswamy et al, 1976) as increased leucine increases the requirement for pyridoxine (vitamin B_6). Several of the enzymes in the tryptophan-nicotinic acid pathway are pyridoxine dependent and, when pyridoxine intake is low and a deficiency is present, disturbances of this pathway lead to deficient nicotinic acid production and, eventually, to pellagra.

The early signs of pellagra are non-specific and include anorexia, weakness, digestive disturbances and, often, irritability, anxiety and depression. As the condition progresses glossitis, stomatitis, diarrhoea and dermatitis develop, the latter usually being found on areas of skin exposed to sunlight. In the early stages the dermatitis resembles sunburn and, as the acute stage passes into a chronic phase, skin changes include thickening, scaling, hyperkeratinization and pigmentation. Psychic and emotional changes occur during early pellagra which progress to disorientation, delirium and hallucination. The patient may become hyperactive and manic or apathetic, lethargic and stuporous. Anaemia from associated deficiencies is a common occurrence.

The treatment involves provision of a diet adequate in both nicotinic acid and tryptophan, combined with supplementation with these. Such treatment is most effective when it is combined with administration of other vitamins, as patients with pellagra are usually suffering from multiple deficiencies.

Acute symptoms improve within a few days but several weeks of treatment are necessary for full recovery. Iron therapy or folic acid supplementation may be required to cure the associated anaemia.

Fat soluble vitamins

Vitamin A. The best known effect of a

deficiency of vitamin A (retinol) is a loss of night vision (night blindness) which arises from a failure to regenerate rhodopsin, the light sensitive pigment present in the rods of the retina (also known as visual purple).

Xerophthalmia, a drying of the conjunctiva and later the cornea, is associated with atrophy of the periocular glands, and leads finally to keratomalacia and blindness. The condition may progress rapidly, particularly in children, once a deficiency becomes severe.

Characteristic changes of skin texture are found. Follicular hyperkeratosis (toad skin) or xeroderma (alligator skin) are common. Xeroderma represents a dryness of the skin with an associated fine layer of dandruff. Follicular hyperkeratosis represents a condition in which the hair follicles become blocked with keratin and the skin becomes dry, scaly and rough.

Treatment. Treatment is dependent on the administration of therapeutic doses of the vitamin and is combined with a correction of the dietary pattern and, where necessary, treatment of any underlying disease.

If the deficiency is associated with a protein deficiency, dietary protein alone may result in an improvement provided that hepatic stores of the vitamin are adequate. Protein repletion will ensure the appropriate transport protein is available.

Vitamin D. Rickets, a nutritional and metabolic disorder, is primarily a disease of infants and children in which calcification of the bones fails to occur normally. Osteomalacia is a disease of adulthood which is similar to the rickets seen in children.

Rickets normally results from a vitamin D deficiency and a corresponding disturbance of the calcium:phosphorus ratio. However, a diet lacking adequate calcium and/or phosphorus, or part absorption of these minerals, may also result in rickets.

Vitamin D is known as the antirachitic vitamin as it controls the absorption of calcium and phosphorus and the reabsorption of these substances from bone. Thus, a deficiency of the vitamin has three main effects:

- it impairs intestinal calcium absorption
- it reduces the responsiveness of the osteoclasts to parathyroid hormone
- it leads to defects in osteoblast activity and retards their activity.

The decreased sensitivity to parathyroid hormone is compensated for by an increase in the size of the parathyroid glands and a subsequent increase in secretion. This results in an enhanced response from the renal tubules and a decreased excretion of calcium accompanied by an increase in phosphate clearance.

Osteomalacia is attributed to one of five causative factors:

- a defect in renal tubular reabsorption
- a failure to respond to vitamin D
- a deficiency of vitamin D
- an inadequate calcium intake
- an excessive loss of calcium in the faeces.

It is characterized by softening of the bones and deformities especially of the spine, thorax, pelvis and limbs. General weakness and 'rheumatic' pain are typical symptoms, although there may also be a waddling gait and tetany. Secondary hyperparathyroidism, due to constant hypocalcaemia, may accompany osteomalacia. Pseudofractures may occur in association with severe muscle weakness and bone pain.

Treatment. This is directed both at correction of the vitamin D deficiency and at the underlying gastrointestinal disease (which is the usual cause of the deficiency). Exposure to ultraviolet light may be beneficial in patients with malabsorption, as skin manufacture of the vitamin will help to overcome the effects of the intestinal block.

However, it must be remembered that the most common bone disease resulting from malabsorption is osteoporosis and not osteomalacia. Osteoporosis is a metabolic disorder defined as a reduction in the amount of bone without any changes in its composition (deossification). Table 23.7 shows the differences between these two conditions.

Table 23.7 Differential diagnosis of osteoporosis and osteomalacia (based on Davidson et al, 1979)

Presentation	Osteoporosis	Osteomalacia
Clinical features		
Bone pain	Episodic — normally associated with a fracture	Persistent
Muscle weakness	Absent	Common — causes disability and characteristic 'waddling' gait
Fractures	Common presenting feature often following minimal trauma	Uncommon Healing delayed when occurs
Skeletal deformity	Follows fractures	Common
Radiological features		
Loss of bone density	Rare — most marked in spine	Widespread
Loss of bone detail	Not normally present	Characteristic
Histological changes	Reduced quantity of bone but composition is normal	Normal bone quantity but excess osteoid tissue present
Biochemical features		
Plasma calcium and phosphate	Normal	Frequently low
Plasma alkaline phosphatase	Normal	Often elevated
Urinary calcium	May be normal or high	Often depressed
Response to vitamin D	No response	Dramatic

Some examples of mineral deficiencies

Calcium and phosphorus. The majority of the body calcium is in bone, and a significant deficiency results in bone disease. The extraosseus fraction (about 1%) is of great importance because of its effects on neuromuscular excitability and cardiac muscle. Most calcium salts also contain phosphate, which is important in its own right for its buffering power and its ability to form 'high energy' phosphate bonds, as well as for its association with calcium.

Calcium intake depends on both the dietary intake (of which approximately 30% is absorbed) and on the level of vitamin D and the synergistic effect of parathyroid hormone, which is necessary for adequate absorption. Within the intestine calcium may be rendered insoluble by phosphate, fatty acids or phytate, which bind the mineral preventing absorption and promoting its excretion. A diet which is otherwise satisfactory is unlikely to be deficient in phospate (Baron, 1973). However, phosphate absorption may be reduced by giving antacids containing aluminium hydroxide, as this forms the insoluble salt, calcium hydroxide. Excess calcium in the intestine will cause precipitation of calcium phosphate; thus when calcium absorption is defective, inadequate phosphate absorption commonly occurs.

Calcium absorption commonly decreases with age when it may result from either inadequate vitamin D or from vitamin D 'resistance' (Nordin, 1973). This results in an elevation of serum calcium, particularly if it arose from an increased sensitivity of bone to parathyroid hormone resulting in increased mobilization of calcium. This raised serum calcium in turn reduces gastrointestinal absorption. Decreased renal function (also associated with ageing) also results in decreased calcium reabsorption.

Hypocalcaemia. Hypocalcaemia may be due to deficient calcium absorption, to hypoparathyroidism or to excessive renal losses, and causes hyperexcitability of the nervous system.

Such enhancement of neuromuscular excitability gives rise to tetany. Other effects include cataract formation and depression.

Hypercalcaemia. This usually arises from excess breakdown of bone from hyperparathyroidism or malignant disease (such as myeloma). It rarely arises as a result of excessive absorption, except where there is overdosage of vitamin D or hypersensitivity to the vitamin. Hypercalcaemia results in muscle weakness, gastrointestinal symptoms, dizziness, polydipsia and lassitude. Metastatic calcification may occur when plasma phosphate is raised, as calcium phosphate is formed and deposited at various sites in the body (e.g. renal calcification).

Changes in phosphate levels have few harmful effects in themselves except where they affect calcium distribution.

Osteoporosis, the deossification of bone, is often confused with osteomalacia (see Table 23.7). This is a reduction in the amount of bone which is not accompanied by any changes in the composition. As bone loss proceeds, skeletal strength is lost and fractures may occur following even minimal stress. The disease may be idiopathic or secondary to a known disorder when it is usually induced by endocrine, gastrointestinal or renal factors.

It is not entirely clear whether a calcium deficiency is a factor in the aetiology of osteoporosis, although Nordin (1973) has shown the condition to be associated with a negative calcium balance which, over a prolonged period, would result in a significant loss of skeleton. However, the ratio of calcium to phosphorus in the diet does appear to be a factor in the development of the condition. In the adult diet this ratio should be 1 although it is believed to be 1:4 at present (Lutwak, 1974). The phosphate intake is high as many popular foods — cereal, meat, potatoes — contain phosphate but very little calcium.

Osteoporosis develops slowly over a period of years and is, initially, manifested by weakness, anorexia and pain which may be associated with fractures which occur easily. As bones become involved pain, tenderness and muscle cramps occur, and bowing develops as the bone is unable to support the body weight. Stooped posture and a decrease in height are common due to spinal collapse.

An increase in both vitamin D and calcium intake is indicated and calcium infusions may be used to improve calcium retention, enhance formation of bone and reduce bone resorption. Sufficient vitamin D must be available to enable calcium taken into the body to be adequately utilized. Jowsey at al (1973) have found beneficial effects from concurrent administration of fluoride, although this is a controversial approach to treatment. Bone formation is stimulated although some workers feel that the bone thus formed is of an inferior quality. However, it has also been found that when fluoride intake is optimal, calcification of the aorta is much less common (Hegsted, 1967).

During treatment, exercise is indicated to prevent atrophy of bone.

Iodine. Body iodine is stored by the thyroid gland in which it is used for synthesis of the thyroid hormones. A deficiency of ingested iodine results in goitre, an enlargement of the gland. Goitrogens in food can also cause goitre by their inhibition of the thyroid function.

The iodine content of food is an important factor which determines the incidence of goitre, and its incidence can be correlated with the intake of iodine from water or food in a particular region. The iodine content of animals or plants is determined by the environment in which they grow, and the amount of iodine in the drinking water may be regarded as a measure of the content of the soil and therefore of the foodstuffs grown in that region. However, drinking water per se contributes little iodine to the total intake (Murray et al, 1948).

Iodine in food and water is rapidly absorbed from the gastrointestinal tract, mostly as inorganic iodide, and taken up by the thyroid gland where it is oxidized to iodine and immediately bound to tyrosine with the formation of mono-iodotyrosine and di-iodotyrosine and the subsequent conversion of these into the hormones tri-iodothyronine and thyroxine.

The thyroid hormones determine the metabolic rate of body cells, and if secretion is deficient basal metabolism falls, circulation is reduced and the patient generally 'slows down' (see myxoedema — Ch. 19).

When iodine is not available for hormone production, the pituitary responds by increasing its secretion of thyroid stimulating hormone (TSH), thus plasma TSH concentration is abnormally high. This in turn stimulates the gland to increase its uptake of iodine and normally leads to an enlargement of the gland.

In most cases of simple goitre there are few clinical manifestations other than an enlargement of the gland, but this may require surgical treatment either for aesthetic reasons or as a result of serious respiratory embarrassment or other effects of retrosternal growth.

Nutrients and anaemia

Macrocytic anaemia accompanied by a megaloblastic bone marrow results from a deficiency of folic acid or vitamin B_{12}, whereas iron deficiency results in microcytic, hypochromic anaemia. Deficiencies of all three nutrients will result in anaemia showing features of both those mentioned above.

Macrocytic anaemia is seen in tropical sprue or following resection or disease of the terminal ileum, when vitamin B_{12} is inadequately absorbed. When bacterial overgrowth occurs in the upper small intestine this type of anaemia may occur, and administration of a broad spectrum antibiotic may be all that is required to restore normal absorption. In contrast to pernicious anaemia, absorption is not increased by the concurrent administration of the intrinsic factor and vitamin B_{12}.

Megaloblastic anaemia may, rarely, be seen in patients with adult coeliac disease (gluten sensitive enteropathy) when absorption of B_{12} is impaired.

Megaloblastosis and anaemia may also be seen in folic acid deficiency but, as there is frequently an associated deficiency of B_{12}, diagnosis depends on the findings of a low serum or erythrocyte folate level or the response to administration of the vitamin.

Iron absorption is often subnormal except when malabsorption results from an uncomplicated pancreatic insufficiency. Mucosal disease or the inability to release organic iron from inorganic compounds are the usual causes, although occult blood losses may contribute to anaemia.

As incorporation of iron into erythrocytes is dependent on both folic acid and vitamin B_{12}, iron deficiency may not become apparent until deficiencies of these have been corrected. Iron deficiency is common in gluten sensitive enteropathy and in the advanced stages of tropical sprue.

INTERACTION BETWEEN NUTRITION AND CERTAIN PATHOLOGICAL STATES AND TREATMENT MODALITIES

Drug-nutrient interactions

The interrelationship between drugs and nutritional status is a factor which must be considered when studying the nutrient supply. Both the therapeutic and side-effects of prescribed drugs may affect nutrient intake, metabolism or requirements (Table 23.8). Drug induced malnutrition most commonly develops in patients receiving long-term drug therapy.

Effects of drug therapy on nutrient metabolism

Change in carbohydrate metabolism. Marks (1974) has divided drugs affecting carbohydrate metabolism into 2 categories:

- those tending to lower fasting blood sugar with little or no improvement in glucose tolerance
- those tending to raise fasting blood sugar levels and reduce glucose tolerance (Table 23.8).

D'Arcy & Griffin (1979) have shown the thiazide diuretics to be potentially diabetogenic when given in high doses to recently developed diabetics, to those with a family history of diabetes or to those with hypertension, and therefore recommend that carbohydrate tolerance be estimated prior to commencing such therapy.

Diazoxide inhibits insulin release and is

Table 23.8 Possible effects of drugs on nutritional status

Changes in nutritional status	Effect	Drugs (examples only)
Alterations of food intake		
Changes in appetite	Increased	Alcohol, insulin, steroids, Biguanides,
	Decreased	Indomethacin, Morphine
Changes in taste sensation	Decreased sweet	Amphetamines
	Decreased sensitivity	Phenytoin
	Nausea and vomiting	Many cancer chemotherapeutic agents
Alteration of nutrient absorption		
Luminal effects:		
Changes in GI motility	Reduction in transit time	Cathartic agents
Changes in bile acid activity	Inhibition of fat digestion and absorption	Neomycin Clofibrate
Drug nutrient complexes	Binds pyridoxine (vitamin B_6) so that absorption inhibited	Isoniazid
Mucosal effects:		
Inactivation of absorptive enzyme systems	Malabsorption of fat and vitamin B_{12}	Colchicine
	Decreased absorption of sucrose and xylose	Neomycin
Damage to mucosal cells	Malabsorption	Neomycin, cathartic agents
Alteration of nutrient metabolism	Folate antagonism	Methotrexate
	Interference with vitamin D metabolism	Phenytoin
Alteration of nutrient excretion	Excretion of folate, hypercalcuria	Aspirin Frusemide
Drugs causing hyperglycaemia		Phenothiazines, Probenecid, Phenytoin,
Drugs causing hypoglycaemia		Sulphonamides, Aspirin, Barbiturates,
Drugs increasing plasma lipids		Corticosteroids, Chlorpromazine,
Drugs reducing plasma lipids		Phenformin Colchicine, Phenindione

therefore a potent diabetogenic agent (Okun et al, 1963), particularly when combined with a thiazide diuretic.

A number of patients undergoing corticosteroid therapy will develop hyperglycaemia (Schubert & Schulte, 1963) and diabetic patients receiving even topical applications of steroids may absorb sufficient to disturb their management.

The therapeutic effect of the sulphonylureas is to control hyperglycaemia, but their use may cause serious hypoglycaemia. This commonly occurs as a result of an interaction with another drug (e.g. warfarin, phenylbutazone) when these displace sulphonylureas from their binding sites on plasma proteins, thus greatly increasing the amount of drug reaching the tissues. Other drugs may compete for the hepatic drug metabolizing enzymes, decreasing their rate of degradation and thus potentiating their hypoglycaemic effect (Marks, 1974).

Effect on lipids. A number of drugs affecting the absorption of fat have been identified (Truswell, 1973). These include neomycin, which creates morphological changes in the jejunal villi and therefore causes fat malabsorption; phenindione, para-amino-salicylic acid (PAS) and aspirin may produce similar effects.

Other drugs lower plasma lipid concentration by decreasing lipolysis and may be used clinically in the treatment of hyperlipidaemia. Cholestyramine, the treatment of choice in Type II hyperlipidaemia, will lower plasma cholesterol but, in large doses, induces steatorrhoea with its attendant problems. Clofibrate, used to treat Types IIb, III, IV and V hyperlipidaemia, reduces plasma cholesterol, VLDL (very low density lipoproteins) and triglycerides.

Some drugs (e.g. oral contraceptives, large doses of corticosteroids and ethanol) raise plasma triglyceride concentrations, and oral contraceptives also raise plasma cholesterol levels. Phenobarbitone has been found to raise both triglyceride and cholesterol concentrations (Miller & Nestel, 1973).

Effect on protein metabolism. A number of drugs cause negative nitrogen balance by increasing the urinary excretion of nitrogen (e.g. thyroid hormones, corticosteroids). Others, such as the anabolic steroids, have the opposite effect and stimulate protein synthesis.

Alterations in minerals and vitamin metabolism. Drugs interfering with the action of a vitamin, or the enzymes dependent upon it, include antimetabolites (e.g. mercaptopurine), antivitamins (e.g. methotrexate), and enzyme inducers (e.g. anticonvulsants).

Antimetabolites and antivitamins block enzymatic reactions as the enzyme takes up these substances instead of the actual vitamin or its metabolites. This action forms the basis of some cancer chemotherapeutic agents, which are taken up by rapidly dividing cells which die when the antivitamin does not function in the same way as the real vitamin. Methotrexate, for example, is a folic acid analogue which prevents folic acid binding to the enzymes so that it is excreted. Without folic acid, DNA synthesis is inhibited, cell replication ceases and the cells die. This induced folic acid deficiency will lead to macrocytic anaemia if the folic acid is not replaced once treatment is completed.

Other drugs may affect metabolism of a nutrient by forming a complex with it and making it unavailable for use by the body. An example is isonicotinic acid hydrazide (isoniazid), used in the long term treatment of tuberculosis, which binds pyridoxine (vitamin B_6) so that it is excreted in the urine (Vilter, 1964).

Long-term anticonvulsant therapy may result in clinical rickets or osteomalacia due to increased induction of the hepatic enzymes, which in turn interfere with vitamin D metabolism so that there is a smaller amount of the active vitamin available (Matheson et al, 1976). Low serum folate levels and, on occasions, macrocytic anaemia occur in many patients undergoing long-term anticonvulsant therapy (Reynolds, 1974).

Effects of nutrient deficiency on drug metabolism

The metabolism of drugs may be altered in nutritional deficiency as the activity of hepatic drug metabolizing enzymes depends on an adequate intake of protein, lipids, carbohydrate and certain trace nutrients, notably riboflavin (vitamin B_2), ascorbic acid (vitamin C), zinc and magnesium (Basu & Dickerson, 1974). Other factors influencing drug metabolism include the rate of absorption and transport to the liver, the presence of disease, liver function and concurrent administration of other drugs which may alter the rate of metabolism of the first drug. Such effects may be of particular clinical significance and may increase or decrease the toxicity of a drug.

Nutrient supply can affect drug metabolism in one of two ways. First, when the dietary intake of energy is low, tissue protein is catabolized to provide energy, thus fewer amino acids are available for protein synthesis and the levels of the necessary enzymes are reduced. Second, there may be competition between the metabolism of drugs and the needs of the tissues for particular nutrients.

However, when studying drug-nutrient interactions, it must be remembered that clinical nutritional deficiencies normally result from a combination of factors and are more likely to occur in patients having marginal nutritional status before a drug is prescribed.

Surgery and trauma

Effects of surgery and trauma on metabolism

Surgery and trauma have profound effects on metabolism and, in Britain, approximately half of the patients who have a major abdominal operation suffer from malnutrition (Klidjian, 1981). Yet nutrition is often neglected in the care of such patients, particularly in the unconscious patient who is unable to voice his discomfort or to adjust to his changed needs (Hitchcock & Masson, 1970).

The problem was first recognized by Cuthbertson (1930) and later by Studley (1936), who showed that the most important single factor affecting morbidity was pre-operative weight loss, and those patients losing one-quarter of their weight had a 30% mortality rate.

Moore (1959) has summarized these effects as a four phase response:

- the injury phase — an acute catabolic phase lasting between 2–4 days
- the turning point — (about one week after injury) when the body changes from a catabolic to an anabolic state
- protein anabolism — restoration of the lean cell mass (muscle) taking 3–4 weeks (may be longer depending on the severity of the injury)
- fat anabolism — replacement of the body storage fat and return to pre-trauma weight: this takes approximately 6 weeks and corresponds to the usual period of convalescence

Obviously these stages may be modified by the severity of the injury and by postoperative complications (Smiddy, 1976).

The injury (catabolic) phase is the most important, as once the patient is over this, recovery is on the way. The most readily available energy source, liver glycogen, is rapidly depleted and the breakdown of lean body mass and fat begins. Thus, during this phase, protein catabolism exceeds protein synthesis and muscle protein is used to supply energy via gluconeogenesis and nitrogen excretion (as urea) rises. The extent of protein degradation can, therefore, be estimated by the net loss of nitrogen in the urine, 10g being lost daily following moderate trauma. This is equivalent to 25g protein or 250g muscle tissue (Bucknall, 1979). Oxidation of peripheral fat stores accounts for 70–80% of the energy in the postoperative phase (Lee, 1978) and blood levels of free fatty acids (FFA) and triglycerides rise. The FFA are either utilized directly in the peripheral tissue or converted into acetoacetate and β-hydroxybutyrate (the ketone bodies) to provide an energy substrate, whilst glycerol is transported to the liver and converted to glucose. These changes are mediated by the catabolic hormones, adrenaline, cortisol and glucagon, which predominate over insulin, the main anabolic hormone.

During the injury phase, therefore, there is a net loss of protein with a negative nitrogen balance, and an associated retention of water and sodium with a net loss of potassium (due to aldosterone secretion). The breakdown of body tissue leads to an increase in body water, which may mask weight loss, and the increase in water results in dilution of serum sodium so that a homeostatic release of antidiuretic hormone occurs, creating further water retention. At the same time, energy requirements are markedly increased as both the metabolic rate and resting energy expenditure rise. This can, in part, be explained by the increased requirement for water loss by evaporation and can be reduced by nursing the patient in a higher ambient temperature. However, energy reserves tend to be utilized at 4 times the normal rate (Bucknall, 1979) and, if energy is not supplied, the body will exhaust its stores in about 10 days.

Losses of 4–8% body weight often follow even uncomplicated surgery, although it is generally agreed that losses of up to 10% can be sustained without prejudice to convalescence (Dickerson, 1982).

The failure to feed a normally well-nourished individual for the first few days is of little significance. However, when injury is severe or when patients cannot take adequate oral feeding, a failure to take corrective action will ensure that the patient continues to starve and can only be detrimental to his recovery.

Management. The alimentary tract provides the most satisfactory route by which to instigate feeding, provided that it is functional, as this avoids the problems associated with parenteral nutrition (see Ch. 14). For intragastric feeding a nasogastric or fine bore feeding tube is passed through the nose into the stomach (see discussion on tube feeding, Ch. 14). Gastric emptying may be delayed following surgery, thus tube feeds must be given with caution and certainly not until bowel sounds are heard. Gastric aspiration must be carried out prior to every feed to ensure that the stomach is emptying. It is usual to start the feeding regime with saline or glucose solutions, giving 30ml/hr initially and increasing to 90ml/hr if this can be tolerated (Bucknall, 1979). Half strength milk, glucose and water may be given on the second day, increasing the quantity given, but by the third day the energy content must be increased by giving the appropriate tube feed formula. The energy requirement may be as much as 12.6 – 25.2MJ (3000–-6000 kcal) daily and the protein 1g/kg body weight, but during the catabolic phase this may be greatly increased and the need to provide a high protein diet cannot be overemphasized (Hitchcock & Masson, 1970).

When oral intake is inadequate and tube feeding unsatisfactory, parenteral nutrition must be instigated.

Cancer and cancer therapy

Effect on the patient

Many patients with cancer lose weight at some point during their illness, the degree and severity depending to some extent on the site of the tumour and the type of malignancy involved. Subsequent treatments, surgery, chemotherapy or radiotherapy, may limit the patient's food intake for prolonged periods of time, compromising both the patient's condition and his response to treatment (Holmes, 1983). A growing neoplasm will extract nutrients from its host (Copeland et al, 1979) exacerbating malnutrition, particularly when the host is unable to ingest nutrients in amounts large enough to supply the demands of both host and tumour. Table 23.9 indicates possible nutritional problems in these patients.

Table 23.9 Consequences of malnutrition

Weight loss
Muscle wasting
Hypoproteinaemia
Oedema
Anaemia — iron, folic acid or vitamin B_{12} deficiency
Haemorrhage or other bleeding disorders
Increased susceptibility to infection due to decreased immunocompetence
Delayed wound healing
Increased toxicity of drugs
General debility, apathy and depression

Chemotherapeutic agents, in general, act by interfering with cellular function and replication thus causing cell death. They are, however, unable to discriminate between normal and malignant cells and their effects are seen first on rapidly replicating cells such as those of the tumour, but also those of the bone marrow and gastrointestinal tract. The effects on the latter are commonly the most dramatic and, as they include nausea, vomiting, diarrhoea, stomatitis and mucositis, may have significant implications for the nutrient supply (Holmes, 1983). The profound effects of these agents on the intestinal mucosa and/or the major secreting organs, coupled with the effects of the disease process itself, may result in the development of the malabsorption syndrome.

Radiation therapy, particularly if directed at any portion of the gastrointestinal tract, may also result in malabsorption and serious nutritional disturbances (Donaldson, 1977), even in patients receiving only low dose radiation (Trier &

Browning, 1966). Diarrhoea, which frequently occurs during or following radiation therapy, further contributes to malabsorption and has been attributed to a significant net movement of sodium and water from the blood into the lumen of the irradiated bowel (Goodner et al, 1955). The net result of radiation enteritis is that the patient eats less food and is less able to digest and absorb those nutrients reaching the small intestine (Trier & Browning, 1966; Terpila, 1971; Jervis et al, 1969).

A serious degree of associated malnutrition may deny some patients sufficient therapy and nutritional support is clearly a necessary adjunct to cancer therapy. Many workers (De Wys et al, 1980; Lanzotti et al, 1975) have shown this to be the case and patients who are nutritionally depleted tend to show a poorer response to chemotherapy. However, nutritional repletion of cancer patients has been criticized on the basis that it might increase tumour growth. There is, at present, little evidence to support this and Copeland et al (1979) have found no evidence of increased tumour growth in studies involving over 1000 patients.

Studley (1936) was amongst the first to recognize the importance of nutritional status in determining the clinical outcome. It has since been recognized that increased morbidity and mortality are consequent upon protein and calorie malnutrition.

Management. Early in the management of the disease a nutritional history should be obtained, which allows the monitoring of changes in weight, food consumption and meal composition (Ch. 14).

Anorexia, a common side effect of cancer and its treatment, must receive special attention from the nurse; efforts to encourage the patient to eat should be aggressive, persevering and compassionate, yet all steps must be taken to ensure that the oral intake is adequate (Holmes, 1983). Changes in taste sensation, experienced by many patients, may mean that food tastes excessively bitter or sweet or, in some cases, has no taste (hypogueutsia). These can make feeding the patient more difficult, and considerable ingenuity may be needed to find suitable foods. Many patients continue to enjoy their favourite dishes but such changes in taste or the presence of stomatitis or mucositis may make even these unpalatable.

Control of the symptoms limiting food intake (nausea and vomiting, pain) or absorption (diarrhoea) will play a valuable role in overcoming many of the problems, and may pave the way for periods of comparatively good health and significantly affect the patient's quality of life. Thus, local anaesthetic mouthwashes or sucking crushed ice may help those with pain or discomfort on eating or swallowing. Liquids given with a meal may make eating easier but may limit the intake of solids. Appetite may be stimulated by alcohol when this is given before meals.

Early satiety is another common problem. When this occurs frequent small meals are often better tolerated and, to ensure nutritional requirements are met, nutritional supplements may be required.

When the oral intake is insufficient to maintain weight, additional measures may be required which may include tube feeding or parenteral nutrition.

Failure to maintain body weight is indicative of nutritional failure which may, in turn, lead to all the effects of malnutrition (Table 23.9) which, when superimposed upon the effects of the disease and its treatment, clearly show the need for nutritional support and the role of the nurse in this area of patient care.

Infection

The severity and outcome of infection are frequently worsened by malnutrition, and patients fed on a diet low in protein may develop a lowered resistance to infection as a result of decreased immunocompetence. In turn, infection may precipitate nutritional disease in the malnourished.

Effect of infection on nutritional status

The most common effect of infection is anorexia, accompanied by a change to a liquid diet based on carbohydrate at the expense of other nutrients — particularly protein. In addition,

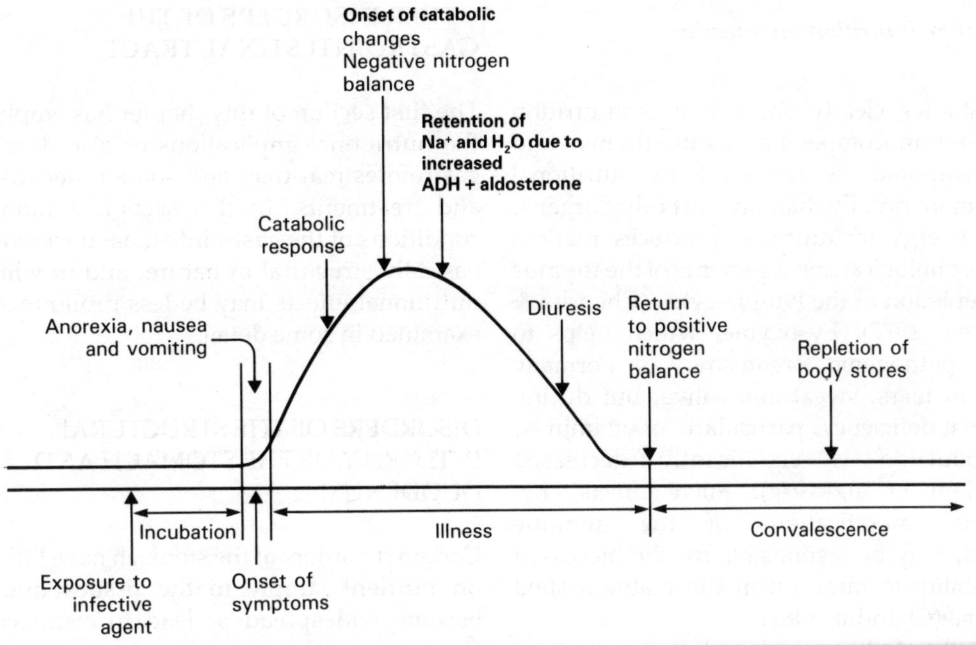

Fig. 23.2 The catabolic response to infection (based on Beisel, 1976)

therapeutic agents (e.g. antibiotics, purgatives) may have effects on absorption or on the intestinal flora and therefore on the synthesis of some nutrients. In addition, the effects of fever will increase both basal metabolism and the loss of nutrients in the sweat.

An acute infection will result in a response which is similar to that discussed under surgery and trauma and is mediated by cortisol and insulin. This results in a mobilization of amino acids from the body tissues to be used, through gluconeogenesis, to maintain blood glucose levels. Nitrogen losses during infection, even when this is mild and asymptomatic, result in a negative nitrogen balance (Scrimshaw, 1965) even when the patient is receiving an adequate protein intake.

The catabolic response (Fig. 23.2) commences with the onset of fever and, in addition to a negative nitrogen balance, results in disturbances of potassium, magnesium, zinc, phosphate and sulphate balance, all of which may continue into convalescence. When infection is severe or prolonged, muscle wasting and weight loss will occur. Hyperglycaemia results from a decreased insulin secretion combined with a tissue resistance to insulin, which explains why normally well-controlled diabetics require more insulin during an infective illness.

The duration of this response is dependent upon the nature and extent of the cause but will normally last for several days. The following anabolic phase, when protein requirements are high to allow tissue repletion, is generally twice as long (Scrimshaw, 1975).

Infection associated with vomiting or diarrhoea will add to the nutritional stress by reducing absorption and therefore the availability of nutrients.

Vitamin deficiencies are common during acute infective episodes. For example, the synthesis of the B vitamins by the intestinal flora may be affected by intestinal infections as well as by drugs used in its treatment. In addition, an infective episode will precipitate a decrease in blood levels of zinc and of iron (Scrimshaw, 1975) and may be associated with losses of sodium, chloride, potassium and phosphorus, particularly when diarrhoea is present.

Effects of malnutrition on infection

Many studies clearly show that malnutrition affects immunocompetence, as the thymus and other lymphoid tissues react to nutritional deficits more rapidly than do most other organs. Protein energy malnutrition produces marked histomorphological derangements of the thymus and a depletion of the lymphocytes (Chandra & Newberne, 1977). Lysozyme, which helps to destroy pathogenic organisms, is normally present in tears, sweat and saliva, but during nutritional deficiency, particularly of vitamin A, its production is significantly decreased (Mohanram et al, 1974). Such effects, i.e. nutritional modifications of the immune response, may be responsible for the increased susceptibility to infection in the malnourished individual (Chandra, 1981).

The cells of the reticuloendothelial system, macrophages amongst others, normally play an important role in protecting the body against bacterial invasion, but in protein and vitamin deficiency states their activity is reduced. Tissue changes and alterations in cilial movement and in the mucus trapping of infecting agents are all altered by malnutrition (Chandra, 1981).

Nutritional deficiencies also affect tissue integrity and wound healing. The integrity of epithelial tissues (the skin and mucus membranes) is altered by certain pathologic changes, thus mucus secretion may be reduced, mucosal surfaces become permeable, oedema of the underlying tissue may occur and the accumulation of cellular debris provides a favourable medium for the growth of infecting organisms. Deficiencies of vitamin A, ascorbic acid, thiamin, riboflavin, niacin and protein are likely to produce such effects (Scrimshaw, 1975).

The effects on wound healing result from changes in the fibroblastic response and collagen formation, and arise particularly from protein deficiency. Ascorbic acid deficiency will result in a failure to synthesize the particular amino acids from which collagen is made.

OTHER DISORDERS OF THE GASTROINTESTINAL TRACT

The first section of this chapter has emphasized the nutritional implications of disorders of the gastrointestinal tract and some other disorders and treatments. In this section a number of conditions of the gastrointestinal tract which are basically structural in nature, and in which the nutritional effects may be less pronounced, are examined in some detail.

DISORDERS OF THE STRUCTURAL INTEGRITY OF THE STOMACH AND DUODENUM

Certain disorders of the stomach have little effect on nutrient supply to the tissues until they become widespread or lead to complications. Carcinoma of the stomach and gastric ulceration are the obvious examples. As the causes and management of gastric and duodenal ulcers are so similar they will be examined together as peptic ulcers.

Peptic ulceration

A peptic ulcer is a distinct break in the continuity of the mucosa of the stomach or duodenum.

Incidence

Langman et al (1983) review recent advances in knowledge about the stomach and duodenum. They cite a number of studies indicating that the incidence of peptic ulceration, as indicated by admission and mortality rates, has dropped over the past 20 years. While men are affected more frequently than women, most of the drop in incidence has been amongst the male section of the population. These changes were beginning before the development of new and more effective methods of medical treatment.

Peptic ulceration appears to be more common in urban than in rural parts of England and Wales and is the cause of considerable loss of working days, even though this has dropped from 64.8 to 37.1 days per 100 workers per year between 1954

Table 23.10 Social class and ulcer frequency (Registrar General, 1971). Standardized mortality ratio in England and Wales by social class, 1959–63

Type of ulcer	Social class				
	I	II	III	IV	V
Gastric ulcer	46	58	94	106	109
Duodenal ulcer	70	84	113	102	136

and 1979 (Wells 1981). Gastric ulceration is less common than ulceration of the duodenum but both are more common in unskilled than in skilled or professional workers (Table 23.10) (Registrar-General, 1971).

Aetiology

In both gastric and duodenal ulceration the balance between the potentially damaging effects of the gastrointestinal secretions and the protective properties of the mucosa is disturbed. It is suggested by Feldman & Sabovich (1980) that peptic ulcer disease is a 'heterogenous group of disorders with a common final pathway leading to a "hole" in either the gastric or duodenal mucosa'.

Jones (1979) reviews factors involved in the pathogenesis of gastric ulcers but also indicates the 'essential unity between gastric and duodenal ulcers which may be dependent on vascular mechanisms'. Figure 23.3 shows factors which may be involved in the development of ulceration.

Presentation of disease

In both types of peptic ulceration the major symptom is pain, usually epigastric. The pain is often related to food intake, but not necessarily so, and frequently occurs at night particularly in those with duodenal ulceration (Baron et al, 1980). The pain is relieved by antacids. Because the pain is often related to food intake some patients with gastric ulcers may have been restricting their dietary intake for some time and will report marked weight loss.

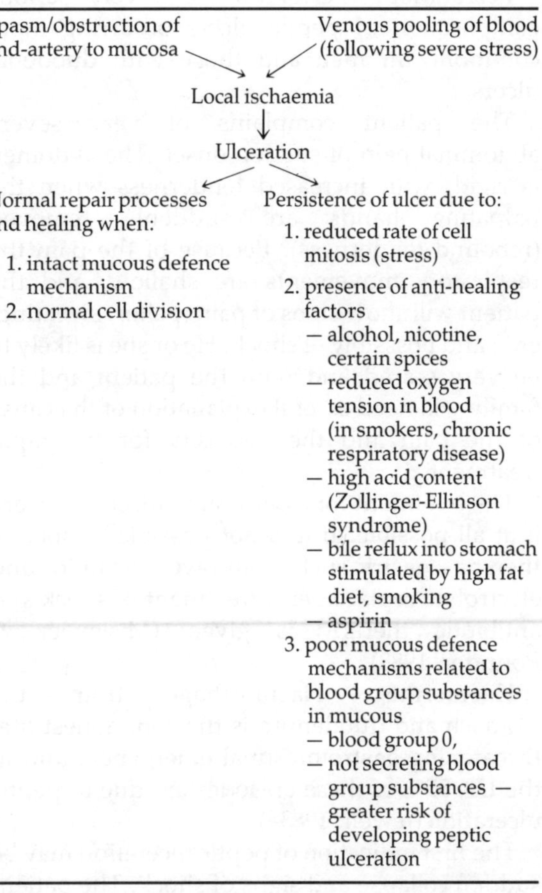

Fig. 23.3 Possible development of peptic ulceration (adapted mainly from Jones, 1979 and Wastell, 1979)

A barium meal may be used to outline the ulcer on X-ray, but fibreoptic endoscopy is the best method for diagnosing peptic ulceration. Apart from allowing direct inspection of the ulcer it also facilitates the taking of biopsies from the ulcer for histological examination for malignant cells. The care of patients undergoing diagnostic procedures is discussed in Chapter 11.

Although pain is the commonest symptom of peptic ulceration, it does not invariably occur and some patients do not go for medical help until complications of ulceration occur. It is these complications which are the major causes of morbidity and mortality. These complications are of three types:

- perforation
- haemorrhage
- fibrosis.

Perforation. Perforation is a very serious complication of peptic ulcers occurring more commonly in men and those with duodenal ulcers.

The patient complains of very severe abdominal pain of sudden onset. The abdomen is rigid, with increased tenderness when the palpating hands are suddenly removed (rebound tenderness). Because of the pain the respiratory movements are shallow, and the patient will show signs of pain (pallor, sweating, etc.) and posssibly of shock. He or she is likely to be very scared and both the patient and the family will need careful explanation of the cause of the pain and the necessity for the rapid treatment.

The treatment for a perforated ulcer is surgery if at all possible. If it is not possible to operate then nasogastric suction, intravenous fluids and electrolyte replacement, treatment of shock and antibiotic therapy is given (Misiewicz & Pounder, 1983).

Haemorrhage. Haemorrhage from the stomach and duodenum is the commonest life-threatening gastrointestinal emergency, and in the UK 55% of these episodes are due to peptic ulceration (Jewell, 1983a).

The first indication of peptic ulceration may be sudden collapse and signs of shock. The patient may vomit blood (haematemesis) or increased bowel activity may lead to lower abdominal colic followed by the defaecation first of normal stools and then of melaena, which is dark red or black in colour due to partial digestion of the blood. Spontaneous cessation of bleeding is common, but the amount of blood lost will usually result in a varying degree of anaemia.

On admission to hospital the patient is likely to be very frightened and, although the urgency of the technical management is necessary, it is possible and important to give some information and emotional support at the same time.

Medical management of the patient following such haemorrhage has three phases (Misiewicz & Pounder, 1983):

- resuscitation
- exact diagnosis
- treatment.

Resuscitation. If in a state of shock the patient will need the volume of blood restored by the intravenous administration of blood, (when cross-matched) plasma or colloidal volume expander. In the elderly or those with cardiac or renal disease a central venous line is inserted to allow monitoring of the central venous pressure during the rapid transfusion.

Even if not in a state of shock an intravenous infusion will be set up to allow rapid treatment should another haemorrhage occur, and to allow the correction of anaemia as soon as blood has been cross-matched. This will enable the patient to withstand further bleeding if it should occur.

Diagnosis. Exact diagnosis is necessary so that the appropriate treatment can be given, and the methods discussed previously are used. Endoscopy is the most effective aid to diagnosis but does carry with it certain risks, as it is an invasive procedure. However, it enables precise location of the bleeding site and some degree of prediction of rebleeding (Langman et al, 1983).

Treatment. The aim of treatment is to ensure survival but the mortality rate remains at approximately 10%. As the age of patients is increasing and, therefore, the risk associated with operation is greater, it appears that some improvement in treatment has occurred (Langman et al, 1983).

Drug therapy is sometimes used but its effectiveness in preventing further haemorrhage is not yet proven. Similarly, laser and electrocoagulation methods of haemostasis to prevent rebleeding have been tried, but again the results are mainly inconclusive.

Surgery is carried out when haemorrhage continues or when a number of high risk factors indicate that further haemorrhage is likely. These patients are often elderly and require skilled medical and nursing care to minimize the risk of postoperative complications and reduce the mortality rate.

Fibrosis. The fibrosis resulting from long-standing ulceration near to the pyloric sphincter of the stomach can result in pyloric stenosis and the onset of vomiting as pyloric obstruction increases. Weight loss is common and dehydration and electrolyte imbalance may develop.

The treatment of this condition is surgical following correction of fluid, electrolyte and nutritional disturbances.

Management

The aim of management of patients with peptic ulceration is to enhance healing of the ulcer by:

- relieving pain
- reducing the development of complications
- enabling an adequate nutritional intake.

Management may be either through medical or surgical treatment, although rarely would an operation be performed before medical treatment had been attempted, unless the patient has not presented until complications have developed.

Whatever the medical intervention being used, there are certain principles underlying the care of these patients which are of major concern to nursing. Factors identified in Figure 23.3 as implicated in the persistence of ulcers fall into three groups. Two of these can be modified by nursing intervention with patients:

- reduced rate of cell mitosis due to stress
- presence of anti-healing factors.

Minimizing stress. This is discussed in detail in Chapters 8 and 12. The patient with a peptic ulcer may or may not need to be in hospital for treatment, but one of the aims of nursing management is to help the patient to minimize stress resulting from physical or mental stimuli. Helping the patient to identify those factors which he or she perceives as stressful and to plan methods of coping adequately is an important part of the nursing management necessary for long-term benefit.

If the patient is in hospital, the resulting uncertainty and feelings of loss of control may increase stress. The nurse needs to involve the patient in the planning of care so that disruption to the normal pattern of daily activity is minimal and the feeling of control is enhanced.

Rest is a major aspect of the management of patients with peptic ulceration and advice on curtailing unnecessary activity, getting adequate rest during the day and a good night's sleep should be given. Usually bed rest is not necessary except in those 'with intractable symptoms, in labourers and in certain anxious individuals' (Marks, 1979). Teaching methods of relaxation may be helpful.

Minimizing anti-healing factors. Until recently regular feeding and taking antacids, along with bed rest, were the standard treatments for peptic ulceration. These still play an important part in raising the pH in the stomach by buffering the acid secreted and thus enhancing healing. Buchman et al (1969) found that this treatment resulted in 101 of 103 patients becoming asymptomatic within 2 days. They also found that whether a bland or the standard hospital diet was given was immaterial. Patients should be advised, therefore, to eat small meals at frequent intervals and to avoid only those foods which exacerbate their symptoms.

They should also be advised to restrict their alcohol intake and to avoid taking aspirin, as these are known to disturb the integrity of the gastric mucosa (Geall et al, 1970). Smoking should be restricted or stopped in order to enhance the oxygen supply to the stomach lining and enhance healing.

Medical treatment. Rest, frequent feeding and antacids are the mainstay of treatment. Antacids such as magnesium trisilicate or aluminium hyroxide are usually given in 15–30ml doses ½ to 1 hour after meals, at night and when needed to relieve pain. Antacid tablets are often convenient to use and can be taken liberally (see earlier).

Anticholinergic drugs are frequently used, although these cause side-effects such as dry mouth and, sometimes, difficulty in micturition. They are avoided in the elderly and when gastric emptying is slowed. A number of newer drugs have been developed which act in various ways on the cortico-hypothalamic pathways which regulate gastric activity, on acid-pepsin levels or mucosal resistance, or which increase gastric emptying. The effectiveness of many of these drugs has not yet been clearly demonstrated (Marks, 1979).

Cimetidine, a H_2-receptor antagonist, causes a considerable reduction in acid secretion and appears to enhance ulcer healing with relatively few side-effects. However, there is a high incidence of recurrence, although it is not entirely clear whether this is higher following treatment with cimetidine than following other medical treatment (Marks, 1979).

Medical treatment will result in healing of 80% of all peptic ulcers, and more of those without complication (Marks, 1979), but some patients will continue to require surgery.

Surgical treatment. Surgical treatment of peptic ulceration aims:

- *either* to remove the ulcerated part of the stomach
- *or* to reduce acid secretion by cutting the vagus nerve, while minimizing the risk of recurrence and reducing after-effects of the operation due to interference with gastric motility or nutrient absorption.

A range of operations has been developed that reduce acid secretion through division of the vagus nerve, modify drainage of the stomach which may have been altered by vagotomy, or resect part of the stomach (Fig. 23.4 also shows total gastric resection used in treatment of carcinoma of the stomach). Kennedy (1979) critically discusses the range of operations used and reviews the evidence of their effectiveness in achieving the above aims. He concludes that, although there is a wide range of possible operations for patients with duodenal ulcers, a proximal gastric vagotomy (highly selective vagotomy) without drainage is probably the best choice. In this procedure only the vagus nerve supply to the acid-secreting part of the stomach is severed. Thus, the secretion of acid is reduced but the motor activity of the antrum and pylorus is not affected, and gastric emptying continues with little or no alteration. The mortality rate is very low (0.5%) but the recurrence rate may be higher than for some other types of surgery, although it has not been performed long enough for the evidence about this to be available.

In gastric ulceration, Kennedy suggests that the operation of choice is a Bilroth I gastrectomy. The part of the stomach liable to ulceration, the antrum, is excised and the remainder anastomosed end-on to the duodenum. This operation has a low rate of recurrence of ulceration (1.5%) and a low mortality rate (1.8%).

Following gastric surgery the patient will have a nasogastric tube in position and an intravenous infusion running. The nasogastric tube will be used to remove gastric secretions until normal motility returns, and intravenous fluids will be given until oral fluids can be tolerated. The length of time for which these are needed will vary depending on the operation performed and the time taken for gut motility to return, indicated by bowel sounds being heard and flatus passed.

Complications of gastric surgery. The major complications following gastric surgery are of four main types:

- recurrence of ulceration
- nutritional deficiences
- disturbed motility leading to 'dumping syndrome', or diarrhoea
- hypoglycaemia.

Recurrence of ulceration will usually need to be treated by re-operation of a more radical type. Thus a highly selective vagotomy may be converted to another type. Results are usually good but the mortality rate is higher than for the original operation. In some cases treatment with cimetidine results in healing and surgery can be postponed and possibly avoided.

Iron-deficiency anaemia can result from loss of the hydrochloric acid needed to convert ferric to ferrous iron which can be readily absorbed in the gut. This occurs more frequently after partial gastrectomy (Kennedy, 1979) and these patients should be advised about an appropriate diet containing adequate amounts of iron in the ferrous form. Osteomalacia due to lack of calcium absorption occasionally occurs and can be treated with oral calcium and vitamin D.

'Dumping syndrome' is a term used to describe the condition which occurs because of the rapid movement of gastric contents into the small bowel following gastric drainage operations or partial gastrectomy. It occurs during or shortly after a meal and lasts 1 or 2 hours. The hyperosmotic contents of the jejunum attract fluid from the circulation and the distention of the small intestine leads to feelings

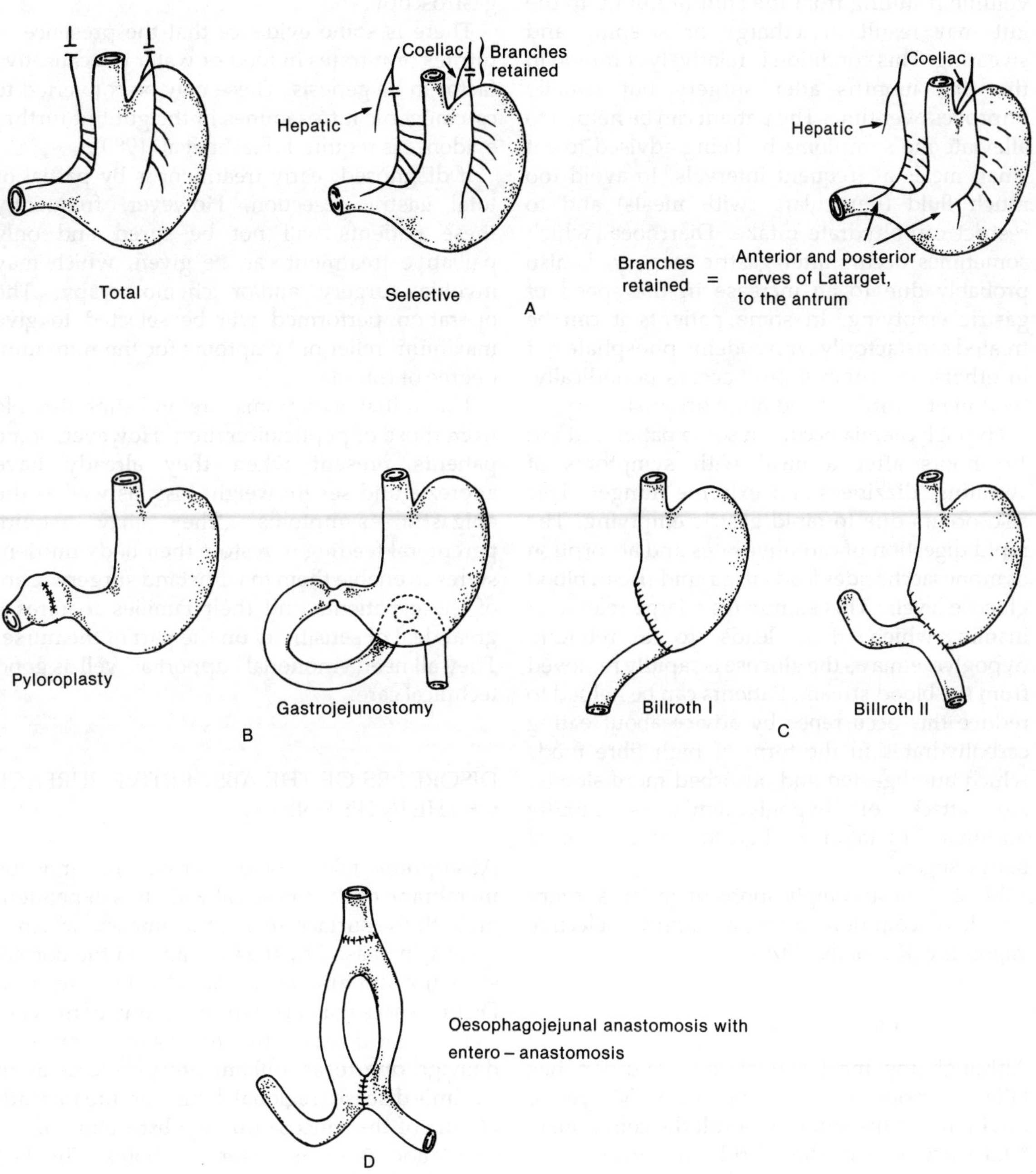

Fig. 23.4 Gastric operations (A) Different types of vagotomy (B) Types of gastric drainage (C) Partial gastric resection (D) Total gastric resection. (McFarland, 1980).

of fullness, often nausea and occasionally vomiting and/or diarrhoea. The fall in the blood volume resulting from the shift of fluid into the gut may result in lethargy or sleeping and sweating. This condition is relatively common in the first months after surgery but usually improves over time. The patient can be helped to alleviate the symptoms by being advised to eat small meals at frequent intervals, to avoid too much fluid (particularly with meals) and to restrict carbohydrate intake. Diarrhoea, which sometimes occurs after gastric surgery, is also probably due to an increase in the speed of gastric emptying. In some patients it can be treated satisfactorily with codeine phosphate but in others, in whom it only occurs periodically, treatment is difficult and often unsatisfactory.

Hypoglycaemia occurs in some patients about 1½ hours after a meal with symptoms of sweating, dizziness and extreme hunger. This also occurs due to rapid gastric emptying. The rapid digestion of carbohydrates and absorption of monosaccharides leads to a rapid rise in blood glucose levels. This stimulates a large release of insulin which then leads to a rebound hypoglycaemia as the glucose is rapidly removed from the blood stream. Patients can be helped to reduce this occurrence by advice about eating carbohydrates in the form of high fibre foods which are digested and absorbed more slowly. An attack of hypoglycaemia is rapidly terminated by taking oral glucose in the form of barley sugar.

Most of these complications of gastric surgery are less common after a highly selective vagotomy (Kennedy, 1979).

Gastric carcinoma

Although the incidence of this condition has fallen considerably in the past 50 years, carcinoma of the stomach is still the commonest fatal carcinoma in the world. In Europe most patients are not usually diagnosed until the disease is already advanced and the results of treatment are poor, only a 20% 5-year survival rate (Doll, 1978). However, Japanese results reported by Muto et al (1968) demonstrate clearly that 5-year survival rates can be considerably improved (from 23 to 44%) by early diagnosis through effective and widespread use of gastroscopy.

There is some evidence that the presence of nitrites or nitrates in food or water is a causative factor in its genesis. These may be converted to carcinogenic nitrosamines in the gut but further evidence is required (Fraser et al, 1980).

If diagnosed, early treatment is by partial or total gastric resection. However, frequently these patients will not be cured and only palliative treatment can be given, which may involve surgery and/or chemotherapy. The operation performed will be selected to give maximum relief of symptoms for the minimum degree of trauma.

The initial symptoms are indistinguishable from those of peptic ulceration. However, some patients present when they already have anorexia and severe weight loss, as well as the epigastric symptoms. They may require parenteral feeding to restore their body nutrient stores to enable them to withstand surgery. Care of these patients and their families requires a great deal of sensitivity on the part of the nurse. They all need emotional support as well as good technical care.

DISORDERS OF THE ABSORPTIVE SURFACE OF THE INTESTINE

Absorption takes place across the mucous membrane of the intestinal wall. It is dependent on both the surface area of the mucosa, which is greatly increased by the villi, and on the normal structure and function of the cells of the mucosa. Disturbances may arise from atrophy of the villi, as in coeliac disease, from more general mucosal damage due to an inflammatory process as in Crohn's disease (regional ileitis), or due to death of part of the mucosa due to obstruction of the circulation as in mesenteric embolus. This last condition will also lead to infarction of the musculature of the gut and result in symptoms of intestinal obstruction.

Coeliac disease

In coeliac disease the patient may have the classic

Table 23.11 Incidence of Crohn's disease per 100 000 population (Jewell, 1983b)

Aberdeen	1955–61	1.7
	1964–66	3.3
	1967–69	4.5
	1970–72	4.3
	1973–75	2.6
Cardiff	1934–70	1.1
	1971–77	4.6
Malmo	1958–65	3.5
	1966–73	6.0
Uppsala	1955–61	1.7
	1962–67	3.1
	1968–73	5.0
Stockholm	1955–59	1.5
	1960–64	2.2
	1965–69	3.6
	1970–74	4.5
	1975–79	4.1

signs and symptoms of malabsorption, although some patients have less severe symptoms. Some children affected may be diagnosed only after investigation for failure to thrive and grow and, unless diagnosed and treated, they may fail to reach puberty.

In this condition the mucosal surface is flat due to villous atrophy and there are abnormalities, including the presence of inflammatory cells, in the epithelium. There is a familial susceptibility to this condition which may be due to an enzyme deficiency. However, the favoured theory is that it results from an immunological reaction against gluten which causes damage to the intestinal mucosa.

The disturbances found in this disease are reversible if the patient ingests no gluten in the diet. Gluten is found in bread and other wheat products — which includes anything made with flour. The necessity for a gluten-free diet will result in additional expense for the patient and family and the need to acquire expertize in cooking with gluten-free flour. As the basic disturbance is permanent, a gluten-free diet is needed for the rest of the individual's life if symptoms are to be avoided (Losowsky, 1983).

Crohn's disease

Crohn's disease is a chronic inflammatory condition and, although sometimes known as regional ileitis, it can affect any part of the gastrointestinal tract in a discontinuous fashion. It tends to lead to the development of fistulae (Jewell, 1983b). It is not certain whether patients with the inflammatory bowel diseases of Crohn's disease and ulcerative colitis are suffering from two separate conditions or different manifestations of the same disease.

The incidence of Crohn's disease has changed considerably in Europe and Scandinavia since 1950 (Table 23.11) although the reasons for this are not clear. The incidence of ulcerative colitis has remained unchanged during this period (at 10–12 per 100 000) so it is unlikely that the rise in incidence of Crohn's disease is due to more accurate diagnosis (Jewell, 1983b). It occurs most commonly in young adults, although it can affect any age group.

Aetiology

Crohn's disease appears to have a multifactorial aetiology. A genetic contribution to its aetiology is indicated by a higher than usual incidence of this condition and ulcerative colitis among the family of patients with Crohn's disease (Allan & Hodgson, 1983). The environmental factors which trigger the development of the disease are not certain but diet, infective agents and immune mechanisms are all possible factors.

Thornton et al (1979) carried out a small study comparing the previous diet of 30 patients who developed Crohn's disease with that of 30 controls. They suggested that a diet high in refined sugar and low in fruit and vegetables preceded, and may favour, the development of Crohn's disease. Further work is needed in this area.

The possibility that some specific infective agent leads to Crohn's disease has not been confirmed, although extracts from affected tissue can cause pathogenic changes in tissue cultures.

It is also possible that this condition results from a disturbance of the normal immune response, but no basic defect has yet been identified (Jewell, 1983b).

Table 23.12 Major clinical features of Crohn's disease (from Jewell, 1983)

Feature	Frequency %
Diarrhoea	70–90
Abdominal pain	45–66
Weight loss	65–75
Fever	30–40
Rectal bleeding	in 50% of those with colonic disease
Perianal disease	in 30% of those with colonic disease
Signs of anaemia	Common
Signs of malabsorbtion of vitamins/minerals	Infrequent
Extra–intestinal manifestations	
Aphthous ulceration	20
Erythema nodosum	5–10
Acute arthropathy	6–12
Eye complications	3–10
Sacro-iliitis	15–18
Ankylosing spondylitis	2–6
Pericholangitis	5–6
Gallstones	Very common
Chronic active hepatitis	2–3
Cirrhosis	2–3
Fatty change of liver	6
Amyloidosis	Rare

Pathological changes

The changes in Crohn's disease occur most commonly in the ileum and/or colon although involvement of other parts of the gut is occasionally seen. Histological and enzyme studies suggest that the whole of the gastrointestinal tract may be abnormal, even though only parts of it may be affected at any one time. The lesions may occur in parts of the gut separated by apparently normal tissue.

In the affected parts of the gastrointestinal tract the mucosa is ulcerated and deep, fissuring ulcers may develop in oedematous, inflamed mucosa leading to a 'cobblestone' appearance. The mesentery becomes oedematous and the serosa may become inflamed and adhere to adjoining parts of the intestine, or other organs such as the bladder or vagina, and fistulae may develop. Fibrosis of the submucosal tissue frequently leads to the development of strictures and stenosis of the gut (Jewell, 1983b).

The effect of these changes on the patient varies according to the part of the gastrointestinal tract affected, the major manifestations of this disease are shown in Table 23.12. A few patients with disease of the terminal ileum present with symptoms similar to those of appendicitis, while some present with fever, weight loss and anaemia but no gastrointestinal symptoms.

A number of nutritional deficiencies can result and anaemia is common. This may be due to iron deficiency from blood loss, deficiency of vitamin B_{12} (particularly in disease of the terminal ileum) or of folic acid. Osteomalacia may occur when calcium absorption is restricted by extensive small bowel disease. Vitamin K deficiency may lead to a tendency to bleed.

Complications

The commonest complications of this disease are intestinal obstruction due to fibrosis, and the development of fistulae. These may be between parts of the gastrointestinal tract or between the gut and the bladder (leading to faeces passed in the urine and a high risk of infection passing up to the kidneys) or the gut and vagina (and a faecal vaginal discharge). The development of a fistula between parts of the gastrointestinal tract can lead to malabsorption as nutrients bypass areas of the absorptive surface or as a result of bacterial growth in the ileum. Severe malnutrition due to malabsorption may develop in patients who have had large parts of their ileum resected due to widespread, severe disease.

Perforation and haemorrhage can occur, and carcinoma of the colon develops in 3–5% of patients with Crohn's disease of the colon (similar to patients with ulcerative colitis).

Diagnosis

X-ray with contrast medium will show discrete and fissure ulcers, long ulcers, sinuses and possibly adhesions. When appropriate, endoscopy and histological examination of biopsy specimens will help to confirm the diagnosis.

Management of the patient with Crohn's disease

The clinical management of the patient with Crohn's disease divides into the management of an acute attack in order to achieve a remission, and the long term management to prevent recurrence. Active treatment is only required during the acute phase of the condition. Management of Crohn's disease is through drug therapy, nutritional care and sometimes surgery.

Drug therapy. Allan & Hodgson (1983) discuss various drug regimes that have been used in the treatment of Crohn's disease. They conclude that corticosteroids are of value while sulphasalazine is useful in acute colonic disease, but not when only the small bowel is affected. Prednisolone is the corticosteroid often used. It is given in high doses (60–80mg daily or 20–40 mg if the disease is less severe) for 4 to 6 weeks; the dose is then reduced over a period of another 4 to 6 weeks and then stopped (Jewel, 1983b).

Nutritional management. During an acute exacerbation, energy requirements are considerably increased due to a raised temperature, the inflammatory process itself and the increased catabolism due to steroids (Stotts et al, 1984). Nutritional support may be needed and an elemental diet or parenteral nutrition may be given. However, this does not appear to affect the outcome of the attack (Powell-Tuck, 1980). Deficiencies of folic acid, vitamins B_{12}, B complex, C and D and iron must be corrected and disturbances of fluid and electrolytes treated.

Parenteral nutrition may also be used during the pre- operative period to enhance the patient's ability to withstand surgery. It is suggested that parenteral nutrition, in conjunction with surgery, is valuable in the treatment of fistulae (Royle, 1980).

Certain patients with this condition end up with 'short bowel syndrome' when only small lengths of the small intestine remain following extensive, often repeated, surgery. The ability to absorb nutrients is obviously greatly reduced and their lives may be maintained by home parenteral nutrition (Rault & Scribner, 1977).

Permanent changes in the diet may be recommended in order to reduce the risk of recurrent attacks. Heaton et al (1979) suggest that a diet high in unrefined carbohydrate and low in sugar may reduce the relapse rate. They found that, over a period of 4 years and 4 months, 32 patients on such a diet had 111 days in hospital and one required surgery, compared to 533 days in hospital and five needing surgery among 32 control patients continuing with their normal diet. However, this work involved the retrospective matching of controls and the findings need to be confirmed in further work.

Surgery. Most patients (70–80%) will undergo at least one operation due to this disease when symptoms fail to respond to medical treatment, or if intestinal obstruction due to strictures, perforation, fistulae, abscesses or other complications develop (Jewell, 1983b).

Irving (1981) emphasizes that the small bowel is valuable and therefore only grossly diseased areas should be removed in order to conserve as much absorptive surface as possible. While surgery will not cure the disorder, it is nearly always necessary in order to cure fistulae arising from the affected bowel.

Caring for the patient with Crohn's disease

The nurses' role in caring for a patient with Crohn's disease involves the provision of physical care, emotional support and teaching.

During an acute exacerbation the patient may become very debilitated and weak and will require assistance with activities of daily living. He or she is at risk of developing pressure sores due to dehydration, weight loss, immobility and sweating. The patient should be taught to relieve the pressure frequently, or, if unable to do so unaided, should be turned regularly (2- hourly).

Diarrhoea is one of the major symptoms of this disease and the frequency, consistency and amount should be assessed as one indicator of the patient's response to treatment. The patient is likely to be distressed by the smells and sound of bowel movements and will be less embarrassed if he or she can be wheeled out to the toilet, even if a commode has to be used there so that faeces can be observed. If this is not possible then particular care should be taken to keep the environment free of odour by the frequent use of deodorant aerosols. The speed with which requests for toilet facilities are met will be of considerable importance to these patients.

Particular areas of the skin will need special attention. Diarrhoea can result in irritation and soreness of the perianal area and anal fissures and fistulae are not uncommon. The patient should be taught to keep this area clean, by frequent sitz baths if necessary, and the application of a barrier cream around the anus may help to prevent some discomfort.

They may also have fistulae opening onto the abdomen, and the skin will need protection against the irritant drainage in order to prevent excoriation. The application of Stomahesive or karaya gum and a stoma bag to collect the drainage will help to protect the skin, and will also allow accurate measurement of the fluid lost.

During an acute exacerbation the patient will need emotional support, which should be supplemented by the necessary teaching as the patient recovers and is able to understand the dietary recommendations to minimize the recurrence of the condition.

OBSTRUCTION OF THE INTESTINE

Whatever the cause, intestinal obstruction has considerable effects on the physiological status of the individual affected. The severity of the condition leads to considerable anxiety both in the patient and the relatives.

Intestinal obstruction can be acute or chronic, complete or incomplete, intermittent or continuous and in less severe forms it has to be distinguished from constipation (Macleod, 1984).

Table 23.13 shows a classification of intestinal obstruction. Whatever the original cause, paralysis of the gut may become superimposed on a mechanical obstruction.

Presentation of intestinal obstruction

The patient presents initially with abdominal pain, vomiting and failure to pass gas or faeces rectally; later abdominal distension develops. The acute condition rapidly becomes life-threatening due to the severity of the fluid and electrolyte disturbances.

Fluid and electrolyte disturbances. Large quantities of fluid are lost from the circulation, most of which progressively accumulates in the bowel above the obstruction. Normally there is a balance between fluids absorbed from the intestine and fluid secreted into the gut. However, Shields (1965) found that within 12 hours of an artificially induced obstruction in dogs, the ileum above the obstruction was no longer absorbing water but was secreting fluid at an increasing rate. Eventually the whole of the bowel above the obstruction becomes distended and up to 50% of the plasma volume may be within the gastrointestinal tract (Groer & Shekleton, 1983).

As the volume of the extracellular fluid diminishes, the patient's blood becomes more concentrated and hypovolaemic shock will lead to death unless treatment is instituted. Potassium, released by cell catabolism, is lost in the urine and metabolic acidosis commonly develops due to the combined effects of loss of alkaline secretions from the gut and ketosis due to starvation (Schwartz & Storer, 1984).

Vomiting. Reflex vomiting occurs almost immediately after obstruction of the intestine. This is followed by a quiescent period which is short in high bowel obstruction but may last up to 2 days in low small bowel obstruction. In colonic obstruction, vomiting does not occur until the small bowel becomes distended and may not happen at all if the ileocaecal valve is competent (Schwartz & Storer, 1984).

Failure to pass gas and faeces. This is a major diagnostic symptom, although in a high bowel obstruction gas and faeces below the obstruction may be passed. In partial obstruction, explosive diarrhoea may follow severe pain caused by increased intestinal contraction which forces faeces past the obstruction.

Pain. In an acute mechanical obstruction, violent peristalsis occurs in an 'attempt' to overcome the obstruction. This gives rise to severe cramping pain. Initially the pain is constant but after a short time it occurs in waves interspersed by periods without any pain. The bouts of pain occur every 4–5 minutes in high intestinal obstruction and at longer intervals, 10–20 minutes, with lower obstructions.

Table 23.13 Classification of intestinal obstruction (adapted from Schwartz & Storer, 1984)

I	Simple	
	Strangulated	Interference to blood supply Gangrene, perforation and peritonitis
II	Mechanical obstruction	
	Blocking of the lumen	Gallstones Impaction of faeces Intussusception
	Lesions of bowel	
	Congenital	Atresia and stenosis Imperforate anus Meckel's diverticulum
	Traumatic	
	Inflammatory	Crohn's disease Diverticulitis Chronic ulcerative colitis
	Neoplastic	
	Miscellaneous	Radiation stricture Endometriosis Potassium induced stricture
	Lesions extrinsic to bowel	
	Adhesion	Constriction or angulation of gut
	Hernia	
	Extrinsic masses	Neoplasms Abscesses etc
	Volvulus	
III	Paralytic obstruction	
	Neuromuscular defects	
	Megacolon	
	Paralytic ileus	Abdominal causes — intestinal obstruction peritonitis retroperitoneal lesions Systemic causes — electrolyte imbalance toxaemia
	Spastic ileus	
	Vascular occlusion	
	Arterial	
	Venous	

In a paralytic obstruction such pain does not occur, but generalized abdominal discomfort due to distension develops. A steady, severe continuous pain is usually due to strangulation (Schwartz & Storer, 1984).

Strangulated obstruction

In this condition the blood supply is obstructed and, in addition to the other effects of obstruction, haemoserous fluid leaks into the gut and peritoneal cavity. As the bowel becomes gangrenous and permeable, toxins produced by bacteria in the intestine leak into the peritoneal cavity causing peritonitis, which must be treated with antibiotics.

Management

The management of the patient with postoperative paralytic ileus is discussed in Chapter 17. For other patients the aims of management are:

- to achieve normal fluid and electrolyte balance
- to decompress the gut
- to operate to relieve the obstruction (except in postoperative paralytic ileus).

Fluid and electrolyte balance. This is discussed in detail in Chapter 26. In this situation if possible, surgery will be undertaken before major disturbances have developed. If derangements of fluid and electrolyte balance have already occurred then surgery will be delayed to enable restoration to normality, except in those with a strangulated obstruction. In these patients immediate operation is essential and, while vigorous attempts will be made to improve fluid and electrolyte status, time is not available to restore them to normal.

Postoperative fluid and electrolyte management must take into account the altered fluid distribution in the body due to the excessive secretion of fluid into the gut. This usually corrects itself by about the third postoperative day, and as this fluid becomes reabsorbed the patient is at risk of becoming overhydrated. Electrolyte levels must be closely monitored, as both hyponatraemia and hypokalaemia can develop in prolonged paralysis of the gut (Schwartz & Storer, 1984).

Gut decompression. Gastrointestinal aspiration is always instituted in these patients before operation, and continued postoperatively until normal gut motility has returned. Either a nasogastric tube which only aspirates the stomach, or one such as the Miller-Abbott tube, which enters the upper part of the small intestine, is used. This tube has a mercury weight on the tip which enables gravity to help pull the tube through the pylorus. The patient lies on the right side with feet slightly elevated. A small balloon at the end of the tube is inflated when it reaches the intestine and peristalsis then carries it onwards.

Gastrointestinal suction may need to be continued for some time postoperatively, as the return of normal gut motility is often delayed till the fifth or sixth postoperative day after relief of intestinal obstruction (compared to about the third day after abdominal operation).

Surgery. Surgery should be performed as soon as possible, except in those patients with simple mechanical obstruction when there has been a delay in reaching appropriate medical help. In these patients operation can be postponed until fluid and electrolyte normality is achieved.

The type of operation performed for intestinal obstruction falls into one of five categories (Schwartz & Storer, 1984):

- Procedures not requiring opening of the bowel
  - lysis of adhesions
  - manipulation-reduction of intussusception
  - reduction of incarcerated hernia.
- Enterotomy for removal of obstruction material
  - gallstones, bezoar (a ball of hair, vegetable fibres, etc.).
- Resection of the obstructing lesion or strangulated bowel with primary anastomosis.
- Short-circuiting anastomosis around an obstruction.
- Formation of a cutaneous stoma proximal to the obstruction
  - caecostomy
  - transverse colostomy.

Obviously both the cause of the obstruction and the operation performed have implications for the patient. While the surgeon will normally give the patient this information it is important that the nurse has the knowledge to help the patient clarify any misunderstandings. Sometimes a stoma is only a temporary measure, although temporary can sometimes be a considerable number of months, and this must be explained.

Caring for the patient with intestinal obstruction

Much of the care of the patient with intestinal obstruction is similar to that of any patient undergoing surgery, as discussed in Chapter 17.

In intestinal obstruction the patient is unable to absorb nutrients or fluids and is indeed losing electrolyte-rich fluid into the gastrointestinal tract. After operation the gut may take 5 to 6 days to begin functioning normally again. During the entire period the patient will be given intravenous fluids and electrolytes. Serum electrolytes will be monitored and the patient must be observed for signs of fluid overload, especially around the third postoperative day as discussed above. Total parenteral nutrition may be used to restore nutritional status.

Once the gut is functioning normally again, fluids, an easily digested and then a normal-type diet is progressively given as the patient can tolerate it. During this illness a considerable degree of catabolism occurs and a high protein, high energy diet during convalescence will help in the regeneration of tissue.

The patient with complete intestinal obstruction is not passing faeces or flatus per rectum, while the patient with only partial obstruction may have episodes of diarrhoea preceded by severe, cramping pain.

Once the obstruction is relieved and the gut is functioning normally, elimination of faeces will resume. The patient is asked regularly whether flatus has been passed as this is an important indication of returning function of the gastrointestinal tract. Those patients who have had a stoma formed will need to learn how to deal with this, and this topic is discussed in Chapter 25.

The abdominal distension which develops, due partly to the accumulation of gas in the intestine, can cause respiratory embarrassment and the patient will probably be more comfortable sitting in an upright position in bed. Postoperatively the abdominal incision will inhibit deep breathing, and breathing and coughing exercises should be encouraged and an explanation of the reason given.

DISORDERS OF THE HEPATIC PORTAL SYSTEM

The hepatic portal system transports nutrients absorbed from the gut to the liver where storage, transformation and controlled release into the blood stream takes place. Fibrosis of the liver, which can result from a number of conditions, constricts the blood vessels, leading to obstruction of the flow of blood and a rise in the blood pressure — portal hypertension.

Portal hypertension

Severe fibrosis of the liver, from whatever cause, compresses the blood vessels in the liver and reduces the entry of blood from the low-pressure portal system. Blood from the high-pressure arterial system will still be able to enter the liver and will increase the back pressure on the hepatic portal system. Abnormal connections between the hepatic artery and the portal vein may develop and contribute to the development of portal hypertension (Groer & Shekleton, 1983).

This high pressure within the portal system will lead to the development of collateral blood vessels, which allow blood from the now high-pressure portal system to pass into the low-pressure systemic venous circulation. This occurs mainly at the lower end of the oesophagus resulting in oesophageal varices, at the anus and lower rectum resulting in haemorrhoids, through the normally-obliterated embryological circulation through the falciform ligament resulting in visible, dilated veins on the abdomen, and between the splenic vein and the left renal vein (Groer & Shekleton, 1983; Macleod, 1984).

The dilated veins are not strong and haemorrhage from oesophageal varices and haemorrhoids is not uncommon. Because the pressure within them is so high, the volume of blood lost can be very large and haematemesis from ruptured oesophageal varices may be fatal. A number of techniques have been used to achieve haemostasis and are discussed by Pennington & Bouchier (1983). A Sengstaken tube, which has balloons at the tip which are inflated and used to apply direct pressure to the bleeding points, is often used to achieve primary haemostasis. Operative techniques which obliterate the varices reduce considerably the risk of rebleeding.

The portal hypertension itself can be lowered by the surgical formation of a portal-systemic shunt, thus allowing the high pressure blood in the portal circulation to move directly into the systemic circulation. One of the complications that occurs more frequently after this operation is hepatic encephalopathy, discussed on page 765.

Ascites

Ascites is frequently associated with portal hypertension, and results in part from the portal hypertension and obstruction to lymphatic drainage so that the fluid produced cannot be reabsorbed. It is this mechanism which determines that the fluid will accumulate within the abdominal cavity. However, other changes contribute to the accumulation of fluid within the body. When the liver is not producing adequate amounts of albumin, the plasma osmotic pressure is low and the reabsorption of fluid into the capillaries is reduced. In addition, the diseased liver may not inactivate aldosterone and antidiuretic hormone, so that excessive amounts of sodium and water are reabsorbed by the kidneys.

Ascites is treated by giving a low sodium diet and potassium-sparing diuretics are often used (sometimes abdominal paracentesis will be performed to drain off the accumulated fluid). A diet with a moderate amount of protein (20–40g) is given in order to replenish the serum albumin levels, but without precipitating hepatic encephalopathy.

DISORDERS OF THE LIVER

The liver is the most metabolically active organ in the body and the range of activities in which it is involved indicates the scale of the disturbances which may develop in liver disease. These activities are:

- *metabolism of*
  — carbohydrates
  — proteins
  — lipids
  — vitamins A, D, K
  — iron

  also has role in temperature regulation
- *storage of*
  — glycogen
  — vitamins
  — iron
- *detoxification of*
  — drugs
  — endotoxins
  — alkaloids
  — hormones
- *excretion of*
  — bile salts
  — bile pigments
  — heavy metals, dyes etc.
- *protection of individual by*
  — Kupffer cells which remove specific pathogens
  — preventing haemorrhage and intra-vascular coagulation by formation of clotting factors dand of heparin
- *circulatory functions*
  — blood transfer between portal and systemic circulation
  — regulation of blood volume
  — fluid transfer via lymph production (Groer & Shekleton, 1983)

However, it is protected to a considerable extent by two factors:

- It has a considerable functional reserve, and it has been suggested that approximately 80% must be damaged before symptoms of liver failure appear (Beland & Passos, 1975).
- It has the ability to regenerate completely, even when up to 70% of the liver is destroyed (Groer & Shekleton, 1983).

Causes of liver disease

The liver is exposed to a wide variety of disease-creating conditions because of:

- its function in the detoxification and

Table 23.14 Types, causes, clinical features and specific management of liver disease

Disease			Clinical features	Management
Hepatitis — inflammation of parenchymal cells of liver				
Acute	viral	e.g. serum hepatitis	Liver enlarged and tender, jaundice if severe, serum aminotransferase ↑, Australia antigen in serum	no alcohol
	bacterial	e.g. pyogenic liver abscess	↑ temperature, rigors, weight ↓, jaundice	drain abscess antibiotics
		e.g. leptospirosis (Weil's disease)	jaundice, bleeding, fever	penicillin
	parasitic	e.g. amoebiasis	amoebic abscess, enlarged liver, systemic disturbances	emetine HCl or chloroquine, aspiration of abscess if necessary
	toxins	e.g. acute alcoholic hepatitis	large tender liver, vomiting, confusion, jaundice, aminotransferase ↑	withdraw alcohol
Chronic	?follows acute viral hepatitis	chronic persistent hepatitis	fatigue, aminotransferase ↑, excess mononuclear cells on biopsy, eventually recovers within 2 years.	no treatment
	?auto-immune	acute chronic hepatitis	similar to acute viral hepatitis which recurs at intervals *or* presents with jaundice, portal hypertension and cirrhosis: shows ↑ aminotrans-ferase, ↑ immunoglobulin G, ↑ alkaline phosphatase	corticosteroids
Cholangitis — inflammation of intrahepatic bile ducts				
Acute	infective	following partial obstruction e.g. by gallstones	mild — intermittent fever, rigors, obstructive jaundice extension to acute supperative cholangitis — increasing jaundice, septicaemia, shock, renal failure, ?hepatic abscesses	antibiotics drainage of biliary tree
Chronic	?cause	destructive, non-supperative (primary biliary cirrhosis)	itching, jaundice, steathorrhoea →osteomalacia & osteoporosis, alkaline phosphatase ↑, amino-transferases ↑ x ⅔, high gamma globulin, ↑ immunoglobulin M	symptomatic
	secondary	sclerosing cholangitis 2° to e.g. ulcerative colitis		
	primary	sclerosing cholangitis	painless, increasing jaundice. ↑ alkaline phosphatase	? corticosteroids

contd overleaf

Table 23.14 continued

Disease		Clinical features		Management
Cirrhosis — necrosis of liver cells, fibrosis and nodular regeneration				
Toxins	alcohol	alcoholic cirrhosis	variable signs and symptoms	abstain from alcohol
	copper	hepatolenticular degeneration (Wilson's disease)	liver, small or large, smooth or knobbly infertility, impotence, testicular atrophy	chelating agent to increase excretion
Infection		post-necrotic cirrhosis	jaundice — sometimes	
Cholestasis	— small duct damage	primary biliary cirrhosis (see above)	oesophageal varices, ascites encephalopathy may occur in severe cases or following portal-caval shunt	
	— large duct obstruction	secondary biliary cirrhosis		
Venous out-flow block	large veins	congestive cardiac failure	liver function tests may be normal or show only limited changes	treat C.C.F.
	small veins	veno-occlusive veins		
Unknown		active chronic hepatitis		
Vascular disorders				
Occlusion of large veins	sudden	Budd-Chiari syndrome	abdominal pain, large tender liver, ascites. liver failure and death common, or hepatic fibrosis and portal hypertension	treat obstruction
	slow	often associated with polycythaemia	large liver, chronic ascites, oedema	venesection if polycythaemia
Venous congestion		congestive cardiac failure		
Portal or splenic vein obstruction		from infection, tumours, etc.	portal hypertension	portal-systemic shunt
Tumours				
Primary	benign	haemangiomata	enlarged, pulsating liver	radiotherapy, steroids or ligation of hepatic artery
	malignant	hepatoma	more common in cirrhotic liver: weight loss, ascites, jaundice, pain, enlarging tender liver	occasionally, resection possible; chemotherapy
Secondary	malignant	from breast, stomach, large bowel, pancreas and kidney	as above	occasionally resection of primary and single secondary tumour
Miscellaneous				
Amyloidosis		2° to e.g. rheumatoid arthritis Crohn's disease	enlarged liver, normal liver function tests except for ↑ alkaline phosphatase	
Sarcoidosis				
Malignant reticuloses		i.e. Hodgkin's disease		

excretion of toxins

- its position, in that most substances absorbed from the gut go first to the liver
- its very large blood supply.

Table 23.14 indicates the range of disorders affecting this organ and gives some indication of their clinical presentation and management.

Liver function tests

Tests of liver function are carried out for three major reasons (Macleod, 1984):

- to assist in the differential diagnosis of jaundice (see below), with the chief aim of distinguishing between jaundice requiring surgical treatment and jaundice requiring medical treatment
- to obtain confirmation of suspected liver disease
- to estimate hepatic function as a guide to progress and an aid to prognosis.

The tests used examine a variety of different aspects of function of the liver, not all of which may be impaired in any specific disease (Macleod, 1984).

Tests of metabolic functions. These tests examine the function of the parenchymal cells and are not altered in the early stages of obstruction of the biliary system. Various aspects of protein metabolism are assessed through examination of the different plasma proteins. Albumin is lowered and globulin raised in parenchymal liver disease. The prothrombin time may be altered and the fibrinogen content of the blood reduced.

Tests of metabolic function which are dependent upon patent bile ducts. Serum alkaline phosphatase is moderately raised in parenchymal liver disease, but severely increased in obstruction of the biliary system. It can therefore be used in the differential diagnosis of the cause of jaundice. Clearance tests of, for example, bromsulphthalein examine the rate at which the substance is cleared from the blood. Normally 95% of the substance should be cleared from the blood in 45 minutes.

Tests of biliary excretion. These tests will be altered to some extent in disease of the parenchymal cells, but are greatly altered in obstruction of the biliary tract. Estimation of the amounts of total, conjugated and unconjugated bilirubin in the blood is of value in the differential diagnosis of jaundice, discussed below.

Tests of liver cell damage. The cells of the liver contain certain enzymes in large amounts, which are released into the blood stream in cases of cellular damage. The two most important enzymes in the assessment of liver damage are alanine aminotransferase (glutamic pyruvate transferase, GPT) and aspartate aminotransferase (glutamic oxaloacetic transaminase, GOT). These are not raised to any great extent in obstructive jaundice unless there is accompanying cholangitis (Macleod, 1984). Lactic dehydrogenase (LDH) is also released when liver cells are damaged.

Test for immunological disturbance. In a number of liver conditions there seems to be some disturbance of the immune system. Raised levels of plasma globulins are found particularly in chronic liver disease, but changes in the levels of specific immunoglobulins are of limited value in diagnosis. However, one particular α-globulin, alphafetoprotein, normally found only in the embryo, is also found in 30–70% of patients with hepatoma.

Autoantibodies are sometimes found in patients with certain chronic liver diseases and probably indicates that an autoimmune process is involved. Australia antigen is found in the blood of patients with serum hepatitis, and in a few people may remain indefinitely. It is highly infectious and special precautions must be taken when handling blood from these patients (Macleod, 1984).

Miscellaneous tests. A number of other procedures may be used in the diagnosis of liver disease. Liver biopsy, ultrasonic scan and computerized tomography are all used in the diagnosis of structural changes in the liver, while trans-hepatic cholangiography can be used to examine the biliary tract (Pennington & Bouchier, 1983).

Effects of liver failure

Whatever the cause, the effects of liver failure

are similar and cover the range of functions. However, the most important in relation to the management of the patient involve the changes in metabolism (discussed previously), detoxification and excretion.

Changes in detoxification

If the liver is diseased to the extent that detoxification is affected there are two groups of substances whose activity will be altered with potentially severe effects. The normal breakdown of hormones which terminates their activity is carried out by the drug-metabolizing enzymes in the liver. In the absence of an adequate level of activity of these enzymes, the effect of these hormones will be increased and the effects seen in the patient. Increased levels of antidiuretic hormone and aldosterone will result in sodium and water retention and contribute to the development of oedema and ascites. Increased levels of female sex hormones, produced by both sexes in small amounts, can lead to gynaecomastia in some male patients, spider angiomata (spider-shaped arterial dilation in the skin) and telangiectasis (capillary dilatations in the skin).

Changes in excretion — jaundice

The main indication of disturbance in the excretory function of the liver is the development of jaundice, which is a yellow colouration of the skin and eyes due to increased levels of bilirubin in the blood. Bilirubin, which is produced as a result of haemoglobin and myoglobin breakdown, is transported to the liver bound to albumin and is conjugated in the liver and excreted through the biliary tract. Jaundice can occur because of a disruption at any of these points and an accurate diagnosis is necessary to ensure that the correct treatment can be given.

Haemolytic jaundice. This is due to excessive breakdown of haemoglobin, producing bilirubin in amounts greater than the liver can deal with. The patient is likely to be anaemic, the degree depending on the severity of the haemolysis, and mildly jaundiced. The amount of stercobilinogen and stercobilin in the faeces is large, so they are brown or orange, and some of it is reabsorbed and excreted in the urine as urobilinogen. The urine is normal in colour when passed but darkens as the urobilinogen is oxidized to urobilin.

Hepatocellular jaundice. This is due to damage to the parenchymal cells of the liver by infections, toxins or possibly deficiencies of specific food factors, or is due to immaturity or congenital defect of the mechanisms for conjugation and/or transport of bilirubin. The degree of jaundice may be mild or severe, showing first as yellowing of the sclera of the eyes and bile in the urine. As liver inflammation increases and obstruction to the bile ducts develops the jaundice deepens, the stools become pale and the urine darker.

Obstructive jaundice. In this condition there is some block between the parenchymal cells, where the bilirubin is conjugated, and the duodenum. Conjugated bilirubin and other bile components then enter the bloodstream. Obstructive jaundice falls into two categories:

- extrahepatic cholestasis, where the obstruction is of the main ducts, most commonly caused by gallstones or carcinoma of the head of the pancreas
- intrahepatic cholestasis, where the blockage occurs in the biliary canaliculi. This has many causes including intrinsic disease of the liver and some drugs. Drugs may cause jaundice through a sensitivity reaction or through direct toxicity leading to inflammation and oedema in the canaliculi.

These patients will be severely jaundiced, will have pale, fatty stools and dark urine. They suffer from pruritus, anorexia and a metallic taste in the mouth. The lack of bile in the gut leads to impaired absorption of fat-soluble vitamins. The lack of vitamin K will lead to an increased coagulation time and a tendency to bleed. In long-standing obstructive jaundice, damage to the parenchymal liver cells occurs, leading to all the effects of liver disease discussed above.

Hepatic encephalopathy and hepatic coma

The terminal stages of liver disease are hepatic encephalopathy and hepatic coma. The initial symptoms include euphoria, confusion, drowsiness, dysarthria, and a coarse tremor of the outstretched hands. Sometimes epileptic fits occur. In the later stages the patient is restless and excitable before progressing to stupor and coma. An unpleasant, musty odour (foetor hepaticus) is smelt on the breath (Mann, 1975). The precise biochemical cause is not clear, but blood ammonia levels are usually raised and it may be due to the effects of this and other products of protein metabolism, alkalosis and electrolyte disturbances.

Hepatic encephalopathy occurs when the levels of these substances in the blood are raised. This can happen after a portal-systemic shunt has been formed, as the substances absorbed from the gut now by-pass the liver and can reach the brain directly. It can also develop after a high-protein meal or after bleeding from oesophageal varices.

The treatment of a patient with hepatic encephalopathy is difficult as most drugs are metabolized in the liver and some, e.g. morphine, can precipitate coma. However, some short-chain barbiturates which are long-acting are excreted by the kidney and can be used (Groer & Shekleton, 1983). Measures are taken to reduce the amount of ammonia absorbed by giving a low protein diet (and aspirating any blood in the stomach) and by giving neomycin to sterilize the gut.

The level of mental functioning may vary considerably from time to time. Treatment may lead to a patient recovering from coma and having no signs of hepatic encephalopathy.

Care of the patient with liver or gall bladder disease

The patients suffer from a number of problems which are similar in disorders of the two organs.

Respiratory problems

The tenderness or pain of an inflamed liver or diseased gall bladder and the ascites of some liver disease restrict diaphragmatic and chest movements, thus reducing lung expansion and increasing the risk of chest infections. Similarly, the site of the upper abdominal incision for surgery to the gall bladder increases the difficulty of respiration. An upright position in bed will help lung expansion, and patients should be taught deep-breathing exercises and coughing and encouraged to perform these hourly. Surgical patients should be taught how to splint the wound and must be given adequate analgesia.

Nutritional modifications

Both liver and gall bladder disease require dietary modification.

The necessity for a low protein diet for a patient with hepatic encephalopathy has already been discussed. Such patients may well have ascites and need a low sodium diet to reduce fluid retention. In some other conditions, such as cirrhosis of the liver, a high protein, high energy diet will assist liver regeneration. Malnutrition is relatively common in patients with cirrhosis due to excessive alcohol consumption and a high calorie, high protein diet with vitamin supplements is required. Such a patient will have an additional problem as he will be advised to give up alcohol and may need support and help to do this.

Patients with liver disease are often nauseated and anorexic, and careful thought and imagination will be needed in providing attractive food in quantities they are able to tolerate, while ensuring that the nutritional intake is adequate to promote recovery.

In patients with disease of the gall bladder, nausea, abdominal discomfort and flatulence will cause anorexia. In some patients symptoms can be controlled by a low fat diet which reduces the activity of the gall bladder. They may need guidance in how to modify their diet to reduce the fat content but still have an enjoyable diet with adequate amounts of all other nutrients. About 25% of the total calories should be given as fat. It is undesirable to have too strict a limitation, as some fat is important in allowing some gall bladder drainage into the duodenum. Patients who are obese may be advised to lose weight for two reasons. It may help to reduce their symptoms and, if they do undergo surgery, the risk of chest infection will be reduced and their wound will heal more readily (adipose tissue heals slowly).

Pre-operatively these patients are often given IM vitamin K to ensure adequate blood clotting. As a fat-soluble vitamin, its absorption will have been restricted. Postoperatively an intravenous infusion will be given and possibly gastric aspiration performed until fluids can be tolerated. After a cholecystectomy many people continue to need a fairly low fat diet.

Pain and pruritus

While patients with liver disease may have some pain, it tends to be less severe than in those with gall bladder disease or biliary colic. Adequate management of pain is essential and is discussed in Chapter 9 and in the Appendix. Phenazocine is the analgaesic of choice for relief of biliary colic as it has less tendency to increase biliary pressure than other narcotic analgaesics (BMA and Pharmaceutical Society of Great Britain, 1985).

Pruritus results from high levels of bilirubin in the blood, and the itching of the skin may be very severe and cause considerable distress to the jaundiced patient. It can be eased by using antihistamines such as Piriton, and cholestyramine can also give relief of the symptom by reducing the level of bilirubin in the blood. This drug is a basic anion-exchange resin which is not absorbed from the gut; it binds with the bilirubin entering the gut and thus prevents its reabsorption. It cannot be used in complete biliary obstruction (Rogers et al, 1981).

Nursing measures can help to relieve the constant irritation and help the patient to get some rest. The room should be kept cool with a fairly high humidity, and light cotton clothing should be worn. The nails should be kept short so that skin damage from scratching is minimized. Tepid baths and application of calamine or emollient preparations will help to soothe the skin. Soaps and detergents will dry the skin and should be avoided, although bath oils can be used.

Psychological problems

During phases of hepatic encephalopathy, the confusion, drowsiness and tremor will reduce the ability to move and protect oneself and a patient in this condition will need to be protected from harm. Cotsides may be used, but the psychological effect of this must be assessed. It may upset the patient and thus increase agitation and cause further harm.

Some patients may have difficulty in integrating changes in body function and appearance into their body image. Ascites, gynaecomastia, spider angiomata and telangiectasis all alter one's appearance and may be difficult to accept. For some men gynaecomastia may be particularly problematical. The yellow coloration of jaundice is clearly visible in those with white skins, but also results in an alteration of skin colour in those with brown, black or yellow skins and is visible in the sclera of the eyes.

These patients may be inhibited in interaction and upset by their changed appearance. Explanation of the cause of changes and the expected effect of treatment may help both patient and family to accept them.

CONCLUSION

Disturbances of nutrient supply to the cells of the body can arise from a number of different causes. Inadequate food available in the environment or inappropriate selection of food are perhaps the primary causes of failure of nutrient supply. Some of the factors involved in food selection are discussed in Chapter 14.

Dysfunction of the mechanisms controlling feeding behaviour or disorders of the gastrointestinal tract or accessory organs of digestion — the pancreas, gall bladder and liver — can also result in disturbances in nutrients entering the body. Metabolic disturbances will affect the controlled supply of nutrients to the cells of the body, and the effect of liver dysfunction on nutrient supply and use has been discussed. The effects of disorders of hormonal regulation on nutrient use are discussed in Chapter 19, while the effects of inborn errors of metabolism mainly present during infancy and childhood are not discussed in detail in this text.

Failure to maintain a satisfactory nutrient supply leads to malnutrition and all its attendant complications. However, an overabundant supply of certain nutrients, notably fat, sugar and salt, is also implicated in the aetiology of certain diseases — this too is discussed in Chapter 14. Nurses who understand this, together with the many reasons for a failure of the nutrient supply, are better able to integrate nutrition into the total care of their patients.

REFERENCES

Albrink M 1975 Diseases of obesity. In: Beeson P B, McDermott H W (eds) Textbook of medicine, 14th edn. Saunders, Philadelphia

Allan R N, Hodgson H J F 1983 Inflammatory bowel disease. In: Bouchier I A D (ed) Recent advances in gastroenterology 5. Churchill Livingstone, Edinburgh

Baron D N 1973 A short textbook of clinical pathology, 3rd edn. Hodder and Stoughton, London

Baron J H, Langman M J S, Wastell C, 1980 Stomach and duodenum. In: Bouchier I A D (ed) Recent advances in gastroenterology 4. Churchill Livingstone, Edinburgh

Bass L 1977 More fibre — less constipation. American Journal of Nursing 77:254–255

Basu T K, Dickerson J W T 1974 Interrelationships of nutrition and the metabolism of drugs. Chemico-Biological Interactions 8:193–206

Beisel W R 1976 The influence of infection or injury on nutritional requirements during adolescence. In: McKigney J I, Munro H N (eds) Nutrient requirements in adolescence. MIT Press, Cambridge, Mass.

Beland I L, Passos J Y 1975 Clinical nursing — pathophysiological and psychosocial approaches. Macmillan, New York

Bistrian B R, Blackburn G L, Hallowell E, Heddle R 1974 Protein status of general surgical patients. Journal of the American Medical Association 230:858–860

British Medical Association and The Pharmaceutical Society of Great Britain 1985 British National Formulary Number 9

Brobeck J R 1948 Food intake as a mechanism of temperature regulation. Yale Journal of Biology and Medicine 20:545–552

Bruch H 1974 Perils of behaviour modification in treatment of anorexia. Journal of the American Medical Association 230:1419–1422

Bruch H 1977 Anorexia nervosa. Dietetic Currents 4(2)

Buchman E, Kaung D T, Dolan K, Knapp R N 1969 Unrestricted diet in the treatment of duodenal ulcer. Gastroenterology 56:1016–1020

Bucknall T E 1979 Nutrition in the severely injured patient. Mead Johnson Nutritional News, December

Cahill G F, Herrrera M G, Morgan A P 1966 Hormone fuel interrelationships during fasting. Journal of Clinical Investigation 45:1751–1769

Chandra R K, Newberne P M 1977 Nutrition, immunity and infection. Mechanism of interaction. Plenum Press, New York

Chandra R K 1981 Immunocompetence as a functional index of nutritional status. British Medical Bulletin 37:89–94

Cockel R 1971 Antiemetics. The Practitioner 206:56–63

Copeland E M, Daly J M, Ota D M, Dudrick S J 1979 Nutrition, cancer and intravenous hyperalimentation. Cancer 43 (suppl 5): 2108–2116

Cuthbertson D P 1930 The disturbance of metabolism produced by bony and non bony injury with a note on certain abnormal conditions of the bone. Biochemical Journal 24:1244–1236

D'Arcy P F, Griffin J P 1979 Iatrogenic diseases, 2nd ed. Oxford University Press, London

Davidson S, Passmore R, Brock J F, Truswell A S 1979 Human nutrition and dietetics, 7th edn. Churchill Livingstone, Edinburgh

De Wys W D, Begg C, Lavin P T et al 1980 Prognostic effect of weight loss prior to chemotherapy in cancer patients. American Journal of Medicine 69:491–497

Dickerson J W T 1982 Personal communication

Dickerson J W T, Lee H A (eds) 1978 Nutrition in the clinical management of disease. Edward Arnold, London

Dietz F 1979 Radiation therapy: external radiation. Cancer Nursing 2:233–244

Doll R 1978 Epidemiology. In: Truelove S C, Heyworth M F (eds) Topics in gastroenterology 6. Blackwell Scientific, Oxford

Donaldson S S 1977 Nutritional consequences of radiotherapy. Cancer Research 37:2407–2413

Edholm O G, Adam J M, Healy M J 1970 Food intake and energy expenditure of army recruits. British Journal of Nutrition 24:1091–1107

Exton Smith A N 1978 Nutrition in the elderly. In: Dickerson J W T, Lee H A (eds) Nutrition in the clinical management of disease. Edward Arnold, London

Feldman E J, Sabovich K A 1980 Stress and peptic ulcer disease. Gastroenterology 28:1087–1089

Felig P, Owen O E, Wahren J 1969 Amino acid metabolism during prolonged starvation. Journal of Clinical Investigation 48:58– 94

Flack R, Grayer E A 1975 Consciousness raising group for obese women. Social Work 20:484–487

Fraser P, Chilvers C, Beral V, Hill M J 1980 Nitrate and human cancer: a review of the evidence. International Journal of Epidemiology 9:3–11

Geall M G, Phillips S F, Summerskill W H J 1970 Profile of gastric potential difference in man: effects of aspirin, alcohol, bile and endogenous acid. Gastroenterology 58:437–443

Golden S 1975 Cancer chemotherapy and management of patient problems. Nursing Forum 14:279–303

Goodner C J, Moore, T E, Bowers J Z, Armstrong W D 1955 Effects of whole body X-irradiation on the absorption and distribution of Na^{22} and H^3OH from the gastrointestinal tract of the fasted rat. American Journal of Physiology 183:475–484

Grande F 1968 Energy balance and body composition changes. A critical study of three recent publications. Annals of Internal Medicine 68:467–475

Greenberger N J, Isselbacher K J 1977 Disorders of

absorption. In: Thorn G W, Harrison T R (eds) Harrison's principles of internal medicine 8th edn. McGraw-Hill, New York

Groer M E, Shekleton M E 1983 Basic pathophysiology: a conceptual approach 2nd edn. C V Mosby, St Louis

Gull W W 1874 Anorexia nervosa (apepsia hysterica, anorexia hysterica). Transactions of the Clinical Society of London 7:22

Guyton A C 1981 Textbook of medical physiology, 6th edn. Saunders, Philadelphia

Harper A E, Benevenga N J, Wohlheuter R M 1970 Effects of ingestion of disproportionate amounts of amino acids. Physiological Reviews 50:428–558

Heaton K W, Thornton J R, Emmett P M 1979 Treatment of Crohn's disease with a unrefined carbohydrate, fibre rich diet. British Medical Journal 2:764–766

Hegsted D M 1967 Nutrition, bone and calcified tissue. Journal of the American Dietetic Association 50:105–111

Henderson V 1960 Basic principles of nursing care. International Council of Nurses, Geneva, Switzerland

Hill G L, Blackett R L, Pickford I, Burkinshaw L, Young G A, Warren J V, Schoran C J, Morgan O B 1977 Malnutrition in surgical patients: an unrecognized problem. Lancet (8013):689– 692

Hitchcock E R, Masson A H B 1970 Metabolism in management of the unconscious patient. Blackwell Scientific, Oxford

Holmes S 1983 Dietary problems in the cancer patient. Nursing Mirror 157(2):27–30

Irving M 1981 Inflammatory bowel disease 1, with special reference to the small bowel. In: Lumley J S P, Craven J L (eds) Surgical review 2. Pitman Medical, Tunbridge Wells

Irving W J, Cullen D R, Ewart R B L, Baird J D, Harcourt Webster J N 1975 Diseases of the endocrine glands. In: Passmore R, Robson J S (eds) A companion to medical studies, vol 3. Blackwell Scientific, Oxford

Jacobs P, Bothwell T, Charlton R W 1964 Role of hydrochloric acid in iron absorption. Journal of Applied Physiology 19:187–194

Janowitz H D, Hollander F, Orringer D, Levy M H, Winklestein A, Kaufman M R, Margolin S G 1950 A quantitative study of the gastric secretory responses to sham feeding in a human subject. Gastroenterology 16:104–116

Jefferies G H 1975 Disease of the liver II. In:Beeson P B, McDermott W (eds) Textbook of medicine, 14th edn. Saunders, Philadelphia.

Jervis H R, Donati R M, Stromberg L R, Sprinz H 1969 Histochemical investigation of mucosa of exteriorized small intestine of the rat exposed to X-radiation. Strahlentherapie 137:326–343. cited by Copeland E M, Souchou E A, MacFadyen B V, Rapp M A, Dudrick S J 1977. Intravenous hyperalimentation as an adjunct to radiation therapy. Cancer 39:609–616

Jewell D P 1983a Symptomatology of gastrointestinal disease. In: Weatherall D J, Ledingham J G G, Warrell D A (eds) Oxford textbook of medicine. Oxford University Press, Oxford

Jewell D P 1983b Crohn's disease. In: Weatherhall D J, Ledingham J G G, Warrell D A (eds) Oxford textbook of medicine. Oxford University Press, Oxford

Jones F A, 1979 Pathogenesis of gastric ulcer. In: Truelove S C, Willoughby C P (eds) Topics in gastroenterology 7. Blackwell Scientific, Oxford

Jowsey J, Riggs B L, Kelly P J 1973 Long term experience with fluoride and fluoride combination treatment of osteoporosis. In: Kuhlencordt F, Kruse H (eds) Calcium metabolism, bone and metabolic bone disease. Springer Verlag, New York

Jung R 1981 Annual Review — Nutrition, Hospital Update 7/883–898

Keele C A, Neil E, Joels N 1982 Samson Wright's applied physiology, 13th edn. Oxford University Press, Oxford

Kennedy K 1979 A critical appraisal of surgical treatment. In: Truelove S C, Willoughly C P (eds) Topics in gastroenterology 7. Blackwell Scientific, Oxford

Keys A, Brozek J, Henschel A, Mickelson O, Taylor H L 1950 The biology of human starvation, vols 1–11. University of Minnesota Press, Minneapolis

Klidjian A M 1981 Problems of nutrition in surgical patients, Part 1 and 2. Update 22:1101–13, 1449–53

Krause M V, Mahan L K 1984 Nutritional care in conditions of overweight and underweight. In: Food, nutritition and diet therapy, 7th edn. Saunders, Philadelphia

Krishnaswamy K, Rao S B, Raghuram, T C et al 1976 Effects of vitamin B_6 on leucine induced changes in human subjects. American Journal of Clinical Nutrition 29:177–181

Langman M J S, Pounder R E, Wastell C 1983 The stomach and duodenum. In: Bouchier, I A D (ed) Recent advances in gastroenterology 5. Churchill Livingstone, Edinburgh

Lanzotti V J, Copeland E M, George S L, Dudrick S J, Samuels M L, 1975 Cancer: Chemotherapeutic response and intravenous hyperalimentation. Cancer Chemotherapy Report 59:437–439

Larsson S 1954 On hypothalamic organisation of nervous mechanism regulating food intake. Acta Physologica Scandinavica 32 (suppl 115):1–63

Leahy D, St Germain J, Varrichio C 1979 The nurse and radiotherapy. CV Mosby, St Louis

Lee H A 1978 Parenteral nutrition. In: Dickerson J W T, Lee H A (eds) Nutrition in the clinical management of disease. Edward Arnold, London

Lepkovsky S 1977 The role of the chemical senses in nutrition. In: Kare M R, Maller O (eds) The chemical senses and nutrition. Academic Press, New York

Losowsky M S 1983 Malabsorption. In: Weatherall D J, Ledingham J G G, Warrell D A (eds) Oxford textbook of medicine. Oxford University Press, Oxford

Lutwak, L 1974 Dietary calcium and reversal of bone demineralisation. Nutrition News 37(1)

Macleod J (ed) 1984 Davidson's principles and practice of medicine, 13th edn. Churchill Livingstone, Edinburgh

Mann W N 1975 Conybeare's textbook of medicine, 16th edn. Churchill Livingstone, Edinburgh

Marks I N 1979 A sceptical view of medical treatment. In: Truelove S C, Willoughby C P (eds) Topics in gastroenterology 7. Blackwell Scientific, Oxford

Marks V 1974 Effects of drugs on carbohydrate metabolism Proceedings of the Nutrition Society 33:209–214

Matheson R T, Herbert J J, Jubix W 1976 Absorption and biotransformation of cholecalciferol in drug–induced osteomalacia. Journal of Clinical Pharmacology 16:426–432

Mayer J, Monella J F, Seltzer C C 1965 Hunger and satiety in man. Postgraduate Medicine 37A:97–102

Mayer-Gross W, Walker J W 1946 Taste and selection in hypoglycaemia. British Journal of Experimental Pathology 27:297–298

McFarland J 1980 Basic clinical surgery for nurses and medical students, 2nd edn. Butterworths, London

McMichael H B 1975 Chemical studies of carbohydrate digestion and absorption. Biochemical Society Transaction 3(2):223–227

Mecklenberg R S, Loriaux D L, Thompson R H, Anderson A E, Lipsett M B 1974 Hypothalamic dysfunction in patients with anorexia nervosa. Medicine (Baltimore) 53:147–159

Metropolitan Life Insurance Company 1960 Actuarial tables. Statistical Bulletin 41(6):1

Miller D S, Payne P R 1962 Journal of Nutrition 78:255–262

Miller N E, Nestel P J 1973 Altered bile metabolism during treatment with phenobarbitone. Clinical Science and Molecular Medicine 45:257–262

Minuchin S, Rosman B, Baker 1978 Psychosomatic families: anorexia nervosa in context. Harvard University Press, Cambridge, Massachusetts

Misiewicz J J, Pounder R E 1983 Peptic ulcer. In: Weatherall D J, Ledingham J G G, Warrell D A (eds) Oxford textbook of medicine. Oxford University Press, Oxford

Mohanram M, Reddy V, Mishra S 1974 Lysozyme activity in plasma and leucocytes in malnourished children. British Journal of Nutrition 32:313–316

Moore F D 1959 Metabolic care of the surgical patient. Saunders, Philadelphia

Morgan H G, Russell G F M 1975 Value of family background and clinical features as predictors of long term outcome in anorexia nervosa: four year follow up study of 41 patients. Psychological Medicine 5:355–371

Murray M N, Ryle J A, Simpson B W, Wilson D C 1948 MRC Memo No. 18

Muto M, Maki T, Majima S, Yamaguchi I 1968 Improvement in the end–results of surgical treatment of gastric cancer. Surgery 63:229–235

Neill D J 1972 Masticatory studies. In: A nutrition survey of the elderly. DHSS, HMSO, London

Nordin B E C 1973 Metabolic bone and stone disease. Williams & Wilkins, Baltimore

Okun R, Russell R P, Wilson W R 1963 Use of diazoxide with trichloromethiazide for hypertension. Archives of Internal Medicine 112:882–888

Pennington C R, Bouchier I A D 1983 The liver. In: Bouchier I A D (ed) Recent advances in gastroenterology 5. Churchill Livingstone, Edinburgh

Powell-Tuck K 1980 Nutritional methods (treatment for Crohn's disease). In: Truelove S C, Kennedy H J (eds) Topics in gastroenterology 8. Blackwell Scientific, Oxford

Rault R M, Scribner B H 1977 Treatment of Crohn's disease with home parenteral nutrition. Gastroenterology 73:1077–1081

Registrar General 1971 Registrar General's decennial supplements mortality tables for 1959–69. HMSO, London

Reynolds E H 1974 Iatrogenic nutritional effects of anticonvulsants. Proceedings of the Nutrition Society 33:225– 229

Rogers M J, Spector R G, Trounce J R 1981 A textbook of clinical pharmacology. Hodder and Stoughton, London

Royal College of Physicians of London 1980 Medical aspects of dietary fibre. Pitman Medical, Tunbridge Wells

Royal College of Physicians of London 1983 Obesity. Journal of the Royal College of Physicians 17:3–58

Royle G 1980 Its use in inflammatory conditions (Parenteral feeding). In: Truelove S C, Kennedy H J (eds) Topics in gastroenterology 8. Blackwell Scientific, Oxford

Russell G F M 1982 The treatment of anorexia nervosa and bulimia nervosa. Paper presented at Extremes of Nutrition, First British Society of Gastroenterology/Glaxo International Teaching Day

Russell, G F M 1975 Anorexia nervosa. In: Beeson P B, McDermott W (eds) Textbook of medicine, 14th edn. Saunders, Philadelphia

Schubert G E, Shulte H D 1963 Contributions to the clinical picture of steroid diabetes. Deutsche Medizinische Wochenschrift 88:1175–1188

Schwartz S I, Storer E H 1984 Manifestations of gastrointestinal disease. In: Schwartz S I, Shires G T, Spencer F C, Storer E H (eds) Principles of surgery, 4th edn. McGraw-Hill, New York

Scrimshaw N S 1965 Malnutrition and infection. Borden's Review of Nutrition 26(2):17–29

Scrimshaw N S 1975 Deficiencies of individual nutrients: Hypovitaminosis A (including xeropthalmia and keratomalacia). In: Beeson P B, McDermott W (eds) Textbook of medicine, 14th edn. Saunders, Philadelphia

Sharon I M 1965 Sensory properties of food and their function during eating. Food Technology 19:35–36

Shields R 1965 The absorption and secretion of fluid and electrolytes by the obstructed bowel. British Journal of Surgery 52:774

Simon R I 1963 Obesity as a depressive equivalent. Journal of the American Medical Association 183:208–210

Smiddy F G 1976 Medical management of the surgical patient. Edward Arnold, London

Stedman 1982 Illustrated Stedman's medical dictionary, 24th edn. Williams and Wilkins, Baltimore

Stotts N A, Fitzgerald K A, Williams K R 1984 Care of the patient critically ill with inflammatory bowel disease. Nursing Clinics of North America 19(1):61–70

Studley H O 1936 Percentage of weight loss: basic indicator of surgical risk in patients with chronic peptic ulcer. Journal of the American Medical Association 106:458–460

Terpila S 1971 Morphologic and functional response of human small intestine to ionising radiation. Scandinavian Journal of Gastroenterology (suppl) 6:9–48

Thornton J R, Emmett P M, Heaton K W 1979 Diet and Crohn's disease: characteristics of the pre–illness diet. British Medical Journal 2:762–764

Trayhurn P, James W P T 1981 Thermogenesis — a control mechanism in obesity? 1. Brown fat may play an important role. Nutrition Bulletin 31, British Nutrition Foundation 6(1):15–22

Trier J S, Browning T H 1966 Morphologic response of the mucosa of the human small intestine to X-ray exposure. Journal of Clinical Investigation 45:194–204

Truswell A S 1973 Effects of drugs on nutrients. Update 7; 179–186

Van Itallie T B, Yang M 1977 Diet and weight loss. New England Journal of Medicine 297:1158–1169

Vilter R W 1964 The vitamin B_6–hydrazide relationship. Vitamins and Hormones 22:797–805

Warren M P, Van de Wiele R L 1973 Clinical and metabolic features of anorexia nervosa. American Journal of Obstetrics and Gynecology 117:435–449

Wastell C 1979 Pathogenesis of duodenal ulcer. In: Truelove S C, Willoughby C P (eds) Topics in gastroenterology 7. Blackwell Scientific, Oxford

Way L W 1975 Diseases of the gallbladder and bile ducts. In: Beeson P B, McDermott W (eds) Textbook of medicine 14th edn. Saunders, Philadelphia

Wells N 1981 Sickness absence — a review. Offices of Health Economics Briefing No 16, London

Williams C D 1962 Malnutrition. Lancet 2:342–344
Youmans J B 1964 The changing face of nutritional disease in America. Journal of the American Medical Association 189:672–676
Zilva S F, Pannall P R 1979 Clinical chemistry in diagnosis and treatment. Lloyd Luke, London

24

Disturbances of maintenance of the internal environment — oxygenation and carbon dioxide excretion

INTRODUCTION

One of the most vital factors to be maintained in the internal environment is a supply of oxygen to the tissues. Any deficiency in this may have permanent effects on parts or the whole of the body, and if severe may rapidly prove fatal. As Haldane (1914) said 'Hypoxia not only breaks the machine but wrecks the machinery'. The level of carbon dioxide in the blood similarly has important effects. Perhaps less often considered is the fact that too high a level of oxygenation can be detrimental to health, if not immediately then in the longer term. Yet perhaps because oxygenation and carbon dioxide elimination are so vital, the human body has various ways of adaptation which provide for maintenance of function despite abnormalities in the body or its external environment. From the patient's subjective point of view, disturbance of oxygenation and of breathing, the main mechanism for maintaining it, can lead to some of the most distressing symptoms possible. For many people acute breathlessness and/or difficulty in breathing seems even more distressing and disabling than pain.

STRUCTURE AND FUNCTION

Oxygen is constantly used by the body tissues in metabolic processes (about 200ml/min for an adult at rest) and carbon dioxide is constantly produced. The rate of oxygen utilization and carbon dioxide production are variable. Therefore an efficient system responsive to changing demands is required to maintain the levels required for health and effective function of the body as a whole. This system can be considered in three parts:

1. The structure and function maintaining ventilation, that is the exchange of air between the alveoli and the external environment
2. The gas diffusion and transport system
3. The control mechanism

These will be described here only insofar as is necessary to discuss disturbances and abnormalities. Further information can be found in any good physiology text.

Ventilation

The main essentials for good ventilation are:

- Patent airways
- Distensible (compliant) intact lungs
- An intact thoracic cage and diaphragm which are stimulated to move rhythmically to increase and decrease the size of the thoracic cavity, thus lowering the intrathoracic pressure on inspiration and raising it on expiration.
- A sub-atmospheric pressure between the parietal and visceral layers of the pleura, so that as the chest walls move out the lungs expand drawing in air, which is then expelled when the chest walls move inwards as the intercostal muscles relax (or as the expiratory intercostals cause active expiration)

The diaphragm plays quite an important part in ventilation, particularly if the rib cage is less mobile due to rigidity, heaviness, or weak muscle movements. The amount of air inspired or expired varies under the influence of the control mechanisms, there being an inspiratory reserve of 2.5–3.5 litres from resting volume and approximately 1 litre expiratory reserve, expelled on further forced expiration. However it is important to remember that of the 500ml (approximately) tidal volume of an adult breathing quietly, some 150ml remains in the anatomical dead space at the end of expiration, to be drawn down into the lungs as inspiration recommences. So that the air drawn from the environment reaching the alveoli each inspiration is only 350ml. Since the size of the dead space remains constant, if respiration becomes rapid and shallow the 150 ml of air re-entering the lungs forms a larger proportion of the tidal volume. Thus even with a more rapid rate the actual exchange of air between the environment and the alveoli may be reduced. Conversely with a slower rate and increased tidal volume the exchange may be increased (see Table 24.1).

There are also small areas of alveolar dead space, where air enters the alveoli but the blood supply is inadequate for much diffusion of gases to occur. In normal lungs the area of alveolar dead space is small and unimportant, but in abnormal conditions the imbalance between alveolar ventilation and perfusion can become severe and may even be fatal.

The phospholipoprotein in the fluid which lines the alveolar walls (known as pulmonary surfactant) reduces the surface tension. When pulmonary surfactant is reduced, greatly increased effort is required to distend the lungs with air. One example of this is the respiratory

Table 24.1 Alveolar ventilation at different respiratory rates

Tidal volume		Dead space volume		Respiratory rate		Alveolar ventilation (exchange between alveoli and environment)
500 ml	–	150 ml	×	20	=	7000ml
200 ml	–	150 ml	×	30	=	1500 ml
750 ml	–	150 ml	×	14	=	8400 ml

distress syndrome in premature infants with immature lungs.

Gas diffusion and transport

Gas diffusion depends on the difference in pressure of the gas on either side of the membrane, the area and thickness of the membrane and the density and permeability of the membrane. It is the pressure gradient (difference in pressure) between one side of the membrane and the other which causes diffusion of gases, both across the alveolar membrane in the lungs and across the cell membranes from the interstitial fluid into the cells of body tissues. Since carbon dioxide diffuses more rapidly than oxygen, any reduction in diffusion capacity is likely to affect oxygenation more than carbon dioxide elimination.

For normal gas exchange to occur between the alveoli and the blood there must be both good alveolar ventilation and perfusion. Obviously, where both ventilation and perfusion are absent no gas exchange can take place. When perfusion is deficient but the alveoli are ventilated then the effort of ventilating the alveoli is wasted, but such blood as does pass through the area will be oxygenated. However, good perfusion of an unventilated area results in desaturated blood passing through into the arterial circulation, a situation known as shunting. Ventilation-perfusion imbalance is often referred to as V/Q inequality or imbalance.

Oxygen transport

Comparatively little oxygen can be carried dissolved in the blood, 3ml per litre in arterial blood. But if the haemoglobin level is normal (around 15g/100ml), another 197ml per litre is transported bound to the haemoglobin. As blood passes through the tissues, oxygen is taken up from the plasma by the cells, but as the PO_2 (partial pressure of oxygen dissolved in the plasma) falls, oxygen is released or dissociated from the haemoglobin and passes into the plasma. The rate at which this occurs is altered by various factors. The oxygen dissociation curve (Fig. 24.1) shows that when the temperature is

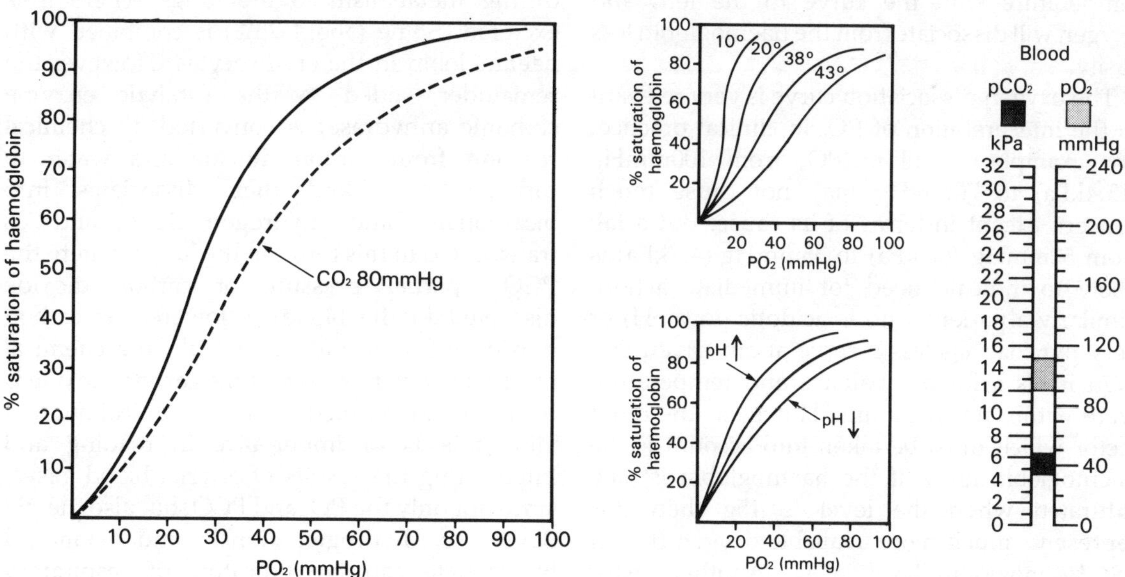

Fig. 24.1 Haemoglobin-oxygen dissociation curve. It can be seen on the graphs that when the body temperature is raised, the pH decreased or the PCO_2 increased, the curve shifts to the right, i.e. oxygen dissociates from haemoglobin more readily for use by the tissues. Since SI units are now in use in many places, these are shown with the equivalents on the scale on the right.

Table 24.2 Disturbances in acid-base balance in respiratory disorders

Condition	pH	PCO_2 mmHg	Standard bicarb. mmol/l	PO_2 mmHg
Normal	7.35–7.45	40	24	100
Respiratory acidosis	↓	↑	normal	normal or ↓
Compensated respiratory acidosis	normal	↑	↑	normal or ↓
Respiratory alkalosis	↑	↓	normal	normal
Compensated respiratory alkalosis	normal	↓	↓	normal
Metabolic acidosis	↓	normal	↓	normal

38°C and the acid base balance normal (pH7.35–7.45), if the PO_2 is 60mmHg (8kPa), 90% of the haemoglobin is saturated or combined with oxygen. A rise to a PO_2 of 100mmHg (13.4kPa) only increases saturation to 97%, so there is a considerable safety factor (Vander et al, 1975). However both a rise in temperature or a fall in pH cause the oxygen to dissociate from the haemoglobin more readily (the curve shifts to the right and downwards), so that for any given PO_2 the percentage of haemoglobin saturated will be lower. Conversely, alkalosis or a fall in temperature shift the curve to the left, and oxygen will dissociate from the haemoglobin less easily.

The oxygen dissociation curve is very relevant to the interpretation of PO_2 in clinical practice. For example, a fall in PO_2 from 100mmHg (13.4kPa) to 70mmHg may not cause much concern except in terms of its cause. But a fall from 50mmHg (6.7kPa) to 35mmHg (4.7kPa) is likely to indicate need for immediate action. Similarly a patient who is acidotic (low pH) or very pyrexial has less reserve at any given PO_2 than if his acid-base balance and temperature were within normal limits. However, the other factor which must be taken into account is the haemoglobin level. If the haemoglobin is 60% saturated when the level is 15g then this represents much more available oxygen than if the haemoglobin level is 8g. Another factor worth noting is that while cyanosis usually becomes evident when the saturation level drops to about 75–80%, this depends on the haemoglobin level. Cyanosis only occurs when there is at least 5g desaturated haemoglobin per 100ml of blood. Therefore if the patient's haemoglobin level is very low cyanosis may never be seen, however hypoxic he becomes. To summarize, haemoglobin is vital to the transport of oxygen from the lungs to the body tissues.

Carbon dioxide transport

As with oxygen, relatively little carbon dioxide can be transported dissolved in the blood. Therefore some other mechanism is necessary for it to pass from the tissues where it is produced during metabolism to the lungs where it is excreted. Some (about 25%) is combined with haemoglobin in the erythrocytes. However the remainder, aided by the catalytic enzyme carbonic anhydrase, is converted by chemical reaction from carbon dioxide and water to carbonic acid, and then dissociates into bicarbonate and hydrogen ions and is transported in this form. In the lungs, where the PCO_2 (partial pressure of carbon dioxide dissolved in the blood) is lowered as carbon dioxide diffuses into the alveoli, the chemical reaction is reversed so that the carbon dioxide is released and excreted. From the clinical point of view this is of importance in reading and interpreting the results of arterial blood gases, since not only the PO_2 and PCO_2 but also the pH (level of hydrogen ions) and standard bicarbonate can be indicative of respiratory function.

Acid-base balance

Respiratory function plays a considerable part in

regulating the acid-base balance, and can cause three of the four major types of imbalance. Respiratory failure and a rise in PCO_2 (hypercapnia) results in respiratory acidosis, unless it is longstanding and compensated, i.e. the standard bicarbonate (base) rises to balance rise in hydrogen ions (acid), thus restoring the pH within normal limits. Conversely hyperventilation and a fall in PCO_2 (hypocapnia) results in respiratory alkalosis. Tissue hypoxia, whether due to respiratory causes or deficient circulation, results in metabolism following the anaerobic path with increased production of lactic acid, thus leading to metabolic acidosis (Table 24.2).

Control of respiration

The respiratory cycle is mainly controlled by the inspiratory neurons in the medulla, the lower portion of the brainstem. These initiate, via the spinal cord and the intercostal and phrenic nerves, contraction of the intercostal inspiratory muscles and diaphragm, causing inspiration. Expiration occurs when these muscles relax and is largely passive, though active expiration can take place involving the expiratory intercostal muscles and controlled by the expiratory neurons in the medulla. But what regulates the rate and depth of respiration? This can be controlled voluntarily to some extent, but not if the involuntary controls are too intensely stimulated. Research over a number of years has shown that the main stimulus to breathing under normal conditions is a rise in hydrogen ions (acidity) of the cerebrospinal fluid which surrounds the brain acting on central chemoreceptors. This is usually caused by a rise in carbon dioxide levels, but metabolic acidosis also causes an increase in ventilation. Hypoxia, a low PO_2, also stimulates respiration by its effect on the chemoreceptors in the aortic and carotid bodies. But this mechanism only becomes important when the response of the respiratory centre to change in the PCO_2 and pH fails. An example is compensated respiratory acidosis, when the PCO_2 is persistently raised but a normal pH is maintained by raised standard bicarbonate level. In this situation it is hypoxia which stimulates ventilation and excessive oxygen administration may lead to bradypnoea or even apnoea. There are other factors which affect the respiratory centre, such as temperature input from the cerebral cortex, adrenaline, reflexes from muscles and joints, baroceptor reflexes, protective reflexes such as coughing, pain and emotion (Vander et al, 1975).

One of the important factors in increase or decrease of the ventilatory volume is the diameter of the bronchi and bronchioles. The walls of each of these contain smooth muscle with a good nerve supply, which is sensitive to hormones such as adrenaline. Flow of air through the air passages and the associated effort to achieve it are considerably affected by their diameter, for example doubling the radius increases the flow sixteenfold for the same effort. Since the radius normally decreases on expiration, any extra decrease will usually cause difficulty on expiration, e.g. when the bronchi are inflamed and thickened in bronchitis wheezing may occur.

HYPOCAPNIA, HYPERCAPNIA AND HYPOXIA

Whatever the cause, the basic signs and symptoms associated with hypocapnia (low PCO_2), hypercapnia (high PCO_2), or hypoxia (low PO_2) remain constant, so these will be described before discussion of the various abnormalities which may cause them. However it must be recognized that hypoxia may occur concurrently with hyper- or hypocapnia, so signs and symptoms may be mixed depending on the predominant factor. Blood gas analysis of an arterial blood specimen is necessary to confirm diagnosis.

Hypocapnia

This causes pallor, lightheadedness, tingling and numbness in the limbs or round the mouth, and if severe may cause carpopedal spasm (tetany). This can be quite alarming to the person concerned even if the cause is psychosomatic. Anxiety then maintains rapid breathing, increasing the problem.

Hypercapnia

This is indicated by flushed, warm skin, and reddened conjunctiva (vasodilatation), sweating, possibly tachycardia, hypertension, headache, and other cerebral signs such as irritability, lack of concentration, confusion, drowsiness and eventually coma. One of the signs of improvement or deterioration sometimes used in assessing patients with chronic respiratory failure and CO_2 retention is the ability to write legibly and intelligibly, this ability increasing as CO_2 retention decreases and cerebral function improves.

Hypoxia

Common signs and symptoms of hypoxia include tachycardia, tachypnoea and a feeling of breathlessness, pallor or cyanosis, and cerebral signs such as lethargy and decreased responsiveness (obtundation), or confusion and sometimes agitation. Cyanosis may be central, visible in all areas of the body in a Caucasian, particularly the mucous membranes of the mouth. (In dark-skinned patients it can only be seen in the mucous membranes or sometimes in the lighter skin, such as the palms of the hands.) It is caused by general deficiency of oxygen in the circulation. Peripheral cyanosis results from decreased perfusion of blood through the peripheries, so that a greater proportion of oxygen is extracted from the blood as it flows through. If the area, e.g. an ear lobe or finger, is rubbed gently circulation increases and the area temporarily becomes pink. Since cyanosis only occurs when there is at least 5g reduced (desaturated) haemoglobin per 100ml blood, it will occur quite readily in a polycythaemic patient and not at all in a very anaemic one, however great the hypoxia.

There are four main types of hypoxia:

1. Hypoxic hypoxia, in which the PO_2 is decreased, due for example to hypoventilation or low environmental oxygen
2. Anaemic hypoxia, in which the haemoglobin is decreased or abnormal and therefore oxygen transport is reduced
3. Ischaemic hypoxia, when perfusion of tissues is poor and therefore little oxygen reaches them, e.g. in shock
4. Histotoxic hypoxia, in which oxygen reaches the tissues but utilization is prevented by a toxic agent such as cyanide

It should be recognized that anything which increases tissue demand for oxygen, e.g. raised metabolic rate or pyrexia, may precipitate a state of hypoxia in a patient whose oxygen supply to the tissues would otherwise be adequate. The metabolic requirement for oxygen increases 12% for each degree Celsius rise in temperature and 7% for each degree Fahrenheit (Aspinall & Tanner, 1981). Poor tissue perfusion which would lead to ischaemic hypoxia has been discussed in Chapter 10. Deficiencies in blood constituents have been discussed elsewhere (Ch. 22), and histotoxic hypoxia is rare. Therefore conditions leading to hypoxic hypoxia will be the main subject of discussion.

RESPIRATORY FAILURE

Causes of respiratory failure are many and can be classified in various ways. Here it is proposed to relate them to the three parts of the system previously described as maintaining normal oxygen-carbon dioxide balance, and to discuss:

1. Abnormalities of the structure and function of the thorax and airways affecting ventilation
2. Abnormalities affecting gas diffusion and transport in the lungs
3. Abnormalities affecting the control mechanisms

Internationally-agreed diagnostic criteria for respiratory failure are an arterial oxygen (PO_2) of less than 8.0kPa (60mmHg) or CO_2 tension (PCO_2) above 6.5kPa (49mmHg) when the patient is breathing room air. Thus a low PO_2 is always present but the PCO_2 may be low, normal or raised (Jones, 1978). The degree of hypercapnia is an indication of the degree of hypoventilation, whatever has caused this.

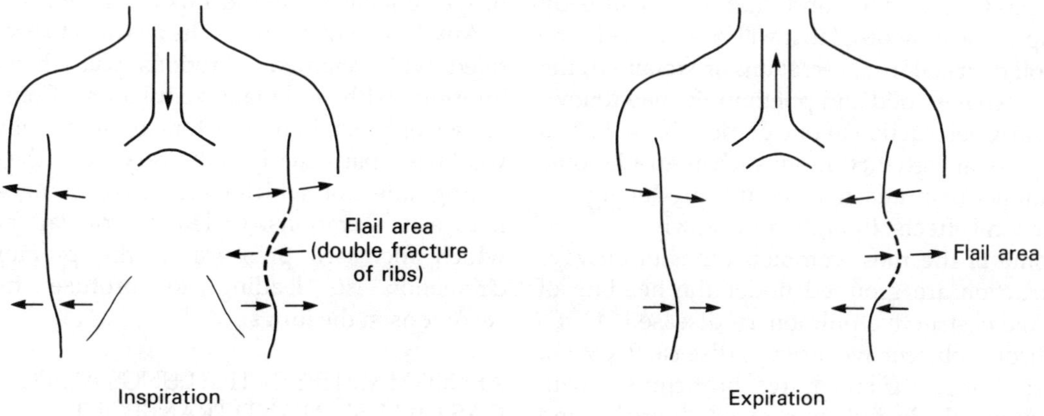

Fig. 24.2 Paradoxical respiration. When there are double fractures of several ribs, the affected area of the chest wall becomes a flail (unsupported) and moves paradoxically, i.e. in the opposite direction to the rest of the chest wall, thus impeding lung function. Fractures of the sternum or costochondral junctions may have the same effect.

CONDITIONS OF THE THORAX AND AIRWAYS REDUCING VENTILATION

Abnormalities of the thorax and pleura

Rigidity of the rib-cage, such as may occur in ankylosing spondylitis or advancing years (Ebersole & Hess, 1981), or abnormal shape such as kyphoscoliosis or pectus excavatum, reduce the vital capacity by limiting expansion of the lungs and so limiting respiratory reserve. Trauma, whether accidental or surgical, may result in restriction of ventilation due to pain or due to a flail segment of chest wall. In this condition a portion of the bony chest wall becomes detached from other bony structures, due either to double fractures of several ribs, or fracture of the costochondral junctions on either side of the sternum. As the chest wall moves out on inspiration the intrathoracic pressure decreases and the loose portion is sucked inwards, conversely it is pushed outwards when the intrathoracic pressure rises on expiration. Thus, as the major portion of the lungs inflates and deflates the portion of lung under the loose (flail) section deflates and inflates; this is known as paradoxical respiration. Consequently air may be moved from one area of the lung to another instead of moving out of the lungs to be replaced by fresh air (Fig. 24.2). If the flail area is large this rapidly results in respiratory failure, with both hypercapnia and hypoxia.

A penetrating injury through the chest wall, rupture of an emphysematous bulla (air cyst), or spontaneous rupture of the pleura overlying the lung will cause pneumothorax. If there is a loose flap of tissue allowing air into the pleural cavity but not out, then a tension pneumothorax will cause increasing compression of the remaining lung. A pleural effusion or bleeding may limit lung expansion, and if chronic or infected (empyema) may cause the pleura to become thickened and less mobile thus permanently restricting lung expansion and respiratory reserve.

Airways obstruction

The most dramatic cause of respiratory failure is airway obstruction due to inhalation of a foreign body, or of some gas or liquid which causes laryngeal spasm. The flow of air in and out of the lungs may cease, in which case the person will soon become unconscious and, within about 4 minutes, will die or sustain permanent hypoxic damage to the brain and other vital organs unless the airway is cleared and ventilation recommenced. If the foreign material passes further down and blocks one of the bronchi then no air can pass beyond it, and that which already occupies the lung distal to it will be absorbed. The alveoli then collapse, secretions are retained, the lung becomes solid and pneumonia may follow. Similarly obstruction of one or more bronchi by a benign or malignant tumour such as an adenoma or adenocarcinoma may occur, producing the same local effects, though more slowly.

Some of the most common types of airways obstruction are grouped under the heading of chronic obstructive pulmonary disease (COPD) or chronic obstructive airways disease (COAD). These range from pure bronchitis, with inflamed, thickened, narrowed bronchi and increased sputum production, to emphysema where the main pathological abnormality is destruction of the alveolar walls and decreasing elasticity of the lungs. Most patients with COPD have a combination of these conditions. Those in whom bronchitis predominates are sometimes referred to as 'blue bloaters' because of the central cyanosis, pulmonary hypertension and general oedema due to sodium and water retention which occur in the advanced stages, in addition to hypercapnia. Those with emphysema as the main pathology are referred to as 'pink puffers' since they are often thin and pink with right ventricular hypertrophy, 'puffing' (expiring through pursed lips) at an increased rate (Leonard, 1981).

Bronchospasm with 'wheezing' on expiration is a common feature of chronic obstructive pulmonary disease, but may also be due to other causes and typically occurs in asthma which affects about 3% of the population in the United Kingdom (Jones & Luksza, 1979). The cause of asthma is unknown, though allergens are sometimes a precipitating factor. The bronchospasm is accompanied by thickening of the bronchial walls due to congestion and oedema, and formation of thick plugs of mucus, leucocytes, serum and shed cells of the ciliated mucous membrane. These plugs obstruct the smaller airways and lead to a mismatch between ventilation and perfusion of some alveoli, resulting in hypoxia and, if the condition is very severe, hypercapnia. Long-term effects include hyperinflation of the lungs, pneumothorax, emphysema and sometimes aspergillosis, a fungus infection (Jones & Luksza, 1979).

Anything which causes the airways to become filled with retained secretions will obviously interfere with adequate ventilation. Common causes or precipitating factors are immobility or weakness, particularly in the very old or the very young, infection which increases or changes the nature of secretions, or left ventricular failure which increases pressure in the pulmonary circulation so leading to profuse frothy secretions in the lungs.

ABNORMALITIES IN THE LUNGS AFFECTING GAS DIFFUSION AND TRANSPORT

Adult respiratory distress syndrome (ARDS)

One of the relatively common causes of respiratory failure due to interference with gas diffusion is a condition now usually referred to as adult respiratory distress syndrome (ARDS), because the eventual pathological effects on the lung (interstitial fibrosis and formation of hyaline membrane) are like those in the lungs of infants with respiratory distress syndrome. It includes those conditions known as 'shock lung', 'pump lung' and 'ventilator lung', amongst others. Wagner (1981), in a review of the literature, lists the many conditions which may be associated with ARDS, which include low perfusion state (shock) from any cause, severe soft tissue injury, inhalation of acid gastric contents (Mendelson's syndrome), fractures leading to fat emboli, sepsis and toxaemia, and cerebral hypoxia. Other causative factors include those related to treatment such as massive transfusion, excessive fluid administration, oxygen toxicity due to prolonged use of high concentrations of oxygen, or prolonged artificial ventilation. For a full review of the condition, treatment and nursing care see Wagner (1981), but the main features of the condition are increasing hypoxia which may become increasingly unresponsive to oxygen therapy, pulmonary oedema associated with increased pulmonary capillary permeability, and decreased pulmonary compliance (stiff lungs). Treatment is more likely to be successful if started early, so any patient with any of the conditions associated with ARDS should be observed for early signs. These include, in the patient breathing spontaneously, increased breathing (with or without the patient feeling breathless), respiratory alkalosis, and possibly some hypoxaemia though initially this may be compensated by the increased breathing. Untreated the condition may progress within a few days to terminal respiratory failure.

Lung fibrosis and emphysema

Fibrosis of the lung with thickening of the alveolar walls, and emphysema, in which the alveolar wall area is decreased by destruction, are both more chronic conditions which reduce the capacity for oxygen and carbon dioxide to diffuse across the alveolar membrane into or out of the circulation. Conditions outside the lung, such as left ventricular failure or electrolyte imbalance, may also result in a diffusion block by causing pulmonary oedema. The increased interstitial fluid increases the alveolar-capillary distance thus reducing gas diffusion.

Disturbed perfusion

Oxygenation of the body tissues requires not only an adequate intake of oxygen but a means of transport, that is adequate perfusion of lung tissue with blood carrying sufficient haemoglobin in the red cells for effective oxygen transport. Any condition which obstructs the circulation to lung tissue will lead to hypoxia if it affects a sufficiently large area. Pulmonary embolism is an example of this. In the case of congenital abnormalities such as pulmonary valve stenosis, the reduced flow of blood through the lungs limits oxygenation, but there may also be the added complication of a shunt of deoxygenated blood from right to left side of the heart through a septal defect. This may result in a sufficient degree of hypoxaemia to cause constant central cyanosis. If the circulating blood is deficient in haemoglobin this will increase susceptibility to tissue hypoxia due to other causes.

ABNORMALITIES OF THE CONTROL MECHANISMS

As previously stated, control over ventilation involves the respiratory centre in the brain, the nerve supply to the diaphragm, chest wall and bronchi, and chemoreceptors in the aortic and carotid bodies. Therefore anything which affects these may alter respiratory function and change the oxygen-carbon dioxide balance in the body.

First, the central respiratory centre. This may be acutely affected by cerebral trauma, haemorrhage or tumours, each of which may cause a rise in intracranial pressure which in turn interferes with normal function of the respiratory centre. Initially the effect may be hyperventilation and respiratory alkalosis or irregular respiration (Bordeaux, 1973), but as the pressure rises the ventilation rate is likely to slow until eventually breathing ceases. Damage deep in the cerebral hemispheres, diencephalon or basal ganglion may cause Cheyne-Stokes respiration. This is rhythmic, respirations increasing in rate and depth to a maximum, then gradually decreasing until the cycle starts again. Apneustic breathing (a pause at full inspiration) may occur with massive lesions in the pons. Hypoglycaemia, hypoxia and cerebral infarction may cause some degree of central neurogenic hyperventilation, since all affect the medulla oblongata and midbrain respiratory centres.

Ingestion of drugs may affect respiration in various ways according to the drug ingested. For example, hypnotics such as the barbiturates or opiates depress the respiratory centre, so that with large doses or a very susceptible patient ventilation decreases in rate and depth and may cease; while acetylsalicylic acid (aspirin) in large doses may cause hyperventilation due to metabolic acidosis. Even in doses normally therapeutic, drugs may cause respiratory difficulties. For example post-operative analgesics such as morphia or pethedine given in doses normal for the size and age of the patient may depress respiration sufficiently to cause hypoxia in a very sick patient or one whose respiratory function was already impaired. Beta receptor blocking drugs given to reduce sympathetic stimulation of a damaged heart may lead to bronchospasm in susceptible people, and of course dramatic respiratory distress and anaphylactic shock may result from a drug to which the patient is allergic.

As already mentioned, in chronic respiratory

failure the central respiratory centre may become accustomed to a higher PCO_2, and stimulation of ventilation then depends on the sensitivity to hypoxia of the chemoreceptors in the carotid bodies and aortic arch.

Any condition which affects the nerve supply to the thoracic wall and/or diaphragm will affect ventilation and may cause respiratory failure which may be permanent or reversible, as in poliomyelitis or myasthenia gravis.

There are also rare conditions, such as the Ondine's Curse syndrome in which the patient simply fails to breathe when asleep (Zeluff et al, 1977).

This is by no means a comprehensive list of conditions which may lead to respiratory failure, hypoxia and hypercapnia, but includes examples of types most commonly encountered.

TREATMENT OF RESPIRATORY CONDITIONS WHICH MAY CAUSE OXYGEN-CARBON DIOXIDE IMBALANCE

The main aims of treatment of respiratory conditions can be summed up as maintaining or restoring clear airways, maintenance of adequate ventilation, and prevention or early detection and treatment of conditions which impair gas diffusion and oxygenation. The most common methods of achieving these aims are discussed below.

REMOVAL OF ANY ACUTE OBSTRUCTION

If a foreign body is inhaled it may be possible to remove it: if a child has the problem, by tipping the child upside down and smacking smartly on the back of the chest; if an adult is in severe trouble, by performing Heimlich's manoeuvre, i.e. abdominal thrusts (Sumner & Grau, 1982). If the obstruction is further down, bronchoscopy or even surgery may be necessary. However, it is better to avoid the problem than treat it, and common causes of obstruction such as the tongue falling back and obstructing the airway, or inhalation of vomit, can usually be prevented by observation and proper management of any very weak or unconscious person. Ideally such patients, or at least the head, should be turned to one side, but if this is not possible then the tongue can be kept forward by support behind the angle of the jaw, keeping the lower jaw forward. A common cause of obstruction in children is inhalation of peanuts. For this reason it is better not to give them to small children, or if they are given, then to insist that the children do not run around or laugh and talk while eating them.

FACILITATION OF REMOVAL OF SECRETIONS

Normally the mucus produced in the tracheobronchial tree can be moved upwards by the cilia until it enters the pharynx, occasionally aided by a slight cough, and is swallowed. The failure of this mechanism usually results from one or a combination of three factors:

- Change in the amount of secretions
- Change in the viscosity of secretions
- Change in the activity of the cilia and/or ability to cough

Change in the amount and viscosity of the secretion may be due to infection, the sputum becoming thick and viscid at first, then looser, purulent and sometimes copious. In infections such as bronchitis there is the added problem of inflamed and consequently narrowed airways, particularly on expiration, which makes it difficult to expectorate secretions. Dehydration will make any secretions more viscid and difficult to expectorate, while in asthma the added leucocytes and shed ciliated epithelium causes the secretions to form plugs which block the smaller bronchioles. In pulmonary oedema it is the copious amount of frothy secretions which is the problem, rather than the consistency. Cigarette-smoking is a common cause of impaired function of the cilia.

The measures directed at clearing secretions therefore include adequate but not excessive hydration; cessation of smoking; medications which may loosen secretions, relieve bronchospasm, or decrease infection or pulmonary oedema; good positioning to facilitate good lung function, and promotion of effective breathing. Hydration includes not only an adequate fluid intake but sometimes added local hydration by humidifiers, nebulizers or other inhalations (Levi, 1979). While technicians are now sometimes responsible for the maintenance and sterilization of such equipment, it remains the responsibility of any nurse using such equipment to ensure that she or he uses it safely and effectively. This means constant checking that the equipment is working and that it is maintained in a clean condition and disinfected during and after use as appropriate.

Tracheobronchial suction may be necessary if coughing is ineffective. If repeated suction is necessary then usually endotracheal intubation and perhaps tracheostomy is performed. Skilled care is then necessary to avoid the dangers of intubation, or tracheostomy (Leonard, 1981). These include obstruction of the airway by secretions, kinking or malposition of the tube; necrosis of the trachea due to pressure from an overinflated cuff on the tube, or malposition (this may lead to haemorrhage, tracheo-oesophageal fistula or, later, tracheal stenosis); infection, since normal humidifying and protective mechanisms are by-passed, and the mucosal damage during suction and possibly from dehydration. The patient may also suffer frustration from difficulties in communication owing to inability to talk.

DRUG THERAPY

Medications are administered for the purpose of keeping the air passages moist, removal of tenacious sputum, control of coughing, relief of bronchospasm, or eliminating infection (Bailey, 1979). Drugs may be given by inhalation, orally, by injection or occasionally rectally. Those given by steam inhalation include well-tried preparations such as tincture of benzoin compound to soothe and moisten inflamed airways, aerosols such as acetylcysteine or tyloxapol (as in Alevaire), or bronchodilators such as isoprenaline or salbutamol, or sodium chromoglycate to reduce the allergic response in asthma. These latter drugs are usually given via small inhalers which can be carried by the patient. Other medications such as expectorants, antibiotics, bronchodilators, or drugs used to relieve an unproductive and troublesome cough are usually given by mouth, but may be given by injection for very ill patients or those unable to take drugs orally. Some patients such as the severely ill asthmatic may be having a combination of aminophylline and steroids (Jones, 1979) and antibiotics intravenously, in which case it is very important to check which are incompatible and cannot be mixed in one infusion. When the patient cannot take the drugs by mouth and slower absorption is acceptable they may be used in suppository form.

GOOD BODY POSITIONING AND PROMOTION OF EFFECTIVE VENTILATION

Physiotherapists can be invaluable in teaching diaphragmatic and lateral breathing and other breathing exercises, in using or teaching techniques such as percussion or vibration over the rib cage, and for teaching positioning to drain specific areas of the lung by postural drainage. However, the availability of physiotherapists is very variable between different countries, different parts of a country or area, and even different hours of the day and night. Therefore nurses need to learn enough about these techniques to be able to support the patients in continuing their exercises, and to maintain adequate respiratory care when no physiotherapist is available. There are books and articles on the subject available (e.g. Brown, 1979), but the best way to learn is to observe and ask questions of good physiotherapists when working with them in patient care.

OXYGEN THERAPY

This is a treatment commonly used and often badly maintained. To be effective the correct amount of oxygen must reach the patient constantly, adequately humidified if necessary to avoid drying and damage to the mucous membranes.

Oxygen equipment

Various kinds of equipment are used to administer oxygen, and each has advantages and disadvantages in different situations. Some of the most commonly used types are face masks, nasal cannulae, tracheostomy masks or T-pieces, and intermittent positive pressure breathing (IPPB) machines or other ventilators. Oxygen tents are less often used now because of the cumbersome nature of the equipment, the difficulty of maintaining adequate oxygenation when the tent is opened for nursing procedures, and patient discomfort. However, incubators and head tents are still used for very young children, and small humidified tents for other children.

Nasal cannulae have the advantage that the patient can eat, drink, talk, and be given nursing care easily while wearing them. With a flow of 1–4l oxygen per minute the inspired oxygen can be 23–50%, although it varies according to the patient's inspiratory flow and whether there is mouth-breathing. Humidification is necessary to prevent soreness of the nose and throat, particularly if higher flow rates are used.

Low-flow oxygen masks such as the Hudson or MC also deliver a variable inspired oxygen percentage (FIO_2) since the patient breathes in some air round the mask, thus decreasing the FIO_2 as the inspiratory flow increases. Like all face masks they make it impossible for the patient to eat or drink normally without moving the mask, and are often disliked by patients who find them hot and uncomfortable. However, an inspired oxygen concentration of 60% or more may be achieved if the mask fits well and a high flow of oxygen is used. It is an adequate means of delivering oxygen when the lungs are normal and oxygen is given for a relatively short time, e.g. after non-thoracic surgery, but unsafe for anyone known to have chronic bronchitis in case the concentration becomes too high and depresses respiration, which could decrease the inspiratory flow, increase further the FIO_2 and lead to increasing hypercapnia.

High-flow oxygen masks were originally designed to deliver a safe and constant FIO_2 to patients with chronic respiratory disease. They work on the Venturi principle, i.e. the oxygen flows at high velocity through a small orifice entraining a fixed amount of air according to the design and size of lateral openings in the base of the mask. Masks are now available to deliver various stated percentages of inspired oxygen, from 24% to 60%, and some have interchangeable parts which allow the same mask to be used to deliver various percentages. High-flow systems do tend to dry the patient's mucous membranes unless the gas is humidified. Most masks are now disposable. Face tents (Levi, 1979) can be useful for humidification but cannot be used to increase the FIO_2 although they may be tolerated by the patient better than a mask. To ensure adequate oxygenation in some conditions, such as the respiratory distress syndrome, it may be necessary to deliver the oxygen via an endotracheal tube with intermittent positive pressure ventilation.

Dangers of oxygen administration and excessive oxygenation

The most common hazard in oxygen administration, apart from obvious dangers like fire, is with the patient with a chronically raised PCO_2, for example the chronic bronchitic, for whom slight hypoxia is necessary to stimulate ventilation. Since the respiratory centre has become insensitive to a rise in PCO_2, the amount of oxygen which can be given without depressing respiration is often 30% or less, and may be finely balanced.

It has been known since 1899 (Lorrain-Smith) that inhalation of high concentrations of oxygen may cause discomfort and lung damage. Breathing 100% oxygen at sea-level may cause retrosternal discomfort after only 6 hours; with 60% oxygen, after 36 hours (Scottish Home and Health Department, 1969). This has become of practical importance with the increased use of artificial ventilation, which makes it possible to administer high concentrations of oxygen over a prolonged period. For this reason the FIO_2 is now usually monitored and kept at 50% or less (Jones, 1978; Wagner, 1981) when possible to avoid pulmonary oxygen toxicity and the adult respiratory distress syndrome (ARDS).

Oxygen toxicity affecting the central nervous system and possibly causing convulsions (the Paul Bert effect) is only a risk in hyperbaric oxygen or diving therapy, since it only occurs when oxygen is breathed at greater than atmospheric pressure (Donald, 1947).

Another hazard is retrolental fibroplasia due to an abnormally raised arterial PO_2 over a period of several hours in premature infants. Since the 1950s, when a number of children became blind through this, it has been recognized that the high concentrations of oxygen necessary to treat the respiratory distress of the newborn syndrome can be safely used if the arterial PO_2 is carefully controlled (Pugh, 1978).

Since intermittent positive pressure breathing, with machines such as the Bird or Bennet ventilator, is used quite frequently in therapy it should be remembered that use of 100% oxygen may actually increase rather than decrease areas of lung de-aeration and collapse. This is because all the oxygen can be absorbed, allowing alveoli to collapse, while if air is used it is not totally absorbable because of the nitrogen content.

The other danger associated with oxygen administration is infection due to contamination or inadequate sterilization of equipment. This is a particular hazard for the very ill or those with respiratory difficulties; the more severe the condition, the more the patient needs prolonged oxygen therapy, with its risks of increasingly contaminated equipment, and the more susceptible the patient's lungs are to infection. Disposable equipment should be used when possible.

ARTIFICIAL VENTILATION

Although ventilation can be maintained by manually squeezing a bag attached to a Waters circuit and mask or endotracheal tube, other mechanical means of ventilation are necessary for prolonged respiratory support. Negative pressure applied to the thorax by a cuirasse or tank (iron lung) respirator is still sometimes used for people with permanent respiratory failure, for example after poliomyelitis. However, intermittent or inspiratory positive pressure ventilation (IPPV) via an endotracheal tube is now much more commonly used since it allows much more sophisticated and effective control of ventilation and oxygenation, as well as control of secretions, particularly when swallowing is impaired. There are numerous types of ventilators of varying degrees of complexity and suitability for different patients. Basically they can be divided into two main types:

1. Pressure controlled, the inspiratory flow being ended when the pre-set pressure is reached, even if the volume is small
2. Volume controlled, the inspiratory flow being ended when the pre-set volume is reached irrespective of the pressure (though most do have a pre-set safety limit); this is more suitable for patients with variable or poor compliance ('stretchability' of the lung)

The ventilation rate may be pre-set, controlled by the patient if the machine has a 'trigger' mechanism which starts the inspiratory flow as the patient starts to breathe and creates a negative pressure, or a combination of these. Intermittent mandatory ventilation (IMV) may be used, usually when re-establishing spontaneous ventilation. The patient breathes on his own but is intermittently forced to take a deeper breath by the machine. Where alveolar collapse is a problem, as in respiratory distress syndrome, positive end expiratory pressure (PEEP) may be used to prevent alveoli collapsing at the end of expiration (Levi, 1979). For the spontaneously breathing patient this is known as CPAP (continuous positive airway pressure) and sometimes for the artificially ventilated patient as CPPV (continuous positive pressure ventilation). Since the airway's pressure never reaches the baseline and the negative inspiratory phase is abolished, this removes the 'thoracic pump' effect whereby return of venous blood to the heart is increased as blood is drawn up into the thorax as the intrathoracic pressure decreases. Therefore hypotension may occur in the ill patient with an unstable circulation. Another facility offered by some ventilators is 'retard', the expiratory phase being prolonged.

Any nurse caring for a patient who is being artifically ventilated should know enough about the machine to detect any malfunction and know what to do about it, and to be confident enough in managing it safely to be able to concentrate on the patient rather than the machine. It is also essential to remember that the presence of an oropharyngeal or tracheostomy tube does not necessarily mean a clear airway. The tube may become displaced from the trachea or down one bronchus, or occluded by kinking (which may not be visible if inside the patient), secretions, or by being clamped between the patient's jaws. Therefore constant observation is necessary, as is recording vital signs and other essential parameters as necessary for safety in the particular situation.

PATIENT EDUCATION

Although left until last, this is often one of the most important yet neglected aspects of treatment and nursing care. Even a very ill artifically ventilated patient usually needs to know enough about his or her condition and care to maintain some understanding and control in his or her mind, even if totally paralysed. The less severely ill patient can only mobilize his forces for recovery and co-operate fully with those who care for him if he understands and knows enough to do so. For the person with a chronic respiratory condition requiring drug and breathing exercise regimes, and possibly oxygen or other therapy at home, education of the patient and if necessary his family is essential to avoid non-compliance and possibly failure of treatment, and to enable as normal a life as possible. Effective learning by patients requires motivation, and the delivery of appropriate information at an appropriate rate and time, by an appropriate method; so a nurse requires skill and knowledge to assess what is needed, deliver it, and assess whether learning has occurred. Since all this occurs within the context of the nurse-patient relationship, good interpersonal skills are often of crucial importance.

NURSING CARE OF PATIENTS WITH ACTUAL OR POTENTIAL PROBLEMS IN MAINTAINING NORMAL LEVELS OF OXYGEN AND CARBON DIOXIDE

Individual factors such as age, gender, psychological differences which affect health, and specific disturbances due to the physical disease may be relevant to the nursing care of a patient with actual or potential difficulties in oxygenation and carbon dioxide elimination, just as such difficulties may affect any or all the activities of living. Therefore each of these must be considered for its relevance in assessment of the person's need for nursing care, in planning, delivering and evaluating care. Being aware of the possible implications of aspects which may not be of outstandingly obvious relevance can enable a nurse to prevent problems from arising, or detect them early and minimize the ill effects as far as possible.

IMPLICATIONS OF OTHER PHYSICAL DISEASES

The relevance of a main diagnosis of respiratory disease or damage to oxygen and carbon dioxide balance is obvious. The relevance of other medical conditions and treatment may not be so obvious. If a patient with COPD has, for example, abdominal surgery, it is probable that with good anaesthetic techniques his respiratory condition can be quite adequately maintained around the time of operation. It may well be in the later postoperative period with limited mobility, incisional pain and some abdominal distension in addition to some weakness, that difficulties develop. The timed vital capacity often falls 30% after lower abdominal surgery and 50% after upper abdominal surgery, and the maximum reduction is most likely around the second postoperative day (Redding, 1977). With this, some areas of alveolar collapse are likely to develop, with ventilation/perfusion imbalance. The patient with normal pre-operative function can tolerate and overcome this, but the patient with COPD or a reduced pre-operative vital capacity, due to a rigid or malformed thoracic cage (e.g. pectus excavatum) or to muscular weakness or obesity, cannot and respiratory distress may follow. There are added potential iatrogenic hazards in that opiate analgesics may be given and depress respiration still further. Or, since it is known that some hypoxaemia may occur after abdominal surgery (SHHD, 1969), oxygen may be administered routinely without adequate monitoring of blood gases and respiratory function, provoking, in a patient with COPD, carbon dioxide retention and narcosis, which will reduce ventilation still further.

Pneumothorax due to a ruptured emphysematous bulla or 'air cyst' is one of the complications of chronic respiratory disease. This may lead to severe carbon dioxide retention and hypoxia, unless underwater seal or valved drainage is soon instituted and maintained patent, so that air can escape from the pleural space, allowing the lung to expand (Fig. 24.3). For the patient with limited respiratory reserve, any change in routine due to admission to hospital may threaten stability of oxygen-carbon dioxide balance, since often such a person has established a routine of life which maintains adequate respiratory function. Assessment and planning to meet the individual's needs is necessary to avoid or cope with such problems.

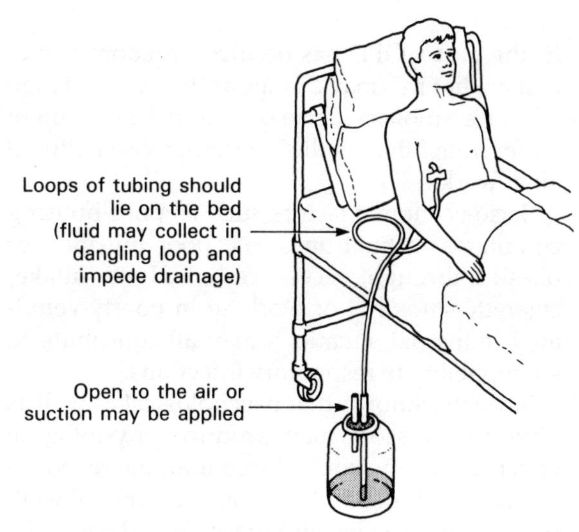
Loops of tubing should lie on the bed (fluid may collect in dangling loop and impede drainage)
Open to the air or suction may be applied

Fig. 24.3 Underwaterseal drainage may be used to drain fluid or air from the pleural cavity. The drain is attached to a rigid tube, the lower end of which should be about 2.5 cm below the fluid level in the bottle. This allows drainage but prevents air entering the pleural cavity. The fluid level rises and falls in the tube with respiration.

FACTORS MODIFYING RESPIRATORY FUNCTION

Age

Age can certainly be a risk factor in relation to oxygenation in that both the very young and the elderly each have some characteristics which may cause problems.

The young

Young children and particularly infants have narrow airways which can easily become blocked either by inhaled foreign bodies or by secretion, and even a small reduction in diameter may affect air flow considerably. Also children may become dehydrated quite quickly if pyrexial, thus making secretions thicker and ill babies particularly may be too weak to cough effectively. The newborn baby also has a lower PO_2, i.e. 75–80mmHg (10–10.7kPa) as opposed to 90–95mmHg (12–12.7kPa) for young adults. However, the young can produce a cardiac response to hypoxia, by increasing the pulse rate in order to transport more oxygen.

The elderly

Changes in 'healthy' elderly people include reduction of the vital capacity by 25%, reduction of maximum breathing capacity (measured by forced expiratory volume) by 50% between 20 and 80 years, increased rigidity of the chest wall and reduction of the intrathoracic area due to a tendency to stoop and perhaps kyphosis and/or scoliosis, small scattered areas of lung tissue destruction, airway collapse, decreased ciliary efficiency and coughing effectiveness, and difficulty in gaseous exchange across alveolar membranes. The PO_2 of the very elderly is usually around 75mmHg (10kPa), so hypoxia can be induced more readily by adverse factors (Ebersole & Hess, 1981; Murray et al, 1980).

Response to illness is often less obvious in old people, and there may be no cardiac response (tachycardia) even when the PO_2 is down to 40mmHg (5.5kPa). The PCO_2 does not increase with ageing unless some pathology is present.

Other characteristics

In the past COPD has occurred predominantly in men, but this may change as the excess of men who are smokers decreases, and less of them suffer from inhaling dusty or otherwise polluted air at work.

Socio-economic factors such as poor housing conditions in built-up areas, poor nutrition or obesity through excess carbohydrate intake, cigarette-smoking, or working in poorly-ventilated industrial situations may all contribute to susceptibility to respiratory infections.

Since it is known that psychological as well as physical stressors may produce physiological effects which include reduced immune response (Selye, 1976), psychological and emotional well-being may also be important in reducing the infections which may lead to chronic respiratory disease.

Personality and emotional factors may not only alter the course of pathological conditions by making it easier or more difficult to comply with required treatment, but also have more direct effects on oxygenation in a person with limited respiratory function. For example, the physical difficulties of a young woman with myasthenia gravis had not been recognized by her doctor for some time as the condition developed. When she was eventually admitted to hospital, she at times became very anxious and if not given immediate attention she began to cry and thrash around the bed. Although adequately oxygenated at first she soon became hypoxic, presumably due to increased use of oxygen and inability to compensate for this. Once she had been calmed down and distracted with other things oxygenation improved again.

Intellectual and physical capacity may be important factors in coping with respiratory abnormalities. The ability to understand the condition and required treatment and to find enjoyable occupations which are not beyond physical capacity may contribute a great deal to effective coping. Good general physical capacity may to some extent compensate for deficiency in one system, but again intellectual ability and understanding may be required to make the best use of it.

When respiratory abnormalities affect or threaten to affect adversely the activities of daily living, all or any of the above factors may increase or decrease these effects. There can be an additive effect when a number of adverse factors are present.

EFFECT OF RESPIRATORY PROBLEMS ON ACTIVITIES OF LIVING

Breathing

Although the function of breathing has been discussed from the pathophysiological point of view, which is relevant to nursing, it is necessary to consider the more specifically nursing aspects in some detail.

What is actually recorded in the nursing assessment may vary to some extent according to what is already recorded in the medical history, since there is no point in repeating information unnecessarily. It is not usually the nurse who does a full chest examination with ausculation and percussion, though she may on occasion use a stethoscope if she suspects abnormalities may have developed or to assess effectiveness of secretion clearance, or percussion if pneumothorax is suspected. However, anything which has implications for nursing care should be included (and Rokosky [1981] suggests some of these factors), as well as any changes from the information recorded by the doctor. Nursing assessment of respiratory function of any patient is not a single episode but an on-going process, and any risk factors identified should increase observation and alertness to problems.

Breathing is one of the most vital functions, and rapid deterioration, or even a quite small decrease in function in the patient with little reserve, may result if unchecked in a downward spiral and serious or even fatal consequences. For any patient, assessment should include the rate, depth, regularity and ease of breathing. Is dyspnoea or cyanosis present on moderate exertion or at rest, and are accessory muscles used? Do both sides of the chest appear to move equally? Exercise tolerance should be noted, whether breathlessness or wheezing occurs other than with vigorous exertion, and if so when, and anything which appears to provoke it. Smoking habits are relevant and, in addition to what the patient says, nicotine staining of fingers plus observation may give some indication of the amount of smoking involved. The type, frequency and apparent provoking factors of any cough or chest pain, and anything used to relieve it, should be noted, as well as the colour, amount and frequency of sputum produced.

When a patient is admitted to nursing care it is useful to find out from him any previous experience with respiratory problems and health care, since it may be very relevant to present or future care. For example, some people find wearing an oxygen mask very distressing, and if so it may be wise to avoid the use of a mask if possible or at least find ways of reducing the distress, which is easier if the problem is known before it occurs.

Lung function tests are usually performed by technicians in a laboratory, however some of the more simple tests may be performed frequently to assess progress and therefore may be done by nurses. In any case the results are likely to be relevant to nursing care. The most common measures used are vital capacity (VC), forced expiratory volume in one second (FEV_1), maximum breathing capacity in litres per minute (MBC), and sometimes peak expiratory flow rate (PEFR) (Legg, 1979). Other more extensive tests may be necessary in some situations, such as bronchospirometry under anaesthesia, when one bronchus is occluded using a double lumen tube while the function of the other lung is checked. Xenon scans may be used to detect diffusion problems or blockage of a pulmonary vessel by an embolus. It is useful for a nurse to be familiar with the features of a normal chest X-ray so that she can interpret X-rays showing major abnormalities, and to have a knowledge of normal and abnormal blood gas values and acid-base balance since it may sometimes be a nurse who sees the results of such tests first when they arrive on the ward, and urgent action may sometimes be needed.

Any nurse caring for patients likely to have respiratory function tests needs to know sufficient about them not only to use the results when relevant to care, but also to prepare the patient adequately (including making sure that he is adequately informed), to assist when necessary, and to make sure that there are no ill effects. For example, unless pressure is maintained over the site for at least 5 minutes after an arterial puncture to obtain specimens for blood gas analysis, severe bruising may occur.

The overall aims of nursing care for any patient include maintaining or improving respiratory function, prevention or reduction of hypoxia or hypercapnia and, subject to these aims, the maintenance of comfort in breathing. More specified aims for those susceptible to respiratory problems may include:

- Adequate airways clearance
- The relief, avoidance or control of bronchospasm, cough or pain
- The best use of his or her physical and mental capacity for the patient to accomplish daily living activities
- The promotion of such autonomy and independence as is possible.

An important part of nursing care for patients with chronic lung disease is to help them to learn to manage their own condition as far as possible, while maintaining daily life which is as far as possible acceptable to them. This requires the use of a variety of coping strategies (Little & Carnevali, 1976). Methods of clearing airways and maintaining respiratory function have already been discussed (p. 780). However, an individual care plan is necessary to ensure that the patient receives all the care and treatment he or she needs, but with adequate rest in between.

Eating and drinking

Eating and drinking are both activities which may be affected by or may affect respiratory function, and nursing assistance may be required to regulate them. Many patients with respiratory problems are overweight. Obesity tends to reduce lung expansion (due to pressure under the diaphragm and the heavy chest wall), thus predisposing the affected person to respiratory problems, and limited mobility due to breathlessness on exertion may increase this.

Some patients may be anorexic due to hypoxia, pyrexia or foul-tasting sputum, or have difficulty eating due to breathlessness. Therefore careful assessment is needed to see whether the patient is taking an adequate and balanced diet, or over-eating. If necessary the help of a dietitian and/or doctor may be enlisted to plan an appropriate diet. But the most essential person to work with is the patient, for no diet can be helpful unless it is adhered to, i.e. the person concerned both can and will follow it. Patients who have a lot of sputum may eat better if encouraged/assisted to practise deep breathing and clear their chests before meals, with a mouthwash before eating if necessary. When the appetite is poor or eating difficult, calorie-rich fluids may be useful. The protein intake should be maintained since protein deficiency may diminish the effectiveness of the immune system, and these people are already susceptible to chest infections.

Fluid balance is important. If fluid intake is too low, any sputum will be thick, viscid and difficult to expectorate. On the other hand fluid intake may be limited deliberately if the patient has cor pulmonale (heart failure secondary to respiratory disease) and general oedema, or a tendency to pulmonary oedema. Nowadays it is usual to try to maintain an intake of at least 2-2.5 litres in 24 hours, and diuretics are included in medical orders if necessary to prevent fluid retention. Fluids the patient likes, kept easily accessible and at the desired temperature (hot or cold), are important for both physical well-being and comfort. Hot drinks can be especially useful either for settling an irritating cough or for aiding expectoration. Pyrexia and/or sweating automatically increase the fluid requirements.

Elimination

Elimination may be disturbed by hypoxia or respiratory disease. Urinary secretion is usually decreased if there is severe hypoxia (often due to the inability of the hypoxic myocardium to maintain the level of renal arterial pressure necessary to maintain filtration), or fluid retention may occur with cor pulmonale. Breathlessness limiting activity and ability to make the effort to defaecate may lead to constipation. This can often be avoided by attention to diet, e.g. ensuring adequate roughage, fruit and fluids and a regular routine, for example a position comfortable for breathing and the opportunity to defaecate just after breakfast.

Movement

Body movement may be limited for a person with respiratory disease, either by the condition or by the equipment used in treatment. Dyspnoea will obviously limit voluntary activity, though a lot of movement and energy may be used in breathing when accessory muscles are used. The ill, weary person may tend to slump into a position which limits lung expansion, which may be dangerous if lung function is poor. Most patients expand their lungs most easily and effectively when sitting propped up (Fig. 24.4) or leaning forward onto a bed-table. But if movement is limited it is usually important to change the position at intervals in order to prevent areas of collapse at the base of the lungs. Most people can be laid on alternate sides intermittently, either flat or semi-reclining with the back straight, but for some only one side would be appropriate, e.g. after pneumonectomy only the operated side. If the patient is very orthopnoeic (cannot breathe unless sitting up), then breathing exercises to expand the lung bases and some means of relieving sacral and other pressure areas become essential. Some of the modern 'arm-chair' or triangular pillows can be very useful for support, with or without a backrest*. If possible the patient and/or his/her family should be taught how and when to change his or her position if it has a long-lasting condition.

Equipment such as drainage or oxygen administration systems may limit movement unless the patient is taught, and if necessary assisted, to manage them safely while moving.

*Alternatively, the patient may find it more comfortable to remain in a chair, particularly if he or she has found it difficult to maintain a sitting position in bed. A roomy, supportive chair with attached leg rest is usually the most appropriate.

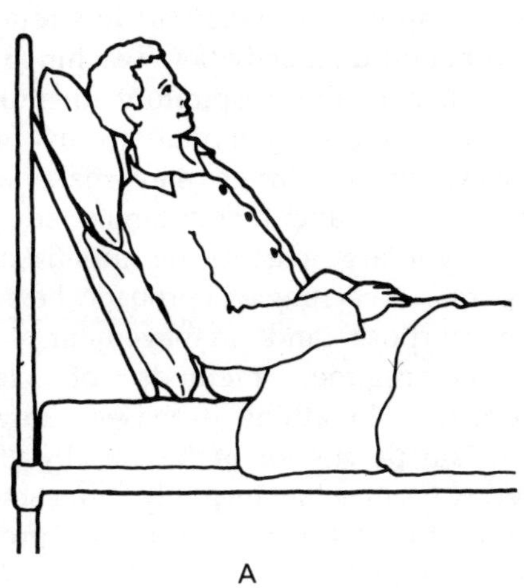

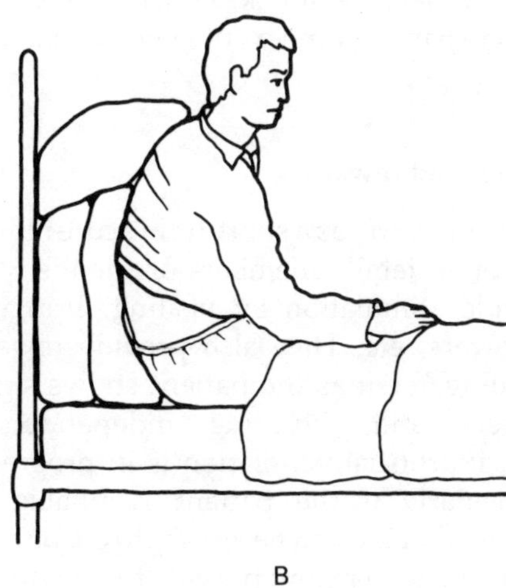

Fig.24.4 Position in bed for optimal ventilation. Lung function is usually more efficient in position A than in B, particularly if the patient is obese.

In many units those with underwater seal drainage are now allowed to walk about once they have learned to keep the tubes unkinked and continuous, and the bottle below chest level. Even a patient on long-term assisted ventilation can often learn to change position safely. Movement may in itself be a protection for people with chronic respiratory disease, since it may stimulate the intermittent increase in rate and depth of breathing necessary to maintain adequate gas exchange. But nursing assistance may be needed to help the patient to match his activities to the oxygen demand his body can meet, while maintaining activity to improve both lung ventilation and quality of life.

Sleep

Sleep may be disturbed by cough, dyspnoea or the need for treatment, so extra care to provide measures such as a comfortable position compatible with good lung expansion, available hot drinks (in a vacuum flask if necessary at home) and adequate warmth (a warm bedroom to avoid provoking bronchospasm when going to bed, or a shawl or jacket round the shoulders when sitting up) as well as fresh air may be necessary. Hypnotics are usually contra-indicated for people with COPD. Even without sedation some symptomless people, as well as those with known lung dysfunction, have periods of apnoea and oxygen desaturation during REM sleep (Block, 1980). Since repeated desaturation seems to be related to development of pulmonary hypertension and cor pulmonale, Block (1981) suggests that many patients with COPD may benefit from 2 l/min of oxygen via a nasal cannula overnight. He provides a review of a number of sleep-related respiratory disorders.

Nursing care should include assessment of the effects of sleep on respiratory function either by observation or, if the patient is at home, by asking anyone who sees him while he sleeps. Teaching the patient to practice deep breathing and clear his chest before sleep and if he wakes in the night, and on waking in the morning, can contribute considerably to his well-being. When there is chest pain, postoperative or other, analgesics should be used with caution. Adequate analgesia to relieve pain is often necessary after surgery or trauma, so that chest movement will not be limited, but if opiates or pethidine are used care must be taken to ensure adequate respiratory function by intermittent deep breathing exercises if the patient is elderly, obese, or is otherwise at risk, which is now true of an increasing number of people having surgery.

Stimulation and reward

For the person who has a short-term acute illness there are often family members or friends who will provide stimulation by visiting, bringing books, flowers, etc. They also provide reward and encouragement as the patient shows signs of recovery and returning independence. However, if artificial ventilation is in progress, and particularly if the patient is unable to respond much, it is often necessary to encourage visitors to talk to them and provide them with as many as possible of the activities which they would normally enjoy, such as listening to music or other tapes or radio programmes. People often do not realize that such an ill patient still may need some kind of enjoyable but not too demanding pastime at times. For a person with chronic lung disease it may become too much of an effort to continue with usual recreational activities, particularly if they are physically demanding or it means going out from home. Sometimes new and less demanding recreations can be found if encouragement is given, but this depends partly on how patients feel about themselves and their current life style.

Self-concept and relationships

The person's self-concept and relationship to others are important in relation to any health problems, but perhaps especially so when he or she has COPD. Many people with this condition have a history of cigarette-smoking as well as obesity. The combination of repeated chest infections, increasing breathlessness and sputum production, limited activity, and requirements to stop smoking and limit eating may cause such people to become depressed, feel that they can no longer play a worthwhile part in life, and just sit around waiting to get worse, which they soon will with this view of the situation. He or she may feel socially unacceptable because of the need to expectorate (particularly if the patient is a woman), and because of his or her inability to tolerate hot, smoky atmospheres or take part in strenous or cold weather outdoor activities. Teaching him or her to manage the respiratory dysfunction actively, and adapt to limitations by finding other ways to do things may make a vast difference, and patient and family education should play a large part in the nursing care of such a person. Teaching will probably be needed on the purpose and management of the medication regime, methods of clearing secretions e.g. breathing exercises, coughing, possibly daily percussion of the chest by a family member, ways of achieving daily living activities with less effort if breathlessness is a problem, and alternating activity with rest. If home oxygen therapy is used then knowledge of the technical aspects is necessary, but also how best to use the oxygen to benefit the person in relation to comfort and lifestyle. For example, a small portable cylinder for the very borderline hypoxic patient may enable him to walk along the road to visit friends or go to the 'pub' for a drink. Encouragement to maintain personal grooming and appearance can be good for morale too, and if a woman is inclined to be cyanosed help on suitable make-up may be appreciated. Overall the emphasis should be on what the person can do, even if in adapted ways, rather than what he or she cannot. People do not suddenly become different people because they are ill, and each may wish to carry on as far as possible his or her previous activities. It is part of nursing care to help them to do this, recognizing that harmful habits may need modifying if the patient agrees.

CARE DURING TERMINAL ILLNESS

For many people respiratory dysfunction is likely to increase as the disease process continues, and they recognize that there will be a continued deterioration in their condition, increasing dependence, and ultimately death. Although everyone knows that death is inevitable, most people do not know how it will come, and therefore can ignore the prospect for most of their lives. For those with chronic respiratory disease, or cardiac conditions where hypoxia causes similar symptoms, evidence of their progress towards death may already be obvious to them and they may need to be able to talk about their fears and thoughts about it. Some may be able to talk to their family or friends, for some 'God is a very present help in time of trouble', and they may have a minister, priest or other religious adviser they can talk to. It is part of nursing to help these patients to find and use their source of support whether the nurse is of the same faith, a different one or none at all. For some, the nurse may provide the support they need, but this requires that the nurse should be able to accept human mortality, including his or her own.

As respiratory failure becomes terminal, decisions may have to be made by doctors, nurses, the patient's family, and where possible the patient, as to whether mechanical ventilatory support should be used to prolong life, or whether the benefit to be gained would be outweighed by the discomforts and deprivations associated with intubation and mechanical ventilation. Both the patient and family may need much support at this time. It is important that nurses should be involved with the doctor in such decisions, since it is they who will spend time with the patient and see the results. In terminal respiratory failure, physical discomforts such as sweating or headaches due to hypercapnia, and severe breathlessness may require nursing care, as may the restlessness and disorientation; the latter may disturb the patient, but may disturb the family even more if the patient is at home. They need reassurance that the aggression, swearing or other uncharacteristic behaviour are part of the illness, due to physical causes. Respiratory distress and disorientation can be distressing to both the sufferer and those who watch. There are many things, sometimes small but important, which a good nurse can find to do to relieve this distress, but perhaps the most essential is just to be there when needed. Both dying and watching with the dying can be a lonely experience.

Nursing has a vital contribution to make to the survival of patients by preventing, or observing and taking prompt action to deal with, any acute oxygen deficit. It also has a large part to play in maintaining respiratory function and quality of life and death for those with chronic respiratory disease.

REFERENCES

Aspinall M J, Tanner C A 1981 Decision-making for patient care. Appleton-Century-Crofts, New York

Bailey R 1979 Drugs and the respiratory system. Nursing (Oxford) First series 7:315–318

Block A J 1980 Respiratory disorders during sleep, Part 1. Heart and Lung 9:1011–1024

Block A J 1981 Respiratory disorders during sleep, Part 2. Heart and Lung 10:90–96

Bordeaux M P 1973 The intensive care unit and observation of the patient acutely ill with neurologic disease. Heart and Lung 2:884–887

Brown S E 1979 Respiratory physiotherapy and the nurse. Nursing (Oxford) First series 6:257–259

Donald K W 1947 Oxygen poisoning in man. British Medical Journal 1:667

Ebersole P, Hess P 1981 Towards healthy aging. C V Mosby, St Louis

Haldane T S 1914 A lecture on symptoms, causes and prevention of anoxaemia. British Medical Journal 2:65

Jones E 1978 Respiratory failure. In: Intensive care. MTP Press, Lancaster

Jones E, Luksza A 1979 Asthma. Nursing (Oxford). First series 6:265– 270

Legg S 1979 Breathlessness — what happens? Nursing (Oxford). First series 6:253–256

Leonard B J 1981 Mechanisms of hypoxia. In: Leonard B J, Redland A R Process in clinical nursing. Prentice-Hall, New Jersey

Levi T 1979 Breathing equipment. Part 1 Nursing 6:260–263; Part 2 Nursing 7:336–339

Little D E, Carnevali D L 1976 Major coping strategies and nursing evaluation criteria. In: Nursing care planning, 2nd edn. J B Lippincott, Philadelphia

Lorrain-Smith T 1899 The pathological effects due to increase of oxygen tension in the air breathed. Journal of Physiology (London) 24:19

Murray R, Huelskoetter M M, O'Driscoll D 1980 Problems of transporting and exchanging oxygen and nutrients in later maturity. In: The nursing process in later maturity.

Pugh R E 1978 Perinatal care. Major hazards ahead — unless. Nursing Mirror 147(17):18–22

Redding J S 1977 Life support. J B Lippincott, Philadelphia

Rokosky J S 1981 Assessment of the individual with altered respiratory function. Nursing Clinics of North America 16(2):195– 208

Scottish Home and Health Department (SHHD) 1969 Uses and dangers of oxygen therapy. HMSO, Edinburgh

Selye H 1976 The stress of life, 2nd edn. McGraw-Hill, New York

Sumner S M, Grau P E 1982 Emergency! First aid for choking. Nursing 82(12):40–49

Vander A J, Sherman J H, Luciano D S 1975 Human physiology, 2nd edn. McGraw-Hill, New York

Wagner Y L 1981 Adult respiratory distress syndrome. In:

Kenner C V, Guzzetta C E, Dossey B M Critical care nursing. Little, Brown & Co, Boston

Zeluff G W, Orman B F, Wilson R K, Carter R E, Dimitrijenc M R, Sharkey P C, Jackson D 1977 Grand rounds in critical care. Ondine's curse. Heart and Lung 6:1057–1063

FURTHER READING

Adams N R 1979 The nurse's role in systematic weaning from a ventilator. Nursing 79 (9):35–41

Breslin E H 1981 Prevention and treatment of pulmonary complications in patients after surgery of the upper abdomen. Heart and Lung 10:511–519

Cline B A, Fisher M L 1982 ARDS means emergency. Nursing 82 (12):63–67

Coady T J, Bennett A 1978 Scan. Technology in nursing. Respiratory function. Monthly series in Nursing Times, 74:Jan–Dec

Erickson R 1981 Chest tubes. They're not really that complicated. Nursing 81 (11):34–43

Evans CC 1979 Pneumonia. Nursing (Oxford) First series 7:320–323

Fournet K M 1974 Patients discharged on diuretics: prime candidates for individual teaching by the nurse. Heart and Lung 3:108–116

Fuchs P L 1979 Understanding continuous mechanical ventilation. Nursing 79 (9):26–33

Goffnett C 1979 Your patient's dying. Now what? Nursing 79 (9):27–33

Hapugoda P A 1981 Infection in specialized areas. Nursing (Oxford) First series 29:1259–1263

Heimlich H J 1976 Death from food-choking prevented by a new life-saving manoeuvre. Heart and Lung 5:755–758

Holloway N M 1979 Aeration assessment (Ch. 9), acute aeration disorders (Ch. 10). In: Nursing the critically-ill adult. Addison-Wesley, California

Jackson H 1979 Nursing care of patients with chest injuries. Nursing (Oxford) First series (7):303–309

Kaufman J S, Woody J W 1980 COPD: better living through teaching. Nursing 80 (10):57–61

Kubler-Ross E 1974 Questions and answers on death and dying. Collier Macmillan, London

Ladyshewsky A 1980 Increased intracranial pressure: when assessment counts. Canadian Nurse 76:34–37

Lance E, Sweetwood H 1978 Chest trauma. Nursing 78 (8):28–33

Meers P D 1980 Hospitals ... should do the sick no harm 9:Respiratory tract infection. Nursing Times 76(38):supplement 1–4

Morrow W F K 1975 Blast injuries to the lungs. Nursing Times 71:1136–1137

Naigow D, Powaser M M 1977 The effect of different endotracheal suction procedures on blood gases in a controlled experimental model. Heart and Lung 6:808–816

Norkool D M 1979 Current concepts of hyperbaric oxygenation and its application in critical care. Heart and Lung 8:728–735

Potter M 1981 Medication compliance — a factor in the drug wastage problem. Nursing Times Occasional Paper 77:17–20

Redman B K 1978 Curriculum in patient education. American Journal of Nursing 78:1363–1366

Redman B K 1980 The process of patient teaching, 4th edn. Mosby, St Louis

Selecky P A 1974 Tracheostomy — a review of present-day indications, complications and care. Heart and Lung 3:272–283

Shrake K 1979 The ABC of ABGs or how to interpret a blood gas value. Nursing 79 (9):26–33

Stoll R 1979 Guidelines for spiritual assessment. American Journal of Nursing 79:1574–1577

Stromborg M F, Stromborg P 1981 Test your knowledge of helping patients cope with COPD. Nursing 81 (11):89–95

Surveyer J A 1980 Smoke inhalation injuries. Heart and Lung 9:825–832

Sweetwood H M 1974 Oxygen administration in the coronary-care unit. Heart and Lung 3:102–107

Tecklin J S 1979 Positioning, percussing and vibrating patients for effective bronchial drainage. Nursing 79 (9):64–71

Wolanin M O, Phillips L R F 1981 Care of the patient with confusion secondary to compromised brain support. Part 1: Hypoxia compromising brain support. In: Confusion. Prevention and care. Mosby, St Louis

Yurick A G, Robb S S, Spier B E, Ebert N J 1980 Assessment base: oxygen and nutrients to support activity. In: The aged person and the nursing process. Appleton-Century-Crofts, New York

25

Disturbances of maintenance of the internal environment – excretion of unwanted substances

INTRODUCTION

As a living organism, man undergoes a constant interaction with his environment in behavioural, mental and physiological contexts. The concept of man as a steady state system maintaining a relatively stable internal environment was first enunciated by Claude Bernard in the late nineteenth century and later developed by Cannon (1939) into the concept of homeostasis familiar to physiologists, doctors and nurses. This term refers to the processes by which the internal environment of the body is maintained within the narrow physiological parameters with respect to pH, temperature, fluid and electrolyte balance and other biochemical substrates necessary for optimal functioning. If man is to be successful in maintaining this internal consistency then it follows that he must extract from the external environment those resources necessary to meet bodily needs. In order to make use of these resources the organs and systems of the body must be working in synchrony. The inevitable result of these processes is that redundant or harmful substances must at some time be eliminated from the body. The action of clearing the body of such wastes may be termed excretion.

It is evident that several organs of the body may be considered to have excretory functions, including the skin and respiratory system. This chapter, however, will deal with the urinary system and lower bowel which handle excretion as a primary function, and whilst the other organs should not be ignored they are dealt with elsewhere.

Few nurses would disagree with the statement that nursing activities associated with the management of excretory functions and related problems are a time-consuming aspect of patient care. Norton et al (1962) found that the treatment of pressure areas and toileting for incontinence required more time than any other single activity for their sample of elderly patients. At the other end of the continuum Wright (1974) summarizes the results of seven investigations into the prevalence of constipation in various subgroups, which produced estimates of between 23% and 60%. The same author also detects inconsistencies between stated and actual practices in the area of bowel care which may suggest a somewhat ad-hoc approach to the management of excretory function. This is particularly significant when one considers that Wright found that, in the 5 days following admission, 54% of patients had a reduction in bowel action and 27% of patients worried about their bowels whilst in hospital.

In the management of urinary excretion, research indicates that there is little room for complacency. Approximately 10% of general hospital patients will have an indwelling urethral catheter inserted at some time during their treatment (Jenner, 1983). Ansell (1962) suggests that a urinary catheter left in situ for 24–48 hours inevitably results in bacteruria, whilst Seal (1982) reports a 3% incidence of bacteraemia in catheterized patients with infected urine. Infections of the urinary tract have been identified as the commonest iatrogenic infection both in the UK and USA, accounting for one third of all infections in hospitalized patients (Beland & Passos, 1975; Meers et al, 1981).

Many, if not most, nurses will have encountered the patient who, because of the development of urinary frequency, commences a regime of self-imposed restriction of fluid intake in order to reduce the demand for bedpans — in doing so exacerbating the original condition. There are also those patients who feel so uncomfortable because of actual or perceived constipation that they resolutely refuse to eat until something is done about it. Clearly, however nurses feel about excretory function, their patients consider it to be of primary importance. In Western society the situation is further complicated by the taboo nature of this subject. From childhood individuals are exposed to training and conditioning with respect to where and when it is socially acceptable to attend to such functions. These internalized values must be considered by nurses and may prove inhibiting when a patient is called upon to urinate whilst in bed, or when in close association with others. In order to manage excretory function intelligently, nurses must consider the relevant anatomy, physiology and pathology as well as the psycho-social and developmental aspects of the presenting problem.

Nurses have a responsibility to their patients to approach the management of excretory functions with sensitivity and a competence based upon a sound knowledge of the first principles involved, and supported by the application of relevant research findings. This belief will be reflected in the presentation of this chapter, and a knowledge of the anatomy and physiology of the systems under discussion is assumed. These areas will only be reviewed where necessary to illustrate a point of practice.

EXCRETORY FUNCTION

Urological nursing is now recognized as a speciality in its own right, and several texts are available which deal with this topic exclusively. A chapter of this length cannot deal with the nursing management of specific disorders such as hydronephrosis and pyelonephritis, for example, and the reader should refer to specialized texts if necessary. This chapter aims to assist the nurse in the assessment and management of excretory function through the application of the principles of applied physiology, general pathology and published research.

When dealing with aspects of excretion even the most junior of nurses very quickly realizes that the associated problems are twofold – output must be maintained, and it must also be controlled! Whilst during an acute illness the maintenance of urinary output will be of obvious importance to the nurse, it is quickly discovered that problems of control may present tremendous difficulties to the patient, and in certain circumstances become a major threat to the individual's physical and psycho-social well-being. The lower urinary system, then, has two functions – to excrete urine and also to store it. A third function also exists which follows logically from the first two, that of body defence. This is not a primary function of the urinary system, but its failure can have serious consequences to the patient and may well be a consequence of nursing intervention, as we shall see.

THE PHYSIOLOGY OF EXCRETION

URINARY FUNCTION

The urinary system

Any assessment or intervention by the nurse must be based upon a sound knowledge of the normal functioning of the urinary system.

The lower urinary system consists of the ureters, urinary bladder, and urethra.

The ureters

Each ureter extends from the renal pelvis to the posterior aspect of the bladder, a distance of 10–12 inches. The passage of urine from the kidney to the bladder is not a passive but an active process, the ureter contracting in a peristaltic wave every 20–60 seconds. This peristaltic activity is initiated by the pressure of collected urine in the renal pelvis and extends towards the bladder. The ureters can exert a pressure of 25–50 mmHg against an obstruction (Guyton, 1981), and their function is influenced by the autonomic nervous system – sympathetic stimulation decreasing and parasympathetic stimulation increasing the frequency of peristaltic action. The ureters enter the bladder posteriorly at an oblique angle, this arrangement serving to prevent the backflow of urine under normal circumstances since the pressure of urine in the bladder will tend to compress the distal ureter.

The bladder

The urinary bladder lies directly posterior to the symphysis pubis. The bladder naturally varies in size according to the urine contained, the mean capacity being approximately 200ml. When distended to an average degree the anterior wall of the bladder may extend above the symphysis pubis for 4 to 6 centimetres. If necessary, up to 500 ml of urine may be stored in the average adult bladder without undue discomfort. At volumes much above this, however, pressures within the bladder begin to rise dramatically resulting in a feeling of urgency and eventually pain as the bladder wall is over-distended. During periods of extreme retention the bladder may be palpable at the level of the umbilicus.

The bladder wall is a three-layered structure consisting of mucous, muscular and serous components. The peritoneal or serous layer extends only over the superior surface. The muscular layer forms the main mass of the bladder, the detrusor muscle, which is again composed of three layers, each of them non-striated muscular tissue. The central muscle layer consists of circularly arranged fibres, sandwiched internally and externally by longitudinal fibres. In the bladder cervix the circular muscle fibres form the sphincter vesicae, or internal sphincter, and surround the urethral orifice (Williams & Warwick, 1980). There is some controversy, however, regarding the exact nature of the innervation of these fibres and their role in micturition and retention (Claridge, 1965). By contrast, the sphincter urethrae, or external sphincter, is composed of striated muscular tissue and is under voluntary control.

The innermost layer of the bladder is the mucous membrane, composed of transitional epithelium. This allows the layer to stretch during bladder filling without being damaged, at least at normal volumes. When the bladder is empty this membrane is thrown into folds or rugae.

The urethra

Urethral structure naturally differs widely between the two sexes. In the male the urethra is approximately 20 cm long, of convoluted course and considered by anatomists to be composed of three distinct parts. The precise structure of these parts need not concern us here, suffice it to say that the diameter and distendability of the urethra varies at different points, the narrowest and least distendable being the portion immediately distal to the prostate, and the external orifice itself (6mm). The mucous membrane which lines the urethra is continuous with the bladder and the tubules of the reproductive system.

The female urethra, by contrast, is only 4 cm long. The mucous membrane lining the urethra is continuous with that of the vulva externally and the bladder internally. Although the diameter of the female urethra is approximately equal to that of the male it is much more distendable (Williams & Warwick, 1980).

Storage of urine and micturition

In striated or skeletal muscle there exists a degree of muscle tone which is a state of partial contraction brought about by nerve impulses from the spinal cord. The detrusor muscle of the bladder is also said to exhibit 'muscle tone' but this is inherently different from that seen in skeletal muscle. The tone of the detrusor muscle (unstriated fibres) is thought to be an intrinsic property of the muscle and does not depend upon an intact nervous supply to the bladder, but instead is related to the normal filling and emptying process which the bladder undergoes in health (Claridge, 1965; Sabetian, 1965).

As the bladder fills with urine, volumes of between 100 and 400ml can be accommodated with relatively little increase in intravesical pressure. At volumes above 400ml bladder pressure begins to rise dramatically (Fig. 25.1). It follows that if urine is to be retained in the bladder then the resistance to the flow of urine must be greater than the pressure within the bladder. There are three interrelated processes involved in maintaining the necessary resistance to outflow from the bladder involving the external sphincter, internal sphincter and detrusor, and pelvic floor muscles. During urine storage there is an inhibition of the detrusor muscle and contraction of the external sphincter and perineal muscles. As stated earlier the precise role of the internal sphincter in urinary control is controversial, with different authorities attributing importance to either the perineal muscles or the so-called internal sphincter.

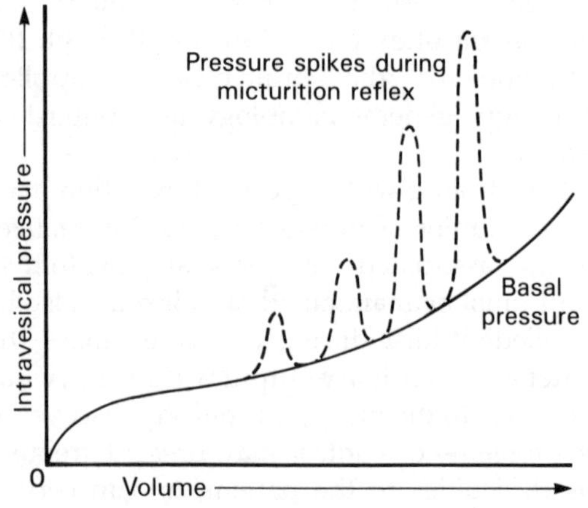

Fig. 25.1 Normal cystometrogram showing gradually increasing basal pressure and the superimposed micturition peaks as the bladder fills.

As the bladder fills, stretch receptors in the detrusor are stimulated which initiate micturition contractions via the sacral segments of the spinal cord. Once initiated the contraction rapidly increases in force until a maximum is reached, held for several seconds, and then lost, the bladder returning to its resting level until the next reflex contraction occurs. This process repeats at ever decreasing intervals and with increasing force until either the outflow resistance is overcome or voluntarily released. Which of these possibilities occurs will depend upon the influence of higher centres. This process of stretching and contracting is the micturition reflex, and central control of urination is achieved by either inhibiting or facilitating this reflex. Higher influences arise from either the brain stem or cerebral cortex and exert their effect by three mechanisms (Guyton, 1981). First, the micturition reflex is partly inhibited at all times when urination is not desired; secondly, the external sphincter is kept in tonic contraction until convenient, and finally, when micturition is desired, central mechanisms can both facilitate the micturition reflex and inhibit the external sphincter.

BOWEL FUNCTION

Just as with urinary excretion the management of bowel function must be based upon a knowledge of normal anatomy and physiology.

Whilst bowel function may be influenced by factors at any level of the alimentary canal, we shall be concerned here with the functioning of the large intestine.

The large intestine — structure

The role of the large intestine is twofold. First electrolytes and water are absorbed from the chyme, and faeces formed. Second, the faeces are stored until such time as they may be expelled from the body. A further function may be attributed to this part of the alimentary canal — that of absorption of vitamins (in particular vitamin K and some of the B vitamins) after production by bacteria in the gut. Our concern, however, is with the primary functions.

For purposes of discussion the large intestine may be divided into three parts: the caecum, including the ileocaecal valve; the colon, composed of ascending, transverse and descending segments; and the rectum.

In common with the rest of the gastrointestinal tract the wall of the large intestine is composed of five layers: an external serous layer, layers of longitudinal muscle, circular muscle and submucosa and, internally, a mucosal layer.

The muscular layers consist of smooth muscle with characteristic properties which account for the movement of the gut. In the colon the longitudinal muscle fibres are gathered together into three strips or bunches running the length of the colon, called taeniae coli. These taeniae are shorter overall than the other layers of the bowel and consequently the colon is pulled into sacs or haustrations. The muscle exhibits a degree of continuous contraction or muscle tone, and also undergoes periods of rhythmical contraction of greater force. The frequency of rhythmical contraction varies in different parts of the alimentary canal and depends upon the influence of other controlling mechanisms; overall control is via an intrinsic nervous pathway which is itself influenced by higher centres. There are two intrinsic neuronal pathways within the gut wall:

- the myenteric plexus, lying between the longitudinal and circular muscle walls and involved principally with the control of movement
- the submucosal plexus, found in the submucosa and concerned with the control of secretion and sensory feedback

The large intestine receives signals from both sympathetic and parasympathetic nervous systems.

The exact origin of the autonomic input varies depending upon the site in question, but generally speaking the parasympathetic fibres arise from either the vagus or pelvic splanchnic nerves, and sympathetic input derives from the coeliac superior mesenteric ganglia or the hypogastric plexus. Generally speaking, sympathetic stimulation decreases the mobility of the gut and parasympathetic increases it, in terms of both strength and frequency of contraction. Strong stimulation of the sympathetic nervous system can bring the gut to a total standstill (Guyton, 1981).

The movement of excreta along the large intestine

Chyme enters the large intestine via the ileocaecal valve in the caecum. This 'valve' has the properties of a sphincter and the degree of tonic contraction exerts a modifying influence over the passage of chyme into the caecum. The ileocaecal valve also prevents backflow of contents back into the ileum. The action of the ileocaecal valve is influenced both by the presence of chyme in the ileum and, in a feedback mechanism, by the degree of distension of the caecum itself. Intense irritation of the caecum will also tend to close the sphincter, thus preventing the backflow of irritants into the ileum.

In comparison with the rest of the gastrointestinal tract, the movements of the colon appear sluggish.

At intervals along the colon the circular muscle layer will begin to contract into a ring-like constriction. This is combined with a contraction of the taeniae coli, or longitudinal muscles, with the effect of rolling and compressing a short portion of the colon and its contents. After a period of perhaps 30 seconds, the contraction gradually subsides before being repeated at intervals of a few minutes in other portions of the colon. This type of action has been termed haustral contraction and has the effect of gradually chopping and rolling the faecal matter within the lumen of the colon, exposing different surfaces to the mucosa. This moves the faeces very slowly along the ascending and transverse colon. Thereafter in the distal transverse and descending colon so called mass movements occur to propel the now semi-solid faeces towards the anus.

Mass movements

A mass movement is initiated by the local dilatation of a portion of colon. This causes a strong contraction of the circular muscle layer in a ring, followed by the rapid contraction of the colon distal to this point for a distance of perhaps 16cm. The net effect of this action is the propulsion of a block of the colonic contents along the colon towards the anus. The movement may be repeated for a period of about ten to fifteen minutes but usually only two or three times a day, commonly following a meal. It is believed that gastrocolic and duodenocolic reflexes help to initiate mass movements via the myenteric plexus in response to the presence of food in the stomach or duodenum. If a mass movement results in faeces entering the rectum then the desire to defaecate will be felt and a defaecation reflex initiated. Ultimate control over the passage of faeces is achieved voluntarily via the external anal sphincter, a ring of striated muscle which surrounds the internal anal sphincter and can thus maintain continence until an opportune moment presents.

The defaecation reflex

There are two components to the defaecation reflex (Fig. 25.2): the intrinsic defaecation reflex, depending upon the myenteric plexus for its action, and the parasympathetic defaecation reflex which involves sacral segments of the spinal cord. The reflex is triggered when faeces are forced into the rectum following a mass movement. Distension of the rectal walls initiates a feedback response via the myenteric plexus which further stimulates peristalsis in the sigmoid colon and rectum. Afferent fibres in the rectum are also stimulated by distension, and these synapse in the sacral segments of the spine with parasympathetic fibres of the nervi erigentes. This parasympathetic input results in powerful peristaltic activity in the descending colon, sigmoid colon and rectum, producing efficient evacuation of faeces. Responses in other parts of the body contribute to the expulsion of faeces. Inspiration, followed by expiration against a closed glottis (Valsalva manoeuvre) greatly increases intra-abdominal pressure. Combined with contraction of abdominal and pelvic floor muscles this action assists in the propulsion of faeces along the colon and rectum. The only method of voluntary control over defaecation is via the muscle of the external anal sphincter which may be kept in a state of contraction by higher centres and prevent defaecation. In this case, the mass movement gradually subsides and may not recur for several hours. Persistent voluntary antagonism of defaecation results in a reduction in force and frequency of the reflexes and can be a cause of severe or chronic constipation.

Absorption and secretion

Up to 1 litre of liquid chyme may pass into the

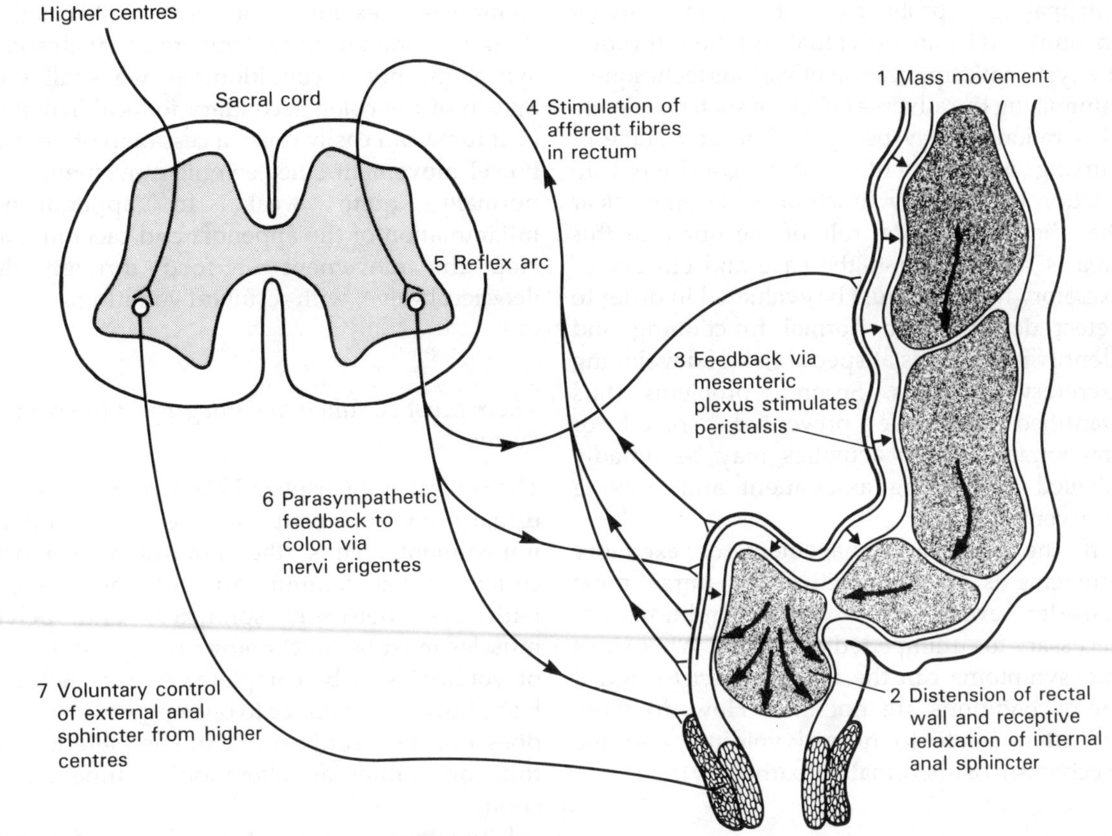

Fig. 25.2 The defaecation reflex

caecum each day. Of this, less than 100ml is normally excreted in the faeces, the rest being absorbed largely in the ascending portion and proximal half of the transverse colon. The absorption of water occurs secondary to the osmotic gradient caused by the active absorption of sodium ions, with chloride ions following across the electrical gradient thus produced. Chloride ions are also actively absorbed in an exchange process resulting in the secretion of bicarbonate ions.

In health, the secretions of the large intestine consist only of mucus, from goblet cells within the mucosa and crypts of Lieberkühn, and the bicarbonate ions mentioned above. These secretions protect the tissues from the irritant and acidic products of bacterial action. The rate of secretion is controlled by intrinsic feedback from sensory stimulation of the surface of the mucosa, and parasympathetic stimulation in the distal portions of the colon, which increases mucus secretion along with motility. Extreme parasympathetic activity can cause over-secretion with the resultant passage of mucus stools. Secretions are also greatly stimulated by local irritation of the mucosa by bacterial action or irritant food products. This action helps to dilute toxins and the local distension thus caused will also stimulate peristalsis, with the effect of quickly washing the irritants through the colon, resulting in diarrhoea.

THE NURSING MANAGEMENT OF EXCRETORY FUNCTION

INTRODUCTION: THE ROLE OF THE NURSE

Nurses are concerned with identifying or

anticipating problems of daily living encountered by an individual and then, through the systematic application of various techniques, minimizing the adverse effects of such problems. This rationale may be applied to any stage of nursing management; if it is considered in relation to excretory function, it becomes clear that the fundamental role of the nurse in this area is twofold. First, the ease and efficacy of excretory function must be evaluated in order to detect deviations in normal functioning and identify individuals at special risk of developing excretory problems. Second, problems thus identified must be prevented, solved or ameliorated. These activities may be broadly labelled as nursing assessment and nursing intervention.

If the nursing management of excretory problems is to be effective the nurse must consider several points. What conditions are necessary for unimpeded excretion? What signs and symptoms can the nurse expect to find if these conditions are not met? How do these indicators relate to normal voiding, and the mechanism of abnormality (pathology)?

Requirements for normal function

By considering the mechanism of excretion the nurse is able to base her management on objective criteria. The prerequisites of normal function may be summarized thus:

There must be anatomical continuity

An unobstructed and intact urinary tract, from renal pelvis to external meatus, is necessary. Obstruction may occur at any of the three levels identified earlier:

- ureters (e.g. calculi, spasm, fibrosis, stenosis)
- bladder (e.g. neoplasm, haematoma)
- urethra (e.g. fibrosis, prostatic enlargement, atresia).

Of course, trauma may damage the urinary tract at any level. The urethra is particularly vulnerable in a displaced pelvic fracture.

Constipation probably represents the commonest example of bowel obstruction though it should be remembered that this is a symptom, not a condition, as we shall see. Spasm of the colon secondary to local irritation or trauma can easily cause a cessation of normal bowel movement since colonic movements are normally quite weak. In appendicitis, inflammation of the appendix and caecum may stop the movement of food through the ileocaecal valve, with resultant vomiting.

There must be functional integrity of the control system

The central and peripheral elements involved in urinary control must be operating without impediment. Thus the brainstem, cerebral cortex, spinal column, afferent and efferent pathways, detrusor, sphincters and pelvic muscles must be functioning normally if control of voiding is to be complete. As we shall see later, however, damage to one or more elements does not necessarily result in complete loss of function, rather an alteration in function or control.

Ultimate control of defaecation also depends upon the intactness of higher centres, but reflex defaecation can occur in the absence of higher influences if the intrinsic and sacral pathways are intact. Loss of parasympathetic input greatly diminishes the strength of bowel movement. A break in the continuity of the myenteric plexus causes severely reduced or absent peristaltic activity. In this condition large amounts of faeces can accumulate in the colon, resulting in megacolon. Suppression of the myenteric plexus by drugs, in particular atropine or sympathomimetics such as noradrenaline, will dramatically reduce effective peristalsis and may even bring about stasis in the gastrointestinal tract.

Perhaps the commonest functional disorder of bowel action results from repeated wilful repression of the defaecation reflex for reasons of convenience or laziness. Eventually this action results in a reduction in frequency and efficiency of defaecation reflexes with resultant constipation.

There must be a suitable environment for voiding to occur

From a very early age members of Western society are taught and conditioned to void only in a limited number of situations and circumstances. When in hospital, or if at home but disabled, the individual may be required to void in situations which would not otherwise be considered 'normal' in terms of either environment (in bed, in the company of others, into strange receptacles) or position (for example, lying). Such constraints can interfere with elimination in two ways: in the case of urination, inhibition due to social or psychological factors may interfere with the production of facilitatory impulses in higher centres, with the result that the detrusor remains inhibited and the sphincters and perineal muscles contracted. This may occur subconsciously, despite the individual's attempts to relax and rationalize the situation. Alternatively, an unusual position, for example balancing on a bedpan for the first time, may make it difficult to relax sufficiently to allow micturition to occur.

Physiologically, the ideal position for defaecation is squatting — lying on a bedpan is therefore far from ideal. Inhibition of the urge to defaecate due to embarrassment, difficulty in getting the attention of a nurse or a wish to minimize discomfort by using the bedpan as infrequently as possible, may result in a reduction in the efficiency of the defaecation reflex as discussed above. This may be a major factor in the development of constipation in bedfast patients. Added to the inhibiting effect of strange environments is the lack of the normal 'triggers' to elimination which are otherwise present. Many nurses will have witnessed the power of such triggers to stimulate micturition when, for example, sitting patients on Ambulifts fitted with 'toilet-style' seats!

Related bodily systems must be operating normally or adequately

Obviously, if little urine is being produced then little will be voided. Urinary excretion therefore depends not only upon the function of the kidney and urinary tract but on other systems too. In particular, the cardiovascular and endocrine systems greatly influence the amount of urine ultimately excreted. In circumstances where the primary pathology involves one of these systems the assessment of urinary function and output can be an important indicator of the efficacy of treatment or course of disease, obvious examples of such disorders being cardiac failure and diabetes insipidus. The failure or weakness of structures which assist in defaecation may result in dyschezia (difficult defaecation). Weakness of abdominal or pelvic muscles due to age or pain following surgery will limit their use during defaecation. Tracheostomy will prevent the expiration against a closed glottis which normally helps expel faeces by raising intra-abdominal pressure. Pain following thoracic surgery may have a similar effect.

The assessment of related physiological systems cannot be covered in this chapter. The possibility that an apparent dysfunction of excretion may in fact be a symptom of disease or deficit elsewhere must, however, be considered by the nurse in her assessment.

Discussion

Difficulties of excretion may develop when factors interfere with one or more of these prerequisites. When an excretory dysfunction occurs then obviously the presenting signs and symptoms will be determined by the underlying causative mechanism. The logical analysis of such signs and symptoms will lead to an insight into the causes of the dysfunction and therefore act as a guide to the nursing management.

An inadequate assessment will lead to the ad hoc management of isolated symptoms and continued discomfort for the patient, coupled with increasing frustration on the part of the nurse as the problem continues despite intervention.

THE ASSESSMENT OF EXCRETORY FUNCTION

Introduction

The apparent obsession which nurses show

when assessing and recording their patients' excretory function has become anecdotal. This may be an inherited attitude from Victorian times when the quality of life was almost considered to be a correlate of bowel function, or it may reflect the difficulties experienced by nurses when helping hospitalized patients maintain normal functions. In either case, as has already been stated, up to 50% of hospitalized patients experience a change in bowel habit on admission (Wright, 1974) and 10% of general hospital patients have an indwelling catheter at some time during their treatment (Jenner, 1983). The incidence of lesser degrees of excretory difficulty must be much higher.

The key to successful management lies in a thorough and careful assessment and the ability of the assessor to extrapolate from this data to gain an insight into causative mechanisms. Only then can active intervention take place (though palliative methods may be employed before this stage).

Nurses are, or should be, concerned with the complete health of an individual. Furthermore, it is usually the case that several patients require care simultaneously and the practising nurse will quickly discover that these two aims conflict. Generally speaking, it is simply not possible to assess every patient with respect to every area, each to the ultimate degree. This fact makes the initial assessment of the patient that much more important since problems, if any, must be recognized and individuals at risk identified for observation. Such information should be tempered with the knowledge of the norm for any particular person. The initial assessment process then has three facets:

- to establish what is 'normal' for an individual
- to identify actual problems of excretion
- to identify potential problems of excretion.

At the completion of this stage of the assessment it is possible to say whether an actual or potential problem exists. If there is no problem, the assessment is completed when a time for re-evaluation has been established. If a problem has been identified the next stage of assessment is the investigation of the problem itself. In this stage, the cause of the dysfunction is considered as the basis for intervention.

Baseline assessment of the patient

Individual variation in excretory function, as with most bodily functions, is wide. On conducting a community survey Connel (1967) found that 'only 1% of the population had bowel habits outside the range of 3 bowel actions per week to 3 per day'. Other authorities quote widely varying figures from 14 times per day to once per year (Keele & Neil, 1961). One dreads to consider the consequences of managing all patients' bowel problems using either of these figures as typical. Obviously, it is foolish to attempt the management of a patient problem with no knowledge of the normal function of the individual concerned. It is the purpose of a baseline assessment to establish such norms.

It would be pointless to reproduce here one of the many patient assessment sheets which have been devised to help collate such information (e.g. Crow, 1977a and 1977b). These are many and the nurse is advised to seek out the standard for her hospital or school of nursing. Often it will be sufficient to ask the patient if he/she experiences any difficulty with his/her bowels or urination and, if so, to go on to assess the problem fully in terms of actual or potential problems whilst in hospital.

Identifying actual patient problems

The signs and symptoms of impaired excretory function may, for convenience, be divided into four categories. This is a functional distinction for the purposes of discussion and as we shall see, a consideration of signs and symptoms alone is rarely sufficient as a guide to intervention, except in emergency cases.

Changes in the quality of excrement. Often the first indicator to the nurse that a patient is developing an excretory problem will be a change in the characteristics of the urine or stool. The normal characteristics of excrement are well documented elsewhere and the nurse is advised to familiarize herself with these if necessary.

Urine. In health, urine is a clear, pale straw yellow colour. The aroma may be described as aromatic, not strong or unpleasant, and the specific gravity lies in the range 1005–1025, pH 4.6–7.5, 6 being typical. Cloudiness is not necessarily pathological but should be investigated more fully. Alkaline urine is commonly cloudy due to the insolubility of urates at high pH. Other causes of turbid urine include pus, bacteria and epithelial cells. In health, fresh urine is practically sterile — culture and/or microscopic examination will confirm the presence of urinary tract infection.

The colour and specific gravity of urine vary with concentration. Very concentrated urine suggests dehydration, whilst large quantities of very pale urine may indicate a forced diuresis or overhydration.

Frank blood in large quantities will be obvious but smaller amounts present as smokey or pink colourations, depending on pH. Note that certain foodstuffs and drugs may also cause a discolouration of the urine, in particular beets, rhubarb and senna. The anti-tubercule drug rifampicin may cause red/orange discolouration, as may the analgesic Pyridium and the popular danthron-based laxatives (Dorbanex, Normax).

Multi-test dip-sticks have simplified the investigation of urine for other constituents which are indicators of systemic disease, but they are not helpful in the assessment of lower excretory function.

Faeces. The normal stool is soft, formed and brown in colour. The colouration of faeces is due to the presence of the bile pigments and their derivatives, stercobilin and urobilin. Changes in colour are due to the constituents of the stool itself. Black or tarry stools (melaena) may be caused by the presence of altered blood from higher levels of the gastrointestinal tract, especially the stomach or duodenum, whilst frank blood or streaks of blood indicate bleeding from lower structures. Pale or clay-coloured stools result from a reduction in the normal pigment content of the faeces, and thus suggest biliary obstruction. Certain foodstuffs and drugs also affect the appearance of the faeces. In particular, iron supplements produce very dark or black stools.

The consistency of the faeces is determined by the speed of passage through the gastrointestinal tract. Stools which remain within the colon for a protracted length of time become dehydrated and hard, due to continual absorption of fluid by the intestinal mucosa. On the other hand, an increase in the speed of passage through the colon reduces the time available for absorption and the result is an unformed or watery stool. This may result from intense local or general irritation of the intestinal mucosa, which causes an increase in intestinal mobility. In severe cases the secretions of the colon also increase - a mechanism which serves to dilute irritants and neutralize low pH by the secretion of bicarbonate. A side-effect of this action is watery or mucous stools.

Changes in the volume of output.

Urine. Urine is typically produced at the rate of 30–50ml per hour. A total output of 720–1200ml per day therefore indicates adequate kidney function. In practice such considerations are problems of fluid balance rather than excretion and, as such, the ideal fluid output for any individual will be affected by many factors, including the overall aims of treatment. The management of fluid balance and electrolyte status is dealt with elsewhere.

Due to the pattern of fluid intake the volume of urine excreted during the day will normally exceed that at night. An exception may occur in cases of reduced kidney perfusion or cardiac failure, when improved renal function due to a supine position increases urine output.

An absolute increase in the amount of urine excreted (rather than a perceived increase due to frequency or other problems of control) is seen in some conditions, but the cause will always lie outside the excretory system itself (which for our purposes does not include the kidney).

Faeces. The difficulty in determining the 'normal' bowel output of an individual has been discussed above. The reader is referred to Wright (1974) Chapter 2 for a full discussion of the literature regarding bowel function. For our purposes Connell's findings (1967), indicating more than three motions per day or less than three per week to be unusual (though not necessarily abnormal), can be accepted as a guide to typical function. At all times the stated norm for any individual patient should be considered.

Constipation may be considered to be a reduction in the frequency of defaecation from what is normal for an individual, with associated difficulty in passing faeces. Conversely, diarrhoea is the increased and repeated passage of loose stools.

The volume of faecal output may occasionally be increased in the absence of diarrhoea. This usually follows a protracted period with no bowel action and may occur in cases of megacolon (Hirschsprung's disease) secondary to psychogenic constipation (Salvati, 1966).

Changes in the ease or control of elimination. As discussed earlier, the urge to micturate will be felt when 200– 450ml of urine has accumulated in the bladder. The reflex arc which is initiated by the stretch of the bladder wall can be inhibited or facilitated by higher centres, as can the tone of the external sphincter. In the case of faecal elimination, relaxation of the external anal sphincter is under voluntary control. Thus, once a certain degree of developmental maturity has resulted in the control of excretion, any subsequent loss of control or ease of function deserves thorough investigation.

Micturition. Micturition commonly occurs 2–10 times per day. In health the process is under voluntary control, though this will eventually be overcome in extreme circumstances. Typically urination is complete within one minute, and is efficient enough to express all but a very small residual volume – usually less than 50ml.

When assessing the control of micturition one must remember the normal variation in voiding patterns. The patient who asks for a bedpan every hour may be demanding of a nurse's time, but this could merely be a reflection of the individual's normal pattern.

Frequency of micturition is said to be present when voiding occurs more often than is normal for the individual, and when this is perceived as a problem. This condition may be a major embarrassment to the patient when dependent upon others for bedpans or assistance. Frequency may be accompanied by urgency, a strong, occasionally uncontrollable desire to micturate. Enuresis refers to the involuntary or unconscious passage of urine, but the term is most commonly used to describe nocturia – nocturnal enuresis, the failure of urinary control at night. Incontinence is a more generic term which describes a loss of control of either urinary or faecal excretion, or both.

At the other end of the continuum, hesitancy is an undue delay in the initiation of voiding once the urge to micturate has been obeyed, the commonest cause of which is outlet obstruction. Strangury is a term used when urination is slow and painful — only small amounts of urine are passed on each occasion.

Defaecation. Just as urinary tract infections or irritations can bring about an alteration of urinary control, so can irritation of the large intestine cause a temporary difficulty of control as the colon reacts with increased peristalsis and secretion. Peristaltic 'rush' can cause extreme urgency and in cases of very severe irritation, such as occurs in ulcerative colitis, mass movements may occur almost continuously. Constipation has been discussed, but it is worth reiterating that there are two elements to constipation: a reduction in the volume of faecal output, and undue difficulty with defaecation.

Generalized signs related to excretory dysfunction. As well as the specific signs and symptoms already discussed excretory problems can also give rise to more generalized sequelae.

The urinary system. Within the urinary system, pain may arise from ureters, bladder or urethra. Ureteral pain is usually severe, radiating to the back, abdomen and thighs. Bladder pain is commonly described as a low abdominal ache, possibly also radiating to the back. The pain of an over-distended bladder, however, is extreme and easily recognized. Spasms of the bladder, due perhaps to irritation from a catheter or infective process, can give rise to urgent, griping pains. Urethral pain may be described as burning or irritating, commonly occurring during micturition.

Gastrointestinal symptoms may develop in some instances due to the anatomical proximity of the kidneys to the peritoneum and colon (Brunner & Suddarth, 1982), and the space occupied by a distended bladder. The peritoneo-intestinal reflex may cause paralysis of the large intestine in response to peritoneal irritation. Similarly, the reno-intestinal and vesico-intestinal reflexes can reduce colonic activity in response to irritation of the kidney or bladder respectively (Guyton, 1981).

The colon. The colon has a large capacity for the storage of faecal material and it may, therefore, be quite some time before generalized signs of gastrointestinal disorders develop. Keele & Neil (1961) cite one example of a man going just over one year with no bowel action. Typically, individuals will complain of vague feelings of malaise, 'fullness' or discomfort. When impaction within the colon is so severe that chyme cannot enter the caecum from the ileum then severe vomiting results.

In contrast to faecal impaction, diarrhoea may rapidly produce severe symptoms due to the loss of large quantities of fluid and electrolytes. In response to irritation of the colon or higher portions of the gastrointestinal tract, motility is increased, with the result that the rate of passage of faeces reduces the time available for absorption. Muscular spasm produces the familiar intestinal colic ('griping' pains) associated with abnormal motility. Local irritation of the colon also produces an increased secretion of water and bicarbonate ions. Severe diarrhoea may lead to dehydration, abnormalities of acid-base balance (due to the loss of bicarbonate ions) and electrolyte imbalances, particularly hypokalaemia due to the loss of intestinal secretions and the potassium they contain.

Psycho-social consequences It is important that nurses consider the social and psychological consequences of their patients' excretory problems. The taboo nature of this subject and the social embarrassment caused may result in the patient reacting in a manner which, to the observer, may appear to be unjustified by the symptoms present. Many nurses have witnessed the severe anxiety felt by female patients suffering from urinary frequency, or the utter dejection and shame felt by adults who suffer an incontinence episode. Such reactions result from values instilled in us all through social conditioning from a very early age, and cannot be treated lightly. In particular, excretory problems can have a crippling effect on the social life of the sufferer. Fear of having an 'accident' in public, not being able to get to a public convenience in time, or of offensive body odours can result in increasing isolation for the sufferer. To the list of signs and symptoms discussed so far we must unfortunately add those of shame, isolation, guilt, depression and anxiety.

Identifying potential patient problems

The process of individual patient care is dependent upon the appropriate assessment of the patient. Since, as we have already discussed, it is rarely possible to assess each patient fully with respect to every area of function, it is necessary that those individuals at particular risk of developing excretory problems are identified for further investigation or observation. How may these patients be identified? The prerequisites of normal excretory function have been outlined above. To recap, these are fourfold and consist of:

- anatomical continuity
- functional integrity of the control system
- suitability of environment
- adequacy of related bodily systems.

Patients at risk due to loss of anatomical continuity. *Urinary system.* Anatomical continuity may be lost due to destructive or obstructive processes, and specific signs and symptoms will depend upon the site and degree of occlusion. Foreign bodies within the urinary tract may cause partial or complete obstruction, and include calculi and blocked catheters. Prolonged periods of immobility (e.g. bedrest) are known to raise the levels of insoluble salts excreted in the urine secondary to increased calcium excretion, increasing the risk of calculi formation (Mitchell, 1977).

Urethral stricture (narrowing) may accompany infective processes, especially venereal disease or chronic urinary infections. Prostatic enlargement can eventually cause partial or complete obstruction in cases of benign prostatic hypertrophy or cancer of the prostate.

Postoperatively, obstruction can occur due to sphincter spasm secondary to sympathetic activity — especially after abdominal, anal or perineal procedures. Localized oedema following surgery may also cause obstruction, as may meatal oedema following childbirth.

Patients who have recently had catheters removed may develop urinary retention due to spasm or loss of detrusor tone. Alternatively dribbling incontinence may be caused due to the prolonged dilatation of sphincters whilst a catheter is in situ.

Obstruction may also originate from outside the urinary tract. Faecal impaction is a cause of urinary retention that every nurse will encounter at some time in her/his career. The pressure of a fully loaded colon compresses the urinary tract causing an obstructive retention. Abdominal or even spinal neoplasms may eventually reach sufficient proportions to cause an obstruction.

Trauma to part of the urinary tract may result in a loss of anatomical continuity. This development is particularly likely in the individual with abdominal injuries, perhaps as the result of a fall or road traffic accident, and patients with pelvic fracture must be assessed and observed carefully for signs of urinary distress.

Urethral or bladder fistulae may result in a diversion of urinary excretion. Destructive neoplasms, vaginal or other abscesses or the prolonged pressure of an indwelling catheter may all cause fistula formation. A fistula may communicate with another body cavity (e.g. vagina or rectum) or with the body surface.

The colon. The occlusion of the colon by hard impacted faeces is a common finding in bowel obstruction. It is apparent, however, that the movement of faeces through the bowel must originally have been embarrassed by some other mechanism, which is why constipation has been identified as a symptom rather than a cause of bowel disorders. Obstruction may occur in the absence of pathology if the normal bowel action is repressed deliberately or reduced in efficacy due to insufficient dietary bulk or aperient abuse. In this latter case, normal defaecation reflexes are disrupted by frequent aperient or enema use. This has the effect of producing a less efficient emptying of the bowel whilst causing a diminution in the strength of subsequent defaecation reflexes. Whilst it appears tautological to consider constipation as a cause of bowel obstruction some individuals, especially the elderly, may present with advanced faecal impaction and nurses should be aware of this at-risk group. The mechanism of such impaction will be discussed in subsequent sections.

The commonest cause of pathological obstruction of the colon is carcinoma (Sabiston, 1981). Volvulus — a twisting and obstruction of a portion of the bowel — will cause obstruction and is more common in the elderly, often affecting the sigmoid loop of the colon (Shafer et al, 1979). Adhesions, which predispose to the development of obstructions, may follow peritonitis or abdominal surgery. Finally, obstruction following herniation of a loop of bowel through the abdominal musculature is a risk in patients with femoral or inguinal hernia and in cases of wound dehiscence following abdominal surgery.

Individuals at risk. Individuals at risk of developing excretory problems due to a loss of anatomical continuity therefore include:

- the elderly, due to increased incidence of prostatic enlargement and gynaecological problems — faecal impaction is more likely to be a problem in the elderly
- patients on prolonged bed rest
- individuals sustaining abdominal or pelvic trauma, or undergoing surgery
- patients with known intra-abdominal pathology, or a history of such conditions.

Patients at risk due to loss of functional integrity. As stated earlier, the faecal and urinary control systems consist of cerebral, spinal and pelvic elements, and interference at any level may cause a change in normal excretory function. The presenting symptoms will depend upon the site of the dysfunction.

Bladder function. With reference to the urinary tract itself, continued control will depend upon the resistance to flow offered by the bladder, internal sphincter and urethra acting in opposition to increasing intravesicular pressure. It has been shown (Claridge, 1965) that if the diameter of the urethra is sufficiently small then the resistance to flow required to maintain continence may be maintained by quite a low degree of tension in the urethral wall. However, damage to the urethra or internal sphincter which reduces the elasticity of the tissues will interfere with this function, as will stretching or loss of tone due to protracted catheterization. Claridge goes on to present evidence to support the theory that the external sphincter is more an accessory structure to maintain continence at times of stress, for periods of a few seconds, than a major factor in long-term control. The pelvic floor muscles similarly act in a supporting role assisting the counteraction of increased intra-abdominal pressure. Thus damage to the external sphincter or pelvic floor muscles, perhaps occurring during pregnancy or childbirth, may result in a loss of secondary control and occasional incontinence at times of stress (e.g. coughing or sneezing). Jeffcote (1965) makes the point however that this could not occur if the internal sphincter and urethra were operating correctly.

Direct irritation of the bladder itself, through infection, trauma or drug action, may lead to spasm of the detrusor with resultant frequency or urgency.

Trauma or other causes of pathology involving the neural pathways for bladder control may occur at any level and have given rise to a confusing array of terms — neurogenic bladder, tabetic bladder, uninhibited bladder and so on. There are two levels of control — the spinal reflexes at levels S2 to S4, and the voluntary facilitatory or inhibitory inputs from the higher centres.

Damage to the sacral spine may result in an interruption or complete loss of spinal micturition reflexes despite the fact that higher centres are intact. The result is that the bladder fails to respond to the increased volume of filling, losing tone and becoming over-extended. This is the atonic or lower motor neurone bladder. Because this was often seen in the later stages of syphilis the term tabetic bladder is sometimes used. The characteristics of this condition are urinary retention with extended bladder and loss of reflex emptying. Note that prolonged catheterization may also cause a reduction in bladder tone due to the disturbance of the normal filling and emptying process, and the relationship of this action to the maintenance of detrusor tone is discussed earlier. There is therefore a risk of urinary retention following catheter removal. We shall return to this point when discussing the management of patient problems in a later section.

In contrast, a lesion above the sacral level which leaves the spinal reflexes intact but prevents the influence of higher centres, will result in a bladder which empties spontaneously in response to filling. However, Guyton (1981) makes the point that initially urinary retention may occur due to loss of facilitatory input. This condition is occasionally referred to as an upper motor neurone bladder. Characteristics of this condition are spontaneous reflex emptying of the bladder with loss of voluntary control, frequency and a raised residual urine volume due to incomplete emptying (Whittington, 1980). Note that in both cases varying degrees of dysfunction may be seen. Thus in cerebrovascular accident, there may initially be a complete loss of higher control which later returns, albeit to a lesser degree. Spinal lesions may result in 'spinal shock' in which the spinal micturition reflex is lost for a period of time but may eventually return if bladder function is supported.

Bowel function. Spinal injuries may also result in a disturbance of bowel function. Damage to the sacral segments of the spinal cord may interfere with the propagation of the parasympathetic defaecation reflex, resulting in a diminution of peristaltic activity in the descending colon, sigmoid colon and rectum, predisposing to constipation. The loss of sensory feedback also makes active participation in defaecation in response to rectal filling impossible. Loss of sphincter control by higher centres completes the picture of inefficient bowel evacuation coupled with faecal incontinence. Disseminated sclerosis and poliomyelitis are further examples of conditions which may interfere with the nervous control of elimination.

Intrinsic factors also affect the control of bowel action. Insufficient bulk in the colon causes a diminution of bowel activity and increased passage time, since tactile stimulation of the mucosa is reduced. Conversely, the presence of irritant substances such as bacterial toxins will increase both the motility of the bowel and the secretion of water and electrolytes (see earlier). The resultant rush of colonic contents may result in diarrhoea and a temporary loss of or reduction in bowel control. Intense irritation of the bladder mucosa similarly results in increased filling sensitivity and detrusor spasm, leading to urinary frequency and in some cases temporary urinary incontinence.

A number of commonly used drug preparations may affect excretory function. In particular, drugs which have anticholinergic effects or side-effects naturally reduce parasympathetic activity. Thus gut motility is reduced causing a tendency to constipation and there is an increased likelihood of urinary hesitancy and retention. It is well known that morphine and its derivatives may cause constipation. These drugs increase the frequency of haustral contractions in the colon. The net effect is an increase in absorption without a corresponding increase in passage, leading to constipation.

Finally, control of elimination may be reduced because of an individual's actions in response to pain experienced when eliminating. Haemorrhoids or anal fissures may cause extreme discomfort during bowel action resulting in a suppression of the urge to defaecate. Pain experienced in accessory musculature or structures, e.g. the abdominal muscles following surgery or the perineum after episiotomy, will have a similar effect. The intense burning irritation of urethritis may result in the sufferer avoiding micturition as long as possible, thereby exacerbating the original condition.

Individuals at risk. Individuals at risk of developing excretory problems due to an interference with control mechanisms therefore include those who:

- sustain abdominal, pelvic or spinal trauma or undergo surgery
- are on opiates or medications with known anticholinergic effects or side-effects
- experience pain or discomfort during elimination, for whatever reason
- have recently had indwelling urinary catheters removed.

Patients at risk due to unsuitability of environment. Admission to hospital inevitably brings about a major change in the circumstances and environmental conditions of an individual, and persons who are least able to adapt to new situations will be at particular risk. This group includes elderly, very young and very ill patients. The failure to adapt or inability to function optimally in a new situation may bring about a change in excretory function in two ways. Brocklehurst (1978) describes the way in which elderly persons may regress behaviourally in the face of intolerable situations such as admission to hospital. Responsibility for everyday function is removed from the person – control over one's life is lost, and the individual becomes dependent upon others for the provision of food and necessities. Familiar clothing and personal objects may be removed for fear of damage or loss. The elderly person may respond with an emotional crisis which results in loss of excretory control.

Restricted facilities. In addition, restrictions may be imposed on the individual in terms of availability, ease of use or quality of facilities which result in the inability or disinclination to make use of them. With reference to the elderly, Brocklehurst (1978) identifies such circumstances as 'precipitating factors' which serve to push the individual beyond the ability to cope, whilst in more favourable circumstances the person manages adequately.

Most individuals learn from an early age to restrict their excretory activities to socially acceptable situations – somewhere private, clean and with the correct facilities. For one reason or another hospitals can fall short of the ideal. This may be due to a lack of suitable facilities (including staff), thoughtlessness on the part of carers, or a combined effect of both. In addition, when one feels at ease in a situation as nurses generally do in hospitals, it is very easy to underestimate the reluctance felt by some individuals to seek out what they require. Norton et al (1962) describe one case of a patient remaining incontinent of urine for 3 days because she was unaware that she was allowed to ask for a bedpan when necessary.

There is some evidence (Wright, 1974) that patients who are dependent upon staff for bedpans or commodes are more likely to experience a change in bowel habit than those who are independent in toilet needs. This cannot be dismissed as the effect of staffing levels alone since in the same study it was shown that both high and low staffing levels were associated with patients having to wait for bedpans, with the least likelihood of this occurring at intermediate staffing levels. The further finding that only 29% of patients were offered hand-washing facilities after using bedpans or commodes for bowel actions is inexcusable. Evidence is also available of shortcomings in provision and distribution of toileting facilities, and the failure of many nurses to make full use of the equipment which is available, to the detriment of patient care (Wells, 1980). This finding is again supported by Wright (1974), who found that the likelihood of complaints about the unsuitable temperature of bedpans was higher where a bedpan warmer was available. Although when taken in isolation, factors such as cold bedpans may seem trivial issues they are in fact representative of the many ways in which hospitals may fall short of the ideal. Cold bathrooms, lack of privacy or hand-washing facilities, long distances to toilet areas from patient areas, difficult clothing, seats which are too high or too low and patient diffidence may all combine to explain those 54% of patients in Wright's (1974) study who experienced a decrease in bowel frequency when admitted to hospital.

Restricted mobility. A second group of at-risk individuals includes those who, by the nature of the illness or treatment, are severely restricted in their ability to move freely and help themselves. Patients on traction, bedrest or following major surgery or stroke are not only dependent on others to meet their needs, but may also have great difficulty positioning themselves correctly and relaxing sufficiently. The natural position for micturition is upright, sitting or standing, and some individuals find it virtually impossible to urinate whilst supine.

The ideal position for defaecation is squatting — lying on a bedpan is therefore far from ideal, and cleaning oneself following bowel action can involve a precarious combination of fine balance and considerable manual dexterity.

Individuals at risk. Individuals at risk of developing excretory problems due to unsuitable environment therefore include:

- those who experience difficulty in adapting to new situations — the elderly, very young or very ill
- patients with restrictions of mobility due to the nature of treatment, illness or pain.

Patients at risk due to dysfunctions of related bodily systems. During an assessment the nurse must consider the possibility that an apparent problem of excretion may actually be precipated by, or be representative of, problems elsewhere in the body. Such influences may be generalized or limited to a particular system. Dehydration is an obvious example of a general state which can greatly influence excretory function, resulting in the increased reabsorption of water from both the renal tubules and colon. Urine output falls and eventually the colonic contents become dry and hard, making propulsion along the colon and defaecation increasingly difficult.

Pain. Pain associated with excretion was discussed earlier, but it should be remembered that generalized pain can also adversely affect excretion. The patient in pain may find it difficult to relax sufficiently to allow urination or defaecation to occur easily, or may defer the need to eliminate because of the effort or discomfort involved, resulting in constipation.

Reduced mobility. Most hospitalized patients suffer a decrease in general mobility due to restrictions imposed by treatment, illness or pain. Holdstock et al (1970) found that propulsive colonic activity following meals was enhanced by bodily activity, and concluded that 'somatic activity is an important factor in the control of colonic transit in health or disease'

The mechanism by which bodily activity enhances bowel function is not clear. It seems likely that, in addition to increased colonic transit, the simple effect of gravity will help propel faeces toward the anus, triggering a defaecation response. Wright (1974) makes the point that inactivity may result in a reduction of muscle tone, and summarizes several empirical studies which confirm the relationship between activity and trouble-free bowel action. We should remember when considering such studies that mobile patients are less likely to be dependent upon help from others to meet their needs.

Pregnancy. During pregnancy physiological changes occur which may result in constipation. Causes include lowered intestinal muscle tone due to raised progesterone levels, increased insensible fluid loss and the pressure of the uterus (Kilner, 1980). There may also be a decrease in general activity and changed dietary habits.

Mental states. Mental states and psychological conditions can greatly influence excretory function. Ultimate control of defaecation and urination is dependent upon the influence of higher centres. The acutely ill or semi-conscious patient may well be temporarily incontinent, as may the confused individual. Transient incontinence may be a feature of acute confusional disorders in the elderly, precipitated by respiratory and urinary infections or other somatic disorders (Brocklehurst, 1978). Sedative abuse or intolerance may have a similar effect.

Nervous tension and unresolved psychological conflict can also interfere with excretion. Almost everyone at some time or other experiences 'nervous diarrhoea' due to excessive parasympathetic arousal in response to stress. Low-Beer & Read (1971) identify irritable bowel syndrome — a disorder with a recognized psychosomatic element — as the commonest cause of chronic diarrhoea. Alternatively, Salvati (1966) describes a study of 76 patients with chronic psychogenic constipation.

Specific disease states which may present as or precipitate alterations in excretory function are many and cannot be covered in detail. The reader is referred to other chapters for further discussion. Urine output ultimately depends upon urine production and this process may be influenced by hormonal, cardiovascular and infective processes. Similarly, bowel function necessarily reflects upper alimentary functions, and is also dependent upon and affected by changes in hormonal, neural and circulatory disorders.

Individuals at risk. Individuals at risk of developing excretory problems due to dysfunction of related systems therefore include:

- severely ill patients, or those with multiple pathology
- individuals suffering from confusion, impaired levels of consciousness or psychological stress
- those experiencing a reduced level of activity or exercise.

Discussion. The comprehensive assessment of excretory function has three elements: the formulation of baseline values or individual norms, the recognition of current problems through presenting signs and symptoms, and the identification of individuals at particular risk of developing new or further problems. Patient assessment may begin with any of the three elements, depending upon the individual and the point at which intervention occurs. Thus, if a patient is admitted following multiple injury then the risk of excretory problems developing may be considered first. If the conclusion was that there is indeed an increased risk, then a baseline assessment of the normal function would be made (to enable deviations in functioning to be recognized), followed by continual observations for signs and symptoms of developing problems, and reassessment of the risk at a stated time. Alternatively, if an individual was admitted through an accident and emergency department with acute, serious excretory problems then emergency palliative intervention may be indicated based on an assessment of signs and symptoms. Once the acute problem had been controlled, baseline assessment of normal function would follow in order to determine realistic treatment outcomes. Assessment would be completed by the evaluation of any continued risk or the probability of problems recurring.

The nurse must be flexible in her approach to patient assessment. Individualized patient management is occasionally criticized as being too intricate or long-winded, involving the nurse in extensive assessment or history-taking at the expense of action and patient care. This should not be so, and assessment should itself be flexible. There is a time to act, and a time to observe and listen. Only education and experience can help the nurse to determine the best approach to each patient.

MANAGING PROBLEMS OF EXCRETION

Introduction

Decision-making in nursing is a complex process. Following observation and assessment, the nurse must make a decision about the patient.

When planning the intervention and management of a patient's problem the nurse has several aspects to consider. In discussing the management process in nursing, Mitchell (1977) identifies four decision criteria which serve as guidelines when selecting interventions:

- The soundness of the theoretical base. How valid are the theories and principles which relate to the decision? The nurse may draw upon scientific evidence, including nursing research, to guide her/his decision. Since it is impossible to be expert in all fields the nurse must maintain a commitment to regular study and supplement her/his knowledge base when necessary.
- Compatibility with the patient's level of functioning. How able is the patient to cooperate in his/her care and is this reflected in the management?
- Compatibility with the patient's beliefs, attitudes and perceptions. Has anyone determined what the patient believes about the problem? If he/she feels that the advice on diet and fibre given is of little value then he/she is unlikely to follow it.
- Feasibility. The apparently ideal solution may not be feasible due, for example, to a lack of equipment, time, expertise or staff. A further aspect to consider is that of risk to the patient — risk of harm, discomfort or embarrassment.

Kelly & Hammond (1964) found the nurses' working environment to be probabilistic and uncertain, and the utilization of textbook patterns of cures inappropriate in clinical situations. In discussing the management of excretory problems, therefore, emphasis will be placed on the techniques and approaches available to the nurse rather than any attempt to offer solutions to specific problems. Since nursing management will normally include referral to the medical team if necessary, medical interventions will also be mentioned, but the reader is referred to specialized texts for detailed discussion.

Many of the techniques available to the nurse should already be apparent. Thus, there are four ways in which the nurse can intervene in excretory problems — by taking measures to restore anatomical continuity, improve the function of control systems, adapt the environment, or improve and support the function of related bodily systems. In most cases nursing action will follow naturally from assessment. For example, if shortcomings in environmental factors are identified then the required intervention will be obvious — though not necessarily easily achieved. Obviously it is impossible to manage a problem intelligently unless a thorough assessment has been made. The management of most problems will require a combination of these methods.

Intervention based upon restoring anatomical continuity

It will be recalled from the discussion of patient assessment that the loss of anatomical continuity usually occurs as a result of serious pathology — occlusion of the urinary tract by calculi, neoplasm or stricture; disruption following abdominal trauma; bowel obstruction due to neoplasm, volvulus or extreme inflammation. Because of this, medical intervention may be the most approporiate course of action. Surgical repair of the urinary tract or bowel or resection of space-occupying lesions may be indicated. In extreme cases a complete alteration of anatomical continuity is necessary. Such procedures include techniques for urinary or faecal diversion and various routes are available to the surgeon. In urinary diversion the ureters may be implanted into a closed section of ileum which is then fashioned into a stoma in the abdominal wall, forming an ileal conduit. Alternatively the ureters may be diverted to the sigmoid colon (ureterosigmoidostomy) and urine drains via the rectum. If the level of obstruction is below the bladder then cystostomy or suprapubic catheterization is possible. Faecal diversion (colostomy) may be undertaken at the level of the ascending, transverse or descending colon. The resultant faecal output will vary in character depending upon the site of the stoma. Diversion of intestinal contents may also be undertaken at higher levels, for example ileostomy. The reader is referred to specialized texts for further discussion of such procedures. The care of patients with stomas is discussed in a separate section at the end of this chapter (p. 822).

Nursing actions which may be taken to restore anatomical continuity are necessarily invasive and may expose the patient to a greater risk or discomfort than other techniques at the nurse's disposal. The use of such methods as urinary catheterization and evacuation of impacted faeces should only be considered when other techniques are not appropriate, or when the presenting problem is so acute that immediate intervention is required to prevent further patient injury.

Urinary catheterization

The insertion of a urinary catheter effectively alters the anatomical continuity of the urinary tract. The normal voiding mechanism is bypassed, allowing the nurse or patient artificial control over urination. Catheterization may therefore be employed in order to ensure urine drainage or to achieve control over it. There are two main aims of care for the catheterized patient:

- to maintain a good, unimpeded urine output, thus keeping the patient dry
- to minimize or prevent the development of adverse complications of catheterization.

The choice of catheter. *Types of catheter.* Patient management begins with the choice of the most suitable catheter. Urinary catheters are made of a variety of materials (Blannin & Hobden, 1980; Blannin, 1982; Kennedy, 1984a), but are of three main types: plastic, coated latex and pure silicone. Plastic catheters have a relatively large lumen and are resistant to kinking, but are stiff and do not conform easily to the contours of the urethra. These catheters are suitable for short-term post-surgical use. Blannin & Hobden (1980) found leakage occurred in 70% of female and 50% of male patients using these catheters, with 15% being rejected within 48 hours. Catheters of a coated latex construction are flexible and designed to be left in situ for longer periods of between 2 and 12 weeks, depending upon the coating material (those with silicone-elastomer coats generally lasting longer than Teflon or siliconized latex). Blannin & Hobden (1980) found that 84% of patients developed problems with latex catheters over a 2 month period. Pure silicone and silicone-coated catheters are designed for long-term use, 70% being in situ for over 2 months without problem in the Blannin & Hobden study. It should be noted that such figures are only guidelines and in practice each patient will differ in his or her tolerance of a catheter, some individuals quickly blocking or rejecting their catheter, irrespective of type. As a general guide, catheters which are intended for short-term use (for example peri-operatively) may be of Teflon or siliconized-coated latex, whereas long-term use calls for one of the more expensive pure silicone or silicone-elastomer varieties. These may cost six or seven times as much as the equivalent latex-based catheter.

Size of catheter. Equally careful consideration should be given to catheter size (McGill, 1982). Kennedy (1984a) recommends that size Ch12 or Ch14 (Charrier) is adequate unless urine is particularly viscous or gritty.

When examining differently sized catheters, Blannin & Hobden (1980) found considerable variation in internal and external diameters of catheters of a given size, and conclude that small variations in size are therefore unlikely to be important. Using stepwise forward multiple regression, Kennedy et al (1983) found a relationship between large catheter size and the incidence of complications, especially bypassing and blocking. Blannin (1982) reports that some patients will inevitably block a catheter irrespective of size and suggests that occlusion may be occurring at the drainage eyelet, the size of which will remain relatively similar in different gauge catheters. In conclusion there is little evidence that large gauge catheters (Ch. 20 and above) have any advantage over smaller sizes and on the contrary they are associated with an increased incidence of side-effects. The general rule should be to use as small a gauge as possible initially (Chs 12–14) and then reassess the patient with the catheter in situ.

Maintaining urine flow. Liquids flow from an area of higher pressure to one of lower pressure at a rate proportional to the resistance to flow. The resistance to flow is determined by the viscosity of the fluid and the diameter and length of the tube. If these simple rules are borne in mind then the guidelines for maintaining trouble-free catheter drainage becomes clear:

- Urine which is gritty or viscous will flow less freely. Therefore maintain an adequate fluid intake. Kennedy (1985) has found a minimum 2000 ml per day to be necessary for the average adult.
- Avoid long catheters and drainage tubing. Short catheters are available for female patients and will offer less resistance to flow. This is an important point since female patients are more likely to suffer adverse effects from their catheters than males (Kennedy et al, 1983) and therefore any measures which will reduce the problems of this group should be utilized. Long lengths of drainage tubing will offer greater resistance to flow than short tubing, and will also tend to hang in dependent loops producing a 'manometer effect' which increases resistance to flow. Ideally the tubing should run continually downhill to discourage pooling and stagnation of urine.
- Ensure that catheters are not kinked or compressed by the patient. The short female catheters are less likely to become coiled or kinked.
- Use drainage tubing which is of the widest diameter practicable (increased catheter sizes have such small differences in lumen size that their benefit is negligible when considered against the disadvantages of large gauge catheters, considered below).
- Ensure that the collection bag is not higher than the bladder.
- The evidence for and against bladder washouts is equivocal. Blannin (1982) concludes that they are only necessary when an adequate flow cannot be maintained by other means. Other studies have produced differing recommendations (Kennedy & Brocklehurst, 1982).

Minimizing the adverse effects of catheterization. Adverse effects of catheterization include urinary tract infection, trauma or discomfort, leakage and post-catheterization difficulties.

Urinary tract infection. As stated in the opening section of this chapter, Ansell (1962) concludes that a urinary catheter left in situ for 24–48 hours will result in urinary tract infection. This statement was made over 20 years ago and referred to open drainage systems, but in a more recent study a pre-trial urinary tract infection rate of 45% was found in catheterized surgical patients (Southampton Infection Control Team, 1982). The literature relating to catheter care and infection is enormous and often conflicting. Trials are often poorly controlled and it is difficult to determine the relative efficacy of the various measures employed to reduce urinary tract infection.

Bacteria can enter a closed catheter system via four routes: via the urethra during catheterization, by ascending the catheter/urethral junction, via the lumen of the catheter and by contamination during circuit breakages (Ansell, 1962; Stamm, 1975). Any attempt to reduce the incidence of bacteruria must therefore consider all of these routes.

THE PREVENTION OF INFECTION DURING CATHETERIZATION. Strict aseptic techniques should be used when inserting catheters (Seal & Ward, 1983). For ethical reasons the benefit of aseptic techniques cannot be proven experimentally but the value of asepsis in invasive techniques should be beyond doubt to all nurses. An antiseptic lubricant may be used to further reduce the likelihood of infection during catheterization.

INFECTION AT THE CATHETER/MEATAL JUNCTION. The probability that bacteruria occurs as a result of bacteria ascending the fluid space between the catheter and urethra was demonstrated in a well-known study by Kass & Schneiderman in 1957, when a species of bacterium which had been applied to the thighs and genitalia of three patients was later identified in the urine. Ansell (1962) points out that this contamination could have occurred via other routes, shedding doubt on the validity of the findings and going on to suggest that the risk of infection via this route is minimal. This may account for the inability of subsequent studies to conclusively demonstrate a difference when comparing routine self-care of catheters by patients and strict aseptic cleansing of catheter sites by nurses. Stamm (1975) concludes that since the incidence of urinary tract infection can be reduced to 15–20% without the use of urethral antiseptics then the peri-urethral route of infection, if present, is of little importance when compared to other routes. This issue remains unresolved. For reasons of patient comfort, catheter care should be adequate to prevent the build-up of secretions and encrustations at the urethral meatus. At the present time the benefits of antiseptic regimes over routine hygiene measures remain unproven.

INFECTION VIA THE CATHETER LUMEN. Urine is an ideal medium for bacterial growth. Stagnant urine in tubing or drainage bags will quickly culture bacteria, which may then ascend to the bladder. This may occur if the bag is raised above the level of the bladder allowing a backflow of urine. The inadvertent compression of bags which do not have non-return valves will force urine up the drainage tube. There are two approaches to the prevention of infection via this route.

Firstly, reflux of urine into the bladder can be prevented. Urine bags which are fitted with non-return valves will prevent collected urine from re-entering the tubing. Tubing and collection bags should be positioned to encourage continual drainage, with no loops for the collection of urine. If a catheter bag has to be lifted above the level of the bladder then the tubing may be pinched momentarily to prevent backflow.

The second approach which has been found to be effective is to prevent the multiplication of bacteria in the urine by adding an antiseptic to the collection bag (Webb & Blandy, 1968; Southampton Infection Control Team, 1982). If this technique is employed then a non-return valve is desirable to prevent accidental reflux of solutions into the bladder. Alternatively, collecting bags may be emptied more frequently to prevent stagnation of urine. This will involve breaking the drainage circuit, which should be done aseptically.

INFECTION DUE TO CIRCUIT BREAKAGE. All catheter drainage should be conducted under 'closed' systems, that is, at no point is the circuit left open to the air, with the exception of a filtered air-inlet on some rigid containers. If this arrangement is used then it follows that external contamination can only occur when the circuit is broken — when the tap is opened, bag changed, etc. Nurses can reduce the incidence of infection via this route by swabbing tubing junctions and taps with antiseptics before opening them, and by wearing sterile gloves during such procedures. There should be careful selection of drainage bags to ensure ease of emptying, preferably with one hand and without contaminating the fingers with urine. Kennedy (1984b) describes a drainage system which allows extension of a leg-bag into a larger night bag, eliminating the need to change bags every evening and morning.

DISCUSSION. It is difficult to estimate the relative value of the management guidelines outlined above. The Southampton Infection Control Team (1982) achieved a reduction in the incidence of bacteruria from 45% to 18% by the utilization of aseptic techniques in catheter care and the instillation of antiseptics in collecting bags. Since the antiseptic prevented infection via the catheter lumen, the authors conclude that the bacteruria that did occur resulted from infection at the urethral junction and suggest therefore that abstaining from showering or bathing may prevent infection during the acute period. However, others have suggested that this route of infection can be minimized by applying an antiseptic cream around the meatus.

It is generally agreed that prophylactic antibiotics are of doubtful or undetermined value in the prevention of urinary tract infection in long-term catheterizations (Cleland et al, 1971; Stamm, 1975; Kennedy & Brocklehurst, 1982) and may in fact result in the selection and subsequent culture of resistant organisms. The probability of bacteruria developing rises markedly as the period of catheterization increases. Stamm (1975) concludes that closed, sterile catheterization will not prevent bacteruria in long-term treatment (2 weeks) and Cleland et al (1971) were 'unaware of any writer ever claiming that bacteruria could be prevented in case of continued use of indwelling catheter.' These authors did find, however, that broad-spectrum antibiotics were effective in reducing the incidence of bacteruria in short-term treatments, 23.7% of patients on antibiotics developing urinary tract infections as compared to 75.6% of those receiving no chemotherapy. These findings compare with the Southampton study (1982) in which 10% of patients on antibiotics developed bacteruria, compared to 24% of those not receiving them.

Minimizing trauma and discomfort. Kennedy et al (1983) found irritation from indwelling catheters to be a problem for 14% of patients in their study, and a frequent or continual problem for 8%. There are several measures which may minimize catheter discomfort. The catheter should be of the appropriate gauge — large catheter sizes are associated with an increased incidence of patient problems. Large size catheters are more likely to traumatize mucosa or obstruct urethral glands. Failure of the catheter to conform easily to the contours of the urethra results in pressure being exerted at the site of the bend, with the possibility of pressure sore, abscess or fistula formation (Brunner & Suddarth, 1982; McGill, 1982). Ensuring that the penis is straight and that the catheter does not exit at an angle from the urethra will reduce the likelihood of pressure trauma. Traction on the catheter itself will irritate the bladder trigone, causing discomfort and increased bladder spasm. This can be minimized by ensuring that the collecting bag and tubing are adequately supported. Similarly, catheter balloons which are filled to maximum capacity may increase detrusor spasm. A 30ml balloon when filled will have a diameter of almost 4cm and weigh 30g (approx 1oz). This volume acts as a foreign body, irritating the bladder and causing abdominal discomfort (McGill, 1982). Nurses who are concerned that the patient may pull out an indwelling catheter unless the balloon is filled to maximum should address themselves to the real problem — that the patient is at risk of injury due to a tendency to pull on the catheter — since it is possible for a determined patient to pull out a catheter despite a 30ml balloon, thereby causing severe trauma to the urethra. In most cases a 5–10ml balloon capacity should adequately secure the catheter in place, but a catheter designed with this size of balloon should be used rather than incompletely filling a larger balloon.

Minimizing catheter leakage. When examining the management of long-term catheterized patients Kennedy & Brocklehurst (1982) found that 40% of patients had problems with catheters bypassing, and that the attempts of nurses to minimize this problem were often misdirected. There is now evidence (Kennedy, 1984a) that the (female) urethra has a slit-like structure on cross-section. The author goes on to suggest that, because of this anatomy, large size catheters will tend to distort the normal shape of the urethra to a greater degree than small gauge tubes. It is postulated that large catheters will cause the appearance of channels at either side of the tube which will predispose to bypassing. This theory is supported by the finding in an earlier study that catheter bypassing is associated with large size catheters (Kennedy et al, 1983). The practice of replacing catheters which are bypassing with one of a larger size to 'plug up the gap' is therefore misguided. The nurse must investigate the problem of bypassing fully to determine the cause, which may be an oversize catheter, blockage or bladder spasm. The common practice of increasing the volume of water in the balloon in an attempt to prevent bypassing can now be seen to be misguided, since if the bypassing is due to detrusor spasm then the increased balloon volume will exacerbate it.

Urinary tract infection will increase the incidence of catheter leakage due to the associated bladder irritation and increase in urinary deposition, especially if the urine pH increases as a result of the infection. In conclusion, catheter bypassing may be minimized by careful selection of catheter size, the control of bladder spasm and the maintenance of a deposit-free lumen by ensuring adequate urine output and preventing urinary tract infection wherever possible. A patient who is troubled by catheter leakage must be adequately reassessed to determine the true cause of the problem.

Minimizing post-catheterization difficulties. An indwelling catheter disrupts the normal anatomy and function of the urinary tract. The filling and emptying cycle which is essential for the maintenance of detrusor tone is disrupted, and the sphincters and urethra are constantly dilated by the presence of the catheter. If a significant loss of detrusor tone occurs then post-catheterization urinary retention may develop. Alternatively, there may be a constant slight urinary leakage until the sphincters and urethra recover their normal anatomy. It would seem logical that this second problem will relate to catheter size, with large gauge catheters distorting the urethra to a greater degree, though no experimental proof is available at the moment. In a study of post-catheterization bladder dysfunction, Williamson (1982) found that dysfunction could be reduced by introducing a simple clamping regime before catheter removal. A group of patients who had undergone a nine-hour period of reconditioning, consisting of a 5-minute clamp release every three hours, regained normal bladder sensation and function more quickly than the control group, who had had no conditioning (mean 1.92 hours compared to 2.75 hours). In conclusion, nurses can attempt to minimize post-catheterization problems by using the smallest appropriate catheter and instituting a catheter clamping regime prior to removal.

Bowel obstruction

If for any reason the transit of faecal matter through the bowel is delayed, then the continual reabsorption of water will result in a dry, hardened stool which is difficult to pass. Constipation occurs when there is a reduction in the frequency of defaecation from what is normal for the individual, combined with a difficulty in passing faeces. This condition is a *symptom* occurring as a result of increased transit time which may occur for a number of reasons related to anatomy, control, environment or other bodily systems. The nursing management of constipation will normally involve more than simply administering an aperient, as we shall see later. However, in constipation a vicious circle often develops in which hardened faeces further impede bowel transit. The first stage may then be to achieve adequate bowel evacuation.

Action of aperients. Aperients (whether taken orally or administered rectally) have three basic modes of action which reflect the physiology of the colon. Volume-forming aperients stimulate peristalsis by distending the bowel wall and initiating mass movements. This effect may be achieved either orally or rectally. Magnesium sulphate (Epsom salts) and phosphate enemas work in this fashion. The osmotic effect of the non-absorbable salt causes water accumulation in the bowel. Lactulose (Duphalac) functions in this way but is a disaccharide which is not absorbed by the digestive tract. Other bulk-forming preparations achieve their effect by providing a volume of non-digestible fibre which will encourage peristalsis and mass movement through tactile stimulation of the mucosa and distension of the bowel wall. Vegetable fibre and bran are common examples of this type of aperient. Hydrophilic substances which swell on contact with water are also employed (Celevac, Cologel).

The drying and hardening of the stool which occurs in constipation impedes easy passage through the colon. A second type of aperient — stool softeners and lubricants — acts on this component of the problem. Liquid paraffin and glycerine suppositories function in a similar fashion to lubricate the stool, making passage easier. Dioctyl sodium sulphosuccinate reduces surface tension allowing faeces to absorb water more readily and thus soften. It may take 24 hours or more to take effect. Soap solution enemas work through a combination of volume effects, lubrication, stool softening and mucosal irritation. Strong solutions can be extremely irritating and Mitchell (1977) describes one case of fetal death following the administration of a strong soap-solution enema to an expectant mother. Such preparations are now losing favour following the advent of pre-prepared enemas.

The last group of aperients all function by stimulating the colon directly in one fashion or another. Turner & Richens (1978) point out that 'irritant' is something of a misnomer since the precise mode of action in each case may differ. Bisacodyl (Dulcolax) acts upon the mucosa of the large intestine, whilst anthraquinone-based aperients such as senna (Senokot) and danthron act directly upon the myenteric plexus of the colon wall to stimulate peristalsis. This action is specific to the colon and does not affect other portions of the digestive tract. Commercial preparations are available which combine an anthraquinone laxative with a stool softener and lubricant (e.g. Dorbanex, Normax). Extremely irritating substances such as jalap, croton oil, aloin and colocynth should be avoided.

Adverse effects of aperient use. As with any drug, individual aperients will have specific side-effects and contra-indications. The nurse is advised to familiarize herself with these before administration.

Aperient abuse may have serious consequences for the individual concerned. Repeated artificially induced defaecation will ultimately cause a weakening of the natural defaecation reflex and disruption of bowel function. Often the individual will fail to realize that there may be no bowel action for 2 or 3 days following the use of a laxative because of the extreme degree of evacuation achieved. This sign is seen as an indication of the need for further medication and so a cycle is initiated in which natural bowel function is totally disrupted. Conversely the carefully planned and systematic use of aperients can be of great value when establishing and maintaining bowel function in the chronically ill, or in cases where normal control mechanisms have been damaged, for example in spinal injury. It is important that the nurse assesses the patient fully and chooses the most appropriate type of aperient. Often a combination of treatments will be required.

Intervention based upon improving or supporting control mechanisms

The control of bladder and bowel function is a complex process involving central and peripheral elements. Problems of excretory function which result in or manifest themselves as an alteration in control must therefore be carefully and fully assessed. It is likely that such problems will be multifactorial in origin, with elements relating to anatomy, environmental influences, related bodily systems and dysfunctions of the control system itself all contributing to the clinical picture.

Before embarking upon any programme to improve excretory control the nurse must ensure that the patient is adequately prepared in order to achieve the maximum benefit possible. For example, there is little point in pursuing a continence programme if the patient is suffering urgency or diarrhoea due to urinary tract or bowel infection. Similarly, Delehanty & Stravino (1970) stress the importance of correct timing and psychological preparation when initiating bladder training programmes following spinal injury.

Any bladder or bowel infection should be assessed and appropriately treated before continuing. Other intrinsic problems such as calculi or urethritis must be eliminated or accommodated within the care plan. When considering bladder control an adequate fluid intake is essential and in some cases an increased intake of up to 3000ml over 24 hours may be necessary (Whittington, 1980; Pratt, 1971a).

Before bowel training programmes begin the patient must be free from faecal impaction or constipation and be established on an appropriately balanced diet containing adequate fibre. The presence of other conditions which may affect bowel action must be ascertained, e.g. haemorrhoids or anal fissure.

Medication regimes must be reviewed and may require adjustment to eliminate the anticholinergic effects or side-effects of some preparations if they are thought to interfere with excretory function. Sedatives may cause constipation and mental clouding in some cases.

Urinary control

It will be recalled that the control of urinary function involves central and local mechanisms. Reflex emptying of the bladder is initiated in response to stretching of the detrusor during filling and mediated via a reflex arc at the sacral level of the cord. Higher centres can inhibit or facilitate this reflex action and exert ultimate control over urination by contraction or relaxation of the external sphincter via the pudendal nerve.

Neurogenic bladder. This term is applied to conditions in which bladder function is altered as a result of nervous damage or interference. The precise underlying pathology may be extremely complex and involve all or part of the upper or lower control pathways or a mixture of both. The reader is referred to Sabiston (1981) for a detailed discussion of such cases. For our purposes three basic types of neurogenic bladder can be identified — those cases resulting from disruption of the sacral or reflex component, those arising following damage to upper spinal or central components, and those involving a mixture of both pathologies (Whittington, 1980). These conditions have been termed lower motor neurone and upper motor neurone bladder respectively, but this terminology is confusing since bladder function is dependent upon sensory as well as motor elements. The aim of the medical and nursing care of these individuals is to support residual function and prevent further injury, for example by preventing urinary retention and bladder distension, and to help the patient regain the fullest possible control of urinary function.

It may take days or weeks for the full nature and extent of the urinary dysfunction to become apparent (Pratt, 1971a). During this period the bladder must be protected from injury due to overdistension whilst detrusor tone is maintained as far as possible. Aseptic intermittent catheterization will prevent bladder distension whilst allowing the normal filling process, which is involved in the maintenance of bladder tone, to continue. Indwelling catheterization in association with intermittent rather than continual drainage may be as effective. The difficulty in keeping such patients free of urinary tract infection has been discussed earlier.

The automatic or reflex bladder. Damage to the control mechanisms above the level of the sacral reflex centres (S2 to S4) will leave the micturition reflex intact but prevent the voluntary modification and control of urination. Thus the bladder will still respond to filling but will empty spontaneously and cannot be controlled by the individual. Initially there may be urinary retention due to the loss of facilitatory impulses. Typically bladder emptying is incomplete with raised residual urine volumes. This condition is sometimes referred to as the automatic or reflex bladder. The individual has no real sensation of bladder filling but can often learn to recognize the presence of a full bladder from other cues such as a feeling of abdominal fullness, sweating or restlessness. In many cases effective control over urination can be achieved by exploiting the effect of 'trigger zones' — areas which, when stimulated, initiate urination. Stimulation of the lower abdomen, inner thighs and genital areas may have this effect, which is explained by the fact that the innervation to these areas involve the same sacral centre (Whittington, 1980). If, as in some cases, the detrusor is hypertonic following the trauma then it may be necessary to reduce detrusor tone by nerve block or section before a satisfactory degree of control and filling volume can be achieved (Sabiston, 1981).

The autonomic or atonic bladder. Damage to the sacral micturition reflex mechanism will prevent the bladder emptying in response to filling. Bladder sensation is usually reduced and the micturition process cannot be initiated. If intervention is not prompt there may be gross distension of the detrusor, with traumatic loss of muscle tone and overflow incontinence when pressures inside the bladder overcome outflow resistance. This condition is often termed the autonomic or atonic bladder since distension of the bladder causes a loss of detrusor tone. If the patient can be taught to recognize the abdominal sensations associated with a full bladder, then it may be possible to empty the bladder by raising the intravesical pressure sufficiently to overcome outlet resistance. This is achieved by pressing the abdominal wall above the symphysis pubis or raising intra-abdominal pressures by contracting the muscles of the abdomen and breathing out against a closed glottis (Valsalva manoeuvre). The success of this procedure will depend upon the patient's ability to overcome the resistance to urine flow presented by the external sphincter. In some cases it is necessary to reduce the tone of the external sphincter by nerve block or section (Sabiston, 1981).

The elderly. The loss of urinary control which is seen in some elderly individuals may have many and complex causes. Environmental factors, reduced mobility, mental clouding or oversedation and a reduction in manual dexterity may all contribute to the apparent urinary incontinence. A thorough assessment of all precipitating factors must be made before intervention is planned. Cerebrovascular pathologies may result in urinary dysfunctions which have much in common with the automatic bladder dysfunctions discussed above, with reduced awareness of bladder filling and the need to void, reduced inhibition, frequency and urgency. The first stage in the management of such conditions is to make a thorough record of the time and frequency of micturition. This will then act as a guide to the planning of regular toileting regimes — up to 2-hourly if necessary. The aim of such toileting regimes is twofold. First, the patient is kept dry and comfortable, which increases self-esteem and establishes hope in the mind of the individual that the problem is not insurmountable. Secondly the association between the sensation of a full bladder and the need to urinate is reinforced. As stated earlier, these measures must be combined with an investigation of the anatomical and psycho-social aspects of the presenting problem.

Bowel control

Difficulty with the control of bowel function, and incontinence in particular, is generally considered to be less common than the equivalent urinary condition (Saxon, 1962; Boore, 1980) but nevertheless is of great importance to the nurse and patient.

Due to the presence of an intrinsic nerve supply bowel function is more resilient than the bladder in the event of nervous damage (Shafer et al, 1979). Guttman (1973) discusses at length the management of intestinal function following spinal injury and concludes that in the majority of cases the patients can adjust to the impairment of bowel function. Since, with skilled intervention and teaching, bowel function can be re-established to a satisfactory degree following severe injury of this sort it may be useful to review the stages of rehabilitation outlined by Guttman. It would be an over-simplification of the complex problems faced by the elderly to conclude that these techniques are directly applicable to the problems of incontinence in elderly patients, since environmental, psychological and social elements of the problem will differ, but parallels may be drawn between the general principles involved.

Damage to the spinal cord at any level initially produces faecal retention (Pratt, 1971b). The retention is due to spinal shock which disrupts the normal defaecation reflexes. During this stage the patient is dependent upon nursing intervention and the use of digital evacuation or enema to empty the bowel until a degree of function returns to the intestinal tract.

Eventually isolated reflex activity will return to the bowel. Guttman (1973) identifies three factors which will affect the efficacy of bowel action at this stage:

- the position of the patient, with prolonged periods in a supine position hindering bowel function
- the qualities of the food eaten, with particular reference to fibre content: an adequate fluid intake is also essential
- characteristics of the reflex activity of the spinal cord.

If the level of the lesion interferes with the action of abdominal muscles then defaecation is adversely affected. If damage to the spinal component of the defaecation reflex occurs, then the response of the sigmoid colon and rectum to distension is lost, and the external sphincter loses tone.

The final stage of management involves the reconditioning of bowel function. Investigations of the bowel are undertaken to detect any long-standing abnormality which may affect the program. The aim during reconditioning is to ensure that the patient has an adequate bowel movement every day, or in some cases every other day. If necessary, bowel function is supported initially by the use of mild aperients and stool softeners. Since the gastrocolic reflex is most effective in the early morning following breakfast, this time is particularly useful during reconditioning. Toiletting is therefore performed after breakfast. The patient is taught to utilize accessory organs to improve bowel action by, for example, gentle massage of the abdomen or stimulation of the perianal area with a protected finger. In this way a regular bowel action is gradually established.

The elderly incontinent patient may well be found to be severly constipated. If faeces accumulate in the bowel then eventually a faecal liquid will bypass the mass and present as a continual incontinence or diarrhoea. Rectal examination reveals a mass of hardened faeces. Naturally a full medical investigation will be undertaken on admission to determine that faecal impaction is the true cause of the dysfunction, and that it is not associated with a more sinister pathology. Other related disorders, such as haemorrhoids or anal fissure should also be noted at this stage.

In this situation it becomes impossible for the individual to empty the bowel effectively. The first stage of management, therefore, will be to achieve bowel evacuation by the controlled use of faecal softeners, enemas and possibly manual evacuation of faeces. It is pointless to attempt further intervention until evacuation is achieved, though attention to diet may begin immediately, with particular reference to fibre and fluid intake.

Once the bowel is empty then a programme of reconditioning can be planned. The presence of any underlying pathology which may affect the intervention should have been determined on admission. After each meal, and particularly breakfast, the patient is encouraged to attempt a bowel action. This timing exploits the action of the gastrocolic reflex in assisting defaecation. Initially it may be necessary to initiate defaecation by the use of a glycerine suppository, but this should be discontinued as a bowel pattern develops. Once regular bowel action is established toiletting may be reduced to reflect the individual's developing habit. The patient may also try to encourage defaecation by gentle massage of the abdomen, leaning forward, and raising intra-abdominal pressure by exhaling against a closed glottis (Valsalva manoeuvre), provided that this action is not contra-indicated (which it may be in cerebro-vascular or cardiac conditions).

It cannot be stated too strongly that it is pointless to consider bowel function in isolation from social, psychological and related physical factors. To do so could well result in the recurrence of the problem on discharge if, for example, the individual is lonely and poorly motivated, has poor home facilities possibly including an outside toilet, or has great difficulty maintaining an adequate diet due to restricted mobility and problems with shopping.

The management of faecal and urinary dysfunctions is time-consuming and difficult, but of inestimable value to the patient concerned. These factors must be recognized during the planning of nursing intervention. An attempt to help every patient simultaneously is impossible and will ultimately fail (Saxon, 1962; Kennedy, 1985), thus reinforcing in the minds of the patients and their carers that the situation is hopeless and the problems insurmountable. Often the task of helping an incontinent patient will be an unpleasant one. Nurses who are troubled by this would do well to note the comment of Joy Bolwell (1982), in her compassionate discussion of the problems of incontinence — it is far worse to *be* wet than to change someone who *is*.

Intervention based upon adapting the environment

We have identified earlier the many ways in which the hospital environment falls short of being ideal. Of course, hospitals are primarily intended to provide facilities for the treatment of the sick, and to an extent, it is inevitable that such aims will be incompatible with the production of 'homely' atmospheres. The truth is, however, that hospitals may have an adverse effect on patient well-being. Hospital patients have been shown to have significantly higher levels of anxiety than individuals in the community (Franklin, 1974). Manifestations of this reaction include unhappiness, loss of interest in the outside world and a preoccupation with bodily processes (Rachman & Philips, 1978).

Factors within the environment which may influence excretory function include facilities and equipment, and the attitudes and skills of staff.

When planning a continence program, Saxon (1962) found that nurses were initially opposed to the treatment regimes. When it was suggested that the use of 'nappy-like' incontinence devices was degrading and should cease both nurses and patients raised objections. It was eventually found, however, that rather than causing increased soilage of clothing, the move to dress patients in their normal clothes increased self esteem and helped reduce incontinence. One of the first steps in reducing incontinence in a ward may therefore be to change staff attitudes.

It would appear that hospital wards are rarely designed with patients in mind. The nurse must therefore consider the abilities of the patient and how these relate to the environment. How far is it to the toilet or bathroom areas? Is there somewhere to rest en-route if the patient is tired? Are the toilets clean and properly equipped, with hand-washing facilities and aids or hand-rails for the infirm? Are toilets draughty and cold or lacking in privacy? Can the patient manage his/her clothing or would he/she benefit from aids or adapted garments?

On the other hand, what facilities *does* the ward have and are they being used effectively? Recall that Wells (1980) found that nurses frequently failed to make full use of special equipment. Are adjustable beds set at the most suitable height so that the patient can get out easily and go to the toilet if necessary? Are lifting aids used if available, or is toiletting delayed because the patient cannot be lifted easily? What facilities are available in terms of staff expertise? Is a continence advisor available and if so has advice been sought?

The intelligent assessment of an individual's problems by an empathetic nurse will often identify many ways in which the ward environment may adversely affect the patient. Such problems are specific to the circumstances and the individual concerned and cannot be fully anticipated here. However, nurses can ask themselves if they would be happy to use the facilities available to patients. If the answer is anything but an unqualified 'yes' then should not something be done?

Intervention based upon supporting related systems

In this chapter we have discussed excretory problems largely in isolation from the rest of the body, with referral to other chapters if necessary. Of course, in reality the body functions as an integrated whole and this fact is reflected in patient assessment using the nursing process.

There are many ways in which related bodily systems can affect excretory function.

The influence upon the patient of levels of mobility and agility have been discussed above. Bowel function is enhanced by bodily activity (Holdstock et al, 1970) and Guttman (1973) reports that regular turning of a bedridden patient will improve bowel function. Restrictions on mobility also affect the positioning of the patient for elimination. The level of general musculoskeletal fitness will affect the stamina of an individual and the actions of specific accessory musculature, for example the abdominal and perineal muscles, will directly affect excretion. Stress incontinence will often respond to exercises aimed at strengthening the perineal muscles. Abdominal or perineal surgery may adversely affect excretion.

Cardiovascular fitness will influence the tolerance of general mobility. Many patients with cardiac problems cannot tolerate the raised intrathoracic pressure associated with straining to evacuate the bowel, and constipation may result if not carefully managed.

Hormonal changes can affect fluid excretion directly. One response to surgery is an increased secretion of antidiuretic hormone, which will reduce urine output. In the elderly female patient oestrogen deficiency may result in urethritis, increased frequency and incontinence (Kennedy, 1985).

The function of the gastrointestinal system above the level of the colon will obviously affect bowel action. Changes in diet due to treatment regimes or any alteration in the method of ingestion must be carefully assessed for the effect on bowel function. Stomatitis or even ill-fitting dentures will affect the ability of an individual to eat certain foods such as fruit or vegetables, which are high in natural fibre.

The functional integrity of the central nervous system is of obvious importance since intracerebral pathologies may affect any other bodily system. Elderly patients may be particularly susceptible to transient confusional states due to somatic disorders, and these may result in temporary incontinence. A dulling of mental ability due to sedative abuse, mismanagement or intolerance will have similar effects. Finally, we should remember that depression, fear and anxiety can manifest themselves in many ways. At the functional level, continuous arousal of the autonomic nervous system will affect both urinary and faecal excretion. At the affective level, individuals may eventually regress or act irrationally in the face of intolerable situations.

CONCLUSION

In order to intervene in problems of excretion the nurse must have an understanding of the mechanisms and systems in question. The acquisition of this knowledge and the skills required to implement such measures are the aims of nurse education, and it follows that a nurse's education can never be complete. It is hoped that the list of references at the end of this chapter will help the nurse to extend her/his knowledge in this area of patient care.

Problems of excretion are amenable to careful assessment and informed, logical intervention. The problems are complex, whilst the functions appear simple. This may lead the nurse into ill-managed or ad-hoc treatments which result in failure, the loss of hope and a loss of dignity on the part of the patient. Poorly managed excretory problems may adversely affect many other aspects of patient care, and will certainly result in a major change in lifestyle for the patient. No individual would ever choose to be incontinent or to rely upon others for the performance of basic needs if offered the opportunity for independence. It is a choice that every nurse should endeavour to offer.

CARE OF THE PATIENT WITH A STOMA

TYPES OF STOMA

In the UK, colostomy, ileostomy and urinary conduit are the most commonly formed stomas. In 1980, over 5000 permanent colostomy operations were performed, 250–300 ileostomies and an estimated 200 urinary conduits (Devlin, 1985).

Colostomy

A colostomy is an artificial opening into any part of the large colon. The stoma formed may be permanent or temporary. The principal indication for permanent colostomy is carcinoma of the rectum, treated either by abdomino-perineal resection or by Hartmann's procedure. Other indications include anal carcinoma, irreparable trauma to the rectum and rectal prolapse. A permanent or end colostomy is most often formed in the descending or sigmoid colon and sited in the left lower quadrant of the abdomen. A temporary colostomy is formed to defunction the portion of the colon distal to it. This type of stoma is raised as an emergency treatment for obstruction or perforation of the left colon. This may be due to carcinoma, diverticular disease, volvulus, or wounds to the colon or rectum. Diversion of the faecal stream through a temporary colostomy also may be a first stage in operations on the left colon or rectum and in repairs of fistulae, allowing subsequent surgery to be undertaken in a clean field. Although a temporary colostomy may be raised at any point on the colon, the site of choice is the right transverse colon which can be mobilized easily. A double barrelled or loop colostomy may be formed. The variety of rods and bridges available to support a temporary colostomy are reviewed by Houghton & Steele (1983).

Ileostomy

An ileostomy is formed from the last part of the small intestine, the terminal ileum, and is usually sited in the right lower abdomen. The major indications for ileostomy are ulcerative colitis and Crohn's disease, but it may be required also in cases of familial polyposis of the colon and malignant and pre-malignant growths in the large intestine. Where these conditions are treated by total colectomy and excision of the rectum (pan-proctocolectomy) the stoma will be permanent. Where it is possible to perform a total colectomy and ileorectal anastomosis, a temporary loop ileostomy may be raised to protect the anastomosis during healing.

Urinary diversion

There are several methods of diverting the flow of urine, with the ileal conduit being described as the least unsatisfactory (Devlin, 1985). Although this is a urinary stoma, it is constructed using part of the small intestine. A portion of the ileum is resected, preserving its blood supply. Both ureters are implanted into the proximal end of the ileal segment. The distal end is brought through the abdominal wall to form a stoma. A full description of the construction of an ileal conduit is given by Hendry (1978). Urinary diversion is required most often due to malignancy. This includes carcinoma of the bladder, of the urethra and, in women, carcinoma of the cervix or uterus. With new developments in reconstructive urology, urinary diversion is performed now only as a last resort for neurological disorders resulting in unmanageable incontinence and for urinary fistulae (Devlin, 1985).

PSYCHOLOGICAL IMPACT OF STOMA SURGERY

Surgery which results in the formation of a stoma is recognized as an event which frequently causes a distortion of body-image (Norris, 1978). The term body-image refers to the unique way each individual has of perceiving his/her physical self (McCloskey, 1976). This perception of self develops from infancy and continues to be revised throughout life to incorporate the physical changes which occur to the body. After stoma surgery, the patient has to contend with a number of disturbances in the relationship of his/her body parts which he/she may not be able to incorporate into his/her self-image. The patient's perception of him/herself as a whole person is altered by the addition of a stoma to the abdominal wall and by the removal or resection of internal organs (Lindensmith, 1977). Also there is the added problem of loss of voluntary control over elimination which the stoma represents (McCloskey, 1976). Such changes in body structure and functioning are very threatening. For the adult patient the return to an incontinent state is seen as a return to the helplessness of infancy. Reactions to stoma surgery of anxiety, fear of rejection and depression are well documented (Sutherland et al, 1952; Dyk & Sutherland, 1956; Druss et al, 1969; Dlin & Perlman, 1973; Eardley et al, 1976). Nurses have an important role to play in helping patients overcome the psychological and practical difficulties involved in having a stoma.

PRE-OPERATIVE CARE

Psychological preparation

During the pre-operative period, the patient is prepared psychologically and physically for stoma surgery. Through a combination of explanation, information giving, and counselling the patient is helped to adjust to an altered method of elimination.

Explanation and information giving

At the outset, Breckman (1978) recommends that the nurse establishes the patient's understanding of the type of surgery to be undertaken. From this basis, and taking account of factors such as age and mental and physical health, the nurse is able to plan the explanation of surgery and of postoperative management required by the patient. A variety of booklets are available from appliance manufacturers which deal with specific types of stoma and these may serve as a useful reinforcement of information given by the nurse. Some patients may wish to see a stoma appliance before surgery. Mahoney (1976) recommends demonstrating the appliance to be used postoperatively to avoid confusing the patient with different types. Pre-operative teaching sessions also may include a family member, as it is recognized that their acceptance of the stoma has a profound effect on the patient's adjustment (Mikolon, 1982).

Counselling

Much emphasis is placed also on the importance of counselling the patient in view of the psychological difficulties, described above, associated with this type of surgery. This begins pre-operatively and continues throughout the postoperative period. Breckman (1981) distinguishes this from any form of teaching or information giving. It is a purposeful conversation in which the patient can express his/her thoughts and fears and is helped to face his/her problems with less anxiety. Rather than giving information, the nurse adopts the role of perceptive listener. Saunders (1976) describes this as vitally important and states that without pre-operative counselling, patients find it harder to come to terms with their stoma. The psychological adjustment of some patients may be helped also by a visit from a former patient who is coping well with their stoma. This can provide reassurance that resumption of a normal lifestyle is possible (Foulkes, 1981).

Physical preparation

In relation to the physical preparation for surgery, much depends on the regime for bowel preparation favoured by the surgeon. This may be total gut irrigation or the combination of restricted intake and administration of enemas and bowel washouts (Royal College of Nursing, 1981). Whichever method is used, its purpose is to clear the bowel completely of faeces. The marking of the stoma site also is carried out pre-operatively, rather than at the time of operation. This allows the site chosen to be reviewed with the patient lying, sitting and standing. The correct placement of the stoma requires a flat area of abdomen, avoiding bony prominences such as hips or ribs and creases such as the umbilicus, old scars or the groin flexure. Foulkes (1981) gives a detailed description of the considerations involved in siting a stoma.

POSTOPERATIVE APPLIANCE MANAGEMENT

In the period immediately following surgery the responsibility for appliance management lies with the nurse. The usual practice is for the patient to return from theatre with a stoma appliance in place. A clear drainable appliance is used most often. This allows observation of the colour and condition of the stoma and permits emptying of its drainage without having to remove the appliance from the skin (Dudas, 1982). With the repeated removal of adhesive appliances the risk of skin damage is increased. For this reason, Mahoney (1976) recommends leaving the original postoperative appliance in place for several days, provided that there is no leakage beneath the adhesive seal. It is of psychological as well as physical benefit to the patient to have the first postoperative week free from leakage and skin irritation (Saunders, 1978).

Changing an appliance

The technique of changing an appliance receives considerable attention in the literature on stoma care. Much of what is written takes the form of recommendations for practice based on the experience of working with stoma patients. In reviewing this as part of a study on the nursing care of stoma patients, the present author was able to distinguish a number of common elements in appliance changes. These were identified as follows:

- preparation of the patient
- preparation of the equipment
- removal of the old appliance
- skin care
- skin protection
- selection of the new appliance
- preparation of the new appliance
- application
- disposal (Ewing, 1984).

These aspects of care are essentially 'principles' or guidelines for management of the stoma appliance, not steps in a standard procedure. Patients differ with regard to the care required in relation to each guideline. Moreover, even with the same patient, care requirements can change throughout their postoperative course. These guidelines, therefore, provide a flexible framework within which the individual needs of the patient can be met.

Preparation for discharge

Although the nurse is responsible for changing the stoma appliance in the early part of the postoperative period, in preparation for discharge the patient needs to assume that responsibility for him/herself. A gradual introduction to managing the stoma is seen as important. The usual practice is to begin by explaining each aspect of care during the appliance change. Lamanske (1977) recommends that this starts from the onset of recovery in order to familiarize the patient with the process. After this the patient is encouraged to perform part of the appliance change him/herself, such as managing the closure clip. Dudas (1982) describes this move to active participation as essential for satisfactory learning of self care. As the patient becomes proficient with one aspect of care, another can be added. This is what Gross (1979) describes as 'Whole — part — whole learning', working on the principle that it is much easier to learn something in parts than in the entirety. As the patient gradually takes over the physical management of the stoma, the nurse relinquishes her/his participant role for a supervisory one (Dericks & Donovan, 1976). In this way, the patient is able to regain independence with regard to elimination which plays a vital part in his/her rehabilitation.

REFERENCES

Ansell J 1962 Some observations on catheter care. Journal of Chronic Diseases 15:675–682

Beland I L, Passos J Y 1975 Clinical nursing, 3rd edn. Macmillan, New York

Blannin J P 1982 Catheter management. Nursing Times 78:438– 440

Blannin J P, Hobden J 1980 The catheter of choice. Nursing Times 76:2092–2093

Bolwell J 1982 Dignity at all times. Nursing Mirror 7(14):50–54

Boore J R P 1980 The elderly. In: Smith J (ed) Evelyn Pearce's A general textbook of nursing, 20th edn. Faber and Faber, London

Breckman B 1978 Rundown on stoma problems. Journal of Community Nursing 1(11):4–6

Breckman B 1981 Psychosocial areas related to stoma care. In: Breckman B (ed) Stoma care. Beaconsfield Publishers, Beaconsfield

Brocklehurst J C 1978 Textbook of geriatric medicine and gerontology, 2nd edn. Churchill Livingstone, Edinburgh

Brunner L S, Suddarth D S 1982 The Lippincott manual of nursing practice, 3rd edn. Lippincott, Philadelphia

Cannon W B 1939 The wisdom of the body. Norton, New York

Claridge M 1965 The physiology of micturition. British Journal of Urology 37:620–623

Cleland V, Cox F, Berggren H, Macinnis M R 1971 Prevention of bacteruria in female patients with indwelling catheters. Nursing Research 20(4):309–318

Connel A M 1967 The physiology and pathophysiology of constipation. Paraplegia 4:244–250

Crow J 1977a How and why to take a nursing history. Nursing Times 73:950–957

Crow J 1977b A nursing history questionnaire for two patients. Nursing Times 73:978–982
Delehanty L, Stravino V 1970 Achieving bladder control. American Journal of Nursing 70:312–316
Dericks V C, Donovan C T 1976 The ostomy patient really needs you. Nursing (Jenkintown) 6(9):30–33
Devlin H B (ed) 1985 Stoma care today. Medical Education Services, Oxford
Dlin B M, Perlman A 1973 Emotional response to ileostomy and colostomy in patients over the age of 50. Modern Geriatrics 3(4):216–219
Druss R G, O'Connor J F,Stern L O 1969 Psychologic response to colectomy II: Adjustment to a permanent colostomy. Archives of General Psychiatry 20(4):419–427
Dudas S 1982 Post operative considerations. In: Broadwell D C, Jackson B S (eds) Principles of ostomy care. C V Mosby, St Louis
Dyk R B, Sutherland A M 1956 Adaptation of the spouse and other family members to the colostomy patient. Cancer 9:123– 138
Eardley A, George W D, Davis F, Schofield P F, Wilson M C, Wakefield J, Selwood R A 1976 Colostomy: the consequences of surgery. Clinical Oncology 2(3):277–283
Ewing G 1984 A study of the post operative nursing care of stoma patients during appliance changes. Unpublished PhD thesis, University of Edinburgh
Foulkes B 1981 The practical management of bowel stomas. In: Breckman B (ed) Stoma care. Beaconsfield Publishers, Beaconsfield
Franklin B L 1974 Patient anxiety on admission to hospital. Royal College of Nursing, London
Gross L 1979 Guiding ostomy patients through the rehabilitation process. In: Gross L, Bailey Z (eds) Enterostomal therapy: developing institutional and community programs. Nursing Resources Inc., Wakefield, Mass.
Guttman L 1973 Spinal cord injuries — comprehensive management and research. Blackwell, London
Guyton A C 1981 Textbook of medical physiology, 6th edn. W B Saunders, London
Hendry W F 1978 Urinary diversion in the adult. In: Todd I P (ed) Intestinal stomas. Heinemann Medical, London
Holdstock D J, Misiewicz J J, Smith T, Rowlands E N 1970 Propulsion (mass movements) in the human colon and its relationship to meals and somatic activity. Gut 11:91–99
Houghton P W J, Steele K V 1983 The immaculate stoma. Nursing Times 79(25):62–63
Jeffcote T N A 1965 The principles governing the treatment of stress incontinence of urine in the female. British Journal of Urology 37:633–643
Jenner E A 1983 Catheterisation and urinary tract infection. Nursing (Oxford)) 2:13 (supplement)
Kass E H, Schneiderman L J 1957 Entry of bacteria into the urinary tracts of patients with inlying catheters. New England Journal of Medicine 256:556–557
Keele C A, Neil E 1961 Samson Wright's applied physiology, 10th edn. Oxford University Press, London
Kelly K, Hammond K R 1964 Approach to the study of clinical inference in nursing. Nursing Research 13(4):314,319–322
Kennedy A 1984a Catheter concepts. Nursing Mirror 159(15):42–46
Kennedy A 1984b Drainage system on trial. Nursing Mirror 158(7):19–20
Kennedy A 1985 Elimination. In: Cormack D (ed) Geriatric nursing – a conceptual approach. Blackwell Scientific, London
Kennedy A P, Brocklehurst J C 1982 The nursing management of patients with indwelling catheters. Journal of Advanced Nursing 7:411–417
Kennedy A P, Brocklehurst J C, Lye M D W 1983 Factors related to the problems of long-term catheterisation. Journal of Advanced Nursing 8:207–212
Kilner M K 1980 Constipation in pregnancy. Nursing (Oxford) Series 1, (17):753
Lamanske J 1977 Helping the ileostomy patient to help himself. Nursing (Jenkintown) 7(1):34–39
Lindensmith S 1977 Body image and the crisis of enterostomy. The Canadian Nurse 73(11):24–27
Low-Beer T S, Read A E 1971 Diarrhoea: mechanisms and treatment. Gut 12:1021–1036
McCloskey J C 1976 How to make the most of body image theory in nursing practice. Nursing (Jenkintown) 6(5):68–72
McGill S 1982 It's the size that's important. Nursing Mirror 154(14):48–49
Mahoney J M 1976 Guide to ostomy nursing care. Little, Brown & Co, Boston
Meers P C, Ayliffe G A J, Emmerson A M 1981 Report on the National Survey of Infection in Hospitals 1980. Journal of Hospital Infection 2:(supplement)23–38
Mikolon S 1982 Psychosocial issues in ostomy management. In: Broadwell D C, Jackson B S (eds) Principles of ostomy care. Mosby, St Louis
Mitchell P H 1977 Concepts basic to nursing, 2nd edn. McGraw-Hill, New York
Norris C M 1978 Body image, its relevance to professional nursing. In: Carlson C E, Blackwell B (eds) Behavioural concepts and nursing intervention. Lippincott, Philadelphia
Norton D, McLaren R, Exton-Smith A N 1962 reprinted 1975 An investigation of geriatric nursing problems in hospital. Churchill Livingstone, Edinburgh
Pratt R 1971a Management of the bladder. Nursing Times, 67:604–607
Pratt R 1971b Bowel management. Nursing Times 67:638–639
Rachman S J, Philips C 1978 Psychology and medicine. Penguin, Harmondsworth
Royal College of Nursing 1981 Stoma care: a team approach. RCN, London
Sabetian M 1965 The genesis of bladder tone. British Journal of Urology 37:424–432
Sabiston D C (ed) 1981 Davis-Christopher textbook of surgery: biological basis of modern surgical practice, 12th edn. Saunders, Philadelphia
Salvati E P 1966 Psychogenic constipation. Diseases of the colon and rectum 9:293–294
Saunders B 1976 Stoma care. Medicine. 2nd series, No. 19. Gastro-Intestinal Disorders Part III:891–896
Saunders B 1978 Principles of stomal care: The ileostomy. In: Todd I P (ed) Intestinal stomas. Heinemann, London
Saxon J 1962 Techniques for bowel and bladder training. American Journal of Nursing 62(9):69–71
Seal D V 1982 Infection in the catheterized patient. Nursing (Oxford) Series 2(8):207–208
Seal D V, Ward K 1983 Catheterization and urinary tract infection. Basic technique for aseptic catheterization of urinary tract infection. Nursing (Oxford) 2(13):5–6
Shafer K N, Sawyer J R, McClusksy A M, Beck E L, Phipps W 1979 Medical-surgical nursing, 6th edn. C V Mosby, London

Southampton Infection Control Team 1982 Evaluation of aseptic techniques and chlorhexidine on the rate of catheter-associated urinary tract infection. Lancet 1:89–91
Stamm W E 1975 Guidelines for prevention of catheter-associated urinary tract infections. Annals of Internal Medicine 82:386–390
Sutherland A M et al 1952 Psychological impact of cancer and cancer surgery. Cancer 5(5):857–872
Turner P, Richens A 1978 Clinical pharmacology, 3rd edn. Churchill Livingstone, Edinburgh
Webb J K, Blandy K P 1968 Closed urinary drainage into plastic bags containing antiseptic. British Journal of Urology 40:585– 588
Wells T J 1980 Problems in geriatric nursing care. Churchill Livingstone, Edinburgh
Whittington L 1980 Bladder retraining. Canadian Nurse, 76(6):26–29
Williams P L, Warwick R (eds) 1980 Gray's anatomy, 36th edn. Churchill Livingstone, Edinburgh
Williamson M L 1982 Reducing post-catheterisation bladder dysfunction by reconditioning. Nursing Research 31(1):28–30
Wright L 1974 Bowel function in hospital patients. Royal College of Nursing, London

26

Disturbances of fluid and electrolyte balance

INTRODUCTION

Water is the most abundant substance in our body and, in association with a variety of solutes, forms approximately 60% of the total body weight in adults. Variations in this total percentage occur in relation to the amount of body fat, i.e. the less fat the greater the proportion of water to total body weight. The human body (unlike the camel!) has no capacity for water storage and therefore the continuance of optimum body functioning is dependent on adequate replacement of lost fluid. Humans are capable of living for a long time without other nutrients, but only a few days without water.

The consequences of water loss are graphically described by Pflaum (1979). A 1% loss of body water stimulates thirst, 5–8% loss will precipitate fatigue, tachycardia, pyrexia and a deterioration in mental function. 11–15% loss results in delirium, deafness, hypovolaemia and consequent renal failure. A 20% loss is usually fatal.

A consideration of water loss alone is unrealistic in view of the fact that our body fluids also contain a whole variety of dissolved substances. These can be divided into two basic kinds, those that dissociate in solution, the electrolytes, and those that do not, e.g. glucose. Electrolytes are so named because they ionize, i.e. develop an electrical charge when dissolved in water. The distribution of these various ions varies between body fluids in different

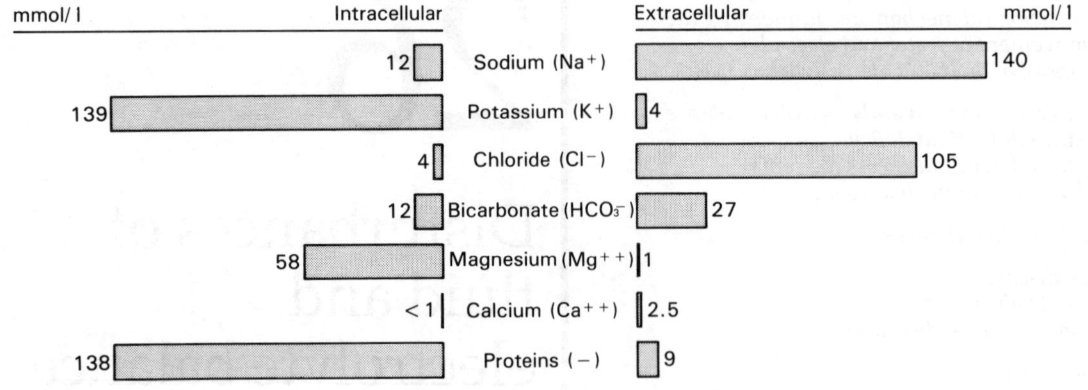

Fig. 26.1 Distribution of major ions between the intra- and extra-cellular fluids.

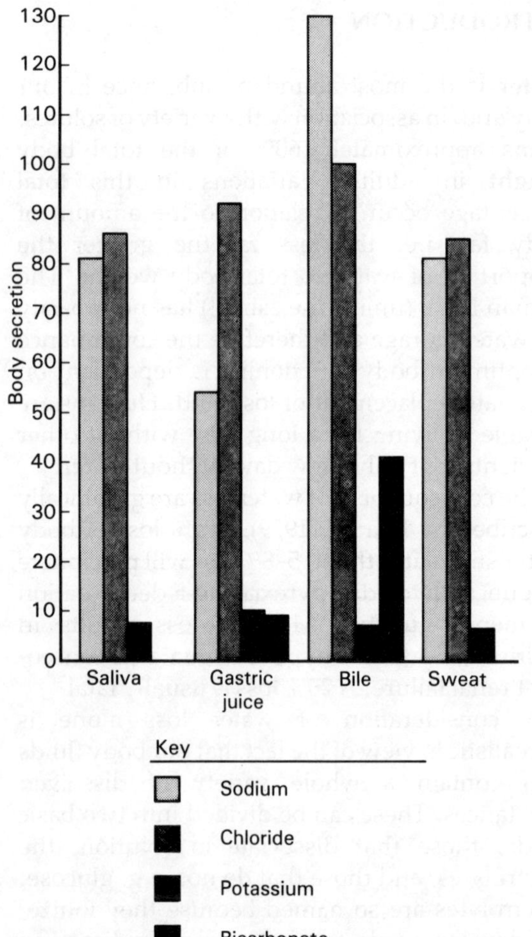

Fig. 26.2 Constituents of body fluids in various body compartments.

compartments and these variations are directly related to the functions which the particular fluids perform. Figure 26.1 illustrates the distribution of major ions between the intra- and extracellular fluids, while Figure 26.2 shows the constituents of body fluids in various body compartments.

The main concern when considering fluid and electrolyte disturbance is the maintenance of correct electrolyte distribution across the cell membrane. The primary difference between the intra- and extracellular fluids is the asymmetric distribution of sodium (Na^+) and potassium (K^+). From Figure 26.1 it is evident that potassium is primarily an intracellular electrolyte and sodium the main extracellular electrolyte. The maintenance of this distribution pattern is vital for the correct functioning of many body processes, e.g. nerve transmission. The extracellular concentration of sodium also has a direct effect on the amount of water present in the body. It is therefore unrealistic to attempt to consider water and sodium as separate entities, as the fate of one directly affects the other. Generally speaking, disturbances of fluid balance will be concomitant with those of sodium imbalance.

Asymmetric distribution of electrolytes across the cell membrane, although most marked, is not exclusive to sodium and potassium. Chloride and bicarbonate are also mainly extracellular. These two ions together compete to combine

Table 26.1 Normal values of main electrolytes (from MacLeod, 1984)

Electrolyte	Symbol	Normal value
Sodium	Na^+	132–144 mmol/l
Potassium	K^+	3.3–4.7 mmol/l
Chloride	Cl^-	95.0–105.0mmol/l
Bicarbonate	HCO_3^-	21–27.5mmol/l
Calcium	Ca^{++}	2.12–2.62mmol/l
Magnesium	Mg^{++}	0.75–1.0mmol/l

with sodium (see Fig. 26.1). This is in order to balance the positive and negative charges between these three ions. It also means that there is a reciprocal relationship between chloride and bicarbonate ions in terms of concentration, i.e. if chloride levels rise, bicarbonate levels fall, and vice versa. This is very important in relation to the body's acid-base balance as bicarbonate forms one of the major buffer systems in our extracellular fluids.

Looking at the value of free calcium ions shown in Table 26.1 gives a rather erroneous view of the total amount of calcium present in our body. 99% of our body calcium is contained within bones and is physiologically inert. Plasma calcium is found partly in combination with plasma proteins and other substances such as phosphate. The value given in this table therefore refers to the tiny proportion of free calcium ion. This value is maintained very efficiently by an exchange system between plasma and bone.

Finally the extra- and intracellular distribution of magnesium, a rarely considered electrolyte of which imbalances are uncommon in clinical practice, is shown in Figure 26.1.

The physiological roles of these electrolytes and the effects of imbalance are considered later in the chapter. Table 26.1 shows the normal values of the major electrolytes.

PHYSIOLOGICAL MECHANISMS INFLUENCING THE MOVEMENT OF WATER AND ELECTROLYTES

Several mechanisms operate which affect the movement and distribution of water and electrolytes in the body. These will be briefly described below.

Osmosis This is defined as the movement of water from a low concentration of a solution towards a high concentration of solution until equal concentrations are obtained. (The easiest way to remember this concept is by the thought that water always moves towards salt). The ability of a solution to cause an osmotic effect is dependent on the number of particles dissolved in it. The number of particles will in turn directly affect the concentration of fluid, a property described by the term osmolality. This term is commonly substituted in clinical practice by the term tonicity. Solutions can then be variously described as isotonic (iso-osmotic) hypotonic (hypo-osmotic) or hypertonic (hyper-osmotic). This property is very important in relation to the range of intravenous fluids in clinical use which will be considered later in the chapter.

Diffusion This is the constant random movement of particles in a solution in order to achieve equal distribution within that solution. Diffusion can and does occur across the cell membrane and the rate and ease with which it occurs is dependent on various factors:

- The relative size of the cell membrane pores and the diffusing particles. Generally speaking the smaller the size of the diffusing particle, the more readily it moves through the cell membrane. Water, urea and chloride are examples of small molecules, but glucose and the amino acids are relatively large and can only diffuse very slowly. In order to aid the movement of these larger molecules, carrier proteins can act as shuttles, a process known as facilitated diffusion.
- The electrical charge of the diffusing particle affects the ease with which it moves across the cell membrane. The pores in the cell membrane tend to be positively charged and ions with a like charge will tend to be repulsed, e.g. Na^+ and K^+. This does not, however, totally prevent movement of these two ions by diffusion.
- Concentration differences on either side

of the membrane can also facilitate movement, i.e. the greater the difference the higher the rate of movement.

- Electrical potential can affect the movement of particles even with a minimal concentration gradient. The net charge inside the cell is negative in relation to the outside and will therefore tend to draw positive ions in.
- A high pressure gradient on one side of the cell membrane intensifies the forces on the membrane pores and 'pushes' particles through.

To summarize, these effects influence the movement of Na^+ and K^+ in particular. The repulsive effect of the positively charged membrane pores is insufficient to overcome the effect of the concentration gradient. As a result Na^+ and K^+ do cross the cell membrane but at a slower rate than would be expected from the concentration gradient. The importance of maintaining high levels of K^+ inside the cell and high levels of Na^+ outside the cell has already been emphasized and a further mechanism helps to counteract the exchange described above.

Active transport. This mechanism is dependent on a supply of energy in the form of adenosine tri-phosphate and utilizes a cell membrane carrier system. The most important feature of this system is that it can and does work against concentration gradients. The maintenance of Na^+ and Ka^+ balance in relation to the intra- and extracellular fluids is achieved by a carrier system called the sodium pump. This pump actively exchanges intracellular Na^+ for extracellular K^+ on a 2:3 ratio, in other words, it pumps Na^+ (2 parts) out of the cell and K^+ (3 parts) into the cell. Active transport mechanisms exist for many other substances, e.g. amino acids and glucose, to ensure that the cell can accumulate essential nutrients for activities such as protein synthesis. The rate of passive movement of ions such as Na^+ and K^+ is far less than the rate at which active transport can work, providing sufficient energy supplies are available.

Filtration. Hydrostatic pressure is the force behind the process of filtration. It is best

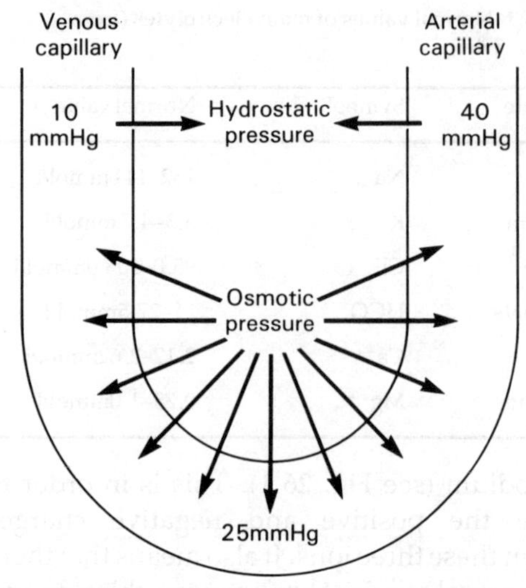

Fig.26.3 Fluid exchange between capillary beds and interstitial fluids.

explained by referral to the fluid exchange which takes place between the capillary beds and the interstitial fluids (Fig. 26.3).

From Figure 26.3 it can be seen that filtration is achieved at the arterial end because the hydrostatic pressure forcing fluid out of the capillary is higher than the intravascular osmotic pressure holding fluid in. The balance between the interstitial fluid and the intravascular fluid is restored at the venous end of the capillary where the intravascular osmotic pressure is higher than the venous capillary pressure. This same process operates within the glomerular capillary network in the kidneys.

In summary, the result of the interplay between these mechanisms is that water is able to move relatively freely between the intracellular and extracellular compartments, in response to osmotic changes. The solutes, including the electrolytes mentioned, are usually confined to one side or the other of the cell membrane by a series of mechanisms including active transport. The major intracellular osmotic solutes are potassium, protein, magnesium and phosphates. The major extracellular osmotic solutes are sodium, which is by far the most important, plus chloride and bicarbonate. Hume et al (1982) stated that the net effect of this

Table 26.2 Main sources of normal fluid loss and fluid gain in a 24-hour period

Gains		Losses	
Liquids	1000 ml	Urine	1500 ml
Food	1200 ml	Perspiration	400–500 ml
Metabolic water	300–500 ml	Lungs	400-500 ml
		Faeces	200 ml
Total	2500–2700 ml	Total	2500–2700 ml

distribution is that 'fluid volume is a function of extracellular fluid tonicity'. In other words, a change in the osmolality of either compartment will result in an adjustment of the water distribution between the compartments.

CONTROL OF FLUID AND ELECTROLYTE BALANCE

Fluid and electrolyte balance is normally in a state of dynamic equilibrium. In other words, fluids and electrolytes are constantly being lost and replaced, but the overall balance and distribution is maintained within fine limits. Table 26.2 illustrates the main sources of fluid loss and gain.

The losses from the lungs, skin and intestine are collectively referred to as insensible loss. Variations in these losses are in direct response to external agents, e.g. during exercise expiration loss and perspiration both increase. The necessary adjustments to overall fluid loss are made via the kidney.

Blood volume, pH, electrolyte concentration and extracellular fluid volume are all dependent on renal control, which is influenced by the interaction of two main hormones, anti-diuretic hormone (ADH), otherwise known as vasopressin, and aldosterone.

Anti-diuretic hormone. This is released from the posterior lobe of the pituitary gland. It is a water-conserving hormone which promotes the reabsorption of water from the distal renal tubule and collecting duct. Urine therefore becomes more concentrated under the influence of this hormone. The release of anti-diuretic hormone is increased by several factors:

- High plasma osmolality due to an elevated level of sodium, glucose or blood urea.
- Low circulating blood volume, hypovolaemia. Secretion is stimulated via stretch receptors in the aortic arch and carotid sinus.
- Low output not related to hypovolaemia, e.g. cardiac failure.
- Stress response — ADH production will increase despite below normal osmolality in patients suffering severe pain, emotion or stress.
- Anaesthetics and certain drugs, e.g. morphine and chlorpropamide, can either increase ADH secretion or augment renal tubular response to circulating hormone.
- Patients receiving positive pressure ventilation have increased ADH secretion.

Aldosterone. Aldosterone is a mineralocorticoid hormone and is released from the adrenal cortex. In response to this hormone the kidneys conserve sodium (and therefore water), and excrete potassium on a direct exchange system. Factors influencing aldosterone release include the following:

- a high serum potassium, hyperkalaemia
- low serum sodium, hyponatraemia
- hypovolaemia, which mediates aldosterone release via the renin-angiotensin system.

DISTURBANCES IN FLUID AND ELECTROLYTE BALANCE

Fluid and electrolyte disturbances can be extremely complex and are certainly quite

Table 26.3 Main causes of extracellular fluid deficit

Deficit	Patient conditions
Inadequate intake	Coma Dysphagia Access problems, e.g. immobility Manipulation difficulties, e.g. arthritis, Parkinson's disease Voluntary restriction, e.g. due to incontinence Depression, confusion Visual impairment Sedation
Excess output	Fever Vomiting, diarrhoea Wound drainage Respiratory loss, e.g. status asthmaticus Specific hormonal problems, e.g. diabetes insipidus Haemorrhage or serum loss from burns Iatrogenic, e.g. diuretics

common. Nurses must be conversant with the 'cues' which may indicate an 'at risk' patient, be able to assess the type and extent of the problem and, finally, monitor the effectiveness of treatment. Fluid balance and electrolyte disturbances may be primary conditions or, more commonly, secondary to other conditions. They can be grouped into three main categories:

- change in extracellular volume of either an excess or a deficit
- movement of extracellular fluid from one body compartment to another
- alterations in electrolyte concentrations.

It must be emphasized at this point that these three groups are not mutually exclusive and an inter-relationship between all three frequently exists. The emphasis is on extracellular fluid changes for two reasons, firstly we have direct access to extracellular fluids and secondly extracellular fluid and electrolyte status also reflects intracellular changes.

EXTRACELLULAR FLUID DEFICIT

The term dehydration is commonly used to describe loss of extracellular fluid. Dehydration actually refers to loss of water only, which is quite rare. The commonest cause of primary water loss is the condition diabetes insipidus (see Ch.19 on hormonal disturbances). Other causes of dehydration (see Table 26.3) are more likely to result in loss of both water and electrolytes. As sodium is the primary osmotic solute in the extracellular fluid, alterations in its concentration largely determine how water will re-distribute between the intra- and extracellular compartment. If losses of sodium and water are equal, the osmolality or tonicity of the extracellular fluid will remain unaltered and therefore intracellular fluid volume will be unchanged. In many of the common causes of dehydration, e.g. excessive sweating, both sodium and water are lost but not in an isotonic concentration. Water loss more commonly exceeds sodium loss. This results in a raised sodium concentration, hypernatraemia, in the extracellular fluid. Osmotic correction between the intra- and extracellular fluid is very rapid (Hume et al, 1982) and the net result is that water moves from the cells into the extracellular fluids. Many of the clinical manifestations of dehydration are due to the intra-cellular dehydration which occurs in these circumstances. Brain cells in particular are very vulnerable to the effects of osmotic dehydration and for this reason do have a protective mechanism. If the onset of dehydration is relatively slow, the brain cells can generate intracellular solutes called 'idiogenic' osmoles (Hume et al, 1982). These protect the brain from dehydration. However, if dehydration is rapid or fluid loss extensive, this mechanism may fail to compensate and mental functioning will deteriorate.

Severe extracellular fluid deficit can result in the clinical syndrome of shock. This is discussed in detail in Chapter 10 and will not be considered further here. Depending on the severity of the fluid and electrolyte loss, two methods of correction may be utilized, oral fluid replacement and/or intravenous fluid replacement. Firstly, however, it is necessary to consider why and which patients may be at risk and how to clinically assess the patient.

Patient assessment and monitoring

Extracellular fluid deficit can occur in patients of all ages and as a result of numerous causes, itemized in Table 26.3.

Table 26.3 clearly indicates the wide range of 'at risk' patients and early identification of these patients is of particular importance. The problem can arise very rapidly, as with acute haemorrhage, or perhaps less obviously over a period of days or weeks. The elderly are particularly at risk of the latter and nurses must be alert to this potential problem and be able to undertake a proper assessment.

Physical observations

- Dry skin, lips and mucosa. In the elderly, reduced skin turgor may be a facet of the normal ageing process rather than dehydration. However, reduced skin turgor in most patients can be deduced by gently pinching the skin. If it remains wrinkled for more than 15 seconds then one plausible reason may be loss of extracellular fluid.
- The tongue will show longitudinal furrows.
- Most patients will complain of thirst but some elderly patients may not. Salivation is also decreased.
- Lethargy, weakness and, in more extreme cases, mental confusion and personality changes may occur.

Table 26.4 Laboratory findings which may support clinical assessment of dehydration

Urine	Specific gravity raised	> 1.030
Serum urea		> 8 mmol/l
Serum sodium		> 150 mmol/l
Haematocrit		> 45
Urine chloride		> 50 mmol/l

- The axilla and groin areas may be dry.
- Blood pressure changes will occur when the intra-vascular volume deficit reaches between 15%–20%. Compensatory mechanisms sustaining systolic pressure begin to fail at this point. The most useful information is obtained by testing for postural changes. A systolic pressure deficit of 10 mmHg between the supine and standing positions could be indicative of fluid loss in an adult patient. The pulse pressure may also be reduced, i.e. the difference between systolic and diastolic pressures.
- Tachycardia may be noted, but this is not a very useful indicator as it could be due to many other causes, e.g. stress or pyrexia.
- Weight loss is a far more useful indicator and a loss of more than 0.5kg per day may well be related to fluid loss.
- Urine output will fall and a flow rate of less than 30 ml/h is indicative of a serious fluid deficit.

These clinical signs may be supported by more objective data from laboratory tests, and nurses must be able to utilize this data source as part of patient assessment. This presumes knowledge of normal values! The tests shown in Table 26.4 may be useful.

Monitoring fluid balance

The fluid balance status of patients is monitored by using the following two means:

- daily weighing
- fluid balance charts.

The use of both these monitoring devices is

widespread on all types of hospital wards. The up-dating of fluid balance charts and 'doing the weighing' is very often one of the pleasanter jobs of the very junior nurses. However, the accuracy and therefore usefulness of fluid balance charts has been seriously questioned. A study by Pflaum (1979) compared the differences in fluid balance assessment of the same patients as shown by intake/output charts and daily weights. Her results revealed a mean error in the intake/output charts of 799.5 ml per day when compared with daily weight calculations. The enormity of the deficit led her to question the use of intake/output charts at all. This may be an extreme reaction but it does serve as a warning about the way in which nurses perform this routine task, and the value of the interpretations placed upon them. The use of daily weights is generally considered to be a more accurate assessment of body fluid balance. This presumes that the patient's dry weight remains stable on a day to day basis, a safe assumption according to Greco, Quiantanilla & Huang (1979). In order to maximize the accuracy of daily weights, the following rules of practice are recommended:

- The patient should be weighed at the same time each day, ideally in the morning before breakfast, although this may not be feasible.
- The patient's bladder (or catheter bag) should be emptied just prior to being weighed.
- The same weight of clothing should be worn on each occasion.
- The same scales should be used each time.

Graphical representation of the daily changes provides an easy method of documentation, as well as being a good way of seeing trends over time.

The use of intake/output charts, as already mentioned, is a questionable method of monitoring accurate fluid balance; however, the charts are extensively used and cannot be ignored. Intake/output charts can become rather complex documents, a factor which may compound the problem of inaccuracy. However, provision should be made for the following columns:

Intake

- Oral and/or nasogastric
- Intravenous or subcutaneous

Output

- Urine output
- One or preferably two columns for other routes of loss, e.g. vomit, wound drainage, aspiration, liquid stools.

Accurate volume totals are obviously very important both for individual columns and total intake/output. Again graphical representation provides an excellent means of identifying trends. It is also very important to note that *content* of lost fluid can be just as important as volume. Content can be vital in relation to diagnostic possibilities and in order to monitor electrolyte losses (see Fig. 26.2). Vomiting 500 ml of fresh blood obviously has different implications to vomiting bile stained or faecal fluid.

Intake/output charts should be and can be a valuable source of information to both medical and nursing staff. Treatment changes are often made on the basis of the information contained on these charts, and, therefore, it is important to minimize any error. Table 26.5 shows some sources of error.

Many of these sources of error are correctable by improved communication, teaching and persistent attention to the accurate measurement of fluids in calibrated containers.

Intervention

Having diagnosed an extracellular fluid defect, either potential or actual, and considered methods of monitoring fluid balance, appropriate nursing intervention must follow. It is always worth bearing in mind the old but wise adage that prevention is better than cure.

Oral intake

Ideally an adequate fluid replacement regime by the oral route is recommended. This is particularly appropriate for patients who are at risk of chronic loss or inadequate intake. Whenever possible the full co-operation of the patient should be elicited, ensuring that they

Table 26.5 Sources of error in intake/output monitoring

Type of error	Source
Intake	Variety of receptacle used for fluid, e.g. cups, glasses, which tend to be assigned a common average volume, e.g. 180ml per glass, 150 ml per cup. No account is taken of how full receptacles were initially or how much residue was left. The recorded amount is therefore a 'guesstimate'
	Use of non-quantified estimates, e.g. sips, for very small quantities
	Reliance on patient's memory and/or honesty for intake over a period of time usually related to shift change-overs
	Variation in practice, and therefore the potential for confusion, in the recording of intravenous fluid intake
Output	Non-quantified entries for urinary incontinence, vomit or wound drainage
	Failure to measure more unusual losses, e.g. liquid faeces
	Not including urine taken for specimens, e.g. M.S.U. or for testing
	Patient goes to the toilet through failure to realize the need for measuring all urine
	Blocked catheters
General factors	Reliance on very junior staff to maintain the charts, who may not appreciate the need for accuracy
	Failure to communicate to all ward staff about which patients are being monitored
	Putting off charting drinks or other fluids until 'later', when there is more time
	Lack of patient co-operation through failure to inform them of the purpose of the chart and how they can help
	Guessing at, rather than measuring, fluid volumes
	Several nurses going round to complete the same charts

understand fully the reasons for the planned fluid intake regime. Patients' normal intake routines should be considered both in terms of volume and type of fluid. Negotiation can then be based on this foundation. Total intake over a 24-hour period will obviously vary according to individual need, but a minimal intake of 2 litres for at risk patients is a reasonable target to aim for, unless there are specific contraindications. The 24-hour intake should then be planned in detail between the nurse and patient.

Meal times, medication administration and patient preferences must be considered in planning fluid intake. Patients' toileting requirements may also need some discussion, voluntary fluid restriction is often related to a dread of using the commode. Once agreement has been reached between patient and nurse, the regime must be communicated to all ward staff and the patient's family. The patient's care plan should be updated and details of the change related verbally during ward report. It is not enough to tell other ward staff to 'push fluids', 'increase intake', or give other equally vague directives. It may also be necessary to include the domestic staff as they are often in charge of the teapot during meal times! A final point from Boylan (1979) is that drinking is often associated with social occasions. This could be particularly important in relation to the elderly at-risk patient.

Nurses must also be very aware of when and how help may be required. Heavy water jugs may be beyond the strength and manipulative skills of the elderly or incapacitated patient. Stroke patients with a hemianopia may not be able to see drinks left far over on their affected side. It may be necessary to help patients to take

Table 26.6 Intravenous fluids in common use — composition, energy content and tonicity

Intravenous fluid	Na^+	CL^-	K^+	HCO_3^-	Calorie/l	Tonicity
Dextrose 5%					200	Isotonic
Dextrose 10%					400	Hypertonic
Dextrose 5% NaCl 0.9%	154	154			200	Hypertonic
Dextrose 5% NaCl 0.45%	75		75		200	Hypertonic
Dextrose 5% KCl 0.15%		20	20		200	Slightly hypertonic
Dextrose 5% KCl 0.3%		40	40		200	Slightly hypertonic
Sodium chloride 0.9%	150	150				Isotonic
Sodium chloride 0.18%	31	31				Very hypotonic
Sodium chloride 0.45%	77	77				Hypotonic
Sodium chloride 1.8%	308	308				Hypertonic
Sodium bicarbonate 1.4%	167			167		Isotonic
Sodium bicarbonate 4.2%	500			500		Hypertonic
Sodium bicarbonate 8.4%	1000			1000		Very hypertonic

the prescribed fluids in which case the following considerations may apply:

- Swallowing is always easier in an upright or semi-upright position; the risk of fluid aspiration is particularly high in patients with dysphagia
- Water can become very boring to drink, particularly for elderly patients, whose sense of taste may be diminished. Sweet fruit juices provide some colour as well as taste. There are several types of very nutritious drinks now available, which may be appropriately included in fluid regimes if patients are underweight or anorexic
- Patients are far more likely to drink if good oral care is maintained. Clean teeth and a healthy oral mucosa improve thirst recognition, taste capacity and therefore likely compliance with fluid intake regimes
- Patients must not be rushed as they may inhale fluid.

Intravenous fluid replacement

Oral fluid replacement may be inadequate or inappropriate in situations where fluid loss has been rapid and/or extensive. Replacement of fluid and/or electrolyte loss by the intravenous route requires careful consideration of exactly how the composition of the extracellular fluid has been disturbed. Many of the common causes of extracellular fluid deficit result in a loss of hypotonic fluid, i.e. proportionally higher water loss than salt loss. In these circumstances, it is important to realize that, although the patient's biochemistry may show a hypernatraemia, there is an overall loss of total body sodium as well as water.

Intravenous fluid replacement in these circumstances has two main objectives:

- to restore circulating volume
- to correct electrolyte balance.

The first objective may be achieved by infusing isotonic saline (see Table 26.6), the second by an infusion of either hypotonic saline or 5% dextrose. The important point about this corrective treatment is that the reversal of hypernatraemia must be undertaken slowly (Hume et al, 1982). This is to prevent neurological complications resulting from cerebral oedema. If corrective treatment is given too quickly, the brain cells will not have time to degrade the idiogenic osmoles generated to protect against dehydration. If extracellular osmolality falls too quickly, the raised osmotic pressure in the brain cells, due to the idiogenic osmoles, will cause the cells to swell.

Patients may well present with far more complex disturbances than those just described. Specific electrolyte abnormalities are considered in some detail later in this chapter. Decisions about how particular fluid and/or electrolyte disturbances are to be treated remain primarily

Table 26.7 Main reasons for use of intravenous therapy

Replacement therapy	Fluids Electrolytes Blood Blood products, e.g. platelets, Factor VIII, albumin, etc.
Drug therapy	e.g. Heparin, cytotoxic drugs, antibiotics
Monitoring	Central venous pressure Pulmonary artery wedge pressure
Hyperalimentation	
Emergency access	'Keeping a vein open'

in the hands of medical staff. However, nurses are very largely responsible for patient welfare during intravenous therapy. This responsibility must encompass an understanding of the objectives of treatment and its possible complications. Table 26.6 shows the common fluids in use and how they relate in terms of tonicity to normal body fluids.

Nurses' role in relation to intravenous therapy. An estimated 12% of inpatients have an intravenous infusion at some time during their hospital stay (Jenner, 1983). The reason for intravenous therapy is frequently but not exclusively related to fluid replacement. Table 26.7 summarizes the main reasons for intravenous therapy.

In the past, the nurse's role in relation to intravenous therapy may well have been confined to knowing 'the contents of the trolley and how to assist the doctor' (Marks, 1981). This is manifestly no longer adequate or desirable. Since the Breckenridge report (1976) more formal recognition of the nurse's role has been made and a recent multidisciplinary conference concluded that nurses could take greater responsibility for intravenous therapy. Considerable interest in this area and the extended role of the nurse has been expressed by Marks and others. At the present time, with the exception of qualified and specially trained nurses working in specialized areas, medical staff are responsible for the insertion of the intravenous cannulae and the prescription of the fluids to be infused. Speechley (1984) suggests that the role of the nurse can be related to three main areas of responsibility:

- maintaining asepsis, both during and after cannulation
- patient safety during fluid administration
- patient comfort, both physical and psychological, during intravenous therapy.

Maintaining asepsis. The natural incidence of intravenous infections is unknown but an estimate as low as 1% would represent approximately 10 000 infections a year in the United Kingdom (Jenner, 1983). The consequences of infection may range from a painful, but relatively innocuous, localized phlebitis to a fatal septicaemia. Sources of infection are twofold:

- intrinsic, that is contained within the apparatus and/or infusion fluid before use
- extrinsic, contaminant introduced into the apparatus and/or patient by the people concerned with setting up and monitoring the system.

Intrinsic sources of infection are rare due to the excellent quality control measures taken by manufacturers. However, transport and ward storage facilities for sterile equipment are not always ideal and the following checks should be made. Intravenous bags should be checked for any damage to the sterile packaging. The fluid should be examined in a good light for any signs of turbidity or particles which could indicate contamination. If contamination is suspected the pharmacist must be informed and microbiological examination of the fluid performed. The expiry date must also be carefully checked and adhered to!

Extrinsic infections are invariably iatrogenic and can be prevented by nurses and doctors employing meticulous aseptic technique whenever they set up and/or handle intravenous equipment. It is often the most junior and inexperienced doctors who are allocated the job of erecting intravenous infusions. They may not only need but be grateful for the experienced guidance of a senior nurse. The following rules, if followed, should greatly reduce the risk of infection:

- use alcohol-based cleansers and the recommended hand washing and drying techniques
- clean bungs or injection access sites with an alcohol based antiseptic, and allow time for it to dry
- infusion bags should be changed as quickly as possible using a non-touch technique for the sterile connection areas
- the fluid container must not hang for longer than 24h, a special risk when intravenous lines are being used to keep the vein patent
- current DHSS recommendations (Rosenheim Report, 1972) state that the giving set should be changed every 24 hours — this may be arguable in the light of research by Buxton et al (1979) which shows that infection risks are not increased if giving sets are only changed every 48 hours
- peripheral intravenous cannulae should ideally be re-sited every 48 hours (Maki et al, 1973), although this may not always be practicable
- the cannula site should be inspected every day for signs of thrombophlebitis, i.e. redness, swelling and tenderness, along the course of the vein
- a sterile gauze dressing should be applied daily and the insertion site kept clean and dry.

If any signs of infection do occur, the infusion should be stopped and ideally re-sited. A swab from the infusion site and the tip of the intravenous cannulae should be sent to the microbiology laboratory for culture and sensitivity testing. If systemic infection is suspected, blood cultures may also be taken. In the unusual circumstances of a suspect intrinsic infection, the infusion fluid and the giving set should also be examined. Pyrogenic reactions of this type, although rare, are often very serious. Patients can develop a hyperpyrexia and rigors (see Ch. 27) and in extreme circumstances septic shock may develop.

Patient safety. The idea that intravenous therapy is prescribed medical treatment can lead to a passive attitude by nurses towards the safety aspects of intravenous fluid administration. The monitoring of intravenous fluids on general wards is often left to the most junior nurses, who know least about possible complications.

Safety begins with the careful checking of the prescription and fluid to be administered by two nurses, preferably one of whom is qualified. Particular care must be taken if any fluid additives, e.g. drugs, have to be administered. All additives must be carefully checked and thoroughly mixed, but particular care needs to be taken with potassium.

Potassium is 'heavy' and will tend to accumulate in the bottom of the fluid, leading to the risk of the patient receiving a concentrated dose which could precipitate a cardiac dysrhythmia or arrest. Drug additives should be treated with extreme caution, any nurses dealing with them must be very aware of any incompatibilities between drug and dilution fluid. Drugs should never be added to parenteral feeding fluids, blood or blood products. All intravenous fluids with drug additives must be clearly labelled and recorded.

The second important consideration in relation to patient safety is regulation of flow. Anyone with even minimal experience of monitoring intravenous infusions will be aware that flow rates can be extremely erratic and difficult to control. The rate at which fluids are prescribed to flow may depend on several factors:

- fluid type and reason for administration
- patient's age and body size
- pre-existing renal or cardiac conditions which will limit tolerance to fast rates or high volumes of infused fluids.

Flow control problems can be caused by multiple factors. These are summarized in Table 26.8.

The use of electronic infusion control devices is becoming increasingly common. Using a traditional gravity system, a fluid container less than three feet above the cannula site is likely to result in a reduced flow rate and potential problems related to cannula patency. Intravenous pumps are not gravity dependent and this problem does not arise. An alarm system

Table 26.8 Factors affecting flow rates (Steel, 1983)

Patient factors	Direct intervention with the clamp Raising or lowering the site High blood pressure slows rate Altering bed height
Obstruction (partial or complete)	Clot formation in cannula Kinked or pinched tubing Venous spasm Phlebitis Clogged filters Air vent obstruction
Miscellaneous	Tissue infiltration Fluid viscosity Needle gauge Solution temperature

triggered by anything occluding the tubing or an empty fluid container will quickly alert nursing staff to any problems. The use of such pumps is strongly recommended with high viscosity fluids or when drugs are being administered (Dunn & Heath, 1981). Any patients particularly at risk from fluid overload would also benefit from the close flow regulation achieved by the many electronic pumps available. Dunn & Heath (1981) showed that the use of an electronic pump greatly improved compliance with prescribed regimes in terms of rate and duration of flow. It also economized on nursing staff time.

Patients at risk of fluid overload include the elderly and anyone with renal or cardiac pathology. This risk may be exacerbated by nurses who indulge in the practice of 'speeding up the drip' when regimes get behind schedule. Table 26.6 shows fluids in common use; those which are iso- or hypotonic are particularly likely to lead to this problem. The problem usually becomes manifest by the patient developing the signs and symptoms of pulmonary oedema. (See section on extracellular fluid excess.)

Nurses are responsible for monitoring patients in relation to these hazards and for knowing which patients are at special risk. Junior nurses should therefore be supervised and taught by senior nurses if they are caring for patients receiving intravenous therapy.

Patient comfort. This is the third aim of successful intravenous therapy and begins with patient preparation. A simple but thorough explanation of the purpose of the infusion and the setting up procedure should be given. Most patients have a 'needle phobia' and may well be afraid of the cannulation process. The use of local anaesthesia is not generally practised and the best approach is to advise the patient on how to assist the doctor to achieve successful cannulation at the first attempt! The patient will be less inconvenienced if the non-dominant arm is used, taking care not to 'trap' tight nightdress sleeves above the insertion site.

The choice of site should avoid joints and flexures if possible as cannulae are more easily dislodged in these areas (Jenner, 1983). If the patient is hirsute, then removal of hair from the area may be necessary. This also reduces the risk of introducing skin flora into the vein. The use of plastic splints and a bulky bandage to secure the cannulae remains widespread but is generally unnecessary. Inspection of the cannulation site is less likely in these circumstances (Jenner, 1983). Splints may be useful if the cannula is in an area of flexion. Patients need the reassurance of a nurse checking the infusion and Steel (1983) recommends every hour. It is very important that the patient does not do any 'self adjusting' in the mistaken hope of getting it over more quickly. The patient should also be advised to report any sensations of burning or actual pain at the cannulation site as this may be indicative of early thrombophlebitis. Oedema at the site of cannulation, wetness of the dressing and/or a persistently slow flow rate may indicate local infiltration of fluid into the subcutaneous tissues. Inflammation along a vein which has been used for intravenous therapy can be soothed by the application of an old-fashioned but effective glycerine of Ichthammol dressing.

Patient comfort can also be enhanced by giving help with the activities of daily living which normally require two hands, such as washing, dressing and eating. Patient condition permitting, there is no *a priori* reason why they should be confined to bed. Supervised activity is desirable for both physical and psychological welfare. Patients may also worry about going to sleep in case they dislodge the cannula or the flow rate changes. It is important that nurses check the infusion, ensure the patient is comfortable and inform them that they will be checking the infusion at regular intervals during the night.

Oral fluid intake should not be ignored unless there are specific reasons why the patient may not drink. This is particularly important if patients are on a fluid replacement regime as the transition from intravenous to oral fluids tends to be rather abrupt.

EXTRACELLULAR FLUID EXCESS (OEDEMA)

Oedema is defined as the presence of excess interstitial fluid (Guyton, 1986). It is, generally speaking, present as a consequence of a traumatic and/or pathological process which has disturbed the normal fluid exchange between the blood and interstitial fluid. This normal process was described at the beginning of the chapter (see Fig 26.3).

Oedema does not become clinically apparent until the volume of fluid in the interstitial spaces has risen to at least 30% above normal. The fact that this large rise in excess volume can occur before oedema is evident implies that some very efficient compensatory mechanisms are at work. The normal pressure of the free interstitial fluid is negative, at about 6 mmHg. Oedema does not occur until the pressure has risen to a positive value. Once the pressure has reached a very minimal positive value, oedema becomes clinically evident very rapidly. Oedema causes stretching of the tissue spaces and is detectable by applying finger pressure to the skin. If a small depression or pit remains, caused by the temporary translocation of fluid, then oedema is present. Occasionally, due to the presence of infection, the fluid coagulates and does not 'pit' on applying finger pressure, this is referred to as brawny oedema.

Three main factors help to provide a safety margin which allows interstitial fluid volume to rise before oedema occurs. Lymph flow increases in response to minimal lowering of the normal negative pressure and therefore helps to remove some excess fluid. Protein is also removed by the lymphatic system therefore helping to lower the colloid osmotic pressure of the interstitial fluid. The summation of these factors is as follows (Guyton, 1986):

Negative interstitial fluid pressure	6.3 mmHg
Increased lymphatic flow	7.0 mmHg
Protein removal via the lymphatics	4.0 mmHg
	17.3 mmHg

This means that, in relation to the figures quoted above, either the capillary pressure must rise by 17 mmHg above its normal value, or, the intravascular colloid osmotic pressure must fall 17 mmHg below its normal value, before oedema will occur.

Causes of oedema

There are four main mechanisms by which oedema can arise:

- increased capillary pressure
- a reduction in intravascular colloid pressure due to a fall in plasma proteins
- obstruction of the lymph vessels
- increased porosity of the capillary walls.

Table 26.9 summarizes the specific causes in relation to these four mechanisms.
The four mechanisms are not mutually exclusive and several may be operating at any one time in relation to a particular pathology.

Signs and symptoms of oedema

Recognition of clinical oedema depends to some extent on the underlying pathology, but the following signs and symptoms may provide a useful guide:

- Obvious swelling in dependent parts such as ankles, if patients are ambulatory, or the scrotum and sacrum if patients are confined to bed. Patients may complain that shoes or rings are very tight.
- 'Pitting' on the application of digital pressure. If the oedema is very gross then it may not be possible to displace the fluid and the skin surface will appear taut and shiny and will feel hard.
- Excessive weight gain will develop and can be correlated directly to the volume of fluid retention. 1 litre of fluid weighs 1 kilogram or 2.2 pounds. Other causes of

Table 26.9 Causes of oedema in relation to the four mechanisms described

Mechanism	Causes
Increased capillary pressure	Venous obstruction, e.g. thrombosis Venous dilatation due to cardiac failure Arteriolar dilatation due to allergic reactions or angioneurotic oedema Loss of muscular pumping action, e.g. paralysed arm following stroke
Decreased plasma proteins	Extensive loss from burns Renal loss — albuminuria Nutritional deficit — starvation Liver disease
Lymphatic obstruction	Lymph gland removal to prevent spread of malignancy Metastatic infiltration Nematode infection — filariasis Elephantiasis
Increased capillary permeability	Trauma — burns Allergic reactions Effect of bacterial toxins

weight gain are unlikely to occur so rapidly and would not be associated with the other clinical signs.

- Jugular venous pressure rises with the intravascular fluid overload. The jugular vein is normally visible no higher than 2cm above the sternal angle when a person is sitting at a 45° angle. Neck vein distension which is apparent above this height is indicative of fluid overload (Folklightly, 1984).
- Elevated blood pressure may occur with fluid overload but is not a reliable indication, as there are many other causes.
- Dyspnoea and/or orthopnoea may be present if the patient has a pleural effusion or pulmonary embolism.

Pathology of oedema

The pathology underlying oedematous states is complex but has its basis in the disruption of the normal sodium and water balance. As previously stated, extracellular fluid volume is a function of the amount of total body sodium. In the two commonest oedematous states, i.e. congestive cardiac failure and hepatic cirrhosis, total body sodium is increased but there is a proportionately greater increase in body water (Hume et al, 1982). This means that plasma sodium levels can appear to be below normal. The conseqence of this hyponatraemic/hypervolaemic state in terms of the body disruption of water means that the circulating blood volume is actually reduced. This reduction in effective arterial blood volume decreases the glomerular filtration rate (G.F.R.), and increases the proximal reabsorption of sodium and water. Further retention of sodium and water is caused by the activation of the renin/angiotensin system and the release of ADH. These patients are thus caught in a vicious circle of increasing oedema due to the compensatory mechanisms set in motion by a reduced arterial blood volume. (Detailed management of a patient with congestive heart failure can be found in Chapter 22.).

The problem of oedema can also manifest itself as a localized problem and can reflect iatrogenic as well as pathological causes. To illustrate these kinds of problems three common examples of how extracellular fluid excess can occur will be discussed: pulmonary oedema, ascites, and peri-operative fluid balance.

Pulmonary oedema

Pulmonary oedema is the presence of excessive quantities of fluid in the alvoeli and/or interstitial spaces of the lungs. It can occur as an acute emergency or develop over a period of time, sometimes as part of the cycle of generalized oedema already described. It occurs as a consequence of raised pulmonary capillary pressure. The lungs have a larger safety margin than other body tissues due to the high colloid pressure of the blood in the lungs which effectively dehydrates the lung tissue. The normal pulmonary capillary pressure is approximately 7 mmHg and the colloid pressure 28 mmHg, which gives an effective safety margin of 23 mmHg. Chronic raised pressure causes pulmonary lymphatic vessels to enlarge and therefore increase their drainage capacity, which affords further protection to the lung tissues.

The onset of pulmonary oedema is marked by increasing respiratory embarrassment. Dyspnoea on exertion is the earliest sign. Paroxysmal nocturnal dyspnoea is a later problem and the patients classically describe being awoken from sleep unable to breathe and needing 'fresh air'. Getting out of bed and opening the window usually relieves the symptoms within a few minutes. If the condition progresses eventually the patient will require several pillows to prop themselves up with in order to sleep, or will even choose to sit in a high-back chair to sleep.

Aims of care are twofold, firstly to relieve the dyspnoea and secondly to maximize alveolar exchange of gases. Most patients will assume an upright position and many are helped by leaning forward supported on a bed table and pillows. If the patient also has peripheral oedema it is not advisable to elevate their legs. Increasing venous return may further embarrass cardiac function and exacerbate the patient's condition. Providing there are no contraindications, e.g. chronic obstructive airways disease, a high percentage of oxygen can be administered. Diuretics are usually the treatment of choice and will be considered later.

Ascites

Ascites is the name given to a collection of fluid in the peritoneal cavity. It is most commonly associated with cirrhosis of the liver or pelvic/abdominal malignancies. Ascites associated with cirrhosis of the liver has a complex pathology which illustrates well how the mechanisms described earlier may interact to produce a situation of abnormal fluid balance.

The liver normally offers resistance to blood flow from the portal system. As the disease process progresses the liver becomes increasingly fibrosed and impedes the portal circulation, particularly the outflow of blood from the liver sinusoids to the vena cava. This mechanical obstruction causes an ultra filtrate of blood to exude from the liver surface. This fluid has a high protein content and therefore a high colloid pressure which draws more fluid from the gut and mesentery. This is exacerbated by low albumin production by the diseased liver leading to an intravascular hypoalbuminaemia. The combination of these factors results in a persistent reduction of effective blood volume. The renal and extra-renal mechanisms for conserving sodium and water are therefore activated. The levels of aldosterone and ADH are elevated by these mechanisms and remain abnormally high because the diseased liver is unable to de-activate them at the normal rate. Generalized oedema as well as ascites eventually develops as a consequence of the interaction of these various mechanisms.

The treatment of choice is usually the diuretic spironolactone (see later section). Occasionally if the ascites does not respond to diuretics a procedure known as paracentesis abdominis is performed. This is a minor surgical procedure in which the ascitic fluid is drained by the insertion of a cannula into the peritoneal cavity. It is extremely important that the patient's bladder is first emptied in order to avoid perforation by the cannula. Ideally the patient should be seated in a chair or in a high Fowlers position. The patient's blood pressure should be checked to ensure that they do not have postural hypotension due to the reduced intravascular volume. The doctor inserts the cannula after first infiltrating the site with local anaesthetic. The ascitic fluid should be drained slowly using a regulator clamp. If the fluid is drained too quickly then the sudden release of pressure from the abdominal vessels may cause collapse due to pooling of the circulating blood in the abdominal vessels.

The procedure is not performed unless there is no other satisfactory solution. The protein loss is heavy and it does carry the risks outlined above. The procedure is only palliative in many cases but can result in an enormous improvement in patient comfort.

Peri-operative fluid balance

The third situation in which patients are at risk of fluid overload, and of which nurses should be aware, is the peri-operative and particularly the postoperative period. Surgery is invariably associated with water and sodium retention, resulting in an 'obligatory oliguria' (Bevan, 1978). The reason for the label of obligatory oliguria is that fluid replacement, however adequate, does not result in normal diuresis. This is due to an increase in plasma anti-diuretic activity during surgery of up to 50–100 times pre-operative levels (Bevan 1978). This begins to fall at the termination of surgery and returns to normal 3–5 days postoperatively. A direct causal relationship between high plasma anti-diuretic activity and oliguria is not, however, that easy to establish. The urine produced immediately postoperatively is not only low in volume but it is poorly concentrated, which suggests that other factors may be involved.

The fluid balance status of the postoperative patient is complex and many factors have to be considered:

- raised levels of A.D.H. result in retention of sodium and water and a postoperative oliguria
- extracellular deficits occur due to two main causes (McAlsan 1980): external losses, including haemorrhage, exudate, vomiting, naso-gastric suction, diarrhoea and fistula drainage; internal losses, due to peritonitis, ascites, surgical injury and sequestration in burns;
- surgical procedures increase capillary permeability and protein loss will reduce the intravascular oncotic pressure; this results in an extracellular transudate into the walls and lumen of the bowel, peritoneal and retro-peritoneal spaces (Rando, 1982).

This redistribution of extracellular fluid into these areas is known as third space loss and reduces the amount of functional extracellular fluid volume. The patient is rendered hypovolaemic in terms of intravascular volume but is in fact suffering from extracellular fluid overload when third space losses are accounted for. It is very important to note that the third space loss is only temporary and begins to be reabsorbed back into the blood stream 2–3 days postoperatively (Folklightly, 1984), thus re-expanding blood volume.

Fluid replacement regimes must therefore be very carefully calculated, as postoperative patients receiving intravenous therapy are very much at risk of fluid overload. The precipitation of pulmonary oedema from fluid overload is usually iatrogenic and any patient with a history of renal or cardiac problems is particularly at risk. Nurses need to be aware of this potential problem and the approximate time factors related to the fluid balance changes described above during the postoperative period.

Nursing responsibilites are three fold:

- Ensuring the smooth running of the intravenous fluid replacement regime (see previous section on intravenous infusions). This particularly applies if normal saline is being infused when the practice of speeding up an infusion which is behind schedule could be especially risky.
- Monitoring the fluid balance status of the patient: Intake/output charts are commonly used in preference to daily weights because of the difficulties and discomfort involved in weighing a postoperative patient with a number of tubes, drains and bulky dressings to manoeuvre. The difficulties involved in maintaining these charts with any degree of accuracy has already been discussed at length. Daily weights are preferable and more accurate if they can be implemented.

Table 26.10 Diuretics and their uses

Type	Example(s)	General uses	Principal side-effects
Loop diuretic	Frusemide Bumetanide Ethacrynic acid	Heart failure — all types Pulmonary oedema Prophylaxis — overload risk Nephrotic syndrome	Dehydration Hypokalaemia
Thiazide	Bendrofluazide Chlorothiazide Triamterene	Hypertension control Mild oedema Adjunct to loop diuretics in heart failure	Raised uric acid and/or glucose — hypokalaemia Hyperkalaemia
Osmotic	Mannitol	Cerebral oedema	Expands blood volume Possible 'overload' effect
Carbonic anhydrase blockers	Acetazolamide	Glaucoma	Hypersensitivity Blood dyscrasias
Mercurial (rarely used)	Mersalyl	Similar to loop diuretics	Alkalosis

- Recognition of actual and potential fluid overload problems. This involves knowing beforehand which patients are at risk. Recognition of the development of and necessary intervention for the onset of acute pulmonary oedema has already been discussed.

Diuretic therapy

Diuretics are one of the commonest groups of drugs to be prescribed. A summary of the types of drugs in common use is shown in Table 26.10.

The main focus of this section will be the consequences of diuretic therapy for the patient and the nurse's role in monitoring treatment. The overall aim of diuretic therapy is to rid the body of excess fluid without disturbing the normal electrolyte composition (Metheny & Snively, 1983). The primary nursing responsibility relates to monitoring fluid loss and checking for the development of side effects. The relative merits of using daily weights or intake/output charts as a means of fluid balance monitoring have been discussed at length. Daily girth measurements may be very useful if patients have ascites. Clinical assessment of the patient is also necessary. The patient should gain progressive release of symptoms and improve in his or her ability to carry out the activities of daily living without becoming exhausted. Blood pressure monitoring 4-hourly is important, particularily for patients with heart failure or low circulating blood volume. These patients may already be relatively hypotensive. Diuretics may exacerbate this situation and the patient can develop postural hypotension. The most serious side effect of diuretic activity is hypokalaemia. This is discussed in detail in the next section. Dehydration may also ensue if diuretic activity is continued for too long at too high a dose. Once weight loss has levelled off and/or urine output has fallen to near normal levels or below then treatment review is necessary.

Diuretic therapy is not always very popular with the patients. Loop diuretics, such as frusemide, are very potent and begin working within half an hour of administration, and a very ill patient rendered immobile by gross oedema may develop iatrogenic incontinence. Non-compliance with treatment then becomes a risk if the patient begins to feel that he/she is losing control. It is essential that the nurse supports the patient by providing information about the drugs, their purpose, how they work and how to cope with them. Practical support in the form of prompt response to urgent calls, and fast and sympathetic intervention should incontinence occur, will help patients over the first few days of treatment. Iatrogenic incontinence is usually only a temporary problem. Continued

Table 26.11 Main causes of hypernatraemia and hyponatraemia

Hypernatraemia	Hyponatraemia
Renal loss of water	Sodium dilution
Diabetes insipidus Osmotic diuresis caused by glucose, urea or mannitol Diuretic and low intake Renal concentrating disorders	Excess ADH secretion Water intoxication, e.g. psychogenic polydipsia, Excess 5% dextrose infusion Hypoalbuminaemia due to malnutrition or renal loss Heart failure
Extra-renal loss of water Insensible loss via respiratory tract or skin	Sodium loss Gastrointestinal losses vomiting, diarrhoea Burns, sweating Third space loss, e.g. ascites Diuretic therapy Renal loss and high oral water intake
Sodium gain	
Hypertonic infusion Hyperaldosteronism Cushing's syndrome High solute intake via tube feeding or $NaHCO_3$ intake	

expressions of complaint about taking diuretics even when the underlying pathology is under control, should be taken very seriously. Acute exacerbation of oedema a short period after discharge can be due to deliberate non-compliance with the prescribed drug regime.

This problem may be offset by a careful assessment of the patient's problem in relation to their home environment. Restricted mobility and difficulty of access to toilet facilities may result in the patient developing iatrogenic incontinence. The problem caused by taking the drug can seem worse than those caused by not taking it. Timing of administration can be vital. The patient should have a good idea of how quickly it will begin to work so that they can be 'ready'. If possible it should be taken early enough in the day for the effect to have worn off by nighttime; nocturia can be very distressing for some patients.

MAJOR ELECTROLYTE DISTURBANCES

Introduction

In order to understand the complexities of electrolyte disturbances it is first of all essential to be fully conversant with certain aspects of normal electrolyte function. Nurses need to know the normal blood values of the major electrolytes (see Table 26.1), their physiological roles and body distribution. Knowledge of the normal routes of intake, excretion and the regulatory mechanisms will help nurses to identify at risk patients. Recognition of abnormal blood values, which is the most usual but by no means exclusive means of identifying imbalances, then becomes relatively simple. Two types of imbalance occur, a higher than normal concentration (hyper...) or a lower than normal concentration (hypo...), each with their own consequences for the patient. The causes of electrolyte imbalances are many, varied and often complex. Knowledge of likely causes enhances the nurse's ability to identify potential disturbances and aid early detection or, preferably, avoid them occurring. Knowing the signs and symptoms will help to direct nursing assessment of the at risk patients and provide a strong base for successful care planning and monitoring of treatment.

Sodium imbalance

It has already been emphasized that sodium and water balance are intricately linked, and

Table 26.12 Less common causes of hypokalaemia

Drug therapy other than diuretics Insulin injection Peptic ulcer therapy Steroids — corticotrophin Chemotherapy — cytarabine, thioguanine, doxorubicin hydrochloride
Urinary losses due to renal disease
Aldosteronism and Cushing's syndrome
Low dietary intake (rare)

imbalances are defined by the relationship between the two in the body. Two of the major causes of sodium and/or fluid imbalance have already been discussed in detail in relation to fluid deficit and fluid overload. Table 26.11 summarizes the main causes of hypernatraemia and hyponatraemia (see Ch. 19 for a discussion of the hormone-related disturbances such as aldosteronism and Cushing's syndrome).

Potassium imbalance

Potassium is the main intracellular electrolyte and its distribution across the cell membrane is maintained by the ion pumps (see Fig. 26.1). Daily ingestion of potassium equals approximately 50–100mmol daily, of which about 85–90% is absorbed (Narins et al, 1982). Intake is balanced almost entirely by renal excretion although very small amounts are lost via the skin, saliva and gastrointestinal tract. Renal excretion is controlled primarily by the hormone aldosterone which causes conservation of sodium and consequent excretion of potassium. An excess or deficit of potassium can be defined by the following serum levels (Felver, 1980).

Hyperkalaemia: Serum K^+ above 5 mmol/l
Hypokalaemia: Serum K^+ below 3.5 mmol/l.

Hypokalaemia

The three commonest causes of hypokalaemia are:

- diuretic therapy (excluding potassium sparing drugs, e.g. spironolactone)
- intravenous fluid therapy with insufficient or no potassium replacement
- gastrointestinal losses (Lawson, 1979).

Other less common causes of hypokalaemia are indicated in Table 26.12.

Hypokalaemia affects the resting potential of muscle cells by prolonging the refractory period following contraction. The effect on the patient can be profound, producing muscle weakness, particularly in the legs, to the extent that the patient may be unable to walk or support body weight. All body muscles may potentially be affected, including the gastrointestinal tract, leading to abdominal distension (Macleod, 1984). The most serious effect is on the cardiac muscle, leading to the development of dysrhythmias and possibly cardiac arrest. Hypokalaemia also potentiates the action of digoxin and, as many patients take both diuretics and digoxin, careful monitoring for signs of digoxin toxicity may also be appropriate. Two of the commonest causes are iatrogenic, and prevention is therefore primarily in the hands of the medical staff. However, gauging adequate replacement therapy is not always straightforward and nurses must be alert to the harbingers of increased risk, e.g. development of diarrhoea or patient non-compliance. Nurses are particularly responsible for educating patients about their drugs and stressing the importance of taking the sometimes unpopular 'Slow K' tablets. When appropriate, the hazards of laxative abuse should also be emphasized. Advice on dietary sources of potassium, e.g. fruit juice, may also be helpful.

Potassium replacement may be oral or intravenous. The use of intravenous potassium carries some risk which has already been alluded to earlier in relation to intravenous therapy. Potassium can accumulate very rapidly in the intravascular compartment and it should always be given diluted and very slowly. 15–20 mmol per hour is the maximum advised rate.

Hyperkalaemia

This is one of the major problems of patients with oliguric renal failure (see the section on renal disease, below). Increased intake, either oral or via intravenous therapy, may cause hyperkalaemia, but normal kidneys can usually cope unless the input is very rapid. Any disorder causing massive cell damage, e.g. burns or crush injury, may result in the rapid release of intracellular potassium. Any condition which decreases either the release of or the effect of aldosterone, such as Addison's disease, can also cause hyperkalaemia.

Muscle cells respond to hyperkalaemia by becoming less sensitive to incoming stimuli, i.e. hyperpolarized. In the gastrointestinal tract this can result in constipation, abdominal distension or even paralytic ileus. Voluntary muscle weakness which begins peripherally and extends towards central muscles can ensue if the imbalance is severe. Cardiac dysrhythmias may also occur.

Treatment for hyperkalaemia is dealt with in detail later in this chapter in relation to oliguric renal failure.

Magnesium imbalance

Magnesium balance, unlike most other important biological cations, is not under direct hormonal regulation. Gastrointestinal absorption is largely unregulated, serum levels being balanced by renal excretion and reabsorption. If serum magnesium levels rise above 2 mmol/l, renal reabsorption is incomplete and the excess is excreted in the urine. Complete reabsorption occurs if serum levels fall below 1.5 mmol/l. Imbalance can be defined by the following blood levels (Felver, 1980):

Hypomagnesaemia: Serum Mg^{++} below 1.5 mmol/l
Hypermagnesaemia: Serum Mg^{++} above 2.5 mmol/l

Hypomagnesaemia

This is the more common of the two disorders and often co-exists with hypocalcaemia and hypokalaemia. Deficiency is more commonly associated with decreased absorption as opposed to insufficient intake, unless the patient is suffering from chronic malnutrition or alcoholism. The effect of hypomagnesaemia is to increase the release of acetylcholine at the neuromuscular junction, thus increasing muscle irritability (Felver, 1980). This manifests in the patient as hyperactive reflexes, insomnia, leg cramps, twitching and, in extreme deficit, tetany, convulsions and cardiac dysrhythmias can ensue. The condition is treated by straightforward intramuscular or intra-venous replacement therapy with magnesium sulphate.

Hypermagnesaemia

This is extremely rare because of the superb capacity of the normal kidney to excrete magnesium (Narins, 1982). Impaired excretion may occur in chronic renal failure or adrenal insufficiency. Manifestations are related to the decreased acetylcholine release at the neuromuscular junctions and subsequent lowering of neuromuscular excitability. Patients have serious and progressive symptoms depending on how high the serum Mg^{++} levels are elevated. Hypotension, flushing, sweating and a feeling of warmth occur with levels of 3–4 mmol/l. Increasing levels produce signs of central nervous system depression, such as lethargy and drowsiness. Deep tendon reflexes weaken, flaccid paralysis occurs and eventually cardiac and respiratory function will diminish. Treatment is difficult; increasing fluid intake may aid renal excretion, and any food or preparations known to contain magnesium, such as antacids, are withheld. The condition is life threatening and life support equipment may well be required.

ACID-BASE DISTURBANCES

Acid-base balance is a complex and intricate matter involving the interplay of several electrolytes. Imbalances can be extremely serious because they disturb the normal pH of the blood. pH refers to the concentration of free hydrogen (H^+) ions and is usually estimated for blood, normal values being between 7.35 and 7.45. The two principal electrolytes involved are hydrogen, H^+, and bicarbonate, HCO_3^-, but others including chloride (Cl^-) and phosphates also have a role to play. Control of acid-base balance is achieved normally by the kidneys and the lungs. The interaction between the two principal electrolytes involved can be seen from the following equation:

$$CO_2 + H_2O \rightleftharpoons H_2CO_3 \rightleftharpoons H^+ + HCO_3^-$$

Carbon dioxide	Water	Carbonic acid	Hydrogen	Bicarbonate

The lungs assist with acid-base balance by adjusting the amount of CO_2 expired, this in turn modifies the amount of carbonic acid in the blood. Renal control mechanisms are complex but, put very simply, consist of two areas of function:

- Bicarbonate ions, HCO_3^-, are reabsorbed from the glomerular filtrate. The tubules can also form new HCO_3^- and bind them to reabsorbed sodium Na^+. The sodium bicarbonate formed then goes back into the plasma.
- Excess hydrogen ions, H^+ are excreted in the urine as acid and ammonium compounds.
- The kidneys can adjust the formation and reabsorption of HCO_3^- according to need.

There are two main disturbances of acid-base balance:

- acidosis, characterized by an increase in acid or decrease in base resulting in a blood pH of 7.35 or below.
- alkalosis, characterized by an increase in base or decrease in acid resulting in a blood pH of 7.45 or above.

Both acidosis and alkalosis can be caused by respiratory or metabolic disturbances.

Acidosis

Respiratory acidosis occurs when carbon dioxide is retained in the bloodstream resulting in an increase in carbonic acid levels. This occurs in relation to many types of lung pathology (which are discussed in Chapter 24).

Metabolic acidosis has many and varied causes. It can be caused by loss of hydrochloric acid from nasogastric suction or vomiting, or excessive production of acidic substances, such as ketones in the ketoacidosis of diabetes mellitus. The effects on the patient are variable in both intensity and duration depending on the cause, e.g. the acidosis related to exercise is due to an oxygen debt and subsequent accumulation of lactic acid. This is quickly reversed by rest and restoration of the oxygen debt. Prolonged and/or progressive acidosis has serious effects on the patient related primarily to the central nervous system, cardiovascular system and the respiratory system. Patients may complain of headaches, lethargy and drowsiness. Stupor and coma may ensue as the condition progresses. Respirations become deep and rapid in an effort to exhale CO_2 and lower carbonic acid levels. The acidosis will eventually impair cardiac function and cardiac output will fall causing hypotension. The cells begin to exchange H^+ for K^+ and the kidneys excrete hydrogen, thus retaining potassium and causing a hyperkalaemia.

Blood gas estimations will help in determining the seriousness of the situation and how well the body's compensatory mechanisms are coping. Treatment must be directed towards replacing HCO_3^- via an intravenous infusion of sodium bicarbonate, and dealing with the underlying pathology.

Alkalosis

Respiratory alkalosis occurs when patients hyperventilate and lower CO_2 levels excessively. This can occur as a response to pain or anxiety. Artificial ventilation via a respirator can also cause respiratory alkalosis. The change in pH leads to a lowering of the level of calcium ions which are free in the blood. Potassium and hydrogen ions also exchange in the cells causing a hypokalaemia. In addition, the kidneys excrete potassium in order to retain hydrogen, also leading to hypokalaemia. Respiratory alkalosis rarely requires medical intervention and is quickly reversed.

Oral ingestion of alkalis, mainly taken for the relief of indigestion, can lead to alkalosis if taken excessively.

The effects on the patient are partly related to the hypocalcaemia which results from the alkalosis. This manifests as twitching and tremors initially developing into tetany, and into convulsions and coma if the condition progresses. Atrial tachycardia commonly occurs with alkalosis. Hypoventilation develops as a compensatory mechanism to retain CO_2 and raise the level of carbonic acid. The condition is corrected by replacing the lost chloride ions via potassium chloride supplements and an infusion of normal saline.

RENAL DISEASE

RENAL FAILURE

Renal nursing has become almost synonymous with the care of patients with end stage renal disease (E.S.R.D.). This area of work does indeed form the major component of their work and never more so than in the last twenty-five years. A new ethos in terms of treatment and attitude of both professional and lay people has developed. Patients designated as having E.S.R.D. twenty-five years ago, who were over forty years of age or unfortunate enough to have co-existent pathology, e.g. diabetes, were almost certain to die. Treatment facilities were in short supply and the era of renal transplants in its infancy. The first successful transplant was in 1956 between identical twins in Boston, Massachusetts. Today renal transplantation and the carrying of kidney donor cards by an informed general public is commonplace. Despite a persistent media campaign to enhance this voluntary donor system and raise funds for dialysis patients, an economic problem still exists in relation to the need for and provision of care for patients with renal disease. In the British population approximately 3500 people each year become potential candidates for some form of treatment. Of these about 1500 are denied access to treatment and consequently die (Gabriel, 1983). Some of these patients will not even be referred to a nephrologist for consideration. The Rosenheim Report in 1972 resulted in most patients of 45 years or under being accepted for treatment. Views on the criteria for being accepted for treatment have become increasingly liberalized since then and the advent of continuous ambulatory peritoneal dialysis (C.A.P.D.) has undoubtedly aided this process.

This part of the chapter will deal primarily with acute and chronic renal failure. The two conditions are not the same but do naturally have features in common. In order to avoid repetition, the pathologies are dealt with separately, and the principles of nursing care, including dialysis, are presented as a general discussion with particular emphasis on the long term management of E.S.R.D. A review of other common renal pathologies will form the end section of this chapter on fluid and electrolyte disturbances.

Acute renal failure

This clinical syndrome is usually characterized by oliguria and an inability to excrete the products of metabolism. The causes of this syndrome can best be summarized in the following three groups:

- *Pre-renal* causes are the commonest and include any condition leading to an abnormal decrease in renal blood flow (hypoperfusion).
- *Intra-renal* causes include those which result in direct damage to the basement membrane of the glomeruli or the tubules.
- *Post-renal* failure is associated with obstructive lesions, of either the renal outflow or urinary tract, which prevent the flow of urine from the kidney to the urethra.

Specific causes related to these three categories are summarized in Table 26.13.

Acute renal failure (A.R.F.) can be classified as either reversible or irreversible. If it is reversible then the common pattern of recovery is via two main stages, the oliguric and the diuretic stage.

The oliguric stage

The first stage, as the name suggests, is characterized by a much reduced urine output, of the order of 50–150 ml in 24 hours. Anuria is

Table 26.13 Causes of acute renal failure

Pre-renal causes	
Hypovolaemia	Haemorrhage Serum loss from burns Severe dehydration
Cardiogenic shock, low output	
Hepato-renal syndrome	
Renal vascular lesions	Thrombosis or emboli of renal artery Dissecting aortic aneurysms Aortic saddle embolus
Postoperative patients	Highest risk following cardiac, aortic and gastrointestinal surgery
Intra-renal causes	
Glomerulonephritis	
Haemolytic blood transfusion reaction	
Nephrotoxins	
Drugs	Phenacetin, sulphonamides, streptomycin, tetracycline, cytotoxic agents
Chemicals	Lead, mercury, carbon tetrachloride, arsenic, paraquat
Post-renal causes	
Prostatic hypertrophy Renal stones or ureteric calculi Carcinoma of cervix, pelvic malignancy Retroperitoneal fibrosis	

rare and is usually associated with post-renal obstruction. Identifying the cause is particularly important for the patient with A.R.F. Obstructive lesions may be dealt with very promptly and rapid restoration of normal renal function is very possible. Hypovolaemia can also be dealt with rapidly and successfully with appropriate fluid replacement. If, however, the oliguria persists for longer than 48 hours then several major problems may arise, the two most immediate and serious ones being hyperkalaemia and fluid overload.

Metabolic problems in acute renal failure.

Hyperkalaemia. Hyperkalaemia can become a serious problem within hours, particularly with patients suffering from severe trauma or any other condition leading to increased catabolism of damaged tissue which increases the amount of potassium in the extracellular fluids. The effects of hyperkalaemia were discussed earlier in the chapter. It is one of the main causes of death due to the onset of cardiac dysrhythmias or arrest in patients with A.R.F.

Temporary measures may be utilized to lower serum potassium levels:

- an intravenous infusion of hypertonic dextrose and insulin will cause a shift of potassium into the cells (rebound hypoglycaemia can complicate this treatment)
- infusion of sodium bicarbonate will again cause a rapid shift of potassium into the cells
- the administration of calcium helps to stabilize the cardiac cell membrane and counteract the effect of raised potassium levels (this treatment does not lower potassium levels)
- the administration of ion-exchange resins.

Long term measures for treating hyperkalaemia involve dialysis, which will be dealt with in detail later in the chapter.

Fluid overload. This can be exacerbated by either excessive oral fluid intake or intravenous therapy. Levine (1983) recommends replacing only half of the estimated deficit in the first 24 hours. Fluid replacement regimes should be based on urine output plus estimated insensible loss. The use of drugs to improve urine output seems to be an area of some contention. Lee (1982) states that there is no evidence that the use of frusemide in A.R.F. is in any way beneficial. Despite this claim, it is evident from the literature that it may be used by some doctors during the oliguric phase of A.R.F. Dopamine or dobutamine are cardiac stimulants which act on sympathetic receptors in cardiac muscle, and can be useful in patients who have a low cardiac output despite a normal circulatory volume. The use of hypertonic mannitol following fluid replacement is considered by some to be useful in the first 48 hours of A.R.F. Generally speaking, any fluid overload has to be treated with very carefully monitored replacement regimes and, if necessary, by dialysis. A useful biochemical indicator of over-hydration is the presence of hyponatraemia. This may also be exacerbated by acidosis which causes a sodium shift into the cells or vomiting and/or diarrhoea. Correction of hyponatraemia is usually achieved by controlling water intake. The use of hypertonic saline is very risky and can precipitate pulmonary oedema and/or heart failure.

Hypocalcaemia and hyperphosphataemia. These become potential problems if the oliguric phase continues for more than 7–10 days. The kidneys normally convert vitamin D into the active compound 1.25-dihydroxycholecalciferol under the influence of parathyroid hormone (see Ch. 19). This hormone promotes the gastrointestinal uptake of calcium. In A.R.F. this mechanism is impaired and may be further compromised if the patient becomes uraemic, as this also decreases calcium absorption by the gastrointestinal tract. The effects of the imbalance between these two electrolytes are mainly attributable to the hypocalcaemia. Calcium and potassium have antagonistic effects on heart muscle and a low calcium level potentiates the effect of the hyperkalaemia. Treatment is usually either the giving of intravenous calcium gluconate or activated vitamin D, 1.25-dihydroxycholecalciferol.

Uraemia. Uraemia is a toxic condition due to the inability of the kidneys to excrete urea, organic acids, potassium and other metabolic waste products. It may progress very rapidly in the first few days of oliguria in hypercatabolic patients. Lee (1982) groups patients with A.R.F. according to the rate of blood urea increases. These groups provide some rough guidelines on which to base nutritional support needs and the frequency of dialysis. Uraemic patients are very susceptible to infection and this is one of the major causes of mortality.

Metabolic acidosis. Metabolic acidosis occurs because the kidneys are unable to excrete the acidic waste products of normal metabolic processes. The net result of these acidic products (H^+) accumulating in the blood stream is a fall in pH. The body's compensatory mechanism will control the pH levels for a while. Sodium bicarbonate will buffer the hydrogen ions until falling bicarbonate levels can no longer prevent a fall in pH. Hyperventilation occurs in an effort to exhale carbon dioxide and therefore lower the level of carbonic acid in the blood. Treatment with intravenous sodium bicarbonate may be sufficient to maintain the patient until or if the diuretic phase is reached.

Anaemia. Anaemia can develop within a few days of the onset of A.R.F. due to a lack of the erythropoietin from the kidney. The anaemia is usually a normochromic normocytic type. The longevity of the red cells may be reduced if the patient is also uraemic, exacerbating the anaemic state. Acidosis may also be enhanced if the patient is anaemic, as haemoglobin also acts as a buffer for the hydrogen ions in the blood. The anaemia is usually left untreated unless other symptoms, such as hypovolaemic angina or active bleeding, occur. Fresh packed cells are given by choice, as the administration of stored blood increases potassium levels. Longer term transfusion risks include the stimulation of antibody formation which may compromise the chances of a successful transplant.

Diuretic phase

Successful management of the above problems will obviously enhance the probability of patients reaching this stage, and being out of danger. As the name suggests, the indicator that the patient has reached this phase is an increase in urine output to at least 400 ml per day. Some patients begin to pass vast quantities of urine and are ironically at risk of dehydration. Initially it is important to remember that although the kidneys are producing urine they may not be able to concentrate it. The patient remains at risk of electrolyte disturbances and possible hypovolaemia. Gradual recovery of renal function can proceed over a short period of a few days or much longer. During this time dialysis may still be necessary.

The prognosis of A.R.F. is just above 60% recovery (Lee, 1982) which is still considered to be quite poor and has not really improved over the last twenty years. However, it must be remembered that patients are now actively treated who would have been left to die twenty years ago due to lack of facilities.

Chronic renal failure

This condition is characterized by a gradual loss of functional nephrons. The main causes are listed in Table 26.14.

Chronic renal failure (C.R.F.) is a complex condition with a varied and changing pattern of problems. The failing kidney becomes progressively less able to deal with the load of electrolytes and waste products being filtered by a decreasing population of functional nephrons. The kidneys nevertheless have a remarkable compensatory capacity. Only one third of the total number of nephrons are required to deal with a normal load of waste products and prevent any harmful accumulation in the body fluids. The failing kidney function in C.R.F. should be seen as a continuum between normal function and end stage renal disease, but stages can be identified along this continuum (Oestreich, 1979).

Tale 26.14 Causes of chronic renal failure

Causes
Glomerulonephritis
Pyelonephritis
Polycystic kidneys
Hypertensive disease
Renal vascular disease
Urinary obstruction
Diabetes mellitus
Idiopathic

Stages in chronic renal failure

Reduced renal reserve. The kidneys cope normally unless some undue physiological stress is placed upon them. Blood urea levels are high normal, but the patient has no other symptoms.

Renal insufficiency. Patients have elevated blood urea levels on a normal diet. Urine concentration is impaired and the patient may be mildly anaemic.

Renal failure. The patient has many of the imbalances associated with failing kidney function. These are severe uraemia, acidosis, hyperkalaemia, anaemia, hypocalcaemia, hyperphosphataemia and impaired urine dilution.

End stage renal disease (E.S.R.D.). Renal function is severely impaired and systemic problems begin to arise in the cardiovascular, neuromuscular and gastrointestinal systems.

The problems which may arise for the patient are very dependent on the stage of the disease. A patient with renal insufficiency may manage very well with some restriction in dietary protein and salt. The major problems, which arise as the patient develops renal failure, are monitored carefully in order to prepare for the onset of E.S.R.D. and the time of decision about dialysis and/or transplantation.

Nursing considerations for the pre-dialysis patient

A detailed and systematic assessment of the patient is essential in order to plan care because of the changing, variable and progressive nature of the condition. These characteristics of the condition can also pose serious psychological and social problems alongside the physical ones. The assessment has to consider specific problems related to failing renal function, and the systemic problems which arise due to progression or inadequate control of the condition.

Fluid balance. The pattern of urinary excretion in terms of volume can vary enormously. Patients in renal failure may present with polyuria, normal volume output or oliguria, and the following information will help to establish the patient's urinary output pattern.

It is very useful to know a patient's normal weight, even approximately, and to ask if they notice any variations. A record of daily weights can be made and the daily recordings kept as a graph. A fluid intake and output chart can provide very useful information. Output recordings must include any diarrhoea, vomit or nasogastric drainage.

Insensible loss, although it cannot be measured, must be considered. An anuric patient will still lose up to 800 ml of fluid per day via perspiration, respiration and in faeces. A pyrexial or dyspnoeic patient may lose much more than this.

Patients with oliguria, i.e. urine output of 400 ml or less per 24 hours, who are drinking an unrestricted amount of fluid, will inevitably be retaining fluid. Patient assessment must include looking for signs of systemic oedema in ankle or sacral areas, and for signs of pulmonary oedema. Polyuric patients may be dehydrated.

Maintaining fluid balance is based on a simple general formula: replacement of estimated insensible loss, i.e. 500–800 ml, plus the total output of the previous 24 hours. On this regime a patient who is anuric can be controlled by replacing estimated insensible loss in every 24 hours. The daily weight recordings will reflect the accuracy of the estimated replacement volume. This kind of restriction is very difficult for patients to come to terms with. The planning of a 'drinks' regime must be done with maximum adherence to the patient's own wishes. Compliance is far more likely if the patient exercises control of his/her intake pattern within the allowance calculated. Non-compliance, which naturally manifests most commonly as excess intake, can quickly be detected by unaccountable weight gain despite a 'model' fluid balance chart. Compliance can also be improved by good oral care. If the patient is uraemic they may suffer from extreme thirst. This is thought to be due to the osmotic effect of high urea causing cellular dehydration (Metheny & Snively, 1983). Thirst cannot, in these circumstances, be taken as a guide to the patient's state of hydration.

Examination of the patient's urine is an integral part of the assessment procedure. Many of the tests form part of the laboratory-based diagnostic procedure. Ward testing by means of the commonly used 'dip stick' tests are relatively useless for renal patients because they do not provide accurate quantified information. Nurses will probably be involved in collecting 24-hour urine samples for protein loss estimation and creatinine clearance tests. A mid-stream urine specimen may also be requested for bacteriological examination.

Nutrition. Dietary restriction is one of the mainstays of treatment for patients with renal failure. Appetite may not be particularly affected if patients have an adequately controlled biochemistry unless their fluid intake is severely restricted. A dry mouth and furred tongue makes eating very difficult and this may be compounded by the fact that the food is also dry. The diet itself will be tailored to the ease with which residual renal function is able to excrete metabolic waste. The general aim of the diet is to decrease endogenous protein catabolism and the subsequent release of nitrogenous products and potassium. A high carbohydrate and high fat diet should be encouraged and, if blood urea and creatinine levels rise, low protein may be necessary. Protein content may be reduced to as little as 20 g a day, sufficient to meet maintenance and body repair needs only. In view of the risk of hyperkalaemia, the dietary potassium content must also be considered. Citrus fruits, fruit juices and bananas are all rich in potassium and should be avoided. It is unfortunate that these are all foods which would provide refreshment for patients on a restricted fluid regime. Patients with fluid overload and an excess total body sodium may also require a low sodium diet. For many this is the final insult to an already strict dietary regime.

In view of the severity of these restrictions it is

not surprising that the patient may take some time to adapt to and accept the new diet. Compliance with these severe restrictions must at times seem an impossible burden. Eating is also a social activity and patients may well feel isolated from other members of their family and friends. Holidays or even eating out will necessitate special arrangements being made and a degree of forward planning not even considered in normal circumstances. These factors can reinforce the sick role and lead to poor dietary compliance. Some patients take a fatalistic view of the situation and feel that they have little or no control over either the disease itself or their own life. The relevance of such dietary restrictions is therefore minimized and non-compliance is the consequence (Salmons, 1980). Dietary abuse has also been interpreted by some researchers as being suicidal in nature (Salmons, 1980).

Gastrointestinal disturbances. More specific gastro-intestinal problems may arise in association with the uraemic syndrome. Anorexia stimulated by the sight and/or smell of food is common. Intractable vomiting and gastritis sometimes associated with haematemesis may occur. The mucous membrane of the mouth becomes irritated and inflamed. Halitosis characterized by the smell of ammonia and a metallic taste in the mouth is also a problem. Resolution of these problems is often dependent on the commencement of dialysis, in order to control the uraemia.

Anaemia. Patients with chronic renal failure invariably suffer from a chronic anaemia with an Hb of 10–11g/dl. Its origin is multifactorial and diet is considered to be one of the components. Low haemoglobin levels will pre-dispose the patient to developing cardiac failure, particularly if he/she also has fluid overload and/or is non-compliant with sodium restriction. Patients' general energy levels will be low and allowance must be made for periods of rest.

Sexuality. Chronic renal failure can have a drastic effect on the patient's normal sexuality. Women often have amenorrhoea and may become infertile. Men may experience loss of libido and even impotence as a consequence of the illness. Over 60% of the patients surveyed by Abram et al (1975) suffered reduced or absent libido; only 20% had no alteration in sexual function.

Loss of sexual function may be related to physical factors such as hyperprolactinaemia, neuropathy and general debility (Auer, 1982). Sexual problems are often dismissed as being organic in nature (Knapp, 1982), and it is, in some instances, these factors which are the primary cause. However, anxiety, depression and the side-effects of drugs are often additive factors. Sexual problems can place a further strain on partners. Auer (1982) feels, however, that estrangement between couples is not always attributable directly to the sexual problem but to the withdrawal of affection and communication which accompanies it. The effect of an illness such as C.R.F. even with its concomitant sexual problems is not necessarily divisive, and many couples may come closer together.

Cognitive – perceptual changes. These changes are probably the most difficult to assess because of the interaction between physical and psychological factors. The degree of uraemia the patient is suffering must be assessed by monitoring the urea and creatinine levels in the blood. Uraemic patients become very apathetic and tired. Irritability and outbursts of temper or irrational behaviour may occur. Disturbances of thinking and depression will ensue as uraemia progresses. Serum urea levels of 30 mmol/l or above impair memory and the ability for abstract thought deteriorates (Salmons, 1980). Hallucinations may also occur during a uraemic phase; these are usually visual but auditory ones are also possible. These manifestations of a physical deterioration may be greatly compounded by fear and/or depression. Behavioural changes which cannot be related to a physical cause must be considered as psychological in origin.

Headaches are a frequent and distressing complaint and are associated with either hypertension and/or anxiety states. Hypertension results from a combination of fluid retention and excess renin production, and 4-hourly blood pressure monitoring is essential. Anxiety headaches are often characterized as being like a tight band around the head and are often frontal or occipital in distribution (Salmons, 1980). Analgesics tend not to be very effective in anxiety states. Nurses must take the time to ascertain the exact nature of the headache and take note of any associations with investigative or treatment procedures, as well as checking the patient's blood pressure.

Depression may also be a complication of anti-hypertensive therapy. e.g. methyldopa or propranolol (Evans & Whitlock, 1978) and this must be considered. If nurses do feel that a patient has evidence of a depressive illness over and above the effect of any biochemical or drug-related disturbances, then expert assessment is essential. The risk of a suicide attempt by a depressed patient is very real as renal patients have a higher rate of suicide than the normal population (Auer, 1982). In a small minority of patients, E.C.T. or a course of drug therapy may be required.

Metabolic acidosis. The development of metabolic acidosis may further impair the patient's neurological status. Respiratory compensation occurs and tachypnoea, worsening to a fast, deep paroxysmal pattern of breathing (Kussmaul respirations) should alert nursing staff to this problem. Blood gas changes, particularly a low pH, low bicarbonate and low PCO_2 will confirm the diagnosis. The PCO_2 level will remain low as long as the respiratory compensation mechanisms are being effective.

Skin care. Chronic anaemia and the accumulation of unexcreted bilirubin give the patient a characteristic pallid, grey-yellow complexion. Pruritus can be a serious problem and skin lesions from scratching at dry, scaly skin are common. The pruritus is probably related to the deposition of phosphate crystals (Stark & Hunt, 1983). The use of moisturizers and specific lotions to relieve the irritation may be prescribed with some effect. The damage from scratching can be minimized by keeping finger nails short, clean and smooth. The skin should also be examined for signs of purpura. This is particularly related to lack of factor III which is associated with chronic glomerulonephritis. Patients with uncontrolled uraemia may begin to excrete urea crystals via the sweat glands; this is particularly evident on the neck, forehead and nose. These patients are at special risk of skin breakdown and a 2-hourly change of position is necessary for anyone who is immobile or confined to bed for long periods. Careful inspection of the skin to ensure early detection of any breaks, due either to scratching or pressure, will enable prophylactic measures against infection to be taken.

Monitoring body temperature. Patients with renal failure have an increased susceptibility to sore throats and pulmonary infections. Four-hourly temperature monitoring will help towards early detection of this potentially serious complication. Other signs may be evident prior to the onset of pyrexia such as cough, tachypnoea of effort and tachycardia. These should be drawn to the attention of medical staff so that appropriate antibiotics can be prescribed.

Patients with uraemia may become hypothermic, even in the presence of an overt infection. This is a serious sign and is often terminal.

Systemic problems. Patients approaching E.S.R.D. may develop two other complications of renal failure. The first is osteoporosis. Hypocalcaemia provokes the release of large quantities of parathyroid hormone (P.T.H.). The high levels of P.T.H. elevate blood calcium by de-calcifying bone. Radiological review of the skeleton is necessary to monitor for this potential problem. The risk of pathological fractures arises if this problem occurs.

The second complication is pericarditis. This is quite common and arises in 30–50% of patients with E.S.R.D. (Stark, 1982).

The patient on dialysis

The time inevitably arises when a patient with renal failure can no longer be maintained on conservative treatment and a decision has to be made whether or not to offer some form of dialysis. It is beyond the remit of this chapter to discuss selection criteria and these may vary from one treatment centre to another. Suffice it to say that they do exist and that more stringent exclusion criteria are applied in relation to situations where availability of resources is sparse. Once the decision to treat a patient has been taken then two basic forms of maintenance therapy are available, peritoneal dialysis and haemodialysis.

Many patients will experience both types of

dialysis during the course of their illness. Both types of treatment can be carried out by the patients in their own homes, providing the facilities, expertise and will are forthcoming. Home dialysis is the ideal goal as it then gives the patients more autonomy, it is cheaper and statistically the patients do better. More home dialysis patients return to full time employment and the five year survival rate of 70–80% is higher in home dialysis patients (Levine, 1983).

The relative merits of the alternative forms of dialysis are not discussed here. Only the patient can determine whether the quality of life treatment offers is worth the problems, both physical and psychological, that inevitably accompany it.

Peritoneal dialysis (P.D.)

The principle underlying peritoneal dialysis was conceived as long ago as 1923 by a physician called Ganter. Its general use as a therapy for the uraemia of E.S.R.D. was not widely accepted until the late 1950s, when dialysate fluid became commercially available (Manis & Friedman, 1979). The simultaneous development of haemodialysis techniques rendered this form of long term treatment a poor relation until relatively recently, when the modified technique of continuous ambulatory peritoneal dialysis was introduced.

Principles of peritoneal dialysis. This form of treatment utilizes the peritoneum as a natural, inert semi-permeable membrane. An artificial idealized extracellular fluid, the dialysate, is instilled into the peritoneum and the toxic solutes which have accumulated in the body then diffuse across the peritoneum to equilibrate in the dialysis fluid. The rate of diffusion is mainly dependent on the concentration gradient between the body fluids and the dialysate. Other factors such as fluid temperature and molecular size also modify rates of diffusion.

The tonicity of the dialysis fluid will also affect how much fluid is withdrawn from the body during the dialysis process. The dialysing fluid is basically an isotonic solution of electrolytes with dextrose added in order to counteract the osmotic pressure of the plasma. Modifications can be made particularly in relation to the potassium and dextrose content. For hyperkalaemic patients the dialysate fluid may contain no potassium or a very low concentration in order to remove potassium from the patient. Fluid overload problems may be dealt with by using a high concentration of dextrose, forming a hypertonic dialysis fluid which will extract extra fluid. Hypertonic dialysis fluid also results in enhanced urea extraction.

Access to the peritoneum is achieved via the Tenckhoff catheter. This catheter is made of flexible silastic with lateral perforations and a hole at the distal end. It can be inserted, under local or general anaesthetic, into the bottom of the peritoneal cavity in order to maximize drainage efficiency. The catheter also has one or two special cuffs which become embedded into the subcutaneous tissues as the wound heals. This forms a very stable bond. It also helps to prevent the migration of bacteria along the outside of the catheter. The catheter exit site on the skin should be treated as a wound site and strict aseptic technique employed to dress around it after each period of dialysis.

During dialysis, 2 litres of warmed sterile dialysate fluid are run into the peritoneal cavity. The length of instillation can vary between 8 hours, if the patient is dialysing overnight, or (more usually) 2–4 hours depending on patient need. The fluid is then drained out using a simple gravity system to complete the cycle. The number of cycles required varies according to individual need.

Intermittent peritoneal dialysis (I.P.D.). Peritoneal dialysis can be used either intermittently (I.P.D.) or continuously (C.A.P.D.). The use of I.P.D. is more commonly confined to the treatment of acute renal failure or for certain types of poisoning. Salicylate and barbiturate poisoning are both amenable to treatment by peritoneal dialysis. Patients with C.R.F. do use I.P.D. as a maintenance treatment but it is the least popular of the three choices. Treatment time, which is between 9–12 hours, three or four times a week, is prohibitive for many patients.

The machine required to undergo I.P.D. independently is small and relatively simple to use without any help. The machine carries a 10 litre can of dialysing fluid and can be set to deliver a 2 litre instillation and initiate drainage on a timed cycle (Smith, 1982). An alarm on the machine will sound if insufficient fluid drains out and it will withhold the next cycle until the alarm has been dealt with, either by manual override or completion of the drainage volume. If the patient chooses to use the manual override, the machine will continue with the next cycle but the patient risks precipitating the effects of over-distension. These may include dyspnoea, nausea, vomiting, abdominal pain, the urge to defaecate and phrenic nerve pain (Ainge, 1981a). If the patient is using a hypertonic dialysis fluid (6.36% dextrose) great care must be taken to monitor fluid loss. Excess fluid and salt loss can lead to muscular cramps, nausea, vomiting and hypotension. The main risk of overnight dialysis is one of disconnection and subsequent flooding of the bed! Restless sleepers may also obstruct the patient line from the machine and prevent instillation of the dialysate. The alarm bell should awaken the patient.

Continuous ambulatory peritoneal dialysis (C.A.P.D.). A popular alternative to I.P.D. was developed 10 years ago at the University of Texas by Moncrief, Popovich and Nolph (1978) and is known popularly as C.A.P.D. This method is based on the simple principle that a continuous dialysis system would simulate more closely the normal physiological functioning of the healthy kidney. The introduction of flexible plastic containers by Oreopoulos & Robson (1978) instead of bottles greatly enhanced the popularity of the system and reduced the risk of the biggest problem with peritoneal dialysis, which is peritonitis.

Generally speaking, most patients with E.S.R.D. are suitable for treatment by C.A.P.D. Table 26.15 itemizes patients who are particularly suitable for consideration.

From Table 26.15 it can be seen that many of the criteria which may previously have been applied to exclude patients from treatment become manageable with C.A.P.D. Unfortunately some patients will continue to be excluded, and Table 26.16 indicates reasons why C.A.P.D. may be unsuitable.

Successful C.A.P.D. patients have to be well motivated, able to follow meticulously an aseptic technique consistently over what may be a very prolonged period of time.

Table 26.15 Special indications for C.A.P.D.

Vascular access problem
Severe hypertension
Impaired cardiac function
Diabetic patients
Patients over 60 years of age
Young patients — neonates
Inability to tolerate haemodialysis, for any reason

Table 26.16 Contraindications to C.A.P.D.

Blind patients	When no help available
Poor muscle co-ordination	
Peritoneal scarring or adhesions	
Abdominal hernias	
Abdominal wounds, colostomy or ileostomy	
Lumbar disk disease or spinal disorders	
Advanced pregnancy	
Impaired pulmonary function	
Lack of interest or commitment	
Poor personal hygiene standards	

The procedure itself and the equipment are the simplest of all the dialysis techniques. The Tenckhoff peritoneal catheter is used as previously described. Two litres of peritoneal dialysis fluid is run into the peritoneal cavity via a simple gravity system and left in place for 4 hours. The empty dialysis bag remains connected to the tubing and can be rolled up and placed in a holder around the patient's waist, underneath their clothing. At the end of 4 hours, the bag is simply unrolled, placed below the level of the abdomen and the fluid allowed to drain out by gravity. After drainage, a fresh bag is connected and the procedure repeated. Instillation takes approximately 10 minutes and drainage 10–20 minutes (Chang, 1981). This procedure has to be repeated 3–5 times a day, seven days a week.

Advantages of C.A.P.D. C.A.P.D. has some very obvious advantages over both I.P.D. and haemodialysis. The main one is that blood chemistry is kept more stable, the peaks and troughs experienced by patients on other forms of dialysis are avoided by its constant nature. The patients generally have a more consistent feeling of well-being and do not complain of the 'washed out' sensation reported so often by haemodialysis patients. An increased haemoglobin and haematocrit add to the patients' feeling of well being. These improved levels are thought to be due to a less restricted diet and the absence of blood loss which can accompany haemodialysis. Diabetics are more stable as they do not have to contend with sudden changes in blood sugar levels.

Protein loss, amounting to 8–12 g/day can be a problem with peritoneal dialysis. However, dietary restrictions on protein intake can be considerably relaxed and 80–100 g/day may be required to replace dialysis loss. Potassium levels need careful monitoring as hypokalaemia can occur if patients require five exchanges per day (Ainge, 1981b). Fluid and sodium intake may also be less restricted unless the patient has a particular problem with oedema and/or hypertension. Water soluble vitamins may also be lost in the peritoneal fluid and oral supplements will be required.

C.A.P.D. requires no special machinery, the patient can be completely independent and therefore in control of his/her treatment. The patient is not immobilized for any length of time and can continue with work and social activities with minimal inconvenience. The patient's home needs no modification unless storage facilities for the dialysing fluid proves to be a problem.

Problems with C.A.P.D. No system is of course problem free, including C.A.P.D. The single biggest risk is that of peritonitis, which is even higher than with the I.P.D. system. Contamination by air or touch during the bag exchange is the usual cause. The commonest organisms involved are the Staphylococcus epidermidis and Staphylococcus aureus, both normal skin flora. Gram negative organisms from the bowel account for approximately 20% of cases (Khanna & Oreopoulos, 1982). Once contamination has occurred, the peritoneal cavity and the dialysing fluid provide an ideal culture medium for the bacteria to multiply. The onset of peritonitis is usually well marked by a pyrexia, abdominal pain and clouding of the drainage fluid. Treatment is usually by lavage with intraperitoneal antibiotics. Repeated attacks of peritonitis must bring into question the suitability of the patient for this form of treatment. A new development which may help to reduce the risk of peritonitis is the germicidal chamber. The chamber uses ultraviolet light to inactivate bacteria and is applied to the connector site that links the transfer set with the outlet part of the dialysate bag.

Drainage of the peritoneal fluid may be a problem for some patients, particularly those who, for unknown reasons, produce a lot of fibrin in the peritoneal cavity which can obstruct the catheter. Drainage can be assisted by positional adjustment and raising intra-abdominal pressure by coughing.

Several more general problems are also coming to light. Obesity from the use of the hypertonic dialysing fluid can ensue due to the patient receiving extra calories. There is some evidence that triglyceride levels are elevated and the high density lipoprotein fraction decreased in some patients, leading to accelerated atherosclerosis (Levine, 1983). A degree of immunosuppression may also occur, and episodes of candida and herpes zoster infections are common. Finally, due to the persistently raised intra-abdominal pressure, abdominal hernias and uterine prolapse with rectocele or cystocele may occur.

Nursing role in relation to peritoneal dialysis. The first and most important contribution nurses have to make is towards the selection of suitable patients for long-term treatment. Nurses are in a unique position to assess patient motivation and commitment toward both learning the technique and maintaining the high standard of care required to ensure success. Once selection has been made then the nurse's aim is to help the patient towards self management and feeling confident enough to cope both physically and psycho-logically at home. Three main areas can be identified on which nurses need to focus their care:

- teaching the techniques required in order to render the patient able to manage the dialysis exchange procedure safely and efficiently
- teaching the broader aspects of self management such as fluid balance, nutritional requirements and how to recognize complications

- providing information, counselling and support to the patient and family in order to help them to cope with the emotional trauma and long-term implications of their condition.

Teaching of techniques. The first need is centred on learning two main procedures, solution exchange and care of the catheter and exit site. The importance of a meticulous and consistently excellent technique must be emphasized as a necessary prophylactic measure against peritonitis.

The principles of dialysis must be outlined and a simple explanation of the equipment and its relationship with the peritoneal cavity should be given. The use of visual aids and allowing the patient to handle the equipment will facilitate its acceptance. The mechanics of the fluid exchange, where the fluid goes to and what happens to the bag will be of particular concern to the patient. As always in these situations, another patient who is well established and coping well can be of enormous help and support to the new patient.

Selection of a suitable environment at home and if appropriate at work should be discussed with the patient and family. A room which is quiet and from which pets can be excluded is ideal. The room should contain an easily cleaned working surface and a comfortable chair which provides firm back support. The details of the exchange procedure may vary slightly from centre to centre.

Care of the catheter and exit site is equally important. Inspection of the site for redness, tenderness, swelling or signs of leakage should be carried out daily. The catheter must be checked for debris, cracks or tears. The ideal time for the patient to do this is whilst bathing or showering. Washing the site with povidone-iodine scrub is generally recommended, followed by careful drying with sterile gauze. Lotions and powders, unless prescribed for a specific purpose, should not be applied to the skin around the site. If the patient is afraid of the catheter pulling then adhesive tape can be used for extra security. Clean clothes should always be worn next to the site. The patient will be

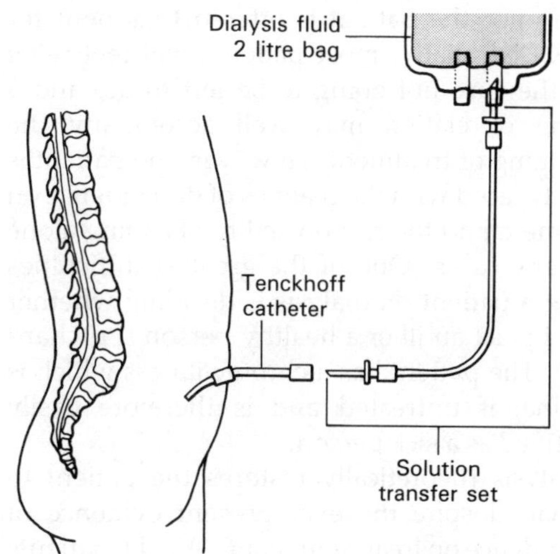

Fig. 26.4 Dialysis with a solution transfer set

required to visit Out-patients every 6 weeks for the solution transfer set to be exchanged by the nurse (see Fig. 26.4).

C.A.P.D. procedures are not complicated or difficult to learn, but they are repetitive, time consuming and demanding of care and attention every time they are carried out. Nurses concerned with teaching these procedures must have time to spend with these patients and a lot of patience. C.A.P.D. units based on general wards with no separate staff are disadvantaged as time may not be as available for patient teaching.

General management. The information the patient requires in relation to general management has already been discussed in detail. Particular care needs to be taken to ensure the patient understands how fluid balance is regulated via the use of isotonic or hypertonic dialysate. The dietician will be closely involved in planning a suitable diet to meet the particular needs of each patient.

The onset of obesity from the use of hypertonic dialysing fluid may need emphasizing if a patient is at special risk. Patient compliance will be considerably enhanced if negotiation rather than dictation is the approach adopted.

Emotional support. The family must not of course be excluded from this patient education programme, and at least one other person close to the patient should be competent to take over if the need arises. Psychological problems do not cease once the patient is offered treatment for E.S.R.D. Initially, most patients will feel relief that they are not going to be left to die and a feeling of elation may well accompany the beginning of treatment. However, the patient is quickly faced with the realities of dependence on treatment and the responsibility of coping alone in many cases. One of the greatest difficulties facing a patient on dialysis is deciding whether he is in fact an ill or a healthy person (Pritchard 1982). The patient has a chronic illness which is terminal if untreated and is therefore easily identified as a sick person.

Dialysis theoretically restores the patient to normal, despite the ever present evidence of dependence on treatment. For C.A.P.D. patients this problem is compounded by the incessant nature of the treatment, with no breaks. A survey of 30 patients after a mean period of seven months on C.A.P.D. showed that 21 could forget they were on treatment most of the time. Women under 30 years had the greatest difficulty forgetting about it (Travenol, 1984). The commonest problem with C.A.P.D. patients is obsessional cleanliness and attention to detail. This may be safer for the patient from the point of view of preventing peritonitis, but could have serious repercussions on family life. Children in particular could be affected by being denied physical contact if they have dirty clothes or hands.

Body image change is also a particular problem for C.A.P.D. or I.P.D. patients, and this may be particularly pertinent to the women under 30 mentioned in the Travenol survey. The patients constantly have an extra two litres of fluid in their abdomen which creates a permanent state of distension. This has a direct and obvious effect on the type of clothes the patient can wear. Patients may well feel that this detracts from their sexual image and could lead to relationship difficulties.

Nursing intervention in these areas has to be directed at building the type of relationship that allows for discussion of these feelings to take place. The nurse dealing with patients in Outpatients should pay attention to the psychological state on each six week visit, and be prepared to offer advice and/or counselling if necessary.

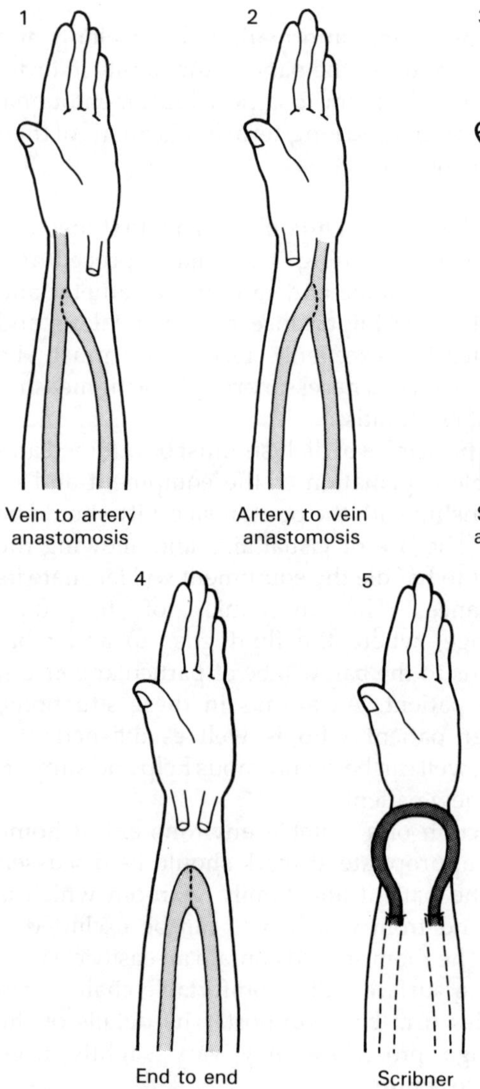

Fig. 26.5 Sites for haemodialysis.

Haemodialysis

This is a process whereby an artificial membrane is used in an external apparatus through which blood is circulated, either via an arteriovenous loop using blood pressure to provide flow or a vein-vein loop with pump-assisted flow. The system delivers the patient's anti-coagulated blood to one side of the artificial membrane and dialysis fluid to the opposite side of the membrane.

Haemodialysis is an expensive form of treatment but time has proven its effectiveness and reliability. Preparation should ideally commence about 3 months before the treatment is actually required. One of the reasons is to allow time for preparation of the vascular access site. The first commonly used device for vascular access was the external arteriovenous shunt developed by Scribner in 1960 (see Fig. 26.5). The shunt is usually placed in the forearm and joins an artery and vein by means of a length of Teflon tubing. It is rarely used now for long-term haemodialysis but may be the first choice for patients with reversible A.R.F. or for those requiring dialysis for self-poisoning. Its use long-term is prohibited by three main complications:

- a tendency to clot
- infection, which is usually confined to a localized cellulitis but may develop into septicaemia
- dislodgement, which can prove life-threatening from arterial bleeding.

The more recent and popular method of vascular access is via an arteriovenous fistula (see Fig. 26.5). The creation of a fistula results in enlargement and arterialization of the anastomosed vein. The vein can then be successfully used as an access site for haemodialysis. The fistula requires 3 to 6 months to mature into a suitable site. The most popular placement sites are the forearm or upper arm on the patient's non-dominant side.

Several complications can occur at the arteriovenous fistula site:

- thrombosis, usually precipitated by extrinsic pressure from bandages which are too tight or from poor positioning
- venous hypertension resulting in the hand swelling—this is generally expected in the early post-formation period but can become debilitating if it continues for a long period: the oedema may be relieved by elevation of the arm and special hand exercises
- ischaemia of the fingers, known as 'steal syndrome' — the incidence of this is less than 2% of the patients with fistulae, but it can be very serious, leading to gangrene in some cases
- aneurysms may develop, which are related to repeated venepunctures at the same site — this can be avoided by the patient rotating sites to allow for healing and to prevent the formation of excessive scar tissue
- haematoma formation at the puncture site
- fistulae result in an increased cardiac output of approximately 10% — this could precipitate cardiac failure in some at risk patients
- infection, most commonly at the puncture site or on the suture line. The incidence is approximately 1% (Lancaster, 1979).

In this immediate pre-dialysis period, ideally the patient should be given the opportunity to look around the haemodialysis unit in which they will start their treatment. Talking to other patients well established on treatment may help them to express any anxieties they may have about venepuncture or seeing their own blood circulate outside their body. Every effort should be made to allay any anxieties they have and to answer all their questions, several times over if need be!

The principle underlying haemodialysis is the same as peritoneal dialysis. The difference lies in the use of an external artificial semi-permeable membrane instead of a natural internal one. The characteristics of the membrane itself are designed to ensure clearance of all toxic solutes. Recent modifications to membrane design have been based on a theory by Scribner's group, called the 'middle molecule theory' (Babb et al, 1971). This theory is based on the idea that the uraemic syndrome may be caused by a molecule other than urea and creatinine, a larger sized molecule known as a 'middle molecule'. Removal of these 'middle molecules', because of their higher molecular weight, requires slower flow rates of blood and dialysate and a larger surface area (Manis & Friedman, 1979). The most recent membranes have been designed to facilitate removal of these middle molecules. This theory is by no means accepted by all nephrologists.

Patients on haemodialysis typically undergo 3 treatments per week for a period of 4–6 hours.

Many patients do successfully transfer to home dialysis but a percentage remain dependent on hospital dialysis care.

Haemodialysis procedure. Before dialysis commences the nurse must undertake a thorough assessment of the patient. All the vital signs are checked. Temperature and pulse recordings are taken to screen for any signs of infection. A hypothermia may be indicative of an elevated blood urea. Patients with E.S.R.D. are particularly susceptible to respiratory infection and therefore special note should be taken of respiratory rate and rhythm, or the presence of a cough and/or wheeze. A lying and standing blood pressure is checked and compared with previous recordings. Hypertension is a common complication of renal failure and medication adjustments may be necessary. The patient's pre-dialysis weight is extremely important and must be compared, ideally, with the patient's known 'dry weight' and previous pre-dialysis weights. Excessive inter-dialysis weight gain could indicate patient non-compliance with fluid regimes and should be explored. Systemic checks for oedema of the feet, ankles, hands and peri-orbital regions should also be made. The patient may have other problems which need discussing such as nausea, headaches or dietary restrictions. The patient's mental state should be carefully noted during this assessment. Depression or inappropriate expressions of anger and defiance could accompany physical evidence of non-compliance and may indicate a maladaptive coping response to the pressures of treatment.

The medical staff will also wish to assess the patient's biochemical status with particular reference to blood urea, creatinine and electrolyte levels. The patient's clotting time should also be checked prior to starting dialysis.

From the results of this assessment a decision will be made on how much weight loss, i.e. fluid removal, the patient requires and the electrolyte adjustments to be made during dialysis. The haemodialyser is then primed with the required dialysate, making sure that all air is removed from the blood and dialysate channels.

During dialysis the blood is anti-coagulated and heparin is used for this purpose. Anticoagulation is most commonly achieved by using a continuous infusion pump attached to the arterial inlet channel. The heparin is then deactivated by protamine sulphate just before the blood is returned to the patient. Blood flow through the dialyser is started very slowly initially and reaches optimum flow within thirty minutes. During this time the nurse must monitor the patient carefully for signs of hypotension. One of the early signs is an increase in diastolic pressure, a compensatory sign which occurs just prior to the development of hypotension. The patient may complain of nausea and feeling faint and thirsty. Restlessness, excessive perspiration and confusion can accompany this state. In order to deal with this problem the blood flow rate through the dialyser should be reduced and the patient's legs elevated. A bolus dose of 100–500 ml of normal saline will help to boost blood volume, but if the condition is severe an intravenous colloid osmotic agent may be required (Lancaster 1979). Following administration of such treatment, a careful watch must be kept for the development of pulmonary oedema.

As dialysis proceeds, the patient's weight must be monitored and this is usually achieved by the use of bed scales. It is essential to note carefully exactly what was on the bed when the pre-dialysis weight was taken. The accumulation of food trays, books or clothes will give erroneous weight results during dialysis and may lead to excess fluid removal! The patient's temperature, pulse, blood pressure and respiratory status are checked at pre-determined intervals during the dialysis period. It is quite acceptable for patients to eat and/or drink during their dialysis period. Some treatment centres allow dietary relaxation during the first 2–3 hours so that the patients can indulge in their favourite forbidden food. This policy is severely criticized in other centres and strict adherence to fluid and diet requirements maintained.

One of the greatest problems for the patient is boredom, which is exacerbated by very restricted mobility. Diversionary activities such as television, reading or crafts should be freely allowed, providing they are not a nuisance to other patients. Some activity should be encouraged and a change of position at least every two hours is desirable. The nursing staff should take every opportunity to encourage dialogue not only between themselves and patients, but amongst the patients. Sharing common problems and possible solutions may be very helpful, particularly if the patients are new to the unit and/or treatment regime. The experience may also be one of learning as well as teaching for the doctors and nurses on the units.

Patient medications may be withheld immediately before and during dialysis if they are known to be removed by the treatment. Anti-hypertensive drugs should not be given for a few hours before, during or immediately after dialysis, because of the risk of hypotension. The body's compensatory mechanisms are impaired by anti-hypertensive drugs and will not be able to operate when blood is diverted through the dialyser.

During dialysis, blood tests for urea, creatinine and electrolyte levels will be checked. The patient's clotting time will also be monitored to ensure that the heparin is being inactivated before blood is returned to the patient's circulation.

Termination of dialysis is a quick and straightforward process, providing the nurse and/or patient take meticulous care. The heparin infusion is usually discontinued approximately fifteen minutes before termination, and the patient's clotting time is checked to ensure it is back to normal. The arterial line is connected to a normal saline (0.9%) infusion and the dialyser flushed through to ensure maximum return of blood volume to the patient. If the patient has an arteriovenous fistula, then a pressure dressing must be applied to the venepuncture sites to prevent haemorrhage. Immediately after the termination of dialysis the patient's temperature, pulse and blood pressure are taken for comparison with pre-dialysis levels. The patient's weight is also checked to ensure that fluid balance targets have been met.

Haemodialysis problems. One of the most important jobs of the nurse supervising haemodialysis is to ensure patient safety. The nurse must be aware of the potential complications of this procedure and be able to carry out appropriate actions. The main problems are discussed below:

Hypotension. This is probably the commonest intra-dialysis problem and it has been dealt with in relation to patient care above. Persistent hypotension, after the termination of dialysis is usually related to postural changes and is due to excessive fluid removal. These patients are very sensitive to small volume changes and replacement therapy may not be necessary (Levine 1983). A small bolus intravenous injection of normal saline 100–200ml may be given if the hypotension persists beyond a few hours after dialysis.

Dialysis disequilibrium syndrome. This is a potentially very dangerous problem and patients are most at risk during their first two or three treatment sessions. The cause is thought to be the rapid reduction of serum urea levels during dialysis. The rate of serum removal of urea is faster than the rate at which brain cells can transfer urea to the serum. This results in a urea gradient building up between the brain cells and serum. Urea is an osmotic solute which will cause water to move across into the brain cells, causing cerebral oedema.

The patient will initially complain of headaches, nausea and vomiting. A bradycardia and hypertension develop as intracranial pressure rises. If no treatment is given the condition will culminate in convulsions, coma and death.

Prevention is obviously the primary aim in dealing with a condition of this seriousness. The use of a hypertonic dialysate may help to prevent the rapid fall in urea which is thought to precipitate this condition. Shorter and more frequent periods of dialysis may be necessary to prevent high blood urea levels occurring. The underlying cause of high urea levels may need investigating, particularly if dietary non-compliance is a possible cause. Patient education and counselling is essential if this proves to be the case. Prophylactic anti-convulsant therapy may be considered for patients starting on haemodialysis treatment or for patients at special risk.

Haemorrhage. The patient is at risk of haemorrhage because of two main factors: heparinization of his/her blood, and equipment connecting circulatory access to the haemodialyser. Dislodgment of needles from access sites, separation of blood lines or rupture of the dialyser membrane can all lead to serious and rapid blood loss. Meticulous checking of the equipment in the pre-dialysis preparation and firm strapping of needles in the circulatory access sites is essential. The patient must take great care not to move too far, trap or tangle the lines. The risk from heparinization is related to inadequate deactivation by protamine sulphate. If the patient is also hypertensive, then they may be vulnerable to intracerebral haemorrhage or development of a subdural haematoma following minimal trauma (Levine, 1983). Table 26.17 summarizes other potential problems.

Home dialysis. Approximately two-thirds of the patients who are on a haemodialysis programme carry out their treatment at home. This is very desirable for two main reasons, it is less costly and patient mortality is reduced. More patients on home dialysis return to full time employment and the risk of hepatitis is considerably reduced.

Patient selection for home dialysis is dependent on three main factors:

- suitable home facilities and/or the availability of grants to make any alterations necessary to facilitate home dialysis
- willingness of the patient and family to take on the responsibility of home care — evidence of coercion by the patient or the family must be carefully examined
- the patient and family must be able to master the practical skills involved and understand potential problems which may occur.

Learning the practical skills involved demands time, patience and repetition and can be mastered successfully by most patients. Dealing with the complex psychological reactions which may accompany the idea of home dialysis is less straightforward.

Reactions to the thought of home dialysis can vary enormously. Unwillingness to learn, 'indifference' to treatment or even denial of the need are not uncommon reactions (Auer, 1982). Defiance and resentment towards renal unit staff may be the outward manifestations of quite normal fears. Anxieties over the reliability of the machine, handling the apparatus and performing self-venepuncture in the absence of professional support may well affect willingness to learn (Pritchard, 1982). These defence mechanisms should not be challenged unless they are leading to serious problems of non-compliance or refusal of treatment. The defence mechanisms will be abandoned as the patient feels ready to face the challenge.

Table 26.17 Potential problems associated with haemodialysis

Problem	Possible causes
Air embolism	Leaks or loose connections in blood lines Retained air in dialyser Blood pump producing suction in arterial line
Pyrogen reactions	Contaminated dialysate Bacteraemia
Haemolysis	Hypo-osmolar dialysis and resultant water intoxication Copper poisoning (rare)
Hyperthermia	Malfunctioning thermostat

The dialysis helper, commonly the patient's spouse, will also be in need of professional support, sometimes even more so than the patient. If the patient has been the dominant partner, he or she may well resent becoming dependent on the helper. The helper's confidence may be sapped by the patient's display of irritation at their clumsiness or slowness to learn (Auer, 1982). The previous relationship may take a dramatic change of course with the patient taking on a dependent, child-like role, particularly within an over-protective family.

One of the factors which may provide an incentive towards self-care is returning to work. This can provide a vital morale booster, restoring self-esteem and confidence. A successful transition to home dialysis can come as an enormous relief to some patients. Dialysis time can be adjusted to suit work and/or family commitments. The patient is no longer tied to the costly and time consuming exercise of travelling to the hospital three times a week.

Renal transplantation

This is the ultimate hope of every patient being treated for E.S.R.D. The success of the transplantation scheme is of course entirely reliant on the supply of transplantable kidneys. There are two potential sources of kidneys, living relative donors (L.R.D.) and cadaver kidneys. Every year an estimated 4,000 cases of brain death occur of which approximately 10% are used as transplant donors (Bradley & Selwood, 1983). The waiting list of potential recipients for these cadaver kidneys doubles every four years. Despite variations in the criteria applied for selecting suitable patients for transplantation, the major limiting factor remains the shortage of transplantable kidneys. This problem is compounded by the fact that a proportion of patients on the waiting list are waiting for a second or subsequent transplant.

The transplantation service is co-ordinated nationally by the United Kingdom Transplant Service (U.K.T.S.), established in 1972. The U.K.T.S. keeps records of all patients awaiting a transplant and provides an organ matching service. Each year it produces the U.K. Transplant Report which details every transplant undertaken for the preceding year. Local contact with the U.K.T.S. is mediated via regional transplant co-ordinators, first introduced in 1979 (Taber, 1982a). This role is fulfilled by a variety of professional health workers, including nurses. Their role includes improving organ procurement by liaison with professional colleagues about the characteristics of potential donors. The medical and nursing profession regard their immediate patient as their priority, quite correctly, but all too often the further possibility of them becoming organ donors is not considered. Doctors and nurses need definitive guidelines about the criteria and procedure involved in organ recovery.

In relation to the general public, the role of the transplant co-ordinator and of other medical and nursing staff is to help to dispel the misconceptions surrounding the issue of organ donors. One of the issues which has caused concern amongst the public, via the media, is the issue of brain death and the subsequent artificial maintenance of 'life' in order to preserve transplantable organs. However, many people do carry kidney donor cards and the Kidney Patients Association has helped to raise the conscience of the general public.

The use of living relative donors poses an entirely different set of ethical issues. Matches between identical twins are ideal and success is almost 100% in these cases. However, great care must be taken to ensure that the donor has not been placed under any family pressure or coercion to do something against his or her will. The recipient has also to live with an eternal sense of gratitude and a lifetime of worry about the continued health of the donor. Despite the high success rate of L.R.D. the issues mentioned require very careful consideration. The risk of death to a L.R.D. is very small, approximately 3 per 1000, and life expectancy postoperatively is virtually normal (Levine 1983).

Pre-transplant considerations

Not all patients on long term maintenance dialysis will be considered suitable for transplantation. The selection criteria are becoming more liberal but patients with multiple systemic complications or a concomitant chronic disease, e.g. diabetes, may be excluded. Statistically mortality rates do begin to rise in recipients of 50 years or over, and this must be considered.

Psychological stability should also be assessed although many problems generated by the stress of chronic dialysis may be improved by transplantation (Cianci et al, 1981).

Once a potential donor has been identified, then tissue typing is the first major step. This procedure is more accurately known as HLA (Human Leucocyte Antigens) typing. There are five main HLA loci on chromosomes for the A,B,C,D and DR loci. Until 1981 the U.K.T.S. matched donors and recipients for the HLA A and B loci only. This, however, despite seemingly good matches, still produced inconsistencies in the predicted survival rates. Since July 1981 the DR locus has also been included in the matching procedure by the U.K.T.S. However, it is technically more difficult to perform and not all tissue typing laboratories are able to perform the test (Tate, 1982). One further vital test must be performed and that is to see if antibodies against donor lymphocytes are circulating in the recipient's serum. If they are present then transplantation is contraindicated.

Once a suitable match has been made then the potential recipient has to be informed and prepared. The renal transplant recipient may experience many emotions when the moment he or she has been waiting for, sometimes for several years, finally arrives. Fear as well as excitement must colour this time. If the patient has been properly prepared he or she will be aware that success is by no means guaranteed and some doubts about going through the whole traumatic procedure must arise. Prior to surgery every effort should be made to ensure that the patient is in an optimum physical and mental condition. A series of checks and tests are necessary, which are itemized in Table 26.18. The exclusion of an infective locus is of particular importance because of the immunosuppressive therapy required postoperatively. In some cases elective bilateral nephrectomy may be carried out. This includes patients with polycystic kidneys, uncontrollable hypertension or kidney infection. Dialysis may be indicated prior to surgery to improve the patient's biochemical status. Pre-transplant transfusion may also be carried out as there is evidence to suggest that graft survival is thereby enhanced. The reason for this is unknown.

The immediate pre-operative care is similar to any standard preparation and will not be detailed further.

Table 26.18 Pre-transplant medical checklist

Exclusion of malignant disease — the one absolute contraindication to transplantation
Barium meal and/or endoscopy to exclude peptic ulceration
Urological survey to exclude or identify obstructive lesions or polycystic disease
Skeletal survey to assess for osteoporosis
Cardiovascular assessment for cardiac or peripheral vascular disease due to atherosclerosis

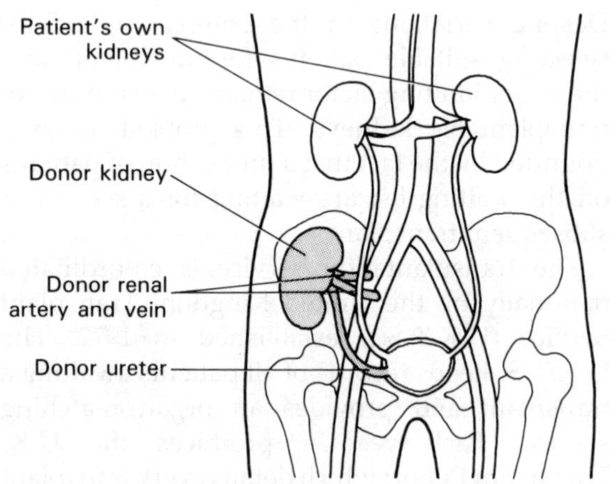

Fig. 26.6 Position of transplanted kidney.

Transplant procedure and postoperative care

The new kidney is placed in the right or left iliac fossa, outside the peritoneal cavity. The renal vessels of the donor kidney are anastomosed to the patient's iliac artery and vein and the ureter into the patient's bladder (see Fig. 26.6). The transplanted kidney can and sometimes does begin producing urine even before the patient leaves the operating table. Particular care has to be taken in the intra-operative period to ensure that the patient does not become hypovolaemic.

The early postoperative period is particularly critical as the patient will be receiving high doses of immunosuppressive drugs. The treatment is started as soon as the operation is completed to try and prevent graft rejection. Table 26.19 gives an indication of the range of drugs commonly used for immunosuppression therapy (Taber, 1982b).

There are four main aims of postoperative care (Maguire, 1982):

- prevention of infection
- on-going management of renal failure
- diagnosis and treatment of rejection
- preparation for discharge.

Prevention of infection. The patient is reverse barrier nursed as soon as the operation is over in order to protect him or her against infection. A minimal number of doctors and nurses should be involved in carrying out care

Table 26.19 Immunosuppressive drugs

Drug	Action	Side-effects
Azathioprine	Anti-metabolite: interferes with the synthesis of nucleic acid bases and therefore DNA and RNA	Leukopenia Toxic hepatitis Stomatitis Alopecia Gastrointestinal disturbances
Steroids	Lympholytic agent: combats cellular rejection	Pituitary-adrenal suppression Peptic ulcers Osteoporosis Cushing's syndrome Increased infection risk
Cyclosporin	Fungal metabolite: effective in host versus graft reactions	Hepatoxic Gum hyperplasia Hirsutism
Anti-lymphocyte serum	Inhibits lymphocyte function	Thrombocytopenia Fever Anaphylactic reactions
Plasmaphoresis	Vascular graft rejection, plasma exchange regimen not of proven value	

during any one shift. Any nurses with a cold or other minor infection should not be allowed near the patient. Visitors must also be restricted for several days and likewise not allowed to see the patient if they have had contact with or have signs of any infection. Wound care should be minimal and it should only be redressed if evidence of excess leakage or infection occurs. The patient will be catheterized for the first few days postoperatively and this forms an obvious focus for infection. Meticulous aseptic technique must be employed for catheter care, bladder irrigation, specimen collecting and emptying and/or changing catheter bags. Bacteriological screening may be carried out at pre-determined intervals on wound swabs, urine samples, blood cultures and other susceptible sites.

On-going management of renal failure. It is important that the patient fully understands that the transplanted kidney may not start working immediately. Even if it does produce urine its concentrating capacity will be imperfect initially. This means that the patient must continue all the care necessary for someone with E.S.R.D. Fluid balance especially must be very carefully monitored. The patient should be weighed, using bed scales, immediately postoperatively. Fluid replacement will be intravenous initially and is calculated on urine output volume and estimated insensible loss. Urine output should be measured hourly and the catheter carefully checked for patency if the patient appears anuric.The urine is likely to be bloodstained for the first 24–48 hours postoperatively and clot formation may cause urinary retention and strain on the bladder anastomosis. If catheter irrigation is considered necessary it must be done very carefully, with a low volume input in order to avoid over-distension of the bladder. Oral fluid replacement should be possible within 2–3 days and the catheter removed as soon as possible after this. Renal function tests will be monitored daily and dialysis may well be necessary in the early postoperative phase. A restricted protein, high calorie diet will be continued, with possible sodium and potassium restriction. The patient may well find the continuation of this treatment very depressing after the initial elation over receiving a transplant. Acute tubular necrosis may complicate renal transplantation and this may necessitate the continuation of dialysis for up to four weeks (Levine 1983).

Diagnosis and treatment of rejection. Recognition of the early signs of rejection is vital if treatment is to be effective. Acute rejection may occur anytime between 0–30 days after the transplant. The signs include tenderness and enlargement of the graft accompanied by pyrexia and hypertension. Urinary output falls and laboratory tests usually confirm rising blood urea and creatinine levels. The patient feels ill, lethargic and, not unreasonably, very anxious. Steroids form the mainstay of treatment for acute rejection. Infection is the major threat to all transplant patients at this time and is the main cause of death during the first three post-operative months (Bradley & Selwood, 1983).

Preparation for discharge. Assuming all goes well in the early postoperative period the patients are usually mobile, eating and drinking by the third or fourth day. Reverse barrier nursing can be stopped when sutures, drains and catheter have all been removed and the patient is apyrexial and feeling well.

The psychological well-being of the patient must not be ignored. Most patients feel quite elated in the early postoperative phase. Some patients may feel very anxious if they have received a kidney from a person of the opposite sex; adolescents are particularly prone to this problem (Salmons, 1980). Four stages of reaction to transplant surgery are described by Nelson (1978):

- Foreign body stage. The patients feel that the new kidney 'sticks out' and that it feels funny. They try and protect the new organ from physical trauma and treat it as being very fragile.
- Partial internalization follows, indicated by a falling away of interest and pre-occupation in the transplant.
- Complete internalization is denoted by the fact that the patient is unaware of his new organ unless asked about it. This may take up to two years to achieve.
- Regression to the foreign body stage can occur whenever investigations or checks on the organ's functional status are performed.

These stages form a useful guideline for nurses to assess a patient's level of adaptation to the new organ. Preparation for discharge also requires the patient to relinquish a long standing 'sick role' and face a normal lifestyle.

It is important that nurses help the patient to master certain new self-care skills prior to discharge.

Responsibility for self-medication is one very important aspect as the patient will be taking low dosage immunosuppressive therapy for the life-span of the kidney. Recognition of the signs of rejection must be taught, without making the patient too afraid of every minor ache and pain. The need for dietary restrictions is dependent on the adequacy of renal function and whether or not the patient is hypertensive. Generally speaking it will be far more liberal a diet than the pre-transplant one. Patients are taught how to take their own temperature and are advised to monitor this and their weight daily after discharge.

Survival rates following transplantation vary from centre to centre. In 1980, 680 cadaveric transplants were carried out, of which 61% of first grafts and 52% of second grafts survived 6 months (Bradley & Selwood, 1983). There is little doubt that the improved quality of life following successful kidney transplant far outweighs the risks for the majority of patients with E.S.R.D.

COMMON RENAL DISORDERS

Renal pathology can be studied in relation to the three main causative catagories, inflammatory, infective and obstructive disorders.

Inflammatory renal disease

Nephritis is the global term used to cover the spectrum of inflammatory conditions which can affect the kidney. The area of the kidney most commonly affected is the glomeruli, although the tubules can also be involved.

Glomerulonephritis may be a primary condition or one which is secondary to a systemic disease. The primary form of the disease shows a complex variety of pathological features which have many presenting symptoms in common. Children as well as adults may be susceptible to this condition and it is one of the commonest causes of renal failure.

The majority of these patients present with what is known as the nephrotic syndrome. The main features of this syndrome are proteinuria and consequent hypoalbuminaemia, oedema and hyperlipidaemia.

Nursing care considerations

Patient assessment usually reveals a lethargic, anorexic and sometimes pyrexial patient. A proportion of these patients will have had a streptococcal throat infection approximately two weeks prior to the onset of renal symptoms. The renal response is not due directly to the bacteria but is associated with an antigen-antibody reaction. Oedema becomes clinically manifest very rapidly and is present in the patient's face, ankles and legs. In extreme cases ascites may also occur. Urinalysis will reveal a heavy proteinuria and in some cases a haematuria. Urine output is markedly decreased. Hypertension may occur as a consequence of the salt and water retention.

Bed rest is important in the initial stages as it appears to aid recovery. The oedema and oliguria make fluid balance one of the major nursing problems. Fluid restriction may not necessarily be imposed immediately, this is dependent on the degree of oedema and response to treatment. Daily weights and/or an intake/output chart need to be recorded. Daily girth measurements may be taken to assess the effectiveness of oedema control. Blood pressure recording should be made at least once daily and more frequently if it continues to rise. Antihypertensive therapy is sometimes necessary to achieve adequate control. Dietary considerations are dependent on the degree of protein loss in the urine and the patient's blood urea levels. Initially a high protein diet may be given in order to replace urinary loss and correct hypoalbuminaemia. However, if blood urea levels rise and the patient's condition does not resolve then protein restriction may become necessary. A no-added-salt diet will help to resolve the oedema.

Medical treatment revolves around the use of steroid therapy, which is not always effective. The prognosis is uncertain, some patients will respond quickly within a week and recover completely. Others will apparently recover only to suffer recurrent relapses, and the remainder develop renal failure.

Infective renal disease

The renal tract is normally sterile, free from all commensal bacteria, but it remains the commonest area of bacterial infection in our society (Levine 1983). There are two main clinical problems: pyelonephritis and cystitis.

Pyelonephritis

This may be an acute or chronic condition and is probably much more common than the rate of diagnosis may suggest. It is thought that a large number of sufferers remain either asymptomatic or have symptoms not commonly associated with a typical renal infection.

Patients with pyelonephritis usually present with high pyrexia, often above 40°C, loin pain, nausea and vomiting. Urine output may be low and urinalysis usually shows albuminuria and haematuria. The patient feels ill and frequently complains of all the general symptoms associated with fever e.g. weakness, malaise, aching joints and anorexia. Rigors are not uncommon if patients develop hyperpyrexia. A mid-stream specimen of urine for culture and sensitivity is necessary in order to determine the most appropriate antibiotic to be used.

Nursing strategies are primarily related to the care of a pyrexial patient, which is discussed in Chapter 27. Fluid balance is particularly important due to the risk of dehydration from insensible loss and from the point of view of renal function. The majority of patients fully recover and experience no further problems.

Repeated infections may lead to chronic pyelonephritis and the formation of scar tissue in the renal tissue. An obstructive lesion may occur as a consequence and a few patients will eventually develop renal failure.

Cystitis

This condition causes inflammation of the urinary

bladder and is more common in women than men. The most common cause is urinary contamination from the enteric bacteria Escherichia coli. Incidence is extremely high and an estimated 25 to 35% of the female population in the childbearing years will experience an attack of cystitis. Potential sufferers are particularly at risk with the onset of sexual activity and pregnancy (Sheahan & Seabolt, 1982).

Onset of the condition is characterized by dysuria, frequency of micturition, urgency often accompanied by stress incontinence, and occasionally haematuria. These symptoms can be extremely incapacitating and their disruptive effect on the patient's lifestyle should not be underestimated.

Most cases respond well to antibiotics. Various medications are also available which alter the pH of the urine and help to alleviate the dysuria. Copious fluids are also advisable, although sometimes patients resist this suggestion because of the resulting frequency of micturition and accompanying pain.

The main focus of care should be preventative, as many attacks of cystitis are avoidable with revised personal hygiene habits. After micturition women should be very careful to clean themselves by wiping anterior to posterior, and therefore avoid transferring organisms from the rectum to the urethra. Wipes should of course only be used once. Lubrication during intercourse may also be advisable to prevent trauma.

Obstructive renal disease

Obstructive lesions of the urinary tract may occur at almost any level. Common areas are the urethra, bladder neck, ureter and renal pelvis. Table 26.20 summarizes the main causes. The patient may present with a variety of symptoms depending on the cause and severity of the condition. Some patients may present for the first time with acute or chronic renal failure if the obstruction is bilateral. More common complaints are related to problems with micturition, frequency, difficulty in voiding, dribbling and nocturia. Unilateral obstruction can be more difficult to detect as it can remain

Table 26.20 Obstructive lesions of the urinary tract

Level of obstruction	Type of obstructive lesion
Kidney	Renal calculi Tumour Multicystic disease
Ureter	Stricture Tumour Adynamic segment Blood clots Calculi
Bladder	Tumour Blood clots Neurogenic bladder
Urethra and bladder neck	Enlarged prostate (benign or malignant) Stricture Phimosis
Extra-renal causes	Disease of female reproductive tract: tumours of cervix, uterus or ovary Retroperitoneal fibrosis Haematoma Malignancy Aortic aneurysm

unsymptomatic for some period of time. The first indication of a problem may be loin pain or the onset of renal colic. Untreated obstructive lesions may become complicated by a superimposed infection resulting in pyelonephritis.

Renal calculi

Renal calculi are a common cause of unilateral obstructive renal disease. There are various types of renal calculi, the commonest being formed from calcium. They may be present for some time with the patient remaining asymptomatic. This situation is dramatically altered if the stone moves from the renal pelvis down the ureter. If the stone is wider in diameter than the ureter then the patient will develop acute renal colic. This presents as an excruciating spasmodic pain which begins in the loin and spreads or moves down to the groin area as the stone is pushed down the ureter by strong peristaltic waves. Patients are very restless, pale and sweaty during an attack and frequently have nausea and vomiting due to the pain.

Management. Immediate care is obviously related to pain relief and a strong analgesic, such as pethidine 100mg, plus an antispasmodic drug may be required. If the nausea and vomiting are severe an anti-emetic may be administered and the patient carefully observed for signs of dehydration. Bilateral obstruction from the movement of renal calculi is uncommon but possible and can lead to the onset of acute renal failure. Careful check must be kept on urinary elimination patterns. Any urine which is passed should be strained in order to detect any stones passed. Most renal stones are passed within one week of the onset of problems (Levine, 1983). Surgical intervention is indicated in the remainder of cases.

Prior to surgery it is obviously important to locate exactly where the stone is and to assess renal function. The patient will require abdominal X-rays and specific renal radiological assessment by intravenous pyelogram or retrograde pyelogram. The non-invasive investigation of ultrasound may also be useful. If there is a possibility that the stone is in the bladder then a cystoscopy may be performed. Stones can be removed directly if they are quite small, or bigger stones may be crushed and the gravel passed spontaneously in the urine.

Surgical treatment is dependent on the position of the stone:

- renal pelvis — nephrolithotomy
- ureter — ureterolithotomy
- bladder — cystotomy.

Occasionally a nephrectomy is necessary, and it is very important that the patient is reasured that it is quite possible to live a normal life with one kidney.

The care of patients undergoing renal surgery is similar to that of patients having other operations, and is dealt with in Chapter 17.

CONCLUSION

The spectrum of renal disease pathology ranges from the nuisance value of mild cystitis to life-threatening renal failure. Within this spectrum the rapid evolution of treatment for renal failure by dialysis and/or transplantation has resulted in a specialized field of care in which nurses have a major role to fulfil. Working with renal patients demands a range of skills both physical and psycho-social which can only be achieved via a sound knowledge base and high level of commitment and understanding. It demands a level of sharing of technical knowledge and expertise between carers and patients which is difficult to parallel in any other field of care. The future of renal transplantation and dialysis should be an optimistic one as the intricacies of the autoimmune system are understood and the lessons of thirty years of experience are learnt. It is interesting that the major cautionary note is still being generated by the ethical considerations surrounding the whole issue of transplant surgery. The term 'brain death' and the criteria by which it is decided is regularly questioned, both within the health professions and in the media. As indicated earlier, the major limiting factor in the treatment regime is the shortage of transplantable kidneys. The public debate on brain death is not helping to ease this problem. Perhaps the final responsibility of nurses towards their patients is to take an active part in this debate.

REFERENCES

Abram H, Sheridan L R, Epstein W F 1975 Sexual functioning in patients with chronic renal failure. Journal of Nervous and Mental Disorders 160(3):220

Ainge R M 1981a Intermittent peritoneal dialysis. Nursing Times 77(43):1839–1840

Ainge R M 1981b Continuous ambulatory peritoneal dialysis. Nursing Times 77(38):1036–1038

Auer J 1982 Renal replacement therapy 9–1 Psychological problems in long-term care. Nursing Times 78(25):1058–1066

Babb A L, Popovich R P, Christopher T G et al 1971 The genesis of the square- metre-hour hypothesis. Transactions of the American Society of Artificial Internal Organs 17:81–91. Cited by Manis T & Friedman E A, Dialytic therapy for irreversible uraemia. New England Journal of Medicine 301(23):1260–1265

Bevan D R 1978 Intraoperative fluid balance. British Journal of Hospital Medicine 19(5):45–48

Boylan A 1979 Dehydration — subtle, sinister, preventable. Registered Nurse 42(8):37–41

Bradley B A, Selwood N H 1983 The natural history of transplantable kidneys. Health Trends 15:25–27

Breckenridge Report 1976 The addition of drugs to intravenous fluids. DHSS HC (76) 9

Buxton A E, Highsmith A K, Garner J S, West C M, Stamm W E, Dixon R E, McGowan J E Jr 1979 Contamination of intravenous infusion fluid: effects of changing administration sets. Annals of Internal Medicine 90(5):764–768
Chang M 1981 No more needles. Nursing Mirror 153(50):22–25
Cianci J, Lamb J, Ryan R K 1981 Renal transplantation. American Journal of Nursing 81(2):354–355
Dunn S M, Heath G 1981 Intravenous technology and the nurse. Nursing Times 77(12):492–495
Evans L E J, Whitlock F A 1978 Drugs and depression. Drugs 15:53–71
Felver L 1980 Understanding the electrolyte maze. American Journal of Nursing 80:1591–1595
Folklightly M 1984 Solving the puzzles of patients' fluid imbalances. Nursing (Horsham) 14(2):34–41
Gabriel R 1983 A patient's guide to dialysis and transplantation. MTP Press, Lancaster
Greco F del, Quintanilla A, Huang C M 1979 The clinical assessment of fluid balance. Heart and Lung 8(3):481–482
Guyton A C 1986 Textbook of medical physiology, 7th edn. Saunders, London
Hume D, Narins R G, Bremmer B M 1982 Disorders of water balance. Hospital Practice 14(3):133–145
Jenner E 1983 Clinical: Infused with safety. Nursing Mirror 156(14):23–27
Khanna R, Oreopoulos D G 1982 The present and future role of continuous ambulatory peritoneal dialysis (CAPD). American Journal of Kidney Disease 2(3):381–385
Knapp M S 1982 Renal failure — dilemmas and developments. British Medical Journal 284(6314):847–850
Lancaster L E 1979 The patient with end stage renal disease. Wiley, New York
Lawson D H 1979 Severe hypokalaemia in hospitalised patients. Archives of Internal Medicine 139(9):978–980
Lee H A 1982 Renal replacement therapy 5–1 Acute renal failure. Nursing Times 78(21):891–896
Levine D 1983 Care of the renal patient. Saunders, Philadelphia
McAlsan T C 1980 Rational fluid therapy. Refresher Course in Anaesthesiology 80:115–126
Macleod J 1984 Davidson's principles and practice of medicine, 14th edn. Churchill Livingstone, Edinburgh
Maguire K 1982 Renal replacement therapy 6–1 Renal transplanation. Pre- and post-operative care. Nursing Times 78(22):933–934
Maki D, Goldman D A, Rhame F S 1973 Infection control in intravenous therapy. Annals of Internal Medicine 79(6):31–35
Manis T, Friedman E A 1979 Dialytic therapy for irreversible uraemia. New England Journal of Medicine 301(23):1260–1265
Marks M 1981 Intravenous therapy: the extended role of the nurse. Nursing Focus 2(7):377–381
Metheny D, Snively W 1983 The nurse's handbook of fluid balance. Lippincott, Philadelphia
Moncrief J W, Popovich R P, Nolph K D 1978 Theoretical and practical implications of continuous ambulatory dialysis. Nephron 21:117–122
Narins R G, Jones E R, Stom M C et al 1982 Diagnostic strategies in disorders of fluid, electrolyte and acid-base homeostasis. American Journal of Medicine 72(3):496–520
Nelson B 1978 A nursing approach to patients with long-term renal transplants. Nursing Clinics of North America 13:157–169
Oestreich S J K 1979 Rational nursing care in chronic renal disease. American Journal of Nursing 79(6):1096–1099
Oreopoulos D G, Robson M D 1978 Continuous ambulatory peritoneal dialysis: a revolution in the treatment of chronic renal failure. Dialysis Transplant 7:799- -800
Pflaum S S 1979 Investigation of intake/output as a means of assessing body fluid balance. Heart and Lung 8(3):495–498
Pritchard M 1982 Psychological pressures in a renal unit. British Journal of Hospital Medicine 23(5):512–516
Rando J T 1982 Fluid and electrolyte management of the adult surgical patient. Journal of the American Association of Nurse Anaesthetists 50(1):49–54
Rosenheim Report 1972 Hepatitis and the treatment of chronic renal failure. Report of the Advisory Group, DHSS, London
Salmons P H 1980 Psychosocial aspects of chronic renal failure. British Journal of Hospital Medicine 21(6):617–622
Sheahan S L, Seabolt J P 1982 Understanding urinary tract infection in women. Nursing (Horsham) 12(11):68–70
Smith T 1982 A cycler for one. Nursing Mirror 154(42)56–57
Speechley V 1984 The nurse's role in intravenous management. Nursing Times 80(18):28-32
Stark J L 1982 How to Succeed against acute renal failure. Nursing (Horsham) 12(7):26–33
Stark J L, Hunt V 1983 Helping your patient with chronic renal failure. Nursing (Horsham) 13(9):51–63
Steel J 1983 Too slow or too fast: the erratic I.V.I. American Journal of Nursing 83(6):898–901
Taber S 1982a Renal replacement therapy 6–2 Other aspects of renal transplantation — donor procurement, preservation and alternative rejection therapy. Nursing Times 78(22):935–939
Taber S 1982b Renal replacement therapy 7 The role of the transplant co- ordinator. Nursing Times 78(23):973–978
Tate D G 1982 Renal replacement therapy 8–1 Tissue-typing and its role in transplantation. Nursing Times 78(24):1017–1019
Travenol Survey of CAPD in Britain Today 1984 Research survey into continuous ambulatory peritoneal dialysis. Travenol Laboratories Ltd, Egham, Surrey

27

Disturbances of temperature control

INTRODUCTION

The enzyme activity regulating all chemical reactions within the body, and thus all cellular function, is optimal within the narrow definition of normal body temperature. Deviations above or below this normal range, therefore, affect total body function.

Normal body temperature is maintained by the balance which exists between heat gain and heat loss. This balance is finely controlled and has to be maintained for the enzyme action necessary for normal cellular function to continue. In the early part of this century, Barbour's (1912) research into the control of body temperature established that the hypothalamus is the vital control centre for thermoregulation of the internal environment. The anterior section of the hypothalamus, in conjunction with the parasympathetic system, produces an action termed thermolysis which controls heat loss. The posterior section, whose function is mediated by the sympathetic system, produces an action termed thermogenesis which conserves body heat (Castle, 1979) (Fig. 27.1). As human beings are homeothermic, that is they maintain their body temperature within narrow limits, health and actual survival depend on the maintenance of the equilibrium between thermolysis and thermogenesis. The equilibrium is achieved by the interaction of the systems regulating the body temperature.

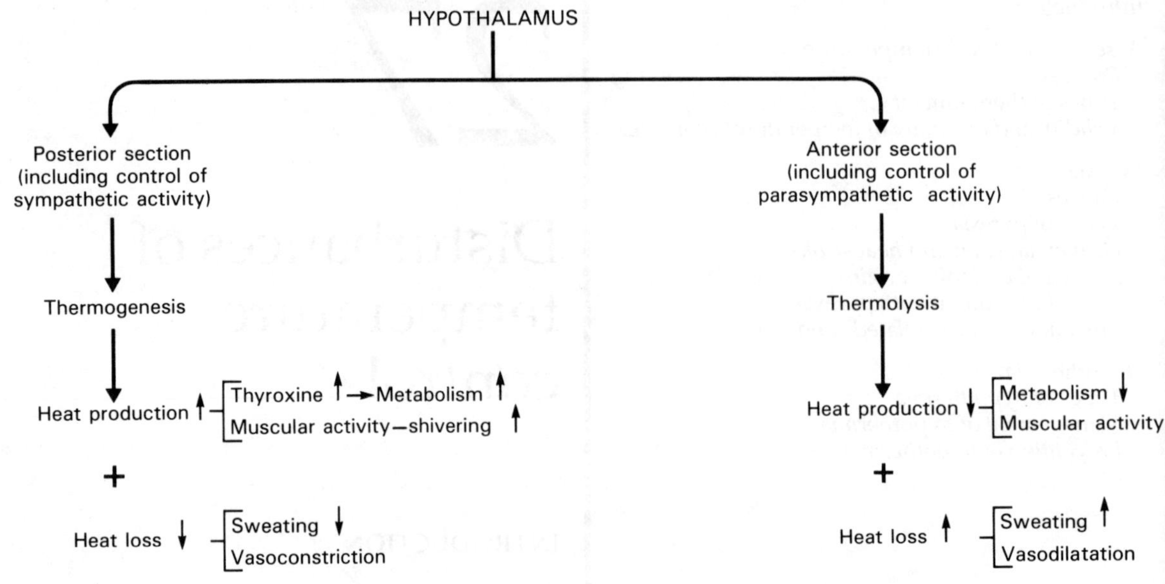

Fig. 27.1 Diagrammatic representation of thermogenesis and thermolysis.

Environmental conditions are not always favourable to human beings. While there are physiological mechanisms to modify heat gain and loss, people have also learned to modify their immediate surroundings to effectively reduce the demand for physiological adaptation. If people are cold, they wear extra clothing; if they are too hot, they wear less clothing or turn on a fan. It is only when external conditions become extreme or when disease jeopardizes the balance of homeostasis that effective temperature control is threatened.

In human beings, whereas shell temperature involves the skin, subcutaneous tissue and the superficial surface of muscle, central core temperature is related to the deep underlying structures of the body such as the brain, the heart and the liver. By its insulating effect, the shell assists the hypothalamus in maintaining central core temperature. Changes in vasodilatation effectively alter the depth of the shell, thereby adjusting heat loss.

The central core temperature of the body is regulated within normal limits close to 37°C. Slight variations due to circadian rhythm do occur (Minor & Waterhouse, 1981). This biorhythm causes marginal fluctuations of temperature throughout the day, reaching a maximum in the afternoon and a minimum in the early hours of the morning. When oral and rectal temperatures are monitored, differences of 0.5–1.5°C may be recorded between early morning and afternoon. It should, however, be noted that this temperature curve is not characteristic of all individuals and it may be found that a person's temperature is higher in the morning than in the afternoon or evening.

An individual's biological rhythms serve to co-ordinate physiological functions with social processes. In a society which is orientated to working during the day and sleeping at night the circadian rhythm allows optimal efficiency, but temperature levels may be affected by various factors which can disrupt this biological process. Nurses and others who work during the night, and pilots and air hostesses who travel by jet across time zones, can experience an alteration in their biorhythms and may show less typical temperature recordings. Environmental factors may also cause mild to moderate variations in body temperature. If the ward temperature is not controlled on a hot summer day, the patient's temperature may show evidence of heat gain to the level of 1–2°C. In the adult, exposure to a cold environment results in only a slight loss of heat; in the elderly, where the ageing process slows down internal body activity, thermoregulation also becomes less effective. This accounts for the tendency of the older person to develop hypothermia and, during the summer months, to show an increased susceptibility to develop heat stroke (Ellis et al, 1980).

Muscular activity in the form of exercise can create a considerable rise in body temperature. People chewing gum (necessitating the use of muscles in the mouth), athletes taking strenuous exercise, soldiers marching with heavy packs and women in the second stage of labour have all shown rises in oral and rectal temperature recordings (MacBryde & Blacklow, 1970). Community jogs and 'fun runs' are now extremely popular. The individual who has had a limited amount of physical training, or even one who trains to run, may suffer heat exhaustion or heat stroke necessitating admission to hospital (Hughson & Sutton, 1978).

Temperature ranges can therefore be seen to fluctuate normally during circadian rhythms, in certain environmental conditions and in heightened activity. Deviations from this 'normal' temperature pattern, however, may indicate abnormal processes such as infection, injury to the body or the presence of a disease. As man is susceptible to numerous factors which may upset his central core temperature, it is vital that the physiological and environmental conditions are controlled to assist maintenance of the balance which exists between heat gain and heat loss.

ASSESSMENT OF BODY TEMPERATURE

Recording the body temperature is an important technique in assessing an individual's state of health. Measurement, interpretation and evaluation of temperature ranges are fundamental nursing skills. These skills depend on the nurse's theoretical and clinical expertise, on her assessment of the patient's physical and emotional status at the time of the procedure, and on her knowledge of the patient's medical condition. The sites most frequently used are the oral and rectal routes, axillary skin fold placement and the abdominal skin area when thermometer tape is used. Additionally, the body temperature may be measured using an oesophageal or gastric probe. Occasionally it may be useful to measure the temperature of urine which has been freshly voided (Edholm, 1978). Also, although not practical in the ward area, laboratory tests on temperature ranges taken next to the tympanic membrane record hypothalamic changes more accurately than do those at oral and rectal sites. Where patients have problems in maintaining thermoregulation, normally it is the oral and rectal sites which are selected. Of these, the oral route, using the sublingual pocket, is preferable because of its close proximity to the central thermoreceptors which respond rapidly to change in the central core temperature (Blainey, 1974).

ROUTES

Oral

When using the oral route, to record a range of temperature as close to the central core temperature as possible, more accurate readings are achieved if the thermometer is placed in the sublingual pocket (Erickson,1976). This 'heat pocket' is situated near rich blood supplies. The lingual artery supplies blood to the floor of the mouth and to the undersurface of the tongue, as far as its tip. It is necessary that care should be taken to note any injury or abnormality in this area before inserting the thermometer into the mouth. It is recommended that an interval of at least 15 minutes should be allowed to elapse after drinking hot or cold drinks, chewing gum or smoking (Kozier & Erb, 1983).

Rectal

Adult patients may be embarrassed or experience discomfort when temperature is recorded by the rectal route. It is important in using this route that the thermometer bulb is inserted firmly against the rectal mucosa with its rich blood supply, rather than into soft faeces. The rectal route is not recommended in patients who suffer from haemorrhoids or who have had anal surgery. It is also evident that using this route can cause cardiac arrhythmias. Bradycardia may occur due to vagal response to anal stimulation in the patient with myocardial infarction (Gruber 1974), and tachycardia may occur in the emotional patient (Blainey, 1974).

Axillary

Axillary recordings have been found to vary between right and left arm in elderly patients so that the same arm should always be used (Howell, 1972). The armpit should be dry, and care should be taken to insert the thermometer into the centre of the axilla in contact with the skin surfaces. This site is commonly used with children, confused patients, those unable to hold the instrument in the mouth for long enough, those with sore or injured mouths and those who might, deliberately or inadvertently, bite off the thermometer bulb.

Selection

Whichever route is used for recording body temperature the site should be consistent, and if a change is required this alteration should be noted on the temperature chart. The administration of oxygen by face mask does not alter the temperature recorded orally, so the site of measurement need not be changed if a patient requires oxygen (Hasler & Cohen, 1982; Lim-Levy, 1982). While it is sometimes assumed that rectal temperature is about 0.5°C higher and axillary recording 0.5°C lower than oral measurements, research does not support these assumptions (Seller & Yoder, 1961; Nichols et al, 1966). Individual variations were so pronounced that no acceptable formula for comparing temperatures recorded in different sites could be suggested.

TYPES OF THERMOMETER

The thermometers in use today consist of numerous types. Some thermometers are extremely sophisticated, with chemical dots which change colour according to temperature range, whilst others contain an electronic sensor probe attached to a battery unit with a visible dial. The clinical glass thermometer with oral and rectal bulb is probably still the most extensively used type of thermometer. Moorat (1976) compared the cost-effectiveness of taking temperatures using three different types of thermometers: the clinical glass thermometer, the heat sensitive strip and the electronic thermometer. The authors suggest that the use of electronic calculating thermometers would reduce the cost of routine temperature taking by at least 300%, largely due to the time saved.

VALIDITY AND RELIABILITY OF TEMPERATURE RECORDINGS

Whatever route and whichever type of thermometer is used, valid, reliable temperature measurements will only be obtained if a number of factors are taken into account.

Time in position of thermometer

The importance of careful positioning has already been mentioned, but the length of time the thermometer is left in position is also of great importance. Many workers have examined this question and suggested various times for the different sites used. Nichols and her colleagues have undertaken some of the most comprehensive work in this area (Nichols et al, 1966; Nichols, 1972; Nichols et al, 1972). It was found that it took between 1–12 minutes for oral or axillary placements and 1–9 minutes for rectal placements to record the maximum temperature measurement. The commonly used 3-minute timing led to marked inaccuracy. It was recommended that the thermometer should be left in position for 7–8 minutes in the mouth, 9 minutes in the axilla or 2 minutes in the rectum. The use of these timings will mean that in 90% of the recordings made, the reading will be within 0.1°C of the maximum reading which could be achieved. Electronic thermometers only take approximately 30 seconds to record temperature accurately.

Time of day

If the aim of temperature recording is to identify those patients with an elevated temperature, then the time of day when the recording is taken is important. Temperature recordings between 4–8 pm coincide with the highest point in the circadian rhythm of body temperature (Schmidt, 1972). Angerami (1980) found that recordings at 7 pm were most likely to identify pyrexial patients.

Other factors

As discussed previously, activity and a too-warm environment will both cause a perfectly normal rise in temperature which may be above the limit usually considered as 'normal', i.e. about 37.2°C. Clearly the interpretation of any temperature recording must take into account such factors. If a patient regularly attends the physiotherapy department, his/her temperature may well appear elevated if recorded immediately on his/her return to the ward. The difficulty in interpreting the meaning of a temperature measurement is increased if it is an isolated recording. Each individual has a characteristic body temperature and, for most people, that lies within the normal range of 36.3–37.2°C. However, some people will have a characteristic temperature slightly outside this range. If the usual temperature is slightly below normal, then a rise in temperature to 'only' 37.2°C may cause malaise and all the other effects of pyrexia.

In the interpretation of any temperature recording, other signs and symptoms of an elevated temperature must be noted. Indeed, signs or symptoms of a raised temperature such as tachycardia or sweating, or indications of a disorder which results in pyrexia, should lead the nurse to record the patient's temperature as part of her fuller assessment.

PYREXIA

CAUSES

Pyrexia, or a significant rise in body temperature, can occur in a number of ways.

Fever

A fever results when the 'thermostat' in the hypothalamus is reset to maintain the body at a temperature higher than normal. The mechanics involved in control of body temperature function as usual but at a higher level than normal (Davis-Sharts, 1978). This resetting of the 'thermostat' results from the action of pyrogens on the thermoregulatory centre in the hypothalamus. The endogenous pyrogens involved are released mainly from leucocytes as a result of cell damage (Hensel, 1981). This is presumably the route by which a number of diverse conditions such as infections, thrombosis, autoimmune disorders and malignancy result in pyrexia. It is not clear how these pyrogens influence hypothalamic function but it has been suggested that prostaglandin E is involved. There is some support for this hypothesis, as an injection of prostaglandin E into the hypothalamus causes a rise in temperature and antipyretics such as salicylates (aspirin) inhibit the synthesis of prostaglandins (Hensel, 1981). However, the evidence is not conclusive.

When the temperature rises due to the resetting of the thermostat it may do so slowly, or through a rigor. In a rigor the temperature rises quickly through the 'normal' physiological responses to cold. The shivering and vasoconstriction lead to production of heat and retention of heat within the body. At the onset of the rigor, when shivering is marked, the patient appears pale and complains of feeling cold. During this stage peripheral thermoreceptors in the skin are stimulated to produce gross vasoconstriction which reduces the rate of heat loss through conduction and convection, resulting in a skin surface which is pale and cold to touch. Eccrine sweat gland activity is reduced to minimize evaporation of fluid from the body surface. Normally muscular activity results from smooth co-ordination of muscle contraction followed by a period of relaxation. In shivering, the smooth control is lost and the muscles contract and relax out of sequence with each other. These abnormal bursts of action may present in a mild form when the patient complains of feeling cold and there are visible signs of tremor or spasm. In a more serious condition shivering may take the form of violent body movements with chattering teeth. During this period of muscular activity the body increases catecholamine and thyroxine levels in an attempt to raise the body temperature. All these factors contribute to the rise in the rate of metabolism resulting in an increased production of the waste products, carbon dioxide and water. Because of the increase in carbon dioxide the patient's respirations are increased in rate and depth, which in turn leads to the loss of fluid, and the patient experiences an awareness of thirst and feeling of exhaustion. To compensate for the rise in metabolism there is also an increase in the need to supply oxygen and glucose to the tissues, which becomes evident in the recording of a rapid and full pulse rate.

When the body temperature reaches the new 'set point' there again exists a balance between heat gain and heat loss; muscular activity halts and vasodilatation occurs. Although the skin appears flushed and warm to touch the patient does not complain of feeling hot or cold. At this stage of the pyrexia the high temperature level produces a rapid heart beat. Further loss of fluid is evident due to an increase in both respiration rate and insensible loss through peripheral vasodilatation. There may also be headache or photophobia. The patient may enter a period of mental confusion and disturbance of sensory perception.

Body temperature may return to normal by lysis, over a period of time, or by crisis, when it falls rapidly as body function returns to normal. During this period the patient will feel hot and heat is lost through sweating and vasodilatation.

Other causes of pyrexia

Fever can be distinguished from other causes of hyperthermia when the control of body temperature is no longer functioning (Hensel, 1981). The thermoregulatory centre in the hypothalamus may be damaged by trauma or infarction. The balance between heat production and heat loss is no longer controlled and body temperature rises.

In extremely hot environmental conditions, particularly if associated with high humidity, the body's normal mechanisms for heat loss may be overwhelmed and heat exhaustion followed by heat stroke may develop.

A rather different cause of a rise in body temperature occurs in thyrotoxicosis, where the increased metabolic rate leads to a rise in heat production.

Finally, malignant hyperthermia is a condition which occurs in susceptible people and is triggered by potent inhalation anaesthetics or muscle relaxants. There is a rapid rise in body temperature, muscular rigidity and severe metabolic acidosis develops. The hypothalamic regulating centre is overwhelmed (Davies, 1981).

TYPES OF PYREXIA

In clinical terms the rise in temperature is classified into different grades of pyrexia. In practice these terms seem to be used for patterns of pyrexia and are useful in indicating possible causes. Low grade pyrexia is normally defined as a temperature above normal but not exceeding 38.5°C. This may be indicative of an inflammatory response due to a mild infection, allergy, disturbance of body tissue by trauma, thrombosis or infarction, malignancy or an autoimmune response. Moderate to high grade pyrexia (38–40°C) may be caused by wound, respiratory or urinary tract infection. Hyperpyrexia occurs when temperatures are elevated to approximately 40°C and above, exposing the body to severe stress. A pyrexia in this range may arise because of bacteraemia, damage to the hypothalamus or high environmental temperatures.

Various typical fever patterns (e.g. constant, remittent) were of importance before the widespread use of antibiotics but are now of little relevance. However, there are certain patterns of pyrexia which are typical of certain conditions. For example, after an operation it is common to find a low grade pyrexia for 1–2 days as a normal response to tissue damage. After this a low grade to moderate pyrexia may indicate a deep vein thrombosis or a wound infection. A moderate pyrexia due to infection treated by antibiotics quickly resolves about the second day, but may re-occur on the fourth or fifth day due to the development of strains of bacteria resistant to the antibiotics prescribed. Non-completion of the course of antibiotics encourages this development.

A long-lasting, low grade pyrexia with general malaise may be indicative of such conditions as glandular fever (infectious mononucleosis), brucellosis or tuberculosis. Factors such as environment, age or occupation may suggest the most likely diagnosis. For example, a veterinary surgeon or farm worker is more likely than a city dweller to contract brucellosis, which also occurs in animals. Glandular fever is commonest among young people in their teens and 20s, while tuberculosis may be associated with poor living conditions or recent immigration.

The temperature rise may be modified by the action of certain drugs. The antipyretics, salicylates, paracetamol or indomethacin all reduce a high temperature caused by pyrogens, possibly by their affect on the hypothalamus. Steroid hormones minimize the inflammatory response and antibiotics combat infection, thus both minimize the release of pyrogens.

HEAT EXHAUSTION AND HEAT STROKE

A hot, humid environment can only be tolerated for short periods and in some instances for seconds or minutes. After this time the body suffers severe consequences such as heat exhaustion and/or heat stroke. Air which is inspired is hot and if there is the added problem of high humidity, preventing fluid evaporation from the skin surface, the balance between heat gain and heat loss is unstable and leans in favour of heat gain. The body temperature will rise to an alarming level resulting in the individual entering a state of collapse or unconsciousness.

Heat exhaustion

Heat exhaustion can either be predominantly due to water depletion or to sodium depletion.

Water depletion

Water depletion occurs when water lost through prolonged sweating is not adequately replaced. It can develop over a period of several days if fluid lost is only partially replaced because palatable drinking water is not readily available (Leithead & Lind, 1964). In early water depletion the body weight is reduced by about 2% (equivalent to 1.5l in a 70kg man). Thirst may be the only symptom at this stage. In the moderately severe state there is a deficit of approximately 6% of body weight (4.2l in a 70kg man). This individual will suffer intense thirst and a dry mouth, will have a rapid pulse and a rectal temperature elevated by about 2°C. Urine production will be low. A patient with very severe water depletion will show weight loss of more than 7% (equivalent to 5-10l in a 70kg man). In addition to the other signs and symptoms, the patient will show marked impairment of physical and mental capacities. Cyanosis and circulatory failure are followed by coma and death when fluid loss is approximately 20%.

Water depletion heat exhaustion is diagnosed largely by the circumstances in which it arises, on clinical grounds and by finding a high serum sodium concentration. Management is by rest in a cool well-ventilated room and by the intake of a high fluid volume. In the first 24 hours, 6–8 litres of fluid should be taken and then modified according to the patient's condition (Leithead & Lind, 1964).

Sodium depletion

Sodium depletion heat exhaustion is due to inadequate replacement of salt lost through prolonged sweating. The water lost through sweating is replaced, but without the additional salt the extracellular fluid (ECF) becomes hypotonic. Water moves into the cells increasing the volume of the intracellular fluid compartment and reducing the ECF volume. The condition occurs most commonly in those who have not yet adapted to a considerable increase in environmental temperature. This adaptation is normally achieved by a reduction in the amount of sodium lost in sweat. This patient will be fatigued with profound weariness and muscular weakness. Headache, constipation or diarrhoea and fainting are fairly common while nausea, vomiting and severe muscle cramps sometimes occur. Because the extracellular fluid is not hyperosmotic but hypo-osmotic, the patient does not suffer from thirst. In the very severe state the patient will go into a state of shock. This condition develops insidiously over several days but, because it causes incapacity at an early stage, it is usually diagnosed and treated promptly. Management is by rest in a cool room and by taking large amounts of a high intake of salt and water. Fluids such as consommé or tomato juice can contain fairly large amounts of salt without being unpalatable. When food can be taken in adequate amounts then salt should be added in measured quantities. About 20g of salt in a day should be taken (Leithead & Lind, 1964).

Heatstroke

Heatstroke may develop from heat exhaustion, but more commonly appears to develop rapidly in subjects exposed to high temperatures who are not yet acclimatized to heat. It is a serious condition in which the temperature rises above 40.6°C, partly due to generalized cessation of sweating. It results in central nervous system disturbances such as convulsions or coma which may terminate in death. The patient may show cyanosis of the face and petechiae are fairly common. Incontinence of watery faeces, often with some fresh blood, and vomiting sometimes occurs and exacerbates any fluid and electrolyte imbalance already present.

At risk groups

Runners

It is evident that the popular sport of long-distance running, whether taking place in a hot, humid environment or a temperate climate, can cause heat exhaustion and heat stroke. In Sydney (Lancet, 1979) the city-to-surf-fun-run race has enabled doctors to investigate the hazards of this strenuous exercise by identifying and examining the environmental, medical and physical factors accompanying this event. Biochemical and haematological values of those runners who had not trained and who had collapsed were contrasted with those runners who had trained. The serum bicarbonate of the collapsed runners was lowered and they also had higher creatinine, urea nitrogen and uric acid levels than those runners who had trained for the race. It is interesting to note that Hughson & Sutton (1978), in a letter to the British Medical Journal relating to a run-for-fun race held in Waterloo, Ontario in 1978, found that none of the experienced competitive runners were admitted to hospital and very few suffered even minor heat-related problems. Nicholson & Somerville (1978) reported the effects of a run-for-fun exercise organized in Auckland in the late summer of 1977. The run was 11 km long, began at 10 am, the temperature being 21.3°C, humidity 73% and wind velocity 9 knots. Of the 20 000 runners taking part, 200 were given first aid and 16 were admitted to hospital. The latter were men aged between 20–44 years of age and all were not only highly motivated to finish but were active in another sport and had trained for the run. On admission to hospital the runners presented with vomiting, faecal incontinence, delirium, apathy, coma and a mean rectal temperature of 39.1°C. A 22-year-old contestant was admitted with convulsions and a rectal temperature of 41.6°C and his condition necessitated the use of positive pressure ventilation. The runners continued to suffer for a week after the event with complaints of muscular cramps, nausea and lethargy.

The elderly and adults

The effects of raised environmental temperature on the elderly have received minimal attention compared to the hazards of low environmental temperature. The United Kingdom experienced a heat wave in 1976 which lasted approximately from mid-June to mid-July during which time Birmingham recorded mean daily temperature of 22°C from 24 June–8 July. During this 2 week period the coroner reported an increase in mortality rates of 20% and during the brief period from 3–5 July an increase in mortality rates of 30%. The elderly who died during these hot weeks were mainly those who suffered from cerebrovascular or cardiovascular disease (Ellis et al, 1980). Heatstroke and heat exhaustion were never reported as the primary cause of death and 'effects of heat' were only reported as a contributory cause on three death certificates. Concerning morbidity rates in Birmingham during the heatwave, the claims for sickness benefit in workers were not significantly raised, but nine people were admitted to various hospitals with illness due to heat stress and a moderate increase in visits to two large general practitioner units was noted.

PYREXIA OF UNKNOWN ORIGIN

When a patient develops a pyrexia, careful history-taking, physical examination and laboratory tests should establish a diagnosis and the problem causing the pyrexia can be dealt with by prescribing the appropriate treatment. However, pyrexia as such may occasionally be the reason for admission to hospital and even after exhaustive clinical and laboratory tests the cause remains undetermined. Pyrexia of unknown origin (PUO) requires meticulous recording of the patient's history, with daily physical assessment and laboratory investigations. The time lapse between investigations and the final diagnosis can be exhausting for the patient because of the numerous tests and examinations involved. Waiting for the results can cause great anxiety for both the patients and those who are concerned about them (see Ch. 11).

Most cases of PUO are eventually found to be due to infection (40%), or neoplastic disease (20%) or collagen-vascular disorders (15%) (Jacoby & Swartz, 1973).

A spurious pyrexia may be due to the patient's own manipulations resulting in inaccurate recordings. This may lead to exhaustive investigations to find the cause of this pyrexia of unknown origin. In the patient who feels the need to mislead in this way, the psychological or social help necessary to solve the problem cannot be made available until the evidence of spurious recordings has been established. Petersdorf & Bennet (1957) stressed that the patient's chart is an essential tool in diagnosing this condition. They reasoned that a meticulously kept chart would show that the temperature recordings failed to follow the normal circadian pattern and that the rise in temperature levels would not correspond with the patient's pulse rate. Lee & Atkins (1972), investigating the methods used by patients to manipulate thermometers in order to record an apparently high temperature, provide some interesting material. A hot external source was often used when the bulb of the thermometer was immersed within a liquid or held against the object, so rapidly producing an elevated reading on the thermometer scale. Poor results were obtained from the friction method involving the tongue or anal sphincter, but a high recording was produced when the bulb of the thermometer was rubbed against the skin, between the palms of the hands or against hospital linen.

If, on several recordings, there appears to be a spurious pyrexia, the patient's actions should be discreetly observed and evaluated. Lee & Atkins (1972) suggest that a second temperature recording should be taken after an inexplicably raised temperature has been reported. A new thermometer is then used and it should be inserted and its position observed by the nurse throughout the stated time for insertion at the selected site. The nurse should be aware of the possibility of this type of pyrexia and should therefore assist, guide and support the patient during this period. The patient is usually well aware of the intention and meaning of the nurse's actions in checking the repeated recordings. It may be appropriate for someone other than the nurse to work with the patient in helping the expression of any anxieties. Simply ignoring the incident will leave the patient with heightened anxieties, and possibly also shame and embarrassment for having acted in a way which he/she may feel is condemned by those caring for him/her.

CARE OF THE PATIENT WITH PYREXIA

The care of the patient with pyrexia involves

first, the identification and treatment of the cause. This is primarily the concern of the medical staff, although the nursing observations will be of the utmost importance. Secondly the care involves dealing with the effects on the patient of a rise in temperature. Thirdly, it may also be necessary to take steps to bring down the body temperature.

Dealing with the effects of pyrexia

The effects of pyrexia are due to the increase in the rate at which all chemical reactions in the body occur. This manifests as an increase in the metabolic rate of about 14% for each 1°C rise in temperature (Ganong, 1981). In severe infection the metabolic rate may be increased by 20–40% (Wannemacher & Beisel, 1977). As a result, all the body cells require an increased supply of nutrients and oxygen, indicated by a rise in the pulse and respiratory rates. These, and body temperature, will need to be recorded at regular intervals to monitor the course of the illness. In many cases 4-hourly recordings will be adequate, but in a patient with a particularly high temperature or in whom it is changing rapidly, hourly or even half-hourly recordings will be required.

Breathing

The increased metabolic rate results in a rise in the production of carbon dioxide, leading to a tendency to develop acidosis. This stimulates the rate and depth of respiration in order to remove the excess carbon dioxide, and also brings more oxygen into the body. However, a more important factor in increasing oxygen supply to the tissues is the greater than usual dissociation of oxyhaemoglobin. Release of oxygen from the haemoglobin is increased by a rise in temperature and carbon dioxide concentration, as well as by the reduced oxygen tension in the tissue fluid.

Eating and drinking

A patient with pyrexia often also suffers from general malaise, anorexia and possibly nausea. Because of this, food intake is likely to be reduced, but nutritional requirements are increased due to the increased metabolic rate. In order to supply energy to the tissues the body stores of nutrients, glycogen and fats, are broken down. In addition, protein may need to be catabolized as an energy source (Wannemacher & Beisel, 1977).

In the course of one research project, stimulation of a pyrexial state was induced in healthy and nutritionally sound individuals (Beisel et al, 1968). The results produced an increased level of nitrogen and potassium in the urinary output which continued 24 hours after the temperature returned to the volunteer's normal level. As about 40% of body protein is contained in skeletal muscle, this body tissue is the principal source for protein catabolism during the pyrexial state in an acute infection. It therefore follows that if the patient's nutritional intake is not maintained, negative nitrogen balance will occur with evidence of wasting of body tissue. When the patient is not enthusiastic or is unable to take food, there is now a vast variety of palatable liquid feeds available to supply nutrients in an easily digestible form. These supply the body with all the necessary substances to maintain or stabilize the patient's nutritional status, and can be given to supplement any normal or light diet the patient is able to manage.

A rise in temperature is accompanied by an increase in insensible fluid loss through the skin, possibly by visible sweating, and through the increased respiration rate. The amount of the insensible loss by breathing depends on the depth and rate of respiration and on the humidity of atmospheric air. The healthy individual loses approximately 350 ml of water in 24 hours through breathing. In pyrexia, when respirations are increased both in depth and rate, there is more fluid lost from the body. Although sweat is hypotonic and its electrolyte content is lower than plasma, body fluid and sodium levels can be greatly depleted by sweating. This depletion of fluid depends on the individual's tolerance to heat and the environmental temperature. In a normal situation fluid loss may vary from 300–700 ml per day, but in the pyrexial state, when there is visible sweat on the body and the bed linen contains enough moisture to warrant a change of linen, there may be a loss of 1000 ml or more of fluid from the body. This increase in loss of fluid and electrolytes will normally cause thirst resulting in replacement of fluid by drinking. If adequate replacement does not occur the signs of dehydration will develop, including oliguria and concentration of urine. In an acute infection which also includes involvement of the bowel, there may be excessive fluid loss from the gastrointestinal tract in the form of vomiting and diarrhoea. This may require intravenous replacement.

A variety of oral fluids can be offered and the nurse should ask the patient what drinks he/she enjoys. It is important not only to give alternatives to assist oral intake, but that the fluid given can contribute toward the maintenance of the electrolyte balance and nutritional levels. For example, protein is contained in milk, potassium and sodium in drinks such as tomato juice and meat extracts, while sugars are present in most fruit juices. It is necessary to encourage the patient to take at least 2–3 litres of oral fluids in every 24 hours. The patient's intake and output should be carefully recorded and urine specific gravity measured, in order to monitor the adequacy of fluid intake. If the patient is unable to take enough fluid by mouth then intravenous fluids may have to be administered.

Excessive mouth breathing and generally inadequate hydration results in deterioration of the oral mucosa, with the presence of halitosis, dry furred tongue and mouth infection. These conditions will add to the problems of the patient who may already be anorexic. Oral fluids and sections of fruit such as pineapple and orange to eat will help to minimize the discomfort and unpleasant taste. Frequent mouth washes will also be useful. As these patients are usually receiving antibiotics they are also at risk of thrush (Candida albicans) which further adds to their mouth discomfort.

Eliminating

The importance of recording urine output in order to measure hydration status has already been mentioned. A patient who is dehydrated, unable to eat normally, and taking little exercise is likely to become constipated. Bowel actions should be recorded and the abdomen examined at intervals for distension. Laxatives or suppositories may have to be used to prevent prolonged constipation and discomfort.

Moving and protecting self

The patient will be confined to bed during the period when his/her temperature is elevated and, because metabolism is increased, there is an increased risk of pressure sore development. The patient is also likely to be sweating considerably. Skin care, therefore, is very important and the condition of pressure areas must be checked at least twice a day. If possible patients should be taught to change their position frequently. If they are unable to do this for themselves, their position should be changed at least 2-hourly.

Resting and sleeping

The environment in which the patient is being cared for should be well-ventilated and quiet. It is essential that the patient is allowed to rest as this helps to decrease the metabolic demand. Also, a peaceful room is necessary to protect the patient from any stimuli which might cause cerebral irritation. Anxiety detracts from the ability to rest, and the patient may feel anxious if the thermometer continues to record pyrexia, particularly if this is delaying surgery or discharge from hospital. The nurse can help to minimize further anxiety by anticipating the patient's needs and by giving a full explanation of nursing procedures carried out. In some instances it may help the patient to understand the mechanism of pyrexia, the probable course of the infection or disease and the reason for prescribing medication. Giving the patient details and results of tests is clearly important. These measures make the patient far less vulnerable by giving him/her a sense of security, and a stronger rapport is established between the staff and patient.

If the patient is restless or feels hot and

uncomfortable a bed bath with change of night clothes, clean bed linen and change of position may help to relax him/her and will promote rest and sleep.

During a rigor the patient will feel cold and a flannelette blanket tucked around him/her and additional blankets on the bed will be needed. Violent shivering and chattering of teeth may cause anxiety, therefore the nurse should remain with the patient and protect him/her from self injury. Shivering, whether appearing in a mild or severe form, utilizes a great deal of energy and the patient may be exhausted after this stage of a rigor. As soon as the shivering stops the temperature must be recorded and the extra blanket or blankets removed to permit heat loss from the body surface.

Lowering body temperature

Antipyretics

In 1970, Milton & Wendlant noted that prostaglandins increased body temperature by acting on the heat regulating centre of the hypothalamus. It is hypothesized that this occurs in the pathological state but at present there is no evidence to suggest that prostaglandins are involved in the normal state of thermoregulation (Cox, 1978). Antipyretics in the form of tablets or suppositories are useful in reducing high temperature levels. By using animal studies Vane (1978) produced evidence to suggest that aspirin-like drugs caused a marked fall in temperature and it is evident that these drugs inhibit the inflammatory action of prostaglandins. Treatment with aspirin is effective for about 2 hours and probably reduces pyrexia by acting on the hypothalamus to temporarily reset the thermostat to normal. This causes vasodilatation and sweating to lose the excess heat contained in the body. Some patients find the sweating involved very unpleasant and prefer to remain pyrexial. While most pharmacology books state that antipyretics do not affect the body temperature in the normothermic subject, Cox (1978) suggests that some antipyrexial drugs, namely paracetamol and indomethacin, may create a loss of core temperature when given to an apyrexial patient. Therefore careful assessment of vital signs is necessary before the administration of these drugs.

Tepid sponging and fanning

When the temperature remains elevated or continues to rise and the skin is hot to touch, various methods to aid cooling of the body surface and lowering of temperature levels can be utilized. The patient who has a moderate to high pyrexia may benefit from a tepid sponge or use of a fan.

Lowering of temperature levels by 1–2°C may be achieved by a tepid sponge 'bath' which assists heat loss by means of conduction, convection and evaporation. It must be remembered that the patient should be cooled and not chilled, as the latter will cause re-activation of the shivering process resulting in the temperature increasing once more. To evaluate the results of this procedure it is necessary to take the temperature before and after tepid sponging. Sponges are partially wrung from a basin containing water at a temperature of 27–30°C. The skin surface is bathed with long even strokes, allowing some of the moisture to evaporate, and the excess is dried with gentle patting movements. Drying by towel friction is not recommended as this creates more heat gain. To assist further cooling whilst the sponge bath is taking place, cloths or sponges that have been wrung out can be placed on areas which receive a rich blood supply such as the groin, axillae and wrists.

Another aid to cooling is an electric fan. The patient can be placed naked on the bed with a modesty garment over the groin. A wet sheet may also be placed over the patient and a fan, positioned safely, is permitted to transmit air over the sheet, thereby cooling the surface of the body. Again, to evaluate the results it is necessary to take the temperature before and after this procedure.

Other methods

In hyperpyrexia, cooling can be achieved by the

use of a hypothermic blanket or a body cooling unit. The hypothermic blanket is covered by a sheet which is more comfortable for the patient and allows absorption of sweat. Rectal or oesophageal probes monitor the patient's temperature continually. The blanket reduces the core temperature until the level has fallen by several degrees; it is then switched off, allowing the body to return to its normal thermal state naturally. Alternatively, the blanket may continue to assist loss of temperature until a mild (30–35°C) or moderate (24–30°C) induced hypothermia has been reached. Whilst lying on the cooling blanket the limbs lose heat more readily than the rest of the body. This produces a reduction in peripheral sensitivity and lack of awareness of pressure, therefore increasing the risk of pressure sore formation. Peripheral vasoconstriction and reduced metabolic rate due to excessive cooling also increases the risk of skin breakdown, particularly over bony prominences. Frequent inspection of these areas, together with position change, is therefore essential. Frostbite is also a possibility. To prevent shivering or cardiac arrhythmias occurring, care must be taken to reduce the temperature level slowly. If the patient is fully conscious the treatment should be explained in appropriate terms. Not only will this relieve the patient's anxiety, but if he understands the use of the blanket the conscious patient can help prevent undesirable consequences by informing the nurse when, for example, he loses the sensation of touch in his limbs or feels discomfort on the bony prominences.

Heat stroke rarely occurs conveniently close to medical services. Patients with heat stroke should immediately be taken into a shady, cool environment and their clothes removed. They should be placed in the prone position with limbs spread apart to create an increased surface area to assist heat loss. Any other actions such as fanning which may increase heat loss should be taken. As soon as is humanly possible the temperature should be recorded and the patient taken to a hospital centre where treatment may be given to replace fluid, to restore electrolyte balance and to reduce body heat. In an attempt to reduce temperature levels some hospitals instil iced saline into the stomach or rectum. Animal studies (Bynum et al, 1978) have produced evidence that the use of peritoneal lavage-cooling lowered rectal temperature more effectively than the use of slush baths, and this may become used more frequently.

Weiner & Khogali (1980) developed a body-cooling unit which is successful in the rapid lowering of core temperature without creating problems of shivering, cardiac arrhythmias and dehydration. This body-cooling unit consists of a mesh bed draped across a water bath. Warm air at a temperature of approximately 30–35°C circulates around the patient and sprays of cold water are projected onto the body surface, allowing the transfer of heat from core to shell thus promoting heat loss. This cooling unit keeps the body surface moist and maintains skin temperature at about 32°C. As the patient is more accessible in the mesh bed as compared with other methods of cooling, e.g. a cold water immersion bath, recording the vital signs and other nursing care actions are less difficult to manage.

PREVENTION OF HEAT-RELATED CONDITIONS

Many of the conditions associated with exposure to high environmental temperature can be prevented by recognition of those at risk and the giving of appropriate care or advice.

During heat waves the elderly in particular are at risk, as their adaptive abilities are less than in younger adults. Therefore careful monitoring of body temperature is needed and an adequate fluid intake, cool, loose clothing and a cool, well-ventilated environment should be provided. In a letter to the British Medical Journal, Goldfrank et al (1979) suggested that medication such as diuretics and alcohol (which increase fluid loss) and anti-cholinergics (which block some of the heat-losing mechanisms) should be either reduced or stopped during hot periods.

Those taking part in competitive or other runs should be taught about the signs and symptoms of heat exhaustion, should train beforehand and should have ample electrolyte-containing fluids provided both before and during the race.

When an individual is exposed to his/her first experience of living and working in a hot environment, his/her general activities should initially be limited and then gradually increased over a 2–3 week period. This allows acclimatization to take place, although Sodeman & Sodeman (1979) state that this achieved tolerance can be halted and reversed under certain conditions: for example, if alcohol is taken in excess causing a fall in ADH secretion and there is an increased fluid loss; if oral intake is unduly limited; if systemic illness is present, or if the individual becomes particularly fatigued. Sodeman & Sodeman also mention the physiological changes that occur during the process of acclimatization. Profuse sweating occurs and the electrolyte content of sweat falls. The cardiac output gradually returns to the previous baseline rate and postural hypotension, which may have occurred when the individual was first subjected to the hot environment, is halted.

HYPOTHERMIA

In the normal physiological state, when the body is cooled the internal regulating mechanisms endeavour to maintain body temperature. This is done by increasing the heat produced through a rise in the metabolic rate, caused by increased secretion of thyroid hormones and adrenaline and by shivering. At the same time heat loss is reduced through vasoconstriction. In addition, behavioural changes to regulate body temperature are employed.

If these mechanisms are ineffective, body temperature drops. As the condition of hypothermia develops the metabolic rate drops and all bodily activities become sluggish. Hypothermia can be classified according to severity and according to length of time it takes to develop. Mild hypothermia is when the core body temperature is 34–35°C. Intense vasoconstriction and shivering still function to try to maintain body temperature but muscular weakness and incoordination are developing. The mental state becomes dulled (Collins 1983).

Moderate hypothermia is when the core temperature falls to between 30–34°C. This is the transitional zone between the mild condition, when body mechanisms for maintaining core temperature are still working, and the severe state when they mainly cease. Shivering usually ceases but vasoconstriction remains. Pulse and respiratory rates drop and consciousness is lost between 30–32°C (Collins, 1983).

In severe hypothermia the core temperature is below 30°C and the patient is very cold to touch. The skin may have blue patches and become oedematous. Breathing may be almost imperceptible. The reduced oxygen supply to the myocardium increases the heart's susceptibility to cardiac arrhythmias (Rae, 1980) and ventricular fibrillation may develop around 28°C (Allan, 1974). Below a body temperature of about 25°C the mechanisms for maintaining body temperature are lost and heat loss to the surroundings occurs passively (Collins, 1983).

Hypothermia can be induced as a method of treatment in neurological conditions or to increase the safety margin in performing some neurosurgical or cardiac operations. The metabolic rate is lowered and, therefore, the nutritional and oxygen requirements of the tissues are reduced. The period when the circulation to the brain can be disrupted is thus extended. Body temperature is monitored closely throughout the procedure.

TYPES OF HYPOTHERMIA

Acute hypothermia

Accidental hypothermia can be described as acute, subacute or chronic. In acute hypothermia the patient's temperature is 30°C or below and he is unconscious. This description has also been applied when hypothermia develops in less than 6 hours and 'immersion hypothermia' is the classical case. Immersion in very cold water will lead to rapid heat loss accompanied by extensive shivering. Consciousness may be lost fairly quickly and the subject thus drowns. The rate of heat loss is greater in colder water but is modified by a number of factors. Individuals with a low surface to volume ratio, i.e. of a short, stocky build and with a thick subcutaneous fat layer, lose heat more slowly. If the surface area can be reduced by curling up, then again heat loss is slowed. The shivering response is very variable and good shiverers maintain their body temperature for longer than others. As alcohol consumption increases vasodilatation, this increases the rate of cooling. Physical activity counteracts vasoconstriction and heat loss is increased by one third when an individual is moving, e.g. swimming, rather than staying still and shivering (Hayward, 1983).

Subacute hypothermia

When body temperature is above 30°C and the patient is still conscious the condition is described as subacute. This situation may take 6–24 hours to develop and 'exhaustion hypothermia' is an example of this, although this condition may become more severe with time. Exhaustion hypothermia often develops when the subject has been hurrying and sweating. The sweating and vasodilatation both increase heat loss and, as clothing becomes wet, heat loss occurs even faster. The fluid loss also causes some degree of dehydration, and blood glucose levels may fall as glucose is utilized in metabolism, or rise if gluconeogenesis due to hormonal changes is considerable (Kuehn, 1983).

Chronic hypothermia

Chronic or subclinical hypothermia develops over a lengthy period of exposure to a cool environment and is most common among the elderly. Social conditions such as inadequate heating, or money to pay for it, and insufficient clothing and intake of nutrients, are often associated with the development of hypothermia among this group of people. The condition is suspected when the patient's skin, even in areas such as the abdomen, feels cold to the touch. The skin is usually pale and waxy in appearance and consciousness is often impaired. The diagnosis can only be confirmed by measuring the body temperature, usually by the rectal route. A low-reading thermometer which can record temperatures down to 24°C is used (Wollner & Spalding, 1978).

Predisposing factors

A number of physiological changes which are more common in the elderly predispose them to the development of this condition. Fox et al (1973) found that 10% of the elderly people that they examined had abnormally low body temperatures. Over a period of 4 years, Collins et al (1977) examined thermoregulation in 47 elderly individuals. They found that although there was no change in the general life-style there was evidence of a continuing decline in their thermoregulatory function. In a cold environment vasoconstriction was less noticeable than in the healthy adult and this resulted in excessive loss of body heat. A number of studies indicate that at least some elderly people have reduced sensitivity to temperature change (Horvath et al, 1955; Watts, 1972; Collins et al, 1977) and therefore do not take appropriate action to keep warm.

There is also evidence that thermogenesis becomes less efficient with age (Cooper & Ferguson, 1983). MacMillan et al (1967) described differences found between a group of elderly subjects who had recovered from an episode of accidental hypothermia and a control group. The group who had previously been hypothermic did not respond to cold by shivering, by an increased metabolic rate (as shown by oxygen consumption) or by vasoconstriction.

Cooper & Ferguson (1983) have classified some of the conditions that predispose the elderly to the development of hypothermia:

- changes in perception of environmental temperature, for example, without obvious disease or as a result of neurological disease (e.g. stroke).
- changes in the ability to generate heat in the cold, for example, minute but unrecognized brain lesions, immobilization (severe arthritis, stroke), myxoedema or panhypopituitarism, coma (diabetes, cerebral vascular accident, use of alcohol, use of street drugs, trauma), or subclinical malnutrition.

- failure of behavioural responses to cold, e.g. senility, mild confusion, or Alzheimer's disease.
- effects of prescription drugs, e.g. drugs used to treat high blood pressure (e.g. Aldomet, sympathetic transmitter modifiers), drugs used to alter mood (e.g. imipramine) or unrecognized myxoedema psychosis treated with chlorpromazine or tranquillizers and barbiturates.
- simple exposure (e.g. falling into cold water, being caught in a vehicle in a blizzard) which could happen at any age.
- severe autonomic dysfunction that prevents control of blood vessels in the skin, (e.g. Shy-Drager syndrome, intermediolateral column degeneration, or hypothalamic tumours).

MANAGEMENT OF HYPOTHERMIA

There is still no consensus on the best method of rewarming a hypothermic individual. Although results have improved in the past 20 years there is still a high mortality rate. Kuehn (1983) quotes results including 49% (Bowman, 1977) and 60% (Ledingham & Mone, 1980) overall mortality rate, this rate being lower in the milder cases of hypothermia.

Certain principles of rewarming can be identified. Methods of rewarming can be divided into surface methods and core techniques. Table 27.1 shows a list of methods used and the ease with which they can be implemented. Whatever method is used, the aim is to achieve a normal body temperature while preventing, or minimizing, the complications which may occur.

Complications of hypothermia and rewarming

All systems of the body are involved in hypothermia and may show signs of impaired function during rewarming. Some of these will be life-threatening and the early recognition and treatment of them are essential for successful resuscitation.

Cardiovascular problems

In patients where hypothermia has developed slowly fluid appears to leak out of the circulation into the tissues, leading to a fall in plasma volume and blood pressure. When vasodilatation occurs as a result of surface rewarming there may be a further fall in blood pressure leading to rewarming shock (Kuehn, 1983). If the blood pressure falls as the patient is rewarmed he or she should be rapidly cooled again and gradually rewarmed after stabilization of the blood pressure (Wollner, 1967). Frequent monitoring of the blood pressure will be essential. Cold blood which has been trapped in the peripheral tissues will be released back into the body core when vasodilatation occurs. The resulting drop in core temperature can lead to cardiac dysrhythmias and arrest. Cardiac monitoring will greatly ease the observation of the patient.

The circulation is slowed and haematocrit raised because of the reduced plasma volume. The risk of blood clotting would seem to be increased and has been reported (Bunker & Goldstein, 1958), but thrombocytopenia is also relatively common (Wessel & Bigelow, 1959). Observation for both bleeding and clotting will therefore be necessary. Passive, and later active, leg exercises should be carried out. The blood volume will be restored by administration of intravenous fluids (warmed to room temperature) but it is particularly important that overloading of the circulation be avoided. Central venous pressure measurements are valuable in monitoring the fluid volume status of the body, and fluid intake and output must be measured. Oliguria is common.

Metabolic disturbances

While body temperature is low, metabolic rate is also reduced, but will increase as rewarming occurs. With an inadequate circulation this will lead to tissue anoxia and metabolic acidosis (McNichol & Smith, 1964). In hypothermia the blood glucose level may rise as insulin is inactive, but on rewarming glucose enters the cells and hypoglycaemia may develop. Changes in insulin

Table 27.1 Comparison of methods of rewarming (from Kuehn, 1983)

Method	Rate of core-temperature increase (°C per hour)	Ease of implementation Field	Hospital
Surface techniques			
Blanket insulation in warm room	0.5–1.0	Good	Good
Body-heat rewarming	Low	Good	Superfluous
Radiation treatment (heat cradle)	0.5–1.0	Poor	Good
Hot-bath rewarming	3–4	Good	Good
Hot-water suit, blanket, mattress	1–2	Good	Good
Hot-water showers	1–2	Good	Superfluous
Electric blanket, heat pack	Approx 1	Good	Good
Core techniques			
Respiratory rewarming	0.5–2.0	Good	Good
Peritoneal dialysis	0.5–4.5	Poor	Good
Mediastinal irrigation	8.0	Poor	Good
Extracorporeal circulation	7.0–10.5	Poor	Good
Haemodialysis	0.5	Poor	Good
Intragastric lavage	2–3	Poor	Good
Colonic lavage	Low	Good	Good
Diathermy (Microwave)	4.7	Poor	Good
Food and drink	Negligible	Good	Good

activity also lead to changes in serum potassium concentrations (Beisel et al, 1968). Blood glucose levels, serum electrolytes and blood gases will all need to be monitored. The metabolic disturbances will increase the vulnerability of the tissues and regular, frequent turning of the patient is essential.

Respiratory problems

Respiration is slow and shallow in hypothermia and therefore the patient is at risk of developing a chest infection. Signs of bronchopneumonia are often minimal and intravenous antibiotics are often given routinely (Wollner & Spalding, 1978). Position changing and physiotherapy will help to reduce this risk. While the patient is unconscious he/she must be positioned to prevent inhalation of vomit. This is a marked risk because dilation of the stomach is common in hypothermia. If possible, an endotracheal tube is not used as the insertion may invoke cardiac dysrhythmias.

Surface rewarming

As the name indicates, surface rewarming involves allowing heat to enter the body from the surface, eventually leading to an increase in core body temperature. To reduce the risk of a large volume of cold blood re-entering the body and affecting heart function, heat should be applied to the head, trunk, neck and groin but active warming of the limbs should be omitted.

People exposed to extreme cold who are otherwise fit can be warmed fairly quickly by surface rewarming (Keatinge, 1969). However, surface rewarming is not recommended unless the hot bath method can be used. This is because the application of heat to the skin prevents the shivering response and so reduces heat produced by the body.

Kaufman (1983) recommends that, in those with subacute hypothermia, action should be taken to minimize further heat loss and energy expenditure until help can be obtained. The individual affected should be wrapped in warm, dry clothing, if available, and sit on a non-conducting surface such as wood. Heat loss through respiration can be reduced by covering the head, mouth and nose with a cap and scarf. Heat loss by evaporation must be minimized. Unless plenty of dry clothing is available it is better simply to cover the wet clothing. The heat required to warm 1kg of water from 4°C to 34°C is only 30kcal, and the wet, warmed clothes will reduce heat loss. In the mildly hypothermic patient exercise can be helpful in increasing heat production.

Elderly patients with hypothermia must be rewarmed slowly as they are more likely to succumb to complications (Wollner & Spalding, 1978). Emslie-Smith (1981) recommends that the elderly should be placed in a warm room with the environmental temperature kept between 20–30°C. The patient's temperature should be continually monitored by an electronic rectal probe and the body temperature allowed to rise by about 0.5°C an hour. Blood pressure must be recorded half-hourly.

Core rewarming

As can be seen from Table 27.1, a number of techniques are available for directly raising the temperature of the body core. If such techniques are available, the problems associated with this type of rewarming are shock and cardiac dysrhythmias due to cold blood re-entering the body core. However, most of these methods require sophisticated equipment and medically qualified personnel. In addition, these methods expose the patient to the risk of infection.

Ledingham et al (1980) have produced a method of rewarming hypothermic patients which may solve many problems which arise from attempts to raise central core temperature. With the use of a modified Sengstaken tube, rewarming of the patient can take place without physiological complications occurring, for example, dysrhythmias and hypotension. Once the tube is passed, Ringer's lactate solution at a temperature of 41°C is allowed to pass through the apparatus resulting in the central structures of the body being warmed before the shell. With the use of gastric lavage, Ledingham suggests that this method of rewarming would be of use in patients who have central core temperatures of 32°C and below.

PREVENTION OF HYPOTHERMIA

Hypothermia will continue to occur in those who expose themselves to harsh environmental conditions for work or sport. However, some actions can be taken to avoid or minimize the risk. Wearing special survival garments when there is a risk of submersion in cold water can reduce the dangers involved (Hayward, 1983). Knowledge of the factors which increase the risk of 'exhaustion hypothermia' should enable those who climb or hike to avoid becoming overheated and thus reduce heat loss.

With the elderly there is much that can be done to reduce the risk of developing hypothermia (BMA, 1964). Elderly people and their relatives should be taught about the importance of a warm environment at night as well as during the day. Advice on nutrition, clothing and bedding may all be of value, and monetary assistance can be organized for extra fuel. Community health and social work staff have an important role to play in identifying those at risk due to environmental and social factors, and in taking action to reduce that risk. In addition, all health care professionals should be alert to the possibility of this condition and be able to identify it. Exton-Smith (1968) recommended that a low-reading thermometer should be carried by every general practitioner, health visitor and district nurse.

REFERENCES

Allan E T 1974 Hypothermia: prolonged immersion in cold water. Nursing Times 70:1928–1929

Angerami E L S 1980 Epidemiological study of body temperature in patients in hospital. International Journal of Nursing Studies 17:91–99

Barbour H G 1912 In: MacBryde C M, Blacklow R S (eds) 1970 Signs and symptoms: applied pathologic physiology and clinical interpretation, 5th edn. Lippincott, Philadelphia

Beisel W R, Goldman R F, Joy R J T 1968 Metabolic balance studies during induced hyperthermia in man. Journal of Applied Physiology 24:1–10

Blainey C G 1974 Site selection in taking body temperature. American Journal of Nursing 74:1859–1861

Bowman W 1977 Medical aspects of mountain nursing. Journal of Winter Emergency Care 2:31–47

British Medical Association Special Committee 1964 Accidental hypothermia in the elderly. British Medical Journal 2:1255–1258

Bunker J P, Goldstein R 1958 Coagulation during hypothermia in man. Proceedings of the Society for Experimental Biology and Medicine 97:199–202

Bynum G, Patton J, Bowers W, Leav I, Hamlet M, Marsili M, Wolfe D 1978 Peritoneal lavage cooling in an anaesthetized dog heatstroke model. Aviation Space and Environmental Medicine 49:779–784
Castle M 1979 Fever: understanding a sinister sign. Nursing (Horsham) 9(20):26–33
Collins K J 1983 Hypothermia: the facts. Oxford University Press, Oxford
Collins K J, Dore C, Exton-Smith A N, Fox R H, McDonald I C, Woodward P M 1977 Accidental hypothermia and impaired temperature homeostasis in the elderly. British Medical Journal 1:353–356
Cooper K E, Ferguson A V 1983 Thermoregulation and hypothermia in the elderly. In: Pozos R S, Wittners L E (eds) The nature and treatment of hypothermia. Croom Helm, London
Cox B 1978 Pharmacology of the hypothalamus. Macmillan, London
Davies D M (ed) 1981 Textbook of adverse drug reactions, 2nd edn. Oxford University Press, Oxford
Davis-Sharts 1978 Mechanisms and manifestations of fever. American Journal of Nursing 78:1874–1877
Edholm O G 1978 Man — hot and cold. Edward Arnold, London
Ellis F P, Prince H P, Lovatt G, Whittington R M 1980 Mortality and morbidity in Birmingham during the 1976 heatwave. Quarterly Journal of Medicine 49(193):1–8
Emslie-Smith D 1981 Hypothermia in the elderly. British Journal of Hospital Medicine 26:442,448–50,452
Erickson R 1976 Thermometer placement for oral temperature measurement in febrile adults. International Journal of Nursing Studies 13:199–208
Exton-Smith A N 1968 Accidental hypothermia in the elderly. Practitioner 200:804–812
Fox R H, MacGibbon R, Danes L, Woodward P M 1973 Problem of the old and the cold. British Medical Journal 1:21–24
Ganong W F 1981 Review of medical physiology, 10th edn. Lange Medical, Los Altos, California
Goldfrank L, Davis R, Dunford M 1979 Heatwave deaths and drugs affecting temperature regulation. Letter, British Medical Journal 2(6188):494–495
Gruber P A 1974 Changes in cardiac rate associated with the use of the rectal thermometer in the patient with acute myocardial infarction. Heart Lung 3:2
Hasler M E, Cohen J A 1982 The effect of oxygen administration on oral temperature assessment. Nursing Research 31:265–268
Hayward, J S 1983 The physiology of immersion hypothermia. In: Pozos R S, Wittmers L E (eds) The nature and treatment of hypothermia. Croom Helm, London
Hensel H 1981 Thermoreception and temperature regulation. Academic Press, London
Horvath S M, Radcliffe C E, Hatt P K, Spurr G B 1955 Metabolic responses of old people in a cold environment. Journal of Applied Physiology 8:145–148
Howell T H 1972 Axillary temperature in aged women. Age and Ageing 1:250–254
Hughson R L, Sutton J R 1978 Heat stroke in a 'run for fun'. Letter, British Medical Journal 2(6145):1158
Jacoby G A, Swartz M N 1973 Fever of undetermined origin. New England Journal of Medicine 289:1407–1410
Kaufman W C 1983 The development and rectification of hiker's hypothermia. In: Pozos R S, Wittmers L E (eds) The nature and treatment of hypothermia. Croom Helm, London
Keatinge W R 1969 Survival in cold water. Blackwell Scientific, Oxford
Kozier B, Erb G L 1983 Foundations of nursing: concepts and procedures. Addison-Wesley, London
Kuehn L A 1983 Introduction. In: Pozos, R S, Wiltmers L E (ed) the nature and treatment of hypothermia. Croom Helm, London
Lancet 1979 Running repairs. 2(8156):1344
Ledingham I, Mone J 1980 Treatment of accidental hypothermia: a prospective clinical study. British Medical Journal 2:1102– 1105
Ledingham I McA, Douglas I H S, Routh G S, Macdonald A M 1980 Central rewarming system for treatment of hypothermia. Lancet 1(8179):1168–1169
Lee R V, Atkins E 1972 Spurious fever. American Journal of Nursing 72:1094–1095
Leithead C S, Lind A R 1964 Heat stress and heat disorders. Cassell, London
Lim-Levy F 1982 The effect of oxygen inhalation on oral temperature. Nursing Research 31:150–152
MacBryde C M, Blacklow R S 1970 Signs and symptoms: applied pathologic physiology and clinical interpretation, 5th edn. Lippincott, Philadelphia
MacMillan A L, Corbett J L, Johnson R H, Smith A C, Spalding J R K, Wollner L 1967 Temperature regulation in survivors of accidental hypothermia of the elderly. Lancet 2:165–169
McNichol M W, Smith R 1964 Accidental hypothermia. British Medical Journal 1(5374):19–21
Milton A S, Wendlant S 1970 A possible role for prostaglandin E1 as a modulator for temperature regulation in the central nervous system of the cat. Journal of Physiology 207:76–77
Minor D G, Waterhouse J M 1981 Circadian rhythms and the human. Wright, Bristol
Moorat D S 1976 The cost of taking temperatures. Nursing Times 72:767–770
Nichols G A 1972 Time analysis of afebrile and febrile temperature readings. Nursing Research 21:463–464
Nichols G A, Ruskin M M, Glor B A K, Kelly W H 1966 Oral, axillary and rectal temperature determinations and relationships. Nursing Research 15:307–309
Nichols G A, Kucha D H, Mahoney R P 1972 Rectal thermometer placement times for febrile adults. Nursing Research 21:76–77
Nicholson M R, Somerville K N 1978 Heat stroke in a 'run for fun' race. British Medical Journal 1:6126
Petersdorf R G, Bennet I L 1957 cited in Lee R V, Atkins E 1972 Spurious fever. American Journal of Nursing 72:1094–1095
Rae D 1980 Accidental hypothermia: emergency rewarming techniques. Canadian Nurse 76(2):28–30
Schmidt A J 1972 TPRs: an old habit or a significant routine? Hospitals 46(2):57–60
Seller J H, Yoder A E 1961 A comparative study of temperature readings. Nursing Research 10:43–45
Sodeman W A, Sodeman T M 1979 Pathologic physiology: mechanisms of disease, 6th edn. Saunders, Philadelphia
Vane J R 1978 In: Cox B et al (eds) Pharmacology of the hypothalamus. Macmillan, London
Wannemacher R W, Beisel W R 1977 Metabolic response of the host to infectious disease. In: Richards, J R, Kinney, J M (eds) Nutritional aspects of care in the critically ill.

Churchill Livingstone, Edinburgh
Watts A J 1972 Hypothermia in the aged: a study of the role of cold sensitivity. Environmental Research (New York) 5:119–126
Weiner J S, Khogali M 1980 A physiological body-cooling unit for treatment of heatstroke. Lancet I(8167):507–509
Wessel R H, Bigelow W G 1959 The use of heparin to minimize thrombocytopenia and bleeding tendencies during hypothermia. Surgery 45:223–228
Wollner L 1967 Accidental hypothermia and temperature regulation in the elderly. Gerontologia clinica 9:347–359
Wollner L, Spalding J M K 1978 The autonomic nervous system. In: Brocklehurst J C (ed) Textbook of geriatric medicine and gerontology. Churchill Livingstone, Edinburgh

Appendix

The physiology of pain

INTRODUCTION

Pain is a complex psychological and physiological phenomenon which is usually initiated by the activation of pain receptors (nociceptors) in cutaneous and visceral tissues. Specialist sets of afferent units transmit nerve impulses, which encode nociceptive information, from the periphery to the dorsal horn of the spinal cord (or the trigeminal complex in the brain stem).

Neurons arising from the spinal cord project to supraspinal centres via several complex and divergent routes. Activity in these multiple ascending pathways results in the activation of medullary, midbrain, thalamic and cortical structures. Central processing of nociceptive information in these regions generates the sensory-discriminative, cognitive-evaluative and motivational-affective components of the pain experience. In addition autonomic and motor responses may be evoked.

Modulation of pain transmission at spinal (and possibly other) levels of the neural axis may occur due to segmental mechanisms or as a consequence of the influence of descending pathways originating from the brain stem or possibly cortical structures.

From this brief introduction it can be seen that the physiology of pain can be divided into three major study areas: peripheral mechanisms, central mechanisms and the modulation of pain transmission. This is the approach which will be

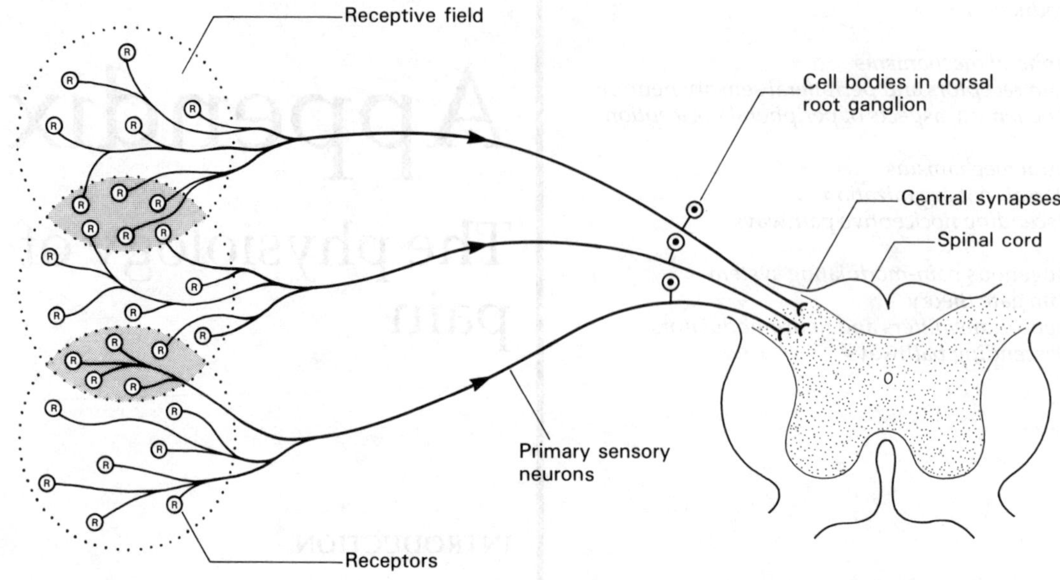

Fig. A 1 Organization of peripheral sensory units

adopted in the following sections, and although it is not the intention to consider physical and pharmacological aspects of analgesia in depth, they will be cited whenever considered appropriate.

PERIPHERAL MECHANISMS

PAIN RECEPTORS AND PERIPHERAL SENSORY NEURONS

Sensory information generated by the activation of sensory receptors is conveyed to the central nervous system (CNS) by peripheral sensory neurons whose cell bodies are located in the dorsal root ganglion of the spinal cord or the trigeminal complex. The receptors and their associated sensory neurons constitute a primary sensory unit (Fig. A1). It must be noted that Figure A1 is a simplification of the existing organization that takes no account of the extensive peripheral and central branching which occurs in certain primary afferents. This gives rise to the innervation of structures other than the skin (Fig. A2) and central input into more than one cord segment.

The sensory neurons together with motor neurons have been classified on the basis of their cross-sectional diameter and conduction velocity as indicated in Table A1. Proprioceptive information from the musculoskeletal system, light touch and tactile discrimination are transmitted in the rapidly conducting myelinated A alpha (Aα) and A beta (Aβ) fibres, while information transduced by nociceptors (pain receptors) is carried by small, slowly conducting, finely myelinated A delta (Aδ) fibres or the even smaller, very slowly conducting, non-myelinated C fibres.

Nociceptors are generally regarded as being simple free or undifferentiated nerve endings which are present in the dermis and epidermis. Although nociceptors are structurally similar they differ with respect to their *thresholds* — the minimum stimulus which activates them — and their *specificity* for transducing both noxious (tissue damaging) and non-noxious stimuli. Some nociceptors associated with Aδ fibres are unimodal, responding to high threshold mechanical stimulation, while others are bimodal, responding to both noxious and non-noxious thermal stimuli or noxious mechanical and thermal stimulation. The group C

Table A 1 Classification of neurons

Type	Group	Conduction velocity m/s	Diameter nm	Function or associated receptor
A-alpha	I	70–120	12–20	Proprioception; golgi tendon organ and muscle spindle
				Somatic motor
beta		30–70	5–12	Touch, pressure, muscle spindle
gamma	II	15–30	3–6	Motor to muscle spindle
delta	III	12–30	2–5	Pain, temperature (cold)
B		3–15	1–3	Preganglionic autonomic
C	IV	0.5 –2.0	0.2 –2	Postganglionic autonomic
				Pain, temperature (cold and hot), pressure

nociceptors are usually polymodal and are responsive to noxious mechanical, thermal and chemical stimulation but also to gentle mechanical events. The unique area surrounding a sensory receptor within which it is capable of transducing a sensory stimulus and subsequently generating receptor and action potentials is known as the *receptive field* of the sensory neuron. Adjacent receptive fields overlap and therefore stimulation of the overlapping region may excite more than one sensory neuron (Fig. A1). The precision with which the site of stimulus can be located will therefore in part depend on the size of the receptive fields and the extent of the overlap. While some primary sensory neurons are only associated with a single sensory receptor (Aβ, low threshold mechanoreceptor), those conveying information generated by impending or actual tissue damage (Aδ and C fibres) tend to exhibit extensive but variable branching and as a consequence of this have relatively large receptive fields. This, together with the characteristics of the spinal cord organization and the ascending pathways involved in nociceptive transmission within the CNS, accounts for the fact that pain tends to be a poorly localized sensation when compared with tactile sensations. The ability to identify precisely the site of a stimulation will also depend on the density of sensory receptors in a particular region of the body. Nociceptors are found in high concentrations in tissues such as skin, arteries and mucous membranes while neural tissue within the brain and articular cartilage are devoid of nociceptors. This variation in *nociceptor density* accounts for the differences in sensitivity found in these tissues to injury. Furthermore it should be noted that internal organs and tissues may only respond to a certain type of stimulus. Thus it is possible to cut or burn the intestines without mediating pain, but stretching or distension evokes painful responses.

When subjected to repeated stimulation most sensory receptors *adapt* at varying rates, that is they become less responsive to the applied stimulus. In contrast nociceptors either adapt very slowly or they *sensitise,* which is characterized by a a decrease in the stimulus intensity required to reach threshold. In addition this can give rise to prolonged activity in the primary nociceptive unit and a correspondingly persistent sensation characteristic of pain. (Other mechanisms may also be involved — see Central Mechanisms.)

Variations in specificity, thresholds, size of functional receptive fields and rates of adaptation of nociceptors, together with the differing conduction velocities of the nociceptive afferent-fibres, are considered to account at least in part for the sensations experienced when tissue is damaged. The more rapidly conducting Aδ fibres give rise to the perception of immediate, bright, sharp, localized sensations and are responsible for the initiation

Table A 2 Properties of nociceptors and nociceptive afferents

Properties	Aδ units		C units
Diameter nm	1–5		0.2–2
Conduction velocity m/s	5–30		0.5–2
Structure	Myelinated		Non-myelinated
Adaptation	Slow		Sensitize
Receptive fields	Multiple points small*		Single zone large*
Functional classification	Unimodal	Bimodal	Polymodal
Modality transduced	High threshold mechanical stimulation	Noxious and non noxious thermal stimulation or noxious mechanical and thermal stimulation.	Noxious mechanical, thermal and mechanical stimulation.
Regional distribution	Somatic	Somatic	Somatic and visceral
Sensation perceived	Sharp, bright, stabbing. pin prick, fast pain		Dull, aching, burning, sustained, slow pain

*variable, relative

of withdrawal reflexes. The duller, prolonged, delocalized burning sensation which follows the initial response is due to activity in the slower conducting polymodal C fibres. Thus the Aδ units appear to be specialized to detect impending tissue damage and evoke rapid protective responses while the C units detect the presence of actual tissue damage or an inflamed area. Some of the properties of nociceptors and nociceptor afferents are summarized in Table A2.

Most of the information available concerning the properties of nociceptive afferent units has been generated from studies on the innervation of the skin. However, polymodal Aδ units have been found in skeletal muscle, cornea, tooth pulp and periodontium and there is evidence for the presence of specialized Aδ units in skeletal muscle and joints. In addition, C-fibre polymodal units have been identified in skeletal muscle and tooth pulp. All of these structures are frequently subjected to stress and other potentially damaging events, and as a consequence would be expected to contain specialist nociceptive units.

In contrast, for most internal structures, tissue damage and inflammation are unusual events, therefore the evolution of specific nociceptive units in such regions would appear to be unlikely. Nevertheless, thoracic and abdominal structures innervated by both sympathetic and parasympathetic components of the autonomic nervous system can be a source of poorly localized pain. Most afferent fibres running in autonomic nerves are not nociceptive, responding to normal physiological activity in organs and tissues. However, nociceptive afferents have been detected in sympathetic nerves associated with the lower part of the oesophagus, abdomen and heart, while pain originating in the upper part of the oesophagus, the airways and pelvic structures is transmitted through parasympathetic nerves. Although a minority of these efferents appear to be highly specialized nociceptive units, for example units sensitive to ischaemia and bradykinin (possibly originating from damaged tissue) occur in the heart, nociception in most internal organs is mediated via mechanoreceptors which are capable of responding to both normal physiological functions and noxious events. Since the innervation of different regions of the thorax and abdomen shows considerable variation and only a limited number of studies have been undertaken, it is not possible at the present time to offer a concise overall view of visceral nociception.

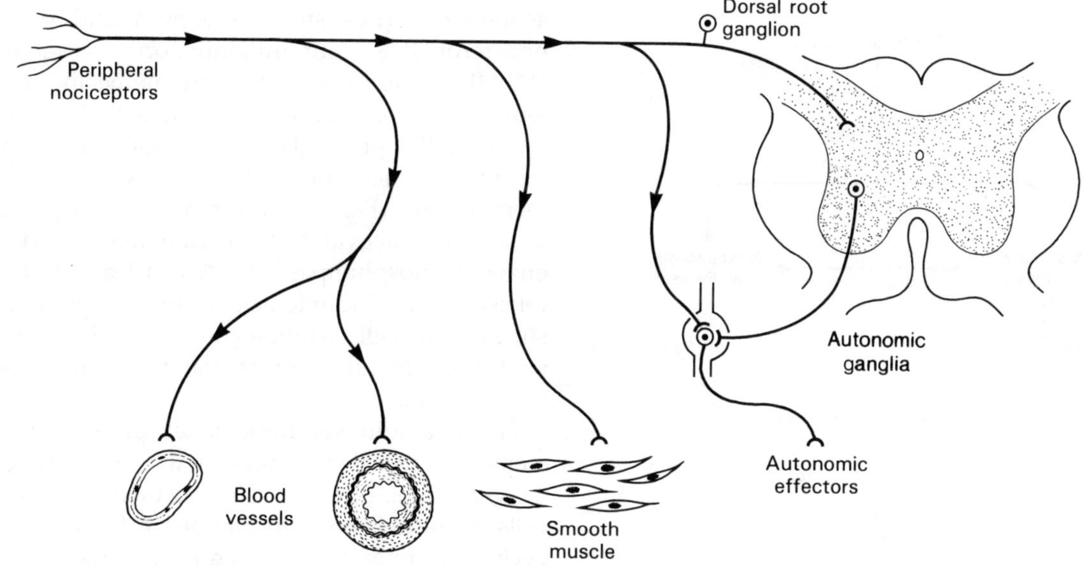

Fig. A 2 Possible organization of substance P, containing C fibres

BIOCHEMICAL ASPECTS OF PERIPHERAL NOCICEPTION

Receptor substances and neurotransmitters

Each functional group of dorsal root cells is thought to synthesize a unique substance which is axonally transported from the cell body to the peripheral nerve ending where it functions as a receptor substance. The release of the receptor substance causes activation of the sensory nerve endings. Transportation of this same substance also takes place into the central terminals of the dorsal root, where it serves as a neurotransmitter for central transmission of afferent information.

The receptor substance/neurotransmitter has not been identified for Aδ fibres, but substance P (SP), a peptide consisting of an 11-amino acid sequence is considered to be a prime candidate for this role in C fibre units. SP is one of a family of biologically active peptides, the tachykinins, which are now known to co-exist in C fibres and possibly other dorsal root neurons. Due to the extensive peripheral branching of C fibres leading to the innervation of blood vessels, various types of smooth muscle and post-ganglionic fibres of the autonomic nervous system, SP and related compounds have been detected in peripheral tissues and organs (Fig. A2). Thus the release of SP as a consequence of tissue damage not only activates nociceptors but due to antidromic stimulation may also elicit inflammatory responses, such as vasodilatation and protein extravasation, together with smooth muscle contraction and autonomic changes.

Although there is strong evidence that SP is a primary neurotransmitter of the first order nociceptive afferents, its role as a receptor substance and the mechanism of nociceptor activation is less clear. Biochemical changes in the microenvironment of nociceptors caused by tissue damage may cause the release of SP with concomitant nociceptor activation. Alternatively, on release from peripheral terminals SP may stimulate nociceptors following the occupation of extracellular receptors.

Tissue damage and nociceptor activation

Tissue damage leads to the rapid release and synthesis of a variety of chemicals which are capable of directly activating pain receptors or lowering their threshold (sensitizing) to the effects of other stimuli such as a second chemical

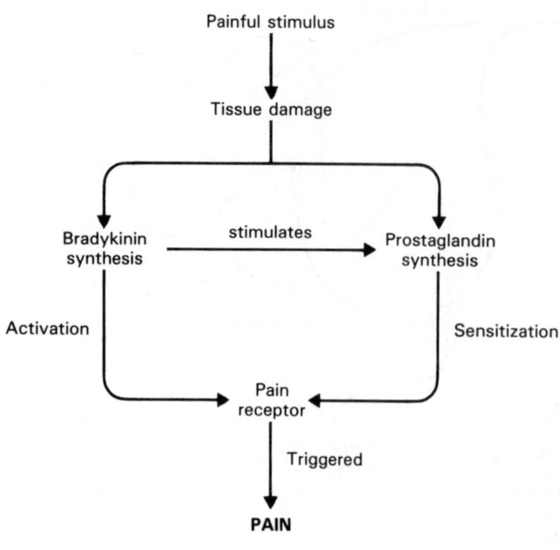

Fig. A 3 Summary of the events associated with receptor activation

factor, heat or mechanical deformation. These algesic substances include intrinsic, preformed mediators such as hydrogen ions, potassium ions, calcium ions, acetylcholine, 5-hydroxytryptamine and histamine. In addition, tissue damage stimulates the formation of bradykinin from inert precursors in plasma and tissue, together with a range of prostaglandins originating from damaged cell membranes.

There is a complex and as yet poorly understood relationship between the various algesic substances. One possible sequence of events involving bradykinin and the prostaglandins which leads to nociceptive activation is illustrated in Figure A3. Prostaglandins are consistently released following tissue damage and are present in all inflammatory exudates. These observations suggest that the synthesis of the prostaglandins and their synergistic interaction with bradykinin (or histamine) may be a common denominator in nociceptor activation. The key role of the prostaglandins in pain and inflammatory responses is reinforced by the demonstration that the analgesic and anti-inflammatory actions of drugs such as aspirin and other nonsteroidal anti-inflammatory agents (NSAIDs) (for example indomethacin and ibuprofen), are at least in part due to their ability to inhibit prostaglandin formation from arachidonic acid derived from damaged cell membranes (Fig. A4). Stimulation of cell membranes activates the membrane bounded enzyme phospholipase A_2, which leads to the release of arachidonic acid from phospholipid stores in the cell membrane and the subsequent synthesis of the prostaglandins and the leukotrienes.

Prostaglandin synthesis takes place in two steps: the initial reactions catalyzed by cyclo-oxygenases are non-specific, occurring in most cells, resulting in the formation of the unstable cyclic endoperoxidases and the damaging superoxides O_2^-. The second reaction is tissue specific and dependent upon the intracellular enzyme involved: the cyclic endoperoxidases can be converted to prostaglandins, PGE_2 and $PGF_{2\alpha}$, prostacyclin (PGI_2) or thromboxane A_2 (TXA_2). PGE_2, $PGF_{2\alpha}$ and possibly prostacyclin are involved in causing pain, erythema and tissue oedema.

Synthesis via the lipooxygenase pathway produces the precursors of the leukotrienes, the chemotactic hydro-peroxy-eicosa-tetraenoic acid (HPETE) and hydroxy-eicosa-tetraenoic acid (HETE), further conversions ultimately producing the leukotrienes. Leukotrienes are chemotactic, pro-inflammatory and are known to play important roles in psoriasis, ulcerative colitis, gout and rheumatoid arthritis.

Cyclo-oxygenases are inhibited by aspirin and other NSAIDS. These drugs are not lipooxygenase inhibitors and may actually divert arachidonic acid into leukotriene synthesis. In contrast, corticosteroids block both prostaglandin and leukotriene synthesis by preventing the activation of the phospholipase A_2 enzyme, so blocking the release of arachidonic acid. This effect has been shown to be due to the ability of corticosteroids to induce the synthesis of lipocortin, an endogenous protein with antiphospholipase A_2 activity (see Fig. A4).

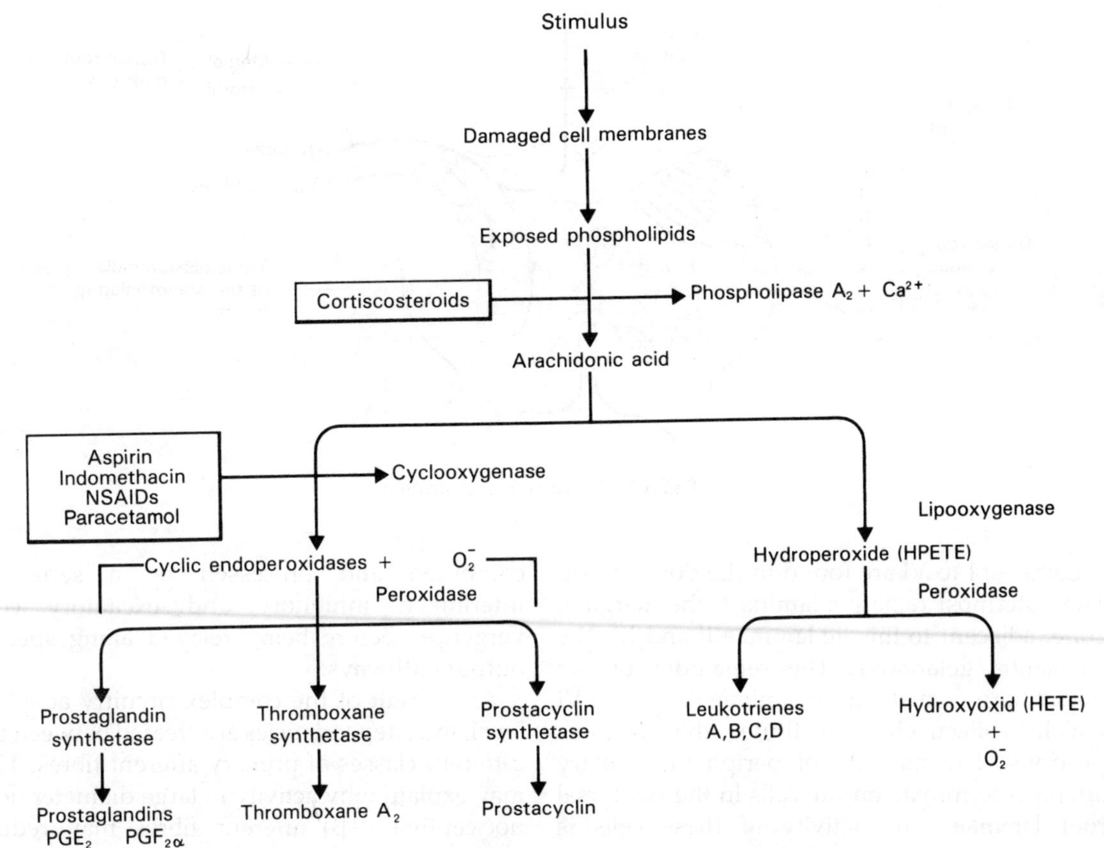

Fig. A 4 Metabolism of arachidonic acid

CENTRAL MECHANISMS

The various classes of nerve fibre are arranged randomly in the peripheral nerves, but as they enter the dorsal roots of the spinal cord they undergo rearrangement and segregation. The large diameter primary afferents assume a medial position — the medial dorsal root division — whereas the small diameter fibres take up a lateral position — the lateral dorsal root division. There is no common pathway for sensory input in the spinal cord, fibres of both types terminating in precise and localized regions.

DORSAL ROOT ORGANIZATION

Dorsal horn cells responding to peripheral input are arranged in an orderly fashion such that their receptive fields form a map of the body. Medial cells respond to distal stimuli and lateral cells to the stimulation of proximal regions. Thus in any cord segment the dermatome is represented transversely. This *somatotopic organization* must be largely due to the orderly input of the primary afferent fibres.

On the basis of cytoarchitectural differentiations the grey matter of the spinal cord can be subdivided into 10 layers or lamina (Fig. A5). It is important to realize that the laminae do not have rigid demarcations and, due to the extensive branching projections of many of these cells, there is a complex interrelationship between adjacent laminae.

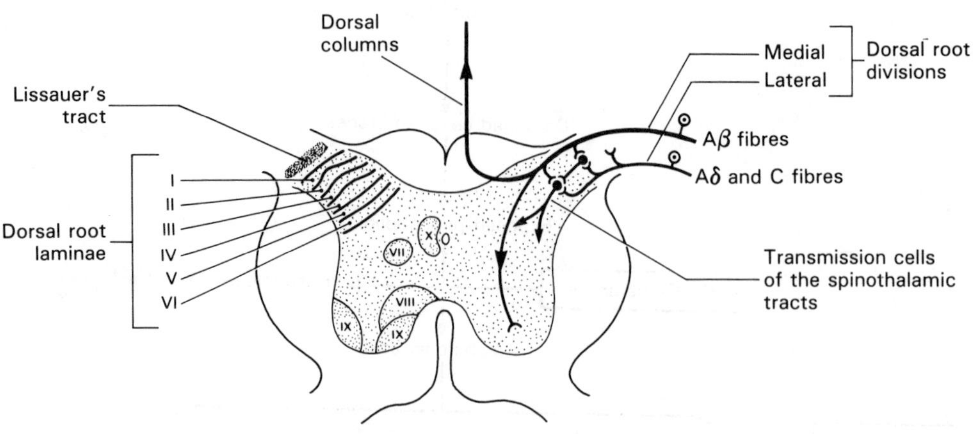

Fig. A 5 Dorsal root organization

Laminae I to VI are found in the dorsal horn. The outermost region is lamina I, the marginal zone, adjacent to this lie laminae II and III, the substantia gelatinosa. The remainder of the dorsal horn is made up of laminae IV, V and VI which collectively constitute the nucleus proprius. The majority of peripheral primary afferents terminate on the cells in the six dorsal root laminae. The activity of these cells is therefore in many cases influenced directly by convergent input from the periphery. This is in contrast to the cells of laminae VII and VIII, the nucleus intermedius, which act as relay neurons, their firing being influenced by input from more superficial dorsal root laminae or supraspinal sources. Lamina IX, found in the anterior horn, contain the cell bodies of the lower motor neurons (LMN) which ultimately control the functioning of peripheral muscle groups. The area around the central canal comprises lamina X.

The input-output characteristics of the spinal cord laminae are illustrated in Figure A6. Before considering them individually it is important at this point to make some general observations.

The complex organization of the spinal cord grey matter, and in particular the dorsal horn, into specialized regions, clearly indicates that the dorsal root cells do not function merely to receive and relay peripheral information to central structures or complete reflex arcs. Information arriving from the periphery is sampled, computed and processed by a series of interlinked inhibitory and excitatory convergences before being relayed along specific output pathways.

As a result of the complex circuitry at spinal level, interdependencies are created between the different classes of primary afferent fibres. This may explain why activity in large diameter non-nociceptive (Aβ) afferent fibres may reduce transmission in nociceptive afferents. Equally it may account for hyperalgesia in clinical syndromes such as causalgia or postherpetic neuralgia where large diameter afferents are selectively deactivated.

There appears to be a general flow of information from dorsally sited laminae to the more ventrally placed ones. A lamina that receives direct peripheral input is dominated by that input, both in respect of internal processing and output characteristics, but these activities are also modulated by converging information from more dorsally placed laminae. Individual cells thus signal increasingly more complex convergences as they are located more and more ventrally. Therefore, cells of lamina 1 are regarded as being relatively specific, while many of the cells found in laminae V, VII and VIII respond to a variety of different sensory modes and are described as wide dynamic range (WDR) cells.

The large diameter, fast conducting Aβ of the

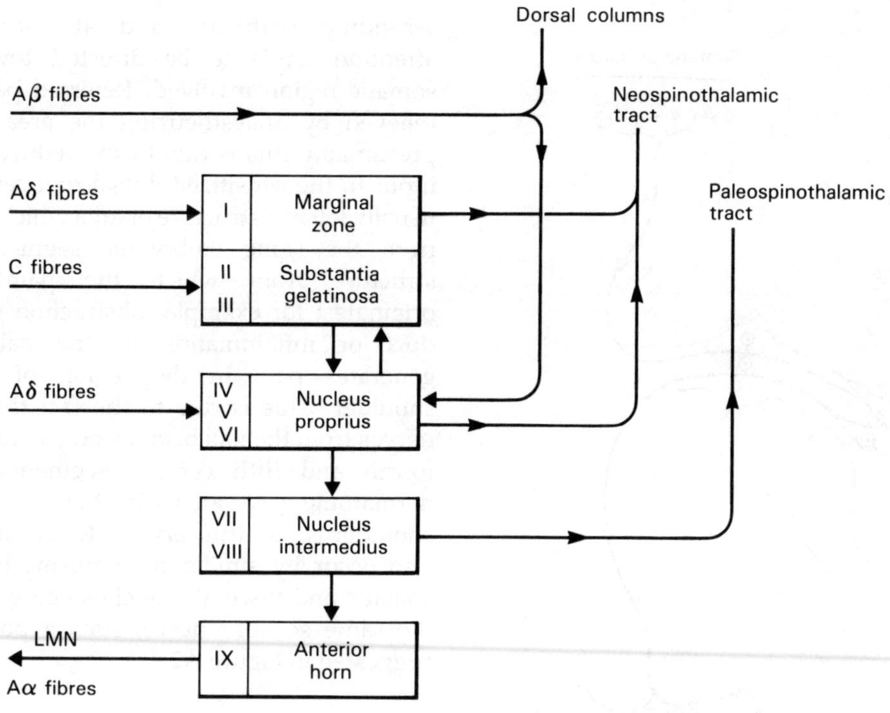

Fig. A 6 The input-output characteristics of the laminae of the spinal cord grey matter

medial dorsal root division course over the medial surface of the dorsal root grey matter and ascend the cord ipsilaterally in the dorsal columns. These large afferent fibres also give off collateral axons which enter the dorsal horn in laminae IV and V, turn back, ultimately terminate in laminae II and may modify transmission in other afferent fibres including those carrying noxious information.

The fibres of the lateral dorsal root division enter the dorsal root laminae at a number of points. The small myelinated Aδ high threshold mechanical and mechanothermal nociceptors terminate in two sites, on the nocispecific cells of lamina I the marginal zone, or deeper in the nucleus proprius, predominantly on the WDR cells found in lamina V.

In contrast, unmyelinated polymodal C fibres terminate exclusively in the superficial layers. Although the precise region of termination remains a matter of debate most studies indicate it to be lamina II, the substantia gelatinosa. While the majority of C fibres make these contacts by direct entry through the dorsal roots, it has been shown that up to 30% of fibres, although their cell bodies are located in the DRG, turn back and enter the spinal cord via the ventral root. This may well help to explain the return of pain following dorsal root rhizotomy.

Damage to tissue or peripheral afferents is often followed by long-term changes in both the discharge patterns and the spinal cord circuitry. After tissue damage the WDR cells, which respond to both noxious and non-noxious stimuli, have their excitability reset such that they respond with a noxious discharge frequency when stimulated by non-noxious input. This change in sensitivity may explain the sustained nature of chronic pain and the hypersensitivity which accompanies it. If a peripheral nerve is cut, new central synapses are established with the nearest intact afferent, thus creating new receptive fields.

Although some of these effects may be

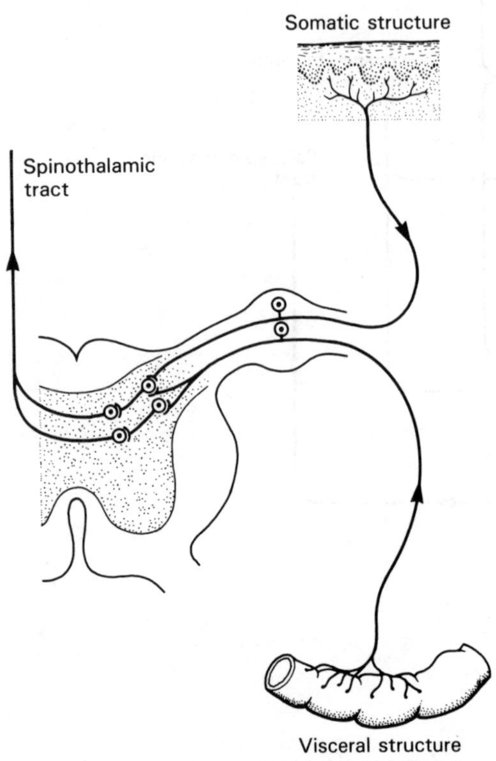

Fig. A 7 The convergence and facilitation theory of referred pain

induced by peripheral changes at the level of the nociceptors, it has been suggested that perhaps more significantly they may be related to the transportation of substances by the peripheral afferents to the central terminals.

Visceral afferents are poorly represented amongst the dorsal root afferents, constituting at the most 10% of the total fibres. Very little is known of their terminations, but there is evidence for the convergence of somatic and visceral afferents in laminae IV to VIII. This convergence may provide a basis for referred pain, whereby pain is not only felt at the site of injury or inflammation, e.g. an internal organ, but also on the surface of the body (Fig. A7).

Facilitation of the dorsal horn cells by the visceral input is thought to lower the threshold for transmission of somatic information. Since visceral structures are poorly represented within ascending pathways and at cortical level, attention tends to be directed towards the somatic region involved. Referred pain can be relieved by anaesthetizing the area involved; presumably this is due to the reduced somatic input to the sensitized dorsal root cells. Pain is usually felt in a structure or area which is derived from the same embryonic segment as the structure from which the painful event originates: for example, obstruction of the bile duct or inflammation of the gall bladder generates pain in the region of the right shoulder. This is due to the fact that afferent nerves from the gall bladder project to the third, fourth and fifth cervical segments and the dermatome associated with the tip of the right shoulder is the fifth cervical. Referred pain may also occur by similar mechanisms but due to somatic and visceral branches being present in the same sensory nerve; such a possibility is suggested in Figure A2.

ASCENDING NOCICEPTIVE PATHWAYS

Nociceptive information is transmitted from the spinal cord to the cortical and subcortical centres by a number of different parallel ascending pathways, the major ones in humans being the spinothalamic tracts. Neurons of these tracts originate from laminae I and V in the dorsal horn and laminae VII and VIII in the intermediate grey matter of the spinal cord. The majority of these fibres decussate at cord level and, having crossed the mid-line, ascend contralaterally in the anterolateral quadrant of the cord. The spinothalamic tracts are frequently divided in the lateral spinothalamic tract or neospinothalamic division and the medial spinothalamic tract or paleospinothalamic division (Figs. A6 and 8).

Neospinothalamic tract (NST)

This tract arises mainly from laminae I and V of the dorsal horn which receive peripheral input from Aδ units. Neurons of lamina I respond only to high threshold noxious mechanical stimulation, whilst those of lamina V respond to

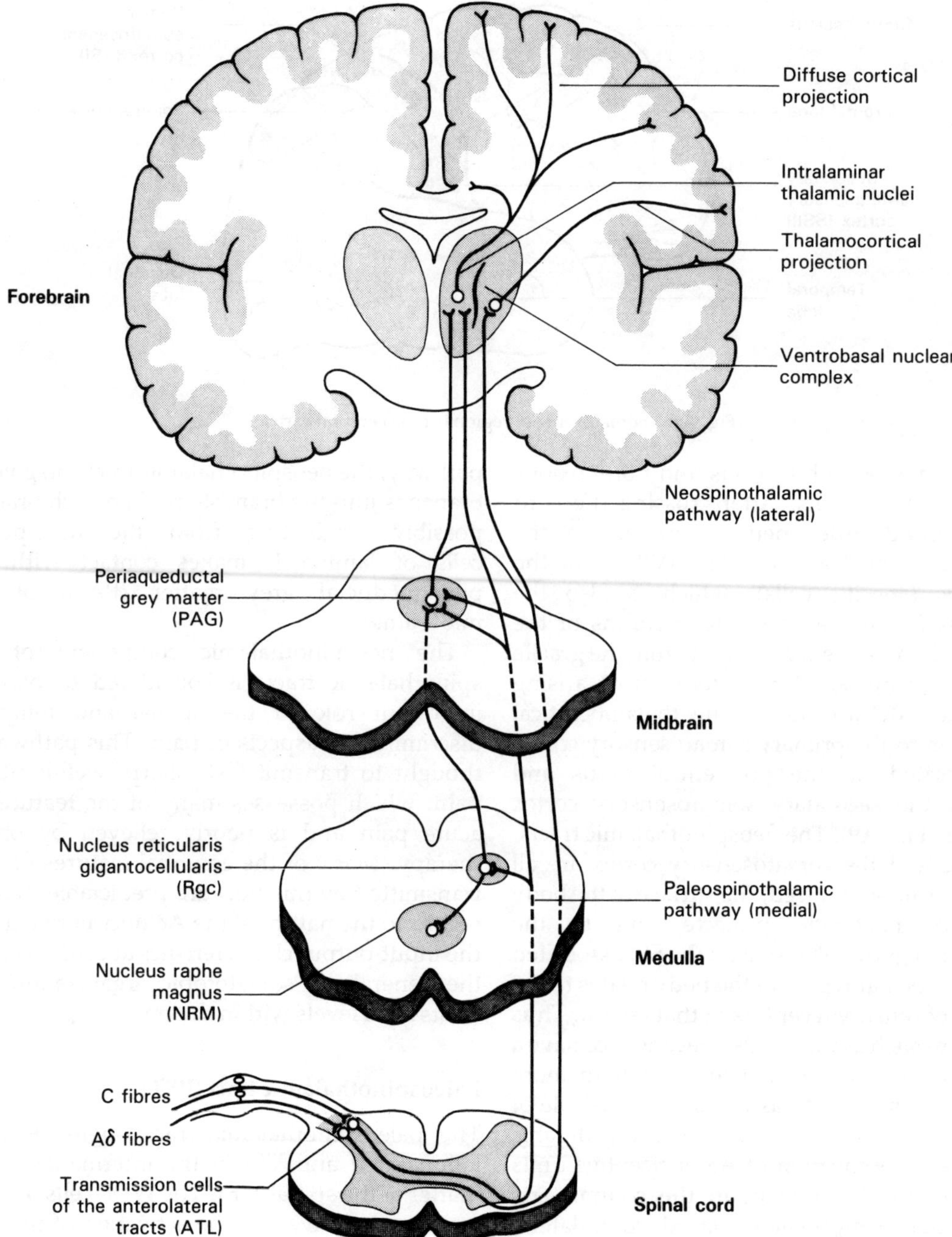

Fig. A 8 Ascending pathways associated with the transmission of nociceptive information

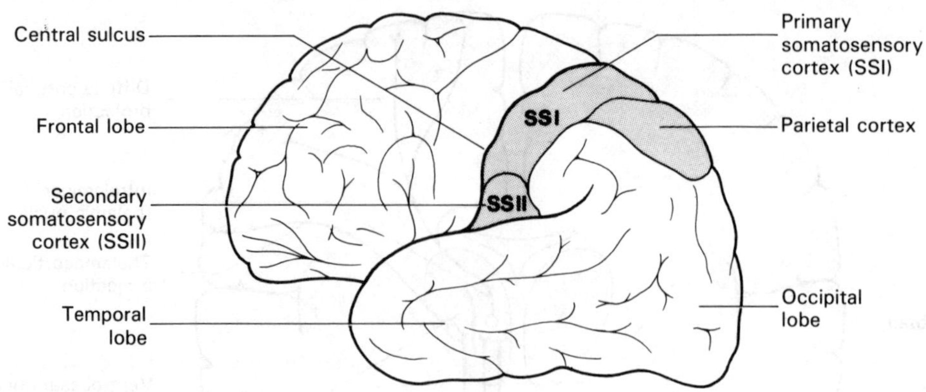

Fig. A 9 Somatosensory regions of the cerebral cortex

a wide range of both noxious and non-noxious stimuli — WDR cells. After crossing the cord these second order neurons project to the ventrobasal nuclear complex (VBC) of the thalamus (specific cells), which is also the terminus for the second order neurons of the dorsal column system after relay from the gracile and cuneate nuclei. Third order neurons arising from the VBC ascend via the thalamocortical projection to the primary somatosensory cortex (SSI) located on the postcentral gyrus and possibly the secondary somatosensory cortex (SSII)(see Fig. A9). The neospinothalamic tracts, the VBC and the somatosensory cortex are all somatopically-organized, the surface of the body being contralaterally projected on to the postcentral gyrus. The area on the SSI associated with a particular region of the body relates to the density of sensory receptors in that region. Thus structures such as the hands, feet and face have a much larger area devoted to them than more proximal regions such as the trunk. The role of the SSI in nociception is a subject of considerable controversy. Activation of Aδ nociceptive units evoke electrical potentials in the contralateral cortex, but appropriately placed contralateral lesions do not eliminate pain, and electrical stimulation of the cortex does not produce pain. It would appear that SSI is not essential for the conscious perception of pain, but it may regulate sub-cortical structures and aid the accurate location of the noxious stimulation. Although primarily regarded as a direct, point-to-point pathway, the neospinothalamic tracts do give off branches into the brain stem. One such branch, possibly originating from the nocispecific cells of lamina I, makes contact with the periaqueductal grey matter (PAG) of the midbrain.

The neospinothalamic component of the spinothalamic tracts is considered to play an important role in the spatial and temporal discriminative aspects of pain. This pathway is thought to transmit fast, sharp, well-localized pain, which possesses many of the features of acute pain and is poorly relieved by opiate therapy. Many of the essential features of pain transmitted by this tract are predictable, having regard to the nature of the Aδ nociceptive units, the input-output characteristics at cord level and the generalized somatotopic organization that exists at all levels within the tracts.

Paleospinothalamic tract (PST)

The paleospinothalamic tract originates from laminae VII and VIII in the intermediate grey matter of the spinal cord. The WDR cells of these laminae are driven by the activation of the cells of lamina II by input from polymodal C fibre units and convergent information from most other laminae. This multisynaptic pathway projects to the intralaminar thalamic nuclei (nonspecific cells) (Figs. A6 and 8). These nuclei are not somatotopically organized; lesioning them relieves the affective components of pain

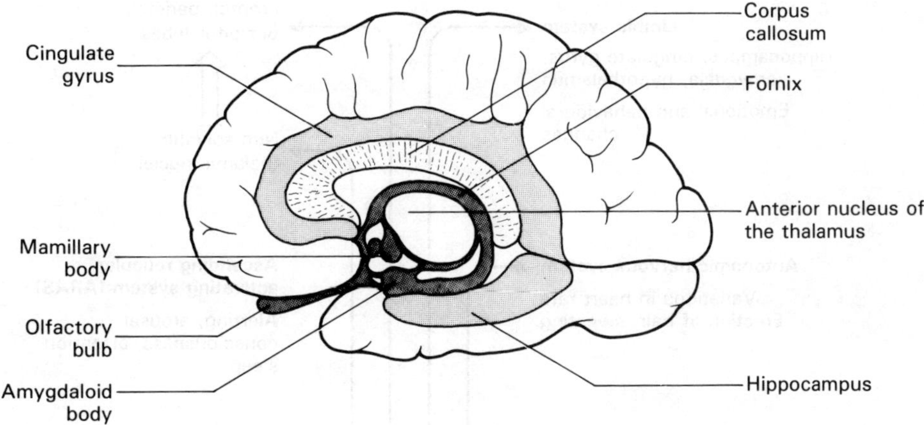

Fig. A 10 Limbic system

while not influencing sensory discriminative aspects. From such observations it is assumed that the paleospinothalamic tracts and their associated structures are likely to play a role in the nondiscriminative features of pain.

During ascent of the neural axis collaterals are given off at many levels, making contact with the major nuclei of the brain stem reticular formation. In the medullary reticular formation this includes the nucleus reticularis lateralis, nucleus reticularis magnocellularis and most significantly the nucleus reticularis gigantocellularis (RgC). Considered to be a major relay nucleus for nociceptive information, neurons of this nucleus have very large, non-somatotropically organized bilateral receptive fields. Projections of these neurons activate the nucleus raphe magnus (NRM) and also ascend into the midbrain. Scattered throughout the medullary reticular formation are the control centres of the autonomic nervous system, which may also receive collateral innervation.

At midbrain level, fibres of the paleospinothalamic tract project to the periaqueductal grey matter (PAG), which in turn projects rostrally to the intralaminar nuclei of the thalamus (some direct spinothalamic tracts are also involved). Axons arising from the intralaminar nuclei form a diffuse series of projections and establish contact with the hypothalamus and thus the limbic system, the frontal, parietal and occipital regions of the cerebral cortex.

These multiple routes and terminations suggest a number of possible roles in the pain experience. The involvement of various cortical regions implies a cognitive-evaluative function where present pain is analyzed in the light of past experiences. This possibility is supported by the responses to pain of patients who have undergone prefrontal leucotomy, who report that they still have pain but it does not concern them anymore. Projections to the hypothalamus and the limbic system — this consists of the limbic cortex (cingulate gyrus, hippocampus and the olfactory bulb) which encircles a number of subcortical structures including the anterior thalamus, parts of the hypothalamus, the amygdaloid nuclei, and the fornix (Fig. A10) — are thought to provide the basis for the aversive motivational and affective aspects of pain.

Stimulation of the brain stem reticular formation with subsequent activation of the non-specific nuclei of the thalamus and the diffuse cortical projections (collectively known as the ascending reticular activating system (ARAS)) serves to alert the whole of the sensory system to incoming signals. Increased activity in the ARAS raises the level of responsiveness of the sensory system and in so doing raises the level of consciousness, alertness and focuses attention. Decreased activity, on the other hand, leads to

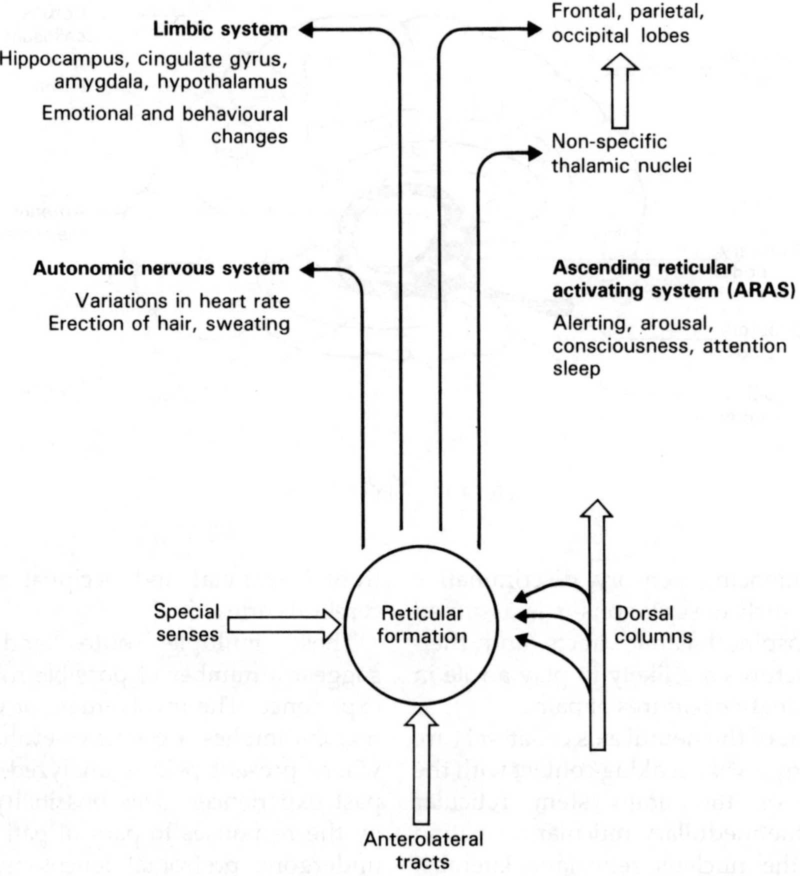

Fig. A 11 Possible roles of the reticular formation in nociception

drowsiness and sleep, mainly due to the inhibitory influences of the sleep centres in the medulla and the pons (see Fig. A11).

Activity within this system gives rise to dull, diffuse, persistent pain, and generates a spectrum of physiological, behavioural and subjective responses. This type of pain has many features which are similar to those of chronic pain, and it also responds to opiate therapy.

Although multiple pathways for nociception do exist and it appears justifiable to segregate them on anatomical, neurophysiological and clinical grounds; it is very likely that interconnections occur, since similar target areas are involved in both pathways.

It is also known that many of the central structures involved in nociceptive transmission, such as the PAG and the NRM, are also implicated in stimulus-produced analgesia and the descending pain control system. This topic will be considered in detail in the next section.

ENDOGENOUS PAIN MODULATING SYSTEM

Unquestionably the postulation by Melzack & Wall in 1965 of the existence of a pain gating mechanism in the dorsal horn of the spinal cord, which could be activated by both segmental and supraspinal influences provided the impetus for stimulating research. The results of which have provided the basis of our current-understanding of the endogenous pain control system.

Over the past two decades through a combination of anatomical, physiological and pharmacological studies knowledge has accumulated of:

- the possible spinal circuitry subserving the gating mechanism. This in turn has spawned a variety of conceptual models of the pain gate
- the presence of pharmacologically discrete descending pathways originating mainly from the brain stem, which if activated inhibit pain transmission at cord level
- the existence of an ever increasing number of endogenous peptides and biogenic amines which function as neurotransmitters and neuromodulators within the endogenous pain control system.

Furthermore these findings have provided a scientific framework for explaining the possible neurophysiological and biochemical mechanisms associated with such techniques as transcutaneous electrical nerve stimulation (TENS), acupuncture analgesia, and stimulus produced analgesia (SPA).* Additionally we now have a better understanding of the mode of action of the existing centrally acting analgesics and new opportunities in drug design based upon their endogenous counterparts. Also, an insight has been provided into why drugs which would not be regarded as first-line analgesics, for example the tricyclic antidepressant drugs and the α adrenergic agonists can provide significant pain relief in specific situations, or act as useful adjuvants to more conventional analgesic therapy.

PAIN GATE THEORY

Melzack & Wall (1965) proposed that the transmission of nociceptive information could be modified during its passage through the dorsal horn of the spinal cord. They suggested a specific circuit within the dorsal horn which could act as a gate; if open it allowed the transmission of nociceptive information and ultimately, after central processing, pain was perceived. Conversely closing the gate reduced or abolished central transmission with an accompanying reduction in pain. The position of the gate is determined by a dynamic interaction between input signals from large diameter Aβ fibres transmitting touch or pressure sensations and the smaller diameter Aδ and C fibres transmitting nociceptive information. Collateral branches from each of these fibre groups terminate on the cells of the substantia gelatinosa (SG) (Fig. A12). The SG cells act as inhibitory

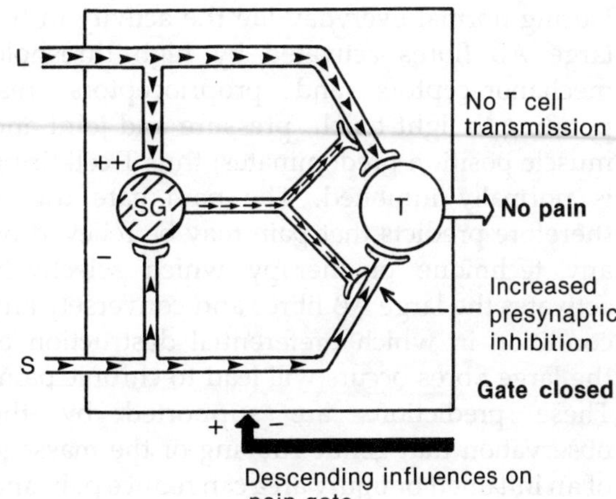

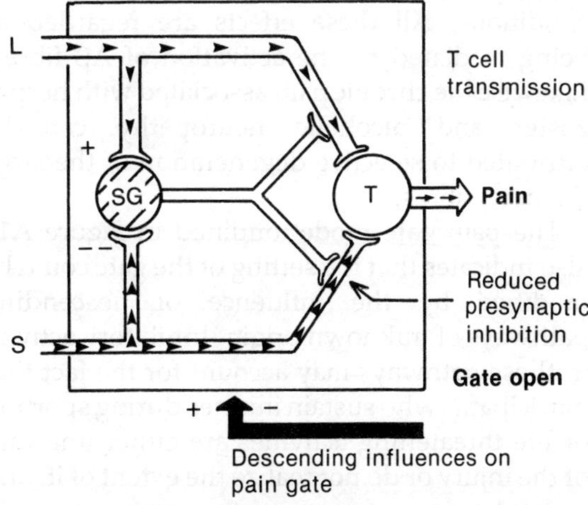

Fig. A 12 Scheme of dorsal horn pain modulating system

* SPA — analgesia produced in animals or man by electrical stimulation of discrete sites in the brain stem

interneurons which, when facilitated, presynaptically inhibit both the large Aβ fibres and smaller Aδ and C fibres, and in so doing ultimately control the firing of the transmission cells (T) of the spinothalamic tracts.

Collaterals of the small diameter fibres are inhibitory causing hypopolarization of the SG cells, thus reducing the presynaptic inhibition. This opens the gate, activating the T cells and the ascending pathways to the brain, allowing pain to be experienced. In contrast the large diameter fibres which are collateral branches of fibres ascending in the dorsal columns facilitate the SG cells causing depolarization thus promoting presynaptic inhibition and closing the gate. Whether the gate is open or shut will depend on the predominant input from peripheral sources. During normal everyday life the activity in the large Aβ fibres activated by high threshold mechanoreceptors and proprioceptors responding to light touch, pressure and joint and muscle position predominates; thus T cell firing is normally inhibited. The pain gate theory therefore predicts that pain may be relieved by any technique or therapy which selectively activates the large Aβ fibres and conversely any condition in which preferential destruction of the large fibres occurs will lead to chronic pain. These predictions are supported by the observation that gentle rubbing or the massage of an inflamed or injury area can reduce pain and the effectiveness of TENS and vibrational techniques in relieving certain painful conditions. All these effects are regarded as being mediated by the activation of Aβ fibres. Likewise the chronic pain associated with herpes zoster and alcoholic neuropathy can be attributed to selective degeneration of the large diameter fibres.

The pain gate model outlined in Figure A12 also indicates that the setting of the gate could be modified by the influence of descending pathways of unknown origin. Inhibitory activity in these pathways may account for the fact that participants who sustain injuries during sporting or life threatening activities are either unaware of the injury or do not realize the extent of it, and certainly do not appear to experience pain commensurate with the nature of the injury.

The gate control theory has over the years since 1965 been subject to both criticism and modification (Melzack & Wall, 1982). Although the existence of a pain gating mechanism at cord level is generally accepted, the precise anatomical and neurochemical organization of it still remains a matter of speculation. Outlined in Figure A13 is one of a number of simplified models which could be proposed from current evidence. As originally stated there is selective peripheral input from C and Aδ nociceptive units to different dorsal root laminae (see Figs A5 & A6). Input from C fibre units causes the release of SP – this facilitates the relay cells of the SG (probably the stalk cells) — which in turn drives the T cells of the paleospinothalamic tracts signalling tissue damage. Activity in the large diameter Aβ fibres presynaptically inhibits C fibre transmission. The neurotransmitter associated with this inhibition is not known and there is also evidence to suggest post-synaptic mechanisms may also be involved. Transmission in the relay cells of the SG may be modified by facilitation of inhibitory interneurons (I), also located in the SG: these constitute a mixed population of cells; some release γ-aminobutyric acid (GABA) others contain enkephalins (En). Collateral branches of Aδ units transmitting sharp pin prick pain entering the dorsal horn at lamina I (or lamina V) may provide one possible source of activation for this inhibitory circuit. Such a circuit may offer an explanation for the possible mechanism by which segmental acupuncture analgesia may occur.

The terminal regions of the C fibres contain a high concentration of opiate receptors but do not appear to be adjacent to any neurons containing opioid peptide neurotransmitters.

This apparant mismatch may indicate non-synaptic transmission involving signals in the medium surrounding the receptors. This phenomenon, known as volume transmission, is thought to exist in other regions of the central nervous system.

Besides the segmental regulatory circuits Figure A13 includes pathways originating mainly from the brain stem and descending via the dorsolateral funiculus (DLF). These pathways inhibit the pain transmitting neurons

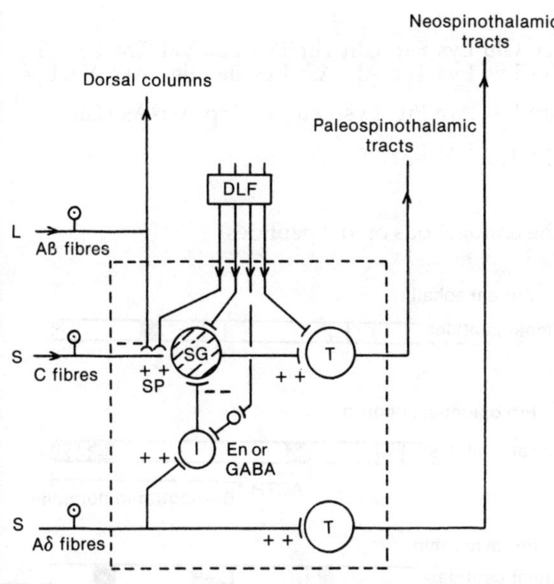

Fig. A 13 Possible pain modulating system of the dorsal horn

SG	Substantia gelatinosa	SP	Substance P
I	Inhibitory inter-neuron	En	enkephalins
T	Transmission cell 2nd order neurons of the spinothalamic tracts	GABA	γ-aminobutyric acid
		DLF	Dorsolateral funiculus

of the superficial dorsal horn. This in theory could occur at a variety of possible sites involving either presynaptic or post-synaptic mechanisms. Some of these theoretical possibilities are shown in Figure A13. Such neurons represent the anatomical substrate for SPA, nonsegmental TENS and acupuncture analgesia. The origins, distribution and neurotransmitter characterising these pathways will now be outlined.

NEUROTRANSMITTERS AND NEUROMODULATORS

Functioning of the endogenous pain modulating system requires the synthesis and release of neurotransmitters and neurohormones. Current research indicates that these are peptides or biogenic amines, although as stated in the previous section amino acids such as γ-aminobutyric acid may also be involved.

Endogenous opioid peptides

The analgesic effects of morphine and other opiates mediated by stereospecific binding to opiate receptors have been recognised since the early 1950s but what was not known was the nature of the endogenous lignands.

In 1975 Hughes et al isolated and characterised the endogenous opioid penta-peptides methionine (met) enkephalin and leucine (leu) enkephalin. Since then a number of related peptides which mimic narcotic analgesics in both bioassays and analgesic tests have been identified. These are collectively referred to as the endogenous opioid peptides.

Properties and distribution

On the basis of differences in both structure and properties the endogenous opioid peptides can be classified into three distinct families, the enkephalins, the endorphins and the dynorphins. Biochemical, immunohistological and pharmacological techniques have been used to indentify the pathways in which they and their associated binding sites (opiate receptors) occur in both the central and peripheral nervous systems (Table A3).

Table A 3 Endogenous opioid petptides and their distribution

a. Enkaphalins	Dorsal horn, medial thalamus, periaqueductal grey matter (PAG), rostral ventromedial medulla (RVM), hypothalamus, adrenal medulla, gastrointestinal tract (myenteric plexus).
b. Endorphins	Anterior and intermediate pituitary, hypothalamus
c. Dynorphins	Dorsal horn, PAG, posterior pituitary, hypothalamus, gastrointestinal tract (submucosal plexus).

The pentapeptides met and leu enkephalin (Fig. A14) are widely distributed throughout the nervous system, often paralleling the location of, the opiate receptors. They are rapidly degraded by nonspecific endopeptidases and are generally

Peptide	Sequence
Leucine-enkephalin	Tyr Gly Gly Phe Leu
Methionine-enkephalin	Tyr Gly Gly Phe Met
β-endorphin	Try Gly Gly Phe Met Thr Ser Glu Lys Ser Gln Thr Pro Leu Val Thr Leu Phe Glu Gly Lys Lys Tyr Ala Asn Lys Ile Ile Ala Asn Lys
Dynorphin	Tyr Gly Gly Phe Leu Arg Arg Ile Arg Pro Lys Leu Lys Trp Asp Asn Glu
α-neoendorphin	Tyr Gly Gly Phe Leu Arg Lys Tyr Pro Lys

Fig. A 14 Amino acid sequences of the endogenous opioid peptides

considered to be inhibitory neurotransmitters. The enkephalins and associated opiate receptors are also found in high concentrations in the vagal nuclei, the area postrema and the parabrachial nuclei, regions of the central nervous system associated with the control of coughing, vomiting and respiration, all of which are known to be influenced by the opiates. Their presence in the gastrointestinal tract may also account for the effects of morphine-like drugs on gastrointestinal motility.

Originally thought to be one of a number of possible cleavage products of the anterior pituitary hormone β-Lipotropin (βLPH), the potent 31 amino acid peptide β-endorphin (BE) has a much more restricted distribution (Fig. A14). BE is found in the anterior and intermediate pituitary, the hypothalamus and also the PAG, although in the latter case this is thought to originate from the hypothalamus. In contrast to the enkephalins, BE has a sustained analgesic effect and may function as a neurohormone rather than a neurotransmitter.

Much less is known about the dynorphin family of peptides. Dynorphin contains 17 amino acids, α-neoendorphin ten, both have quite an extensive distribution and show overlap with the enkephalins in laminae I and II of the dorsal horn and the PAG. The likelihood is that they function as neurotransmitters and may co-exist with the enkephalins in the same neurons. The endogenous opioid peptides are all derived from three large precursor molecules (molecular weight 25 000), proenkephalin, proopiomelanocortin and prodynorphin (proenkaphalin β) (Fig. A15). Within each molecule the active peptide sequences are separated from nonopioid peptide sequences by a pair of basic amino acids which act as markers for specific peptidases

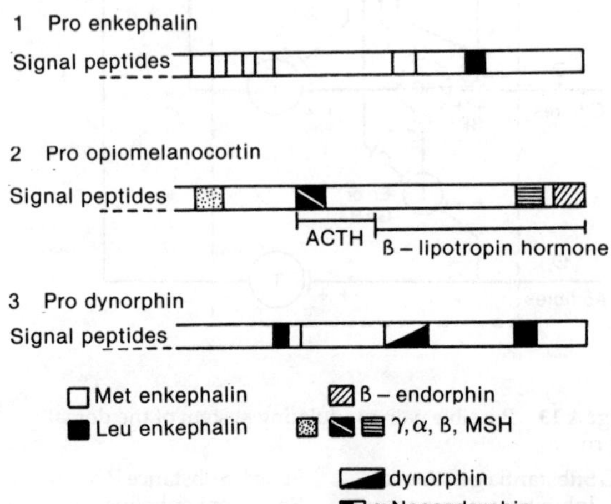

Fig. A 15 Precursor molecules of the endogenous opioid peptides

to cleave the molecules into active fragments. Thus the endogenous opioid peptides are widely distributed throughout the sensory projection system and found in particularly high concentrations in regions associated with pain transmission. That they have a role in pain modulation is strongly supported by the raised levels found in cerebrospinal fluid (CSF) following electrical stimulation of the PAG, low frequency acupuncture, and low frequency-high intensity TENS. Furthermore, intracerebral injections of BE produced profound and prolonged analgesia; reduced levels have also been found in the CSF of patients with chronic pain.

Apart from any established roles the endogenous opioid peptides may have in the modulation of pain transmission, there is evidence to indicate an additional role in the control of the growth and development of neural

Table A 4 Some of the properties and effects of stimulating the opiate receptors

Mu(μ)	Kappa (κ)	Sigma (σ)
Euphoria	Sedation	Delirium
Respiratory depression	Moderate respiratory depression	Respiratory stimulation
Vasomotor depression	No vasomotor effects	Vasomotor stimulation
Miosis	Miosis	Mydriasis
Supraspinal analgesia	Spinal analgesia	?
Naloxone sensitive	Reduced naloxone sensitivity	Reduced nalaxone sensitivity

tissue and possibly the formation of new central synaptic connections following peripheral nerve lesions (see dorsal root organization).

Opiate receptors

In order to explain the differences in the pharmacological profiles of a variety of opiates, Martin (1967) Gilbert & Martin (1976), and Martin (1979) proposed the presence of several types of opioid receptors. The receptors were designated μ-(morphine and morphine like compounds are the typical agonists), κ-(activated by keto-cyclazocine), and σ-(activated by the N-alkyl analogue of α-metazocine) (Table A4). After the discovery of the opioid peptides, it was found that their rank order of potency differed from that of the non-peptide opiates, in both biological systems and binding assays. These observations indicated the existence of a fourth receptor — the delta (δ) receptor. Subsequent investigations into the binding properties of β endorphin (BE) demonstrated that it possessed some unique properties not observed with the other opiate peptides. These findings have been interpreted on the basis of the presence of a further receptor the epsilon (ϵ) receptor.

It has been suggested that β-endorphin is probably an agonist at all classes of receptor, whilst the enkephalins are the natural ligands at the μ and δ receptors and dynorphin and neo-endorphin appear to be the endogenous agonists at κ opiate receptors.

Before considering the biogenic amines associated with the modulation of pain transmission, this is an appropriate point to outline briefly the relationship of the centrally acting analgesics to the opiate receptors.

The centrally acting analagesics are believed to produce their analgesic action and associated side-effects as a consequence of their differing affinities for and intrinsic activities at one or more of the three postulated receptors indicated in Table A5. On the basis of these drug-receptor interactions they have been classified as (1) pure agonists; (2)partial agonists; or (3) mixed agonist-antagonist (see Ch. 15).

Drugs of the morphine type (e.g. morphine, pethidine, dihydrocodeine) are regarded as being pure agonists at the μ and probably also the κ receptor. Partial agonists, for example buprenorphine, act at the μ receptor and have

Table A 5 Centrally acting analgesics and opiate receptor activity

Drug	Receptor activity μ	κ	σ
Morphine	agonist	agonist	–
Buprenorphine	partial agonist	–	–
Pentazocine	antagonist	agonist	agonist

properties that are similar to morphine. Characteristically their dose-response curves reach a plateau at a critical dose level while those of morphine and other pure agonists increase proportionally with dose. Thus in the case of the partial agonists, although they may, for instance, depress respiration, there is a limitation to the degree of depression that they may cause. Agonist-antagonist analgesics include such drugs as nalbuphine and pentazocine, are considered to be agonists at the σ and κ receptors but competetive antagonists at the μ receptor.

Agonists at κ receptors display high analgesic potency in tests for nociception using mechanical stimuli, in contrast μ receptor agonists appear more efficient when heat is used as the test stimulus. It is fascinating to speculate that with the opioid peptides and their receptors there may exist multiple systems each responding to a different noxious challenge.

Finally drugs such as naloxone have affinity for but no intrinsic activity at any of the postulated opiate receptors. Naloxone lacks any significant analgesic activity, does not produce any characteristic symptoms and can, to varying degrees, antagonize the effects of the narcotic agonist, partial agonist and agonist-antagonist analgesics.

Biogenic amines

It is of interest to note that the administration of the opiate antagonist naloxone only partially blocks stimulus produced analgesia (SPA), high intensity-low frequency TENS and acupuncture analgesia. These observations raise the possibility that in addition to the endogenous opiate peptide system, other neurotransmitters or neuromodulators may be components of the endogenous pain modulating system. Recent studies clearly indicate a role for 5-hydroxytryptamine (5HT) and also, possibly, noradrenaline (NA).

5-Hydroxytryptamine (5HT)

Depletion of 5HT with p-Chlorophenylalanine (pCPA), an inhibitor of 5HT synthesis, reduces the effects of SPA. The analgesia can be restored by the administration of 5-hydroxytryptaphan, a 5HT precursor; this is particularly pronounced when the site of SPA is in the nucleus raphe magnus (NRM). Furthermore tricyclic anti-depressant drugs such as amitriptyline which prevent the presynaptic re-uptake of 5HT, can antagonize hyperalgesia produced by pCPA in animals and increase pain tolerance in man. The tricyclic antidepressant drugs also structurally resemble carbamazepine, an antiepileptic drug which is also very effective in some patients with trigeminal neuralgia. This raises the possibility that at least with respect to their analgesic effects they share a common mode of action, i.e. enhancing 5HT transmission. In addition, the possibility that migraine characterised by persistant headaches, relatively resistant to morphine therapy, may be caused by a 5HT deficiency, provides further evidence for a possible role for 5HT in pain modulation. Other studies have shown that 5HT has an inhibitory effect on neurons located in the superficial laminae of the dorsal horn which respond to noxious stimuli.

These observations suggest that 5HT may be a component in an inhibitory pathway originating in the region of the NRM and possibly other medullary regions, which terminates in the dorsal horn of the spinal cord. The situation is complicated by the finding that the opiate antagonist naloxone does not antagonize the analgesia produced by intrathecal administration of 5HT, but the effects of systemic opiates can be blocked by depletion of 5HT using pCPA. This implies a possible interrelationship between the opioid peptides and 5HT at supraspinal levels.

Noradrenaline (NA)

The role of noradrenaline (NA) in the modulation of pain is both complex and controversial. Adrenergic neurons are known to terminate both in the superficial dorsal horn and the NRM, but their origins are yet to be fully established. Furthermore the contribution that noradrenaline makes to analgesia at these two sites appears to be antagonistic.

At the level of the NRM microinjection of the α_1 (postsynaptic) adrenergic blocking agent phentolamine enhances acupuncture analgesia. Also selective degeneration of the adrenergic fibres innervating the NRM using 6-hydroxydopamine results in augmentation of acupuncture analgesia. In contrast to this, intrathecal injections of phentolamine suppress both acupuncture and opiate induced analgesia. Thus NA may have a dual role in the modulation of pain exerting an inhibitory influence in the NRM, while NA projections to the spinal cord inhibit pain transmission, the latter being consistent with the analgesia produced by intrathecally administered NA.

Additionally it has recently been reported that clonidine an α_2 (presynaptic) adrenergic agonist is of benefit in certain patients with deafferentiation pain due to spinal cord injuries. Finally it is worth noting that the tricyclic antidepressant drugs not only block the reuptake of 5HT but also NA, thus their analgesic action may also be associated with the complex effects this may have on pain transmission.

Although they have been considered separately, it is unlikely that the biogenic amines are functionally discrete and furthermore it is known that they both co-exist with other transmitters, for example SP, enkephalins or thyrotropin releasing hormone within the same neuron.

Therefore 5HT and NA can be regarded as neurotransmitters in separate, parallel pathways which transmit inhibitory information from a number of possible locations within the brain stem. At various levels they integrate with the endogenous opioid peptides and collectively provide the means of biochemical control and communication between the different neuronal groups which constitute the descending pain modulating pathways. These in their turn provide the means of supraspinal control of the spinal pain gating mechanisms.

DESCENDING PATHWAYS

Electrical stimulation of sites such as the periaqueductal grey matter (PAG) and the nucleus raphe magnus (NRM) produce analgesia in humans and a reduction in the firing of dorsal horn neurons in animals. Also, lesions of the dorsolateral funiculus (DLF) of the spinal cord will abolish the stimulus produced analgesia (SPA) and also opiate produced analgesia. These findings clearly indicate within the DLF the presence of neurons originating from various brain stem sites that are required for SPA and that can suppress the activity of nociceptive neurons located in the dorsal horn. Furthermore the PAG and NRM receive noxious information transmitted via the spinothalamic tracts either directly or relayed through the nucleus gigantocellularis. This constitutes a closed loop system, the ascending limb being the spinothalamic tracts (STT), the descending or efferent component the inhibitory spinal projections of the DLF (Fig. A16). Such a neuronal organization suggests the possibility of a negative feedback system where the output of the transmission cells, T, are continuously monitored at brain stem level and this in turn regulates the output of the NRM and PAG and the level of inhibitory activity in the efferent-fibres descending in the DLF.

The anatomical, neuropharmacological and physiological basis of such an endogenous pain control system has been studied and extensively reviewed by Basbaum & Fields (1978), Fields & Basbaum (1978), Basbaum & Fields (1984). Some of their findings are outlined in Figure A16 and integrated with a possible dorsal horn gating mechanism (originally presented in Fig. A13) to provide an overall view of pain transmission and its modulation.

Overwhelming evidence now exists of an extensive descending pain modulating system which probably originates in cortical and diencephalic structures and successively involves neurons of the midbrain, medulla and dorsal horn.

The PAG of the midbrain appears to occupy a key position, receiving multiple projections from a wide range of structures within the CNS. These include inputs from more rostrally placed sites such as the frontal cortex, the limbic system and also the hypothalamus. The precise significance of these interconnections are not fully understood, but electrical stimulation of certain limbic regions produces analgesia and the

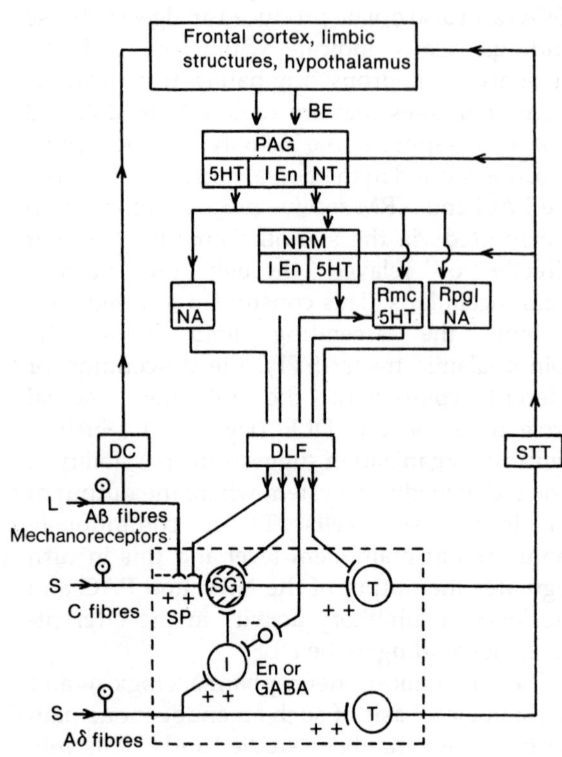

Fig. A 16 Physiological mechanisms underlying the endogenous pain modulating system

SG	Substantia gelatinosa
I	Inhibitory interneurons
T	Transmission cell 2nd order neurons of the spinothalamic tracts STT
DC	Dorsal columns
DLF	Dorsolateral funiculus
PGA	Periaqueductal grey matter
NRM	Nucleus raphe magnus
Rmc	Nucleus reticularis magnocellularis
Rpgl	Nucleus reticularis paragigantocellularis lateralis
SP	Substance P
En	Enkephalins
GABA	γ-Aminobutyric acid
BE	β-Endorphin
NT	Neurotensin
5HT	5-Hydroxytyptamine
NA	Noradrenaline

neurons originating from the hypothalamus, which itself receives projections from the frontal cortex, utilize β-endorphin (BE) as a neurotransmitter-neuromodulator. The involvement of cortical inputs suggests the possibility that cognitive-evaluative and affective components may contribute to pain modulation at this level.

Additional inputs are also derived from the brain stem (not shown in Fig.A16) and, as previously indicated, noxious information being transmitted within the STT is projected via collaterals or relayed through the nucleus reticularis gigantocellularis (RgC) to the PAG (see Fig. A8).

Driven by these diverse inputs the PAG relays information to the nuclei of the rostral ventral medulla (RVM); these include the nucleus raphe magnus (NRM), the adjacent nucleus reticularis magnocellularis (Rmc) and possibly the nucleus reticularis paragigantocellularis lateralis (Rpgl) and medullary adrenergic cellular groups (NA). The neurotransmitters involved in these midbrain-medullary projections are considered to be 5HT or neurotensin (NT). The NRM like the PAG is also activated by transmission in the STT, again relayed via the RgC (see Fig. A8), furthermore it is known that the PGA is reciprocally connected to all the aforementioned medullary structures. Axons of the medullary nuclei project via the DLF to the dorsal horn of the spinal cord, terminating mainly in laminae I, II and V, exerting inhibitory effects on the pain transmitting neurons. The principal neurotransmitters associated with these descending pathways are either NA or 5HT, each appearing to be associated with a specific parallel pathway, but they are both known to co-exist with other transmitters including enkephalins, 5HT and thyrotopin-releasing hormone (TRH). The significance of such coexistence is not known, but one possibility is that the descending pathways, although traditionally thought of as being inhibitory, may also be able to mediate excitatory effects on dorsal horn neurons. Coexistence of neurotransmitters coupled to the possibility of either presynaptic or postsynaptic release just serves to illustrate the complexity of the circuitry which is likely to control the pain modulating system of the dorsal horn. Some of the possible spinal connections are outlined in Figure A16.

In summary, there exists within the peripheral and central nervous systems a neural network which not only contains the structures and mechanisms to allow detection, transmission and perception of pain, but also continuous monitoring and modulation of pain transmission.

This endogenous pain modulating system provides the physiological, anatomical and neuropharmacological basis for the relief of pain mediated by SPA, TENS, acupuncture analgesia and the centrally acting analgesics.

Although considerable advances have been made over the last 20 years in our understanding of pain transmission and its modulation it is clear to all who research, review or merely reflect on the subject, that large gaps still exist in our knowledge of both the fundamental mechanisms involved and those associated with analgesic therapy.

REFERENCES

Basbaum A I, Fields H L 1984 Endogenous pain control systems: Brainstem, spinal pathways and endorphin circuitry. Annual Review of Neuroscience 7:309–338

Basbaum A I, Fields H L 1978 Endogenous pain control mechanism: Review and hypothesis. Annals of Neurology 4:451–462

Gilbert P E, Martin W R 1976 The effects of morphine and nalorphine-like drugs in, the non dependent, morphine dependent and cyclazocine dependent chronic spinal dog. Journal of Pharmacology and Experimental Therapeutics 198:66–82

Fields H L, Basbaum A I 1978 Brain stem control of spinal pain-transmission neurons. Annual Review of Physiology 40:193–221

Hughes J, Smith T W, Kosterlitz H W, Fothergill L A, Morgan B A, Morris H R 1975 Identification of two related pentapeptides from brain with potent opiate agonist activity. Nature 258:577–579

Martin W R 1967 Opioid antagonist. Pharmacological Reviews 10:463–521

Martin W R 1979 History and development of mixed opioid agonists partial agonist and antagonist. British Journal of Clinical Pharmacology 7:2735–2795

Melzack R, Wall P D 1965 Pain mechanisms: A new theory. Science 150:971–979

Melzack R, Wall P D 1982 The challenge of pain. Penguin, Harmondsworth

BIBLIOGRAPHY

The author acknowledges the use of the following publications in preparing the text and recommends them for further reading:

Agnati L F, Fuxe K, Zoli M, Ozini I, Toffano G, Ferraguti F 1986 A correlation analysis of the regional distribution of central enkephalin and β-endorphin immunoreactive terminals and of opiate receptors in adult and old male rats. Evidence for the existence of two main types of communication in the central nervous system: the volume transmission and the wiring transmission. Acta Physiologica Scandinavica 128:201–207

Anonymous 1981 How does acupuncture work? British Medical Journal 283:746–748

Brown A G, Rethélyi M (eds) 1981 Spinal cord sensations. Scottish Academic Press, Edinburgh

Gersh M R, Wolf S L 1985 Applications of transcutaneous electrical nerve stimulation in the management of patients in pain. Physical Therapy 65(3):314–336

Ghynn C J, Teddy P J, Jamous M A, Moore R A, Lloyds J W 1986. Role of spinal noradrenergic system in transmission of pain in patients with spinal cord injuries. Lancet 2:1249

Han J S, Terenius L 1982 Neurochemical basis of acupuncture analgesia. Annual Review of Pharmacology and Toxicology 22:193–220

Houde R W 1979 Analgesic effectiveness of the narcotic agonist-antagonists. British Journal of Clinical Pharmacology 7:2975–3085

Hua X–Y 1986 Tachykinins and calcitonin gene-related peptide in relation to peripheral functions of capsaicin-sensitive sensory neurons. Acta Physiologica Scandinavica Supplement SS1

Hughes J (ed) 1983 Opioid peptides. British Medical Bulletin 39:1–106

Jessell T M 1982 Neurotransmitters and CNS disease pain. Lancet 1084–1088

Kelly D D 1985 Central representations of pain and analgesia. In: Kandel E R, Schwartz J H (eds) Principles of neuroscience, 2nd edn. Elsevier, New York, p 331–343

Leek B F Abdominal and pelvic visceral receptors. British Medical Bulletin 33:163–168

Lyn B 1983 Cutaneous sensations. In: Goldsmith L (ed) Biochemistry and physiology of the skin. Oxford University Press, Oxford Vol 1, p 654–684

Lyn B 1984 The detection of injury and tissue damage. In: Wall P D, Melzack R (eds) Textbook of pain. Churchill Livingstone, Edinburgh

Morley J S 1986 New drug opportunities based on neuropeptides? A personal view. Drug Design and Delivery 1(1):47–50

Nathan P W 1976 The gate-control theory of pain: A critical review. Brain 99:123–158

Newburger P E, Sallan M D 1981 Chronic pain principles of management. Journal of Pediatrics 98(2):180–189

Paintal A S 1977 Thoracic receptors connected with sensations. British Medical Bulletin 33:169–174

Simon L S, Mills J A 1980 Drug Therapy: nonsteroidal anti-inflammatory drugs, (2 parts). New England Journal of Medicine 302:1179,1237

Wall P D 1984 The dorsal horn. In: Wall P D, Melzack R (eds) Textbook of pain. Churchill Livinsgtone, Edinburgh

White J C, Sweet W H 1969 Pain and the neurosurgeon. C C Thomas, Springfield, Illinois

RECOMMENDED FURTHER READING

Royal Society of Medicine 1983 Advances in morphine therapy. International Congress and Symposium Series 64. London

Katzung B G 1984 Basic and clinical pharmacology, 2nd edn. Lange Medical Publications, Los Altos, California

Mannheimer J S, Lampe G N Clinical transcutaneous electrical nerve stimulation. F.A. Davis, Philadelphia

Zygmunt L K, Pycock J 1983 Neurotransmitters and drugs, 2nd edn. Croom Helm, London

Index